47-59

92-

237

248 - 253

ADLER'S PHYSIOLOGY OF THE EYE

Tenth Edition

ADLER'S PHYSIOLOGY OF THE EYE

Clinical Application

Edited by

Paul L. Kaufman, MD
Professor and Director of Glaucoma Services
Department of Ophthalmology and Visual Sciences
University of Wisconsin–Madison
School of Medicine
Hospital and Clinics
Madison, Wisconsin
USA

Albert Alm, MD, PhD
Professor
Department of Neuroscience, Ophthalmology
University Hospital
Uppsala, Sweden

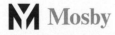 **Mosby**

An Affiliate of Elsevier Science
St. Louis   London   Philadelphia   Sydney   Toronto

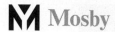

An Affiliate of Elsevier Science

11830 Westline Industrial Drive
St. Louis, Missouri

ADLER'S PHYSIOLOGY OF THE EYE   ISBN 0-323-01136-5
Copyright © 2003, Mosby, Inc. All rights reserved.

NOTICE

Ophthalmology is an ever-changing field. Standard safety precautions must be followed, but as new research and clinical experience broaden our knowledge, changes in treatment and drug therapy may become necessary or appropriate. Readers are advised to check the most current product information provided by the manufacturer of each drug to be administered to verify the recommended dose, the method and duration of administration, and contraindications. It is the responsibility of the licensed prescriber, relying on experience and knowledge of the patient, to determine dosages and the best treatment for each individual patient. Neither the publisher nor the authors/editors assume any liability for any injury and/or damage to persons or property arising from this publication.

Previous editions copyrighted 1950, 1953, 1959, 1965, 1970, 1975, 1981, 1985, 1992

Library of Congress Cataloging-in-Publication Data

Adler's physiology of the eye—10th ed. / [edited by] Paul L. Kaufman, Albert Alm.
      p. ; cm.
   Includes bibliographical references and index.
   ISBN 0-323-01136-5
      1. Eye—Physiology. I. Title: Physiology of the eye. II. Kaufman, Paul L. (Paul Leon),
   1943– III. Alm, A. IV. Adler, Francis Heed, 1895-
      [DNLM: 1. Ocular Physiology. WW 103 A238 2002]
   RE67 .A32 2002
   612.8′4—dc21   2002071828

Acquisitions Editor: Natasha Andjelkovic
Developmental Editor: Kimberley Cox
Publishing Services Manager: Deborah L. Vogel
Project Manager: Claire Kramer
Book Design Manager: Gail Morey Hudson

GW/MVY

Printed in the United States of America

Last digit is the print number: 9   8   7   6   5   4   3   2   1

CONTRIBUTORS

Albert Alm, MD, PhD
Professor
Department of Neuroscience, Ophthalmology
University Hospital
Uppsala, Sweden

Francisco H. Andrade, PhD
Department of Neurology
Case Western Reserve University
Cleveland, Ohio
USA

Sten Andreasson, MD, PhD
Department of Ophthalmology
University Hospital of Lund
Lund, Sweden

Robert S. Baker, MD
Robert Bergen Professor of Ophthalmology
Professor of Pediatrics, Neurology, and
    Neurosurgery
University of Kentucky
Lexington, Kentucky
USA

David C. Beebe, PhD
Jules and Doris Stein RPB Professor
    of Ophthalmology and Visual Sciences
Professor of Cell Biology and Physiology
Washington University School of Medicine
St. Louis, Missouri
USA

David A. R. Bessant, FRCoOphth
Clinical Research Fellow
Department of Molecular Genetics
Institute of Ophthalmology
University College London
Moorfields Eye Hospital
London, England

Shomi S. Bhattacharya, MD
Department of Molecular Genetics
Institute of Ophthalmology
University College London
Moorfields Eye Hospital
London, England

David G. Birch, PhD
Research Director
Retina Foundation of the Southwest
Adjunct Professor
Department of Ophthalmology
University of Texas Southwestern Medical Center
Dallas, Texas
USA

Jamie D. Boyd, PhD
Post-Doctoral Fellow
Department of Biological Sciences
Simon Fraser University
Burnaby, British Columbia
Canada

Vivien A. Casagrande, PhD
Professor
Department of Cell Biology, Psychology,
    and Ophthalmology and Visual Sciences
Vanderbilt University Medical School
Nashville, Tennessee
USA

George A. Cioffi, MD
Director, Glaucoma Service
Department of Ophthalmology
Devers Eye Institute
Chairman
Department of Ophthalmology
Legacy Health System
Portland, Oregon
USA

Briggs E. Cook, Jr., MD
Charlotte Ophthalmology Clinic
Charlotte, North Carolina
USA

Darlene A. Dartt, PhD
Acting Director of Research
Senior Scientist
Schepens Eye Research Institute
Associate Professor
Department of Ophthalmology
Harvard Medical School
Boston, Massachusetts
USA

Henry F. Edelhauser, PhD
Professor of Ophthalmology
Director of Ophthalmic Research
Department of Ophthalmology
Emory University Eye Center
Atlanta, Georgia
USA

Berndt E.J. Ehinger, MD, PhD
Professor
Department of Ophthalmology
University of Lund Hospital
Lund, Sweden

B'Ann True Gabelt, MS
Department of Ophthalmology
    and Visual Sciences
University of Wisconsin–Madison
School of Medicine
Hospital and Clinics
Madison, Wisconsin
USA

Roberta E. Gausas, MD
University of Pennsylvania
Scheie Eye Institute
51 North 39th Street
Philadelphia, Pennsylvania
USA

Adrian Glasser, PhD
Assistant Professor
College of Optometry
University of Houston
Houston, Texas
USA

Elisabet Granstam, MD
Department of Neuroscience, Ophthalmology
University Hospital
Uppsala, Sweden

Qiang Gu, PhD
Assistant Professor
Department of Ophthalmology
University of British Columbia
Investigator
Brain Research Center
Vancouver Hospital and Health Sciences Center
Vancouver, British Columbia
Canada

Ronald S. Harwerth, OD, PhD
John and Rebecca Moores Professor of Optometry
College of Optometry
University of Houston
Houston, Texas
USA

Jennifer M. Ichida
Department of Psychology
Vanderbilt University
Nashville, Tennessee
USA

Chris A. Johnson, PhD
Director of Diagnostic Research
    and Senior Scientist
Department of Ophthalmology
Discoveries in Sight Research Laboratories
Devers Eye Institute
Portland, Oregon
USA

Randy Kardon, MD, PhD
Associate Professor
Director of Neuro-Ophthalmology
Department of Ophthalmology
    and Visual Sciences
University of Iowa Hospitals & Clinics
Iowa City, Iowa
USA

Paul L. Kaufman, MD
Professor and Director of Glaucoma Services
Department of Ophthalmology and Visual Sciences
University of Wisconsin–Madison
School of Medicine
Hospital and Clinics
Madison, Wisconsin
USA

Shalesh Kaushal, MD, PhD
Assistant Professor
Department of Ophthalmology
University of Minnesota
Medical School
Minneapolis, Minnesota
USA

Don O. Kikkawa, MD
Chief of Ophthalmic Plastic and Reconstructive
   Surgery
Associate Professor
Department of Ophthalmology
University of California, San Diego
School of Medicine
La Jolla, California
USA

Morten la Cour, MD
Consultant
Eye Department
National University Hospital, Rigshospitalet
Copenhagen, Denmark

Bradley N. Lemke, MD
Clinical Professor of Ophthalmic Facial Plastic
   Surgery
Department of Ophthalmology and Visual
   Sciences
University of Wisconsin–Madison
School of Medicine
Hospital and Clinics
Madison, Wisconsin
USA

Leonard A. Levin, MD, PhD
Associate Professor
Department of Ophthalmology and Visual Sciences
University of Wisconsin–Madison
School of Medicine
Hospital and Clinics
Madison, Wisconsin
USA

Mark J. Lucarelli, MD
Associate Professor
Director, Oculoplastics Service
Department of Ophthalmology
   and Visual Sciences
University of Wisconsin–Madison
School of Medicine
Hospital and Clinics
Madison, Wisconsin
USA

Henrik Lund-Andersen, MD
Professor
Department of Ophthalmology
Herlev University Hospital
Herlev, Denmark

Ruth E. Manny, OD, PhD
Professor
College of Optometry
University of Houston
Houston, Texas
USA

Joanne A. Matsubara, PhD
Director of Research, Basic Sciences
Department of Ophthalmology
The University of British Columbia
Vancouver, British Columbia
Canada

Allison M. McKendrick, PhD
Department of Psychology
University of Western Australia
Crawley, Australia

David Miller, MD
Associate Clinical Professor of Ophthalmology
Department of Ophthalmology
Harvard Medical School
Massachusetts Eye and Ear Infirmary
Boston, Massachusetts
USA

Anthony M. Norcia, PhD
Smith-Kettlewell Eye Research Institute
San Francisco, California
USA

Lance M. Optican, PhD
Research Biomedical Engineer
Laboratory of Sensorimotor Research
National Eye Institute
Bethesda, Maryland
USA

Serge Picaud, PhD
Directeur de Recherche INSERM
Physiopathologie Cellulaire e Moleculaire
   de la Retine
INSERM EM-igg-18
Strasbourg, France

Vesna Ponjavic, MD, PhD
Associate Professor
Department of Ophthalmology
University of Lund
University Clinic of Lund
Lund, Sweden

John D. Porter, PhD
The Carl F. Asseff Professor
Department of Ophthalmology
Case Western Reserve University
Scientist
The Research Institute
University Hospitals of Cleveland
Cleveland, Ohio
USA

Christian Quaia, PhD
Post-Doctoral Fellow
Laboratory of Sensorimotor Research
National Eye Institute
Bethesda, Maryland
USA

David Regan, PhD, DSc
Industrial Research Professor in Vision
    and Aviation
Department of Psychology and Biology
York University
Professor
Department of Ophthalmology
University of Toronto
Ontario, Canada

Thomas P. Sakmar, MD
Acting President
The Rockefeller University
Senior Physician
The Rockefeller University Hospital
New York, New York
USA

Pamela A. Sample, PhD
Professor/Director
Visual Function Laboratory
Glaucoma Center
Department of Ophthalmology
University of California, San Diego
La Jolla, California
USA

Birgit Sander, PhD
Department of Ophthalmology
Herlev Hospital
University of Copenhagen
Copenhagen, Denmark

Clifton M. Schor, OD, PhD
Professor of Optometry, Vision Science
    and Bioengineering
Department of Optometry
School of Optometry
University of California at Berkeley
Berkeley, California
USA

Rajesh K. Sharma, MD
Department of Ophthalmology
University of Lund Hospital
Lund, Sweden

Joseph P. Shovlin, MD
Associate in Ophthalmology
Department of Ophthalmology
Geisinger Medical Center
Danville, Pennsylvania
Associate in Ophthalmology
Department of Surgery
Princeton Medical Center
Princeton, New Jersey
USA

Bryan S. Sires, MD, PhD
Associate Professor and Vice Chairman
Department of Ophthalmology
University of Washington
Seattle, Washington
USA

Rebecca C. Stacy
Department of Anatomy and Neurobiology
Washington University School of Medicine
St. Louis, Missouri
USA

John L. Ubels, PhD
Department of Biology
Calvin College
Grand Rapids, Michigan
Adjunct Professor
Department of Ophthalmology
Wayne State University School of Medicine
Detroit, Michigan
USA

Gerald Westheimer, PhD
Professor of Neurobiology
University of California
Berkeley, California
USA

Rachel O. Wong, PhD
Associate Professor
Department of Anatomy and Neurobiology
Washington University School of Medicine
St. Louis, Missouri
USA

Samuel M. Wu, PhD
Professor
Department of Ophthalmology
Cullen Eye Institute
Baylor College of Medicine
Houston, Texas
USA

PREFACE

We are honored to have the opportunity to edit the tenth edition of *Adler's Physiology of the Eye*. During the last decade there have been many developments in most of the areas usually covered by this classic textbook. Not only has the amount of available information increased dramatically, but there is no longer a sharp dividing line between classical physiology and cell or even molecular biology. For a textbook with the subtitle *Clinical Application*, the development of techniques for noninvasive studies of the morphology and the physiological responses of the eye is especially relevant. These are likely to make significant contributions to our understanding of the biology of vision and to the pathophysiology of many eye diseases. This book is designed to provide a reference text for preclinical scientists as well as for clinicians. We believe that a major goal for preclinical research is, ultimately, a better understanding of eye diseases and that the best clinical care is not possible without an understanding of basic principles of the function of the eye and the entire visual system.

The eye is a highly specialized organ that contains tissues with considerable variations in structure and function, designed to respond to a variety of specific demands. The orbit and the eyelids provide protection against trauma, and the latter help lubricate the ocular surface. Light rays are focused on photoreceptors in the macula of the two eyes through the contributions of several tissues: cornea, lens, iris, aqueous humor, vitreous, and extraocular muscles, each with its specific contribution. An internal circulation of aqueous and a unique arrangement of highly different vascular systems within the eye solve the need for nutrition of transparent tissues. The transfer of light into an image of our surroundings involves sophisticated processing of the signals that originate in the photoreceptors; this processing starts already in the retina and involves the dorsal lateral geniculate nucleus and several cortical areas apart from the visual cortex of the brain.

Such a compendium can only be assembled by combining the expertise of a large number of talented individuals. We have divided the book into sections and have given the section editors a fairly free hand in selecting content. The book would not have been possible without their enthusiasm and engagement and that of all the contributing authors. We hope that this current volume is a worthy successor to those that have preceded it in this venerable series.

ACKNOWLEDGMENTS

To all the authors, past and present, who have made *Adler's* the beloved bible of ocular physiology.

Paul L. Kaufman, MD
Albert Alm, MD

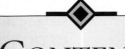

CONTENTS

SECTION 1
THE OCULAR SURFACE
Bradley N. Lemke

 1 Orbit, 3
    Bryan S. Sires, Roberta Gausas,
    Briggs E. Cook, Jr., and Bradley N. Lemke

 2 Ophthalmic Facial Anatomy and
    Physiology, 16
    Don O. Kikkawa, Mark J. Lucarelli,
    Joseph P. Shovlin, Briggs E. Cook, Jr.,
    and Bradley N. Lemke

 3 The Lacrimal System, 30
    Mark J. Lucarelli, Darlene A. Dartt,
    Briggs E. Cook, Jr., and Bradley N. Lemke

SECTION 2
CORNEA AND SCLERA
Henry F. Edelhauser and John L. Ubels

 4 Cornea and Sclera, 47
    Henry F. Edelhauser and John L. Ubels

SECTION 3
LENS
David C. Beebe

 5 The Lens, 117
    David C. Beebe

SECTION 4
OPTICS AND REFRACTION
David Miller

 6 Physiologic Optics and Refraction, 159
    David Miller

SECTION 5
ACCOMMODATION AND PRESBYOPIA
Adrian Glasser and Paul L. Kaufman

 7 Accommodation and Presbyopia, 197
    Adrian Glasser and Paul L. Kaufman

SECTION 6
AQUEOUS HUMOR HYDRODYNAMICS
B'Ann True Gabelt and Paul L. Kaufman

 8 Aqueous Humor Hydrodynamics, 237
    B'Ann True Gabelt and Paul. L. Kaufman

SECTION 7
VITREOUS
Henrik Lund-Andersen

 9 The Vitreous, 293
    Henrik Lund-Andersen and Birgit Sander

SECTION 8
RETINA
Albert Alm and Berndt E.J. Ehinger

10 Development and Structure of the
    Retina, 319
    Rajesh K. Sharma and Berndt E.J. Ehinger

11 The Retinal Pigment Epithelium, 348
    Morten la Cour

12 Genetics and Biology of the Inherited
    Retinal Dystrophies, 358
    David A.R. Bessant, Shalesh Kaushal,
    and Shomi S. Bhattacharya

13 Retinal Biochemistry, 382
    Serge Picaud

14 Electrophysiology and Retinal
    Function, 409
    Vesna Ponjavic and Sten Andréasson

15 Intracellular Light Responses
    and Synaptic Organization
    of the Vertebrate Retina, 422
    Samuel M. Wu

SECTION 9
VISUAL PERCEPTION
Pamela A. Sample and Chris A. Johnson

16 Entoptic Phenomena, 441
    Gerald Westheimer

17 Visual Acuity, 453
    Gerald Westheimer

18 Early Visual Processing of Spatial
    Form, 470
    David Regan

19 Binocular Vision, 484
    Ronald S. Harwerth and Clifton M. Schor

20 Temporal Properties of Vision, 511
    Allison M. McKendrick and Chris A. Johnson

21 Development of Vision in Infancy, 531
    Anthony M. Norcia and Ruth E. Manny

22 Perimetry and Visual Field Testing, 552
    Chris A. Johnson and Pamela A. Sample

23 Color Vision, 578
    Thomas P. Sakmar

24 Visual Adaptation, 586
    David G. Birch

SECTION 10
OPTIC NERVE
Leonard A. Levin

25 Optic Nerve, 603
    Leonard A. Levin

SECTION 11
CENTRAL VISUAL PATHWAYS
Joanne A. Matsubara

26 Overview of the Central Visual
    Pathways, 641
    Jamie D. Boyd, Qiang Gu, and
    Joanne A. Matsubara

27 Activity-Dependent Development
    of Retinogeniculate Projections, 646
    Rachel O. Wong and Rebecca C. Stacy

28 The Lateral Geniculate Nucleus, 655
    Vivien A. Casagrande and Jennifer M. Ichida

29 The Primary Visual Cortex, 669
    Vivien A. Casagrande and Jennifer M. Ichida

30 Extrastriate Visual Cortex, 686
    Jamie D. Boyd and Joanne A. Matsubara

31 Visual Deprivation, 697
    Qiang Gu, Joanne A. Matsubara, and
    Jamie D. Boyd

SECTION 12
PUPIL
Randy Kardon

32 The Pupil, 713
    Randy Kardon

Section 13
CIRCULATION
Albert Alm

33 **Ocular Circulation,** 747
  *George A. Cioffi, Elisabet Granstam,
  and Albert Alm*

Section 14
**EXTRAOCULAR MUSCLES/EYE
MOVEMENTS**
Lance M. Optican

34 **The Extraocular Muscles,** 787
  *John D. Porter, Francisco H. Andrade,
  and Robert S. Baker*

35 **Three-Dimensional Rotations
  of the Eye,** 818
  Christian Quaia and Lance M. Optican

36 **Neural Control of Eye Movements,** 830
  Clifton M. Schor

ADLER'S PHYSIOLOGY OF THE EYE

SECTION 1

THE OCULAR SURFACE

BRADLEY N. LEMKE

CHAPTER 1

ORBIT

Bryan S. Sires, Roberta Gausas, Briggs E. Cook, Jr., and Bradley N. Lemke

EMBRYOLOGY

The bony orbit is formed from the mesenchyme surrounding the early optic vesicle. Two types of bone formation or ossification occur during the genesis of the orbit: endochondral and membranous. Endochondral bones are preformed in cartilage and ossify secondarily. Membranous bones ossify directly from connective tissue.

The orbital walls are derived from cranial neural crest cells. Early in development, the lateral nasal process migrates and fuses with the maxillary process to form the medial, inferior, and lateral orbital walls. The capsule of the forebrain forms the orbital roof. As the globe enlarges, the surrounding connective tissue condenses and thickens, and it is within these fibrous plates that the bones surrounding the orbit develop.[1]

The first bone to develop embryologically is the maxillary bone, recognizable at the 6-week embryonic stage. The maxillary bone is membranous in origin and develops from elements in the region of the canine tooth. Secondary ossification centers follow in the adjacent orbitonasal and premaxillary regions. The frontal, zygomatic, and palatine bones develop as intramembranous ossifications at approximately the 7-week embryonic stage.[4]

In contrast to other bones, the sphenoid bone has both endochondral and membranous origins. The lesser and greater wings of the sphenoid bone form spatially and temporally separate. The lesser wing of the sphenoid and the optic canal begin as cartilaginous structures at the 7-week embryonic stage; the greater wing of the sphenoid, preformed in cartilage, begins to ossify at approximately the 10-week embryonic stage. The optic strut ossifies at 11 weeks. The lesser and greater wings of the sphenoid join together at 16 weeks.[4] Several weeks later the sphenoid bone expands to contact the frontal bone. Ossification of the orbital walls is complete at birth, except for the orbital apex.[14]

OSTEOLOGY/FRACTURES

The bony orbit is designed to support and provide protection to the orbital soft tissues. These tissues consist of the globe and its supporting adnexa. The orbit consists of seven individual bones, which combine to make up the four surrounding walls. They are the sphenoid, frontal, ethmoid, maxillary, zygomatic, palatine, and lacrimal bones. The walls consist of the orbital roof, the orbital floor, and the lateral and medial orbital walls. Each wall has characteristic structural dimensions that provide specific functions.[4,21]

The adult orbit is roughly shaped like a pyramid (Figure 1-1). The orbital rim is thick and rounded at its anterior aperture, providing a hard tissue shield to protect the eye and adnexa from traumatic impacts. The rim is a discontinuous circle with overlap at the nasolacrimal drain. The anterior overlapping circle is the anterior lacrimal crest, and the posterior overlapping circle is the posterior lacrimal crest. The lacrimal fossa, made up of the maxillary and lacrimal bones, sits between the two crests and is the location of the nasolacrimal sac. The medial one third of the superior orbital rim contains a supraorbital notch 75% of the time, whereas a supraorbital foramen is present 25% of the time. The supraorbital neurovascular bundle passes through these structures. The prominence of the medial brow, called the *supraorbital ridges,* is present mostly in males and meets in the midline in an area called the *glabella.* Their presence is the result of the expanding underlying frontal sinus during development. The rim is thickest laterally and is formed by the zygomatic bone and the zygomatic

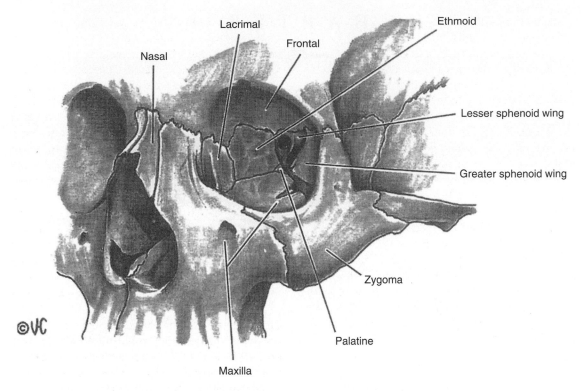

FIGURE 1-1   Osteology of the orbital bones and orbital apex. (Copyright Virginia Cantarella.)

process of the frontal bone. This is the strongest portion of the orbital rim. The lateral rim is a posteriorly directed concavity, which increases the lateral visual field but makes the eye prone to injury. Just inside the lateral orbital rim is the orbital tubercle of the zygomatic bone. This is the attachment point of the lateral canthal ligament along with the lateral rectus muscle check ligament, Whitnall's ligament, and the aponeurosis of the levator palpebrae superioris muscle. The infraorbital foramen, found in the maxilla, sits 4 to 12 mm below the inferior orbital rim. The orbit attains its widest diameter 1 cm behind the orbital rim.

The orbital floor is thin and mainly consists of the orbital plate of the maxillary bone. It also has contributions from the zygoma anterior laterally and the palatine bone posteriorly. The floor is triangular in shape, and it extends from the maxillary-ethmoid buttress to the inferior orbital fissure. This buttress is also referred to as the *medial strut.* The posterior limit of the floor coincides with the posterior wall of the maxillary sinus. The floor does not extend to the apex and is 35 to 40 mm long. A depression lateral to the nasolacrimal fossa exists in the anteromedial orbital floor and is the fossa for

the inferior oblique muscle origin. The infraorbital foramen extends posteriorly through the infraorbital canal to the infraorbital sulcus at the posterior aspect of the orbital floor. This leads to the posterior aspect of the inferior orbital fissure. The floor provides support to the eye and adnexal tissues and separates them from the maxillary sinus.

The maxillary-ethmoid buttress and the infraorbital sulcus/canal provide support to the floor. However, between these structures the floor easily deforms to blunt trauma. The thin bone and relative lack of support of the floor lead to a high rate of fractures compared with the other walls. The floor acts like a release valve to increased orbital pressure and blows out into the maxillary sinus, providing protection to the eye and adnexal soft tissues.[20] The floor can also buckle from a direct blow to the inferior orbital rim.[6] The patient with a blow-out fracture may experience loss of vision, diplopia, enophthalmos, or a numb cheek.

The medial wall is the smallest of the orbital walls. The medial walls are parallel to each other in the midsagittal plane and are 45 to 50 mm in length from the rim to the orbital apex. The medial wall is formed by the maxillary, lacrimal, ethmoid, and sphenoid bones. Posteriorly, the palatine bone can extend onto the medial wall. The lacrimal fossa is anterior, and its thickness is determined by the location of the lacrimal-maxillary suture. In 90% of people the suture is anterior and the fossa is composed more from the thinner lacrimal bone. Rarely, the suture is posterior, and the fossa is composed of the thicker maxillary bone. Behind the posterior lacrimal crest is the lamina papyracea of the ethmoid bone. This structure is extremely thin but is uniformly supported by the honeycombed structure of the ethmoid sinus bony lamina. This structure explains why the medial wall is fractured less than the orbital floor despite both walls being extremely thin. The anterior and posterior ethmoidal foramen lie at the superior aspect of the ethmoid bone along the frontoethmoidal suture. This is approximately at the level of the frontal cranial fossa, and the crista galli can extend 5 to 10 mm below this suture. The anterior ethmoidal foramen lies about 20 mm from the orbital rim, and the posterior ethmoidal foramen lies an additional 10 to 15 mm posteriorly. Posterior to the lamina papyracea is the sphenoid bone. The body of the sphenoid bone is situated between the two orbital apices, and the sphenoid sinus is contained within it. The optic canal is enclosed by the body of the sphenoid, the lesser wing of the sphenoid, and the optic strut.

The orbital roof boundaries form an isosceles triangle and are made up of the orbital plate of the frontal bone with a minor contribution from the lesser wing of sphenoid posteriorly. The anterior third of the roof is the thickest portion. The anterolateral extreme contains a slight depression called the *lacrimal gland fossa*. Overall, the roof is concave, but the fossa is deeper. The medial roof, 3 to 5 mm behind the rim, contains a small depression called the *fovea trochlearis*. This is where the fibrocartilaginous trochlea for the superior oblique tendon resides. The frontal sinus is contained within the frontal bone superior to the roof. The frontosphenoidal suture crosses the orbital apex from the anterior end of the superior orbital fissure to the posterior ethmoidal foramen. This is not usually obvious in the adult orbit. The lesser wing of the sphenoid contributes a portion of the optic canal. The optic canal is separated from the superior orbital fissure by a bridge of bone arising from the lateral portion of the lesser wing of the sphenoid, called the *optic strut*. The canal is nearly in a line with the two ethmoidal foramina. The distance from the posterior ethmoidal foramen to the optic

canal is 4 to 9 mm. The two canals in a skull travel superior, medial, and posterior to meet at the center of the dorsum sellae. The canal houses the optic nerve and ophthalmic artery. A keyhole groove can be seen in the floor of the canal where the ophthalmic artery runs.

The lateral orbital wall is the thickest and strongest wall. The superior and inferior orbital fissures form the boundary. The two walls are at right angles to each other and are about the same length as the medial orbital wall. The wall is thinnest at the zygomaticosphenoidal suture and is a convenient location to perform a lateral orbitotomy. Two other sutures, the zygomaticofrontal and the frontosphenoidal sutures, are also contained in the lateral orbital wall. The three sutures meet just superior to the center of the lateral wall. About 40% of individuals have a meningeal foramen in the frontosphenoidal suture just anterior to the anterior extent of the superior orbital fissure. This foramen transmits an anastomotic branch between the lacrimal artery and the middle meningeal artery. The superior orbital fissure separates the roof and the lateral wall. The lateral rectus spine, the origin of the lateral rectus muscle, sits at the inferior medial aspect of the superior orbital fissure across from the optic strut. The superior orbital fissure transmits nerves for periorbital sensation, lacrimation, and internal and external ocular movement along with orbital venous return. The inferior orbital fissure separates the floor and the lateral orbital wall. The foramen rotundum opens into the posterior inferior orbital fissure and transmits the maxillary nerve through the inferior orbital sulcus to the infraorbital foramen. Nerve fibers from the sphenopalatine ganglion and the inferior orbital vein on its way to the pterygoid plexus also pass through the inferior orbital fissure. The zygomaticotemporal and zygomaticofacial neurovascular bundles pass through the lateral wall just anterior to the inferior orbital fissure and exit just behind the lateral rim, providing sensation to the lateral midface.

Blunt trauma to the cheek can result in a tripod fracture. The fracture points include the zygomaticomaxillary suture, frontozygomatic suture, and zygomatic arch. This complex rotates medially and inferiorly and is caused by muscle contracture across the fracture. Clinically, the cheek is noted to be depressed, and the patient may experience trismus from the coronoid process of the mandible hitting the rotated zygomatic arch. These fractures need to be reduced and fixated at a minimum of two locations. When reduced, the orbital floor may be involved with the fracture and requires appropriate repair to prevent enophthalmos and/or restrictive strabismus from orbital soft tissue prolapse through the fracture defect.

GLOBE: SIZE, POSITION, AND RELATION TO HEAD

Early in human development, the optic vesicles point in different directions, approximately 180 degrees apart, but this angle decreases as the eyes become situated more anteriorly with growth. The adult lateral orbital walls are approximately 90 degrees from each other, and the parallel medial orbital walls are nearly straight anteroposteriorly (Figure 1-2). Therefore the divergent axis of the orbit becomes half of 45 degrees, or approximately 23 degrees.[14] Because of the temporal location of the fovea, the visual axis is not the same as the optic or orbital axis.

At birth, the anteroposterior diameter of the globe is approximately 16 mm, and the globe reaches 90% of its adult size when an infant is 20 months of age.[14] According to studies of Hertel exophthalmometry measurements, the globe becomes relatively more proptotic until an adult is 20 years of age.[5] Adult orbit dimensions are variable.

In the adult the globe measures approximately 24 mm in anteroposterior diameter, although the length may vary from 20 to 30 mm. The vertical diameter is approximately 23 mm, and the horizontal diameter is approximately 23.5 mm. The volume of the globe is 7 cm³, and that of the orbit is 30 cm³.

The globe does not rest completely within the bony orbit. The cornea and portions of the globe anterior to the equator are exposed beyond the edges of the bony orbital rim. Because the vertical height of the orbital rim is approximately 35 mm and the horizontal length approximately 40 mm,

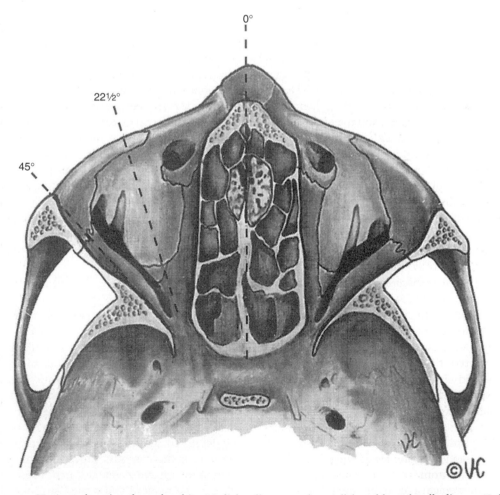

FIGURE 1-2   Horizontal section through orbits. Medial walls are nearly parallel, and lateral walls diverge 45 degrees from midline. (Copyright Virginia Cantarella.)

the globe is slightly more vulnerable to trauma along its lateral aspect.

EXOPHTHALMOS

Because the bony orbit is incapable of acute expansion except anteriorly, any displacement of the eye causes the globe to move forward, resulting in exophthalmos. The term *exophthalmos* is specific for forward displacement of the globe, whereas the term *proptosis* refers to the forward displacement of any object. Therefore the term *exophthalmos* should be used in reference to the globe and orbit. Enophthalmos is the retrodisplacement of the globe posterior into the orbit.

The most common cause of unilateral and bilateral exophthalmos in adults is thyroid eye disease. The mass effect is caused by an inflammatory reaction of an unknown cause. Factors such as glycosaminoglycans collect in the extraocular muscles and/or connective tissue and fat and lead to swelling. This swelling is eventually replaced by chronic scar. Other common causes of exophthalmos include hemangiomas, inflammatory pseudotumors, benign and malignant lymphoid lesions, craniostenoses and the craniofacial dysostosis, and other orbital mass lesions. Enophthalmos resulting from trauma, surgery, previous irradiation, or metastatic lesions may lead to pseudoexophthalmos of the contralateral eye. Severe myopia and buphthalmos may simulate exophthalmos because of the elongated globe associated with these conditions. However, the orbit is normal in size with an enlarged, protruding globe.

The amount of protrusion of the normal eye can be an important clinical marker. The amount of protrusion is typically measured from the deepest part of the lateral orbital rim to the corneal apex. The Hertel exophthalmometer is the most accurate exophthalmometer; it can measure both eyes with a system of mirrors, crosshairs to correct for parallax, and a superimposed millimeter scale. The base distance between the lateral orbital rims can be recorded and used to standardize the measurements of the patient on repeat visits. The Naugle exophthalmometer is a similar device but uses the supraorbital ridges and the malar prominence as the reference point.

Migliori and Gladstone[15] studied 681 adults, ranging in age from 18 to 91 years. They determined the average and upper limit of normal amounts of protrusion in different sexes and races. The 327 Caucasian and 354 African-American sub- jects had no history of orbital or endocrine disease, severe myopia, or buphthalmos. The mean normal protrusion values were 16.5 mm in Caucasian men, 18.5 mm in African-American men, 15.4 mm in Caucasian women, and 17.8 mm in African-American women. The upper limits of normal were 21.7 mm for Caucasian men, 24.7 mm for African-American men, 20.1 mm for Caucasian women, and 23.0 mm for African-American women. No individual had more than 2 mm of asymmetry between eyes. Values greater than the upper limits of normal may indicate orbital disease.

FASCIAL SYSTEM AND FAT

The orbital fascial tissue is a large, single interconnecting network emanating from the periorbita externally.[13] The fascia or connective tissue is intimately associated with the orbital adipocytes and fat. The connective tissue and fat provide support and insulation to the orbital soft tissue structures and assist with free, unimpeded movement of the globe and other orbital soft tissues (Figures 1-3 and 1-4).

The periorbita lines the bones of the orbit and completely encloses all of the orbital soft tissue contents except for the lids, globe, and conjunctiva anteriorly. The densest connection to the orbital bones is along the arcus marginalis. The periorbita is made up of collagen and contains no elastic tissue because it is rigidly fixed to the bone, which requires no elasticity. The connective tissue projects from the periorbital anchor into the orbital soft tissue compartment to envelop all of the orbital soft tissue structures. Also, the connective tissue divides the orbital fat into lobules.

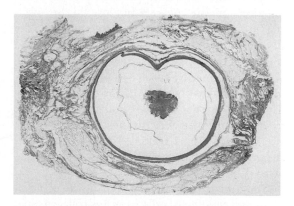

FIGURE 1-3 Coronal histologic section of the right anterior orbit. Note the dense connective tissue in the region of the canthi. Definable fat regions can be identified. (From Sires BS et al: *Ophthal Plast Reconstr Surg* 14:403, 1998.)

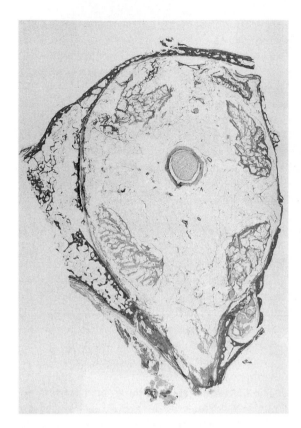

FIGURE 1-4   Coronal histologic section of the right posterior orbit. Note that the connective tissue is sparse and no distinct regions are seen. (From Sires BS et al: *Ophthal Plast Reconstr Surg* 14:403, 1998.)

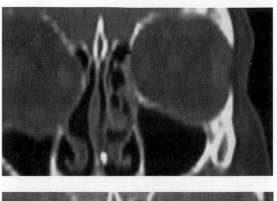

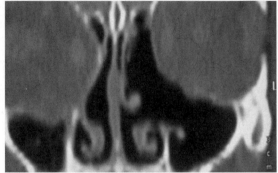

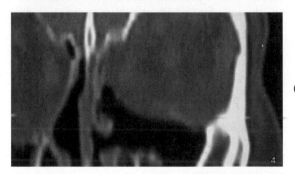

FIGURE 1-5   Intraoperative computed tomography scan of a left orbital decompression before bone removal (**A**) and before (**B**) and after (**C**) opening of the periorbita. Note how the intact periorbita (**B**) holds the orbital soft tissue contents in place after bone removal.

The connective tissue is regionalized, with it being anatomically more complex in the anterior orbit. There are more septa, and the individual septa are more dense anteriorly. Distinct regions in the anterior orbit are apparent but lose this organization in the posterior orbit. Four regions can be defined.[18] Two are located in the inferior orbit; and the lateral one extends into the retrobulbar space, where the connective tissue becomes scant. The regions are divided by the inferior oblique muscle. The medial inferior orbital region includes the area external to the medial rectus muscle. There are also two superior orbital regions; one is situated over the trochlea, and the other is over the top of the levator palpebrae superioris muscle.

The orbital connective tissue consists of fibroblasts and endothelial cells, as well as collagen types I, III, and IV. Collagen type I is a protein that provides structural integrity. Collagen type III is a cellular adhesion molecule between the connective tissue and adipocytes. Collagen type IV is associated with the basement membranes of the vessels found in the connective tissue. Veins tend to run in the connective tissue, whereas arteries are found more randomly. No elastin is present in the fine orbital connective tissue, except for in the elastic lamina of arteries. The collagen density is greatest around the globe in the regions of the medial and lateral canthal ligaments, as well as in the area of Whitnall's ligament. Elastin is associated with the dense collagen of the canthal ligaments and the beginning of the nasolacrimal drain. This area supports the globe and adnexa but allows free, unim-

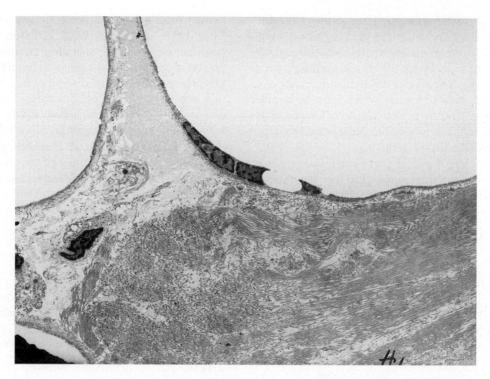

FIGURE 1-6 Electron micrograph of the orbital connective tissue with an adipocyte. Note the fibroblast adjacent to the dense collagen arrangement. (From Sires BS et al: *Ophthal Plast Reconstr Surg* 14:403, 1998.)

peded movement around the axes of Fick. Support of the globe and adnexa by the periorbita is demonstrated during orbital decompression for thyroid eye disease (Figure 1-5). Bone removal of the orbital floor and medial wall can occur with little change in the position of the globe until the periorbita is opened and the dense connective tissue planes are lysed.

The space within the orbital fine connective tissue septa is occupied by adipocytes and fat (Figure 1-6). The plasma membranes of the adipocytes interface with the connective tissue. The collagen type I–collagen type III–adipocyte plasma membrane complex forms a sandwich by means of the adherence function of the collagen type III. Small fatty vacuoles exist at the sandwich interface, and this may be a transport mechanism for the fatty acids. The adipocyte nuclei are thin, flat, eccentrically displaced, and parallel the plasma membrane. Most of the adipocyte volume is the cytoplasm filled with fat.

The fatty acid amounts found in the fat are similar no matter which orbital region is sampled, despite the color differences, which range from white to yellow, of the orbital fat regions.[18] The fat in the orbit is made up of fatty acid chains of variable length, ranging from 14 to 18 carbons long with

variable amounts of unsaturated double bonds. The most common orbital fatty acids are oleic acid (18:1), palmitic acid (16:0), and linoleic acid (18:2). When compared with fatty acids from other body regions, orbital fat is more unsaturated, which may be an advantage for extraocular motility.

The preaponeurotic fat is yellow; the remainder of the orbital fat is white. Carotenoids explain this color difference.[19] These substances are 40-carbon chain tetraterpenoids. They scavenge free radicals, stabilize cell membranes, and assist in transmembrane transport. There is a twofold to fourfold excess of carotenoids in the preaponeurotic fat. Lutein and beta-carotene account for most of this difference. The specific advantage of the carotenoid excess in the preaponeurotic fat is unknown, but possibilities include differences in development, motility mechanisms, free radical scavenger function, and depot support to other structures like the retina.

VASCULATURE

Interal Carotid Arterial Supply

The vascular supply to the orbit is a complex anastomotic network that receives input from both the internal and external carotid artery circulation. The internal carotid artery gives rise to the ophthalmic artery, which provides the primary blood supply for the orbit, including the globe. Although the ophthalmic artery has a rich anastomotic connection to the external carotid circulation, many of its branches are end vessels, which must be handled cautiously during orbital surgery. Damage to the central retinal artery or choroidal vessels results in blindness and ocular ischemia.

The internal carotid artery enters the cavernous sinus and middle cranial fossa via the foramen lacerum. Within the cavernous sinus, the abducens nerve lies along its lateral side and it is surrounded by sympathetic fibers of the carotid plexus derived from the superior cervical ganglion. Several branches are given off, including the meningohypophyseal artery.[9] These cavernous branches play a potential role in carotid-cavernous fistulas.[3] Low-flow fistulas typically form in the posterior cavernous sinus, whereas high-flow fistulas tend to form in the anterior cavernous sinus.[8] Increased pressure in the cavernous sinus causes reversal of flow in the ophthalmic veins and the classic findings of orbital congestion and retinal ischemia.

As the internal carotid travels forward in the cavernous sinus it makes an S-shaped turn along the

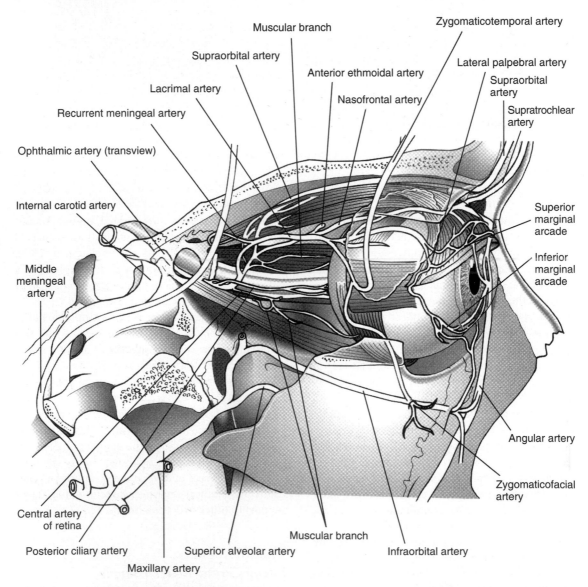

FIGURE 1-7 Direct lateral view of the arteries of the orbit. (From Albert DM [ed]: *Ophthalmic surgery: principles and techniques,* Malden, Mass, 1999, Blackwell Science.)

lateral wall of the sphenoid sinus, indenting the bone (i.e., the carotid siphon). The internal carotid artery emerges from the anterior cavernous sinus medial to the anterior clinoid process and dips inferior to the optic nerve. It is at this point that its first major branch, the ophthalmic artery, is given off. Rarely, the ophthalmic artery may arise from the carotid artery while still within the cavernous sinus and enter the orbit through a separate bony passage, or it may arise from the middle meningeal artery and enter the orbit through the superior orbital fissure.[16]

Having emerged from the carotid inferior artery to the optic nerve, the ophthalmic artery joins the nerve along its inferomedial surface and enters the optic canal. The ophthalmic artery travels through the optic canal within the dural sheath of the optic nerve and shifts to a lateral position. The artery penetrates the outer layers of dura and emerges from the optic foramen along the inferolateral aspect of the optic nerve (Figure 1-7).

In approximately 80% of individuals, the ophthalmic artery then crosses from its lateral position to the medial portion of the orbit by traveling over the optic nerve. In approximately 20% of individuals, it crosses under the optic nerve.[16] On the medial side of the orbit, the artery travels anteriorly between the superior oblique muscle and the optic nerve, until 10 to 15 mm posterior to the trochlea, where it exits the muscle cone.[3] The artery lies close to the medial orbital wall as it approaches the trochlea, most commonly passing between the medial rectus and superior oblique muscles.[2] It exits the orbit inferior to the trochlea and emerges at the superomedial orbital rim.

In 96% of individuals, the ophthalmic artery provides the primary blood supply to the orbit. However, in 3% of individuals the middle meningeal artery contributes equally through an accessory ophthalmic ("recurrent meningeal") branch, and in 1%, the middle meningeal artery is the primary source.[3]

There is variability in the orbital course of the ophthalmic artery and even greater variability in the order of its branching. Hayreh[10] and Hayreh and Dass[11,12] have described the major distribution and anatomic variations of the ophthalmic artery. The most common branching orders of the ophthalmic artery are listed in Table 1-1.[10] Because the branching sequence varies considerably, it is easier to view the branches of the ophthalmic artery based on the anatomic region they supply, namely, ocular, orbital, or extraorbital, rather than based on their order of origin. Branches to ocular structures include the central retinal and posterior ciliary arteries. Branches to orbital structures include the lacrimal and muscular arteries. Branches to extraorbital sites include the

TABLE 1-1

ORDER OF ORIGIN OF BRANCHES OF OPHTHALMIC ARTERY

	OPHTHALMIC ARTERY CROSSED	
ORDER OF ORIGIN	OVER OPTIC NERVE	UNDER OPTIC NERVE
1	Central retinal and medial posterior ciliary	Lateral posterior ciliary
2	Lateral posterior ciliary	Central retinal
3	Lacrimal	Medial muscular
4	Muscular to superior rectus or levator	Medial posterior ciliary
5	Posterior ethmoid and supraorbital, jointly or separately	Lacrimal
6	Medial posterior ciliary	Muscular to superior rectus and levator
7	Medial muscular	Posterior ethmoid and supraorbital, jointly or separately
8	Muscular to superior oblique and medial rectus, jointly, or separately, to either	Muscular to superior oblique and medial rectus, jointly or separately, to either
9	To areolar tissue	Anterior ethmoid
10	Anterior ethmoid	To areolar tissue
11	Medial palpebral or inferior medial palpebral	Medial palpebral or inferior medial palpebral
12	Superior medial palpebral	Superior medial palpebral
Terminal	1. Dorsal nasal	1. Dorsal nasal
	2. Supratrochlear	2. Supratrochlear

From Hayreh SS: *Br J Ophthalmol* 46:212, 1962.

ethmoidal, palpebral, supraorbital, supratrochlear, and dorsal nasal arteries.

Ocular Branches of the Ophthalmic Artery

The first branch of the ophthalmic artery is usually the central retinal artery, which is an end artery to the retina. It typically arises before or as the ophthalmic artery bends medially and travels lateral or inferior to the optic nerve. It penetrates the dura of the optic nerve at a level 5 to 16 mm behind the globe, entering the subarachnoid space and then the substance of the nerve. Within the nerve it courses in a canal toward the disc, where it branches into several arterioles, which supply the retina.

The two posterior ciliary arteries, lateral and medial, are end arteries to the choroid. They too arise near the medial bend in the ophthalmic artery and course anteriorly, dividing into numerous short ciliary branches and two long ciliary branches. Fifteen to twenty short posterior ciliary arteries pierce the sclera in a ring around the optic nerve to supply the optic nerve head and the choroid. The long posterior ciliary arteries run within scleral canals, noticeable as gray channels, and supply the ciliary muscle, iris, and anterior choroid.

Orbital Branches of the Ophthalmic Artery

Intraorbital structures other than the globe are supplied by the orbital branches of the ophthalmic artery. The extraocular muscles are supplied by two main muscular branches: the lateral and the medial. The lateral muscular artery supplies the lateral rectus, superior rectus, superior oblique, and levator palpebrae superioris muscles. The medial muscular artery supplies the medial rectus, inferior rectus, and inferior oblique muscles. As the arteries travel within each rectus muscle, they divide into anterior ciliary branches. Each rectus muscle has two anterior ciliary arteries associated with it, except for the lateral rectus muscle, which has one. At the tendinous muscle insertions, these arteries penetrate the sclera and anastomose with the long posterior ciliary arteries to supply the anterior globe.

The lacrimal artery arises from the ophthalmic artery in close proximity to the origin of the central retinal artery. It courses superolaterally within the orbit near the superior border of the lateral rectus muscle to reach the lacrimal gland. The lacrimal artery branches into the zygomaticotemporal and zygomaticofacial arteries, which exit through the lateral orbital wall via the zygomaticotemporal and zygomaticofacial foramina. It has additional branches that supply the gland and form the superior and inferior lateral palpebral arteries.

The supraorbital artery is given off more distally from the ophthalmic artery and may be absent in 10% to 20% of individuals.[4] It exits the orbit at the supraorbital notch or foramen. It contributes small branches to the superior rectus, superior oblique, and levator muscles, although its main supply is to the eyebrow and forehead.

The intraorbital structures receive additional blood supply from numerous small vessels derived from the cavernous branches of the internal carotid artery, which enter the orbit through the optic canal or superior and inferior orbital fissures.

Extraorbital Branches of the Ophthalmic Artery

Structures outside of the orbit are supplied by the extraorbital branches of the ophthalmic artery. The smaller posterior ethmoidal artery branches medially and exits the orbit through the posterior ethmoidal foramen, located 5 to 10 mm anterior to the optic canal. It supplies posterior nasal and sinus mucosa. The larger anterior ethmoidal artery exits the orbit through its canal, approximately 15 mm anterior to the posterior ethmoidal foramen, and supplies the anterior sinus mucosa, nose, and septum.

The nasofrontal artery is the anterior continuation of the ophthalmic artery in the superomedial extraconal space. Posterior to the trochlea it divides into the supratrochlear artery, which supplies the medial forehead and scalp, and the dorsal nasal artery, which supplies the nasal bridge, forehead, and midline scalp. The dorsal nasal artery also gives rise to the medial palpebral artery, which divides into superior and inferior branches that anastomose with the lateral palpebral vessels to form the marginal and peripheral arterial arcades.

External Carotid Arterial Supply

An extensive anastomotic connection exists between the internal and external carotid systems; this connection brings collateral blood supply to the orbit. The external carotid supplies the orbit via three major branches: the facial (medially), the superficial temporal (laterally), and the maxillary (deep) arteries.

The facial artery arises from the external carotid artery in the carotid triangle below the angle of the jaw. It travels over the mandible, across the cheek, and along the side of the nose toward the medial canthus as the angular artery. This angular branch anastomoses with the dorsal nasal and infraorbital arteries to provide collateral blood flow to the eyelids and anterior part of the orbit. The external carotid artery then divides behind the neck of the mandible into the internal maxillary and superficial temporal arteries. Among the many branches given off by the internal maxillary artery are the middle meningeal and the infraorbital arteries. The infraorbital artery arises in the pterygopalatine fossa at the inferior orbital fissure, travels through the orbit within the infraorbital canal adjacent to the infraorbital nerve, emerges on the face via the infraorbital foramen, and anastomoses with branches of the facial artery. Its branches supply the inferior rectus and inferior oblique muscles, lower eyelid, upper cheek, lacrimal sac, orbital fat, and lacrimal gland.[3] The middle meningeal artery enters the skull base through the foramen spinosum and anastomoses with the lacrimal artery through a recurrent meningeal or meningolacrimal branch.

The other terminal branch of the external carotid is the superficial temporal artery, which gives rise to the frontal, zygomatic, and transverse facial arteries. From its origin anterior to the bony external auditory canal, it crosses the zygomatic process and travels superiorly in front of the ear, where a biopsy sample can be taken in cases of suspected temporal arteritis. Its frontal branch supplies the forehead and anastomoses with the supraorbital and supratrochlear arteries. The zygomatic branch anastomoses with lacrimal and palpebral branches of the ophthalmic artery. The transverse facial branch, supplying the parotid gland and masseter muscle, anastomoses with the infraorbital artery.

Venous Drainage

The venous drainage from the orbit follows a different course than that of the arterial system. Except for the lacrimal and ethmoidal veins, orbital veins do not parallel orbital arteries. Veins closely follow and lie within the complex connective tissue septa of the orbit, whereas the arteries pass through the septa. Venous outflow from the orbit follows three main pathways: posteriorly through the ophthalmic veins into the cavernous sinus, inferiorly into the pterygoid plexus through the inferior orbital fissure, or anteriorly by free communication into the angular vein into the facial system.[4] Orbital veins do not possess valves.

The superior and inferior ophthalmic veins provide the primary outflow for the venous system (Figure 1-8). The superior ophthalmic vein is formed by the confluence of the supraorbital, nasofrontal, and angular veins at the superomedial orbital rim. It can be viewed as having three sections. The first section runs posteriorly in the orbit adjacent to the trochlea and medial to the superior

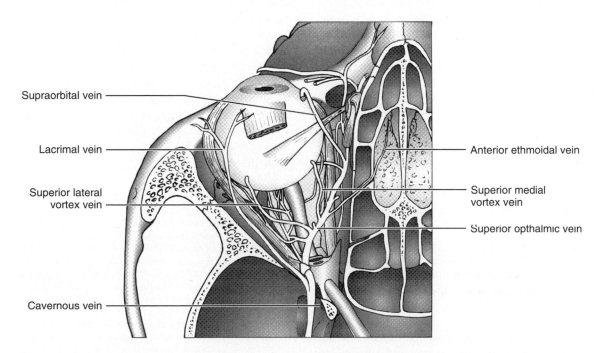

Supraorbital vein

Lacrimal vein

Superior lateral vortex vein

Cavernous vein

Anterior ethmoidal vein

Superior medial vortex vein

Superior opthalmic vein

FIGURE 1-8 Superior view of orbital veins. (From Albert DM [ed]: *Ophthalmic surgery: principles and techniques,* Malden, Mass, 1999, Blackwell Science.)

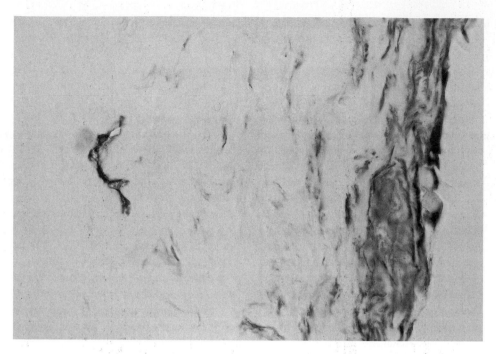

FIGURE 1-9   Thin-walled, partially collapsed lymphatic capillary within mid dura mater of optic nerve stains positive for 5′-nucleotidase.

rectus muscle. Behind the globe, in the second section, it shifts below the superior rectus muscle into a more lateral position. The third section of the superior ophthalmic vein runs along the lateral edge of the superior rectus muscle into the superior orbital fissure above the annulus of Zinn, where it drains into the cavernous sinus venous plexus.

The inferior ophthalmic vein originates as a diffuse venous plexus in the orbital fat beneath the globe.[21] It receives tributaries from the inferior oblique and medial and inferior rectus muscles, lower eyelid, and lacrimal sac. The inferior ophthalmic vein runs posteriorly in the orbit along the lateral border of the inferior rectus muscle and anastomoses with the superior ophthalmic vein, ultimately draining into the cavernous sinus. Inferiorly, it also communicates with the pterygoid plexus through the inferior orbital fissure.

Anteriorly, venous outflow may occur through the angular vein medially and a plexus from the inferior ophthalmic vein to the facial vein laterally.

Lymphatic Drainage

Whereas lymphatic drainage of the eyelids and conjunctiva into the preauricular and submaxillary lymph nodes has been well documented, the orbit has traditionally been believed to be devoid of true endothelial cell–lined lymphatic vessels. However, studies suggest that lymphatic vessels exist in the orbit. Early studies using interstitial injection of dyes, carbon, or fluorochromes failed to identify a lymphatic system. With enzyme histochemistry, more recent studies have identified lymphatic vessels in the orbit of the cynomolgus monkey.[17] Similar studies have identified true endothelial cell–lined lymphatic vessels in the human orbit[7] (Figure 1-9). They were isolated to the lacrimal gland and the dura mater of the optic nerve. Future investigation may delineate a lymphatic pathway throughout the human orbit.

REFERENCES

1. Blechschmidt E, Gasser RF: *Biokinetics and biodynamics of human differentiation,* Springfield, Ill, 1978, Charles C Thomas.
2. Ducasse A et al: Anatomical basis of the surgical approaches to the medial wall of the orbit, *Anat Clin* 7:15, 1985.
3. Dutton JJ: Arterial supply to the orbit. In *Atlas of clinical and surgical orbital anatomy,* Philadelphia, 1994, WB Saunders.
4. Dutton JJ: Osteology of the orbit. In *Atlas of clinical and surgical orbital anatomy,* Philadelphia, 1994, WB Saunders.
5. Fledelius HC, Stubgaard M: Changes in eye position during growth and adult life based on exophthalmometry, interpupillary distance, and orbital distance measurements, *Acta Ophthalmol (Copenh)* 64:481, 1986.
6. Fujino T: Experimental "blow-out" fracture of the orbit, *Plast Reconstr Surg* 54:81, 1974.

7. Gausas RE et al: Identification of human orbital lymphatics, *Ophthal Plast Reconstr Surg* 15:252, 1999.

8. Halbach VV et al: Carotid cavernous fistulae: Indications for urgent treatment, *AJR Am J Roentgenol* 149:587, 1987.

9. Harris FS, Rhoton AL: Anatomy of the cavernous sinus, *J Neurosurg* 45:169, 1976.

10. Hayreh SS: The ophthalmic artery: III. Branches, *Br J Ophthalmol* 46:212, 1962.

11. Hayreh SS, Dass R: The ophthalmic artery: I. Origin and in tracranial and intra-canalicular course, *Br J Ophthalmol* 46:65, 1962.

12. Hayreh SS, Dass R: The ophthalmic artery: II. Intraorbital course, *Br J Ophthalmol* 46:165, 1962.

13. Koornneef L: Details of the orbital connective tissue system in the adult. In *Spatial aspects of orbital musculo-fibrous tissue in man*, Lisse, 1977, Swets & Zweitlinger.

14. Lemke BN, Lucarelli MJ: Anatomy of the ocular adnexa, orbit, and related facial structures. In Nesi FA, Lisman RD, Levine MR (eds): *Smith's ophthalmic plastic and reconstructive surgery*, St Louis, 1998, Mosby.

15. Migliori ME, Gladstone GJ: Determination of the normal range of exophthalmometric values for black and white adults, *Am J Ophthalmol* 98:438, 1984.

16. Rootman J: *Diseases of the orbit*, Philadelphia, 1988, JB Lippincott.

17. Sherman DD et al: Identification of orbital lymphatics: enzyme histochemical, light microscopic and electron microscopic studies, *Ophthal Plast Reconstr Surg* 9:153, 1993.

18. Sires BS et al: Characterization of human orbital fat and connective tissue, *Ophthal Plast Reconstr Surg* 14:403, 1998.

19. Sires BS et al: The color difference in orbital fat, *Arch Ophthalmol* 119:868, 2001.

20. Smith B, Regan WF Jr: Blow-out fracture of the orbit: mechanism and correction of internal orbital fracture, *Am J Ophthalmol* 44:733, 1957.

21. Whitnall SE: Osteology. In *Anatomy of the human orbit and accessory organs of vision*, Huntington, NY, 1979, Krieger.

CHAPTER 2

OPHTHALMIC FACIAL ANATOMY AND PHYSIOLOGY

DON O. KIKKAWA, MARK J. LUCARELLI, JOSEPH P. SHOVLIN, BRIGGS E. COOK, JR., AND BRADLEY N. LEMKE

Clarity and integrity of the ocular surface can in large part be attributed to the eyelids. This is evidenced by the degree of corneal and conjunctival disease noted even with minor eyelid abnormalities. The capacity of greater functioning eyelids is inherent in higher mammals. The main purposes of the eyelids in humans are to protect, lubricate, and maintain the ocular surface.

However, the eyelids are just one aspect of ocular adnexal physiology. To attempt to understand the full function of the eyelids, one must study them in the context of the overall face.

EMBRYOLOGY OF EYELIDS

In their splendor the eyelids are as functionally complex as they are anatomically. The intricacies of eyelid anatomy, however, are rooted in embryonic development.

The upper and lower eyelids develop from a complex inductive interaction between surface ectoderm and mesoderm. Mesenchymal condensations located inferior and superior to the optic cup, referred to as the *frontonasal* (paranasal) and *maxillary* (visceral) *processes,* give rise to upper and lower eyelids respectively.[49] The development of the eyelids can be divided into three stages: growth, differentiation, and maturation.

The stage of growth begins with the initial ectodermal proliferation forming of the lid folds and continues until the time of eyelid fusion. During this time the conjunctiva and the conjunctival fornix develop anatomically. Differentiation begins in the fourth to fifth week of gestation and continues into the second month of gestation, when both the upper and lower eyelids are visible. By the sixth week the invagination of the optic cup has been completed. The lens vesicle has formed and separated from the surface ectoderm.[9] Two layers of surface ectoderm cover the optic cup and lens vesicle. At 7 to 8 weeks gestational age the eyelids begin to project from the surface as the apical surface ectoderm proliferates (Figure 2-1). The underlying mesoderm proliferates most actively at the apex of the eyelid fold, and the lid folds grow toward one another. Two layers of epithelium line the anterior surface, and a single layer lines the posterior surface of the eyelid fold.[56] The posterior layer becomes the palpebral conjunctiva, and the anterior layers become the eyelid skin. At 9 weeks of gestation the eyelids fuse along the eyelid margin, isolating the future conjunctiva from the amniotic fluid and ending the stage of growth. Fusion occurs by means of desmosome epithelial bridges and may protect the developing cornea and conjunctiva.[16] Failure of the eyelids to fuse during the third month can lead to epibulbar dermoid formation.

The conjunctiva develops from surface ectoderm concurrent with the embryologic growth of the eyelids. The intimate anatomic association of the eyelids and conjunctiva necessitates the formation of the conjunctiva during the growth of the eyelids. During the stage of differentiation the mesoderm underlying the conjunctiva develops into the tarsus, orbital septum, canthal ligaments, Tenon's capsule, Müller's muscle, levator palpebrae superioris, lower lid retractors, extraocular muscles, and suspensory ligaments of the conjunctival fornix.

During the early period of extraocular muscle differentiation, there is no evidence of condensa-

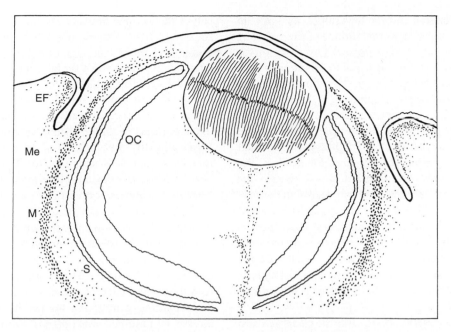

FIGURE 2-1 Artist's depiction of the development of the orbit, connective tissue, extraocular muscles, eyelids, and conjunctival fornix at 7 weeks gestational age. The invagination of the optic cup has been completed, and the lens vesicle has separated from the surface ectoderm. The eyelids begin to project from the surface as the surface ectoderm and underlying mesoderm proliferate. The conjunctiva rests on a bed of mesoderm destined to produce the connective tissues of the eyelids, sclera, orbit, and extraocular muscles. *EF,* Eyelid fold; *M,* muscle; *Me,* mesoderm; *OC,* optic cup; *S,* developing sclera.

tion of the mesoderm destined to become the sheaths of the extraocular muscles.[19] The sclera and Tenon's capsule are first recognized in the anterior portion at 8 weeks of gestation. Muscle sheaths form from fibers within the perimysium and travel outside the muscle to form the intramuscular membrane. This membrane extends anteriorly and divides at the conjunctival fornix to form Tenon's capsule and the fascial attachments to the eyelids. The development of the eyelids, extraocular muscles, and muscle sheaths proceeds concurrently and invests the conjunctiva and conjunctival fornix with their attachments.

Eyelid development continues, with hair follicles developing on the eyelid surface in an anterior-to-posterior direction, and the glands in the eyelid develop during the third to fourth months. The glands of Zeis and Moll arise from their respective epithelial cells, and the meibomian glands develop from downgrowth of basal cells in the posterior margin of the eyelids.[64] Separation of the eyelids, stimulated by function of the meibomian glands and development of the cornea, occurs during the fifth and sixth months of gestation in an anterior-to-posterior direction.[5] Failure of proper separation of the eyelids results in varying degrees of ankyloblepharon.

The medial and lateral parts of the frontonasal mesenchymal condensations fuse loosely to form the upper eyelid fold; maxillary mesenchymal condensations form the lower lid fold. The surface ectoderm covers both sides of the eyelid folds to form the skin on the outer surface and conjunctiva on the inner surface of the eyelids.

Separation of the eyelids is complete at 7 or 8 months of gestation. Muscle cells are derived from the mesoderm of the second visceral arch that surrounds the eye. Continuity of this facial muscular development from common mesoderm is evident in the structure and function of the face (discussed later in this chapter).

EYEBROWS AND FOREHEAD

Cilia of eyelids and eyebrows serve a protective function. Cilia are to be distinguished from fine lanugo hairs that are remnants from embryonic development. Cilia form the outermost barrier of the ocular surface and help protect the globe from larger airborne particles. Lid margin cilia are highly sensitive and, when stimulated, elicit a blink reflex.

Eyebrow cilia grow in different directions depending on their position.[44] The upper rows grow down and lateral, and the lowermost cilia grow up and lateral, meeting in the midline of the eyebrow.

The position of the eyebrows forms one of the foundations for human expression. Elevation of both medial and lateral portions of the eyebrows gives rise to the look of surprise. Depression of the medial portion of the eyebrow depicts anger or concern.

Eyebrow position is functionally dependent on an interplay of elevators and depressors.[40] The main elevator of the eyebrows and forehead is the frontalis muscle. The frontalis muscle elevates the forehead and eyebrows primarily medial to the conjoined fascia of the superficial temporalis fascia and the temporalis fascia proper. Laterally, the brow is supported by fascial attachments to the temporalis fascia. Depressors of the eyebrow medially are the corrugator supercilii, procerus, and orbicularis muscle; laterally, the main depressor is the orbicularis muscle.

Eyebrow elevation helps clear the visual axis and is a natural compensatory response to the forehead sagging and dermatochalasis that occur with aging. In maximal upgaze, the eyebrows also elevate to provide maximal clearance of the visual axis in coordination with lid and globe elevation.

EYELIDS

The normal interpalpebral fissure in adults is 10 to 12 mm, and the average horizontal palpebral fissure length is approximately 30 mm. Between the ages of 12 and 25 years, the horizontal fissure width increases by 10%; conversely, after middle age the fissure shortens by the same amount.[67] The upper eyelid margin rests at approximately the superior limbus in children and 1.5 to 2.0 mm below the superior limbus in adults; the lower eyelid margin rests at approximately the inferior limbus.[16]

The eyelid margin is divided into anterior and posterior lamellas. The anterior lamella is composed of skin, muscle, and associated glands, whereas the posterior lamella is composed of the tarsal plate, conjunctiva, and associated glands (Figure 2-2).

The anterior lamella functions as a single anatomic unit. Underlying the skin is the orbicularis oculi muscle. The pretarsal orbicularis muscle originates medially from the medial canthal tendon via separate superficial and deep heads. As they pass toward the medial canthus, the superficial pretarsal heads of the orbicularis muscle expand into C-shaped cones that envelop and surround the canaliculi of the lacrimal drainage system. Therefore contraction of the orbicularis muscle aids in the lacrimal pump mechanism. The superficial heads of the pretarsal orbicularis muscle then insert onto the anterior arm of the medial canthal tendon. The deep heads of the pretarsal orbicularis muscle emerge in the same region as the superficial heads and surround the posterior portions of the canaliculi. Near the common canaliculus, the deep heads fuse to form Horner's muscle, which travels behind the medial canthal tendon and inserts onto the posterior lacrimal crest. Laterally, the pretarsal orbicularis muscle inserts onto the lateral canthal tendon, and fibers also pass into the subcutaneous tissue to help maintain the normal appearance of the lateral canthal angle.

The glands of Zeis and Moll are located in the anterior lamella of the eyelid and are associated with the eyelash cilia. The glands of Zeis are modified sebaceous glands, and the glands of Moll are eccrine, or modified sweat glands. Both glands secrete their contents around the lash follicle shaft.

Thin horizontally oriented muscle fibers, termed the *muscles of Riolan,* travel between the pretarsal orbicularis muscle and the tarsal plates in the upper and lower eyelids (Figure 2-3). Along the eyelid margin the muscles of Riolan are separated from the pretarsal orbicularis muscle by a small gap, in which lie the eyelash bulbs.[16] Because of their varying orientation in the eyelid, the muscles of Riolan may help rotate the eyelashes toward the eye during closure. The small muscles may also help propel glandular contents during blinking. Clinically, the most anterior aspect of the muscles of Riolan can be recognized along the eyelid margin as the gray line that is distinct in youth but becomes less apparent with age.[70]

The posterior lamella of the eyelid margin is defined by the tarsal plates and conjunctiva. The tarsal plates consist of dense fibrous tissue approximately 1 to 1.5 mm thick. The tarsal plates measure approximately 25 mm in length and vary in height; the tarsal plate in the upper eyelid is between 8 and 12 mm tall, and the tarsal plate in the lower eyelid is between 3 and 4 mm tall. Both tarsal plates taper medially and laterally to conform to the globe.

The tarsal plates contain the meibomian glands in the upper and lower eyelids. The upper eyelid contains approximately 25 meibomian glands, and the lower eyelid contains approximately 20. The meibomian glands are holocrine sebaceous units not associated with lash cilia. The meibomian glands open into central ductules that drain onto

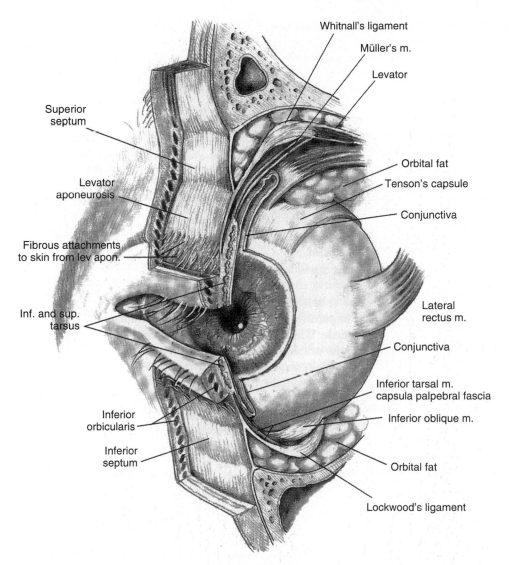

Whitnall's ligament
Müller's m.
Levator
Superior septum
Orbital fat
Tenson's capsule
Conjunctiva
Levator aponeurosis
Fibrous attachments to skin from lev apon.
Lateral rectus m.
Inf. and sup. tarsus
Conjunctiva
Inferior tarsal m. capsula palpebral fascia
Inferior oblique m.
Inferior orbicularis
Inferior septum
Orbital fat
Lockwood's ligament

FIGURE 2-2   Cross section of the eyelid. (From Lemke BN, Lucarelli MJ: Anatomy of the ocular adnexa, orbit, and related facial structures. In Nesi FA, Lisman RD, Levine MR [eds]: *Smith's ophthalmic plastic and reconstructive surgery*, ed 2, St Louis, 1998, Mosby.)

---

the posterior lamella of the eyelid margin posterior to the eyelash cilia. The meibomian glands produce the lipid layer of the tear film.

Distichiasis is an anomaly in which a partial or complete accessory row of eyelashes emerges adjacent to or from the openings of the meibomian glands. In congenital distichiasis this defect may result when a primary epithelial germ cell destined to differentiate into a specialized meibomian sebaceous gland of the tarsus develops into a complete pilosebaceous unit. Acquired distichiasis, on the other hand, usually occurs in the setting of chronic inflammation, such as ocular cicatricial pem-

phigoid or Stevens-Johnson syndrome. Whereas the eyelashes in congenital distichiasis may not irritate the globe for a while, those in acquired distichiasis typically cause significant ocular irritation. It has been postulated that under certain stimuli, including immunologic and chemical stimuli, the meibomian glands may occasionally revert to a pilosebaceous structural unit, producing cilia.[7,55] Distichiasis should be distinguished from trichiasis, a condition in which normal hairs (in the anterior lamella) have assumed an abnormal orientation.

In addition to distichiasis, the meibomian glands of the posterior lamella may also become impacted

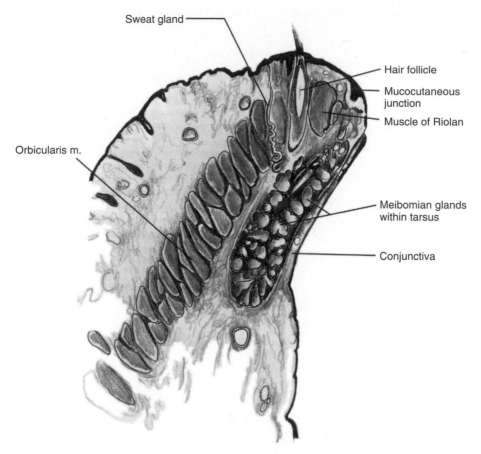

Sweat gland

Hair follicle

Mucocutaneous junction

Muscle of Riolan

Orbicularis m.

Meibomian glands within tarsus

Conjunctiva

FIGURE 2-3   Saggittal section of the eyelid margin. (From Lemke BN, Lucarelli MJ: Anatomy of the ocular adnexa, orbit, and related facial structures. In Nesi FA, Lisman RD, Levine MR [eds]: *Smith's ophthalmic plastic and reconstructive surgery,* ed 2, St Louis, 1998, Mosby.)

with lipid and cellular debris or abnormalities of keratinization may develop; if this occurs, lipogranulomatous inflammation may develop, forming the clinical hordeolum or chalazion.[28]

Eyelid Movement

Eyelid movements can be broadly classified as opening and closing movements. Opening of the eyelids depends on the levator palpebrae superioris muscle, the lower lid retractors, and the smooth muscles of Müller. Eyelid closure is brought about by the orbicularis oculi muscle, which surrounds the palpebral fissure circumferentially.

Opening.   Contraction of the levator palpebrae superioris muscle elevates the upper eyelid. Hence, it is known as the *chief retractor of the upper eyelid.* This action takes place against gravity. The levator is innervated by the superior division of the oculomotor nerve, which also supplies the superior rec-

tus muscle. The muscle is tendinous in its distal 14 to 20 mm and muscular in its proximal part. The aponeurosis inserts onto the anterior tarsal, passes through the orbicularis muscle fibers, and inserts into the dermis to form the upper eyelid skin crease. With age the levator aponeurosis sometimes disinserts from it tarsal insertion, causing ptosis. However, its skin attachments remain intact and cause the eyelid crease to appear higher.

Clinically, it is possible to quantitate the lifting power of the levator by measuring in millimeters the excursion of the upper eyelid from downgaze to upgaze after fixing the frontalis action at the brow. Normal excursion generally measures 14 to 17 mm. Excursion of less than 4 mm is classified as poor. However, a more accurate measurement of muscle function is levator force generation.[21] This test involves attaching a force transducer to the eyelashes and recording the maximum force generated during upgaze. This test can also help one differentiate

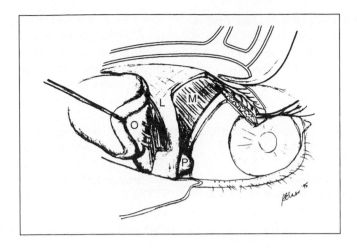

FIGURE 2-4 Lateral extensions of Müller's muscle. (From Morton AD et al: *Arch Ophthalmol* 114:1488, 1996.)

between types of ptosis, such as aponeurogenic, myogenic, neurogenic, and mechanical. Magnetic resonance imaging (MRI) measurements of healthy subjects have shown that lid elevation of 1 cm corresponds to levator shortening of 1.4 cm.[18]

Because of the close anatomic and developmental relationship that the levator shares with the superior rectus muscle, the upper eyelid generally follows the globe in its movements. Both muscles share a common fascial sheath and co-contract on upgaze. Similarly, on downgaze, both the superior rectus and levator relax and the upper lid follows the downward movement of the globe.

Innervation to the levator palpebrae superioris muscle follows Hering's law.[8] That is, synergistic extraocular muscles receive simultaneous and equal innervation. Motor neurons for the levator muscle arise from a single unpaired central caudal nucleus of the oculomotor complex, and single motor neurons may innervate the levator muscle bilaterally. Hence, any supranuclear input into the motor neuron nucleus influences both levator muscles.

The minor retractor of the upper eyelid is Müller's muscle. It accounts for about 2 mm of upper lid lift. Müller's muscle consists of smooth muscle fibers arising from beneath the levator, 15 mm from the upper tarsal border, and inserting on the superior tarsal border. It is innervated by the sympathetic nervous system. Studies have shown that the main subtype of adrenergic receptors in Müller's muscle is α_2. In contrast, β_1-adrenergic receptors were found on the levator muscle.[17] Levator adrenergic receptors are thought to play a role in controlling tonic eyelid position during states of

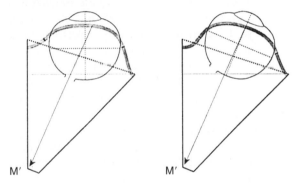

FIGURE 2-5 Lateral accentuation of lid retraction in proptotic globes. (From Lemke BN: *Ophthal Plast Reconstr Surg* 7:1627, 1991.)

arousal, in which serum levels of catecholamines are higher.[17]

Lateral extensions of the levator muscle have been shown to pass between the orbital and palpebral lobes of the lacrimal gland. Anatomic studies have also shown that Müller's muscle sends lateral extensions between the two lacrimal gland lobes[48] (Figure 2-4). This may accentuate the lateral flare seen in thyroid related orbitopathy. Lateral canthal advancement may aid in the treatment of upper lid retraction in cases in which the horizontal length of the tarsoligamentous band cannot cover the lateral aspect of the exophthalmic globe[42] (Figure 2-5).

The lower eyelid retractors depress the lower eyelid in downgaze. As in the upper lid, they are closely linked with the depressors of the eye and the inferior rectus and inferior oblique muscles. They consist of the capsulopalpebral fascia, which is a palpebral fascial extension from the inferior rectus muscle, and the inferior tarsal muscle, which is analogous to Müller's muscle in the upper eyelid. High-resolution MRI has demonstrated that vertical depression of the lower lid in downgaze moves in tandem with the inferior oblique.[26] Attenuation or disinsertion of the lower lid retractors causes vertical instability of the lower eyelid and contributes to both entropion and ectropion.

Closure. The main eyelid protractor is the orbicularis oculi muscle, innervated by the seventh cranial nerve. It is primarily responsible for eyelid closure and blinking. Anatomically, it is broadly divided into three parts: pretarsal, preseptal, and orbital. Deep and superficial heads of the pretarsal orbicularis oculi muscle contribute to the lacrimal pump mechanism.

The orbicularis myofibers have the smallest diameter of any skeletal muscle, including other facial muscles. The orbicularis muscle has relatively short overlapping individual myofibers and, in different portions of the muscle, varies in length.[41] The differing lengths may contribute to the variety of complex movements in facial expression and eyelid function.

Eyelid closure can be divided into blinking, winking, and spasm. The pretarsal and preseptal parts of the orbicularis muscle are responsible for the blink reflex and unforced eyelid closure. The orbital portion is recruited for forced closure.

Blinking. There are three types of blinking: spontaneous, reflex, and voluntary. Spontaneous blinking is the most common form. Although the exact mechanism of spontaneous blinking is debatable, studies have now shown that the preliminary change occurring in a spontaneous blink is contraction of the orbicularis rather than relaxation of the levator palpebrae superioris.[29] The lower lid remains stationary. Lid closure occurs from the lateral canthus toward the medial canthus, forming an integral part of the lacrimal pump mechanism. Studies of all three types of blink have shown that quantitative electromyographic (EMG) readings for spontaneous blinks had the smallest value.[37] Blink rate varies among individuals and is dependent on environmental factors.

Reflex blinking is elicited by sensory stimulation. This can consist of different types of stimuli, such as cutaneous touch, auditory signals, bright visual stimuli, and corneal or ocular irritation. Reflex blinking operates at high speeds and is man-

ifested by simple neural circuits. The neural pathway of reflex blinks consists of both the trigeminal nerves as the afferent nerve and the facial nerve via the polysynaptic connection in the brainstem as the efferent nerve. Cortical input is required for some visual stimuli–evoked reflex blinking. Unexpected or threatening objects cause blinking (the menace reflex), which requires cortical input, whereas blinking in response to bright lights (the dazzle reflex) is subcortical. The afferent pathway for both is through the optic nerve.

Few studies have investigated voluntary blinking. EMG studies reveal that the recorded amplitude and duration for voluntary blinking were larger than those for spontaneous and reflex blinks.[37] Although muscular contraction time is easier to control compared with other blinks, contraction potential amplitude required to generate voluntary blinks was much higher than that needed for other blinks. Preseptal and pretarsal portions of the orbicularis muscle are recruited to complete this action. A form of voluntary blinking is winking, a learned response that dissociates bilateral closure of the two eyes (i.e., closure of one eye only). This involves the simultaneous contraction of the orbital and palpebral portions of the orbicularis.

Eyelid kinematics have been studied in patients who have had blepharoplasty.[2] In such studies, amplitude, velocity, duration, and blink waveforms were studied and compared with preoperative measurements with the use of magnetic search coils. No alterations in blink dynamics were noted.

Pathways for Eyelid Movement. Cortical control of eyelid opening and closing resides in the frontal cortex. The cortical center for eyelid elevation lies close to the oculogyric centers. Stimulation of this area may cause elevation of one or both upper eyelids, with the higher eyelid being on the contralateral side. The caudal central nucleus, a part of the ocular motor nuclear complex, supplies the levator palpebrae superioris muscle. The region of the motor cortex responsible for the eyelid closure is close to the representation for the thumb. The intermediate part of the motor nucleus of the seventh nerve, situated in the lower part of the pons, supplies the orbicularis oculi muscle.

Blepharospasm

Blepharospasm is a bilateral, involuntary, intermittent or persistent spasmodic closure of the eyelids with active contraction of the orbicularis muscles and the brow depressor muscles (i.e., the procerus and corrugator muscles). Blepharospasm can be idiopathic (BEB) or drug induced may be caused by ocular disease or certain neurodegenerative disorders, such as Parkinson disease.[46]

Some patients with benign essential blepharospasm also exhibit dystonic movements of facial, oral, mandibular, or cervical muscles (Meige syndrome). The exact cause of this disease is unknown, but the common pathophysiology in several studies point toward overactivity in the basal ganglia. A significant number of patients with BEB are also unable to initiate eyelid opening or have apraxia of eyelid opening. Frontal lobe involvement is common in patients with eyelid apraxia who do not have blepharospasm.[1] In patients with BEB, chronic inhibition of the levator muscle accompanied by sustained contraction of the orbicularis muscle may play a role. Botulinum A toxin injections help tremendously in the management of this disease. In patients with eyelid apraxia, levator advancement or frontalis suspension is often helpful.

Hemifacial Spasm

Hemifacial spasm results from irritation of the seventh cranial nerve as it exits from the brainstem by the posterior cerebellar artery. Hemifacial spasm is almost always unilateral and remains present even during sleep. The spasms are intermittent and progressive. Of these patients, 90% may have an aberrant artery compressing the facial nerve as it exits the brainstem. Rarely, posterior fossa tumors can cause hemifacial spasm; hence, it is advisable to consider obtaining imaging studies on these patients.

CONJUNCTIVA

Morphology

Together, the corneal epithelium and the conjunctiva form the ocular surface. Nonkeratinizing squamous epithelium, five to seven layers thick, covers the cornea as the corneal epithelium. At the corneoscleral limbus the corneal epithelium blends with the conjunctival epithelium as the compact Bowman's layer of the cornea gives way to the loose vascular stroma of the bulbar conjunctiva. The stem cells of the corneoscleral limbus provide the source to replenish and renew the corneal epithelium. The conjunctiva consists of cuboidal stratified epithelium, which rests on a thin basement membrane. The epithelium is two to three cell layers thick and packed less regular than the corneal epithelium. The cell membranes contain infoldings and microvilli. The conjunctival cells harbor many organelles, particularly mitochondria. The conjunctiva performs two major functions: It provides mucus for the tear film, and it protects the ocular surface from pathogens, both as a physical barrier and as a source of inflammatory cells.

The palpebral conjunctiva lines the inner surface of the eyelids, whereas the bulbar conjunctiva covers the surface of the globe. The conjunctiva contains a surface epithelium and a substantia propria throughout all regions. The connective tissue of the substantia propria contains immune cells and is highly vascular. The substantia propria harbors mast cells, plasma cells, and neutrophils, thus facilitating the cellular portion of the immune response. The reflection of the conjunctiva at the junction of the bulbar and palpebral portions forms the conjunctival fornix. The tarsal conjunctiva is a unique portion of the palpebral conjunctiva that adheres firmly to the underlying tarsus and cannot be separated, even with sharp dissection. Inferior to the tarsus in the lower lid and superior to the tarsus in the upper lid, the palpebral conjunctiva adheres to the lower eyelid retractors and Müller's muscle, respectively. The bulbar conjunctiva lines the surface of the globe and loosely adheres to the underlying sclera. Parallel connective tissue fibers of Tenon's capsule insert obliquely into the bulbar conjunctiva and separate the conjunctiva from the underlying globe. This anatomic arrangement allows the ocular surface to be covered by a continuous smooth mucosal surface while allowing for motility of the globe.

The tear film constitutes a vital component of the ocular surface. The tear film separates into three distinct layers that have three distinct functions. The mucous layer adheres most closely to the corneal and conjunctival epithelium. The mucus in the tear film binds to the microvilli of the corneal and conjunctival epithelium and significantly improves the wetability of the ocular surface.[33] Human tears demonstrate shear thinning. The viscosity of the tears is low at high shear rates but very high at low shear rates. The variation in viscosity minimizes drag during the blink while resisting gravitational drainage in the open eye.[66] The mucus in the tear film produces the shear thinning characteristic and provides the main defense mechanism against microtrauma during the blink.[61] Goblet cells of the conjunctiva produce the mucopolysaccharides that form the mucous layer. The apical cytoplasm of the goblet cell contains membrane-bound mucin granules manufactured in the Golgi complex. The goblet cells release the mucin into the surrounding area by means of apocrine secretion. The concentration of the goblet cells varies depending on the location in the conjunctiva. The goblet cells concentrate in the inferonasal fornix, near the inferior canalicular system, and on the bulbar conjunctiva, particularly the temporal bulbar conjunctiva.[24]

The accessory glands of Krause and Wolfring, along with the lacrimal gland, produce the aqueous layer of the tear film. The aqueous layer is the thickest layer of the tear film and binds to the hydrophilic portions of the mucopolysaccharides of the mucous layer. The concentration of the accessory lacrimal glands also varies depending on the area of the conjunctiva. The glands of Krause are concentrated in the fornix, whereas the glands of Wolfring predominate near the tarsal conjunctiva. The glands of Zeis and the meibomian glands lining the eyelid margin produce the sebaceous secretion that becomes the outer lipid layer of the tear film. The lipid layer improves the stability of the tear film, decreases evaporation, and increases tear break up time.

Stem Cells of the Ocular Surface

The epithelium of the conjunctival and corneal surface is in a constant state of renewal. The corneal epithelium is renewed approximately every 7 to 10 days. Stem cells provide the source for mitotic activity to replenish the conjunctival and corneal epithelium. Stem cells are present in all self-renewing tissues, are long lived, and have a great potential for clonic cell division.[4] Stem cells must be capable of error-free proliferation, and they accomplish this through low mitotic activity and asymmetric deoxyribonucleic acid (DNA) segregation. Asymmetric DNA segregation allows the stem cell to retain its original DNA while the new copy is passed to the daughter cell. Stem cells are poorly differentiated and are also under significant anatomic protection. Studies have demonstrated that the stem cells responsible for replenishing the corneal epithelium are located at the corneoscleral limbus. Histologically, the limbal epithelium is unique, consisting of 10 cell layers compared with 2 to 3 cells layers for the conjunctival epithelium and 5 to 7 cell layers for the conjunctival epithelium. Limbal epithelium is considered an intermediate between corneal and conjunctival epithelium based on the keratin-like protein contents.[39]

The concept of stem cell repopulation of the corneal epithelium has replaced the theory of conjunctival transdifferentiation as the accepted source

of corneal epithelium. The limbal conjunctival cells normally do not serve to repopulate the corneal epithelium. Conjunctival epithelium cannot transdifferentiate into phenotypic corneal epithelium. In disease states manifested by stem cell damage, conjunctival epithelial cells can repopulate the cornea; however, these cells continue to be phenotypically conjunctival in nature and are always associated with corneal neovascularization.

Bulbar and palpebral conjunctivas are two independent cell kinetic systems that originate in two stem cell regions. The bulbar system begins at the limbus, and the palpebral system begins at the mucocutaneous junction.[51] Each system contains two compartments: a progenitor where cells proliferate and a compartment of nonproliferating cells. Stem cells that repopulate the palpebral conjunctiva originate at the mucocutaneous junction and stream toward the inferior fornix.[69] Slow-cycling cells produce transient amplifying cells that undergo division before becoming mature conjunctival epithelial cells. The undetermined limbus stem cells generate two epithelial cell lines: a corneal and a conjunctival. Ultimately, the nonproliferating mature end cells die in the fornix. Conjunctival keratinocytes and goblet cells derive from a common bipotent progenitor.[52] Goblet cell differentiation can occur late in the life of a single conjunctival clone.

The concept of corneal and conjunctival stem cells has revolutionized the treatment of ocular surface disease. Conditions such as Stevens-Johnson syndrome and ocular cicatricial pemphigoid result in both conjunctival and limbal stem cell deficiencies. Surgical procedures have now been designed to replace the stem cells, which then provide replenishment for the conjunctival and corneal epithelium. Conjunctival and corneal autographs and allografts, limbal transplantation, and amniotic membrane grafting have been developed to treat the underlying stem cell deficiency.[32] The disease process and whether it is bilateral or unilateral determines the ideal procedure and the likelihood of maintaining a clear cornea after surgical intervention.

The Dynamics of the Conjunctiva during Ocular Movements

The conjunctiva provides a mucosal barrier lining the eyelids and the bulbar surface. The conjunctiva associates intimately with the underlying connective tissue of the eyelids and orbits to form a system that allows movement of the globe without prolapse of redundant conjunctivas. The fascial extensions of the recti muscles create a dynamic system whereby the conjunctiva and the conjunctival fornix move in unison with the globe.

The suspensory apparatus of the conjunctival fornix can be divided into bulbar and palpebral portions. The inner capsular portion of the capsulopalpebral heads of the recti muscles form the bulbar portion. These connective tissue fibers insert obliquely into the overlying conjunctiva and loosely attach the conjunctiva to the globe. The firm adherence of the palpebral conjunctiva to underlying connective tissue of the eyelid produces the palpebral portion of the suspensory apparatus of the conjunctival fornix. The attachments of the palpebral conjunctiva to the underlying eyelid determine the location and depth of the conjunctival fornix. The connective tissue underlying the palpebral conjunctiva forms the bulk of the suspensory apparatus of the conjunctival fornix and originates as the anterior division of the capsulopalpebral heads of the recti muscles (see Color Plate 1). Attachments of the conjunctiva to the medial and lateral canthal ligaments, connections with the trochlea, and the suspensory ligaments of the lacrimal gland also contribute to the suspensory apparatus of the conjunctival fornix. The system allows for extensive movement of the globe without prolapse and blocking of the visual axis with redundant conjunctiva.

FACE

The eyelids are not isolated structurally or functionally from the adjacent brow, forehead, and midface. Thus proper understanding of periocular anatomy and dynamics requires knowledge of broader facial structure and function. The embryologic development of the eyelids from the mesenchymal, frontonasal, and maxillary processes underscores this close relationship and has been covered previously.

The superficial musculoaponeurotic system (SMAS) was originally described by Mitz and Peyronie[47] (Figure 2-6). This landmark anatomic work described a fibromuscular network that divides the subcutaneous fat in the parotid and cheek regions into two layers. The SMAS lies between the dermis and the deeper facial muscles and is continuous with the superficial facial muscles (frontalis muscle in the upper face and platysma in the lower face). The motor branches of the facial nerve lie deep to the SMAS. Mitz and Peyronie understood

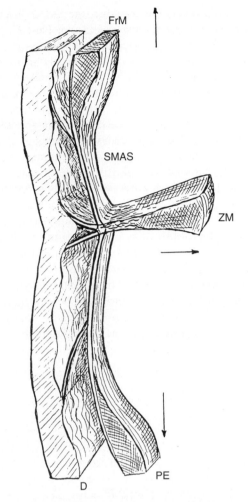

FIGURE 2-6 Schematic view of the superficial musculoaponeurotic system (*SMAS*) showing relation to frontalis muscle (*FrM*), zygomatic muscle (*ZM*), dermis (*D*), and platysma (*Pl*). (From Mitz V, Peyronie M: *Plast Reconstr Surg* 58:80, 1976.)

the SMAS as a distributor of facial muscular contractions to the skin.

Others have further characterized the relationships of the SMAS with the temporal, forehead, malar, nasal, and lip regions.[*] The details of this structure in both the temporoparietal and parotid areas have been controversial. Kikkawa, Lemke, and Dortzbach[38] describe the orbital and eyelid relationships of the SMAS. The SMAS was found to be continuous with the anterior and posterior orbicularis fascia. Thus, analogous to its relationship to

---

*References 10, 12, 27, 36, 38, 53, 54, 62, 65, 68.

the frontalis and the platysma, the SMAS invests the orbicularis oculi muscle (see Color Plate 2).

The SMAS is supported by both soft tissue and bony attachments. The SMAS is typically firmly attached to the parotid fascia. In addition, fibrous attachments can be found extending from the masseteric fascia to the SMAS (masseteric cutaneous ligaments)[45,62] (Figure 2-7). The platysma auricular ligaments and anterior platysma cutaneous ligaments provide similar support.[22] The zygomatic major and minor muscles also penetrate through the SMAS, providing dynamic attachments supported by the osseous origins of the zygomatic muscles.

A few key points of direct osseous attachment support the SMAS. Mitz and Peyronie[47] note attachment of the SMAS to the periosteum at the zygomatic arch. Furnas[22] describes both the zygomatic ligaments and the mandibular ligaments. The zygomatic ligaments originate behind the insertion of the zygomatic minor muscle approximately 4.5 cm anterior to the tragus.[22] Others have

further characterized this important source of midfacial support.[45,62] The mandibular ligaments can be found approximately 1 cm above the mandibular border on the anterior third of the mandible.[22]

The orbitomalar ligament, a bony attachment of the SMAS to the inferior orbital rim, was recently characterized.[38] The cutaneous attachments of this structure correspond to the malar and nasojugal skin folds. A stout lateral component of the orbitomalar ligament is found approximately 5 mm lateral to the lateral orbital rim[45] (Figure 2-8). This structure is distinct from the insertion of the lateral canthal ligament that anchors the lateral commissure of the eyelids just inside the lateral orbital rim at Whitnall's lateral orbital tubercle.

The mimetic muscles are crucial to facial support and expression. The lamellar anatomic arrangement of the mimetic muscles has been reported in detail by Freilinger et al.[20] (Figure 2-9). The most superficial layer contains the orbicularis oculi, the zygomatic minor, and the depressor an-

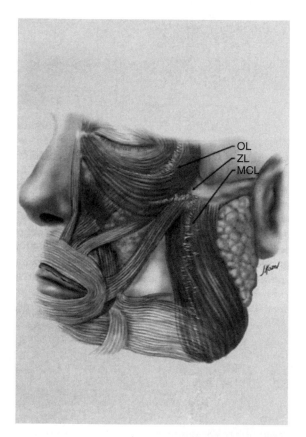

Figure 2-7   Ligamentous support of the midface. *MCL,* Masseteric cutaneous ligaments; *OL,* orbitomalar ligament; *ZL,* zygomatic ligaments. (From Lucarelli MJ et al: *Ophthal Plast Reconstr Surg* 16:1, 2000.)

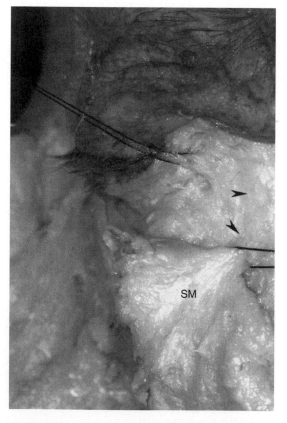

Figure 2-8   Lateral component of orbitomalar ligament. *SM,* Superficial musculoaponeurotic system; *arrows,* inferolateral orbital rim. (From Lucarelli MJ et al: *Ophthal Plast Reconstr Surg* 16:1, 2000.)

guli oris. A second layer includes the zygomatic major, the levator labii superioris alaeque nasi, the depressor labii inferioris, and the platysma. The levator labii superioris and the orbicularis oris make up the next layer. The deepest layer of the mimetic muscles includes the mentalis, the levator anguli oris, and the buccinator. The musculature of the first three layers is innervated on the deep surfaces by the facial nerve. The deepest layer is innervated from the outer surface. The importance of the facial musculature to periocular soft tissue support and to facial expression can easily be seen in patients with Bell's palsy or other disorders causing facial paralysis.

The fatty layers in the periocular region and face are of considerable clinical interest. Aesthetically important orbital fat pads are present in the upper and lower eyelids posterior to the orbital septum. The orbital fat has been characterized extensively by Sires et al.[58] These fat collections may be debulked or redistributed during blepharoplasty. The eyebrow fat pad is present within the posterior layer of the galea and adds support to the eyebrow.[43] The major fat pad in the midface is the malar fat pad. This structure is found subcutaneously and is continuous with jowl fat below the jaw line. Beneath the orbicularis oculi, near the inferior orbital rim, is the suborbicularis oculi fat[3,31] (Figure 2-10). The sub-SMAS fat in the malar region is continuous with the submuscular fat in the eyebrow region.[38] The buccal fat resides deeper in the face, with buccal, temporal, and pterygoid extensions.[15,63]

Significant involutional changes occur in the periocular and facial anatomy with aging. These include skin changes, brow ptosis, blepharoptosis, dermatochalasis, orbital fat prolapse, lower lid entropion and ectropion, midfacial ptosis, increased prominence of the nasolabial fold, and jowl formation. Some of these involutional changes cause functional problems; others result in cosmetic concerns. The underlying causes of many of these entities have been elucidated with anatomic and histologic studies.*

---

*References 6, 11, 13, 14, 23, 25, 30, 34, 35, 43, 45, 50, 57, 59, 60.

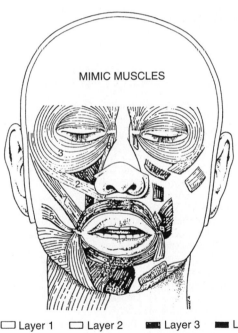

MIMIC MUSCLES

☐ Layer 1   ☐ Layer 2   ▨ Layer 3   ■ Layer 4

Layer 1
M. depressor anguli oris	1
M. zygomaticus minor	2
M. orbicularis oculi	3

Layer 2
M. depressor labii inf.	4
M. risorius	5
Platysma	6
M. zygomaticus major	7
M. lev. lab. sup. alaeque nasi	8

Layer 3
M. orbicularis oris	9
M. levator labii sup.	10

Layer 4
M. mentalis	11
M. levator anguli oris	12
M. buccinator	13

FIGURE 2-9 Four layers of mimic muscles (muscles of facial expression). (From Freilinger G et al: *Plast Reconstr Surg* 80:686, 1987.)

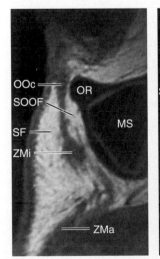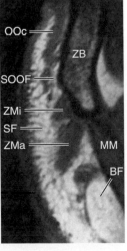

FIGURE 2-10 High-resolution magnetic resonance image of the midface showing through the center of the lower eyelid. *MS,* Maxillary sinus; *OOc,* orbicularis oculi; *OR,* orbital rim; *SF,* subcutaneous fat; *SOOF,* suborbicularis oculi fat; *ZMa,* zygomaticus Major; *ZMi,* zygomaticus minor. (From Lucarelli MJ et al: *Ophthal Plast Reconstr Surg* 16:1, 2000.)

REFERENCES

1. Abe K et al: Eyelid "apraxia" in patients with motor neuron disease, *J Neurol Neurosurg Psych* 59:629, 1995.
2. Abell KM et al: Eyelid kinematics following blepharoplasty, *Ophthal Plast Reconstr Surg* 15:236, 1999.
3. Aiache AE, Ramirez OH: The suborbicularis oculi fat pads: an anatomic and clinical study, *Plast Reconstr Surg* 95:37, 1995.
4. Akpek EK, Foster CS: Limbal cell transplantation, *Int Ophthalmol Clin* 39:71, 1999.
5. Anderson H, Ehlers N, Mattheissen M: Histochemistry and development of the human eyelids, *Acta Ophthalmol* 43:642, 1965.
6. Anderson RL, Beard C: The levator aponeurosis: attachments and their clinical significance, *Arch Ophthalmol* 95:1437, 1977.
7. Anderson RL, Harvey JT: Lid splitting and posterior lamellar cryosurgery for congenital and acquired distichiasis, *Arch Ophthalmol* 99:631, 1981.
8. Averbuch-Heller L et al: Hering's law for eyelids: still valid, *Neurology* 45:1781, 1995.
9. Barishak YR: Embryology of the eyelid and adnexa, *Dev Ophthalmol* 24:1, 1992.
10. Barton FE: The SMAS and the nasolabial fold, *Plast Reconstr Surg* 89:1054, 1992.
11. Berke RN, Wadsworth JAC: Histology of the levator muscle in congenital and acquired ptosis, *Arch Ophthalmol* 53:413, 1955.
12. Bosse JP, Papillon J: Surgical anatomy of the SMAS at the malar region. In *Transactions of the 9th International Congress of Plastic and Reconstructive Surgery,* New York, 1987, McGraw-Hill.
13. Dagleisch R, Smith JLS: Mechanics and histology of senile entropion, *Br J Ophthalmol* 50:79, 1966.
14. Dortzbach RK, Sutula FC: Involutional blepharoptosis: a histopathological study, *Arch Ophthalmol* 98:2045, 1980.
15. Dubin B et al: Anatomy of the buccal fat pad and its clinical significance, *Plast Reconstr Surg* 83:253, 1989.
16. Dutton J: The eyelids and anterior orbit. In Dutton J, Waldrop T (eds): *Atlas of clinical and surgical orbital anatomy,* Philadelphia, 1994, WB Saunders.
17. Esmaeli-Gutstein B et al: Distribution of adrenergic receptor subtypes in the retractor muscles of the upper eyelid, *Ophthal Plast Reconstr Surg* 15:92, 1999.
18. Ettl A et al: Dynamic magnetic resonance imaging of the levator palpebrae superioris muscle, *Ophthalmic Res* 30:54, 1998.
19. Fink WH: The development of the orbital fascia, *Am J Ophthalmol* 42:269, 1956.
20. Freilinger G et al: Surgical anatomy of the mimic muscle system and the facial nerve: importance for reconstructive and aesthetic surgery, *Plast Reconstr Surg* 80:686, 1988.
21. Frueh BR, Musch DC: Evaluation of levator muscle integrity in ptosis with levator force measurement, *Ophthalmology* 103:244, 1996.
22. Furnas DW: The retaining ligaments of the cheek, *Plast Reconstr Surg* 83:11, 1989.
23. Furnas DW: Festoons, mounds, and bags of the eyelids and cheek, *Clin Plast Surg* 20:367, 1993.
24. Gipson IK, Joyce NC: Anatomy and cell biology of the cornea, superficial limbus and conjunctiva. In Albert DM, Jakobiec FA (eds): *Principles and practice of ophthalmology,* Philadelphia, 2000, WB Saunders.
25. Glogau R: Physiologic and structural changes associated with aging skin, *Dermatol Clin* 15:555, 1997.
26. Goldberg RA et al: Physiology of the lower eyelid retractors: tight linkage of the anterior capsulopalpebral fascia demonstrated using ultrafine surface coil MRI, *Ophthal Plast Reconstr Surg* 10:87, 1993.
27. Gosain AK et al: Surgical anatomy of the SMAS: a reinvestigation, *Plast Reconstr Surg* 92:1254, 1993.
28. Gutgesell VJ, Stern GA, Hood CI: Histopathology of meibomian gland dysfunction, *Am J Ophthalmol* 94:383, 1982.
29. Hammond G et al: Functional significance of the early component of the human blink reflex, *Behav Neurosci* 110:7, 1996.
30. Hawes MJ, Dortzbach RK: The microscopic anatomy of the lower eyelid retractors, *Arch Ophthalmol* 100:1313, 1982.
31. Hoenig JA, Shorr N, Shorr J: The suborbicularis oculi fat in aesthetic and reconstructive surgery, *Int Ophthalmol Clin* 37:179, 1997.
32. Holland EJ: Epithelial transplantation for the management of severe ocular surface disease, *Trans Am Ophth Soc* 94:677, 1996.
33. Holly FJ, Lemp MA: Wetability and wetting of the corneal epithelium, *Exp Eye Res* 11:239, 1971.
34. Huang TT, Amayo E, Lewis SR: A histologic study of the lower tarsus and the significance in the surgical management of an involutional senile entropion, *Plast Reconstr Surg* 67:585, 1981.
35. Jones LT, Quickert MH, Wobig JL: The cure of ptosis by aponeurosis repair, *Arch Ophthalmol* 93:629, 1975.
36. Jost G, Lamouche G: SMAS in Rhytidectomy, *Aesth Plast Surg* 6:69, 1982.
37. Kaneko K, Sakamoto K: Evaluation of three types of blinks with the use of EOG and EMG, *Percept Mot Skills* 88:1037, 1999.
38. Kikkawa DO, Lemke BN, Dortzbach RK: Relations of the superficial musculoaponeurotic system to the orbit and characterization of the orbitomalar ligament, *Ophthal Plast Reconstr Surg* 12:77, 1996.
39. Kinoshita S et al: Keratin like proteins in the conjunctival and corneal epithelium are different, *Invest Ophthalmol Vis Sci* 24: 577, 1983.
40. Knize D: An anatomically based study of the mechanism of eyebrow ptosis, *Plast Reconstr Surg* 97:1321, 1996.
41. Lander T, Wirtschafter JD, McLoon LK: Orbicularis oculi muscle fibers are relatively short and heterogeneous in length, *Invest Ophthalmol Vis Sci* 37:1732, 1996.
42. Lemke BN, Khwarg SI: Adjuvant lateral canthal advancement in the surgical management of exophthalmic eyelid retraction, *Arch Ophthalmol* 117:274, 1999.
43. Lemke BN, Stasior OG: The anatomy of eyebrow ptosis, *Arch Ophthalmol* 100:981, 1982.
44. Lemke BN, Stasior OG: Eyebrow incision making, *Adv Ophthalmic Plast Reconstr Surg* 2:19, 1983.
45. Lucarelli MJ et al: The anatomy of midfacial ptosis, *Ophthal Plast Reconstr Surg* 16:7, 2000.
46. Mauriello JA et al: Drug-associated facial dyskinesias—a study of 238 patients, *J Neuro-Ophthalmol* 18:153, 1998.
47. Mitz V, Peyronie M: The superficial musculoaponeurotic system (SMAS) in the parotid and cheek area, *Plast Reconstr Surg* 58:80, 1976.
48. Morton A et al: Lateral extensions of Müller's muscle, *Arch Ophthalmol* 114:1486, 1996.
49. Ozanics V, Jakobiec F: Prenatal development of the eye and its adnexa. In Jakobiec F (ed): *Ocular anatomy, embryology, and teratology,* New York, 1982, Harper and Row.
50. Paris GL, Quickert MH: Disinsertion of the aponeurosis of the levator palpebrae superioris muscle after cataract extraction, *Am J Ophthalmol* 81:337, 1976.

51. Pe'er J et al: Streaming conjunctiva, *Anatomic Rec* 245:36, 1996.
52. Pellegrini G et al: Location and clonal analysis of stem cells and their differentiated progeny in the human ocular surface, *J Cell Bio* 145:769, 1999.
53. Pensler JM, Ward JW, Parry SW: The superficial musculoaponeurotic system in the upper lip: an anatomic study in cadavers, *Plast Reconstr Surg* 75:488, 1985.
54. Ruess W, Owsley JQ: The anatomy of the skin and fascial layers of the face in aesthetic surgery, *Clin Plast Surg* 14:677, 1987.
55. Scheie HG, Albert DM: Distichiasis and trichiasis: origin and management, *Am J Ophthalmol* 61:718, 1966.
56. Sevel D: A reappraisal of the development of the eyelids, *Eye* 2:23, 1988.
57. Shore JW, McCord CD: Anatomic changes in involutional blepharoptosis, *Am J Ophthalmol* 98:21, 1984.
58. Sires BS et al: Characterization of human orbital fat and connective tissue, *Ophthal Plast Reconstr Surg* 14:403, 1998.
59. Sisler HA, Labay G, Finlay J: Senile ectropion and entropion: a comparative histopathological study, *Ann Ophthalmol* 8:319, 1976.
60. Stefanyszyn MA, Hidayat AA, Flanagan JC: The histopathology of involutional ectropion, *Ophthalmology* 92:120, 1985.
61. Stern ME et al: A unified theory of the role of the ocular surface in dry eye, *Adv Exp Med Bio* 438:643, 1998.
62. Stuzin JM, Baker TJ, Gordon HL: The relationship of the superficial and deep facial fascias: relevance to rhytidectomy and aging, *Plast Reconstr Surg* 89:441, 1992.
63. Stuzin JM et al: The anatomy and clinical applications of the buccal fat pad, *Plast Reconstr Surg* 85:29, 1990.
64. Tarbet K, Lemke B: Anatomy of the eyelids and lacrimal drainage system. In Albert DM, Jakobiec FA (eds): *Principles and practice of ophthalmology,* Philadelphia, 2000, WB Saunders.
65. Thaller SR et al: The submuscular aponeurotic system (SMAS): a histologic and comparative anatomy evaluation, *Plast Reconstr Surg* 86:690, 1990.
66. Tiffany JM, Pandit JC, Bron AJ: Soluble mucin and the physical properties of tears, *Adv Exp Med Bio* 438:229, 1998.
67. Van dern Bosch WA, Leenders I, Milder P: Topographic anatomy of the eyelids, and the effects of age and sex, *Br J Ophthalmol* 83:347, 1999.
68. Wassef M: Superficial fascial and muscular layers in the face and neck: a histologic study, *Aesth Plast Surg* 11:171, 1987.
69. Wirtshafter JD et al: Palpebral conjunctival transient amplifying cells originate at the mucocutaneous junction and their progeny migrate toward the fornix, *Tran Am Ophtho Soc* 95:417, 1997.
70. Wulc A, Dryden R, Khatchaturian T: Where is the gray line? *Arch Ophthalmol* 105:1092, 1987.

CHAPTER 3

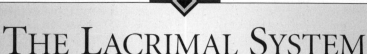

THE LACRIMAL SYSTEM

MARK J. LUCARELLI, DARLENE A. DARTT,
BRIGGS E. COOK, JR., AND BRADLEY N. LEMKE

LACRIMAL GLAND EMBRYOLOGY

The lacrimal gland is first seen during the 25-mm embryonic stage as solid epithelial buds arising from the conjunctiva of the lateral superior fornix. Mesenchymal condensation around these buds forms the secretory gland. The early epithelial buds form the orbital lobe, and the secondary buds, which appear somewhat later (40- to 60-mm stage), develop into the palpebral lobe.[12] The developing tendon of the levator palpebrae superioris muscle divides the gland into two parts. Canalization of the epithelial buds to form ducts begins at the 60-mm stage. The developing orbital lobe of the lacrimal gland becomes isolated from the globe by the developing lateral horn of the levator aponeurosis and the thickened superolateral intermuscular septum during the fifth month of gestation. Full development of the gland does not occur until 3 to 4 years postnatally.[45]

LACRIMAL GLAND AND ACCESSORY GLAND ANATOMY

The main lacrimal gland provides the principal aqueous secretory component to the tear film. The gland is situated within a shallow concavity within the frontal bone (i.e., within the lacrimal gland fossa), under the superolateral orbital rim. The lacrimal gland is divided by the lateral horn of the levator and extensions of Müller's muscle into an orbital lobe above and a palpebral lobe below.[13,42]

The orbital lobe is the larger of the two lobes and lies behind the orbital septum and above the levator aponeurosis.[13] The orbital lobe is approximately 20 mm long, 12 mm wide, and 5 mm thick.[70] The orbital lobe is bound anteriorly by the orbital septum and the preaponeurotic fat pad, medially by the intermuscular septum between the superior and lateral rectus muscles, and laterally by bone.[35]

The palpebral lobe of the lacrimal gland lies underneath the lateral horn of the levator aponeurosis, inferior to the orbital lobe. On upper eyelid eversion, the palpebral lobe may be visualized in the superolateral fornix on the conjunctival surface of the eyelid.

The lacrimal gland appears as a pinkish gray collection of lobules surrounded by connective tissue in the lateral portion of the eyelid. The gland is made up of many acini that drain into progressively larger tubules. These tubules are tributaries of larger ducts. The acini are made up of a basal myoepithelial cell layer with inner columnar secretory cells. The myoepithelial cells help force secretions into the tubular drainage system with contracture.[35]

Ductules and tubules from the orbital lobe of the lacrimal gland pass through its substance and either through the substance of the palpebral lobe or along its fibrous capsule. These ductules and tubules are joined by similar drainage pathways from the palpebral lobe to form 6 to 12 tubules that empty into the superolateral conjunctival fornix, 4 to 5 mm above the tarsus.[35] Injudicious removal of the conjunctiva in this area can lead to impaired secretory function and dry eye.[60]

In addition to the main lacrimal gland, accessory lacrimal glands are found in the conjunctival fornices and along the superior tarsal border. There are approximately 20 to 40 accessory glands of Krause in the superior conjunctival fornix. Fewer accessory glands are present in the lower eyelid. There are typically several accessory lacrimal glands of Wolfring along the superior tarsal border in the upper eyelid. The main lacrimal gland and the accessory lacrimal glands of Krause and Wolfring provide the aqueous component of the tear film.

The arterial supply to the lacrimal gland comes from the lacrimal branch of the ophthalmic artery, from a branch of the infraorbital artery, and often from a contribution from the recurrent meningeal artery. Branches of the lacrimal artery continue through the gland and provide blood supply to the temporal portions of the upper and lower eyelids. The venous drainage of the eyelids follows approximately the same course as the arterial supply and drains into the superior ophthalmic vein.

The lacrimal branch of the trigeminal nerve carries sensory stimuli from the lacrimal gland. The lacrimal nerve travels supertemporally in the orbit and enters the lacrimal gland with the lacrimal ar-

terial vessels. Branches of the lacrimal nerve travel through the lacrimal gland to supply sensation to the superficial temporal eyelid and skin structures.

The course of the parasympathetic secretomotor innervation to the lacrimal gland is more complex (Figure 3-1). Parasympathetic secretomotor fibers originate in the lacrimal nucleus of the pons. These fibers exit at the cerebellopontine angle as the nervus intermedius with fibers from the motor division of the facial nerve. The nervus intermedius travels in the auditory canal to the geniculate ganglion, where it combines with sensory neurons to form the greater superficial petrosal nerve. The greater superficial petrosal nerve travels through the middle cranial fossa, where it unites with the deep petrosal nerve, which carries postganglionic sympathetic fibers from the superior cervical ganglion.[13] Together, these two nerves form the nerve of the pterygoid canal (vidian nerve). The vidian nerve travels through the pterygopalatine fossa and synapses in the pterygopalatine ganglion.

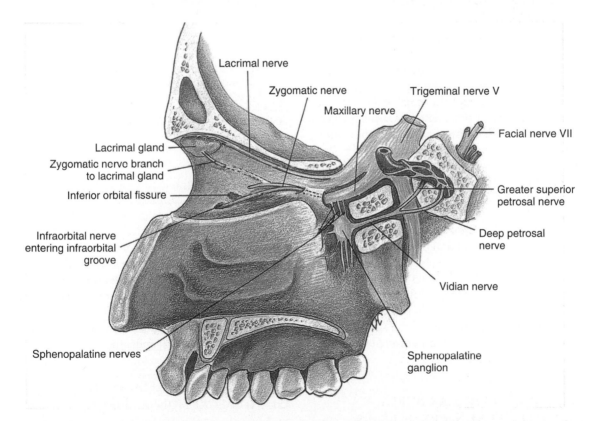

FIGURE 3-1 Parasympathetic innervation of lacrimal gland. Fibers from the facial nerve emerge from the temporal bone as the greater superficial petrosal nerve. They pass through the vidian canal of sphenoid bone as the vidian nerve to enter the sphenopalatine ganglion, communicate with the maxillary nerve via the sphenopalatine nerves, leave the maxillary nerve shortly thereafter as the zygomatic nerve. The zygomatic branch to the lacrimal gland usually joins the lacrimal nerve before entering the gland, but in this specimen, the zygomatic branch was seen entering separately. (From Lemke BN, Lucarelli MJ: Anatomy of the ocular adnexa, orbit, and related facial structures. In Nesi FA et al [eds]: *Smith's ophthalmic plastic and reconstructive surgery,* St Louis, 1998, Mosby.)

Postganglionic parasympathetic fibers leave the pterygopalatine ganglion via the pterygopalatine nerves. Ruskell[52,53] has demonstrated, both histologically and physiologically, the direct passage of parasympathetic fibers from the pterygopalatine ganglion to the lacrimal gland in monkeys. Axons pass through a fine network of orbital nerve fibers (the rami orbitales) or via the retroorbital autonomic plexus. In addition, some fibers may join the zygomatic nerve as it branches from the maxillary division of the trigeminal nerve and enters the orbit through the inferior orbital fissure. The zygomatic nerve gives off the zygomaticotemporal and zygomaticofacial nerves, which penetrate the orbital wall and travel laterally. One or more of the branches of the zygomatic nerve may ascend and enter the posterior surface of the lacrimal gland either alone or in combination with the lacrimal nerve.[13]

STRUCTURE AND FUNCTION OF THE TEAR FILM

The tear film covers the ocular surface, which consists of the cornea and conjunctiva. This fluid is a complicated three-layered structure. It consists of an outer lipid layer, a middle aqueous layer about 7 to 10 mm thick, and the mucous layer that is about 0.2 to 1.0 mm thick. The tear film has several functions that are essential to the health, maintenance, and protection of the ocular surface.[33] First, the tear film contributes to the smooth optical properties of the corneal surface. In addition, tears are the primary source of oxygen to the avascular cornea.[65] They also serve as a lubricant between the lids and the ocular surface. The movement of tears across the ocular surface and their drainage into the nasolacrimal duct help remove foreign bodies, debris, and exfoliated cells.[10] Tears contain many antibacterial proteins that protect the cornea and conjunctiva from bacterial infection.[15] Through these functions the tear film protects the surface of the eye from the external environment and helps maintain the optical surface of the cornea.

GLANDS AND OCULAR SURFACE EPITHELIA THAT SECRETE TEARS

Several different tissues secrete each of the three layers of the tear film (Figure 3-2). The outer lipid layer is produced primarily by the meibomian glands, which are located within the upper and lower eyelids, and to a lesser extent by the glands of Zeiss and Moll. The middle aqueous layer is secreted predom-

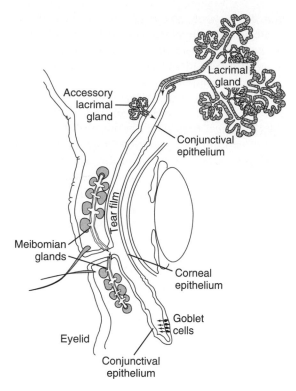

FIGURE 3-2   Schematic showing the glands and epithelia of the eye and ocular surface that contribute to the tear film. Shown are the meibomian glands, which secrete the outer lipid layer; the main and accessory lacrimal glands, as well as the conjunctival and corneal epithelia, which secrete the middle aqueous layer; and the conjunctival goblet cells, which secrete the inner mucous layer. (From Dartt DA, Sullivan DA: Wetting of the ocular surface. In Albert D, Jakobiec F [eds]: *Principles and practice of ophthalmology,* ed 2, Philadelphia, 2000, WB Saunders.)

inantly by the main lacrimal gland. Additional contributors to this layer are the accessory lacrimal glands (glands of Krause and Wolfring) and both the corneal and conjunctival epithelia. The inner mucous layer is elaborated by the conjunctival goblet cells and by the stratified squamous cells of the corneal and conjunctival epithelia.

REGULATION OF MEIBOMIAN GLAND SECRETION OF LIPID

Meibomian glands are sebaceous glands that secrete a complex mixture of lipids onto the tear film. The types of lipids include wax monoesters, sterol esters, hydrocarbons, triglycerides, diglycerides, free sterols (including cholesterol), free fatty acids, and polar lipids (including phospholipids).[43,66] The meibomian glands lie in a parallel row in the upper and lower eyelids. The main duct of these glands opens onto the eyelid margin and is a straight duct from which smaller ducts branch.[64] The smaller ducts each terminate in a single alveolus composed of several layers of epithelial cells. The outer layer of cells is the germinal basal layer, whose cells do not contain lipid droplets (the secretory product). As the cells proliferate and migrate toward the center of the alveolus, they mature. They develop an endoplasmic reticulum that begins to synthesize the lipids that are stored in droplets surrounded by a membrane (secretory granules). The more mature the cell is, the more lipid droplets are generated and the closer it is to the center of the alveolus. Secretion occurs when the innermost cells rupture, releasing lipid droplets and cell debris (meibomian gland secretion) into the ducts. This type of secretion is known as *holocrine secretion.* The meibomian material is stored in the ducts until it is released onto the tear film by the mechanical action of the blink.

Aside from the finding that blinking releases stored material from the ducts, it is not known what regulates meibomian gland secretion. There are at least two possible steps in the secretory process at which secretion can be regulated. The first possible step is by controlling the rate of lipid synthesis in the endoplasmic reticulum; the second possible step is by regulating the rupture of alveolar cells. Androgen sex steroids may regulate lipid synthesis and secretion.[46,62] Neurotransmitters released from nerves surrounding the acini can alter lipid synthesis or cell rupture. Parasympathetic nerves are the predominant innervation of the meibomian gland alveoli and contain acetylcholine, vasoactive intestinal peptide (VIP), and neuropeptide Y (NPY).[7] Sympathetic and sensory nerves are also present, but they are sparsely distributed and usually identified surrounding the vasculature. Thus acetylcholine, VIP, and NPY are primary candidates for neural regulation of meibomian gland secretion. More research into the neural and hormonal regulation of meibomian gland secretion is needed.

REGULATION OF MAIN LACRIMAL GLAND SECRETION OF PROTEINS, ELECTROLYTES, AND WATER

The main lacrimal gland (referred to hereafter as the *lacrimal gland*) is a tubuloacinar exocrine gland that secretes the major portion of protein, electrolytes, and water into the tear film. A variety of proteins are secreted by the lacrimal gland, including antibacte-

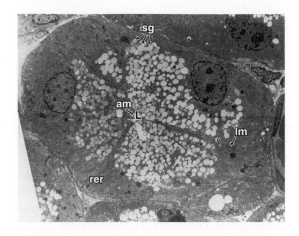

FIGURE 3-3 Transmission electron micrograph of the acinar cells of the main lacrimal gland. Acinar cells are pyramidal cells that are joined together by tight junctions that separate the apical membrane (*am*) from the lateral membrane (*lm*). Secretory proteins are synthesized in the rough endoplasmic reticulum (*rer*), stored in the clear secretory granules (*sg*), and then secreted into the lumen (*L*). (Hematoxylin-eosin stain; ×4000.) (Courtesy Dr. Kenneth R. Kenyon and Ms. Laila Hanninen.)

rial proteins, immunoglobulins, and growth factors. A few of these proteins are lysozyme, lactoferrin, lipocalin, secretory immunoglobulin A (SIgA), epidermal growth factor, several types of transforming growth factors (TGFs), and interleukins. A more extensive list of proteins is found elsewhere.[9] Lacrimal gland fluid electrolyte concentration varies with flow rate. At low flow rates the fluid is hypertonic, and as the flow rate increases, it becomes isotonic.[18] Lacrimal gland fluid contains Na^+, K^+, Cl^-, HCO_3^-, Ca^{2+}, and trace amounts of other ions in the same concentration as plasma, except K^+ and Cl^-, which are present in higher concentrations.[40]

The predominant cell type in the lacrimal gland is the acinar cell that secretes protein, electrolytes, and water (Figure 3-3). These cells form the secretory end pieces, or acini, which are grapelike or tubular (depending on species) structures consisting of acinar cell clusters.[25,68] In the cross section the acini contain a ring of pyramidal-shaped acinar cells that are joined at the lateral side by tight and gap junctions. These junctions make the acinar cells polarized and ensure unidirectional secretion. Secretory proteins are synthesized in the endoplasmic reticulum, modified in the Golgi apparatus, and packaged in secretory granules. There are two types of protein secretions in the lacrimal gland: constitutive and regulated. Constitutively secreted proteins are sorted into secretory granules that are not stored, but immediately fused with the apical plasma membrane and released into the acinar lumen. SIgA is secreted using this pathway.[61] Proteins secreted by the regulatory pathway are packaged into secretory granules that are stored on the apical side of the acinar cell. Fusion of these granules with the apical membrane is controlled and occurs only when the appropriate stimulus is generated. The stimulus is typically produced when neurotransmitters released from nerves or peptide hormones in the blood interact with the basolateral plasma membranes of acinar cells. Most proteins produced by the lacrimal gland are secreted through the regulated pathway. Only about 5% of the total amount of regulated proteins are released upon stimulation. This is known as *merocrine secretion.*

Secretion of lacrimal gland electrolytes and water occurs in two stages.[40] First, the acinar cells secrete a fluid that has an electrolyte composition similar to that of plasma. Then, as this fluid passes through the duct system, the ductal cells modify this fluid by secreting a fluid rich in potassium chloride (KCl). Acinar cell electrolyte secretion is driven by Na^+-K^+-ATPase pumping Na^+ out of the cell and K^+ into the cell (Figure 3-4). On the basolateral side of the cell, Na^+ enters the cell down a favorable electrochemical gradient. Cl^- enters the cell against its electrochemical gradient as its transport is coupled to Na^+ movement via a common ion transporter. K^+ exits the cell down its electrochemical gradient. On the apical (luminal) side of the cell, Cl^- and K^+ leave the cell, entering the secretory fluid down their electrochemical gradients. Na^+ enters the secreted fluid through the paracellular pathway (between the cells), following a favorable electrochemical gradient produced by Cl^- secretion. Water enters the secretory fluid using water channels known as aquaporins.[49] Similar mechanisms are used for duct cell electrolyte and water secretion, except that K^+ and Cl^- are the predominant ions secreted.

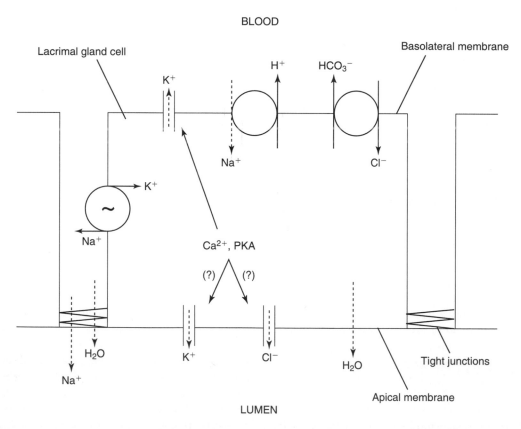

FIGURE 3-4   Schematic of lacrimal gland acinar cell showing the mechanism of electrolyte and water secretion. Possible roles of Ca^{2+} and protein kinase A (*PKA*) in activating ion movements are also indicated. , Na^+-K^+-ATPase; *dashed arrows,* passive ionic movements; *solid arrows,* active ionic movements. (From Dartt DA: Physiology of tear production. In Lemp MA, Marquardt R [eds]: *The dry eye,* Berlin, 1992, Springer-Verlag.)

To a large extent, lacrimal gland secretion is regulated by the nerves that innervate the secretory cells and by peptide and steroid hormones present in the blood. Nerves and peptide hormones stimulate secretion of electrolytes, water, and the regulated proteins. Steroid hormones stimulate the secretion of the constitutive proteins. The lacrimal gland is innervated by parasympathetic, sympathetic, and sensory nerves.[23] The parasympathetic nerves, which predominate, surround the acinar and duct cells and contain the neurotransmitters acetylcholine (a muscarinic cholinergic agonist) and VIP. Sympathetic nerves, releasing norepinephrine, are sparsely distributed and primarily surround the vasculature. Sensory nerves are the least prevalent and contain the neurotransmitters substance P and calcitonin gene-related peptide. The parasympathetic and sympathetic nerves are the efferent portion of a reflex arc that is stimulated by sensory nerves in the cornea and conjunctiva that form the afferent part of the reflex. Stimulation of sensory nerves in the ocular surface by mechanical, thermal, or chemical stimuli activates the parasympathetic and sympathetic nerves to stimulate lacrimal gland protein, electrolyte, and water secretion. Stimulation of the optic nerve by bright light also induces reflex lacrimal gland secretion. Acetylcholine and VIP are potent stimuli of regulated protein and electrolyte and water secretion. Norepinephrine stimulates protein secretion. Each of these stimuli induces secretion by binding to a specific receptor on the lacrimal gland cells and initiating a cascade of intracellular events known as a *signal transduction pathway*. In the lacrimal gland, each of these agonists uses a different cellular signaling pathway to stimulate secretion.

Activation of the cholinergic agonist-dependent pathway requires that acetylcholine be released from parasympathetic nerves and bind to muscarinic acetylcholine receptors of the M_3 subtype[37] (Figure 3-5). These receptors, which are located in the basolateral cell membrane, then activate a guanine nucleotide-binding protein (G protein).[39] The activated G protein turns on the enzyme phospholipase C, which breaks down a membrane phospholipid, phosphatidylinositol 4,5-bisphosphate, into a water-soluble molecule, 1,4,5-inositol triphosphate, and a lipid-soluble molecule, diacylglycerol.[4] 1,4,5-Inositol triphosphate interacts with specific receptors on intracellular organelles to open Ca^{2+} channels that release Ca^{2+} into the cytoplasm. Depletion of the intracellular Ca^{2+} stores further elevates intracellular Ca^{2+} by increasing the influx of Ca^{2+} across the plasma membrane. Ca^{2+}, either by itself or its activation of Ca^{2+}/calmodulin–dependent protein kinases to phosphorylate specific protein substrates, stimulates secretion. Diacylglycerol activates protein kinase C, which is a family of 11 different isoforms that phosphorylate specific protein substrates.[44] Ca^{2+}, Ca^{2+}/calmodulin-dependent protein kinases, and protein kinase C stimulate protein secretion by causing fusion of the secretory granule membranes with the apical plasma membrane to release the stored secretory proteins into the glandular lumen. These stimuli cause electrolyte and water secretion by activating the ion channels, ion pumps, and ion cotransport proteins in the basolateral and apical membranes, thereby increasing the rate of ion movement (see Figure 3-4). Ca^{2+} works by activating enzymes that are Ca^{2+}-dependent; the protein kinases work by phosphorylating and thus activating specific proteins (as yet unidentified) that are part of the protein secretory machinery or are ion transport channels and pumps.

A second cellular signaling pathway is activated by norepinephrine released from sympathetic nerves. This agonist can activate both α_1- and β-adrenergic receptors on lacrimal gland cells. Activation of β-adrenergic receptors induces a cyclic adenosine monophosphate (cAMP)–dependent pathway, which is described subsequently. In most tissues studied, activation of α_1-adrenergic receptors stimulates the same signaling pathway as cholinergic agonists.[21] In contrast, in the lacrimal gland, α_1-adrenergic agonists stimulate a different pathway. α_1-Adrenergic agonists do not stimulate phospholipase C, but they do activate protein kinase C, which results in secretion. These agonists also cause a small increase in intracellular Ca^{2+}. Increasing Ca^{2+} and activating protein kinase C stimulate secretion through the mechanism described for the cholinergic agonist-dependent signaling pathway.

A third signaling pathway, which is cAMP dependent, is activated by VIP released from parasympathetic nerves, by α-melanocyte–stimulating hormone and adrenocorticotropic hormone that are peptide hormones present in the bloodstream, and by norepinephrine activating β-adrenergic receptors[22] (Figure 3-6). These agonists bind to their specific receptors on the basolateral plasma membrane activating them. The activated receptors stimulate G proteins of the $G_{s\alpha}$ subtype, which activate adenylyl cyclase. This enzyme causes the production of cAMP from adenosine triphosphate (ATP). cAMP induces protein kinase A to phosphorylate and thus activate a specific set of protein substrates (as yet

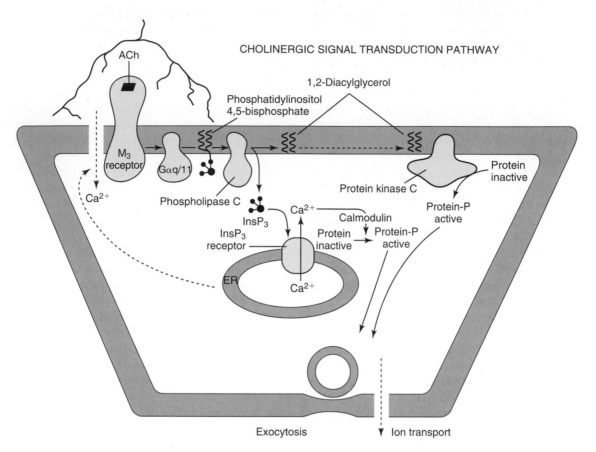

FIGURE 3-5 Schematic of signal transduction pathway activated by cholinergic agonists in lacrimal gland acinar cells to stimulate protein and electrolyte/water secretion. *ER,* Endoplasmic reticulum; *Gαq/11,* q/11 subtype of α subunit of a guanine nucleotide-binding protein; *InsP₃,* inositol triphosphate; *M₃,* subtype 3 of muscarinic receptors; *protein-P,* phosphorylated protein. (From Dartt DA, Hodges RR, Zoukhri D: *Adv Exp Med Biol* 438:113, 1998.)

unidentified) that are part of the protein secretory machinery or are ion transport channels and pumps. The cAMP signal is terminated by increased activity of cAMP phosphodiesterase, which breaks down cAMP into 5′-AMP.

A pathway that inhibits lacrimal gland secretion is also present. Enkephalins, present in nerves, inhibit secretion by preventing the action of cAMP[8] (see Figure 3-6). Enkephalins bind to specific receptors that activate the $G_{i\alpha}$ protein, which prevents activation of $G_{s\alpha}$ by the stimulatory agonists and thus inhibits production of cAMP.

The three stimulatory pathways and one inhibitory pathway are the major mechanisms that nerves use to regulate electrolyte and water, as well as regulated protein, secretion. A different mechanism is used for secretion of constitutive proteins. SIgA is the major constitutive protein secreted by the lacrimal gland and is regulated by the androgen

steroid hormones[61] (Figure 3-7). SIgA consists of polymeric IgA coupled to J chain and secretory component. Androgens regulate the secretion of SIgA by controlling the rate of synthesis of secretory component. Androgens from the bloodstream diffuse into the cell and then into the nucleus, where they bind to their receptors. These receptors are transcription factors that are activated by the androgen binding.

REGULATION OF ACCESSORY LACRIMAL GLAND SECRETION OF PROTEINS, ELECTROLYTES, AND WATER

The accessory lacrimal glands are mini-lacrimal glands located in the conjunctiva of the eyelids, and they are minor contributors to the aqueous layer of the tear film. There has been limited research on the accessory lacrimal glands because they are difficult

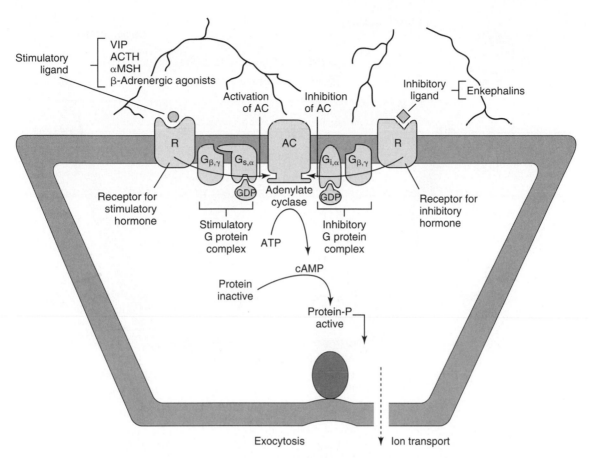

FIGURE 3-6 Schematic of lacrimal gland acinar cell showing the signal transduction pathway activated by stimulatory and inhibitory cAMP-dependent agonists for protein, electrolyte, and water secretion. *ACTH,* Adrenocorticotropic hormone; *5′ AMP,* 5′ analog of adenosine monophosphate; *ATP,* adenosine triphosphate; *cAMP,* cyclic adenosine monophosphate; *Gα, β, and γ,* subunits of a guanine nucleotide binding protein; $G_{s\alpha}, G_{i\alpha}$, α subunits of stimulatory and inhibitory (respectively) subunits of guanine nucleotide binding proteins; *GDP,* guanine diphosphate; *α-MSH,* α-melanocyte-stimulating hormone; *protein-P,* phosphorylated (activated protein); *VIP,* vasoactive intestinal peptide. (Modified from Dartt DA: *Adv Exp Med Biol* 350:5, 1994.)

to isolate. Several proteins secreted by these glands have been identified, and all are the same as those secreted by the main lacrimal gland.[2] Electrolyte and water secretion by the accessory lacrimal glands has not been studied.

Accessory lacrimal glands consist of a single excretory duct that branches into smaller ducts that are surrounded by a single lobule.[56] The ducts are lined by one to two layers of cells and either end blindly or terminate in secretory end pieces that are not acinar cells. Accessory lacrimal glands are well innervated, suggesting that their secretion can be neurally regulated and calling into question the view that these glands contribute only to basal tear secretion. Indirect evidence suggests that most of these nerves are parasympathetic.

REGULATION OF CORNEAL EPITHELIAL CELL ELECTROLYTE AND WATER SECRETION

The corneal epithelium is a minor contributor to the aqueous layer of the tear film. It does not secrete proteins but can secrete electrolytes, such as Na+ and Cl−, and water into tears. Sympathetic nerves releasing norepinephrine, which activates β-adrenergic receptors, are the primary regulators of corneal electrolyte and water secretion.[31] β-Adrenergic agonists bind to their receptors located on the apical membrane of the corneal epithelial cells (Figure 3-8). This interaction activates the cAMP-dependent signaling pathway described for VIP stimulation of the lacrimal gland (see Figure 3-6). The mechanism of electrolyte and water secretion caused by the

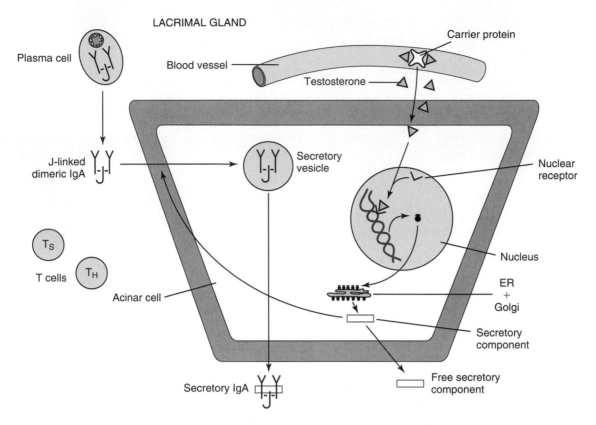

FIGURE 3-7 Schematic of lacrimal gland acinar cell showing the classic mechanism for androgen (indicated here by testosterone) regulation of secretory immunoglobulin A (secretory IgA) secretion. *ER,* Endoplasmic reticulum; T_H, helper T cell; T_S, suppressor T cell. (From Dartt DA, Sullivan DA: Wetting of the ocular surface. In Albert D, Jakobiec F [eds]: *Principles and practice of ophthalmology,* ed 2, Philadelphia, 2000, WB Saunders.)

corneal epithelium is similar to that in the lacrimal gland.

REGULATION OF CONJUNCTIVAL EPITHELIAL CELL ELECTROLYTE AND WATER SECRETION

The conjunctiva is the final source of electrolytes and water in the aqueous layer of the tear film. Because the conjunctiva occupies a portion of the ocular surface much larger than the cornea, it is a potentially significant source of tear electrolytes and water.[69] Like the corneal epithelium, the conjunctiva secretes Na^+, Cl^-, and water.[58] Electrolyte and water secretion by the conjunctiva has only recently begun to be investigated. The information to date indicates that sympathetic nerves can stimulate this secretion. Epinephrine applied to the basal side of the conjunctiva stimulates Cl^- secretion.[32,58] This secretion is mediated by cAMP using the pathway described for VIP in the lacrimal gland (see Figure 3-6), which implies that β-adrenergic receptors are being used. The mechanism for conjunctival electrolyte and water secretion is similar to that described for the lacrimal gland (see Figure 3-4) and for the corneal epithelium (see Figure 3-8). Conjunctival Cl^- secretion into tears accounts for approximately 60% to 75% of the active transport of the conjunctiva. The remainder comes from Na^+-glucose absorption from the tears, indicating that the conjunctiva can also absorb electrolytes and water. The relative contribution of secretion compared with absorption to the volume of tears is unknown.

REGULATION OF CONJUNCTIVAL GOBLET CELL MUCIN SECRETION

One of the major sources of the mucous layer of the tear film is the conjunctival goblet cells. Goblet cells are distributed throughout the conjunctiva and secrete mucins.[28] Mucins are a heterogeneous collection of high-molecular-weight glycoproteins that

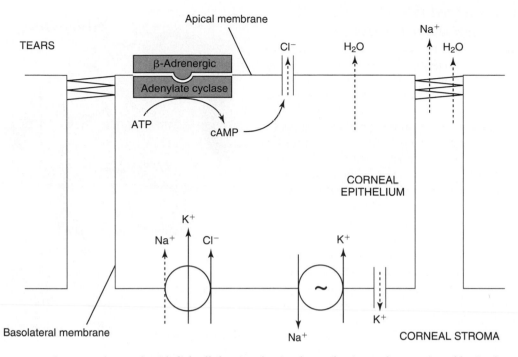

FIGURE 3-8 Schematic of corneal epithelial cell showing the signal transduction pathway activated by β-adrenergic agonists to stimulate electrolyte and water secretion into tears. ∼, Na^+-K^+-ATPase; *dashed arrows,* passive ionic movements; *solid arrows,* active ionic movements. (Modified from Dartt DA: Physiology of tear production. In Lemp MA, Marquardt R [eds]: *The dry eye,* Berlin, 1992, Springer-Verlag.)

consist of a protein backbone with side chains of variable numbers of carbohydrates.[18] Because the carbohydrate side chains are heterogeneous, the genes that synthesize the protein backbone have been used to characterize the mucins. There are nine types of mucin genes *MUC1* to *MUC8*. Conjunctival goblet cells secrete *MUC5AC,* but the other cells in the ocular surface do not secrete this mucin.[24] Goblet cells also secrete other proteins, such as peroxidase.

Goblet cells are highly polarized, with their basolateral membrane on the basal aspect of the conjunctival epithelium and their apical membrane abutting the tear film. Goblet cells are connected to neighboring stratified squamous cells through tight junctions at the apical membrane interface with the lateral membrane. The basal region of the goblet cell contains the nucleus, endoplasmic reticulum, and Golgi apparatus. The apical region contains a large volume of secretory granules that give the cell its unique shape. The protein core of mucins is synthesized in the endoplasmic reticulum and modified by glycosylation in the Golgi apparatus. Mucins are tightly packaged into the secretory granules, where they are stored until they are secreted as regulated

proteins. Upon the appropriate signal, the secretory granules fuse with each other and with the apical membrane, releasing the contents into the tear film. All the secretory granules within the cell are released upon stimulation. The mucin is released in an explosive fashion as the mucin rapidly hydrates with the water of the tear film.

Goblet cell secretion is stimulated by activation of the sensory nerves in the conjunctiva and cornea. By a reflex action, these nerves stimulate the parasympathetic and sympathetic nerves around the goblet cells.[30] The former nerves contain acetylcholine and VIP; the latter contain norepinephrine and NPY. Cholinergic agonists such as acetylcholine and VIP stimulate goblet cell secretion by activating M_2 and M_3 muscarinic acetylcholine receptors and VIP2 receptors, respectively.[50] The signaling pathways activated by these receptors have not yet been published but are probably the same as those used in the lacrimal gland.

A second source of mucins in the tear film is the stratified squamous cells of the corneal and conjunctival epithelia. The relative contribution to the tear film of goblet cell mucins compared with stratified squamous cell mucins is unknown.

EXCRETORY SYSTEM

Embryology and Development

In the 7-mm embryo a depression termed the *naso-lacrimal groove* develops between the lateral nasal and maxillary processes. The ectoderm in this area thickens and becomes buried to form a rod. Canalization of this nasolacrimal ectodermal rod begins at the 32- to 36-mm stage of development.[5] The central cells of the rod degenerate, forming a lumen closed at the cephalad end by conjunctival and canalicular epithelium and closed at the caudad end by nasal and nasolacrimal epithelial components. The superior membrane is normally open by birth, whereas the inferior membrane often persists in newborns.[15,47] Congenital absence of any segment of the nasolacrimal system, supernumerary puncta, and lacrimal fistulas demonstrates abnormalities of development in this region.[5,30,36,57] The membranous bones surrounding the lacrimal excretory system are well developed at 4 months and ossify by birth.

Anatomy and Function of the Lacrimal Excretory System

The lacrimal excretory pathway begins at a 0.3-mm opening on the medial portion of each eyelid, termed the *punctum*. The lower eyelid punctum is located slightly lateral to the upper eyelid punctum. The puncta are the openings of the canaliculi, delicate drainage structures approximately 10 mm in length and 0.5 to 1.0 mm in diameter; they traverse the medial eyelids and enter the nasolacrimal sac (Figure 3-9). The canaliculi are lined with stratified squamous epithelium and surrounded by orbicularis muscle. In approximately 90% of individuals the superior and inferior canaliculi merge to form a common canaliculus before entry into the nasolacrimal sac.[34] The common canaliculus angles anteriorly at approximately 118 degrees and enters the lacrimal sac at mean angle of 58 degrees.[67] This angulation may produce a valvelike effect, preventing retrograde flow from the sac.

The nasolacrimal sac and duct are named portions of the same continuous structure. This portion of the outflow system is lined by nonciliated columnar epithelium. The sac measures approximately 12 mm in vertical length and 4 to 8 mm anteroposteriorly; it rests in the lacrimal sac fossa formed by the lacrimal and maxillary bones. The lower nasolacrimal fossa and the nasolacrimal duct are narrower in females,[19] possibly accounting for the female predominance of nasolacrimal obstruction. The nasolacrimal duct extends through the

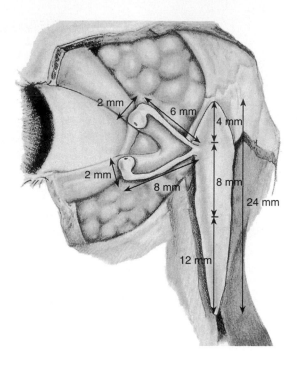

FIGURE 3-9 Approximate dimensions of nasolacrimal excretory system. In the adult the length of system is about 35 mm; in the newborn the system measures about 25 mm. (From Lemke BN, Lucarelli MJ: Anatomy of the ocular adnexa, orbit, and related facial structures. In Nesi FA et al [eds]: *Smith's ophthalmic plastic and reconstructive surgery,* St Louis, 1998, Mosby.)

lacrimal, maxillary, and inferior turbinate bones for a distance of approximately 2 mm to reach the inferior turbinate. A mucosal flap, Hasner's valve, may be present at the opening of the duct into the nose.

From 10% to 25% of secreted tear volume is lost to evaporation under normal conditions.[41] The remaining tears are drained through the lacrimal excretory system into the nose. Some of the tear volume may be absorbed in the nasolacrimal system.[6,59,63]

The most important mechanism of lacrimal drainage is the dynamic effect of the eyelids and medial canthal apparatus. The canaliculi are encased in superficial pretarsal orbicularis oculi muscle as they traverse the medial eyelids and medial canthal region. The anterior and posterior crura of the medial canthal ligament straddle the lacrimal sac before they insert onto the lacrimal crests. Firm fixation of the orbicularis muscle via the medial canthal ligament results in medial displacement of the lower (and to a lesser extent, the upper) eyelids with each blink. In addition, the nasolacrimal sac is ensheathed in a fibromuscular lacrimal sac fascia.

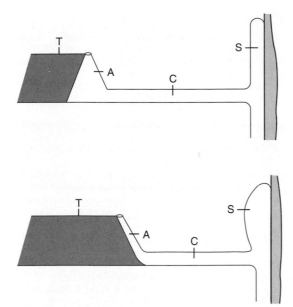

FIGURE 3-10 Jones' lacrimal pump theory. The upper diagram represents eyelids open; the lower diagram shows with eyelids closed. Contraction of the pretarsal orbicularis muscle fibers during eyelid closure narrows the ampulla and shortens the canaliculus pumping tears toward the lacrimal sac. In addition, the theory proposed negative sac pressure during eyelid closure from contraction of the deep heads of the preseptal orbicularis. (From Jones LT, Wobig JL: *Surgery of the eyelids and lacrimal system,* Birmingham, 1976, Aesculapius.)

The deep portion of the pretarsal orbicularis muscle (Horner-Duverney muscle) inserts onto the posterior lacrimal crest and is thought to be important in lacrimal outflow.[1,14,26,27] Similarly, the deep head of the preseptal orbicularis muscle inserts onto the nasolacrimal sac.

On the basis of extensive anatomic dissections, Jones[26] and Jones and Wobig[27] popularized the lacrimal pump theory (Figure 3-10). Jones proposed that contraction of the pretarsal orbicularis muscle fibers during eyelid closure compresses and shortens the canaliculi, pumping tears toward the lacrimal sac. Furthermore, he proposed that simultaneous, lateral movement of the lateral wall of the lacrimal sac from contraction of the deep heads of the preseptal orbicularis muscle generates a negative pressure within the lacrimal sac, siphoning or drawing tears from the canaliculi into the sac. In this theory, with relaxation of the orbicularis muscle, the lacrimal sac collapses, driving tears into the nasolacrimal duct.

Other anatomic and physiologic studies[1,3,11,38,51] have confirmed positive-pressures pumping of the

canaliculi during eyelid closure. However, considerable research has called into question the hypothesis of lacrimal sac negative pressure with eyelid closure.[11,20,48,51] Rosengren[51] intubated the lacrimal sac via the nasolacrimal duct to measure intrasac pressures. He observed increases in sac pressure with eyelid closure and decreases in pressure with eyelid opening. Similarly, Maurice[30] and Ploman, Engel, and Knutsson[48] measured intrasac pressure via the canalicular system, finding positive pressure with eyelid closure.

Doane[11] used high-speed photography to assess the role of blinking in lacrimal drainage. Movements of the tear fluid were made visible by instilling carbon black into the tear film. Doane emphasized compression of the canaliculi and the lacrimal sac during eyelid closure. He suggested that a pressure increase occurs in the canaliculi and, to a lesser extent, in the nasolacrimal sac during eyelid closure. In Doane's model (Figure 3-11), siphoning by the lacrimal sac occurs during relaxation of the blink, rather than during closure as suggested by Jones.

The successful drainage of tears typical after dacryocystorhinostomy suggests that the positive-pressure pumping of tears along the canaliculi is more important than intrasac negative pressure. The consistent problem of epiphora in the setting of facial paralysis underscores the important contribution of the orbicularis muscle to lacrimal outflow. In fact, temporary paralysis of the medial orbicularis oculi muscle with botulinum toxin has been shown to reduce lacrimal outflow and has been suggested as a possible adjunctive therapy for dry eye conditions.[55]

The volume of tears drained per blink has been measured at 1.8 ml by Rosengren[51] and approximately 2.0 ml by Sahlin and Chen.[54] Because a single blink may transport more tears than those produced by basic secretion in 1 minute,[38] the lacrimal excretory system usually functions far below capacity. This would theoretically allow for absorption of some of the volume en route to the nasal cavity. Work by Chavis, Maisey, and Whelham,[6] showing no technetium tracer passing into the nose of one third of subjects under basal secretion rates, lends support to this theory. In a histoanatomic study of the lacrimal drainage system, Thale et al.[63] have demonstrated a plexus of large capacitance vessels surrounding the nasolacrimal sac and duct. These vessels are continuous with the cavernous body of the inferior turbinate. Such vessels may play a role in tear fluid absorption or regulation of tear outflow.

1. Start of blink   Lids open; system filled with fluid

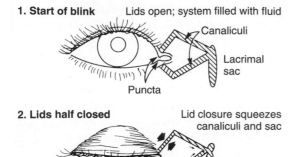

Canaliculi

Lacrimal sac

Puncta

2. Lids half closed   Lid closure squeezes canaliculi and sac

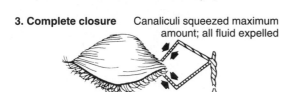

3. Complete closure   Canaliculi squeezed maximum amount; all fluid expelled

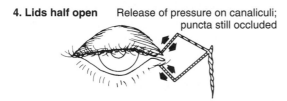

4. Lids half open   Release of pressure on canaliculi; puncta still occluded

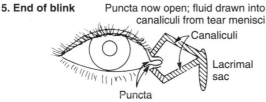

5. End of blink   Puncta now open; fluid drawn into canaliculi from tear menisci

Canaliculi

Lacrimal sac

Puncta

FIGURE 3-11   Doane's model relating blinking and tear drainage. (From Doane MG: *Adv Ophthal Plast Reconstr Surg* 3:49, 1984.)

Lacrimal drainage capacity has been shown to be correlated to the blink rate when the naso-lacrimal duct is in a horizontal position.[54] Sahlin and Chen[54] showed that gravity tended to increase lacrimal drainage. Capillarity may assist tear flow within the canaliculi. Also, the Venturi effect and Bernoulli's principle may aid in lacrimal drainage.[19]

Both adequate secretion and drainage of tears are necessary for optimal visual function. The anatomy and physiology of tear secretion and drainage are complex. Recent developments in the understanding of the physiology of tear secretion may allow improved therapy for patients with the common malady of dry eyes. Similarly, research advances in lacrimal outflow may lead to new medical or surgical therapies for patients with epiphora.

REFERENCES

1. Ahl NC, Hill JD: Horner's muscle and the lacrimal system, *Arch Ophthalmol* 100:488, 1982.
2. Allansmith MB et al: Plasma cell count of main and accessory lacrimal glands and conjunctiva, *Am J Ophthalmol* 82:819, 1976.
3. Becker BB: Tricompartment model of the lacrimal pump mechanism, *Ophthalmology* 99:1139, 1992.
4. Berridge MJ: Inositol triphosphate and calcium signaling, *Nature* 361:315, 1993.
5. Cassady JV: Developmental anatomy of nasolacrimal duct, *Arch Ophthalmol* 47:141, 1952.
6. Chavis RM, Maisey MN, Whelham RA: Quantitative lacrimal scintillography, *Arch Ophthalmol* 96:2066, 1978.
7. Chung C, Tigges M, Stone RA: Peptidergic innervation of the primate meibomian gland, *Invest Ophthalmol Vis Sci* 37:238, 1996.
8. Cripps MM, Bennett DJ: Inhibition of lacrimal function by selective opiate agonists, *Adv Exp Med Biol* 350:127, 1994.
9. Dartt DA, Sullivan DA: Wetting of the ocular surface. In Albert DM, Jakobiec FA (eds): *Principles and practice of ophthalmology: the Harvard system,* ed 2, vol 2, Philadelphia, 2000, WB Saunders.
10. Doane MG: Interactions of eyelids and tears in corneal wetting and the dynamics of the normal human eyeblink, *Am J Ophthalmol* 89:507, 1980.
11. Doane MG: Blinking and the mechanics of the lacrimal drainage system, *Ophthalmology* 88:844, 1981.
12. Duke-Elder SS, Cook C: *System of ophthalmology: normal and abnormal development. Part 1: Embryology,* St Louis, 1963, Mosby.
13. Dutton JJ: The lacrimal systems. In *Atlas of clinical and surgical orbital anatomy,* Philadelphia, 1994, WB Saunders.
14. Duverney M: *Oeuvres anatomiques,* Paris, 1761, Biblioteque Nationale de France.
15. Ffooks OO: Dacryocystitis in infancy, *Br J Ophthalmol* 46:422, 1962.
16. Fullard R: Interactions of eyelids and tears in corneal wetting and the dynamics of the normal human eyeblink, *Am J Ophthalmol* 89:507, 1994.
17. Gilbard J, Dartt DA: Changes in rabbit lacrimal gland fluid osmolarity with flow rate, *Invest Ophthalmol Vis Sci* 23:804, 1982.
18. Gipson IK, Inatomi T: Mucin genes expressed by the ocular surface epithelium, *Prog Retin Eye Res* 16:81, 1997.
19. Groessl SA, Sires BS, Lemke BN: An anatomical basis for primary acquired nasolacrimal duct obstruction, *Arch Ophthalmol* 115:71, 1997.
20. Hill JC, Bethell W, Smirmaul HJ: Lacrimal drainage dynamic evaluation. Part I: Mechanics of tear transport, *Can J Ophthalmol* 9:411, 1974.
21. Hodges RR et al: Adrenergic and cholinergic agonists use separate signal transduction pathways in lacrimal gland, *Am J Physiol* 262:G1087, 1992.
22. Hodges RR et al: Identification of vasoactive intestinal peptide receptor subtypes in the lacrimal gland and their signal transducing components, *Invest Ophthalmol Vis Sci* 38:610, 1997.
23. Ichikawa A, Nakajima Y: Electron microscopy on the lacrimal gland of the rat, *Tohuku J Exp Med* 77:136, 1962.
24. Inatomi T et al: Expression of secretory mucin genes by human conjunctival epithelia, *Invest Ophthalmol Vis Sci* 37:1684, 1996.
25. Jakobiec F, Iwamoto T: The ocular adnexa: lids, conjunctiva, and orbit. In Fine B, Yanoff M (eds): *Ocular histology,* Philadelphia, 1979, Harper and Row.

26. Jones LT: An anatomical approach to problems of the eyelids and lacrimal apparatus, *Arch Ophthalmol* 66:111, 1961.

27. Jones LT, Wobig JL: *Surgery of the eyelids and lacrimal system,* Birmingham, 1976, Aesculapius.

28. Kessing SV: Mucous gland system of the conjunctiva: a quantitative normal anatomical study, *Acta Ophthalmol* 95(suppl):1, 1968.

29. Kessler TL et al: Stimulation of goblet cell mucous secretion by activation of nerves in rat conjunctiva, *Curr Eye Res* 14:985, 1995.

30. Kirk RC: Developmental anomalies of the lacrimal passages: a review of the literature and presentation of three unusual cases, *Am J Ophthalmol* 42:227, 1956.

31. Klyce SD, Crosson CE: Transport processes across the rabbit corneal epithelium: a review, *Curr Eye Res* 4:323, 1985.

32. Kompella UB, Kim KJ, Lee VH: Active chloride transport in the pigmented rabbit conjunctiva, *Curr Eye Res* 12:1041, 1993.

33. Lamberts D: Physiology of the tear film. In Smolin G, Thoft R (eds): *The cornea,* ed 3, Boston, 1994, Little, Brown.

34. Lemke BN: Lacrimal anatomy, *Adv Ophthal Plast Reconstr Surg* 3:11, 1984.

35. Lemke BN, Lucarelli MJ: Anatomy of the ocular adnexa, orbit, and related facial structures. In Nesi FA et al (eds): *Smith's ophthalmic plastic and reconstructive surgery,* St Louis, 1998, Mosby.

36. Masi AV: Congenital fistula of the lacrimal sac, *Arch Ophthalmol* 81:701, 1969.

37. Maudui TP, Jammes H, Rossignol B: M3 muscarinic acetylcholine receptor coupling to PLC in rat exorbital lacrimal acinar cells, *Am J Physiol* 264:C1550, 1993.

38. Maurice DM: The dynamics and drainage of tears, *Int Ophthalmol Clin* 13:103, 1973.

39. Meneray MA, Fields TY, Bennett DJ: Gs and Gq$_{211}$ couple vasoactive intestinal peptide and cholinergic stimulation to lacrimal secretion, *Invest Ophthalmol Vis Sci* 38:1261, 1997.

40. Mircheff A: Water and electrolyte secretion and fluid modification. In Albert DM, Jakobiec F, Robinson N (eds): *Principles and practices of ophthalmology: basic sciences,* Philadelphia, 1994, WB Saunders.

41. Mishima S: Some physiologic aspects of the precorneal tear film, *Arch Ophthalmol* 73:233, 1965.

42. Morton AD et al: Lateral extensions of the Müller muscle, *Arch Ophthalmol* 114:1486, 1996.

43. Nicolaides N: Recent findings on the chemical composition of the lipids of steer and human meibomian glands. In Holly F (ed): *The preocular tear film in health, disease, and contact lens wear,* Lubbock, Tx, 1986, Dry Eye Institute.

44. Nishizuka Y: The role of protein kinase C in cell surface signal transduction and tumor promotion, *Nature* 308:693, 1984.

45. Ozanics V, Jakobiec F: Prenatal development of the eye and its adnexa. In Jakobiec F (ed): *Ocular anatomy, embryology, and teratology,* Philadelphia, 1982, Harper and Row.

46. Perra MT et al: Human meibomian glands: a histochemical study for androgen metabolic enzymes, *Invest Ophthalmol Vis Sci* 31:771, 1990.

47. Petersen RA, Robb RM: The natural course of congenital obstruction of the nasolacrimal duct, *J Pediatr Ophthalmol Strabismus* 15:246, 1978.

48. Ploman KG, Engel A, Knutsson F: Experimental studies of the lacrimal passageways, *Acta Ophthalmol* 6:55, 1928.

49. Raina S et al: Molecular cloning and characterization of an aquaporin cDNA from salivary, lacrimal, and respiratory tissues, *J Biol Chem* 270:1908, 1995.

50. Rios JD et al: Immunolocalization of muscarinic and VIP receptor subtypes and their role in stimulating goblet cell secretion, *Invest Ophthalmol Vis Sci* 40:1102, 1999.

51. Rosengren B: On lacrimal drainage, *Ophthalmologica* 164:409, 1972.

52. Ruskell GL: The orbital branches of the pterygopalatine ganglion and their relationship with internal carotid nerve branches in primates, *J Anat* 106:323, 1970.

53. Ruskell GL: The distribution of autonomic post-ganglionic nerve fibers to the lacrimal gland in monkeys, *J Anat* 109:229, 1971.

54. Sahlin S, Chen E: Gravity, blink rate, and lacrimal drainage capacity, *Am J Ophthalmol* 124:758, 1997.

55. Sahlin S et al: Effect of eyelid botulinum toxin injection on lacrimal drainage, *Am J Ophthalmol* 129:481, 2000.

56. Seifert P et al: Light and electron microscopic morphology of accessory lacrimal glands, *Adv Exp Med Biol* 350:19, 1994.

57. Sevel D: Development and congenital abnormalities of the nasolacrimal apparatus, *J Pediatr Ophthalmol Strabismus* 18:13, 1981.

58. Shi XP, Candia OA: Active sodium and chloride transport across the isolated rabbit conjunctiva, *Curr Eye Res* 14:927, 1995.

59. Sisler HA: Current concepts in the understanding of lacrimal drainage, *Adv Ophthalmic Plast Reconstr Surg* 3:25, 1984.

60. Smith B, Petrelli R: Surgical repair of the prolapsed lacrimal gland, *Arch Ophthalmol* 96:113, 1978.

61. Sullivan DA: Ocular mucosal immunity. In Ogra P et al (eds): *Handbook of mucosal immunology,* ed 2, Orlando, 1998, Academic Press.

62. Sullivan DA et al: Influence of gender, sex steroid hormones, and the hypothalamic-pituitary axis on the structure and function of the lacrimal gland, *Adv Exp Med Biol* 438:11, 1998.

63. Thale A et al: Functional anatomy of the human efferent tear ducts: a new theory of tear outflow mechanism, *Graefe's Arch Clin Exp Ophthalmol* 236:674, 1998.

64. Thody AJ, Shuster S: Control and function of sebaceous glands, *Physiol Rev* 69:383, 1989.

65. Tiffany JM: Physiological functions of the meibomian glands, *Prog Ret Eye Res* 14:47, 1995.

66. Tiffany JM, Marsden RG: The meibomian lipids of the rabbit: II. Detailed composition of the principal esters, *Exp Eye Res* 34:601, 1982.

67. Tucker NA, Tucker SM, Linberg JV: The anatomy of the common canaliculus, *Arch Ophthalmol* 114:1231, 1996.

68. Walcott B: Anatomy and innervation of the human lacrimal gland. In Albert DM, Jakobiec F, Robinson N (eds): *Principles and practice of ophthalmology: basic sciences,* Philadelphia, 1994, WB Saunders.

69. Watsky MA, Jablonski MM, Edelhauser HF: Comparison of conjunctival and corneal surface areas in rabbit and human, *Curr Eye Res* 7:483, 1988.

70. Whitnall S: *The anatomy of the human orbit and accessory organs of vision,* New York, 1932, Oxford University Press.

SECTION 2

CORNEA AND SCLERA

HENRY F. EDELHAUSER AND JOHN L. UBELS

CHAPTER 4

THE CORNEA AND THE SCLERA

HENRY F. EDELHAUSER AND JOHN L. UBELS

Light enters the eye through the transparent cornea, which also forms the major refractive structure of the eye, focusing light onto the retina. The cornea (Figure 4-1) is an excellent example of the unification of structure and function that combine to yield an almost perfectly transparent, avascular, optical tissue that also serves as a barrier between the environment and the inside of the eye. It is made up of an outer layer of epithelial cells that are continuously renewed, differentiating to form a nonkeratinized mucin-expressing superficial layer of cells that interacts with the tear film to form a smooth optical surface.

Most of the cornea is the stroma, made up of collagen fibers and proteoglycans that are synthesized, maintained, and repaired by a system of interspersed keratocytes. The collagen fibers are arranged with respect to one another and interact with the proteoglycans in such a way as to form a mechanically strong extracellular matrix (ECM) that does not scatter light, allowing transmittance of more than 99% of incident visible radiation.

The innermost part of the cornea is a single layer of essentially nonreplicating endothelial cells. These cells, which are essential to maintenance of corneal transparency, form a leaky barrier between the aqueous humor and the stroma. This allows the entry of nutrients into the avascular stroma. In turn, an endothelial system of metabolic pumps, ion transporters, and channels interact to osmotically remove water from the cornea, sustaining a level of stromal hydration compatible with the cornea transparency.

This chapter reviews and explains the anatomic, physiologic, biochemical, and molecular properties of the cornea that account for the characteristics summarized previously, providing a framework for understanding normal corneal function and disease states. The anatomy and permeability of the sclera are also reviewed.

CORNEA

Anatomy and Development

Anatomy of the Epithelium. The corneal epithelium is a stratified, nonkeratinized, nonsecretory squamous epithelium that is five to seven cells thick, consisting of three types of cells; a single layer of basal cells, in which mitosis occurs, adheres to a basement membrane. As cell division occurs, the daughter cells move toward the surface of the cornea and begin to differentiate, forming one to three layers of wing cells. The superficial cells are terminally differentiated squamous cells forming a layer three to four cells thick. These cells finally degenerate and are sloughed from the corneal surface. This process results in turnover of the entire epithelium every 7 days[162] (Figures 4-2 and 4-3). Compared with other epithelia, the cornea is highly regular in its organization, a characteristic important to the optical properties of the cornea.

The single layer of cuboidal basal cells, like the basal cell layer in other squamous epithelia, is the sole source of new cells within the corneal epithelium. No cell division occurs in wing cells or superficial cells. The basal cells originate from stem cells in the basal layer of the limbal epithelium, which is peripheral to the cornea. The basal cells are distinguished from limbal stem cells by the expression of a major keratin pair, the acidic K12 and the basic K3. Keratin K3, with a molecular weight (MW) of 64 kD is considered a specific marker for corneal epithelial differentiation within the ocular surface epithelium[54,389] (Figure 4-4). Mutations of K12 and

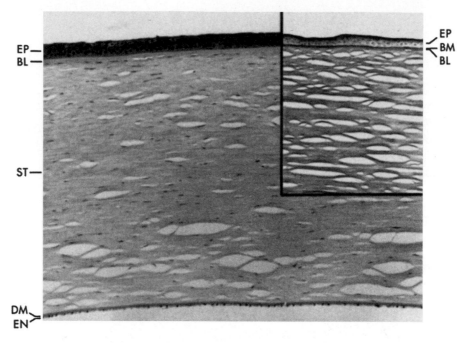

Figure 4-1   Histologic section of a normal human cornea stained with periodic acid–Schiff reveals the outer epithelium (*EP*), basement membrane (*BM*), acellular Bowman's layer (*BL*), stroma (*ST*), Descemet's membrane (*DM*), and endothelial monolayer (*EN*). (Courtesy Dr. Morton E. Smith.)

K3 are present in Meesman's corneal dystrophy, which causes fragility of the corneal epithelium.[197] A minor keratin pair, K14/K5, is also expressed by the these cells.[54,244] Basal cells have a higher level of metabolic and synthetic activity than the more superficial cells and therefore have more prominent mitochondria, endoplasmic reticulum, and Golgi apparatus. They also contain significant stores of glycogen.

The wing cells, named for their characteristic wing-shaped processes, form one to three layers of cells in an intermediate state of differentiation. A prominent characteristic of these cells is an abundance of intracellular keratin tonofilaments. The corneal epithelium is referred to as a *nonkeratinized epithelium* because it normally does not express the cornified cytoskeleton typical of epidermal cells. This situation changes in vitamin A deficiency when the corneal epithelium expresses keratins normally found in the cornified epithelium, or epidermis, of the skin.[245,389,442]

Superficial cells are terminally differentiated and in a process of degeneration, as is evident from the relative paucity of cellular organelles and clumped chromatin in the nucleus. Staining with acridine orange also indicates that these cells have decreased levels of ribonucleic acid (RNA).[126] When examined with scanning electron microscopy, the surface of the cornea is seen as an irregular array of polygonal cells. These cells can be divided into populations of small and large cells or dark and light cells. The smaller, light cells are younger cells that have recently reached the surface of the cornea, whereas the larger, dark cells are mature cells that will be sloughed. Breaks in the epithelium, known as *exfoliation holes,* are also present. These represent areas where a cell is in the process of peeling off the corneal surface, forming a hole through which the underlying superficial cell can be seen (Figure 4-5). The surface cells are covered with a dense coat of microplicae, and dark cells have fewer microplicae than do light cells.[168,344] Adhering to these microvilli is a glycocalyx. This glycocalyx has not been fully characterized; however, it has been shown that the superficial epithelial cells express the MUC1 (Figure 4-6) and MUC4 mucin genes. All corneal epithelial cells express MUC1 messenger ribonucleic acid (mRNA), and the apical membranes of the superficial cells contain the transmembrane MUC1 protein and MUC4 protein.[140,193,347] It has also been shown that the apical membranes of the second and third layers of the superficial cells ex-

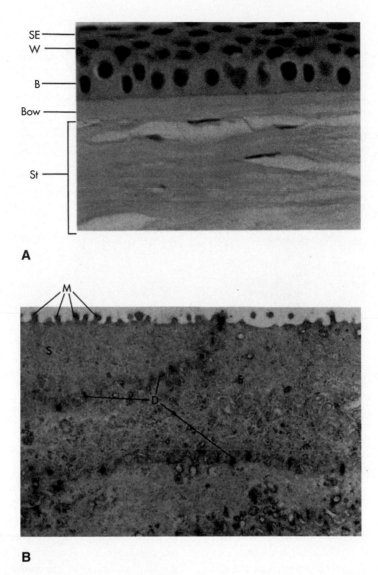

FIGURE 4-2 **A,** Anterior layers of human cornea. *SE,* Surface epithelial cells; *W,* wing cells; *B,* basal epithelial cells; *Bow,* Bowman's layer; *St,* stroma. Basement membrane between basal epithelial cells and Bowman's layer is not visible by light microscopy. (Magnification ×700.) **B,** Surface epithelial cells of human cornea. *D,* Desmosomes; *M,* microvilli; *S,* surface epithelial cell. (Magnification ×18,000.) (**A,** Courtesy Dr. Martha G. Farber. **B,** Courtesy Dr. Adolph I. Cohen.)

press a mucinlike substance when the surface cells are damaged. As discussed in more detail in the following sections, despite the fact that a portion of the superficial cells are dying and will be sloughed, these cells form an essential barrier between the tears and the inner portions of the cornea.

The Basement Membrane and Bowman's Layer. The basal cells of the epithelium rest on a basement membrane, or basal lamina, that is approximately 40 to 60 nm thick. This membrane is similar in structure and composition to the basal laminas of other squamous epithelia. It has been analyzed histochemically and immunologically and contains type IV collagen, laminin, the proteoglycan perlecan, fibronectin, and fibrin.[125,235]

Bowman's layer, which among mammals is found only in primates, lies beneath the basement membrane and is approximately 12 μm thick. It appears to be structureless by light microscopy, but under the electron microscope, it is revealed to be made of randomly arranged collagen fibrils. These are probably,

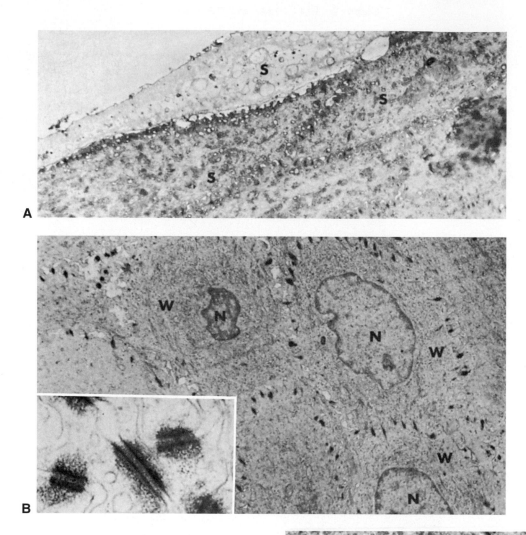

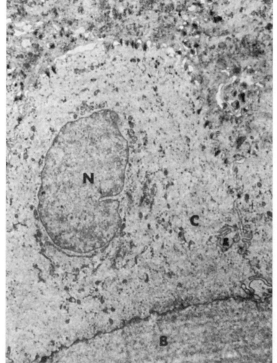

FIGURE 4-3   A, Corneal epithelium, outer surface, shows surface cells (S) without nuclei. (Magnification ×3350.) B, Next layer deeper (wing cells, W) shows much rounder appearance of cells in which nuclei (N) can easily be seen. Note marked interdigitation of cell borders. (Magnification ×3840.) C, Basal cells of corneal epithelium (C) shows nucleus (N) and Bowman's layer (B). (Magnification ×5950.) (B, Courtesy Dr. Jack Kayes.)

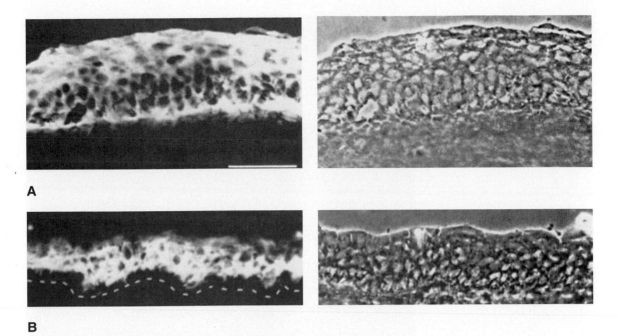

FIGURE 4-4 **A,** Immunofluorescent staining of the 64 K keratin in corneal epithelium with monoclonal antibody AE5. **B,** Immunofluorescent staining of suprabasal cells of the limbal epithelium with monoclonal antibody AE5. Note that the less differentiated basal stem cells do not stain for the 64 K keratin. Photos on *right* are phase-contrast micrographs of the same sections. (Courtesy Dr. Tung-Tien Sun. From Schermer A et al: *J Cell Biol* 103:49, 1986.)

at least in part, type I collagen.[125] Bowman's layer is acellular and may be considered a modified superficial layer of the stroma; the anterior most layer of the stroma is Bowman's layer. The function of this part of the cornea is unknown. It has been suggested that Bowman's layer is a stabilizing element in the cornea; however, results of biomechanical studies do not support this hypothesis.[401]

Cell Adhesion in the Epithelium. The maintenance of the well-organized, stable epithelial structure described previously requires appropriate cell-substrate and cell-cell adhesion. Accordingly, each cell type of the corneal epithelium possesses junctional structures suited to its position and function in the epithelial layer. As stated previously, the basal cells of the epithelium rest on a basement membrane that is approximately 40 to 60 nm thick. This basement membrane is made up primarily of type IV and VII collagen, laminin, fibronectin and the heparan sulfate proteoglycan perlecan.[130] Type XII collagen has also been identified in the basement membrane.[8]

The basal cells, and thereby the entire epithelium, adhere to the basement membrane and stroma via hemidesmosomes, which are integral membrane protein complexes in the basal cell plasma membrane.[145,224] The primary components of the hemidesmosomes that have been identified are the bullous pemphigoid antigen[9] and integrin heterodimer, which is a laminin receptor.[424] The intracellular domains of the hemidesmosomes are linked to keratin filaments. In the basement membrane, the hemidesmosomes are linked to structures known as *anchoring fibrils,* made of type VII collagen, that pass through Bowman's layer into the stroma (Figure 4-7). The anchoring fibrils penetrate as deeply as 2 μm into the stroma, branching intricately among the collagen fibrils and ending in structures known as *anchoring plaques,* which are composed of laminin.[144,437] It should be noted that this adhesion complex is destroyed during photorefractive keratectomy and must be reassembled during the healing process, as discussed subsequently.

The basal, wing, and superficial cells are linked to one another by desmosomes, which are more numerous among superficial cells than between basal cells.[180] As in other stratified epithelia, the plaque region of these desmosomes contains desmoplakin and plakoglobin. However, the corneal epithelium is unique in that the only members of the cadherin family expressed in the desmo-

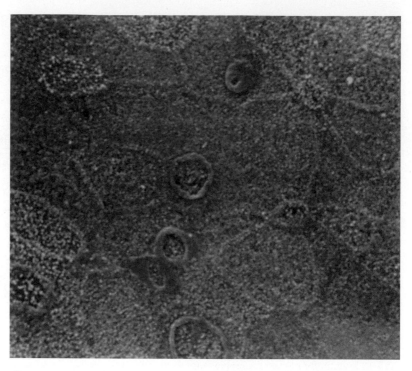

A

FIGURE 4-5   Scanning electron microscopy of the corneal epithelial surface. **A,** Low power (×190) showing light and dark
cells. **B,** High power (×2050) showing microvilli and exfoliation
holes. (Courtesy Dr. Roswell Pfister. From Pfister RR et al: *Cornea*
1:205, 1982.)

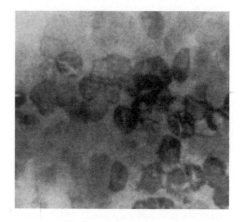

B

FIGURE 4-6   The presence of the membrane-spanning
mucin MUC1 on the apical cells of the human corneal
epithelium, as demonstrated by immunofluorescence microscopy using an antibody designated HMFG-1. (Bar =
13 μm.) (Courtesy Dr. Ilene K. Gipson. See also Inatomi
T et al: Invest Ophthalmol Vis Sci 36:1818, 1995.)

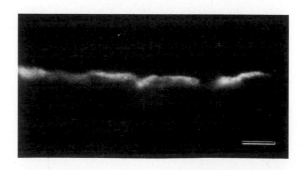

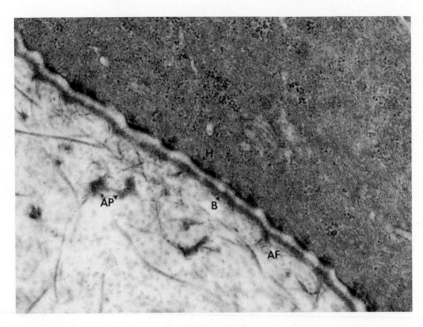

FIGURE 4-7 Adhesion structures of the basal corneal epithelium. *AF,* Anchoring fibrils; *AP,* anchoring plaques; *B,* basement membrane; *H,* hemidesmosomes. (Courtesy Dr. Ilene Gipson.)

somes are desmocollin 2 and desmoglein 2. Desmocollin 1 and desmoglein 1 appear to be specific to cornified epithelia and thus are absent from the ocular surface epithelium.[304]

Of greatest importance to the barrier function of the cornea are the tight junctional complexes that are found only between the superficial cells of the epithelium. These junctions, or *zonula occludens,* completely encircle the cells and represent an actual anastomosis of the lipid bilayer of the adjoining membranes.[300] In this way the superficial cells form a highly effective, semipermeable membrane on the surface of the cornea[193,461] (Figure 4-8, *A*). The presence of the adhesion protein ZO-1 has been demonstrated in the corneal epithelium. Junctions containing this protein completely encircle the most superficial cells, and expression of ZO-1 in wing cells quickly increases when superficial cells are damaged.[461] Focal areas of staining for ZO-1 are also present in adherens junctions between wing and basal cells[428] (Figure 4-9).

The cells of all layers of corneal epithelium are also connected by gap junctions, which are more numerous in the more basal layers than in the superficial cells[300] (Figure 4-8, *B*). The basal cells express the gap junctional protein connexin 43, whereas connexin 50 is found in all cells, again demonstrating the differentiation that occurs in the epithelium. Injection of fluorescent dye demon-

strates that the gap junctions are functional between basal and wing cells but that little dye spread occurs between the terminally differentiated wing cells[476] (Figure 4-10, *A*). This suggests that the basal and wing cells form a functional syncytium, which may be important in coordinating functions such as cell differentiation and migration.

Clinical Manifestations of Abnormalities in Epithelial Structure. Various dystrophies (inherited diseases) and other abnormalities of the corneal epithelium, basement membrane, and Bowman's layer have been described. These diseases often present as deviations from normal corneal structure that interfere with the optical properties of the cornea. The reader is referred to textbooks of ophthalmology for detailed clinical descriptions of these conditions. Especially important are conditions such as epithelial basement membrane dystrophy, which leads to painful recurrent epithelial erosions, making the cornea susceptible to edema and infection. This is apparently caused by abnormal adhesion of the epithelium, and it has been demonstrated that basal cells in this condition have a decreased number of hemidesmosomes.

Reduplication of the basement membrane occurs in aging and diabetic patients.[2,223] This is associated with an increased incidence of epithelial erosions. This abnormality of epithelial adhesion may

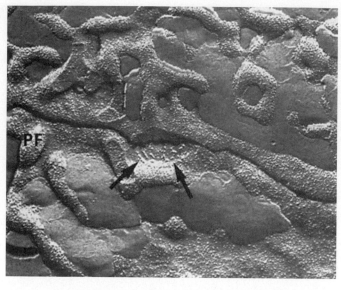

A

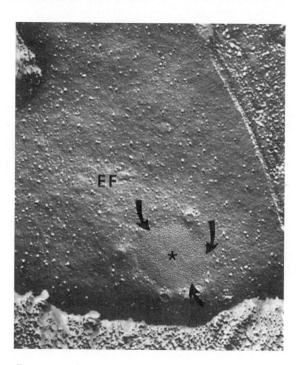

B

FIGURE 4-8   Freeze-fracture electron micrographs of epithelial cell membranes. **A,** Tight junctions that consist of delicate particle strands are present between superficial epithelial cells (*arrows*) on P-face membranes. (Magnification ×60,000.) **B,** Lateral epithelial membranes of cells located deeper in the epithelium are joined by large gap junctional complexes (*arrows* and *). (Magnification ×80,000.) (Courtesy Dr. Barbara McLaughlin. From McLaughlin BJ et al: *Curr Eye Res* 4:951, 1985.)

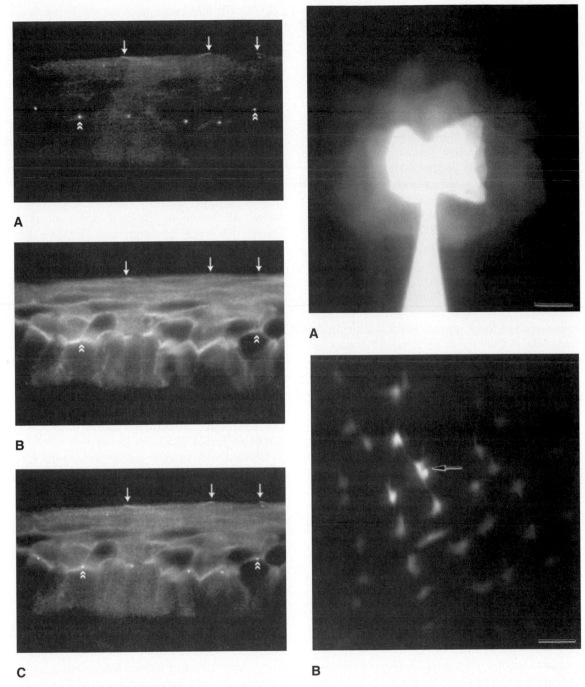

A

B

C

A

B

Figure 4-9 Cryosection of rabbit corneal epithelium immunostained with antibodies to the desmosomal protein ZO-1 (**A**) and the desmosomal-associated protein pinin (**B**). Both proteins are demonstrated in (**C**). Note the presence of ZO-1 along borders of the superficial epithelial cells (*arrows*). The midepithelial staining for ZO-1 can be seen to correspond to basal cell–wing cell junctions, and frequency at sites of confluence of two or more wing cells with a basal cell (*double arrowheads*) demonstrates two distinctly positive locations within the epithelium. (Courtesy Dr. Stephen Sugrue.)

Figure 4-10 **A,** Dye spread through gap junctions between cells in the second layer of the rabbit corneal epithelium. 5,6-Carboxyfluorescein was injected through the micropipette seen in the lower portion of the photograph. **B,** Dye spread through gap junctions among keratocytes in the posterior rabbit corneal stroma after injection of dye into the source cell (*arrows*). (Bars = 25 μm.) (Courtesy Dr. Mitchell Watsky and Dr. Kevin Williams.)

be a result of a reduced depth of penetration of anchoring fibrils through the thickened basement membrane into the stroma.[143]

Stromal Structure. The most important characteristics of the cornea are its transparency and function as a refractive surface, which function to transmit and focus light optimally on the retina. Measured externally, the cornea is oval-shaped, with an average 12.6-mm horizontal diameter and 11.7-mm vertical diameter. The anterior surface of the cornea represents the major refractive component of the eye, contributing approximately 48 diopters of plus power toward the convergence of an image onto the retina. The central third of the cornea is of a generally spherical or toroidal contour, with the radius of curvature of its outer aspect averaging 7.8 mm.[25] The more peripheral portion of the cornea is flatter, radially asymmetric, and thicker (0.65 mm) than the central portion (0.52 mm). The cornea transmits radiation from approximately 310 nm in the ultraviolet to 2500 nm in the infrared.[24] It does not normally absorb light in the visible range, and because of minimal light scattering, more than 99% of incident light above a wavelength of 400 nm is transmitted through the cornea.[110]

These structural and optical characteristics of the cornea are determined primarily by the structure and composition of the stroma, which makes up 90% of the corneal thickness.[217] The stroma is predominantly an ECM comprised of a lamellar arrangement of collagen fibrils running parallel to the corneal surface, with the individual collagen fibrils separated by a matrix of proteoglycans.[62] The collagen fibrils and ECM are maintained by cells called *keratocytes* that lie between the collagen lamellas (Figure 4-11).

The stroma is made up of 200 to 250 lamellas of collagen fibers. The lamellas are formed of bundles of collagen fibers approximately 2.0 μm thick and 9 to 260 μm wide (Figure 4-12). They stretch from limbus to limbus, lying obliquely to one another in the anterior stroma and orthogonally in the posterior stroma.[162,180,302] At the limbus, the collagen fibers turn and run circumferentially forming an annulus 1.5 to 2.0 mm wide around the cornea. It is this annulus of collagen fibers that maintains the curvature of the cornea.[321,322] This has profound implications for possible alterations of stromal structure during refractive or cataract surgery that may lead to postoperative refractive errors.

The collagen fibers are primarily made of type I collagen, with lesser amounts of types V and VI.[320,499] The fibers are approximately 30 nm in diameter and are spaced about 42 to 44 nm apart, yielding a tissue-volume fibril fraction of 28%.[122,301] The collagen fibers have a refractive index of 1.411 compared with the extrafibrillar matrix's refractive index of 1.365.[259] Despite this disparity, minimal light scattering occurs because of the highly uniform size and spacing of the collagen fibers. This is discussed in greater detail in the section on stromal function.

The extrafibrillar material, sometimes called the *ground substance* of the stroma, is largely made up of proteoglycans. The proteoglycans of the corneal stroma all belong to the gene family of small leucine-rich repeat proteoglycans. The core proteins of these molecules have high homogeneity and contain 7 to 10 leucine-rich repeats with the sequences, L-X-X-L-X-L-X-X-N-X-L, where X is any amino acid.[165] These proteoglycans were originally named according to their carbohydrate side chains, and those in the cornea were referred to as *chondroitin sulfate/dermatan sulfate (CD/DS) proteoglycans* and *keratin sulfate (KS) proteoglycans*. The genes for the core protein of these proteoglycans have now been cloned, and the molecules are now named for their core proteins, with decorin, lumican, keratocan, and mimecan having been identified in the cornea.

Decorin is a CD/DS proteoglycan with nine leucine-rich repeats and a single CD/DS side chain that binds to type VI collagen.[165,261,492] It is more abundant in the anterior cornea than in the posterior cornea and is the only CD/DS proteoglycan in the cornea.[50] The cornea contains three closely related KS proteoglycans, which are more abundant in the posterior stroma.[50] The first of these to be cloned and characterized in the cornea was lumican. It is a protein with 342 amino acids (bovine cornea) and 11 leucine-rich repeats, with a single KS side chain.[22,130] This proteoglycan is abundant in the cornea and, as discussed subsequently, is essential to maintenance of corneal transparency, hence the name *lumican*. Keratocan, a second KS proteoglycan in the cornea, has 10 leucine-rich repeats and carries 3 KS side chains.[69,131] It differs from other KS proteoglycans in being an almost exclusively corneal protein.

Finally, a third KS proteoglycan, whimsically named *mimecan*, has been identified in the corneal stroma. This proteoglycan has an MW of 25 kD and five leucine-rich repeats. It carries only one KS chain and is a product of the same gene that codes for the 12-kD glycoprotein osteoglycin, found in bone.[131]

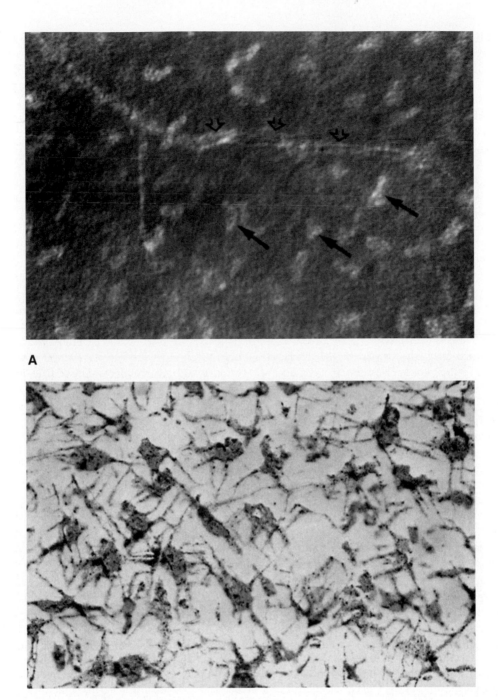

FIGURE 4-11 The corneal stroma observed in vivo by tandem scanning microscopy (TSM) (**A**) compared with conventional light micrograph of fixed, dead specimen stained with 1% gold chloride and cut en face (**B**). Note that in the in vivo image, only the nuclei of the tissue fibrocytes are clearly identified (**A,** *arrows*). Nerves are also detected (*open arrow*) and can be followed throughout the cornea. In the conventional light micrograph, the density of individual stromal fibrocytes appears comparable with that seen in vivo. Note also the thin, filopodial processes that appear to extend from one cell to another. (**A,** TSM, ×220; **B,** 1% AuCl, ×450.) (Courtesy Dr. James V. Jester.)

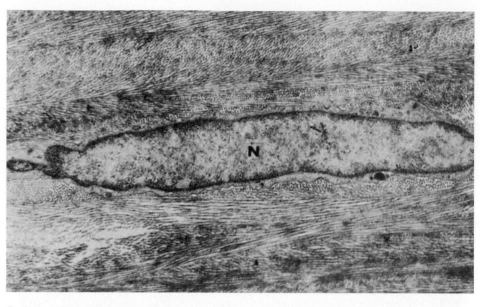

A

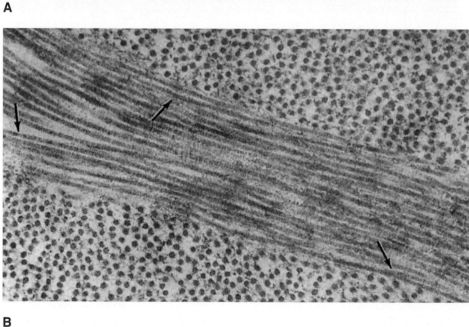

B

FIGURE 4-12   **A,** Nucleus (N) of corneal stromal cell; layers of corneal stromal collagen are seen from various angles. (Magnification ×9000.) **B,** Higher magnification of stromal collagen, showing collagen fibrils cut on end and from side with their 640 A banding visible (arrows). (Magnification ×72,000.) (Courtesy Dr. Jack Kayes.)

Lumican, keratocan, and mimecan are also found in other tissues. They are unique in the cornea compared with these other tissues in that only in the cornea are they present in a highly sulfated form. In other tissues, these core proteins carry no KS side chains or the side chains are present in the nonsulfated form.[69,91,129,165] The sulfation of the side chains in the cornea increases the water-retentive properties of the proteoglycans, which affects hydration of the stroma and hence corneal transparency.

The ECM of the stroma is produced and maintained by cells known as *keratocytes* (not to be confused with the keratinocytes of skin) or *stromal fibroblasts* (see Figure 4-11). These cells make up only 10% of the volume of the stroma. Although these cells are flattened and have sometimes been described as having scant cytoplasm, implying that they are relatively inactive, it is now clear that they are important to the ongoing function of the stroma. The mRNA for lumican, keratocan, and mimecan have all been identified in keratocytes, and these cells also synthesize collagen.[131,165,264,383] The cells are activated when the stroma is damaged and some differentiate into myofibroblasts during wound healing.[203] It also appears that these activities are coordinated via communication among the fibroblasts, which apparently form a syncytium. It has been demonstrated that the cells are connected by gap junctions that contain connexin 43 and that injected dye will spread from cell to cell via these junctions[342,464] (see Figure 4-10, *B*).

Cellular Anatomy of the Corneal Endothelium. A single layer of cells known as the *endothelium* covers the posterior surface of the cornea. This monolayer is formed by a regularly arranged array of polygonal cells, most of which are hexagonal. In general, human corneal endothelial cell density decreases with age. Bourne, Nelson, and Hodge[33] reported a 0.6% decrease in central endothelial cell density per year in typical patients with no history of corneal disease or surgery. Corneas from eyes of newborns can have cell densities greater than 5500 cells/mm². The cell densities range from 2500 to 3000 cells/mm² in adults.[476] This is still well above the minimum level of 400 to 700 cell/mm² required for maintenance of normal corneal function, indicating that adequate cells are available for a lifetime of well over 100 years.[31] Endothelial cells are approximately 20 μm in diameter and 4 to 6 μm thick. With use of an transmission electron microscope, it is evident that these cells, although essentially cuboidal in cross section, adjoin one another in tortuous interdigitations resulting in lateral borders with a length 10 times the cell thickness.

The endothelial cells contain a large nucleus that fills a significant portion of the cell and, as seen by scanning electron microscopy, causes the apical membrane to bulge outward. The cells contain numerous mitochondria, a prominent endoplasmic reticulum, and Golgi apparatus. This is typical of a cell that is metabolically active in transport, synthesis, and secretory function (Figure 4-13).

Endothelial cells are interconnected by tight junctions and gap junctions (Figure 4-14). The apical tight junctional complexes, first demonstrated by transmission electron microscopy, have now been shown by freeze-fracture techniques to be macula occludens rather than zonula occludens in that they do not completely encircle the cells.[300] This results in the endothelium forming a "leaky" barrier between the aqueous humor and the stroma, which, although impeding the free flow of water and solutes, does not form the more effective barrier seen in epithelia with zonular junctions.

The gap junctions are numerous and are observed primarily on the lateral membranes of the cells, although some are also present at the junctions of the apicolateral membranes. The gap junctions do not contribute to the endothelial barrier, but they function in intercellular communication. Fluorescent dye injected into a single endothelial cell quickly spreads to adjacent cells.[369] Unlike the basal cells of the corneal epithelium, the basal membranes of the endothelial cells have no specialized adhesion complexes.

Endothelial Morphometry

The development of the contact specular microscope and its adaptation for use in humans made feasible studies of endothelial functional morphology in vivo.[31,249] With the original technology, analyses were limited to studies of cell density (number of cells per unit area) and detailed statistical studies were limited by the small number of cells visible in the narrow field of view. The wide-field specular microscope, through which several hundred cells can be photographed in a single frame, and the introduction of computer software used to digitally analyze cell area and shape have made detailed morphometry of the endothelium possible[240] (Figure 4-15). It has been shown that there is a significant correlation of histologic corneal endothelial cell counts with specular microscopic high-power field cell density[477] (Figure 4-16).

In addition to having an adequate cell density to maintain corneal function, a stable corneal endothelium has cells of relatively uniform size and shape. The degree of uniformity of cell size is determined by measuring the areas of the apical membranes of a population of cells and calculating the coefficient of variation (CV) of cell size (standard deviation [SD] of mean cell area/mean cell area). The normal endothelium has a CV of approximately 0.25. An increase in this value means that cell size is variable, known as *polymegathism*. This may be indicative of a stressed or unstable endothelium in which cell volume is not adequately regulated or in which the cytoskeleton is abnormal. Figure 4-17 shows that corneas with equal cell density may have widely varying degrees of polymegathism, so

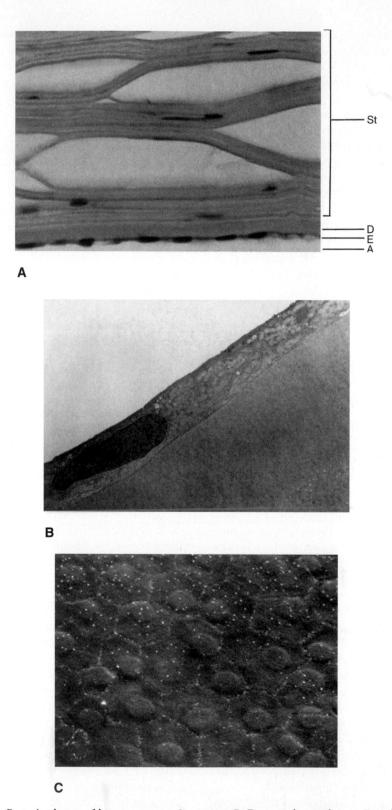

FIGURE 4-13   A, Posterior layers of human cornea: *St,* stroma; *D,* Descemet's membrane; *E,* endothelial cell layer; *A,* space occupied by aqueous humor. Large open spaces in stroma are artifacts of histologic preparation. (Magnification ×1000.) **B,** Transmission electron micrograph of the human corneal endothelium. (Magnification ×3950.) **C,** Scanning electron micrograph of human corneal endothelium. (Magnification ×1000.) (**A,** Courtesy Dr. Martha G. Farber. **B** and **C,** Courtesy Dr. Henry Edelhauser.)

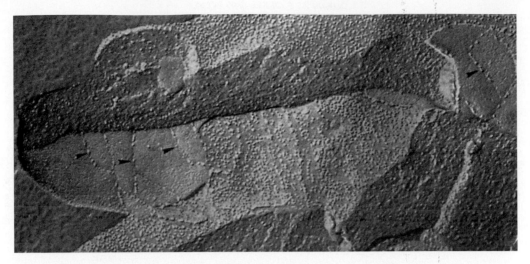

FIGURE 4-14   Freeze-fracture electron micrograph of the rabbit corneal endothelial cell membrane demonstrating tight junctional strands (*arrows*). (Magnification × 8400.) (Courtesy Dr. Monica Stiemke.)

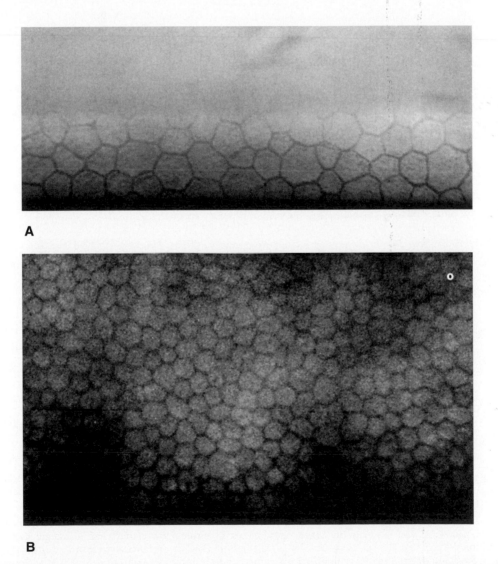

A

B

FIGURE 4-15   Narrow (**A**) and wide-field (**B**) specular micrographs of the human endothelium. Note the regular mosaic of polygonal cells. (Courtesy Dr. Henry Edelhauser.)

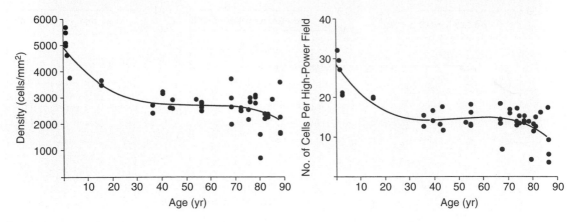

FIGURE 4-16   *Left,* Cell density determined by specular microscopy as a function of age. *Right,* Corresponding number per high-power field as a function of age. Note that the lines for the respective cell count methods (based on the independent variable, age) are nearly superimposable. (Redrawn from Williams K et al: *Arch Ophthalmol* 110:1146, 1992.)

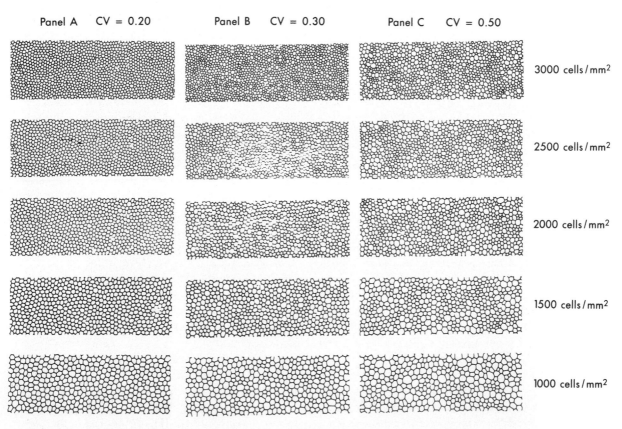

FIGURE 4-17   Morphometric analysis of the corneal endothelium demonstrating variability in cell density and coefficient of variation of cell size. Note that cell size can vary significantly with no change in cell density. *CV,* Coefficient of variation. (From Yee RW et al: *Curr Eye Res* 4:671, 1985.)

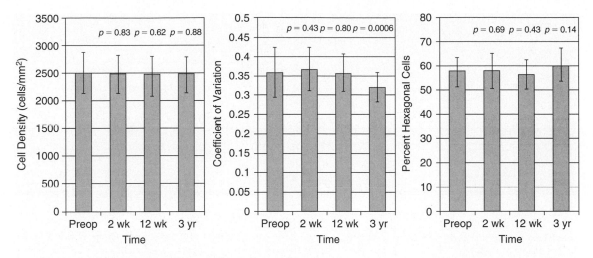

FIGURE 4-18 Changes from preoperative values at 2 weeks, 12 weeks, and 3 years after laser in situ keratomileusis (LASIK). Bars show 1 standard deviation. The only statistically significant change is the coefficient of variation (*middle*) at 3 years. (Redrawn from Collins MJ et al: *Am J Ophthalmol* 131:1, 2001.)

measurement of cell density alone is not an adequate measure of corneal endothelial stability.[489]

A mosaic of hexagonal structures, which is often found in nature, is geometrically and thermodynamically stable. The apical surfaces of the corneal endothelial cell form a mosaic that in the healthy, young cornea consists of 70% to 80% of hexagonal cells. A decrease in hexagons with a concomitant increase in numbers of cells with more than or fewer than six sides is known as *pleomorphism* and may also be a sign of endothelial stress.

The principles of polymegathism and pleomorphism can best be illustrated by a discussion of the effects of aging, disease, surgery, and contact lens wear on these parameters. However, morphometric analysis has shown that polymegathism and pleomorphism increase significantly with aging.[488] Corneal thickness does not increase with age, but these changes in endothelial morphology may render the aged cornea more vulnerable to the stress of intraocular disease or surgery.

The effects of surgery on endothelial morphology have also been documented. Laser in situ keratomileusis (LASIK) is a currently used technology in which corneal stroma is ablated by an excimer laser underneath a lamellar flap, which places the laser closer to the endothelium than does photorefractive keratectomy (PRK). In humans, LASIK has been shown that for the correction of 2.25 to 14.5 diopters of myopia, the procedure has no significant effect on corneal endothelial cell density or the percentage of hexagonal cells 3 years after surgery. The

CV of cell size improved significantly 3 years after surgery[65] (Figure 4-18). This change in CV was likely the effect of contact lens removal because 91% of the patients had a history of contact lens wear.

With few exceptions,[199,339] results of studies of PRK in humans, in which corneal stroma is ablated by an excimer laser for the correction of refractive errors without the use of a lamellar flap, have shown no damage to the corneal endothelium.* In 1999, KeraVision (Fremont, California) received U.S. Food and Drug Administration approval for the intrastromal corneal rings (Intacs) to correct myopic patients from 1.0 to 3.5 diopeters.[388] Based on the specular microscope analysis of the corneal endothelium at the 1-year time frame, there appears to be minimal stress to the endothelium from the Intacs.[13]

Kim, Jean, and Edelhauser[228] showed that there must be a residual corneal thickness of 200 μm of stroma above the corneal endothelium after refractive surgery that should not be ablated to protect the corneal endothelial structure and barrier function. Figure 4-19 illustrates the alizarin red–stained endothelial cells after PRK in a rabbit. In control corneas without PRK (Figure 4-19, *A*), the endothelial cell pattern is normal. After laser ablation of the stoma with a residual thickness of 177, 130, and 91.25 μm from the endothelium, the endothelial cells lose their hexagonal shape. Structurally, excimer laser ablation also stimulates the corneal en-

---

*References 3, 50, 52, 53, 200, 219, 409, 412, 430.

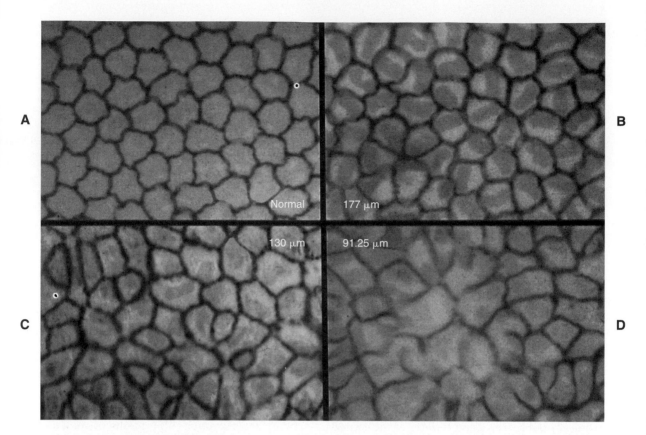

A   B   C   D

FIGURE 4-19   Alizarin red–stained rabbit corneal endothelium 3 days after excimer laser ablation. Normal (**A**). Residual corneal thickness of 177 μm (**B**), 130 μm (**C**), and 91.25 μm (**D**). There is loss of the endothelial hexagonal cells, and the endothelial barrier function has been compromised. (From Edelhauser HF: *Cornea* 19:263, 2000.)

dothelial cells to secrete an amorphous granular material, which is deposited in Descemet's membrane (Figure 4-20).

Initial studies using the clinical specular microscope documented the cell loss that occurs in the graft after penetrating keratoplasty (PK) (Figure 4-21). In corneal grafts after PK, manual counting by an experienced examiner helps minimize falsely high values. In a recent study on long-term follow-up of clear grafts 15 to 33 years after PK, endothelial cell counts ranged from 575 to 1243 cells/mm².[246] Bourne, Nelson, and Hodge[33] reported an endothelial cell loss rate of 7.8% per year from 3 to 5 years after PK, 13 times the rate of decrease in normal corneas (0.6%).

It is well known that cataract extraction with intraocular lens (IOL) implantation can lead to endothelial cell loss. In a study of endothelial cell loss after phacoemulsification with IOL implantation using retrobulbar anesthesia, the mean overall central endothelial cell loss was 8.5% after 12 months.[460] The risk factors found to be significant for higher endothelial cell loss were shorter axial lengths and longer phacoemulsification time. In another study of endothelial cell loss after phacoemulsification with IOL implantation using intracameral 1% preservative-free lidocaine for anesthesia, the mean decrease in cell density was 5.5% after 1 month.[196] CV increased 12.52% and hexagonality decreased 4.7%.

Lidocaine 1% used as intracameral anesthesia readily diffuses through the corneal endothelium, resulting in stromal uptake and endothelial cell swelling (Figure 4-22). With phacoemulsification, however, the washout of lidocaine from the cornea (half-life, 5 minutes) and iris (half-life, 9 minutes) occurs quickly.[7,229] In a study of intracapsular extraction with IOL implantation, the mean endothelial cell loss was 20.3% at 1 year.[416]

Morphometric analysis of corneas of patients with keratoconus or diabetes has clearly shown that

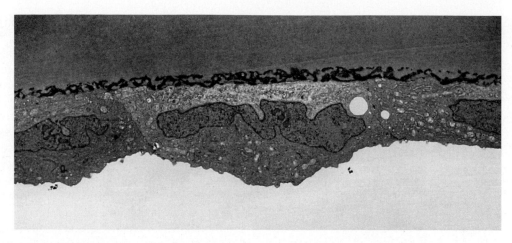

FIGURE 4-20   Rabbit corneal endothelium 6 days after photorefractive keratectomy (PRK) with a residual corneal thickness of 150 μm. Transmission electron micrograph shows a dark amorphous material in Descemet's membrane adjacent to the endothelium. (Magnification × 4600.)

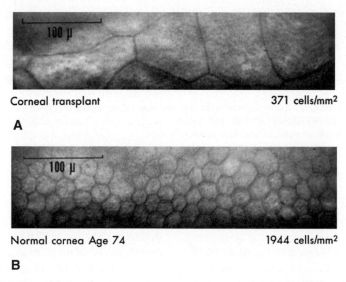

FIGURE 4-21   Specular photomicrographs demonstrating the effect of penetrating keratoplasty on endothelial cell density. **A,** Normal endothelium. **B,** Graft endothelium. (Courtesy Dr. William Bourne. From Bourne WM et al: *Am J Ophthalmol* 81:319, 1976.)

endothelial morphology may change without a decrease in cell density. Keratoconus corneas have a normal cell density, but the CV of cell size is significantly increased and the percentage of hexagonal cells drops from a normal 70% to 50%, showing that the stress placed on the cornea in this disease causes endothelial remodeling.[294] In patients with type 2 diabetes of 10 years' duration or longer, cell density is normal, whereas CV is increased and the percentage of hexagonal cells decreases to 50%. Similar changes are seen in patients with type 1 diabetes, and patients with disease of long duration also demonstrate a decrease in cell density.[396]

The changes in endothelial morphology in the patient with diabetes are related to changes in cellular metabolism. In experimental models of diabetes, these changes can be reversed or prevented by aldose reductase inhibitors, indicating an in-

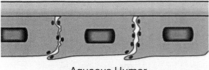

Intracameral 1% Lidocaine HCl
Will Cause Endothelial
Cell Edema

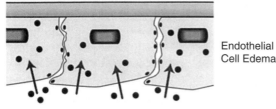

Aqueous Humor

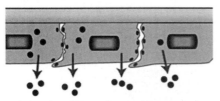

Endothelial
Cell Edema

1% Lidocaine

Lidocaine diffuses from endothelial cells

Figure 4-22 Diagram illustrating the lidocaine diffusion into the corneal endothelium, endothelial cell edema, and the washout of lidocaine from the cornea during phacoemulsification. (From Edelhauser HF: *Cornea* 19:263, 2000.)

volvement of the polyol pathway.[305] It appears that cell volume regulation may be affected by osmotic effects of sugars such as sorbitol or perhaps by inhibition of the Na^+-K^+ pump resulting from alteration in myoinositol metabolism. Given the endothelial changes that result from surgery, the diabetic patient may be at greater risk during surgery than the nondiabetic patient.

In a study of patients suspected to have glaucoma with elevated intraocular pressure (IOP) (no optic nerve damage or visual field loss), it was reported that, in all decades beyond 40 years, there is a significant decrease in endothelial cell density compared with a nonglaucomatous population.[12,488] Even though there is a decrease in endothelial cell density in the patients suspected of having glaucoma, the CV and percentage of hexagonal cells were normal, which indicates endothelial stability. Because of the corneal endothelial changes in the patients with diabetes and glaucoma, special care should be used

when cataract surgery is performed to minimize the surgical stress to the endothelium.

A particularly interesting change in endothelium morphology occurs during long-term contact lens wear (Figure 4-23). Morphologic abnormalities of the corneal endothelium, specifically polymegathism, have been reported with long-term use of rigid polymethylmethacrylate lenses, as well as with daily-wear and extended-wear soft contact lenses.[183,251,271,427] The absence of morphologic abnormalities of the endothelium in eyes wearing highly oxygen-permeable silicone elastomer lenses suggests that contact lens–induced hypoxia is responsible for the observed effects on the endothelium.[390] MacRae et al.[271] have coined the term *CLUE syndrome,* or contact lens–use endotheliopathy syndrome, to describe these effects.

Descemet's Membrane. The corneal endothelium rests on a basement membrane, known as *Descemet's membrane,* which, in the adult eye, is 10 to 15 μm thick. This membrane is secreted by the endothelial cells and increases in thickness throughout life. The basement membrane components, type IV collagen, laminin, and fibronectin, are present in Descemet's membrane, and it has been suggested that the fibronectin functions in adhesion of endothelial cells to the membrane.[154,463] Descemet's membrane may remain intact in cases of severe corneal ulceration, forming a descemetocele after destruction of the epithelium and stroma. This shows that the membrane is highly resistant to proteolytic enzymes.

Fuchs' endothelial dystrophy is a disease of the endothelial cells in which an abnormal Descemet's membrane is secreted. Wartlike excrescences of collagenous material known as *guttata* form on the posterior surface of the membrane, causing thinning and enlargement of the overlying endothelial cells. In the specular microscope, the guttata are seen as black, acellular areas because of the loss of specular reflection from these areas (Figure 4-24). As the disease progresses, endothelial cell function is decreased, cells are lost, and the cornea decompensates.[463]

Corneal Nerves. The cornea is richly supplied with sensory nerves. It is innervated by the ophthalmic division of the trigeminal nerve, via the anterior ciliary nerves, and those of the surrounding conjunctiva. Nerves enter the cornea in the middle third of the stroma and run forward and anteriorly in a radial fashion toward the central area, giving rise to branches that innervate the anterior stroma

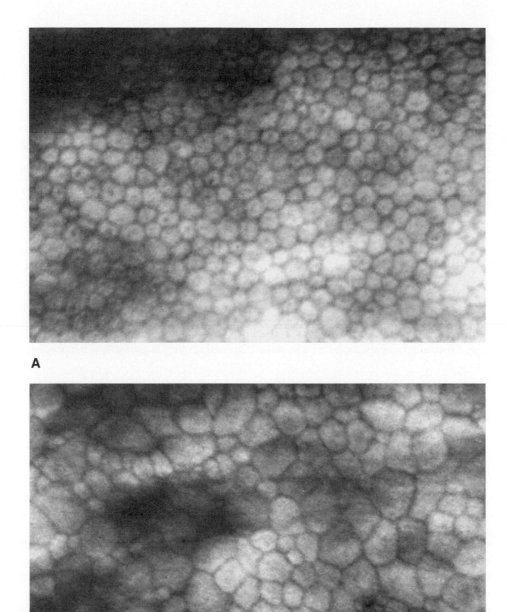

FIGURE 4-23   Endothelial polymegethism and pleomorphism caused by 27 years of contact lens wear. **A,** A 46-year-old non–contact lens wearer. Cell density = 3086 cells/mm²; coefficient of variation (CV) = 0.27; hexagonality = 63%. **B,** A 46-year-old who has worn hard contact lenses for 27 years. Cell density = 1449 cells/mm²; CV = 0.59; hexagonality = 22%. (Courtesy Dr. Scott MacRae.)

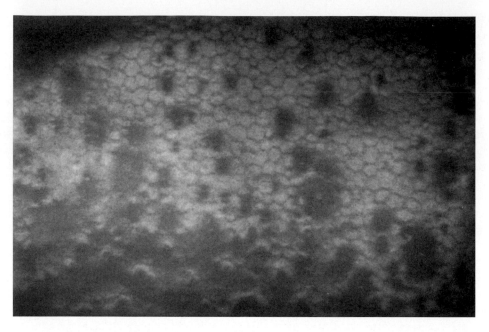

FIGURE 4-24   Specular micrograph showing extensive (dark appearing) corneal guttata, which in areas are confluent.

and midstroma. In the interface between Bowman's layer and the anterior stroma, the stromal nerves form the subepithelial plexus. They then perforate Bowman's layer and form the subbasal epithelial nerve plexus, providing innervation to the basal epithelial cell layer and terminating within the superficial epithelial layers.[331] Some controversy exists regarding whether there is innervation to the posterior stroma. Despite this, it is clear that Descemet's membrane and the endothelium are not innervated in humans.[90,180]

The cornea is one of the most sensitive tissues of the body, and this sensitivity serves a protective function. Accordingly, most of the receptors in the cornea fall into the classification of nociceptors, with simulation resulting in the perception of pain. The A-δ fibers and C fibers that supply the cornea are primarily polymodal fibers responding to mechanical, thermal, and chemical (low pH and hypertonic saline) stimuli. These receptors usually have the lowest threshold for mechanical stimulation. It is extremely painful when these nerves are stimulated by corneal abrasions, ulcers, or bullous keratopathy.

In addition to serving as sensory receptors, it is evident that corneal nerves also serve a trophic function. Patients with sensory denervation of the cornea caused by stroke, diabetic neuropathy, or herpes simplex infections have a high incidence of epithelial erosions and ulcerations known as *neurotrophic ulcers.* This may in part be a result of loss of foreign body sensations, which can lead to mechanical damage to the cornea. However, neuropeptides, including substance P and calcitonin gene-related peptide, are present in corneal nerves and appear to have a direct but poorly understood trophic effect on the epithelium. Retrobulbar or trigeminal injection of capsaicin depletes the nerves of these peptides, resulting in delayed epithelial wound healing. The role of sympathetic nerves in the cornea is controversial. It has been suggested that they are involved in modulation of ion transport or mitotic activity. Stimulation of the sympathetic nerves inhibits corneal epithelial wound healing.[133,448]

Decreased corneal sensitivity has been associated with LASIK. In one study, both corneal and conjunctival sensitivity were noted to be significantly decreased from preoperative levels at 1 week, 1 month, 12 months, and 16 months postoperatively.[15] In addition, contact lens wear has shown decreased corneal sensitivity. Murphy, Patel, and Marshall[317] reported that both soft and rigid gas-permeable lens wear produce a similar type of corneal sensitivity loss. Others have reported that the extent of corneal sensitivity loss varied with the lens material, daily wearing time, number of years of wear, and the lens type (daily or extended wear).[250,307,308]

EMBRYOLOGY AND DEVELOPMENTAL ANOMALIES

Ocular development begins with an outpouching of the diencephalon. This protuberance, called the *optic vesicle,* communicates with the third ventricle of the brain by means of the optic stalk. The optic vesicle, as well as the entire embryo, is covered with a sheet of surface ectoderm. The ectodermal cells overlying the hollow optic vesicle thicken to form the lens placode. The optic vesicle invaginates to form the optic cup, and the lens placode develops a pit. This pitted structure then itself invaginates to become the lens vesicle, which has an anatomic relationship with the optic vesicle resembling a ball in the pocket of a baseball glove. At 5 to 6 weeks of gestation, the lens vesicle detaches and the adjacent surface ectoderm from which it has budded gives rise to the corneal epithelium, which is 1 to 2 cells thick with a gossamer underlying basement membrane. There is a loose, acellular layer destined to become corneal stroma comprised of collagen fibrils. Early on, a population of mesodermal-derived cells accumulates circumferentially around the optic cup under surface ectoderm. However, cumulative evidence indicates that it is a later wave of neural crest–derived perilimbal mesenchymal cells that migrate between the lens and the acellular stroma at 6 weeks of gestation, forming the corneal endothelium. Unlike vascular endothelium, the neural crest–derived corneal endothelium is factor VIII negative.[7] Neural crest cells from this primary wave also form the trabecular meshwork. A second wave of neural crest–derived mesenchymal cell invasion gives rise to corneal fibroblasts (keratocytes), and the crest cells from a third wave contribute to the anterior iris.

Between 6 and 8 weeks, the eyelid folds develop, during which time the corneal epithelium is exposed to amniotic fluid. Between 8 weeks and 5 months, the lids meet and fuse, separating again around 6 months.[204] The corneal epithelium goes through many changes during this period. The number of epithelial cell layers increases from 1 to 2 at 8 weeks to 3 to 4 at 19 weeks, and to 4 to 5 at 27 weeks (around the time of lid separation), increasing to the adult level of 6 to 7 layers by 36 weeks of gestation. The basal lamina is the first component of the epithelial adhesion complex to appear at 8 to 9 weeks. At 13 weeks, hemidesmosomes, anchoring fibrils, and type VII collagen have been observed. There is an increase in the number of hemidesmosomes following week 27, when the eyelids open, which is perhaps in some way associated with lid movement over the epithelium. At 13

weeks, in addition to anchoring fibrils and hemidesmosome formation, a palisade of fine filaments are observed extending perpendicular to the basal lamina into the anterior stroma. This may be a precursor to Bowman's layer, which is 3.8 μm thick at 19 weeks and continues to thicken thereafter.[210] Concomitant with the developmental changes in the epithelial anchoring complex are varying patterns of keratin localization in the corneal epithelium during embryogenesis. A monoclonal antibody (AE5) to a basic 64-kD keratin does not stain the single-layered corneal epithelium at 8 weeks of gestation. At 12 to 13 weeks, the superficial cells of the three to four layered epithelium become AE5 positive, providing an early sign of epithelial differentiation. At 30 weeks, the AE5 antikeratin antibody elicits a suprabasal staining pattern, in contrast to the adult epithelium, which centrally is AE5 positive in all epithelial layers.

With use of immunofluorescence techniques, type I collagen has been detected in the epithelial basement membrane, stroma, and Descemet's membrane from 8 weeks of gestation through postnatal life. Type III, but not type II, collagen is found in these same structures in early fetal life (between 8 and 20 weeks of gestation) but cannot be demonstrated at 27 weeks or thereafter. Type IV collagen is synthesized by epithelial and endothelial cells and is localized in the epithelial basement membrane as early as 8 weeks of gestation and in Descemet's membrane at 9 weeks of gestation and beyond. Bullous pemphigoid antigen, a component of the adult corneal epithelial basement membrane, was localized in the epithelial basement membrane starting at 10 to 15 weeks of gestation. Staining for fibronectin is positive at 11 weeks of gestation in Descemet's membrane and decreases thereafter, whereas the corneal stroma and epithelial basement membrane show staining in early fetal life up to 30 weeks of gestation for both laminin and fibronectin.[19] At 10 to 12 weeks of gestation, keratan sulfate, a major component of the corneal ECM, has been immunologically localized in the stroma and endothelial layer.[192]

The corneal diameter enlarges from 4.2 mm at 16 weeks of gestation to between 9 and 10.5 mm at term. This 5-fold increase in area and 2.3-fold increase in corneal diameter is accompanied by approximately a 2.3-fold decrease in endothelial cell density. At 16 weeks of gestation, there are 11.32 endothelial nuclei per 100 μm, and at term there are 5.61 nuclei per 100 μm. There also appears to be a rapid decrease in cellular density following birth up to age 2 years, with a decline in endothelial cellularity from 6.09 nuclei per 100 μm to 3.93 nuclei per 100 μm (36% change). At the same time, the corneal diameter increases by a factor of 1.2 (from 9.8 mm at birth to 11.75 mm at age 2 years) while endothelial density declines by 1.55. This reflects an increase in endothelial cell size, which becomes stable by age 2 years. After 2 years of age, endothelial cell loss occurs at an annual rate of approximately 0.56%.

The important contribution of neural crest cells to the development of the anterior segment provides a framework for understanding a variety of congenital developmental anomalies. Abnormal neural crest cell migration may result in sclerocornea, Peters anomaly, and Axenfeld and Rieger anomalies and syndromes, as well as posterior embryotoxon and some forms of congenital glaucoma.[221,243] Abnormalities in crest cell terminal induction may underlie congenital hereditary endothelial dystrophy, posterior polymorphous dystrophy, and Fuchs' endothelial dystrophy. Descemet's membrane may give important clues regarding the nature and timing of some of these disorders. Descemet's membrane is composed of a 3-μm anterior banded layer that forms before birth (with a collagen periodicity of 110 μm) and a postnatal posterior nonbanded portion. Whereas the anterior banded portion appears stable with aging, the posterior nonbanded layer thickens with age after birth, increasing from approximately 2 μm at age 10 years to 10 μm at age 80 years. In some disorders, such as congenital hereditary endothelial dystrophy, the fetal anterior banded portion of Descemet's membrane is formed, thus indicating that fetal endothelium was initially present and suggesting a defect in final differentiation of these neural crest–derived cells. This contrasts with sclerocornea and Peters anomaly, in which gross defects or attenuation of the fetal anterior portion of Descemet's membrane centrally suggest a fetal absence of endothelial cells more consistent with an arrest in neural crest cell migration.

Physiology, Cell Biology, and Biochemistry

Maintenance of the Corneal Epithelium and Its Response to Wounding

The corneal epithelium is maintained by a constant cycle of shedding of superficial cells and proliferation of cells in the basal layer. The fact that mitosis is limited to the basal layer was well documented many years ago by observations of mitotic figures and tritiated thymidine labeling of proliferating cells.[123,162,163] The mitotic rate is approximately 10% to 15% per day.

It is apparent that the epithelium is also maintained by a slow migration of basal cells toward the center of the cornea. Evidence for this centripetal cell migration first came from observation of corneal transplants, which showed that donor epithelium was slowly replaced by recipient epithelium and that pigmented cells from the recipient epithelium migrate toward the center of the graft.[230] It has also been demonstrated that India ink particles phagocytosed by basal cells of normal corneas migrate centripetally at approximately 123 μm per week.[40] The source of the new basal cells is the limbal epithelium, a band of cells 0.5 to 1 mm wide at the periphery of the cornea. The limbus contains stem cells, which differentiate into basal cells and migrate onto the cornea, constantly renewing the supply of basal cells. These stem cells are located in the basal layer of the limbus and do not express the 64-KD keratin typical of corneal epithelium[389]; as they migrate upward and onto the corneal basement membrane, the cells begin to express the 64-KD keratin (see Figure 4-4). These data support the hypothesis that the corneal epithelium is maintained by a balance of cell shedding, basal cell division, and renewal of basal cells by centripetal migration of new basal cells originating from the limbal stem cells (Figure 4-25). A disease process or corneal stress that upsets this balance through an increase in cell loss or a decrease in mitosis or migration leads to epithelial breakdown.[404,436]

The primary function of the corneal epithelium is to form a barrier to invasion of the eye by pathogens and to uptake of excess fluid by the stroma. Accidental or iatrogenic abrasion of the corneal epithelium demands a prompt healing response to recover the exposed basement membrane with cells. After abrasion, mitosis ceases and the cells at the wound edge retract, thicken, and lose their hemidesmosomal attachments to the basement membrane. The cells enlarge, and the epithelial sheet begins to migrate by ameboid movement to cover the defect. The edges of the cell membranes ruffle and send out filopodia and lamellipodia toward the center of the wound[345] (Figure 4-26). Staining with fluorescent probes reveals actin stress fibers oriented in the direction of migration[419] (Figure 4-27). The leading edge of the migrating cells is only one cell thick, but the wound is actually covered by a multilayered sheet made up of both basal and squamous cells.[60] After wound closure, mitosis resumes to restore the epithelium to its normal configuration. The

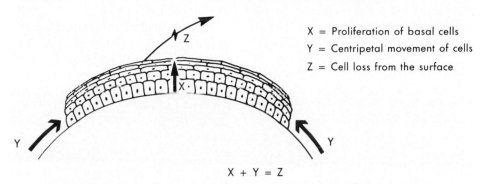

X, Y, Z Hypothesis of corneal epithelial maintenance

X = Proliferation of basal cells
Y = Centripetal movement of cells
Z = Cell loss from the surface

X + Y = Z

FIGURE 4-25   The corneal epithelium is maintained by a balance among sloughing of cells from the corneal surface, cell division in the basal layer, and centripetal migration of cells from the limbus. (Courtesy Dr. Richard Thoft. From Thoft R, Friend J: *Invest Ophthalmol Vis Sci* 24:142, 1983.)

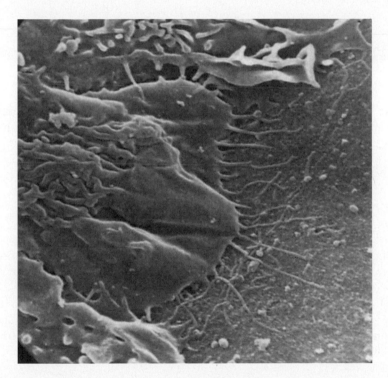

FIGURE 4-26   Scanning electron micrograph of corneal epithelial cells migrating to cover an epithelial abrasion. (Courtesy Dr. Roswell Pfister. From Pfister RR: *Invest Ophthalmol* 14:648, 1975.)

healing process occurs rapidly. An experimental epithelial wound 6 mm in diameter is closed within 48 hours, and the rate of epithelial cell migration is 60 to 80 μm/hr[72,288,337] (Figure 4-28).

Because of the clinical problems of persistent or recurrent corneal epithelial erosions, as well as the advent of refractive surgical procedures such as PRK, there is strong research interest in the study of heal-ing of corneal epithelial wounds. Most of this work has been conducted using experimental wounds in rodents and rabbits or corneal epithelial cells from various species, including humans, in culture. These studies have focused on mechanisms of cell migration, the role of cellular enzymes during the healing response, synthesis and actions of growth factors, intracellular signaling molecules, and control of the

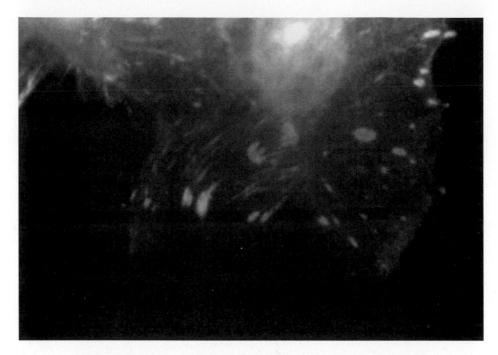

A

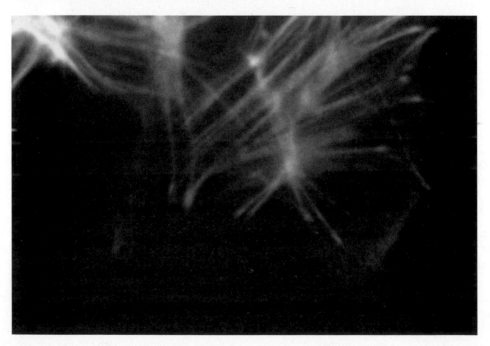

B

FIGURE 4-27   Immunofluorescent staining of vinculin (**A**) and rhodamine phalloidin staining of actin stress fibers (**B**) of rat corneal epithelial cells migrating in vitro. (Courtesy Dr. H. Kaz Soong.)

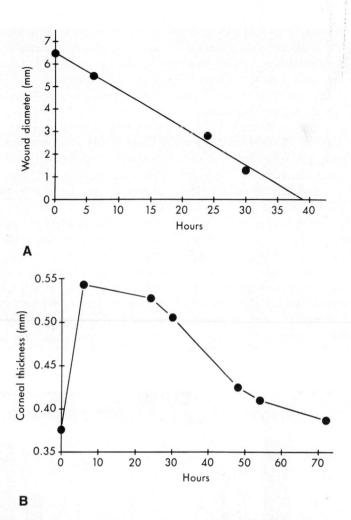

A

B

FIGURE 4-28 Changes in corneal wound diameter (**A**) and thickness (**B**) during healing of a 6.5-mm-diameter epithelial wound in the rabbit. The cell migration rate is 0.8 µm/hr. The cornea swells as a result of uptake of fluid from the tears and then returns to normal thickness as the barrier is reestablished.

cell cycle. The literature in this field is voluminous, and what follows is by no means an exhaustive treatment of the subject. The interested reader is directed to the original literature.

An early observation in studies of the cell biology of corneal epithelial wound healing was that protein synthesis by epithelial cells increases during cell migration.[142,500] This can now be accounted for by numerous events that occur in the healing process. Synthesis of proteins involved in cell adhesion increases during healing. As described previously, the focal adhesion component, vinculin, appears in migrating corneal epithelium. Vinculin is apparently synthesized de novo during the healing process because there is an increase in the amount of this 110-kD protein in migrating cells compared with control.[497] The formation of these focal adhesions includes the pres-

ence of integrins, such as β_1, and the intracellular protein, paxillin, which are important not only in attachment of the cells to substrate but also in activation of various intracellular signaling pathways that control events such as release of calcium and mitosis.[141] A second adhesion protein known to increase in wound healing is the cell surface glycoprotein CD44, which is important in both cell-cell and cell-substrate adhesion. CD44 mRNA transcripts increase in epithelial cells within 3 hours of wounding of rat corneas, peaking at 18 hours. Elevated CD44 protein levels are detected in all layers of the corneal epithelium from wound edge to limbus during cell migration, with a decline toward control levels during the proliferative phase of healing.[493]

The process of cell migration requires energy, and one of the earliest changes observed during the healing process is a decrease in glycogen levels in the migrating cells.[248] The response of the epithelial cells to this glycogen depletion also accounts for the increase in protein synthesis. Corneal epithelial cells are dependent on anaerobic glycolysis and glycolytic activity increases during cell migration.[248] The glycolytic enzyme α-enolase has been identified in the basal epithelium.[503] Expression of this enzyme increases during cell migration and remains elevated in peripheral basal cells for as long as 4 weeks during corneal remodeling.[57] An increase in glycolytic activity obviously requires an increased supply of glucose to the cells. Following wounding of rat corneas, increased expression of glucose transporter GLUT1 mRNA is detectable by 2 hours after wounding, and GLUT1 protein levels increase by 4 hours, peaking at 24 hours after wounding and remaining elevated for at least 2 weeks[430] (Figure 4-29). By this mechanism, an adequate supply of glucose for support of the healing response is maintained.

The cellular events involved in control of cell migration and the cessation and resumption of mitosis during corneal epithelial healing are apparently under autocrine and paracrine control by peptide growth factors. Synthesis of the growth factors and their receptors increases after corneal wounding, again accounting for the increase in protein synthesis after wounding. Soon after the discovery of epidermal growth factor (EGF), it was shown that this peptide can enhance corneal cell migration and corneal epithelial cell proliferation.[387,440] EGF is present in tear fluid, and EGF mRNA is expressed by corneal epithelium, whereas keratocyte growth factor (KGF) and hepatocyte growth factor (HGF) are synthesized by stromal keratocytes.[420,480] Corneal wounding causes an increase in expression of KGF mRNA and HGF mRNA by keratocytes and an accompanying increase in KGF-receptor mRNA and HGF-receptor mRNA in corneal epithelial cells.[481] Expression of

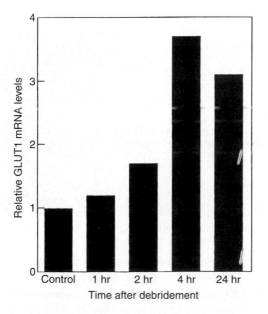
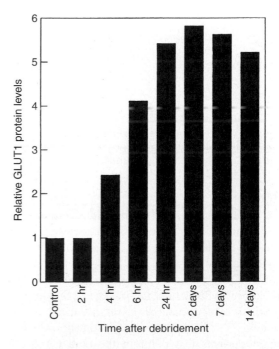

FIGURE 4-29   Increased expression of glucose transporter 1 (GLUT1) in corneal epithelium during wound healing. Three-millimeter debridement wounds were made on central rat cornea and allowed to heal from 1 hour to 21 days. To quantitate changes in GLUT1 messenger ribonucleic acid (mRNA) and protein levels, whole corneal epithelium was harvested and analyzed by reverse transcription–polymerase chain reaction, Northern blot, and Western blot analysis. Expression of GLUT1 protein rapidly increased after wounding and was 2.4-fold higher than that of control at 4 hours after debridement. GLUT1 protein levels continued to increase even after epithelial wound closure (24 hours) and peaked at 2 days after debridement, 5.8-fold higher than that of control. The increase in GLUT1 protein levels coincided with enhanced GLUT1 mRNA levels (3.7-fold higher than that of control at 4 hours after debridement). (Courtesy Dr. James Zieske. From Takahashi H et al: *Exp Eye Res* 63:649, 1996).

basic fibroblast growth factor (bFGF) and transforming growth factor-β (TGF-β) by wounded corneal epithelium have also been reported.[480]

The many processes involved in the migration and mitotic responses to corneal wounding require the activation of numerous intracellular signaling pathways. Recently, it has been demonstrated that EGF receptors are activated in corneal epithelial cells after wounding (Figure 4-30), as evidenced by phosphorylation of this tyrosine kinase receptor.[504] This activation is apparently by means of endogenous EGF and is required for the healing response because cell migration is decreased by inhibitors of EGF-receptor activation. Activation of EGF receptors leads to activation of numerous intracellular signaling proteins, including Ras, the mitogen-activated protein (MAP) kinase cascade, phospholipase C (PLC), and phosphatidylinositol (PI) 3-kinase.

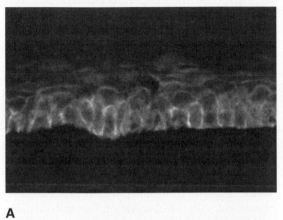

A

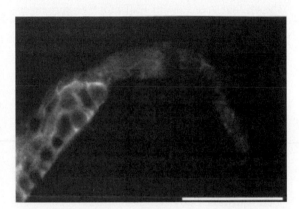

B

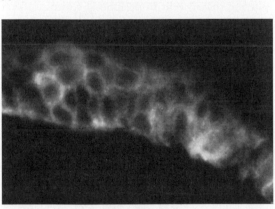

C

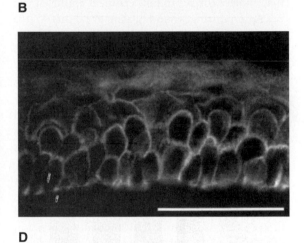

D

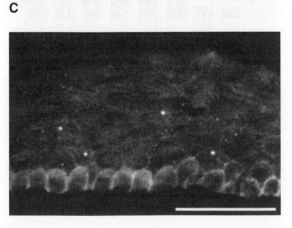

E

FIGURE 4-30 Immunolocalization of epidermal growth factor receptor in rat corneal epithelium during healing of a 3-mm epithelial wound, demonstrating changes in expression levels during the healing process. **A,** Unwounded central corneal epithelium. **B,** Migratory epithelium at the leading edge 1 hour after wounding. **C,** Migratory epithelium at the leading edge 3 hours after wounding. **D,** Epithelium peripheral to the wound area 3 hours after wounding. **E,** Central corneal epithelium 48 hours after wounding. (Bars = 50 μm.) **A, B,** and **E** and **C** and **D** are at the same magnifications. (Courtesy Dr. James Zieske. From Zieske JD et al: *Invest Ophthalmol Vis Sci* 41:1346, 2000.)

One result of activation of the MAP kinase cascade, which is known to be activated by EGF in corneal epithelium, is activation of the immediate early genes *c-fos* and *c-jun*.[214] These transcription factors, which are also activated by corneal wounding, in turn activate many genes involved in protein synthesis and cell proliferation and differentiation.[329] As stated previously, activation of EGF receptors can also activate PLC and PI pathways. This leads to activation of protein kinase C (PKC). It has been shown that activators of PKC promote corneal epithelial wound healing, whereas inhibition of PKC inhibits epithelial cell migration.[55,176] One result of activation of this pathway is the release of intracellular calcium, which is essential for cell migration.[420] It should also be noted that the corneal epithelium is rich in acetylcholine receptors.[457] Acetylcholine can activate the PLC, PI, PKC pathway through a G protein–coupled receptor, also leading to activation of calcium-mediated events.

Corneal wound healing is also controlled by cyclic adenosine monophosphate (cAMP)–mediated pathways. Early evidence for this response was that cholera toxin promotes corneal epithelial cell migration during wound healing in rabbits.[210] It is now known that cholera toxin prevents breakdown of guanosine triphosphate by G proteins, leading to prolonged activation of adenylyl cyclase.[265] G proteins are activated by numerous signaling molecules that bind to G protein–coupled receptors. For example, there are α-adrenergic receptors in corneal epithelium, and norepinephrine, which actives this pathway, stimulates migration and proliferation of human corneal epithelial cells in culture.[316,458]

Inflammatory cytokines are also expressed by wounded corneas, especially after alkali burns. These include interleukin (IL)-1, IL-6, IL-10, and tumor necrosis factor-α. IL-6 stimulates expression of integrin α5β1, which is important in cell migration because of its presence in adhesion plaques. IL-6 is synergistic with EGF and also stimulates HGF and KGF expression.[420] It has also been reported that 8(S)hydroxyeicosatetraenoicacid [8(S)HETE], an arachidonic acid metabolite, promotes corneal epithelial cell migration.[483]

Normally, a simple corneal epithelial abrasion heals quickly and without complication. In conditions such as basement membrane dystrophy, diabetes, persistent or recurrent epithelial defects, and severe injuries (e.g., alkali burns), healing is delayed or normal epithelial adhesion is not established. Because of the importance of growth factors and other signaling molecules in the healing response, several agents, including EGF, KGF, TGF-β, IL-6, fibronectin, retinoids, and sodium citrate, have been studied for their potential as topical drugs for promotion of corneal healing.* In most cases, experimental work has produced a mixture of promising and contradictory results. Results of clinical trials have been inconclusive, and as yet, no drug has been identified that will consistently stimulate corneal epithelial healing and adhesion in humans.

As stated previously, corneal epithelial wounding causes mitosis in migrating basal epithelial cells to stop, followed by resumption of mitosis when the wound closes. The cell cycle is controlled by cyclins and cyclin-dependent kinases, which control the progression of the cell through the G_1, S, G_2, and M phases. The reader is referred to any current cell biology text for details of cell cycle control.[265] In normal human corneas, all epithelial cells stain for cyclin-dependent kinases (cdk2 and cdc2) and cyclin B1. Terminally differentiated, suprabasal cells do not stain for cyclins D, E, and A. However, these cyclins are expressed in basal cells, with increased levels in the peripheral epithelium.[209] This is in agreement with the observation that transient amplifying (basal) cells in peripheral cornea undergo more rounds of proliferation than those in the central epithelium.[256] When wounding occurs, the length of the cell cycle in the peripheral epithelium and limbus decreases and the number of rounds of replication of transient amplifying cells in the limbus and peripheral cornea increases.[256] In the peripheral cornea the G_1/S transition of the basal cells is synchronized and cyclins D and E locate to the nucleus, with increases in their expression 8 to 12 hours after wounding.[58] In contrast, when wounding occurs, expression of EGF receptors is decreased in cells at the wound margin.[504] This leads to a decrease in expression of cyclin D and E, which are normally synthesized in response to EGF. At the same time, the number of receptors for TGF-β increases in the migrating cells. TGF-β causes an increase in expression of cyclin-dependent kinase inhibitors.[495,496] These events arrest the migrating cells in G_1 until wound closure is complete.

The wound healing response also involves the ECM, especially that of the basement membrane. It is apparent that epithelial function under normal conditions and during wound healing, in part, depends on ECM, because the integrins of hemidesmosomes and focal adhesion plaques, which interact with ECM molecules such as fi-

---

*References 79, 310, 326, 325, 340, 346, 405, 440, 443, 446.

bronectin and laminin, influence intracellular signaling pathways with proteins such as paxillin and focal adhesion kinase.[141] Several recent observations support this idea. The inflammatory response to corneal wounding can lead to deposition of fibrin in the wound bed and inhibition of wound healing. It is evident that plasminogen functions to inhibit this response because plasminogen-deficient transgenic mice have a delayed wound healing response and fragile epithelium. Mice that are also fibrinogen deficient have a normal corneal epithelial healing response.[216]

When the corneal epithelium is wounded, laminin 1 disappears from the basement membrane at the wound margin. After wound closure, laminin 1 reappears; it is not until this time that Cx43 and desmoglein reappear in the epithelium.[430] This suggests that laminin 1 provides a signal for reassembly of gap junctions and desmosomes.

It has recently been reported that the proteoglycan lumican is expressed by basal cells and in the basement membrane during corneal epithelial healing. Epithelial healing is inhibited by antilumican antibody and is delayed in lumican-null mice. The lumican may influence wound healing by means of integrin receptors.[385] After wound healing, the adhesion of the epithelium is reestablished by formation of new hemidesmosomes in the basal cell layer. The location of these hemidesmosomes corresponds precisely to the locations of anchoring fibrils in the basement membrane. When a corneal abrasion is limited to the epithelium and the basement membrane is not damaged, a normal epithelium with adhesion complexes is formed soon after healing. In experimental keratectomy wounds of the cornea in which basement membrane is removed, the epithelium must lay down new basement membrane after healing and development of normal adhesion complexes is delayed for more than 12 months.[144,146,224] The importance of these interactions of the epithelial cells with the basement membrane and other ECM proteins cannot be overemphasized, especially in the face of destruction of the basement membrane and superficial stroma in the PRK procedure. LASIK spares these structures and therefore reduces the possibility of epithelial defects complicating recovery from refractive surgery.

Corneal Epithelial Electrophysiology and Ion Transport. In keeping with its function as a barrier, the corneal epithelium is a "tight" epithelium with a relatively low ionic conductance through its apical cell membranes and a high-resistance (12 to 16 kOhm/cm^2) paracellular pathway. It generates a transepithelial potential of 25 to 35 mV as a result of passive diffusion of ions through these resistances.[237] The paracellular resistance and transepithelial potential are dependent on the existence of the apical tight junctions because these values fall to zero when the junctions are disrupted in a calcium-free solution or by exposure of the corneal surface to digitonin.[480] When the resting membrane potential of the superficial cells is recorded by a microelectrode, a potential of approximately −30 mV is recorded. If the electrode is advanced into the wing cells, no change in potential is recorded. This is evidence that the superficial and wing cell layers form a functional syncytium by virtue of the large number of gap junctions connecting these cells. When the electrode enters into a basal cell, an additional voltage drop of approximately 10 to 20 mV is recorded, indicating that a reduced degree of electrical coupling exists between wing cells and basal cells.[234]

The potentials described previously are maintained by epithelial transport of sodium and chloride ions (Figure 4-31). Sodium is pumped from tears to stroma while chloride is transported into the tears. The inward flux of sodium is balanced by the chloride current so that the net flux of solute is zero. Based on studies of corneas mounted in Ussing chambers, it is thought that sodium enters the corneal epithelial cells through channels in the apical membrane of the superficial cells. The sodium permeability of this membrane is lower than that of other epithelia because of a lack of amiloride-sensitive channels, which have a high sodium conductance. However, characteristics of these channels have not been determined by patch recording or cloning. Sodium and chloride also enter the epithelial cells through a basolateral Na-K-2Cl cotransporter. Sodium is then extruded into the stroma by the ouabain-sensitive Na$^+$-K$^+$-ATPase located in the basolateral membranes of the cells[86,237,494] (Figure 4-32).

The maintenance of the inward sodium gradient from the stroma into the epithelial cells by the sodium pump serves as the driving force for transport of chloride into the tears. Chloride moves into the cells against an electrochemical gradient via the Na-K-Cl cotransport mechanism in which sodium moves down its electrochemical gradient, carrying with it the chloride ions.[46] Once inside the cell, chloride diffuses into the tears through channels in the apical cell membrane. This transport of chloride

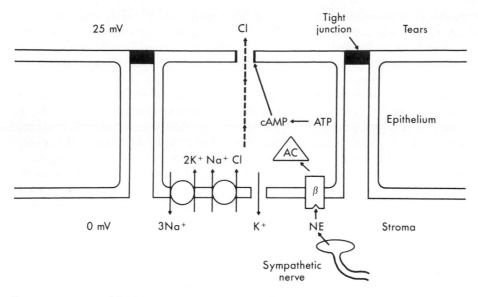

FIGURE 4-31   Model of ion transport, ion channels, and sympathetic neural control of chloride channels in the corneal epithelium. The Na$^+$-K$^+$ pump in the basolateral membrane maintains the Na$^+$ gradient for Na$^+$-Cl$^-$ cotransport. Chloride diffuses down its chemical gradient through apical channels, which are opened by cyclic adenosine monophosphate (cAMP). AC, Adenylate cyclase; ATP, adenosine triphosphate; β, β-adrenergic receptor; *NE*, norepinephrine. (Based on models proposed in Candia OA: *Invest Ophthalmol Vis Sci* 31[suppl]:440, 1990; and Klyce SD: *J Physiol* 321:49, 1981.)

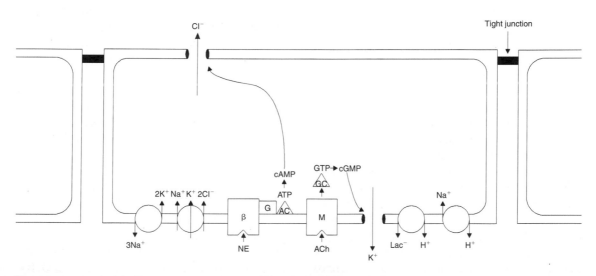

FIGURE 4-32   Model of ion transport in the corneal epithelium. The epithelium is shown as a single cell layer because the cell layers of the epithelium function as a single transporting epithelium. The Na$^+$-K$^+$ pump in the basolateral membrane maintains the Na$^+$ gradient for Na$^+$-K$^+$-2Cl$^-$ cotransport. Chloride diffuses down its chemical gradient through apical channels. Chloride channels are regulated by sympathetic nerves via a cyclic adenosine monophosphate (*cAMP*)–mediated pathway. The large potassium channel is regulated by cholinergic stimulation via a cyclic guanosine monophosphate (*cGMP*)–mediated pathway. This channel also opens in response to decreased extracellular osmolarity and decreased intracellular pH. Intracellular pH is regulated by lactate-H$^+$ cotransport and Na$^+$-H$^+$ exchange. *AC*, Adenylate cyclase; *ACh*, acetylcholine; *β*, β-adrenergic receptor; *G*, heterotrimeric G protein; *GC*, guanylate cyclase; *GTP*, guanosine triphosphate; *Lac*, lactate; *M*, muscarinic receptor; *NE*, norepinephrine.

accounts for 50% of the short-circuit current across the corneal epithelium; its essential coupling to sodium transport is evident from the fact that the chloride secretion is blocked when the sodium pump is inhibited by ouabain. Evidence for the presence of these chloride channels comes primarily from recordings made in Ussing chambers; however, an apical anion conductance has also been measured in corneal epithelium in culture.[283] With use of whole-cell recording techniques, an outward rectifying chloride current has been detected in freshly isolated human corneal epithelial cells and a ClC-3 chloride channel has been identified in a cyclic deoxyribonucleic acid (cDNA) library from rabbit corneal epithelium.[404,465]

Epithelial chloride transport can be regulated, perhaps allowing the cornea to respond to stress.[237] Epithelial chloride transport is stimulated by catecholamines, which act through the second messenger cAMP to increase the apical chloride conductance.[239] Release of catecholamines from sympathetic corneal nerves can be regulated by serotonergic nerves that end on sympathetic nerve terminals, and serotonin also stimulates chloride secretion by the cornea.[236,237] On the basis of these observations, it has been suggested that sympathetic nerves can regulate epithelial ion transport.

The transport processes of the corneal epithelium result in chloride-activated osmotic transport of water out of the cornea, and under certain experimental conditions, this can promote dehydration of a swollen cornea. In vivo the importance of this transport in maintenance of normal corneal thickness and transparency is minimal compared with that of the corneal endothelium, suggesting that this water flux is primarily involved in epithelial homeostasis. Osmotic flux of water through a tight epithelium implies the presence of water channels. Indeed, abundant aquaporin-5 and aquaporin-3 have been identified in rat and bovine corneal epithelium.[160]

The presence of the Na^+-K^+ pump in the corneal epithelium implies an outward K^+ flux. In addition to the leak current typical of most cells, a large-conductance (167 ps in 150 mm KCl) outward rectifying channel has been identified in rabbit and human corneal epithelial cells.[23,366,367] This channel is open at resting membrane potential and is weakly voltage dependent, increasing its open probability at depolarizing voltages.[367] Several characteristics of this K^+ channel indicate that it is important in regulation of epithelial cell function. Current through this channel is stimulated by cyclic guanosine monophosphate and carbachol,

suggesting that it is under muscarinic parasympathetic control[111] (see Figure 4-32). This channel also appears to be mechanosensitive and is activated by stretch.[367,463] When cells are exposed to hyposmotic solutions that cause cell swelling, the current through these channels increases; conversely, hyperosmotic solutions cause a decrease in the current as the cell shrinks.[112] It has also been reported that these K^+ channels are lost during corneal epithelial healing, with an accompanying increase in cell surface area.[283] On the basis of these observations, it is tempting to suggest that this stretch-activated K^+ channel serves a regulatory function allowing the epithelial cells to respond to changes in osmolarity and cell volume by regulating the osmotic flux of water, which may occur in response to changes in K^+ conductance. In this context the loss of K^+ channels during wound healing could explain the increases in cell volume known to occur during cell migration because a loss of K^+ conductance inhibits Cl^- secretion by the cells. This large K^+ channel is also pH sensitive, with acidification increasing the outward K^+ current by increasing the open probability of the channel.[375] This regulation of K^+ conductance by pH has important clinical implications in that hypoxia causes decreased intracellular pH and pH affects a large number of cellular processes, including cell volume and osmolarity. It is well known that contact lens wear causes hypoxia and acidification of the cornea. Stimulation of K^+ transport by a decrease in pH could compensate for the osmotic effects of hypoxia by increasing osmotic efflux of water. Thus it appears that the large K^+ channel, along with the lactate-H^+ cotransporter and Na^+-H^+ exchanger known to be present in corneal epithelium, is important in pH regulation and response to acidification of the cell[26] (see Figure 4-32).

Two other ions important in cellular function are calcium and bicarbonate. Corneal epithelial cells apparently do not have voltage-gated Ca^{2+} channels. Whole-cell recording has provided evidence for a non–voltage-dependent Ca^{2+} influx and the presence of a Na^+-Ca^{2+} exchanger.[375] An L-type calcium channel and a Na^+-Ca^{2+} exchanger have been identified in a cDNA library from rabbit corneal epithelium.[404]

An HCO_3^- current exists across the apical membrane of the corneal epithelium. Measurements of CO_2 and HCO_3^- fluxes across the cornea suggest the presence of carbonic anhydrase in the cornea epithelium and the presence of a basolateral Na^+-HCO_3^- cotransporter.[46] Indeed, this cotransporter, as well as a Cl^--HCO_3^- exchanger, are also present in a cDNA library from rabbit corneal epithelium.[404]

Although a complete, unified model of corneal epithelial transporters and channels, with their regulation and interactions, has not yet been constructed, available information suggests that these systems work homeostatically to maintain conditions in the corneal epithelium conductive to the processes of cell division, migration, differentiation, stratification, and senescence that maintain the corneal epithelial barrier.

Corneal Transparency and Stromal Function

The corneal stroma scatters less than 10% of normal incident light. This is an unexpected property of the cornea given the disparity in refractive index between the collagen fibrils and the proteoglycan matrix. Maurice[292] proposed that corneal transparency is a consequence of a crystalline lattice arrangement of collagen fibrils within stromal lamellas (Figure 4-33) and that light scattered by individual fibrils of uniform diameter is canceled by destructive interference with scattered light from adjacent fibers; therefore light is scattered only in the forward direction.

Such an arrangement requires that all collagen fibrils be of equal diameter and that all fibrils be equidistant from each other. Subsequent studies showed that these conditions are not satisfied in the cornea.[71,110] First, as described previously, the sizes of collagen fibers do vary, albeit within a relatively small range. Although the collagen fibers vary in diameter, they remain weak scatterers of light because their diameter is a small fraction of the wavelengths of visible light. Second, analysis of the spacing of collagen fibers in the cornea shows that the fibers are not arranged in a lattice but rather that they are arranged in a quasirandom configuration. It has been shown that there is a local ordering of the fibrils extending to approximately 200 nm from individual fibrils and that distribution of the fibrils is adequately uniform to account for the transparency of the cornea. However, to maintain this transparency, it is required that the distance between the collagen fibrils be less than one half the wavelength of visible light. Light scattering is wavelength dependent (Figure 4-34). Light transmittance through the cornea decreases slightly as the wavelength decreases from 700 to 400 nm.[110]

This dependence of corneal transparency on the distribution and size of collagen fibrils is supported by observations of swollen corneas and by the structure of the opaque sclera. When the epithelial or endothelial barrier of the cornea is damaged, the stroma imbibes water and swells, leading to a loss of

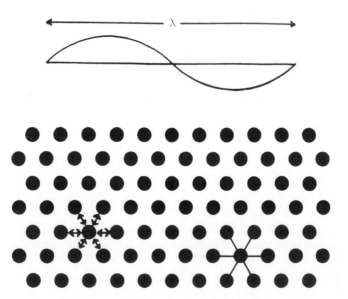

Figure 4-33 Cross-sectional view of fibrils arranged in lattice. Size of wavelength shown above for comparison. Forces of repulsion and rigid links between fibrils shown schematically. (From Maurice D: The physics of corneal transparency. In Duke-Elder S [ed]: *Transparency of the cornea*, Oxford, 1960, Blackwell Scientific.)

corneal transparency. This uptake of water causes formation of "lakes" devoid of collagen fibers within the stroma. This causes increased divergence of refractive index within the stroma, as well as an increase in distance between collagen fibrils, leading to a wavelength-dependent loss of light transmittance that increases with the amount of corneal swelling.

Further support for the theory of cornea transparency is found in examination of the ultrastructure of the sclera. In this tissue the collagen fibers are large and of greatly varying diameter. In addition, their distribution lacks the relative order and close spacing seen in the cornea, leading to the light scatter that renders this tissue nontransparent.

The concept that light scattering in the cornea is dependent on the spacial ordering of the collagen fibrils is also supported by a study of differences in light scattering by the anterior and posterior cornea.[122] It was found that fibril diameter is greater in the anterior cornea than in the posterior cornea

and that the density of fibrils is lower in the anterior cornea than in the posterior cornea in both rabbits and humans. This leads to a twofold (in humans) and threefold (in rabbits) increase in light scatter by the anterior cornea as compared with the posterior cornea.[122] For a more technical and mathematical treatment of this subject, the reader is referred to the original literature.[71,110,122]

Interactions between Proteoglycans and Collagen in the Stroma. Given the importance of uniform, small-diameter collagen fibrils and their close spacing in maintaining corneal transparency, the question arises concerning the mechanisms by which these conditions are maintained. Evidence is mounting that lumican, with its keratin sulfate side chains, is responsible for corneal transparency by interacting with collagen and its hydration characteristics.

When corneas, made edematous by perfusion with a calcium-free solution in vitro, are examined by electron microscopy, it is observed that the di-

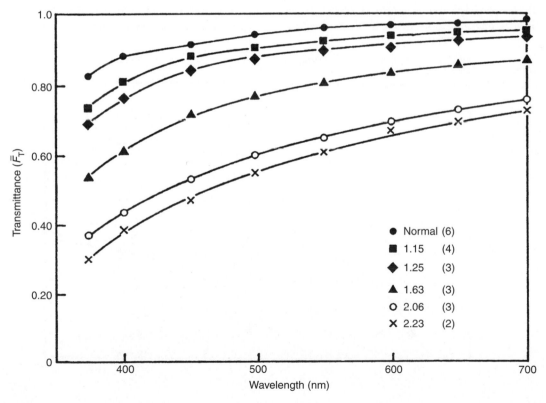

FIGURE 4-34 Experimental values for the fraction of light transmitted through normal and swollen rabbit corneas as a function of wavelength. The ratio of thickness of swollen corneas to initial (normal) thickness and the number of corneas used for each curve are given in the key. As the cornea swells, light transmittance is reduced and at any thickness light transmittance decreases at lower wavelengths. (Courtesy Dr. Richard Farrell. From Farrell RA et al: *J Physiol [Lond]* 233:589, 1973.)

ameter of the collagen fibers increases. This change appears to be caused by lateral aggregation of the collagen fibers, possibly resulting from loss of proteoglycans from the stroma.[218] It was subsequently shown that when perfusate is collected during perfusion of corneas with a calcium-free solution, the swelling of the cornea is accompanied by loss of glycosaminoglycans (GAGs) that can be detected in the perfusate. These corneas were incubated with ^{3}H and ^{35}S-sulfate before perfusion so that the GAGs were radiolabeled. Subsequent enzymatic digestion of the labeled GAGs and analysis by chromatography showed that their composition was primarily keratin sulfate.[215] This suggests that the GAGs were lost from lumican and that lumican is therefore at least partly responsible for control of collagen fiber diameter in the cornea.

When purified type I collagen is incubated in vitro under appropriate physiologic conditions, the collagen forms fibrils similar to those found in vivo. When the collagen is incubated with decorin or lumican, the rate at which fibrils form is reduced and the final diameter of the fibrils that form is also smaller than in the absence of proteoglycan.[358] The inhibitory effect of lumican on fibril formation is greater than that of decorin. If keratin sulfate is removed from lumican, the lumican core protein is as effective as the intact proteoglycan in inhibiting the rate of fibril formation but the final fibril diameter is smaller than that of fibrins that form in the presence of the intact proteoglycan. It was concluded from this study that both decorin and lumican can control the formation and diameter of collagen fibrils, that lumican has a greater influence on fibril diameter than does decorin, and that the core protein alone is sufficient to inhibit fibril formation.[358] The keratin sulfate side chains of lumican may limit the influence of the core protein on fibril diameter (Figures 4-35 and 4-36).

The importance of lumican for control of collagen fibril diameter and corneal transparency has been confirmed in vivo using a lumican knockout mouse.[53] In this study, 44 of 51 mice had bilateral corneal clouding. Electron microscopy showed an increase in mean corneal collagen fibril diameter from 30.2 nm in normal mice to 47.3 nm in lumican knockout mice. Variation in diameter of collagen fibrils of the lumican-deficient mice also increased dramatically. These observations clearly demonstrate a relationship between proteoglycans,

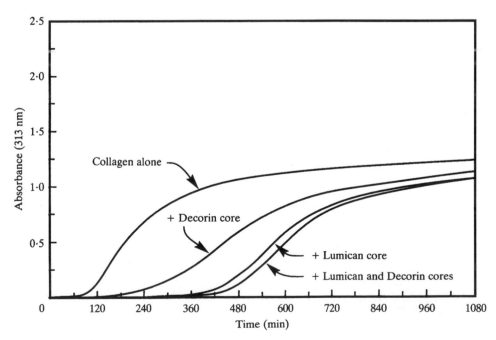

Figure 4-35   When collagen is incubated in vitro in an appropriate buffer, fibrillogenesis occurs, as indicated by an increase in absorbance of the assay mixture at 313 nm. When the core proteins of the proteoglycans decorin or lumican are added to the mixture, collagen fibril formation is inhibited. The effect of lumican is greater than that of decorin, suggesting a role of lumican in regulation of collagen fibril formation in the corneal stroma. (Courtesy Dr. Jody Rada. From Rada JA et al: *Exp Eye Res* 56:635, 1993.)

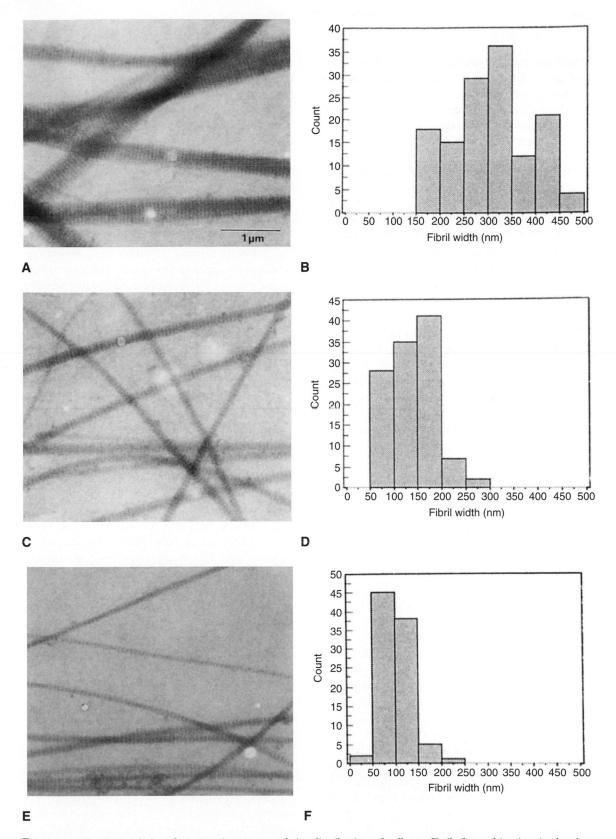

FIGURE 4-36   Transmission electron microscopy and size distribution of collagen fibrils formed in vitro in the absence or presence of lumican or lumican core protein. The size and range of size distribution of the fibrils is reduced in the presence of lumican and lumican core protein. **A** and **B,** Collagen fibrils formed in the absence of lumican. **C** and **D,** Fibrils formed in the presence of intact lumican. **E** and **F,** Fibrils formed in the presence of lumican core protein, without keratan sulfate side chains. The data suggest that formation of small, uniform diameter collagen fibrils in the corneal stroma is controlled by lumican. (Courtesy Dr. Jody Rada. From Rada JA et al: *Exp Eye Res* 56:635, 1993.)

especially lumican, and changes in collagen fiber size and arrangement that lead to corneal clouding in the intact cornea.

The experimental observations discussed previously are also important for the understanding of human corneal dystrophies that lead to a loss of corneal transparency. Corneal dystrophies are inherited disorders that may result from abnormal cellular metabolism. These conditions are usually bilateral and symmetric and lack signs of inflammation or neovascularization.[382] Common stromal dystrophies include granular dystrophy, an autosomal dominant disorder in which microfibrillar deposits lead to corneal opacification. This process is thought to reflect altered phospholipid metabolism. Lattice dystrophy is a stromal disorder that results from the localized accumulation of amyloid. Macular dystrophy is a heterogeneous recessive disease of two subtypes and appears to be the result of abnormal keratan sulfate synthesis.[135,484] Type I macular dystrophy is characterized by a defect in the synthesis of keratan sulfate proteoglycan, leading to an absence of sulfated keratan sulfate in the cornea and serum.[100,232] These abnormalities in the corneal ECM are associated with more proximal spacing of collagen fibrils, which may account for the corneal thinning observed clinically in these patients. In addition, in corneas with macular dystrophy, there are many regions where the normal collagen structure is disrupted and numerous lacunas are seen within the matrix.[363] It has been reported that type I macular dystrophy corneas synthesize lactosaminoglycan-proteoglycan rather than keratan sulfate proteoglycan (lumican) because of a lack of a sulfotransferase.[306] This abnormal keratan sulfate is localized in deposits in the corneal stroma and is not associated with collagen.[260] Although these observations appear to explain the corneal opacity that occurs in macular corneal dystropy type I, interpretation of these data is complicated by the fact that macular dystrophy maps to chromosome 16q22, whereas lumican maps to 12q21.3-q22.[53] Although it is evident that loss of corneal transparency is related to abnormalities in collagen and its relationship to lumican and other proteoglycans, the sugar side chains of proteoglycans also interact with water; it is also well known that corneal transparency is also dependent on stromal hydration.

Stromal Hydration and Proteoglycans. Stromal hydration is normally approximately 3.5 g H_2O/g dry weight and increases linearly with increasing corneal thickness. The relative resistance of the nonedematous epithelium, stroma, and endothelium to diffusion of electrolytes is 2000:1:10, thereby restricting electrolytes and associated water to the stromal compartment.[103,171,295] The corneal stroma has an inherent tendency to imbibe water and to swell. This property reflects the water-binding capacity of the proteoglycans in the ECM.[84,113,309]

Studies have shown that swelling by direct immersion in the distilled water and bathing solutions with different ionic strengths and pH levels caused a significant loss of soluble protein and proteoglycans from the stroma.[188] Studies have shown that equilibrating the tissue to a given hydration by the use of a bounding membrane essentially prevents the loss of proteoglycans.[127,456] This allows for an improved method for assessing the swelling behavior and structure of the tissue. Within a physiologically relevant pH range and at a physiologically relevant temperature, it has been shown that pH changes in the physiologic range can have a small but reproducible effect on the swelling kinetics of isolated mammalian corneal stroma ex vivo.[87]

Stromal edema occurs in the proteoglycan matrix between the collagen fibers, leading to increased spacing of collagen fibrils. In corneas of normal thickness, the swelling pressure is approximately 55 mm Hg (i.e., 80 g/cm²). Swelling pressure is inversely related to corneal thickness. For example, a cornea of 150% normal thickness has a swelling pressure of only 15 mm Hg, compared with 55 mm Hg in the nonedematous cornea. Conversely, compression of the cornea by any means is associated with an increase in stromal swelling pressure.[124,170] The swelling pressure of the stroma is related to the electrostatic repulsion of the negatively charged proteoglycans. Corneal proteoglycans contain chondroitin/dermatan sulfate and keratan sulfate, which belong to the leucine-rich proteoglycan gene family.[92] The major proteoglycan in the corneal stroma is keratan sulfate, which consists of three distinct proteins: lumican, keratocan, and mimecan. These three proteins are found in a number of connective tissues but are expressed at much higher levels in the cornea than in noncorneal tissues.[266] Expression of keratan sulfate proteoglycan appears closely linked to the stromal environment, with FGF-2 promoting its expression in vitro.[266]

Proteoglycans are responsible for maintaining the regular spacing and packing of the collagen fibrils, which is the basis for corneal transparency.[292,400] Lumican may contribute to corneal transparency.

Mice homozygous for a null mutation in lumican develop bilateral corneal opacification.[53] In contrast, mice expressing a mutation in the gene for decorin, the major chondroitin/dermatan sulfate proteoglycan, maintain clear corneas.[53,74] In addition, during development of the chick cornea, the onset of corneal transparency was correlated when lumican switched from a nonsulfated to a sulfated form.[68] Keratocan and mimecan are less well studied.

In addition, the macromolecular structure of proteoglycans increases fluid viscosity and defines the colloid osmotic characteristics of the stroma. The actual concentrations of Na^+ and K^+ are higher in the stroma than in the aqueous humor.[338] However, the ionic activity, which determines the osmotic and diffusional gradients for Na^+, is less in the stroma than in the aqueous humor, reflecting cationic binding by anionic sites on stromal GAGs.[38,169,424] This binding decreases the effective osmolarity of Na^+ in the corneal stroma and favors movement of water from the stroma to the aqueous humor. As discussed in a subsequent section, active dehydration of the cornea is a consequence of the osmotic gradient established by the corneal endothelial metabolic pump, compensating for the leakage of fluid from the aqueous and limbus into the stroma as a consequence of swelling pressure.

Water evaporates from the corneal surface at a rate of 2.5 $\mu l/cm^2/hr$.[335] Evaporation accounts for a 5% thinning of the cornea during the day, compared with the corneal thickness measured when the eyelids open in the morning after nighttime closure.[275] In patients with compromised endothelial metabolic pump function, such as in Fuchs' endothelial dystrophy, epithelial edema is worse in the morning when arising as a result of lack of evaporation at night when the lids are closed. Localized areas of corneal drying and evaporation may result in focal corneal thinning, known as *dellen*. The persistence of dellen may reflect the decrease in stromal fluid flow facility when stromal hydration is abnormal in addition to minimal lateral flow of water in the cornea.[291]

The normal cornea maintains a constant thickness in the presence of IOP up to 50 mm Hg.[492] This is because the stromal swelling pressure is also in a similar range. However, in eyes with IOP higher than 50 mm Hg or in those with abnormal endothelial function, there will be resultant epithelial edema and increased stromal thickness. The relationship between IOP and stromal swelling pressure is IP = IOP − SP, where *IP* is stromal imbibition pressure and *SP* is stromal swelling pressure. In rabbits in which the central corneal stroma was implanted with a saline-filled cannula, the suction on the cannula necessary to prevent the stroma from drawing fluid from the tube is the imbibition pressure.[171] As discussed previously, stromal swelling pressure decreases precipitously with increased corneal thickness. Thus mild corneal edema (e.g., in a marginally functioning corneal transplant) combined with slightly elevated IOP can lead to high imbibition pressures and subsequent microbullous epithelial edema.

Stromal Wound Healing. Stromal wound healing involves the resynthesis and cross-linking of collagen, alterations in proteoglycan synthesis, and gradual wound remodeling leading to the restoration of tensile strength. Within hours, polymorphonuclear cells appear around areas of cellular necrosis in a penetrating corneal wound, followed thereafter by monocytes. Adjacent corneal cells are seen to undergo a process of transformation, leading to an accumulation of fibroblasts. TGF-β significantly reduce corneal fibrosis in vivo.

It has been shown that fibroblasts and myofibroblasts have the ability to establish and maintain intercellular communication with themselves and nonactivated keratocytes, which may be critical in the wound healing process.[466] Stromal keratocytes, which normally form a syncytium, may begin to lose their interconnections and go through morphologic changes, some undergoing hypertrophy, proliferation, and finally, reformation of cellular processes and connecting gap junctions.[257]

Activated corneal cells involved in stromal healing may transiently express fetal antigens, and these scars may have a decrease in the concentration of sulfated epitopes of keratan sulfate and an increase in dermatan sulfate.[10,59,153,273] Following excimer laser keratectomy or mechanical keratectomy in monkeys, fibrinogen is detected at 1 month in the underlying corneal stroma, but not in the overlying healed region, which contains newly synthesized type III collagen, poorly sulfated keratan sulfate, fibronectin, and laminin.[153] Type VI collagen is present uniformly in both untreated and healed corneal stroma, suggesting that newly formed collagen may interdigitate with the old in corneal scars.[77]

Tensile strength in corneal wounds increases gradually up to the fourth postoperative year. Incisions in avascular cornea far from the limbus heal more slowly than peripheral cornea wounds or in chronically inflamed corneas with neovascularization.[155] Studies of delayed corneal wound healing following radial keratotomy showed evidence of epithelial plugs in the incision site up to 47 months postoperatively, along with gaping keratotomy incisions and a malposed Bowman's layer.[78] The use of potent topical steroids may delay the early phases of corneal wound healing.

Endothelial Physiology. As described previously, the stroma tends to imbibe water as a result of the charge characteristics of the proteoglycans of the stromal ground substance. Despite the swelling pressure of the stroma, it does not swell in vivo under normal conditions. Two factors contribute to the prevention of stromal swelling and the maintenance of its water content at 78% (3.8 mg H_2O/mg dry weight): These are the barrier and pump functions of the endothelium. The barrier is incomplete compared with the epithelial barrier.

This is illustrated by comparing swelling rates of the cornea in vitro after removal of the endothelium or inhibition of the metabolic pump (see following discussion). When the endothelium is disrupted, the cornea swells at 127 μm/hr, clearly demonstrating the importance of this cell layer as a barrier. When the metabolic pump is inhibited, the cornea swells at approximately 33 μm/hr; this swelling represents the movement of fluid and solutes from the aqueous humor into the stroma through the incomplete barrier of the intact cell layer[464] (Figure 4-37). This normal leakage of fluid into the cornea serves a vital function; because of the avascularity of the cornea, this fluid is the source of nutrients, including glucose and amino acids, for the cornea.

The continual movement of water into the stroma leads to stromal swelling and loss of transparency if mechanisms are not present to remove fluid from the stroma. Early studies of corneal hydration showed that maintenance of the normal corneal thickness and water content is temperature dependent. The cornea swells when cooled and returns to normal thickness when returned to its normal temperature[164] (Figure 4-38). This phenomenon is known as *temperature reversal* and is clearly demonstrated by eye bank corneas, which swell during refrigeration and return to normal thickness and transparency after grafting.

This temperature reversal clearly shows that the maintenance of corneal hydration is a metabolic, energy-dependent process, and it was subsequently shown that 6 to 8 ml/hr of water is moved by the endothelium from stroma to aqueous humor.[82,293] It was initially suggested that water itself was actively transported by the cornea, leading to the use of terminology describing a corneal "fluid pump." It is now known that cell membranes contain transporters for ions, amino acids, and sugars, but no active transport mechanism that directly transports water molecules is known to exist.

Rather, water moves osmotically down gradients set up by active transport of ions. Therefore the term *metabolic pump* rather than *fluid pump* should

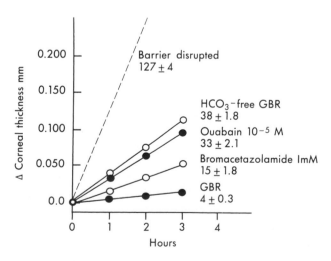

FIGURE 4-37   Maintenance of corneal thickness requires an intact barrier and metabolic pump. Inhibition of the Na^+-K^+-ATPase with ouabain, inhibition of carbonic anhydrase with bromacetazolamide, or lack of bicarbonate all result in swelling. Numbers indicate swelling rates in micrometers per hour. *GBR,* Glutathione bicarbonate Ringer's solution. (Courtesy Dr. Henry Edelhauser. From Waring GO et al: *Ophthalmol* 89:531, 1982.)

be used. The concept has developed that normal corneal hydration represents a balance between the leak across the corneal endothelium and the extrusion of ions and fluid via the endothelial metabolic pump, with the major driving force being the osmotic gradient established by the aqueous humor sodium concentration for corneal deturgescence and transparency.[424]

Endothelial Ion Transport. Several ion transport systems have been identified or postulated to exist in the corneal endothelium. Each of these mechanisms is characterized and then placed into a unified model of the endothelial metabolic pump.

During the initial studies of Na^+-K^+-ATPase, the enzyme was shown to be present in cat cornea, and it is now the most completely characterized of the endothelial ion transporters.* The Na^+-K^+ pump is located in the basolateral membrane of the endothelial cell and is present in normal humans at approximately 1.5×10^6 pump sites per cell and in rabbits at 3×10^6 pump sites per cell.[137,139] These values may be compared with levels of 4 to 5×10^6 sites per cell in the renal tubule and ventricular muscle. The activity of Na^+-K^+-ATPase is vital to the maintenance of normal corneal hydration. Inhibition of the pump with the specific inhibitor ouabain stops sodium transport, causes corneal

---

*References 27, 36, 114, 138, 187, 262, 473.

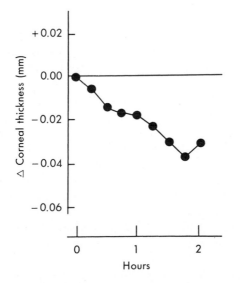

FIGURE 4-38   Temperature reversal in a human cornea during in vitro perfusion. (Courtesy Dr. Henry Edelhauser.)

swelling, prevents temperature reversal, and eliminates the transendothelial potential difference. It also appears that the sodium pump can respond to increases in endothelial permeability, because human corneas with guttata have pump site densities of 6×10^6 sites per cell, which suggests a greater capacity for the endothelial pump to counteract the leak across the barrier.[139] In contrast, the inflamed, edematous cornea has decreased endothelial pump sites despite increased permeability. These responses appear to be mediated by the cyclooxygenase pathway of the arachidonic acid cascade.[270] The basolateral membrane of the endothelial cell also contains an amelioride-sensitive Na^+-H^+ exchanger. It moves sodium into the cell and hydrogen ions outward.[202]

Bicarbonate is also essential to the maintenance of corneal thickness.[178] Removal of bicarbonate from the solution irrigating the endothelium of the isolated, perfused cornea results in corneal swelling, and a net flux of bicarbonate from stroma to aqueous humor has been demonstrated.[190] This transport of bicarbonate is apparently responsible for the -500 μV (aqueous humor negative to stroma) potential across the endothelium.[242] The bicarbonate transported by the endothelium is generated intracellularly by the action of carbonic anhydrase. Carbon dioxide diffuses into the cells from the extracellular space and combines with water in a reaction catalyzed by carbonic anhydrase to form carbonic acid. The carbonic acid readily dissociates into hydrogen and bicarbonate ions. Inhibition of this reaction by carbonic anhydrase inhibitors can result in corneal swelling in vitro.[190] The effect is not as great as that seen when Na^+-K^+-ATPase is inhibited, and it is also interesting that systemic treatment with acetazolamide has no effect on corneal hydration.[242] The transport of bicarbonate across the apical membrane of the cells is energy dependent, but the transporter is not well defined.[178,473] Electrophysiologic evidence points to the existence of an electrogenic HCO_3^--Na^+ cotransport, which moves these ions out of the cell in a 2:1 ratio in a process that is inhibitable by stilbene.[202] This type of transport has not been identified in other cell types, and evidence also exists to indicate that bicarbonate and sodium transport are not directly coupled.[242]

Although the details of endothelial transport are not yet fully elucidated, the components of the system, as described previously, can be assembled into a model that explains ion transport and osmotic water flow across the endothelium[242,292]

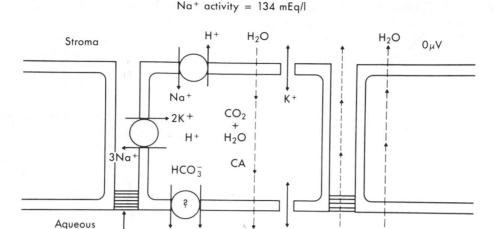

Na⁺ activity = 134 mEq/l

FIGURE 4-39   Model of ion and water movements across the corneal endothelium. Activity of the metabolic pump sets up an osmotic gradient, resulting in movement of fluid from the stroma to the aqueous humor balancing the leak of fluid from the aqueous humor into the stroma. *CA,* Carbonic anhydrase. (Based on models proposed in Jentsch TJ et al: *Curr Eye Res* 4:361, 1985; and Kuang K et al: *Exp Eye Res* 50:487, 1990.)

(Figure 4-39). The Na^+-H^+ exchanger acidifies the extracellular fluid, increasing the level of carbon dioxide that diffuses into the cell. Carbonic anhydrase converts carbon dioxide to hydrogen ion and bicarbonate, which are transported out of the cell by the basolateral Na^+-H^+ exchanger and the apical bicarbonate transport, respectively. As suggested previously, sodium may accompany the bicarbonate with the stoichiometry favoring the anion, setting up the aqueous-negative transendothelial potential. Central to the entire system is the sodium pump, which maintains the sodium gradient required for Na^+-H^+ exchange, thereby promoting bicarbonate production. Transport of sodium into the lateral space may also contribute to the transendothelial potential. Given the apical location of the functional complexes the path of least resistance for sodium movement is into the stroma; therefore the negative potential of the aqueous humor may also result in movement of sodium ions from the lateral spaces into the aqueous humor. Potassium and sodium channels required for the function of this model have also been identified.[242,364]

Although not shown in the model, chloride transport is also required for correct stoichiometry, but this has not yet been adequately identified.

Essential to the function of an endothelial metabolic pump capable of fluid transport is the existence of an osmotic gradient that favors the movement of water from the stroma to the aqueous humor. The sodium concentration of aqueous humor is 143 mEq/L, all of which is osmotically active. The sodium concentration of the stroma is more than 160 mEq/L, which implies a gradient favoring inward movement of water. A large portion of this sodium is bound by the stromal proteoglycans, leaving an osmotically active sodium level of only 134 mEq/L in the stroma. This results in an osmotic pressure of 163.8 mm Hg drawing water out of the cornea.[424] Although incomplete, the metabolic pump model described previously is clearly able to set up the ionic gradient required to counteract the leak of fluid into the cornea. It is evident that the bulk of water movement occurs through the cells. Blockers of glucose transport, such as phloretin, also block water movement across the endothelium.

Endothelial Function and Intraocular Irrigating Solutions. An ideal irrigating solution should contain an energy source (e.g., glucose), an adequate buffer (e.g., bicarbonate), and a substrate (e.g., calcium, glutathione) to maintain junctional stability

TABLE 4-1
THE COMPOSITION OF AQUEOUS HUMOR AND GLUTATHIONE-BICARBONATE RINGER'S SOLUTION (GBR) (ALL CONCENTRATIONS IN MMOL/L)

	AQUEOUS HUMOR	GBR	BSS PLUS*
Sodium	162.9	160	160.0
Potassium	2.2-3.9	5	5.0
Calcium	1.8	1	1.0
Magnesium	1.1	1	1.0
Chloride	131.6	130	130.0
Bicarbonate	20.15	25	25.0
Phosphate	0.62	3	3.0
Lactate	2.5	—	—
Glucose	2.7-3.7	5	5.0
Ascorbate	1.06	—	—
Glutathione	0.002	0.3	0.3
pH	7.38	7.2-7.4	7.4
Osmolarity (mOsm/kg)	304	305	305

*The irrigating solution curently being used for intraocular surgery (phacoemulsification and vitrectomy).

and the blood-aqueous barrier.[6] The pH of the solution should be between 6.7 and 8.1, with an osmolality between 270 and 350 to maintain endothelial cell ultrastructure.[93,468] These observations concerning the physiologic requirements of the corneal endothelium clearly illustrate that any irrigating solution introduced into the anterior chamber of the eye should closely resemble the aqueous humor in composition because the normal environment of the intraocular fluid provides for all of these requirements (Table 4-1).

When the corneal endothelium is exposed to an environment outside this range, cells swell and become vacuolated, functional breakdown occurs, and corneal thickness increases. The cellular swelling that occurs suggests impaired metabolic pump function, which indicates that the corneal edema is caused not only by increased leak as cells degenerate but also by decreased ion and water transport. These factors must be considered when irrigating solutions and drugs are introduced into the anterior chamber.

Bicarbonate is required for the endothelial transport system, and absence of this ion also results in corneal swelling. The endothelial cells of these corneas are swollen and vacuolated, which again is evidence of impaired pump function

(Figure 4-40, *A*). Poorly buffered solutions such as 0.9% saline and lactated Ringer's solution or acidic drug formulations that overcome the buffering capacity of the aqueous humor may expose the cornea to extremes of pH and cause corneal edema[94,97] (Figure 4-41). Normal saline also lacks other components of the aqueous humor known to be required for endothelial function. Irrigation of the endothelium with 0.9% NaCl results in immediate and rapid swelling of the cornea caused by a loss of pump and barrier.[94,152,464] This is clearly the result of a lack of ions essential to endothelial function. The absence of extracellular potassium inhibits the Na-K$^+$-ATPase.

Glutathione, which is present in aqueous humor and endothelial cells, has been shown to promote maintenance of endothelial function in vitro.[82,96,377] This tripeptide is normally present in both its reduced (GSH) and oxidized (GSSG) forms. This balance appears to be important because oxidation of all glutathione by diamide results in breakage of cell junctions.[96] It is suggested that glutathione protects the cell membranes from free radical damage, thereby helping maintain both the pump and the barrier of the endothelium.

Even a short-term, 30-minute irrigation of the cat endothelium in vivo with a balanced salt solution deficient in bicarbonate and glutathione can cause a transient increase in polymegathism and pleomorphism.[147] On the basis of data presented previously, these changes in endothelial cell morphology, as seen enface, are apparently the result of altered cell volume regulation and pump function. This lends support to the earlier argument that pleomorphism and polymorphism are indicative of a physiologically stressed endothelium.

Calcium, which is required to maintain an intact endothelial barrier, requires the presence of this ion because it is always involved in the maintenance of functional complexes. Irrigation of the endothelium with a calcium-free solution causes breakage of the apical junctions.[468] The cells separate and round up, exposing large areas of Descemet's membrane, with a resultant increase of fluid uptake by the stroma. Replacement of calcium in the solution allows re-formation of the junctions. It must be pointed out that not only does loss of intercellular junctions disrupt the barrier, but the separation of the cells from one another also causes a loss of pump polarity; therefore the cells can no longer transport ions vectorially and set up the osmotic and ionic gradients required for movement of fluid into the aqueous humor.[474]

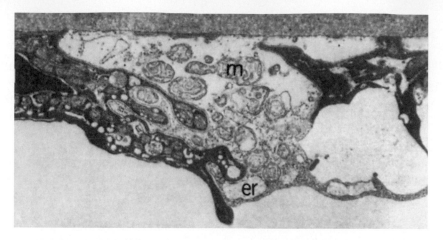

A

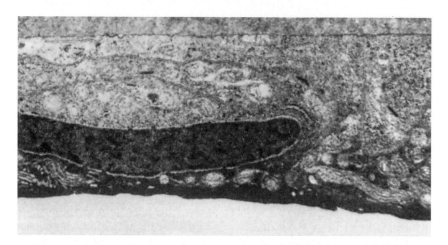

B

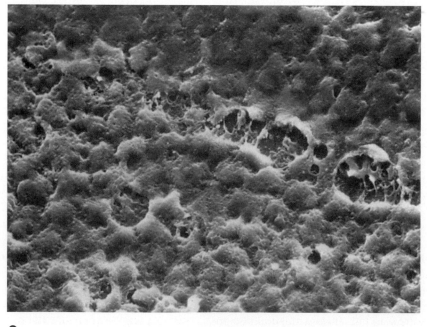

C

FIGURE 4-40 **A,** Transmission electron micrograph of corneal endothelial cells perfused with 0.9% NaCl solution. Note cell swelling and vacuolization indicative of impaired pump function. **B,** Normal corneal endothelium. **C,** Scanning electron micrograph of a corneal endothelium perfused with a calcium-free solution. Note breakage of cell junctions. *er,* Endoplasmic reticulum; *m,* mitochondria. (Magnification ×1000.) (Courtesy Dr. Henry Edelhauser.)

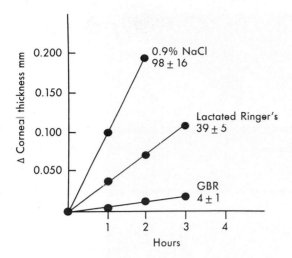

FIGURE 4-41 Changes in corneal thickness of rabbit corneas perfused with three intraocular irrigating solutions. NaCl causes rapid swelling because it lacks calcium, bicarbonate, and other essential ions. Lactated Ringer's solution has a low pH. Glutathione bicarbonate Ringer's (*GBR*) solution resembles aqueous humor and maintains normal corneal thickness. (Courtesy Dr. Henry Edelhauser. From Edelhauser HF et al: *Am J Ophthalmol* 93:327, 1982.)

Epinephrine added to irrigating solutions is used extensively by cataract surgeons to achieve and maintain pupillary mydriasis. When injected into the anterior chamber, intravenous or intracardiac epinephrine have been reported to cause corneal endothelial cell toxicity, likely as a result of a sodium bisulfate preservative and a citrate buffer.[97,189] As a result, 1:1000 preservative-free epinephrine (American Reagant Laboratories, Shirley, New York) currently is available and can be used safely by adding 1 to 500 ml of BSS PLUS, an advanced irrigating, balanced salt solution containing sodium bicarbonate, dextrose, and glutathione (Alcon Laboratories, Inc., Fort Worth, Texas).[94] In addition, phacoemulsification with a high flow of the irrigation solution can alter the endothelial surface glycoprotein layer.

In a study ranking various solutions on their effects to the corneal endothelium in perfusion studies, BSS PLUS and glutathione bicarbonate Ringer's (GBR) solution allowed for the best maintenance of stromal thickness and endothelial permeability.[468] The remaining solutions were SMA2 (Senju Pharmaceutical Co., Ltd., Osaka, Japan), Calcium-free GBR, and Plasma-Lyte (Baxter Healthcare Corp., Deerfield, Illinois). During analysis of glass versus polypropylene bottles for packaging of in-

traocular solutions, it was noted that the latter is permeable to atmospheric gases. This permeability allows for more gas bubbles during phacoemulsification, leading to decreased visibility and increased endothelial cell damage.[468]

The physiologic requirements of the corneal endothelium must also be considered when designing a corneal-preservation medium.[391] The ionic composition of such a solution should be such that the endothelial monolayer is preserved intact for normal barrier function and the transporters will function effectively to promote temperature reversal if the cornea has been stored in the cold.

Endothelial Wound Healing. When endothelial cells are lost as a result of surgical trauma, disease, or the aging process, the defect must be covered primarily by the spreading of cells from areas adjacent to the wound to cover the wounded area. When a single cell is lost, as in aging, the cells immediately surrounding the defect spread to fill in the area left by the missing cell. Over time, this leads to the significant cell enlargement typical of the aged cornea.[31]

When a large defect occurs as a result of surgical insult or a decompensation episode in keratoconus, more extensive cell migration occurs. In experimental wounds, cells as far as 250 μm from the wound edge are involved in migration toward the wound center. Cells near the wound edge migrate at 80 to 100 μm/day in the initial stages of healing, elongating toward the center of the wound, and finally spreading as the wound closes.[289,290] This is followed by remodeling into a more normal hexagonal shape. In vivo the cells do not break contact with one another during spreading and migrating[450] (Figure 4-42). The pump and barrier of the endothelium are reestablished when the confluent monolayer is restored, allowing the cornea to return to normal thickness.[490]

After keratoplasty, the endothelial cells undergo a progressive wound healing response of migration (Figure 4-43) of endothelial cells over the wound edge to the periphery and the development of tight junctions to establish the endothelial barrier. Once the barrier is formed, the endothelial cells increase the number of Na^+-K^+-ATPase pump sites in the lateral membranes of the endothelial cells.[490]

It has been demonstrated that intracellular growth factors released from corneal endothelial cells enhance the migration of surviving cells in vitro.[392] Suramin had a strong inhibitory effect, indicating a major role of heparin-binding growth factors for cellular migration. β-FGF and the regu-

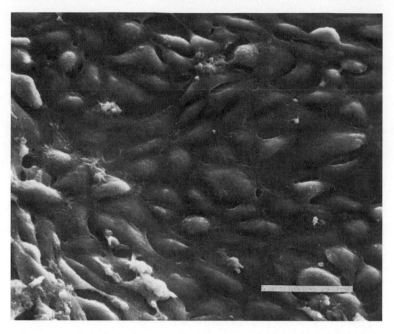

Figure 4-42   Scanning electron micrograph of migrating corneal endothelial cells 2 days after a 2-mm transcorneal freezing. (Bar = 50 μm.)

Corneal button

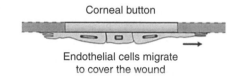

Endothelial cells migrate
to cover the wound

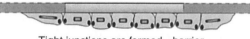

Tight junctions are formed—barrier

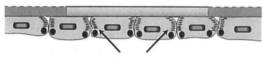

Na$^+$-K$^+$-ATPase pump sites are increased

Figure 4-43   Diagram illustrating the corneal endothelial wound repair after keratoplasty. Migration of endothelial cells to cover the wound edge, development of tight junctions to establish the endothelial barrier, and the formation of Na$^+$-K$^+$-ATPase pump sites on the lateral membrane of the corneal endothelial cells. (Redrawn from Edelhauser HF: *Cornea* 19:263, 2000.)

lation of β-FGF–receptor expression on cells at the wound margin seem to be of crucial importance for the wound healing process.

Schultz et al.[392] and Raphael et al.[370] have shown that cells near the leading edge of the wound incor-

porate 3H-thymidine, whereas cell distal to the wound remain growth arrested in studies of in vivo corneal endothelial wound healing in cats and rabbits. Further data have suggested that cell spreading or migration associated with wound healing is required for entry into the cell cycle for corneal endothelial cells to be capable of proliferating.[184,185,437] In a study of in vivo wound healing of cat corneal endothelium, Petroll et al.[343] reported that proliferation is limited temporally and spatially to spreading endothelial cells within the wound.

The mechanisms of cell migration in the endothelium have not been extensively studied. Actin stress fibers have been demonstrated to be oriented in the direction of cell spreading in cultured cells, and the formation of these fibers and the cell movement can be stimulated by indomethacin.[207,208] The endothelium also contains abundant EGF receptors. Although wound healing can be stimulated by EGF in vitro, its usefulness as a pharmacologic agent to promote endothelial healing has not yet been established.

Corneal Nutrition and Metabolism. Corneal metabolism depends on oxygen derived predominantly from the atmosphere, with minor amounts supplied by the aqueous humor and limbal vasculature.[175,441] The normal amount of oxygen present in the aque-

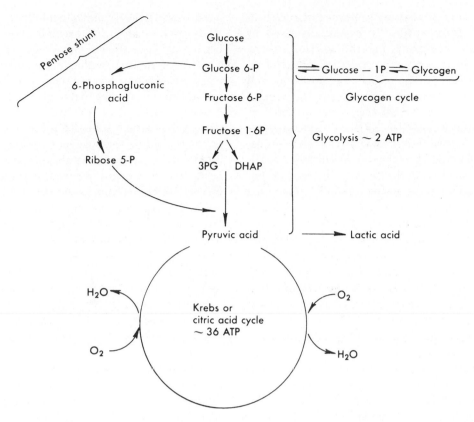

FIGURE 4-44 Metabolism of glucose in cornea. *ATP,* Adenosine triphosphate; *DHAP,* dihydroxyacetone phosphate.

ous humor is low (approximately 40 mm Hg) in comparison with that in tears (155 mm Hg). During sleep or under closed-eye conditions, oxygen is delivered to the cornea by the highly vascularized superior palpebral conjunctivas, albeit at reduced levels (i.e., PO$_2$, 21% with eyelid open; 8% with eyelid closed).[102,181] After cataract removal (i.e., aphakia), oxygen tension may increase in the aqueous humor as a result of decreased oxygen metabolism by the crystalline lens.[182] Thus, in the aphakic eye, oxygen in the aqueous humor may supplement oxygen dissolved in the tears, better meeting corneal oxygen demands and allowing greater tolerance to hypoxic stress such as contact lens use.

The corneal epithelium consumes oxygen at a rate approximately 10 times faster than the stroma does.[376] Several investigators have presented evidence suggesting that there may be a role for intact corneal innervation in maintaining the high metabolic rate of the epithelium.[182,450] Most of the metabolic requirements for glucose, amino acids, vitamins, and other nutrients are supplied to the cornea by the aqueous humor (via the ciliary body), with lesser amounts available in the tears or via limbal

vessels. In addition, glucose can be derived from glycogen stores in the corneal epithelium. Under both hypoxic and normoxic conditions, some glucose is diverted to the hexose monophosphate shunt (Figure 4-44), regulating levels of nicotinamide adenosine dinucleotide phosphate and converting hexoses to pentoses, which are used in nucleic acid synthesis. In addition, glucose derived from the aqueous humor or from epithelial glycogen stores is converted to pyruvate by the anaerobic Embden-Meyerhof pathway (i.e., glycolysis), yielding two molecules of adenosine triphosphate (ATP) per glucose molecule.

Under aerobic conditions, pyruvate is then oxidized in the tricarboxylic acid (TCA or Krebs or citric acid cycle) to yield water, carbon dioxide, and 36 molecules of ATP per cycle. Under hypoxic conditions, such as during contact lens use, increasing amounts of pyruvate are converted by lactate dehydrogenase to lactate, which diffuses from the epithelium into the stroma, osmotically inducing epithelial and stromal edema.[234] Epithelial edema leads to clinical symptoms such as halo and rainbow formation, increased glare sensitivity, and decreased contrast sensitivity. Because the anterior surface of the cornea is structurally fixed by Bowman's membrane and the anterior stroma, stromal corneal edema manifests in a posterior direction, with buckling of the posterior stroma and Descemet's membrane giving rise to vertical striae.[254,350,470] Because of the barrier provided by the superficial epithelial cells, the dispersion of lactate into the tear film is precluded and the elimination of lactate is dependent on slow diffusion across the stroma and endothelium into the aqueous humor. In addition to causing osmotic edema of the epithelium and stroma, metabolic acidosis consequent to lactate metabolism may result in structural and functional alterations in corneal endothelial cells.[490] In the absence of corneal edema, the oxygen permeability of the corneal stroma is somewhat less than 29×10^{-11} ml O_2/cm^2/sec/mm Hg, a value less than that of most high-water-content soft contact lenses.[472]

The oxygen requirements of the cornea have important implications with regard to contact lens use. It has been shown that the cornea can maintain a deturgescent state with sustained oxygen levels as low as 25 mm Hg before edema is induced.[274] For small-diameter hard polymethyl-methacrylate lenses, which are impermeable to oxygen, good lens movement is essential to allow an exchange of tears under the lens with oxygenated tears from the periphery, which is accomplished by the action of the lid blink. For larger-diameter soft lenses, especially those used on an extended-wear basis, oxygen permeability must be sufficient for an adequate supply of oxygen to reach the cornea by diffusion through the lens itself, in addition to the lesser effect of the tear pump exchange with these lenses.

Contact lenses have been shown to induce corneal swelling and the inflammatory response related to the synthesis by the cytochrome P-450 arachidonic acid metabolites.[67] With contact lens wear, there is a time-dependent epithelial increase in the production of 12(R)HETE and 8(R)HETE, which correlates directly to the corneal inflammatory response. The inflammatory response can be reduced after inhibition of the epithelial cytochrome P-450 synthesis of the arachidonic acid metabolites.[66] Thus, when the corneal endothelium is exposed to both metabolites, the endothelial changes that occur are similar to those observed in contact lens–induced hypoxia (e.g., corneal edema, neovascularization, endothelial polymegathism).[76]

Corneal endothelial polymegathism has been widely described in contact lens wearers. One of the underlying mechanisms of polymegathism is re-

lated to 12(R)HETE's ability to inhibit the Na$^+$-K$^+$-ATPase of the endothelial metabolic pump.[396] It has been previously shown that exogenously added 12(R)HETE induces swelling in the isolated rabbit and human cornea when directly perfused to the endothelium, indicating that 12(R)HETE has pharmacologic activity on the corneal endothelium pump mechanism.[98] When 12(R)HETE was placed on the tear side of the isolated rabbit cornea, it was rapidly taken up by the epithelium and metabolized to 8(R)hydroxy-hexadecatrienoic acid [8(R)HHDTrE] (Figure 4-45). Both 12(R)HETE and 8(R)HETE can easily diffuse posteriorly across the cornea through the stroma to the endothelium where further metabolism of 12(R)HETE occurs.[479]

Davis et al.[76] and Conners et al.[67] showed that contact lenses activate the corneal epithelial cytochrome P-450 pathway to produce both 12(R)HETE and 8(R)HHDTrE. Both eicosanoids were sequestered in the cornea as opposed to diffusing into the aqueous environment of the tears and aqueous humor. The eicosanoids can inhibit the endothelial metabolic pump to cause endothelial cellular and corneal stromal swelling.[98] Therefore repeated endothelial cell exposure to 12(R)HETE and 8(R)HHDTrE (e.g., daily contact lens wear) causes endothelial cell swelling, resulting in a permanent change in the cellular cytoskeleton and leading to endothelial polymegathism.[271] It should be noted that corneal endothelial polymegathism occurs only after long-term volume-regulation stress, such as contact lens wear, and in the cornea of a patient with diabetes.[99]

Extended-wear contact lenses alter many aspects of epithelial metabolism. Their use has been associated with a decreased rate of mitosis (possibly contributing to corneal epithelial thinning associated with long-term use), reduced oxygen uptake and glucose utilization, and smaller numbers of intercellular desmosomes (thought to result from prolonged epithelial edema).[21,183,225] The decrease in desmosome malconnections between cells increases the likelihood of abrasions and erosions.[330] This, in concert with the reduced metabolic activity of the epithelium under hypoxic conditions, may compromise the epithelial barrier function and increase the likelihood of ulcerative microbial keratitis.[312]

Vitamin A and the Cornea

The association of malnutrition with corneal ulceration has been recognized for thousands of years. With the discovery of vitamin A, it was determined that this corneal disease is caused by vitamin A deficiency. Lack of vitamin A is responsible for 5 mil-

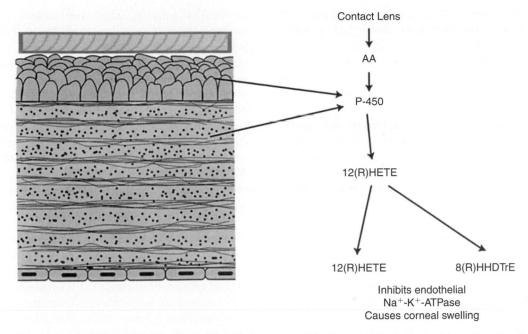

FIGURE 4-45 Contact lenses are capable of stimulating the arachidonic acid (*AA*) cascade in the corneal epithelium directly from the lenses and the protein they absorb from wear. The epithelial cells have a P-450 metabolic pathway that produces two eicosanoids [12(R)HETE and 8(R)HHDTrE] resulting from contact lens wear. These two products have been shown to diffuse across the stroma and inhibit the endothelial Na^+-K^+-ATPase, which causes endothelial cell edema—resulting in polymegethism—and corneal swelling. (From Edelhauser HF: *Cornea* 19:263, 2000.)

lion to 10 million cases of xerophthalmia and 500,000 cases of blindness, primarily in children in developing countries, each year.[416] Lack of vitamin A causes keratinization of the ocular surface epithelium, with the corneal epithelium expressing keratins normally found in skin by terminally differentiated superficial epithelial cells.[442] Vitamin A is also required for mucin production, and it has been shown that expression of MUC1 and MUC4 mRNA and protein by the corneal epithelium is inhibited in vitamin A–deficient rats.[432]

The role of retinoids (compounds with the biologic activity of vitamin A) in control of gene expression is now well understood. The biologically active form of vitamin A is retinoic acid, with its all trans- or a cis-isomers binds to retinoic acid receptors (RAR) or retinoid X receptors (RXR), respectively, in the nucleus. These in turn form heterodimers and homodimers with one another and with thyroid and vitamin D receptors. These bind to response elements on DNA and control gene expression, influencing cell differentiation and protein synthesis.[276,277] The cytoplasmic binding proteins for retinol and retinoic acid that influence intracellular metabolism and transport of retinoids have been identified in the cells of the cornea.[336,444]

It has also been demonstrated that corneal epithelium expresses the RARα, RARβ, and RARγ subtypes and the RXRα and RXRβ subtypes. Stromal fibroblasts also express RARα, RARβ, RARγ, RXRα, and RARβ.[29] The presence of these mediators of retinoid function in the cornea underscores the importance of this vitamin, which now appears to be active almost ubiquitously in the various cell types of the body. Xerophthalmia actually appears late in the progression of vitamin A deficiency, but it is certainly the most obvious and devastating effect of the lack of dietary retinoids. It is obvious that there needs to be a continued fight against the socioeconomic, cultural, and political conditions that often account for this nutritional deficiency that causes childhood blindness.[416]

CORNEAL PHARMACOLOGY

Factors Affecting Drug Penetration

Many factors influence the degree of drug penetration through the cornea. The volume of the normal adult tear film is 7 to 9 µl, and the maximum amount of fluid that the cul-de-sac can maintain is 20 to 30 µl. Thus much of the 50 µl in the average drop of topical medication runs out of the eye immediately after instillation and the remainder is diluted in the preexisting tear film.[294] Reflex tearing caused by irritating or hypertonic solutions results in more rapid tear dilution. Increased protein concentration in tears bathing inflamed or infected eyes may also decrease the bioavailability of drugs that bind to protein.

After topical drug administration, most of the drug enters the aqueous humor by corneal penetration.[83] The corneal epithelium provides an initial barrier to penetration with its tight junctions, thereby limiting adsorption of hydrophilic, ionized substances and favoring the penetration of lipid-soluble hydrophobic compounds. The drug-saturated epithelium may act as a reservoir to release drugs into the hydrophilic corneal stroma. Thus drugs that are delivered at a pH favoring their more lipid-soluble undissociated form more readily enter the epithelium. At the pH of the corneal epithelium, more of the drug dissociates into its water-soluble ionized form, facilitating penetration through the stroma. Loss of the corneal epithelium greatly enhances the penetration of hydrophilic, water-soluble pharmacologic agents, such as gentamicin, that normally traverse the epithelium via transcellular or paracellular routes.

The corneal stroma, comprised of collagen and ECM, allows diffusion of solutes of less than 500,000 MW. The hydrophilic nature of the stroma results in a barrier to lipid-based drugs. Drug penetration through the corneal endothelium is determined mostly by molecular size.

Other means to increase drug penetration through the cornea include increasing the duration of contact of the drug with the ocular surface. This can be accomplished through mechanical means, such as pressing on the lacrimal sac, or by use of viscous drops, suspensions, or ointments; slow-release delivery systems; contact lenses; or porcine collagen corneal shields. The inclusion of surfactants and detergents, such as benzalkonium chloride (BAK) or Tween 20 in topical ocular medications, or the preparation of drug-containing liposomes may also improve drug penetration through the outer epithelial barrier, in addition to the preservative effect inherent to these agents.[295]

Effects of Preservatives Used in Ophthalmic Preparations. Many topical medications are used to treat ocular disease. These include antibiotics, antiviral drugs, glaucoma drugs, antiinflammatory and antiallergy drugs, and artificial tears for treatment of dry eye. To prolong shelf life and protect the eye from infection, these formulations, when packaged in multidose dispensers, must contain preservatives to prevent bacterial growth. These preservatives include BAK, chlorhexidine digluconate, polyquaternium-1, and thimerosal. The most commonly used preservative is BAK, whereas use of thimerosal has been largely discontinued because of allergic reactions. The antibacterial action of BAK is based on the detergent property of the compound, which acts to break down bacterial cell walls. These characteristics of a preservative also render the corneal epithelium and endothelium susceptible to damage when they are exposed to these agents.[42,43,268]

The effects of BAK on the corneal epithelium have been studied extensively. Application of a drop containing 0.01% BAK to the cornea causes an immediate, measurable increase in the permeability of the cornea to fluorescein. This is the result of breakage of junctions between the superficial cells and sloughing of the outer cell layer (Figure 4-46). With prolonged exposure to a preservative, the sloughing of the second layer of superficial cells and possibly some wing cells may also occur. Electrophysiologic experiments have shown that this loss of superficial cells is accompanied by a decrease in the transepithelial voltage resulting from the loss of the high-resistance barrier formed by the apical tight junctions. BAK also inhibits corneal epithelial wound healing. Other preservatives have similar but milder effects on the corneal epithelial surface.

Ophthalmic preparations with preservatives can be used safely by patients with normal corneas, especially when they are used infrequently (i.e., once or twice a day). People with moderate to severe dry eyes have a compromised corneal epithelial barrier, as shown by studies that demonstrate increased corneal epithelial permeability to fluorescein in these patients.[148] If they use tear solutions containing BAK, these patients, who may use artificial tears hourly throughout the day, risk further damage to their corneas and conjunctiva, increasing chances for corneal edema and ocular infection.[447] For this reason, preservative-free tear formulations have been developed and should be used by patients with moderate to severe dry eye disease.[267,446] Ethylenediaminetetraacetic acid (EDTA) is also used to stabilize BAK-containing formulations. EDTA chelates calcium, which is required for maintenance of tight junctions, and artificial tears containing EDTA may increase corneal permeability.[446] Therefore, when possible, ophthalmic products should be formulated without EDTA, and formula-

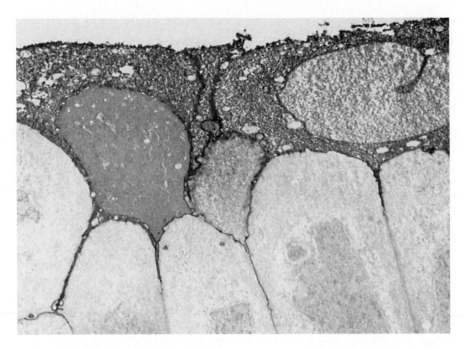

FIGURE 4-46 Corneal epithelium damaged by 0.01% benzalkonium chloride and stained with ruthenium red. The dye penetrates the intercellular space as a result of disruption of the barrier formed by the superficial cells. (Courtesy Dr. Delores López Bernal.)

tions with EDTA should be avoided by patients with dry eyes.

The preservatives BAK and chlorhexidine cause endothelial cell degeneration and corneal edema in vitro.[157,158] Drugs or solutions containing preservatives should never be introduced directly into the anterior chamber of the eye.

SCLERA

Gross and Cellular Anatomy

The sclera, a connective tissue consisting of fibroblasts embedded in an ECM of collagen and elastic fibers interspersed with several types of proteoglycans, provides the structural integrity that defines the shape and axial length of the eye.[70,241,362] The sclera contains approximately 70% water. Scleral collagen fibers, 90% of which are collagen type I, constitute 75% to 80% of the dry weight of the sclera.[89] The sclera is an opaque tissue in stark contrast to the cornea mostly because of the increased water content of the sclera and less uniform orientation of the collagen fibers.

The sclera, like the cornea, is essentially avascular except for the superficial vessels of the episclera and the intrascleral vascular plexus located just posterior to the limbus.[471] The posterior sclera contains the scleral canal and the lamina cribrosa for passage of the optic nerve and contains the sites of perforation by the long and short posterior ciliary arteries, the short ciliary veins, the ciliary nerves, and the vortex veins.[119] The tendons of the rectus muscles insert into the superficial scleral collagen. Overlying the sclera is the episclera, a layer of tissue consisting of a dense vascular connective tissue that merges with the superficial scleral stroma below. The inner layer of the sclera blends imperceptibly with the suprachoroidal and supraciliary lamellas of the uveal tract.[471]

Scleral dimensions are important both surgically and physiologically. The average 17-cm² surface area of the human sclera accounts for 95% of the total surface area of the globe as compared with the 1-cm² surface area of the cornea.[334] Mean scleral thickness ± SD is 0.53 ± 0.14 mm at the corneoscleral limbus, significantly decreasing to 0.39 ± 0.17 mm near the equator, and increasing to 0.9 to 1.0 mm near the optic nerve (Figure 4-47).

The sclera consists of an ECM of collagen and elastic fibers interspersed with several types of proteoglycans. Early biochemical studies demonstrated the presence of types I and III collagen in the hu-

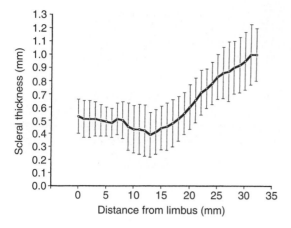

FIGURE 4-47   Line graph comparison of scleral thickness ± standard deviation (y-axis) versus the distance (in millimeters; x-axis) from the surgical limbus (*left*) toward the optic nerve (*right*). (Redrawn from Olsen TW et al: *Am J Ophthalmol* 125:237, 1998.)

man sclera, but not types II and IV.[121,219] With use of immunogold labeling technique, labeling of the striated collagen fibrils suggested colocalization of collagen types I, III, and V.[280] Both types V and VI collagen were localized to filamentous strands in the interfibrillar matrix. Collagen types II and IV were absent from the scleral stroma.

The principal function of type I collagen is an ability to resist tension, and it is found in many tissues, such as bone and tendon.[313] Type III collagen is considered essential in the structural maintenance of expansible organs in which it is present, such as arteries, uterus, and lung.[313] Type V collagen has been implicated in the control of fibril diameter, which may have an anchoring function between basement membranes and the adjacent stromal matrix.[311] This function may be shared with type VI collagen, which has been shown to have a perifibrillar location.[39,220,263]

In another study, collagen fibril bundles were thinner and shorter in the sclera than in the stroma of the cornea.[281,282] However, the important difference between sclera and cornea is that the collagen fibrils in the sclera attained a much larger diameter (up to 10 times) as determined in calibrated morphometric studies.[159] In scanning electron microscopy study of collagen fibrils in human sclera, the diameter ranged from 25 to 230 nm as compared with corneal collagen fibrils, which have a uniform diameter of 25 nm[241] (Figure 4-48). Scleral collagen fibrils formed bundles that were not parallel but were entangled in individual bundles (Figure 4-49). The bundles varied in width and

thickness, with branches that intertwined with each other. Collagen bundles varied from approximately 0.5 to 0.6 μm in thickness.

The external region of the sclera, viewed by scanning electron microscopy, is composed of collagen bundles narrower and thinner than those in the inner region.[241] In the outermost layer, collagen bundles intersect at various angles along the surface of the sclera. Beneath this layer, collagen bundles usually are oriented either meridionally or circularly and are densely interwoven. In the inner layers the bundles tend to be wider and thicker, running in various directions in an intertwined complex fashion.

When viewed by atomic force microscopy (AFM), scleral collagen fibrils have a diameter ranging from 118.3 to 1268.0 nm and show clear banding, with a mean axial D-periodicity of 77.02 nm.[128,303] The mean gap depth between the two overlaps is larger in the sclera than in the cornea. The difference in results between the AFM and electron microscopy may arise because of tissue shrinkage during chemical fixation, dehydration, embedding, and freezing of the electron microscopy specimens.

By conventional electron microscopy, the elastic fiber system, such as the human sclera, consists of three distinct fiber types: elastic, elaunin, and oxytalan. Elastic fibers consist of two components: an amorphous electron-dense core surrounded by a sheath of microfibrils. Oxytalan fibers are collections of typical microfibrils unassociated with amorphous material. Elaunin fibers are intermediate in size between oxytalan and elastic fibers and consist of bundles of typical microfibrils associated with small amounts of elastic-type amorphous material.[279]

In general, an elastic fiber system contains six components (elastin, amyloid P component, laminin, fibronectin, gp115, vitronectin) associated with these three fiber types, as studied by immunogold transmission electron microscopy.[279] In human sclera, both elastic and elaunin fibers contained elastin. The microfibrillar sheaths of elastic fibers labeled for amyloid P component, those of elaunin fibers labeled for amyloid P and laminin, and those of oxytalan fibers labeled for laminin only. No labeling was observed for fibronectin, gp115, and vitronectin in human sclera.[279]

By light microscopic examination of human sclera, Alexander and Garner[1] showed that all three fiber types of the elastic system occurred in the middle and inner layers of the posterior sclera, but only in the inner layer of the anterior sclera. Elaunin fibers extended further forward toward the

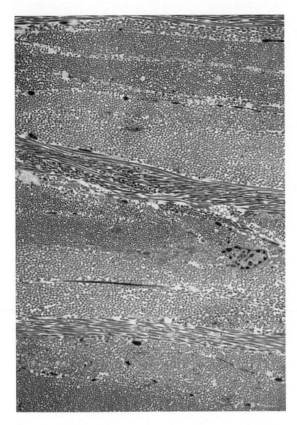

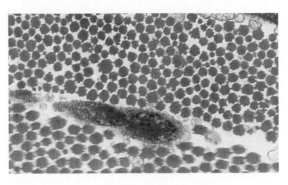

B

FIGURE 4-48 **A,** Lower magnification of collagen fibrils in the sclera (×2945). Scleral collagen fibrils display various diameters. **B,** Higher magnification (×29,450). Scleral collagen fibrils are much larger than those in the cornea.

A

limbus, and oxytalan fibers were the most abundant of the three. An absence of elastic fibers from the outer portion of the sclera has been noted.[1]

Embryology and Development

The sclera is formed by mesenchymal cells that condense around the optic cup during embryogenesis. Most of these cells are derived from the neural crest. However, cells in the temporal region of the sclera are probably derived from paraxial mesoderm that lies juxtaposed to the surface of the optic cup throughout the period of crest cell migration. The sclera develops anteriorly before 7 weeks of gestation and gradually extends posteriorly. The alignment of cells into parallel layers and the deposition of collagen fibrils are evidence of differentiation. Deposits of elastin and GAGs are added to the ECM at a later stage. By 3 months of gestation, some undifferentiated mesenchymal cells have migrated between the nerve fibers in the optic nerve. These cells become oriented transversely and synthesize ECM materials to form the lamina cribosa.[400,471]

Differentiation of the sclera in human embryos and fetuses with a gestational age between 6.4 and 24.0 weeks has been studied by light and electron microscopy.[400] The developmental route was found

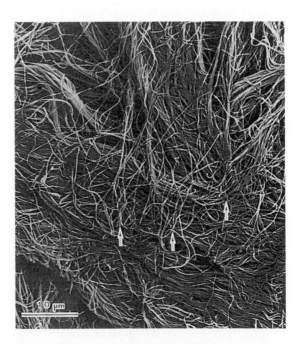

FIGURE 4-49 A tangential view of the collagen bundles in the sclera. Collagen fibrils run in a wavy fashion and intermingle within individual bundles. Note the loose networks of collagen fibrils around the bundles (*arrows*). (Magnification ×2700.) (From Komai Y, Ushiki T: *Invest Ophthalmol Vis Sci* 32:2244, 1991.)

to be anteroposterior and directed from inside outward. Continuous cytologic maturation begins anteriorly during week 7.2, with a loss of free ribosome and polysomes, an increase in the amount of rough-surfaced endoplasmic reticulum and Golgi complex components, and a significant increase in the addition of glycogen and lipid droplets in the choroidal half of the anterior scleral condensation; from there it progresses to the outer (episcleral) half. From the region of the future limbus, these cytodevelopmental events progress posteriorly. By week 13, there are no significant differences between anterior and posterior localization. With the beginning of week 10.9, no more differences were identified between the outer and the inner portions of the sclera. Portions of the endoplasmic reticulum denuded of ribosomes close to the plasmalemma were observed during the whole gestational period studied. In week 24, the diameter of the collagen fibrils had increased more than three times in comparison with week 6.4. Elastic microfibrils were found beginning with week 7.2, whereas the elastic deposits with central electron-translucent cores were characterized for the first time beginning with week 18.[400]

Development and growth of the sclera may be influenced by proteoglycan synthesis. Changes in proteoglycan synthesis in the posterior sclera are closely correlated with changes in ocular size and refraction, suggesting a close relationship between scleral proteoglycan composition and the growth state of the sclera.[361,441] Studies indicate that the synthesis and turnover of scleral proteoglycans is a dynamic process that is dramatically influenced by the visual environment.[284,298,359-361]

Form vision deprivation, either experimentally induced in animals or associated with ocular injury or pathologic conditions in humans, has been shown to result in axial elongation of the ocular globe and subsequent myopia.* Studies using both mammalian and avian models of myopia have shown that changes in the rate of proteoglycan synthesis and accumulation within the sclera are associated with axial elongation and the development of myopia.[327,359,363] In an avian model of form-deprivation myopia in the chick, myopia is clearly established after 1 week of visual deprivation and is accompanied by a larger negative refractive error resulting from an overall increase in globe size that results from an accelerated rate of sclera growth primarily at the posterior pole.[56,247,363]

*References 134, 151, 177, 299, 330, 356, 363, 373, 374, 408, 411, 443, 454, 461, 474, 490.

These changes in proteoglycan synthesis during the induction of and recovery from form-deprivation myopia correspond to periods when the vitreous chamber is rapidly elongating or has temporally ceased to grow, respectively.[156] Studies suggest that the rate of vitreous chamber elongation is directly related to the rate of proteoglycan synthesis within the posterior sclera in the chick eye.[359,360,363] The proteoglycan turnover in the sclera of normal and experimentally myopic chick eyes has been studied.[361] The turnover rate of SO_4-labeled scleral proteoglycans is vision dependent and is accelerated in the posterior sclera of chick eyes during the development of experimental myopia. The loss of proteoglycans from the scleral matrix involves proteolytic cleavage at various sites along the aggrecan core protein through the action, at least in part, of gelatinase A and/or stromelysin.

Scleral Hydration and Proteoglycans

Proteoglycans serve several biologic functions, including in vivo hydration regulation, structural integrity maintenance, growth regulation, matrix organization, and cell adhesion; they also bind certain growth factors.[165] The proteoglycans aggrecan, decorin, and biglycan, with their associated GAG side chains, have been localized to the sclera.

Aggrecan, a proteoglycan typically found in cartilage, is composed of a large (approximately 220 kD) core protein and functions to provide tissue with resilience resulting from the water-binding capacity of its chondroitin and keratan sulfate GAG side chains.[314] Decorin and biglycan, relatively small chondroitin-dermatan sulfate proteoglycans, are present in many connective tissues but differ in distribution and function.

Decorin, with an approximate molecular mass of 120 kD with a core protein of 45 kD, is present in close association with collagen fibrils of many, if not all, connective tissues, where it regulates collagen fibril formation and organization in the ECM.[398,456] Decorin has been shown to suppress cell growth by upregulating the cell cycle inhibitory protein p21, as well as by binding to TGF-β, thereby neutralizing its growth-promoting activity in Chinese hamster ovary cells.[80,486]

Biglycan, with an approximate molecular mass of 200 kD with a core protein of 45 kD, has been found on the surfaces of differentiating cells and is occasionally present in tissue locations in which decorin is completely absent.[201] Although no exact role for biglycan has been confirmed, the core protein of biglycan has been shown to bind TGF-β and to collagen type I, suggesting some functional similarities to decorin.[174,397]

Scleral proteoglycans have been characterized from human donor eyes aged 2 months to 94 years to identify age-related changes in the synthesis and/or accumulation of these ECM components.[363] The relative percentage of newly synthesized and total accumulated aggrecan increased approximately twofold to sixfold from infancy to 94 years. In contrast, the relative percentage of newly synthesized and total accumulated biglycan and decorin decreased by approximately 25%. Chromatography and Western blot results indicated that the absolute amounts of all three proteoglycans significantly increased in concentration within the sclera from birth to the fourth decade. Beyond the fourth decade, decorin and biglycan decreased in all scleral regions and were present in lowest concentrations by the ninth decade. In contrast, aggrecan, which was present in highest concentration in the posterior sclera, was not significantly reduced with increasing age.

Previously reported data on the GAG side chain composition of the human sclera show that it contains chondroitin sulfate (28% to 48%), dermatan sulfate (29% to 49%), heparan sulfate (2% to 12%), and hyaluronan (19% to 33%).[439] The presence of keratan sulfate has been reported by some but not by others.[28,35] Regional analysis of scleral GAGs indicates that the sclera around the optic nerve is the area richest in dermatan sulfate, the sclera around the equator is the richest in hyaluronic acid, and the sclera around the fovea is the richest in chondroitin sulfate.[439]

With increasing age, the sclera undergoes a progressive degeneration of collagen and elastic fibers, a loss of GAGs, scleral dehydration, and an accumulation of lipids and calcium salts.[34,212,452] These changes are associated with increases in tissue density, scleral thinning, yellowing, and decreases in scleral elasticity.[469]

Innervation

The stroma of the sclera is essentially devoid of innervation but allows for passage of nerves such as the optic nerve and ciliary nerves. Research has been conducted to study innervation of the scleral spur. The scleral spur, a wedge-shaped ridge that projects from the inner aspect of the anterior sclera, is composed of circumferentially oriented collagenous and elastic fibers.[200,386,397] The innervation of the presumably contractile, myofibroblast-like scleral spur cells in human and cynomolgus monkey eyes has been studied.[431] The close association of varicose axons with the myofibroblast-like scleral spur cells indicates that nervous signals modulate scleral spur cell tone. A sympathetic scleral spur cell innervation is present only in cynomolgus monkeys but seems to be absent in humans. Conversely, scleral spur axons of presumably parasympathetic origin are absent in the cynomolgus monkey but are present in humans. In both species a cholinergic innervation of the scleral spur seems to be rare or absent.

Wound Healing

A study has investigated the morphologic findings of wound healing in self-sealing incisions using ultrasound biomicroscopy and histology in rabbit eyes.[173] On days 1 and 2 postoperatively, detection of the scleral wound was possible. By day 7 postoperatively, the wound was undetectable. Through light microscopic observation, the scleral wound was open at day 1 postoperatively. On day 2 postoperatively, fibrovascular tissue barely extended into the wound. On day 5 postoperatively, connective tissue extended through the full thickness of the wound. On day 7, the connective tissue became dense and aligned with the lamella. In human eyes, with use of ultrasound biomicroscopy, the scleral incision was detectable until 5 days postoperatively but was undetectable at 7 days postoperatively.

Scleral Permeability

Recently, there has been interest in transscleral delivery of molecules and drugs to potentially treat posterior segment disease because of the difficulty reaching a therapeutic concentration of a drug transcorneally. Intravitreal or intravenous delivery may achieve therapeutic concentration but also may have unwanted side effects. Passive solute diffusion through an aqueous pathway is the primary mechanism of drug permeation across the sclera. The most reasonable diffusion pathway for drugs is through the interfibrillar aqueous media of the gel-like proteoglycans.

Important factors controlling diffusion rates across the sclera are tissue hydration, tissue thickness, and the size and volume fraction of proteoglycans present in the tissue.[101] The sclera has a large and accessible surface area; has a high degree of hydration, rendering it conducive to hydrophilic molecules; is hypocellular with few protein-binding sites; has a paucity of proteolytic enzymes; and has permeability that does not appreciably decline with age.[101,119,333,334]

The influence of scleral composition and hydration on solute transport in the rabbit sclera has been investigated.[30] The permeability coefficient (P, cm · sec^{-1}) is related to the diffusion coefficient (D, cm^2 · sec^{-1}) by the following formula:

$$P = DK/L$$

where K is the partition coefficient and L is the thickness of the sclera across which permeation is measured. The results showed that diffusion and partition coefficients are sensitive to solute MW, decreasing as MW increases. Diffusion and partition coefficients are sensitive to tissue hydration, increasing as hydration increases. Cross-linking of the sclera by glutaraldehyde reduced the partition coefficient significantly for solutes with an MW greater than 3 kD, and removal of GAG side chains has only a small effect on either diffusion or partition coefficients.

The swelling or hydration of the sclera as a function of pH and ionic strength has been studied.[186] The sclera swelled least near a pH of 4, and higher hydrations were achieved with lower ionic strengths. Collagen fibril diameters and D-periodicity were independent of tissue hydration and pH at hydrations higher than 1. Intermolecular spacing in the sclera decreased as ionic strength increased. Results indicated that the isoelectric points of the sclera were close to pH 4.

The effects of age, cryotherapy, transscleral diode laser, and surgical thinning on human scleral permeability showed that age, cryotherapy, and diode laser treatment do not alter scleral permeability, whereas surgical thinning significantly increases permeability.[332] Thermal damage to the human sclera has been studied in relation to temperature and duration of exposure to determine the heat tolerance of the sclera.[373] Results indicated that a temperature of 60° C for 1 minute is well tolerated by human donor sclera.

In addition, the effects of IOP on the permeability of human and rabbit sclera to water, dexamethasone, and carboxyfluorescein have been studied. The results showed that simulated IOP ranging from 15 to 60 mm Hg can decrease scleral permeability to small molecules by half when compared with the sclera with no pressure applied.[381] Scleral permeability to small molecules is thus a weak function of transscleral pressure, over the range of 0 to 60 mm Hg, and a strong function of MW.

The effect of prostaglandins on the permeability of human sclera in vitro showed that there was increased permeability of human sclera exposed to various prostaglandins in organ culture.[227] This increased permeability is accompanied by increased expression of matrix metalloproteinases. The increase in scleral permeability may be one mechanism by which prostaglandins decrease IOP when used topically. In another study the effect of 7-methylxanthine, theobromine, and acetazolamide was evaluated on the ultrastructure and biochemical composition of rabbit sclera.[439] 7-Methylxanthine and theobromine, metabolites of caffeine, increased collagen concentration and the diameter of collagen fibrils in the posterior sclera. There was an apparent loss of collagen induced by chronic treatment with acetazolamide.

The cytostatic substance mitomycin-C (MMC) is used intraoperatively in trabeculectomy as an adjunct therapy to improve outcomes from the surgery. The effect of concentration, time of application, and volumes of MMC on the intrascleral concentration versus the depth profile of MMC in vitro with human sclera showed that the intrascleral MMC concentration increased linearly with increasing concentration and not with increasing volume of the applied MMC solution.[136,453] The superficial concentration of intrascleral MMC decreased with increasing diffusion time as the deep concentration increased. After 30 minutes of diffusion time, equal concentrations of MMC were found in all layers.

A fiber matrix–predictive model of sclera has been developed to describe flux across tissue.[101] All parameters used corresponded to geometric and physiochemical properties of the tissue and of the solutes themselves. The values were obtained from independent measurements reported in the literature and were not derived or fitted. The predicted scleral permeabilities provided by this model showed good agreement with reported experimental data. Changes in the physiochemical parameters of the sclera had rather small effects on the permeability of small compounds, such as most conventional drugs. However, for larger molecules, such as proteins, DNA, virus vectors, and other new products of biotechnology, the model indicates that transscleral delivery could be significantly improved by taking advantage of thinner regions of tissue, by increasing scleral hydration, or by transient modification of the scleral ECM.

The permeability of the sclera has no apparent dependence on distribution coefficient and has a strong dependence on molecular radius.[353] The in vitro permeability of the sclera to high-molecular-weight compounds and the relationship between

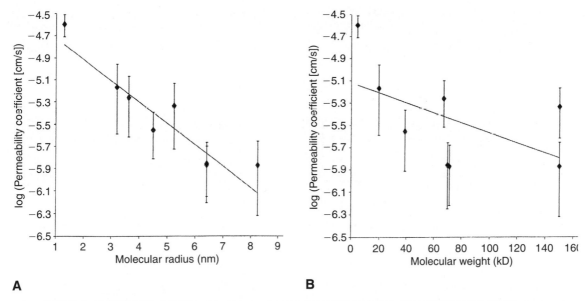

FIGURE 4-50 Scleral permeability versus molecular radius (**A**) and molecular weight (**B**). The least squares regression line is shown for each graph. (Redrawn from Maurice DM, Polgar J: *Invest Ophthalmol Vis Sci* 41:1181, 1977.)

scleral permeability and molecular size has also been investigated.[5] Scleral permeability decreased with increasing MW and molecular radius (Figure 4-50). The sclera was more permeable to globular proteins than to linear dextrans of similar MW. In vitro experiments have demonstrated that the sclera is permeable to molecules ranging from 70 to 150 kD.[296,333]

The transscleral delivery of an anti–intercellular adhesion molcule-1 (ICAM-1) monoclonal antibody (mAb) and its effect on inhibiting vascular endothelial growth factor (VEGF)–induced leukostasis in the choroid and retina as determined by measuring tissue myeloperoxidase (MPO) activity has been studied.[4] Transscleral delivery of anti–ICAM-1 mAb resulted in significant suppression of VEGF-induced leukostasis. This demonstrates that in vivo transscleral delivery is capable of maintaining significant levels of biologically active protein in the choroid and retina of the rabbit eye. The vector provided selective delivery with no measurable systemic absorption. Furthermore, the protein retained its biologic activity. Experimental evidence currently shows that the transscleral delivery of drugs can be accomplished and suggests great promise that this approach will provide new therapeutic options for treatment of diseases of the posterior segment of the eye.

CONCLUSION

In this chapter we presented the cornea as a dynamic organ that is well adapted to its functions of transmission and refraction of light. The cornea can successfully respond to wounding, refractive surgical procedures, and intraocular surgery, yet it is fragile and susceptible to disease and damage. We also presented a review of the sclera, which we hope will provide a greater understanding of this tissue. Research is being performed on this tissue to understand the development and growth of the sclera, which relates to changes in ocular size and refraction. In addition, in the field of transscleral drug delivery, investigators are trying to provide an alternate route of delivery for the treatment of posterior segment disease. We trust the explanation of corneal and scleral structure and function provided in this chapter can provide a point of view from which clinicians and scientists can approach dystrophies and diseases of the eye with deeper understanding and that understanding can form the basis for improved therapeutic and surgical approaches to pathologic conditions in the eye.

REFERENCES

1. Alexander RA, Garner A: Elastic and precursor fibres in the normal human eye, *Exp Eye Res* 36:305, 1983.

2. Alvarado J, Murphy C, Jester R: Age related changes in the basement membrane of the corneal epithelium, *Invest Ophthalmol Vis Sci* 24:1015, 1984.

3. Amano S, Shimizu K: Corneal endothelial changes after excimer laser photorefractive keratectomy, *Am J Ophthalmol* 116:692, 1993.

4. Ambati J, Gragoudas ES, Miller JW: Transscleral delivery of bioactive protein to the choroid and retina, *Invest Ophthalmol Vis Sci* 41:1186, 2000.

5. Ambati J et al: Diffusion of high molecular weight compounds through sclera, *Invest Ophthalmol Vis Sci* 41:1181, 2000.

6. Anderson NJ, Edelhauser HF: Toxicity of ocular surgical solutions, *Int Ophthalmol Clin* 39:91, 1999.

7. Anderson NJ et al: Intracameral anesthesia in vitro iris and corneal uptake and washout of 1% lidocaine hydrochloride, *Arch Ophthalmol* 117:225, 1999.

8. Anderson S et al: Developmentally regulated appearance of spliced variants of type XII collagen in the cornea, *Inv Ophthalmol Vis Sci* 41:55, 2000.

9. Anhalt GJ et al: Bullous pemphigoid autoantibodies are markers of corneal epithelial hemidesmosomes, *Invest Ophthalmol Vis Sci* 28:903, 1987.

10. Anseth A, Fransson LA: Studies on corneal polysaccharides. VI. Isolation of dermatan sulfate from corneal scar tissue, *Exp Eye Res* 8:302, 1969.

11. Avery RL, Connor TB Jr, Farazdaghi M: Systemic amiloride inhibits experimentally induced neovascularization, *Arch Ophthalmol* 108:1474, 1990.

12. Awosika AD et al: Corneal endothelial cell analysis in glaucoma patients, *Invest Ophthalmol Vis Sci* 39:S6, 1998.

13. Azar RG et al: Corneal endothelial evaluation following implanted intrastromal corneal ring segments, *Invest Ophthalmol Vis Sci* 40:S105, 1999.

14. Bahn CF et al: Classification of corneal endothelial disorders based on neural crest origin, *Ophthalmology* 91:558, 1984.

15. Battat L et al: Effects of laser in situ keratomileusis on tear production, clearance, and the ocular surface, *Ophthalmology* 108:1230, 2001.

16. Beebe DC, Masters BR: Cell lineage and the differentiation of corneal epithelial cells, *Invest Ophthalmol Vis Sci* 37:1815, 1996.

17. BenEzra D: Possible mediation of vasculogenesis by products of the immune reaction. In Silverstein AM, O'Connor RG (eds): *Immunology and immunopathology of the eye*, New York, 1978, Masson.

18. BenEzra D, Hemo I, Maltzir G: In vivo angiogenic activity of interleukins, *Arch Ophthalmol* 108:573, 1990.

19. Ben-Zvi A et al: Immunohistochemical characterization of extracellular matrix in the developing human cornea, *Curr Eye Res* 5:105, 1986.

20. Bergmanson JPG: Corneal damage in photokeratitis: why is it so painful? *Optom Vis Sci* 67:407, 1990.

21. Bergmanson JPG, Chu LWF: Corneal response to rigid contact lens wear, *Br J Ophthalmol* 66:667, 1982.

22. Blochberger TC et al: cDNA to chick lumican (corneal keratan sulfate proteoglycan) reveals homology to the small interstitial proteoglycan gene family and expression in muscle and intestine, *J Biol Chem* 267:347, 1992.

23. Bockman CS, Griffith M, Watsky MA: Properties of whole-cell ionic currents in cultured human corneal epithelial cells, *Invest Ophthalmol Vis Sci* 39:1143, 1998.

24. Boettner EA, Wolter JR: Transmission of the ocular media, *Invest Ophthalmol* 6:776, 1962.

25. Bogan SJ et al: Classification of normal corneal topography based on computer-assisted video keratography, *Arch Ophthalmol* 108:945, 1990.

26. Bonano J: Regulation of corneal epithelial intracellular pH, *Optom Vis Sci* 68:682, 1991.

27. Bonting S, Simon K, Hawkins N: Studies on sodium potassium activated adenosine triphosphatase. I. Quantitative distribution in several tissues of the cat, *Arch Biochem Biophys* 95:416, 1961.

28. Borcherding MS et al: Proteoglycans and collagen fibre organization in human corneoscleral tissue, *Exp Eye Res* 21:59, 1975.

29. Bossenbroek NM, Salahian TH, Ubels JL: Expression of nuclear retinoic acid receptor and retinoid X receptor in RNA in the cornea and conjunctiva, *Curr Eye Res* 17:462, 1998.

30. Boubriak OA et al: The effect of hydration and matrix composition on solute diffusion in rabbit sclera, *Exp Eye Res* 71:503, 2000.

31. Bourne WM, Kaufman HE: Specular microscopy of the human corneal endothelium in vivo, *Am J Ophthalmol* 81:319, 1976.

32. Bourne WM, McCarey BE, Kaufman HE: Clinical specular microscopy, *Trans Am Acad Ophthalmol Otolaryngol* 81:OP-743, 1976.

33. Bourne WM, Nelson LF, Hodge DO: Central corneal endothelial cell changes over a ten-year period, *Invest Ophthalmol Vis Sci* 38:779, 1997.

34. Broekhuyse RM: The lipid composition of aging sclera and cornea, *Ophthalmologica* 171:82, 1975.

35. Brown CT et al: Age-related changes of scleral hydration and sulfated glycosaminoglycans, *Mech Ageing Dev* 77:97, 1994.

36. Brown S, Hedbys B: The effect of ouabain on hydration of the cornea, *Invest Ophthalmol* 4:216, 1965.

37. Browning DJ, Proia AD: Ocular rosacea, *Surv Ophthalmol* 31:145, 1986.

38. Brubaker RF, Kupfer C: Microcryoscopic determination of the osmolality of interstitial fluid in the living rabbit cornea, *Invest Ophthalmol* 1:653, 1962.

39. Bruns RR et al: Type VI collagen in extracellular 100-nm periodic filaments and fibrils: identification by immuno-electron microscopy, *J Cell Biol* 103:393, 1986.

40. Buck RC: Measurement of centripetal migration of normal corneal epithelial cells in the mouse, *Invest Ophthalmol Vis Sci* 26:1296, 1985.

41. Burger PC, Chandler DB, Klintworth GK: Corneal vascularization as studied by scanning electron microscopy of vascular casts, *Lab Invest* 48:169, 1983.

42. Burstein NL: Preservative alteration of corneal permeability in humans and rabbits, *Invest Ophthalmol Vis Sci* 25:1453, 1984.

43. Burstein NL, Klyce SD: Electrophysiologic and morphologic effects of ophthalmic preparations on rabbit corneal endothelium, *Invest Ophthalmol Vis Sci* 16:899, 1977.

44. Butterfield CC, Neufeld AH: Cyclic nucleotide and mitosis in the rabbit cornea following superior cervical ganglionectomy, *Exp Eye Res* 25:427, 1977.

45. Candia OA: The flux rates of the Na-Cl cotransport mechanism in the frog corneal epithelium, *Curr Eye Res* 4:333, 1985.

46. Candia OA: Forskolin-induced HCO_3^- current across apical membrane of the frog corneal epithelium, *Am J Physiol* 259:C215, 1990.

47. Candia OA: A novel system to measure labelled CO_2 and HCO_3^- fluxes across epithelia: corneal epithelium as model tissue, *Exp Eye Res* 63:137, 1996.

48. Carlier MF: Control of actin dynamics, *Curr Opin Cell Biol* 10:45, 1998.

49. Carones F et al: The corneal endothelium after myopic excimer laser photorefractive keratectomy, *Arch Ophthalmol* 112:920, 1994.

50. Castaro JA, Bettelheim AA, Bettelheim FA: Water concentration gradients across bovine cornea, *Invest Ophthalmol Vis Sci* 29:963, 1988.

51. Cennamo G et al: Evaluation of corneal thickness and endothelial cells before and after excimer laser treatment, *Refract Corneal Surg* 10:137, 1994.

52. Cennamo G et al: The corneal endothelium 12 months after photorefractive keratectomy in high myopia, *Acta Ophthalmol* 75:128, 1997.

53. Chakravarti S et al: Lumican regulates collagen fibril assembly, skin fragility and corneal opacity in the absence of lumican, *J Cell Biol* 141:1277, 1998.

54. Chaloin-Dufau C et al: Identification of keratins 3 and 12 in corneal epithelium of vertebrates, *Epithel Cell Biol* 2:120, 1993.

55. Chandrasekher G, Bazan NG, Bazan HEP: Selective changes in protein kinase C (PKC) isoform expression in rabbit corneal epithelium during wound healing: inhibition of corneal epithelial repair by PKC-alpha antisense, *Exp Eye Res* 67:603, 1998.

56. Christiensen AM, Wallman J: Evidence that increased scleral growth underlies visual deprivation myopia in chicks, *Invest Ophthalmol Vis Sci* 32:2143, 1991.

57. Chung EH et al: Epithelial regeneration after limbus-to-limbus debridement: expression of alpha-enolase in stem and transient amplifying cells, *Invest Ophthalmol Vis Sci* 36:1336, 1995.

58. Chung EH et al: Synchronization of the G1/S transition in response to corneal debridement, *Invest Ophthalmol Vis Sci* 40:1952, 1999.

59. Cintron C, Covington HI, Kublin CL: Morphologic analysis of proteoglycans in rabbit corneal scars, *Invest Ophthalmol Vis Sci* 31:1789, 1990.

60. Cintron C, Kublin CL, Covington H: Quantitative studies of corneal epithelial wound healing in rabbits, *Curr Eye Res* 1:507, 1982.

61. Cobo LM, Haynes BF: Early corneal findings in Cogan's syndrome, *Ophthalmology* 91:903, 1984.

62. Cogan DG: Applied anatomy and physiology of the cornea, *Trans Am Acad Ophthalmol* 55:329, 1951.

63. Cogan DG, Kinsey VE: The cornea. V. Physiologic aspects, *Arch Ophthalmol* 28:661, 1942.

64. Collin HB, Kenyon KR, Rowsey JJ: Lymphatic vessels in chemically burned human corneas, *Cornea* 5:223, 1986.

65. Collins MJ et al: Effects of laser in situ keratomileusis (LASIK) on the corneal endothelium 3 years postoperatively, *Am J Ophthalmol* 131:1, 2001.

66. Conners MS et al: A closed eye contact lens model of corneal inflammation: part I—increase synthesis of cytochrome R450 arachidonic acid metabolism, *Invest Ophthalmol Vis Sci* 36:828, 1995.

67. Conners MS et al: A closed eye contact lens model of corneal inflammation: part II. Inhibition of cytochrome P450 arachidonic acid metabolism alleviates inflammatory sequelae, *Invest Ophthalmol Vis Sci* 36:841, 1995.

68. Cornuet PK, Blochberger TC, Hassell JR: Molecular polymorphism of lumican during corneal development, *Invest Ophthalmol Vis Sci* 35:870, 1994.

69. Corpuz LM et al: Molecular cloning and tissue distribution of keratocan, *J Biol Chem* 271:9759, 1996.

70. Costar L, Fransson LA: Isolation and characterization of dermatan sulfate proteoglycans from bovine sclera, *Biochem J* 193:143, 1981.

71. Cox JL et al: The transparency of the mammalian cornea, *J Physiol* 210:601, 1970.

72. Crosson CE, Klyce SD, Beuerman RW: Epithelial wound closure in the rabbit cornea, *Invest Ophthalmol Vis Sci* 27:464, 1986.

73. Dabezies OH: *Contact lenses: the CLAO guide to basic science and clinical practice,* Boston, Little, Brown, 1989.

74. Danielson KG et al: Targeted disruption of decorin leads to abnormal collagen fibril morphology and skin fragility, *J Cell Biol* 136:729, 1997.

75. Danjo Y, Gipson IK: Actin 'purse string' filaments are anchored by E-cadherin-mediated adherens junction at the leading edge of the epithelial wound, providing coordinated cell movement, *J Cell Sci* 111:3323, 1998.

76. Davis KL et al: Induction of corneal epithelial cytochrome P-450 arachidonate metabolism by contact lens wear, *Invest Ophthalmol Vis Sci* 33:292, 1992.

77. Davison PF, Galbavy EJ: Connective tissue remodeling in corneal and scleral wounds, *Invest Ophthalmol Vis Sci* 27:1478, 1986.

78. Deg JK, Zavala EY, Binder PS: Delayed corneal wound healing following radial keratotomy, *Ophthalmology* 92:734, 1985.

79. Dellaert MM et al: Influence of topical human epidermal growth factor on postkeratoplasty reepithelialization, *Br J Ophthalmol* 81:391, 1997.

80. De Luca A, Manoranjan S, Baldi A: Decorin-induced growth suppression is associated with up-regulation of p21, an inhibitor of cyclin-dependent kinases, *J Biol Chem* 271:18961, 1996.

81. Deutsch TA, Hughes WF: Suppressive effects of indomethacin on thermally induced neovascularization of rabbit corneas, *Am J Ophthalmol* 87:536, 1979.

82. Dikstein S, Maurice DM: The metabolic basis to the fluid pump in the cornea, *J Physiol* 221:29, 1972.

83. Doane MG, Jensen AD, Dohlman CH: Penetration routes of topically applied eye medications, *Am J Ophthalmol* 85:303, 1978.

84. Dohlman CH, Hedbys BO, Mishima S: The swelling pressure of the cornea, *Invest Ophthalmol Vis Sci* 1:158, 1962.

85. Dong Y et al: Differential expression of two gap junction proteins in corneal epithelium, *Eur J Cell Biol* 64:95, 1994.

86. Donn A, Maurice DM, Mills NL: Studies in the living cornea in vitro: II. The active transport of sodium across the epithelium, *Arch Ophthalmol* 62:748, 1959.

87. Doughty MJ: Re-assessment of the potential impact of physiologically relevant pH changes on the hydration properties of the isolated mammalian corneal stroma, *Biochimica Biophysica Acta* 1472:99, 1999.

88. Duffin RM et al: Flurbiprofen in the treatment of corneal neovascularization induced by contact lenses, *Am J Ophthalmol* 93:607, 1982.

89. Duke-Elder S: *System of ophthalmology,* vol 4, London, 1968, Henry Kimpton.

90. Duke-Elder S, Wybar KC: *System of ophthalmology,* vol II, *anatomy of the visual system,* London, 1961, Henry Kimpton.

91. Dunlevy JR et al: Cloning and chromosomal localization of mouse keratocan, a corneal keratan sulfate proteoglycan, *Mamm Genome* 9:316, 1998.

92. Dunlevy JR et al: Identification of the N-linked oligosaccharide sites in chick corneal lumican and keratocan that receive keratan sulfate, *J Biol Chem* 273:9615, 1998.

93. Edelhauser HF, Gonnering R, Van Horn DL: Intraocular irrigating solutions: a comparative study of BSS PLUS and lactated Ringer's solution, *Arch Ophthalmol* 96:516, 1978.

94. Edelhauser HF et al: Intraocular irrigating solutions: their effect on the corneal endothelium, *Arch Ophthalmol* 93:648, 1975.

95. Edelhauser HF et al: Comparative toxicity of intraocular irrigating solutions on the corneal endothelium, *Am J Ophthalmol* 81:473, 1976.

96. Edelhauser HF et al: The effect of thiol-oxidation of glutathione with diamide on corneal endothelial function, junctional complexes and microfilaments, *J Cell Biol* 68:567, 1976.

97. Edelhauser HF et al: Corneal edema and the intraocular use of epinephrine, *Am J Ophthalmol* 93:327, 1982.

98. Edelhauser HF et al: Swelling in the isolated perfused cornea induced by 12(R) hydroxyeicosatetraenoic acid, *Invest Ophthalmol Vis Sci* 34:2953, 1993.

99. Edelhauser HF et al: The effects of 12(R)HETE and its metabolite 8(R)HHDTrE on corneal endothelial function. In Green K et al (eds): *Advance in ocular toxicology,* New York, 1997, Plenum Press.

100. Edward DP et al: Heterogeneity in macular corneal dystrophy, *Arch Ophthalmol* 106:1579, 1988.

101. Edwards A, Prausnitz MR: Fiber matrix model of sclera and corneal stroma for drug delivery to the eye, *AIChE J* 44:214, 1998.

102. Efron N, Carney LG: Oxygen levels beneath the closed eyelid, *Invest Ophthalmol Vis Sci* 18:93, 1979.

103. Elliott GF, Goodfellow JM, Woolgar AE: Swelling studies of bovine corneal stroma without bounding membranes, *J Physiol* 298:453, 1980.

104. Epstein RJ, Hendricks RL, Stulting RD: Interleukin 2 induces corneal neovascularization in A/J mice, *Cornea* 9:318, 1990.

105. Epstein RJ, Hughes WF: Lymphocyte-induced corneal neovascularization: a morphologic assessment, *Invest Ophthalmol Vis Sci* 21:87, 1981.

106. Epstein RJ, Stulting RD: Corneal neovascularization induced by stimulated lymphocytes in inbred mice, *Invest Ophthalmol Vis Sci* 28:1508, 1987.

107. Epstein RJ, Stulting RD: Lymphocyte-induced corneal neovascularization in inbred mice, *Invest Ophthalmol Vis Sci* 28:61, 1987.

108. Epstein RJ et al: Corneal opacities and anterior segment anomalies in DBA/2 mice, *Cornea* 5:95, 1986.

109. Epstein RJ et al: Corneal neovascularization, pathogenesis and inhibition, *Cornea* 6:250, 1987.

110. Farrell RA, McCally RL, Tatham PER: Wave-length dependencies of light scattering in normal and cold swollen rabbit corneas and their structural implications, *J Physiol* 233:589, 1973.

111. Farrugia G, Rae JL: Regulation of a potassium-selective current in rabbit corneal epithelium by cyclic GMP, carbachol and diltiazem, *J Membr Biol* 129:99, 1992.

112. Farrugia G, Rae JL: Effect of volume changes on a potassium current in rabbit corneal epithelial cells, *Am J Physiol* 264:C1238, 1993.

113. Fair I, Goldstick T: Dynamics of water transport in swelling membranes, *J Cell Sci* 20:962, 1965.

114. Fischbarg J: Active and passive properties of rabbit cornea endothelium, *Exp Eye Res* 15:615, 1973.

115. Folkman J, Klagsbrun M: Angiogenic factors, *Science* 235:442, 1987.

116. Folkman J et al: A heparin-binding angiogenic protein-basic fibroblast growth factor is stored within basement membrane, *Am J Pathol* 130:393, 1988.

117. Folkman J et al: Control of angiogenesis with synthetic heparin substitutes, *Science* 243:1490, 1989.

118. Foster CS, Forstot SL, Wilson LA: Mortality rate in rheumatoid arthritis patients developing necrotizing scleritis or peripheral ulcerative keratitis: effects of systemic immunosuppression, *Ophthalmology* 91:1253, 1984.

119. Foster CS, Sainz de la Maza M: *The sclera,* New York, 1994, Springer-Verlag.

120. Foster CS, Wilson LA, Ekins MB: Immunosuppressive therapy for progressive ocular cicatricial pemphigoid, *Ophthalmol* 89:340, 1982.

121. Freeman JL: Comparative biochemistry of type I collagens from human cornea, sclera and skin. In Hollyfield JG (ed): *Proceedings of the fourth international symposium on the structure of the eye,* Amsterdam, 1981, Elsevier.

122. Freund DE et al: Ultrastructure in anterior and posterior stroma of perfused human and rabbit corneas, *Inv Ophthalmol Vis Sci* 36:1508, 1995.

123. Friedenwald JS, Buscke W: Mitotic and wound healing activities of the corneal epithelium, *Arch Ophthalmol* 32:410, 1944.

124. Friedman MH, Green K: Swelling rate of corneal stroma, *Exp Eye Res* 12:239, 1971.

125. Friend J, Hassel JR: Biochemistry of the cornea. In Smolin G, Thoft RA (eds): *The cornea,* Boston 1994, Little, Brown.

126. Fullard RJ, Wilson GS: Investigation of sloughed corneal epithelial cells collected by non-invasive irrigation of the corneal surface, *Curr Eye Res* 5:847, 1986.

127. Fullwood NJ et al: Synchrotron x-ray diffraction studies of keratoconus corneal stroma, *Invest Ophthalmol Vis Sci* 33:1734, 1992.

128. Fullwood NJ et al: Atomic force microscopy of the cornea and sclera, *Curr Eye Res* 14:529, 1995.

129. Funderburgh JL et al: Arterial lumican: properties of a corneal-type keratan sulfate proteoglycan from bovine aorta, *J Biol Chem* 266:24773, 1991.

130. Funderburgh JL et al: Sequence and structural implications of a bovine keratan sulfate proteoglycan core protein: protein 37B represents bovine lumican and proteins 37A and 25 are unique, *J Biol Chem* 268:11874, 1993.

131. Funderburgh JL et al: Mimecan, the 25-kDa corneal keratan sulfate proteoglycan, is a product of the gene producing osteoglycin, *J Biol Chem* 44:28089, 1997.

132. Gachon AM et al: Immunological and electrophoretic studies of human tear proteins, *Exp Eye Res* 29:539, 1979.

133. Gallar J et al: Effects of capsaicin on corneal wound healing, *Invest Ophthalmol Vis Sci* 31:1968, 1990.

134. Gee SS, Tabarra KF: Increase in ocular axial length in patients with corneal opacification, *Ophthalmology* 95:1276, 1988.

135. Geiger B et al: Immunoelectron microscope studies of membrane microfilament interactions: distributions of alpha-actinin, tropomyosin, and vinculin in intestinal epithelial brush border and chicken gizzard smooth muscle cells, *J Cell Biol* 91:614, 1981.

136. Georgopoulos M et al: In vitro diffusion of mitomycin-C into human sclera after episcleral application: impact of diffusion time, *Exp Eye Res* 71:453, 2000.

137. Geroski DH, Edelhauser HF: Quantitation of Na/K ATPase pump sites in the rabbit corneal endothelium, *Invest Ophthalmol Vis Sci* 25:1056, 1984.

138. Geroski DH, Kies JC, Edelhauser HF: The effects of ouabain on endothelial function in human and rabbit corneas, *Curr Eye Res* 3:331, 1984.

139. Geroski DH, Matsuda M, Edelhauser HF: Pump function of the human corneal endothelium: effects of age and corneal guttata, *Ophthalmol* 92:759, 1985.

140. Gipson IK, Inatomi T: Mucin genes expressed by the ocular surface epithelium, *Prog Retin Eye Res* 16:81, 1996.
141. Gipson IK, Jirawuthiworavong GV: Corneal epithelial wound healing: adhesion during migration. In Nishida T (ed): *Corneal healing responses to injuries and refractive surgeries,* The Hague; New York, 1998, Kugler Publications.
142. Gipson IK, Kiorpes TC: Epithelial sheet movement: protein and glycoprotein synthesis, *Dev Biol* 92:259, 1982.
143. Gipson IK, Spurr-Michaud SJ, Tisdale AS: Anchoring fibrils form a complex network in human and rabbit corneas, *Invest Ophthalmol Vis Sci* 28:212, 1987.
144. Gipson IK, Spurr-Michaud SJ, Tisdale AJ: Hemidesmosomes and anchoring fibril collagen appear synchronously during development and wound healing, *Dev Biol* 126:253, 1988.
145. Gipson IK et al: Hemidesmosome formation in vitro, *J Cell Biol* 97:849, 1983.
146. Gipson IK et al: Reassembly of the anchoring structures of the corneal epithelium during wound repair in the rabbit, *Invest Ophthalmol Vis Sci* 30:425, 1989.
147. Glasser DB et al: Effect of intraocular irrigating solutions on the corneal endothelium after anterior chamber irrigation, *Am J Ophthalmol* 99:321, 1985.
148. Gobbels M, Spitznos M: Effects of artificial tears on corneal epithelial permeability in dry eyes, *Graefes Arch Clin Exp Ophthalmol* 229:345, 1991.
149. Goldman JN, Benedek GB: The relationship between morphology and transparency in the nonswelling corneal stroma of the shark, *Invest Ophthalmol* 6:574, 1967.
150. Goldman JN et al: Structural alterations affecting transparency in swollen human corneas, *Invest Ophthalmol* 7:501, 1968.
151. Gollender M, Thorn F, Erickson P: Development of axial ocular dimensions following eyelid suture in the cat, *Vis Res* 19:221, 1979.
152. Gonnering RS et al: The pH tolerance of the rabbit and human corneal endothelium, *Invest Ophthalmol Vis Sci* 18:373, 1979.
153. Goodman WM et al: Unique parameters in the healing of linear partial thickness penetrating corneal incisions in rabbit: immunohistochemical evaluation, *Curr Eye Res* 8:305, 1989.
154. Gospodarowicz D et al: The identification and localization of fibronectin in cultured corneal endothelial cells: cell surface polarity and physiological implications, *Exp Eye Res* 29:485, 1979.
155. Gosset AR, Dohlman CH: The tensile strength of corneal wounds, *Arch Ophthalmol* 79:595, 1968.
156. Gottlieb MD, Joshi HB, Nickla DC: Scleral changes in chicks with form-deprivation myopia, *Curr Eye Res* 9:1157, 1990.
157. Green K et al: Rabbit endothelial response to ophthalmic preservatives, *Arch Ophthalmol* 95:2218, 1977.
158. Green K et al: Chlorhexidine effects on corneal epithelium and endothelium, *Arch Ophthalmol* 98:1273, 1980.
159. Grignolo A: Studies on the submicroscopical structure of the ocular tissues, *Boll Ocul* 33:513, 1954.
160. Hamann S et al: Aquaporins in complex tissues: distribution of aquaporins 1-5 in human and rat eye, *Am J Physiol* 274:C1332, 1998.
161. Hamano H et al: Effect of contact lens wear on the mitosis of corneal epithelial cells and the amount of lactate in aqueous humor, *Jpn J Ophthalmol* 27:451, 1983.
162. Hanna C, Bicknell DS, O'Brien J: Cell turnover in the adult human eye, *Arch Ophthalmol* 65:695, 1961.
163. Hanna C, O'Brien JE: Cell production and migration in the epithelium layer of the cornea, *Arch Ophthalmol* 64:536, 1960.
164. Harris JE, Nordquist LT: Hydration of the cornea: I. The transport of water from the cornea, *Am J Ophthalmol* 40:100, 1955.
165. Hassell JR et al: Proteoglycan gene families, *Adv Mol Cell Biol* 6:69, 1993.
166. Hay ED: Development of the vertebrate cornea, *Int Rev Cytol* 63:263, 1980.
167. Haynes WL, Proia AD, Klintworth GK: Effect of inhibitors of arachidonic acid metabolism on corneal neovascularization in the rat, *Invest Ophthalmol Vis Sci* 30:1588, 1989.
168. Hazlett CD et al: Desquamation of the corneal epithelium in the immature mouse: a scanning and transmission microscopy study, *Exp Eye Res* 31:21, 1980.
169. Hedbys BO: The role of polysaccharides in corneal swelling, *Exp Eye Res* 1:81, 1961.
170. Hedbys BO, Dohlman CH: A new method for determination of the swelling pressure of the corneal stroma in vitro, *Exp Eye Res* 2:122, 1963.
171. Hedbys BO, Mishima S, Maurice DM: The imbibition pressure of the corneal stroma, *Exp Eye Res* 2:99, 1963.
172. Hendricks RL et al: The effect of flurbiprofen on herpes simplex virus type 1 stromal keratitis in mice, *Invest Ophthalmol Vis Sci* 31:1503, 1990.
173. Hikichi T et al: Wound healing of scleral self-sealing incision: a comparison of ultrasound biomicroscopy and histology findings, *Graefes Arch Clin Exp Ophthalmol* 236:775, 1998.
174. Hildebrand A et al: Interaction of the small interstitial proteoglycans biglycan, decorin and fibromodulin with transforming growth factor beta, *Biochem J* 302:527, 1994.
175. Hill RM, Fatt I: How dependent is the cornea on the atmosphere? *J Am Optom Assoc* 35:873, 1964.
176. Hirakata A, Gupta AG, Proia AD: Effect of protein kinase C inhibitors and activators on corneal re-epithelialization in the rat, *Invest Ophthalmol Vis Sci* 34:216, 1993.
177. Hodos W, Kuenzel WJ: Retinal-image degradation produces ocular enlargement in chicks, *Invest Ophthalmol Vis Sci* 25:652, 1984.
178. Hodson S, Miller F: The bicarbonate ion pump in the endothelium which regulates the hydration of the rabbit cornea, *J Physiol* 236:271, 1974.
179. Hodson SA, Wigham CG: Effect of glutathione on human corneal transendothelial potential difference, *J Physiol* 301:34, 1980.
180. Hogan MJ, Alvarado JA, Weddell E: *Histology of the human eye,* Philadelphia, 1971, WB Saunders.
181. Holden BA, Sweeney DF: The oxygen tension and temperature of the superior palpebral conjunctiva, *Acta Ophthalmol* 63:100, 1985.
182. Holden BA et al: Effects of cataract surgery on corneal function, *Invest Ophthalmol Vis Sci* 22:343, 1982.
183. Holden BA et al: Effects of long-term extended contact lens wear on the human cornea, *Invest Ophthalmol Vis Sci* 26:1489, 1985.
184. Hoppenreijs VPT et al: Effects of human epidermal growth factor on endothelial wound healing of human corneas, *Invest Ophthalmol Vis Sci* 33:1946, 1992.
185. Hoppenreijs VPT et al: Basic fibroblast growth factor stimulates corneal endothelial cell growth and endothelial wound healing of human corneas, *Invest Ophthalmol Vis Sci* 35:931, 1994.
186. Huang Y, Meek KM: Swelling studies on the cornea and sclera: the effects of pH and ionic strength, *Biophys J* 77:1655, 1999.
187. Huff J, Green K: Demonstration of active sodium transport across the isolated rabbit corneal endothelium, *Curr Eye Res* 1:113, 1981.

188. Hughes RA: Biochemistry of the corneal stroma, master's thesis, Milton Keynes, England, 1995, The Open University.

189. Hull DS et al: Effect of epinephrine on the corneal endothelium, *Am J Ophthalmol* 79:245, 1975.

190. Hull DS et al: Corneal endothelial bicarbonate transport and the effect of carbonic anhydrase inhibitors on endothelial permeability, fluxes and corneal thickness, *Invest Ophthalmol Vis Sci* 16:883, 1977.

191. Hyldahl L: Factor VIII expression in the human embryonic eye: differences between endothelial cells of different origin, *Ophthalmologica* 191:184, 1985.

192. Hyldahl L, Aspinall R, Watt FM: Immunolocalization of keratan sulphate in the human embryonic cornea and other fetal organs, *J Cell Sci* 80:181, 1986.

193. Inatomi T et al: Human cornea and conjunctival epithelia express MUC1 mucin, *Invest Ophthalmol Vis Sci* 36:1818, 1995.

194. Ingber D, Folkman J: Inhibition of angiogenesis through modulation of collagen metabolism, *Lab Invest* 59:44, 1988.

195. Inomata H, Smelear GK, Polack FM: Corneal vascularization in experimental uveitis and graft rejection, *Invest Ophthalmol Vis Sci* 10:840, 1971.

196. Iradier MT et al: Intraocular lidocaine in phacoemulsification: an endothelium and blood-aqueous barrier permeability study, *Ophthalmology* 107:896, 2000.

197. Irvine AD et al: Mutations in cornea-specific keratin K3 or K12 genes cause Meesmann's corneal dystrophy, *Nat Genet* 16:184, 1997.

198. Isager P, Hjortdal JO, Ehlers N: The effect of 193-nm excimer laser radiation on the human corneal endothelial cell density, *Acta Ophthalmol* 74:224, 1996.

199. Isager P et al: Endothelial cell loss after photorefractive keratectomy for myopia, *Acta Ophthalmol* 76:304, 1998.

200. Iwamoto T: Light and electron microscopy of the presumed elastic components of the trabeculae and scleral spur of the human eye, *Invest Ophthalmol Vis Sci* 3:144, 1964.

201. Jarvelainen HT et al: Differential expression of small chondroitin/dermatan sulfate proteoglycans, PG-I/biglycan and PG-II/decorin, by vascular smooth muscle and endothelial cells in culture, *J Biol Chem* 266:23274, 1991.

202. Jentsch TJ, Keller SK, Wiederholt M: Ion transport in cultured bovine corneal endothelial cells, *Curr Eye Res* 4:361, 1985.

203. Jester JV, Petroll M, Cavanagh DH: Corneal stromal wound healing in refractive surgery: the role of myofibroblasts, *Prog Retin Eye Res* 18:311, 1999.

204. Jester JV et al: Induction of alpha-smooth muscle actin expression and myofibroblast transformation in cultured corneal keratocytes, *Cornea* 15:505, 1996.

205. Jester JV et al: Inhibition of corneal fibrosis by topical application of blocking antibodies to TGF-beta in the rabbit, *Cornea* 16:177, 1997.

206. Johnson DH, Bourne WM, Campbell RJ: The ultrastructure of Descemet's membrane: I. Changes with age in normal corneas, *Arch Ophthalmol* 100:1942, 1982.

207. Joyce NC, Martin ED, Neufeld AH: Corneal endothelial wound closure in vitro; effects of EGF and/or indomethacin, *Invest Ophthalmol Vis Sci* 30:1548, 1989.

208. Joyce NC, Meklir B, Neufeld AH: In vitro pharmacological separation of corneal endothelial migration and spreading responses, *Invest Ophthalmol Vis Sci* 31:1816, 1990.

209. Joyce NC et al: Cell cycle protein expression and proliferative status in human corneal cells, *Invest Ophthalmol Vis Sci* 37:645, 1996.

210. Jumblatt MM, Neufeld AH: Characterization of cyclic AMP–mediated wound closure of the rabbit corneal epithelium, *Curr Eye Res* 1:189, 1981.

211. Junghaus BM, Collin HB: The limbal vascular response to corneal injury: an autoradiographic study, *Cornea* 8:141, 1989.

212. Kanai A, Kaufman HE: Electron microscopic studies of the elastic fiber in the human sclera, *Invest Ophthalmol Vis Sci* 11:816, 1972.

213. Kang F et al: Cultured bovine epithelial cells express a functional aquaporin water channel, *Invest Ophthalmol Vis Sci* 40:253, 1999.

214. Kang SS et al: Inhibitory effect of PGE2 on EGF-induced MAP kinase activity and rabbit corneal epithelial proliferation, *Invest Ophthalmol Vis Sci* 41:2164, 2000.

215. Kangas TA et al: Loss of stromal glycosaminoglycans during corneal edema, *Invest Ophthalmol Vis Sci* 31:1994, 1990.

216. Kao WW et al: Healing of corneal epithelial defects in plasminogen- and fibrinogen-deficient mice, *Invest Ophthalmol Vis Sci* 39:502, 1998.

217. Kaye G: Stereologic measurement of cell volume fraction of rabbit corneal stroma, *Arch Ophthalmol* 82:792, 1969.

218. Kaye GI et al: Further studies of the effect of perfusion with a Ca^{++}-free medium on the rabbit cornea: extraction of stromal components. In Hollyfield JG, Acosta Vidrio E (eds): *The structure of the eye,* New York, 1982, Elsevier Biomedical.

219. Keeley FW, Morin JD, Vesely S: Characterization of collagen from normal human sclera, *Exp Eye Res* 39:553, 1984.

220. Keene DR, Engvall E, Glanville RW: Ultrastructure of type VI collagen in human skin and cartilage suggests an anchoring function for this filamentous network, *J Cell Biol* 107:1995, 1988.

221. Kenyon KR: Mesenchymal dysgenesis in Peters' anomaly, sclerocornea and congenital endothelial dystrophy, *Exp Eye Res* 21:125, 1975.

222. Kenyon KR: Ocular manifestations and pathology of systemic mucopolysaccharidoses, *Birth Defects* 12:133, 1976.

223. Kenyon KR: Recurrent corneal erosion: pathogenesis and therapy, *Int Ophthalmol Clin* 19:169, 1979.

224. Khodadoust AA et al: Adhesion of regenerating corneal epithelium, *Am J Ophthalmol* 65:339, 1968.

225. Kilp H, Hersig-Salentin B, Framing D: Metabolites and enzymes in the corneal epithelium after extended contact lens wear: the effects of contact lenses on the normal physiology and anatomy of the cornea—symposium summary, *Curr Eye Res* 4:738, 1985.

226. Kim EK et al: Corneal endothelial cytoskeletal changes in F-actin with aging, diabetes, and after cytochalasin exposure, *Am J Ophthalmol* 114:329, 1992.

227. Kim J-W et al: Increased human scleral permeability with prostaglandin exposure, *Invest Ophthalmol Vis Sci* 42:1514, 2001.

228. Kim KS, Jean SJ, Edelhauser HF: Corneal endothelial morphology and barrier function following excimer laser photorefractive keratectomy. In Lass J et al (eds): *Advances in corneal research,* New York, 1997, Plenum Press.

229. Kim T et al: The effects of intraocular lidocaine on the corneal endothelium, *Ophthalmology* 105:125, 1998.

230. Kinoshita S, Friend J, Thoft RA: Sex chromatin of donor corneal epithelium in rabbits, *Invest Ophthalmol Vis Sci* 21:434, 1981.

231. Klintworth GK, Burger PC: Neovascularization of the cornea: current concepts of its pathogenesis, *Int Ophthalmol Clin* 23:27, 1983.

232. Klintworth GK et al: Macular corneal dystrophy: lack of keratan sulfate in serum and cornea, *Ophthalmic Paediatr Genet* 7:139, 1986.

233. Klyce SD: Electrical profiles in the corneal epithelium, *J Physiol* 226:407, 1977.

234. Klyce SD: Stromal lactate accumulation can account for corneal oedema osmotically following epithelial hypoxia in the rabbit, *J Physiol* 321:49, 1981.

235. Klyce SD, Beuerman RW: Structure and function of the cornea. In Kaufman HE et al (eds): *The cornea,* New York, 1988, Churchill Livingstone.

236. Klyce SD, Beuerman RW, Crosson CE: Alteration of corneal epithelium in transport by sympathectomy, *Invest Ophthalmol Vis Sci* 26:434, 1985.

237. Klyce SD, Crosson CE: Transport processes across the rabbit corneal epithelium: a review, *Curr Eye Res* 4:323, 1985.

238. Klyce SD, Dohlman CH, Tolpin DW: In vivo determination of corneal swelling pressure, *Exp Eye Res* 11:220, 1971.

239. Klyce SD, Neufeld AH, Zadunaisky JA: The activation of chloride transport by epinephrine and Db cyclic AMP in the cornea of the rabbit, *Invest Ophthalmol* 12:127, 1973.

240. Koester CJ et al: Wide-field specular microscopy: clinical and research applications, *Ophthalmol* 87:849, 1980.

241. Komai Y, Ushiki T: The three-dimensional organization of collagen fibrils in the human cornea and sclera, *Invest Ophthalmol Vis Sci* 32:2244, 1991.

242. Kuang K et al: Effects of ambient bicarbonate, phosphate and carbonic anhydrase inhibitors on fluid transport across rabbit cornea endothelium, *Exp Eye Res* 50:487, 1990.

243. Kupfer C, Kaiser-Kupfer MI: Observations on the development of the anterior chamber angle with reference to the pathogenesis of congenital glaucomas, *Am J Ophthalmol* 88:424, 1979.

244. Kurpakus MA, Maniaci MT, Esco M: Expression of keratins K12, K4 and K14 during development of ocular surface epithelium, *Curr Eye Res* 13:805, 1994.

245. Kurpakus MA, Stock EL, Jones JRC: Expression of the 55-kD/64-kD corneal keratins in ocular surface epithelium, *Invest Ophthalmol Vis Sci* 31:448, 1990.

246. Kus MM et al: Endothelium and pachymetry of clear grafts 15 to 33 years after penetrating keratoplasty: a report on 20 patients, *Am J Ophthalmol* 127:600, 1999.

247. Kusakari T, Sato T, Tokoro T: Regional scleral changes in form-deprivation myopia in chicks, *Exp Eye Res* 64:465, 1997.

248. Kuwabara T, Perkins DG, Cogan DG: Sliding of the epithelium in experimental corneal wounds, *Invest Ophthalmol* 15:4, 1976.

249. Laing RH, Sandstrom MM, Leibowitz HM: In vivo photomicrography of the corneal epithelium, *Arch Ophthalmol* 93:143, 1975.

250. Larke JR, Hirji NK: Some clinically observed phenomena in extended contact lens wear, *Br J Ophthalmol* 63:475, 1979.

251. Lass JH et al: Morphologic and fluorophotometric analysis of the corneal endothelium in long-term hard and soft contact lens wearers, *CLAO J* 14:105, 1988.

252. Latvala T et al: Distribution of alpha 6 and beta 4 integrins following epithelial abrasion in the rabbit cornea, *Acta Ophthalmol Scand* 74:21, 1996.

253. Lavker RM et al: Relative proliferative rates of limbal and corneal epithelia: implications of corneal epithelial migration, circadian rhythm, and suprabasally located DNA-synthesizing keratinocytes, *Invest Ophthalmol Vis Sci* 32:1864, 1991.

254. Lee D, Wilson G: Non-uniform swelling properties of the corneal stroma, *Curr Eye Res* 1:457, 1981.

255. Lee WR: Immunogold fine structural localization of extracellular matrix components in aged human cornea: I. Types I-IV collagen and laminin, *Graefes Arch Clin Exp Ophthalmol* 229:157, 1991.

256. Lehrer MS, Sun TT, Lavker RM: Strategies of epithelial repair: modulation of stem cell and transit amplifying cell proliferation, *J Cell Sci* 111:2867, 1998.

257. Lemp MA: Cornea and sclera, *Arch Ophthalmol* 94:473, 1976.

258. Lemp MA et al: The precorneal tear film: 1. Factors in spreading and maintaining a continuous tear film over the corneal surface, *Arch Ophthalmol* 83:89, 1970.

259. Leonard DW, Meek KM: Refractive indices of the collagen fibrils and extrafibrillar material of the corneal stroma, *Biophys J* 72:1382, 1997.

260. Lewis D et al: Ultrastructural localization of sulfated and unsulfated keratin sulfate in normal and macular corneal dystrophy type 1, *Glycobiology* 10:305, 2000.

261. Li W et al: cDNA clone to chick corneal chondroitin/dermatan sulfate proteoglycan reveals identity to decorin, *Arch Biochem Biophys* 296:190, 1992.

262. Lim JJ: Na⁺ transport across the rabbit corneal endothelium, *Curr Eye Res* 1:255, 1981.

263. Linsenmayer TF et al: Type VI collagen: immunohistochemical identification as a filamentous component of the extracellular matrix of the developing avian corneal stroma, *Dev Biol* 118:425, 1986.

264. Liu C et al: The cloning of a mouse keratocan cDNA and genomic DNA and the characterization of its expression during eye development, *J Biol Chem* 273:22584, 1998.

265. Lodish H et al: *Molecular cell biology,* ed 4, New York, 2000, WH Freeman.

266. Long CJ et al: Fibroblast growth factor-2 promotes keratan sulfate proteoglycan expression by keratocytes in vitro, *J Biol Chem* 275:13918, 2000.

267. Lopez Bernal D, Ubels JL: Quantitative evaluation of the corneal epithelial barrier: effect of artificial tears and preservatives, *Curr Eye Res* 10:645, 1991.

268. Lopez Bernal D, Ubels JL: Artificial tear composition and promotion of recovery of the damaged corneal epithelium, *Cornea* 12:115, 1993.

269. Lutty GA, Liu SH, Prendergast RA: Angiogenic lymphokines of activated T-cell origin, *Invest Ophthalmol Vis Sci* 24:1595, 1983.

270. MacDonald JM, Geroski DH, Edelhauser HE: Effect of inflammation on the corneal endothelial pump and barrier, *Curr Eye Res* 6:1125, 1987.

271. MacRae SM et al: The effects of hard and soft contact lens wear on the corneal endothelium, *Am J Ophthalmol* 102:50, 1986.

272. Madigan MC et al: Ultrastructural features of contact lens-induced deep corneal neovascularization and associated stromal leukocytes, *Cornea* 9:144, 1990.

273. Malley DS et al: Immunofluorescence study of corneal wound healing after excimer laser anterior keratectomy in the monkey eye, *Arch Ophthalmol* 108:1316, 1990.

274. Mandell RB, Farrell R: Corneal swelling at low atmospheric oxygen pressures, *Invest Ophthalmol Vis Sci* 19:697, 1980.

275. Mandell RB, Fatt I: Thinning of the human cornea on awakening, *Nature* 208:292, 1965.

276. Mangelsdorf DJ: Vitamin A receptors, *Nutr Rev* 52:S32, 1994.

277. Mangelsdorf DJ, Evans RM: The RXR heterodimers and orphan receptors, *Cell* 83:841, 1995.

278. Mardelli PG et al: Corneal endothelial status 12 to 55 months after excimer laser photorefractive keratectomy, *Ophthalmology* 102:544, 1995.

279. Marshall GE: Human scleral elastic system: an immuno-electron microscopic study, *Br J Ophthalmol* 79:57, 1995.

280. Marshall GE, Konstas AGP, Lee WR: Collagens in the aged human macular sclera, *Curr Eye Res* 12:143, 1993.

281. Marshall GE, Konstas AG, Lee WR: Immunogold fine structural localization of extracellular matrix components in aged human cornea: I. Types I-IV collagen and laminin, *Graefes Arch Clin Exp Ophthalmol* 229:157, 1991.

282. Marshall GE, Konstas AG, Lee WR: Immunogold fine structural localization of extracellular matrix components in aged human cornea: II. Collagen types V and VI, *Graefes Arch Clin Exp Ophthalmol* 229:164, 1991.

283. Marshall WS, Hanrahan JW: Anion channels in the apical membrane of mammalian corneal epithelium primary cultures, *Invest Ophthalmol Vis Sci* 32:1562, 1991.

284. Marzani D, Wallman J: Growth of the two layers of the chick sclera is modulated reciprocally by visual conditions, *Invest Ophthalmol Vis Sci* 38:1726, 1997.

285. Matic M et al: Alterations in connexin expression and cell communication in healing corneal epithelium, *Invest Ophthalmol Vis Sci* 38:600, 1997.

286. Matsuda M, Suda T, Manabe R: Quantitative analysis of endothelial mosaic pattern changes in anterior keratoconus, *Am J Ophthalmol* 98:43, 1984.

287. Matsuda M, Suda T, Manabe R: Serial alterations in endothelial cell shape and pattern after intraocular surgery, *Am J Ophthalmol* 98:313, 1984.

288. Matsuda M, Ubels JL, Edelhauser HE: A larger corneal epithelial wound closes at a faster rate, *Invest Ophthalmol Vis Sci* 26:897, 1985.

289. Matsuda M, Ubels JL, Edelhauser HF: Kinetics of corneal wound healing. In Brightbill FS (ed): *Corneal surgery, theory, technique and tissue,* St Louis, 1986, Mosby.

290. Matsuda M et al: Cellular migration and morphology in corneal endothelial wound repair, *Invest Ophthalmol Vis Sci* 26:443, 1985.

291. Maurice DM: The permeability to sodium ions of the living rabbit cornea, *J Physiol (Lond)* 112:367, 1951.

292. Maurice DM: The structure and transparency of the cornea, *J Physiol* 136:263, 1957.

293. Maurice DM: The location of the fluid pump in the cornea, *J Physiol* 221:43, 1972.

294. Maurice DM: Structures and fluids involved in the penetration of topically applied drugs, *Int Ophthalmol Clin* 20:7, 1980.

295. Maurice DM, Mishima S: Ocular pharmacokinetics. In Sears ML (ed): *Pharmacology of the eye,* New York, 1984, Springer-Verlag.

296. Maurice DM, Polgar J: Diffusion across the sclera, *Exp Eye Res* 25:577, 1977.

297. Maurice DM, Polgar J: Diffusion of high molecular weight compounds through sclera, *Invest Ophthalmol Vis Sci* 41:1181, 1977.

298. McBrien NA et al: Structural and biochemical changes in the sclera of experimentally myopic eyes, *Biochem Soc Trans* 19:861, 1991.

299. McKanna JA, Casagrande VA: Reduced lens development in lid-suture myopia, *Exp Eye Res* 26:715, 1978.

300. McLaughlin BJ et al: Freeze fracture quantitative comparison of rabbit corneal epithelial and endothelial membranes, *Curr Eye Res* 4:951, 1985.

301. Meek KM, Leonard DW: Ultrastructure of the corneal stroma: a comparative study, *Biophys J* 64:273, 1993.

302. Meek KM et al: The organization of collagen fibrils in the corneal stroma: a synchrotron x-ray diffraction study, *Curr Eye Res* 6:841, 1987.

303. Meller D, Peters K, Meller K: Human cornea and sclera studied by atomic force microscopy, *Cell Tissue Res* 288:111, 1997.

304. Messent AJ et al: Expression of a single pair of desmosomal glycoproteins renders the corneal epithelium unique amongst stratified epithelia, *Invest Ophthalmol Vis Sci* 41:8, 2000.

305. Meyers LA, Ubels JL, Edelhauser HF: Corneal endothelial morphology in the rat: effects of aging, diabetes and topical aldose reductase inhibitor treatment, *Invest Ophthalmol Vis Sci* 29:940, 1988.

306. Midura RJ et al: Proteoglycan biosynthesis by human corneas from patients with types 1 and 2 macular corneal dystrophy, *J Biol Chem* 265:15947, 1990.

307. Millodot M: Effect of the length of wear of contact lenses on corneal sensitivity, *Acta Ophthalmol* 54:721, 1976.

308. Millodot M: A review of research on the sensitivity of the cornea, *Ophthalmol Physiol Opt* 4:305, 1984.

309. Mishima S, Hedbys BO: The permeability of the corneal epithelium and endothelium, *Exp Eye Res* 6:10, 1967.

310. Mita T et al: Effects of transforming growth factor beta on corneal epithelial and stromal cell function in a rat wound healing model after excimer laser keratectomy, *Graefes Arch Clin Exp Ophthalmol* 236:834, 1998.

311. Modesti A, Kalebic T, Scarpa S: Type V collagen in human amnion is a 12nm fibrillar component of the pericellular interstitium, *Eur J Cell Biol* 35:246, 1984.

312. Mondino BJ, Laheji AK, Adamu SA: Ocular immunity to *Staphylococcus aureus, Invest Ophthalmol Vis Sci* 28:560, 1987.

313. Montes GS, Bezzerra MSF, Junqueira LCU: Collagen distribution in tissues. In Ruggeri A, Motta PM (eds): *Ultrastructure of the connective tissue matrix,* Boston, 1984, Martinus Nijhoff.

314. Muir H: Proteoglycans as organizers of the intercellular matrix: seventeenth CIBA medical lecture, *Biochem Soc Trans* 11:613, 1982.

315. Murphy C et al: Prenatal and postnatal cellularity of the human corneal endothelium: a quantitative histologic study, *Invest Ophthalmol Vis Sci* 25:312, 1984.

316. Murphy CJ et al: Effect of norepinephrine on proliferation, migration, and adhesion of SV-40 transformed human corneal epithelial cells, *Cornea* 17:529, 1998.

317. Murphy PJ, Patel S, Marshall J: The effect of long-term, daily contact lens wear on corneal sensitivity, *Cornea* 20:264, 2001.

318. Muthukkaruppan VR, Auerbach R: Angiogenesis in the mouse cornea, *Science* 205:1416, 1979.

319. Nakazawa K et al: Defective processing of keratan sulfate in macular corneal dystrophy, *J Biol Chem* 259:1351, 1984.

320. Newsome DA, Gross J, Hassell JR: Human corneal stroma contains three distinct collagens, *Invest Ophthalmol Vis Sci* 22:376, 1982.

321. Newton RH, Meek KM: Circumcorneal annulus of collagen fibrils in the human limbus, *Invest Ophthalmol Vis Sci* 39:1125, 1998.

322. Newton RH, Meek KM: The integration of corneal and limbal fibrils in the human eye, *Biophys J* 75:2508, 1998.

323. Niederkorn JY, Ubelaker JE, Martin JE: Vascularization of corneas of hairless mutant mice, *Invest Ophthalmol Vis Sci* 31:948, 1990.

324. Nikolic L et al: Inhibition of vascularization in rabbit corneas by heparin: cortisone pellets, *Invest Ophthalmol Vis Sci* 27:449, 1986.

325. Nishida T et al: Fibronectin: a new therapy for trophic corneal ulcer, *Arch Ophthalmol* 101:1046, 1983.

326. Nishida T et al: Interleukin 6 facilitates corneal epithelial wound closure in vivo, *Arch Ophthalmol* 110:1292, 1992.

327. Norton TT, Rada JA: Reduced extracellular matrix in mammalian sclera with induced myopia, *Vision Res* 35:1271, 1995.

328. Ohashi Y et al: Presence of epidermal growth factor in human tears, *Invest Ophthalmol Vis Sci* 30:1879, 1989.

329. Okada Y et al: Expression of fos family and jun family proto-oncogenes during corneal epithelial wound healing, *Curr Eye Res* 15:1824, 1996.

330. O'Leary DJ, Millodot M: Abnormal oxygen fragility in diabetes and contact lens wear, *Acta Ophthalmol* 59:827, 1981.

331. Oliveira-Soto L, Efron N: Morphology of corneal nerves using confocal microscopy, *Cornea* 20:374, 2001.

332. Olsen TW et al: Effects of age, cryotherapy, transscleral diode laser, surgical thinning, *Invest Ophthalmol Vis Sci* 36:1893, 1995.

333. Olsen TW et al: Human scleral permeability, *Invest Ophthalmol Vis Sci* 36:1893, 1995.

334. Olsen TW et al: Human sclera: thickness and surface area, *Am J Ophthalmol* 125:237, 1998.

335. O'Neal MR, Polse KA: In vivo assessment of mechanisms controlling corneal hydration, *Invest Ophthalmol Vis Sci* 26:849, 1985.

336. Ong DE: Cellular transport and metabolism of vitamin A: roles of the cellular retinoid-binding proteins, *Nutr Rev* 52:S24, 1994.

337. Osgood TB et al: Evaluation of ocular irritancy of hair care products, *J Toxicol Cut Ocular Toxicol* 9:37, 1990.

338. Otori T: Electrolyte content of the rabbit cornea, *Exp Eye Res* 6:356, 1967.

339. Pallikaris IG, Siganos DS: Excimer laser in situ keratomileusis and photorefractive keratectomy for correction of high myopia, *J Refract Corneal Surg* 10:498, 1994.

340. Pastor JC, Calonge M: Epidermal growth factor and corneal wound healing: a multicenter study, *Cornea* 11:311, 1992.

341. Perez E et al: Effects of chronic sympathetic stimulation on cornea wound healing, *Invest Ophthalmol Vis Sci* 28:221, 1987.

342. Petridou S, Masur SK: Immunodetection of connexins and cadherins in corneal fibroblasts and myofibroblasts, *Inv Ophthalmol Vis Sci* 37:1740, 1996.

343. Petroll WM et al: Organization of junctional proteins in proliferating cat corneal endothelium during wound healing, *Cornea* 20:73, 2001.

344. Pfister RR: The normal surface of corneal epithelium: a scanning electron microscope study, *Invest Ophthalmol* 12:654, 1973.

345. Pfister RR: The healing of corneal epithelial abrasions in the rabbit: a scanning electron microscope study, *Invest Ophthalmol* 14:648, 1975.

346. Pfister RR, Haddox JL, Paterson CA: The efficacy of sodium citrate treatment of severe alkali burns of the eye is influenced by the route of administration, *Cornea* 1:205, 1982.

347. Pflugfelder SC et al: Detection of sialomucin complex (MUC4) in human ocular surface epithelium and tear fluid, *Invest Ophthalmol Vis Sci* 41:1316, 2000.

348. Pitts DG: The human ultraviolet action spectrum, *Am J Optom Arch Am Acad Optom* 51:946, 1974.

349. Poggio EC et al: The incidence of ulcerative keratitis among users of daily wear and extended wear contact lenses, *N Engl J Med* 321:779, 1989.

350. Polse KA, Mandell RB: Etiology of corneal striae accompanying hydrogel lens wear, *Invest Ophthalmol* 75:557, 1976.

351. Pouliquero Y et al: Etude analytique et statistique des lamelles, des keratocytes, des fibrilles de collagene de la region de la cornee humaine normale (microscopie optique et electronique), *Arch Ophthalmol (Paris)* 32:563, 1972.

352. Prausnitz MR: Fiber matrix model of sclera and corneal stroma for drug delivery to the eye, *AIChE J* 44:214, 1998.

353. Prausnitz MR, Noonan JS: Permeability of cornea, sclera, and conjunctiva: a literature analysis for drug delivery to the eye, *J Pharm Sci* 87:1479, 1998.

354. Quantock AJ et al: Macular corneal dystrophy: reduction in both corneal thickness and collagen interfibrillar spacing, *Curr Eye Res* 9:393, 1990.

355. Rabin J, Van Sluters RC, Malach R: Emmetropization: a vision dependent phenomenon, *Invest Ophthalmol Vis Sci* 20:561, 1981.

356. Rada JA, Achen VR, Rada KG: Proteoglycan turnover in the sclera of normal and experimentally myopic chick eyes, *Invest Ophthalmol Vis Sci* 39:1990, 1998.

357. Rada JA, Cornuet PK, Hassell JR: Regulation of corneal collagen fibrillogenesis in vitro by corneal proteoglycan (lumican and decorin) core proteins, *Exp Eye Res* 53:635, 1993.

358. Rada JA, Matthews AL, Brenza H: Regional proteoglycan synthesis in the sclera of experimentally myopic chicks, *Exp Eye Res* 59:747, 1994.

359. Rada JA, Thoft RA, Hassell JR: Increased aggrecan (cartilage proteoglycan) production in the sclera of myopic chicks, *Dev Biol* 147:303, 1991.

360. Rada JA, Troilo D: Proteoglycans in the marmoset sclera are affected by form deprivation, *Invest Ophthalmol Vis Sci* 39:S505, 1998.

361. Rada JA et al: Proteoglycans of the human sclera: evidence for an aggrecan-like proteoglycan, *Invest Ophthalmol Vis Sci* 35:S1992, 1991.

362. Rada JA et al: Proteoglycan synthesis by scleral chondrocytes is modulated by a vision dependent mechanism, *Curr Eye Res* 11:767, 1992.

363. Rada JA et al: Proteoglycan composition in the human sclera during growth and aging, *Invest Ophthalmol Vis Sci* 41:1639, 2000.

364. Rae JL, Dewey J, Cooper K: Properties of single potassium-selective ionic channels from the apical membrane of the rabbit cornea endothelium, *Exp Eye Res* 49:591, 1989.

365. Rae JL, Farrugia G: Whole-cell potassium current in rabbit corneal epithelium activated by fenamates, *J Membr Biol* 129:81, 1992.

366. Rae JL et al: Dye and electrical coupling between cells of the rabbit corneal epithelium, *Curr Eye Res* 8:859, 1989.

367. Rae JL et al: Single potassium channels in corneal epithelium, *Invest Ophthalmol Vis Sci* 31:1799, 1990.

368. Rao GN et al: Morphological appearance of the healing corneal endothelium, *Arch Ophthalmol* 96:2027, 1978.

369. Rao GN et al: Morphologic variation in graft endothelium, *Arch Ophthalmol* 98:1403, 1980.

370. Raphael B et al: Enhanced healing of cat corneal endothelial wound by epidermal growth factor, *Invest Ophthalmol Vis Sci* 34:2305, 1993.

371. Rasooly R, Benezra D: Congenital and traumatic cataract: the effect on ocular axial length, *Arch Ophthalmol* 106:1066, 1988.

372. Raviola E, Wiesel TN: An animal model of myopia, *N Engl J Med* 312:1609, 1985.

373. Rem AI et al: Temperature dependence of thermal damage to the sclera: exploring the heat tolerance of the sclera for transscleral thermotherapy, *Exp Eye Res* 72:153, 2001.

374. Rich A, Bartling C, Farrugia G: Effects of pH on the potassium current in rabbit corneal epithelial cells, *Am J Physiol* 272:C744, 1997.

375. Rich A, Rae JL: Calcium entry in rabbit corneal epithelial cells: evidence for a non–voltage dependent pathway, *J Membr Biol* 144:177, 1995.

376. Riley MV: Glucose and oxygen utilization of the cornea, *Exp Eye Res* 8:193, 1969.

377. Riley MV, Meyer RF, Yates EM: Glutathione in the aqueous humor of humans and other species, *Invest Ophthalmol Vis Sci* 19:94, 1980.

378. Rodrigues MM, Krachmer JH: Recent advances in corneal stromal dystrophies, *Cornea* 7:19, 1988.

379. Rodrigues M et al: Suprabasal expression of a 64-kilodalton keratin (no. 3) in developing human corneal epithelium, *Differentiation* 34:60, 1987.

380. Rozenman Y et al: Contact lens-related deep stromal neovascularization, *Am J Ophthalmol* 107:27, 1989.

381. Rudnick DE, Noonan JS, Geroski DH: The effect of intraocular pressure on human and rabbit scleral permeability, *Invest Ophthalmol Vis Sci* 40:3054, 1999.

382. Ruggiero F, Burillon C, Garrone R: Collagen V structural analysis and fibrillar assembly by stromal fibroblasts in culture, *Invest Ophthalmol Vis Sci* 37:1749, 1996.

383. Saika Sh et al: Role of lumican in the corneal epithelium during wound healing, *J Biol Chem* 275:2607, 2000.

384. Salzmann M: *Anatomie und histologie des menschlichen augapfels in normalzustande: seine entwicklung und sein altern,* Leipzig, 1912, Franz Deuticke.

385. Savage CP Jr, Cohen S: Proliferation of corneal epithelium induced by epidermal growth factor, *Exp Eye Res* 15:361, 1973.

386. Schanzlin DJ et al: The intrastromal corneal ring segments: phase II results for the correction of myopia, *Ophthalmology* 104:1067, 1997.

387. Schermer A, Galvin S, Sun T-T: Differentiation related expression of a major 64 k corneal keratin in vivo and in culture suggests a limbal location of corneal epithelial stem cells, *J Cell Biol* 103:49, 1986.

388. Schilling-Schön A et al: The role of endogenous growth factors to support corneal endothelial migration after wounding in vitro, *Exp Eye Res* 71:583, 2000.

389. Schimmelpfennig B et al: Tissue storage. In Brightbill FS (ed): *Corneal surgery: theory, technique and tissue,* St Louis, 1986, Mosby.

390. Schoessler JP, Barr JT, Freson DR: Corneal endothelial observations of silicone elastomer contact lens wearer, *Int Contact Lens Clin* 11:337, 1984.

391. Schonherr E et al: Interaction of biglycan with type I collagen, *J Biol Chem* 270:2776, 1995.

392. Schultz G et al: Growth factors and corneal endothelial cells: III—stimulation of adult human corneal endothelial cell mitosis in vitro by defined mitogenic agents, *Cornea* 11:20, 1992.

393. Schultz RO et al: Corneal endothelial changes in type I and type II diabetes mellitus, *Am J Ophthalmol* 98:401, 1984.

394. Schultz RO et al: Response of the corneal endothelium to cataract surgery, *Arch Ophthalmol* 104:1164, 1986.

395. Schwalbe G: Untersuchungen über die lymphbahnen des auges und ihre begrenzungen, *Arch Mikroskop Anat* 6:1, 1860.

396. Schwartzman ML et al: 12(R) Hydroxyeicosatetraenoic acid: a cytochrome P450-dependent metabolite that inhibits Na^+/K^+ ATPase in the cornea, *Proc Natl Acad Sci USA* 84:8125, 1987.

397. Scott JE: Proteoglycan: collagen interactions in connective tissues—ultrastructural, biochemical, functional and evolutionary aspects, *Int J Biol Macromol* 13:157, 1991.

398. Scott JE, Haigh M: 'Small'-proteoglycan:collagen interactions: keratan sulphate proteoglycan associates with rabbit corneal collagen fibrils at the 'a' and 'c' bands, *Biosci Rep* 5:765, 1985.

399. Seiler T et al: Does Bowman's layer determine the biomechanical properties of the cornea? *Refract Corneal Surg* 8:139, 1992.

400. Sellheyer K, Spitznas M: Development of the human sclera: a morphological study, *Graefes Arch Clin Exp Ophthalmol* 226:89, 1988.

401. Sevel D: A reappraisal of the development of the eyelids, *Eye* 2:123, 1988.

402. Sharma A, Coles WH: Kinetics of corneal epithelial maintenance and graft loss, *Invest Ophthalmol Vis Sci* 30:1962, 1989.

403. Sheardown H et al: A semi-solid drug delivery system for epidermal growth factor in corneal epithelial wound healing, *Curr Eye Res* 16:183, 1997.

404. Shepard AR, Rae JL: Ion transporters and receptors in cDNA libraries from lens and cornea epithelia, *Curr Eye Res* 17:708, 1998.

405. Sher NA et al: The use of the 193-nm excimer laser for myopic photorefractive keratectomy in sighted eyes: a multicenter study, *Arch Ophthalmol* 109:1525, 1991.

406. Sherman SM, Norton TT, Casagrande VA: Myopia in the lid-sutured tree shrew (*Tupaia glis*), *Brain Res* 124:154, 1977.

407. Shi Y, Tabesh M, Sugrue SP: Role of cell adhesion-associated protein, pinin (DRS/memA), in corneal epithelial migration, *Invest Ophthalmol Vis Sci* 41:1337, 2000.

408. Shimizu K, Amano S, Tanako S: Photorefractive keratectomy for myopia: one-year follow up in 97 eyes, *J Cataract Refract Surg* 10:3178, 1994.

409. Simonsen AH, Andreassen TT, Bendix K: The healing strength of corneal wounds in the human eye, *Exp Eye Res* 35:287, 1982.

410. Sliney DH: Eye protective techniques for bright light, *Ophthalmol* 90:937, 1983.

411. Smelser GK, Ozanics V: Importance of atmospheric oxygen for maintenance of the optical properties of the human cornea, *Science* 115:140, 1952.

412. Smith EL III, Maguire GW, Watson JT: Axial lengths and refractive errors in kittens reared with an optically induced anisometropia, *Invest Ophthalmol Vis Sci* 19:1250, 1980.

413. Smolek MK, McCarey BE: Interlamellar adhesive strength in human eyebank corneas, *Invest Ophthalmol Vis Sci* 31:1087, 1990.

414. Snellingen T et al: The South Asian cataract management study: complications, vision outcomes, and corneal endothelial cell loss in a randomized multicenter clinical trial comparing intracapsular cataract extraction with and without anterior chamber intraocular lens implantation, *Ophthalmology* 107:231, 2000.

415. Soirbrane G et al: Binding of basic fibroblast growth factor to normal and neovascularized rabbit cornea, *Invest Ophthalmol Vis Sci* 31:323, 1990.

416. Sommer A, West KP Jr: *Vitamin A deficiency: health, survival, and vision,* New York, 1996, Oxford University Press.

417. Soong HK: Vinculin in focal cell-to-substrate attachments of spreading corneal epithelial cells, *Arch Ophthalmol* 105:1129, 1987.

418. Soong HK, Cintron C: Different corneal epithelial healing mechanisms in rat and rabbit: role of actin and calmodulin, *Invest Ophthalmol Vis Sci* 26:838, 1985.

419. Sotozono C, Kinoshita S: Growth factors and cytokines in corneal wound healing. In Nishida T (ed): *Corneal healing responses to injuries and refractive surgeries,* The Hague; New York, 1998, Kugler Publications.

420. Sotozono C et al: Keratinocyte growth factor accelerates corneal epithelial wound healing in vivo, *Invest Ophthalmol Vis Sci* 36:1524, 1995.

421. Spanakis SG, Petridou S, Masur SK: Functional gap junctions in corneal fibroblasts and myofibroblasts, *Invest Ophthalmol Vis Sci* 39:1320, 1998.

422. Stepp MA et al: α6β4-Integrin heterodimer is a component of hemidesmosomes, *Proc Nat Acad Sci USA* 87:8970, 1990.

423. Stiemke MM et al: Sodium activities and concentrations of the corneal stroma, aqueous humor and plasma in the presence and absence of a transparent cornea, *Invest Ophthalmol Vis Sci* 32(suppl):1065, 1991.

424. Stiemke MM et al: Sodium activity in the aqueous humor and corneal stroma of the rabbit, *Exp Eye Res* 35:425, 1992.

425. Stocker EG, Schoessler JP: Corneal endothelial polymegathism induced by PMMA contact lens wear, *Invest Ophthalmol Vis Sci* 26:857, 1985.

426. Stulting RD et al: The effects of photorefractive keratectomy on the corneal endothelium, *Ophthalmology* 103:1357, 1996.

427. Sugrue SP, Zieske JD: ZO-1 in corneal epithelium: association to the zonula occludens and adherens junctions, *Exp Eye Res* 64:11, 1997.

428. Suvarnamani C et al: The effects of total lymphoid irradiation upon corneal vascularization in the rat following chemical cautery, *Radiation Res* 117:259, 1989.

429. Suzuki K et al: Coordinated reassembly of the basement membrane and junctional proteins during corneal epithelial wound healing, *Invest Ophthalmol Vis Sci* 41:2495, 2000.

430. Takahashi H, Kaminski AE, Zieske JD: Glucose transporter 1 expression is enhanced during corneal epithelial wound repair, *Exp Eye Res* 63:649, 1996.

431. Tamm ER, Koch TA, Mayer B: Innervation of myofibroblast-like scleral spur cells in human and monkey eyes, *Invest Ophthalmol Vis Sci* 36:1633, 1995.

432. Tei M et al: Vitamin A deficiency alters the expression of mucin genes by the rat ocular surface epithelium, *Invest Ophthalmol Vis Sci* 41:82, 2000.

433. Tervo T, Palkema A: Electron microscopic localization of adenosine triphosphatase (Na-K-ATPase) activity in the rat cornea, *Exp Eye Res* 21:269, 1975.

434. Thoft RA, Friend J: Biochemical transformation of regenerating ocular surface epithelium, *Invest Ophthalmol* 16:14, 1977.

435. Thoft RA, Friend J: The X,Y,Z hypothesis of corneal epithelial maintenance, *Invest Ophthalmol Vis Sci* 24:142, 1983.

436. Tisdale AS et al: Development of the anchoring structures of the epithelium in rabbit and human fetal corneas, *Invest Ophthalmol Vis Sci* 29:727, 1988.

437. Treffers WF: Human corneal endothelial wound repair, *Ophthalmology* 89:605, 1982.

438. Trier K, Olsen EB, Ammitzboll T: Regional glycosaminoglycan composition of the human sclera, *Acta Ophthalmol* 68:304, 1990.

439. Trier K et al: Biochemical and ultrastructural changes in rabbit sclera after treatment with 7-methylxanthine, theobromine, acetazolamide, or L-ornithine, *Br J Ophthalmol* 83:1370, 1999.

440. Tripathi RC, Raja SC, Tripathi BJ: Prospects for epidermal growth factor in the management of corneal disorders, *Surv Ophthalmol* 34:457, 1990.

441. Troilo D et al: Late-onset form deprivation in the marmoset produces axial myopia and reduced scleral proteoglycan synthesis, *Invest Ophthalmol Vis Sci* 40:S963, 1999.

442. Tseng SCG et al: Expression of specific keratin markers by rabbit corneal, conjunctival, and esophageal epithelia during vitamin A deficiency, *J Cell Biol* 99:2279, 1984.

443. Twomey JM et al: Ocular enlargement following infantile corneal opacification, *Eye* 4:497, 1990.

444. Ubels JL, Woo EM, Curley RW Jr: N-linked glycoside and glucuronide conjugates of the retinoid, acitretin, are biologically active in cornea and conjunctiva, *J Ocul Pharmacol Ther* 14:505, 1998.

445. Ubels JL et al: The efficacy of retinoic acid ointment for treatment of xerophthalmia and corneal epithelial wounds, *Curr Eye Res* 4:1049, 1985.

446. Ubels JL et al: Effects of preservative-free artificial tear solutions on corneal epithelial structure and function, *Arch Ophthalmol* 113:371, 1995.

447. Ubels JL et al: Conjunctival permeability and ultrastructure: effects of benzalkonium chloride and artificial tears. In Sullivan D et al (eds): *Lacrimal gland, tear film, and dry eye syndromes,* ed 2, New York, 1998, Plenum Press.

448. Uusitalo H, Kootila K, Palkema A: Calcitonin gene–related peptide (CGRP) immunoreactive sensory nerves in the human and guinea pig uvea and cornea, *Exp Eye Res* 48:467, 1989.

449. Van Horn DL et al: Effect of the ophthalmic preservative thimerosal on rabbit and human corneal endothelium, *Invest Ophthalmol Vis Sci* 16:273, 1977.

450. Van Horn DL et al: Regenerative capacity of the corneal endothelium in the rabbit and cat, *Invest Ophthalmol Vis Sci* 16:597, 1977.

451. Vannas A et al: Surgical incision alters the swelling response of the human cornea, *Invest Ophthalmol Vis Sci* 26:864, 1985.

452. Vannas S, Teir H: Observations on structures and age changes in the human sclera, *Acta Ophthalmol* 38:268, 1960.

453. Vass C et al: Intrascleral concentration vs depth profile of mitomycin-C after episcleral application: impact of applied concentration and volume of mitomycin-C solution, *Exp Eye Res* 70:571, 2000.

454. Verbey NL, van Haeringen NJ, de Jong PT: Modulation of immunogenic keratitis in rabbits by topical administration of poly-unsaturated fatty acids, *Curr Eye Res* 7:549, 1988.

455. Von Noorden GK, Lewis RA: Ocular axial length in unilateral congenital cataract and blepharoptosis, *Invest Ophthalmol Vis Sci* 28:750, 1987.

456. Vogel KG, Paulsson M, Heinegard D: Specific inhibition of type I and type II collagen fibrillogenesis by the small proteoglycan of tendon, *Biochem J* 223:587, 1984.

457. Wall RS: A structural and biochemical study of the corneal stroma, Ph.D. thesis, Milton Keynes, England, The Open University.

458. Wallman J, Adams JI: Developmental aspects of experimental myopia in chicks: susceptibility, recovery and relation to emmetropization, *Vis Res* 27:1139, 1987.

459. Walkenbach RJ, Ye GS: Muscarinic cholinoceptor regulation of cyclic guanosine monophosphate in human corneal epithelium, *Invest Ophthalmol Vis Sci* 32:610, 1991.

460. Walkenbach RJ et al: Alpha-adrenoceptors in human corneal epithelium, *Invest Ophthalmol Vis Sci* 32:3067, 1991.

461. Walkow T, Anders N, Klebe S: Endothelial cell loss after phacoemulsification: relation to preoperative and intraoperative parameters, *J Cataract Refract Surg* 26:727, 2000.

462. Wallman J, Turkel J, Trachtman J: Extreme myopia produced by modest changes in early visual experience, *Science* 201:1249, 1978.

463. Wang Y, Chen M, Wolosin JM: ZO-1 in corneal epithelium: stratal distribution and synthesis induction by outer cell removal, *Exp Eye Res* 57:283, 1993.

464. Waring GO et al: The corneal endothelium: normal and pathologic structure and function, *Ophthalmol* 89:531, 1982.

465. Watanabe SI, Tanizaki M, Kaneko A: Two types of stretch-activated channels coexist in the rabbit corneal epithelial cell, *Exp Eye Res* 64:1027, 1997.

466. Watsky MA: Keratocyte gap junctional communication in normal and wounded rabbit corneas and human corneas, *Invest Ophthalmol Vis Sci* 36:2568, 1995.

467. Watsky MA: Loss of fenamate-activated K$^+$ current from epithelial cells during corneal wound healing, *Invest Ophthalmol Vis Sci* 40:1356, 1999.

468. Watsky MA, Edelhauser HF: Intraocular irrigating solutions: the importance of Ca^{++} and glass versus polypropylene bottles, *Int Ophthalmol Clin* 33:109, 1993.

469. Weale RA: *The aging eye,* London, 1963, Harper & Row.

470. Wechsler S: Striate corneal lines, *Am J Optom Physiol Optics* 51:851, 1974.

471. Weingeist TA, Liesegang TJ, Grand MG: *Basic and clinical science course,* section 2, *Fundamentals and principles of ophthalmology,* San Francisco, 1999-2000, American Academy of Ophthalmology.

472. Weissman BA et al: Oxygen permeability of rabbit and human corneal stroma, *Invest Ophthalmol Vis Sci* 24:645, 1983.

473. Whikehart DR, Soppet DR: Activities of transport enzymes located in the plasma membranes of corneal endothelial cells, *Invest Ophthalmol Vis Sci* 21:819, 1981.

474. Wiederholt M, Koch M: Effect of intraocular irrigating solutions on intracellular membrane potentials and swelling rate of isolated human and rabbit cornea, *Invest Ophthalmol Vis Sci* 18:313, 1979.

475. Wiesel TM, Raviola E: Myopia and eye enlargement after neonatal lid fusion in monkeys, *Nature* 266:66, 1977.

476. Wiggert B, Van Horn DL, Fish BL: Effects of vitamin A deficiency on (^{3}H)-retinoid binding to cellular retinoid-binding proteins in the rabbit cornea and conjunctiva, *Exp Eye Res* 34:695, 1982.

477. Williams K et al: Correlation of histologic corneal endothelial cell counts with specular microscopic cell density, *Arch Ophthalmol* 110:1146, 1992.

478. Williams KK, Watsky, MA: Dye spread through gap junctions in the corneal epithelium of the rabbit, *Cur Eye Res* 16:445, 1996.

479. Williams KK, Woods WD, Edelhauser HF: Corneal diffusion and metabolism of 12(R) hydroxyeicosatetraenoic acid (12(R) HETE), *Curr Eye Res* 15:852, 1996.

480. Wilson SE, Lloyd SA, He YG: EGF, basic FGF, and TGF beta-1 messenger RNA production in rabbit corneal epithelial cells, *Invest Ophthalmol Vis Sci* 33:1987, 1992.

481. Wilson SE et al: Expression of HGF, KGF, EGF and receptor messenger RNAs following corneal epithelial wounding, *Exp Eye Res* 68:377, 1999.

482. Wolff CH, Glavan I: Morphologic and fluorophotometric analysis of the corneal endothelium in long-term hard and soft contact lens wearers, *CLAO J* 14:105, 1988.

483. Wolosin JM: Regeneration of resistance and ion transport in rabbit corneal epithelium after induced surface cell exfoliation, *J Membrane Biol* 104:45, 1988.

484. Wu RL et al: Lineage-specific and differentiation-dependent expression of K12 keratin in rabbit corneal/limbal epithelial cells: cDNA cloning and northern blot analysis, *Differentiation* 55:137, 1994.

485. Yamada M, Proia AD: 8(S)-hydroxyeicosatetraenoic acid is the lipoxygenase metabolite of arachidonic acid that regulates epithelial cell migration in the rat cornea, *Cornea* 19:S13, 2000.

486. Yamaguchi Y, Mann DM, Ruoslahti E: Negative regulation of transforming growth factor-beta by the proteoglycan decorin, *Nature* 346:281, 1990.

487. Yang CJ et al: Immunohistochemical evidence of heterogeneity in macular corneal dystrophy, *Am J Ophthalmol* 106:65, 1988.

488. Yee RW, Matsuda M, Edelhauser HF: Wide-field endothelial counting panels, *Am J Ophthalmol* 99:596, 1985.

489. Yee RW et al: Changes in the normal corneal endothelial cellular pattern as a function of age, *Curr Eye Res* 4:671, 1985.

490. Yee RW et al: Correlation of corneal endothelial pump site density, barrier function and morphology in wound repair, *Invest Ophthalmol Vis Sci* 26:1191, 1985.

491. Yinon U et al: Lid suture myopia in developing chicks: optical and structural considerations, *Curr Eye Res* 2:877, 1983.

492. Ytteborg J, Dohiman CH: Corneal edema and intraocular pressure: II—clinical results, *Arch Ophthalmol* 74:477, 1965.

493. Yu FX, Guo J, Zhang Q: Expression and distribution of adhesion molecule CD44 in healing corneal epithelia, *Invest Ophthalmol Vis Sci* 39:710, 1998.

494. Zadunaisky JA: Active transport of chloride across the cornea, *Nature (Lond)* 209:1136, 1977.

495. Zantos SG, Holden BA: Transient endothelial changes soon after wearing soft contact lenses, *Am J Optom Physiol Optics* 54:856, 1977.

496. Zhan Q, Burrows R, Cintron C: Cloning and in situ hybridization of rabbit decorin in corneal tissues, *Invest Ophthalmol Vis Sci* 36:206, 1995.

497. Ziche M, Alessandri G, Gullino PM: Gangliosides promote the angiogenic response, *Lab Invest* 61:629, 1989.

498. Ziche M, Jones J, Gullion DM: Role of prostaglandin E and copper in angiogenesis, *J Natl Cancer Inst* 69:475, 1982.

499. Zieske JD: Regulation of epithelial cell proliferation during corneal repair. In Nishida T (ed): *Corneal healing responses to injuries and refractive surgeries,* The Hague; New York, 1998, Kugler Publications.

500. Zieske JD: Expression of cyclin-dependent kinase inhibitors during corneal wound repair, *Prog Retin Eye Res* 19:257, 2000.

501. Zieske JD, Bukusoglu G, Gipson IK: Enhancement of vinculin synthesis by migrating stratified squamous epithelium, *J Cell Biol* 109:571, 1989.

502. Zieske JD, Bukusoglu G, Yankauckas MA: α-Enolase is restricted to basal cells of stratified squamous epithelium, *Dev Biol* 151:18, 1992.

503. Zieske JD, Gipson IK: Protein synthesis during corneal epithelial wound healing, *Invest Ophthalmol Vis Sci* 27:1, 1986.

504. Zieske JD, Takahashi H, Hutcheon AE: Activation of epidermal growth factor receptor during corneal epithelial migration, *Invest Ophthalmol Vis Sci* 41:1346, 2000.

505. Zimmermann DR et al: Type VI collagen is a major component of the human cornea, *FEBS Letters* 197:55, 1986.

506. Zinn KM, Mockel-Pohl S: Fine structure of the developing cornea, *Int Ophthalmol Clin* 15:19, 1975.

SECTION 3

LENS

David C. Beebe

THE LENS

DAVID C. BEEBE

The lens is a remarkably specialized epithelial tissue that is responsible for fine-tuning the image that is projected on the retina. To perform this function, the lens must be transparent, have a higher refractive index than the medium in which it is suspended, and have refractive surfaces with the proper curvature. The curvature of these surfaces must also be variable to permit the optical system to focus on objects that are far or near.

To maintain transparency and a high refractive index, lens fiber cells are precisely aligned with their neighbors and accumulate high concentrations of proteins, the crystallins. Disruption of the precise organization of the lens fiber cells or damage to the proteins within them can destroy the transparency of the lens, a process known as *cataract formation.* Cataracts are the leading cause of blindness worldwide, and the removal of cataracts is the most common surgical procedure in the aged population.

This chapter provides an overview of the structure, development, biochemistry, physiology, and pathology of the lens. Information about the human lens is emphasized, although studies with animals are included when data for humans are not available. Information is provided on the causes of cataracts and the mechanisms that are thought to protect the lens from cataract. The unsolved issues in the biology and pathology of the lens are highlighted throughout. References to comprehensive reviews and original source material are included to assist the reader. The citations provided are not meant to be inclusive, but rather to highlight articles that are recent or of special relevance, because at the time of this writing, there were nearly 30,000 scientific articles dealing with the lens or cataract in the MEDLINE database. Supplementary information, including a summary of research challenges

relating to the lens and cataract, can be found in the current *Vision Research—A National Plan,* by the National Eye Institute (www.nei.nih.gov/resources/strategicplans/plan.htm).

ANATOMY OF THE ADULT LENS

The lens is formed from two populations of specialized epithelial cells (Figure 5-1). A sheet of cuboidal cells, the *lens epithelium,* covers the anterior surface of the lens closest to the cornea. The bulk of the lens consists of concentric layers of elongated fiber cells. The outer shells of fiber cells extend from just beneath the epithelium to the posterior lens surface, a distance of more than 1 cm in adults. An elastic extracellular matrix, the *lens capsule,* which is secreted by the epithelial and superficial fiber cells, surrounds the entire lens. In the adult lens, most epithelial cells and all fiber cells are not dividing. However, cells near the equatorial margin of the lens epithelium, in a region called the *germinative zone,* proliferate slowly. Most of the cells produced by mitosis in this region migrate toward the posterior of the lens and differentiate into fiber cells at the lens equator.[305] These new fiber cells elongate and accumulate large amounts of crystallins. During elongation the posterior (basal) ends of the fiber cells move along the surface of the capsule and their anterior (apical) ends slide beneath the epithelium until they meet elongating cells from the other side of the lens near the posterior and anterior midlines (see Figure 5-1). The junctions between the apical and basal ends of cells from the opposite sides of the lens are called the *sutures.* Once fiber cells reach the sutures, they stop elongating and their basal ends detach from the capsule (see Figure 5-1, *inset*). Soon after, fiber cells degrade all intracellular membrane-bound organelles, including their nuclei, mitochondria, and endoplasmic reticulum.[11,12,15,209] Mature fiber cells are gradually buried deeper in the lens as successive generations of fibers elongate and differentiate. In this way the lens continues to increase in size and cell number throughout life.[326] Because protein synthesis ceases just before organelle degradation, the components of mature fiber cells must be much more stable than those in cells found in other parts of the body.[334]

The lens is suspended in the anterior of the eye by a band of inelastic microfibrils, the *zonules,* which insert into the lens capsule near the equator (Figures 5-1 and 5-2). These fibrils originate in the nonpigmented layer of the ciliary epithelium, a tis-

sue that is located just posterior to the iris. They consist of the protein fibrillin, one of the components of elastic fibrils in many connective tissues throughout the body.[254,399] However, the zonules do not contain most of the other components of elastic fibers, and the zonular microfibrils do not stretch appreciably. Changes in the tension applied to the zonules are responsible for the alterations in lens curvature during accommodation.

BASICS OF LENS REFRACTION AND TRANSPARENCY

The refractive properties of the lens are the result of the high concentration of crystallins in the cytoplasm of the lens fiber cells and the curvature of the

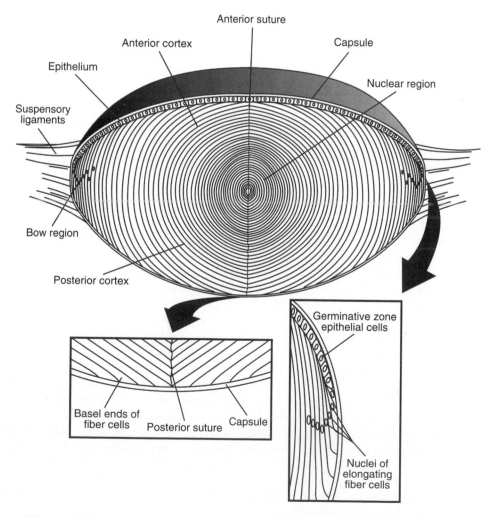

FIGURE 5-1   Diagram of the adult human lens. The expanded regions show the relationships between the elongating lens fiber cells and the posterior capsule as the basal ends of the fibers reach the posterior sutures and the changes in cell shape and orientation that occur as lens epithelial cells differentiate into lens fibers at the lens equator.

lens surfaces. Lens crystallins accumulate to concentrations that are three times higher than in typical cells.[96] This gives the fiber cells a significantly higher refractive index than the fluids around the lens. In the emmetropic eye the curvature of the anterior and posterior surfaces of the lens focuses light at the photoreceptors of the retina. The curvatures of the lens surfaces are the result of the tension on the zonules, the elasticity of the capsule, and the growth properties of the lens fibers and epithelial cells. In younger individuals, refractive error is often caused by abnormalities in corneal curvature or the length of the globe, but rarely by defects in the curvature or refractive index of the lens.

Transparency depends on minimizing light scattering and absorption. Light passes smoothly through the lens as a result of the regular structure of lens fibers (Figure 5-3), the absence of membrane bound organelles, and the small and uniform extracellular space between the fiber cells. Paradoxically, the high crystallin concentration of the lens fiber cell cytoplasm is an essential component of lens transparency. Reduced light scattering results from short-range interactions between the highly concentrated crystallins.[83,385] Although it absorbs increasing amounts of the shorter wavelengths of visible light as it ages, the young human lens is nearly colorless.[157,379]

EARLY DEVELOPMENT

The cells that form the lens are originally part of the surface ectoderm covering the head of the embryo. Interactions between the future lens cells and nearby tissues during early development give these cells a "lens-forming bias."[145] As a result of these interactions, patches of cells that lie on either side of the head express the transcription factor *Pax-6*.[221] At the same time, neural epithelial cells on either side of the diencephalon in the embryonic forebrain bulge laterally to form the optic vesicles,

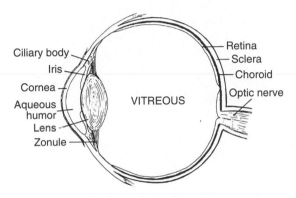

FIGURE 5-2 Diagram showing the relationship of the lens and zonules to the other structures in the adult eye.

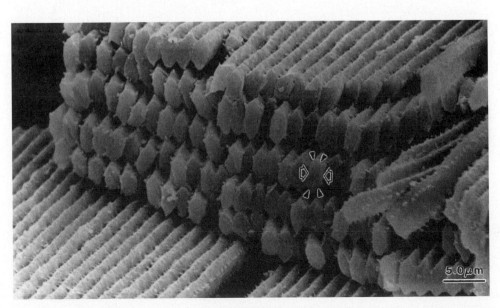

FIGURE 5-3 Scanning electron micrograph showing the orderly arrangement of hexagonal lens fibers (*arrows*) in the vertebrate lens. (Courtesy Dr. J. Kuszak.)

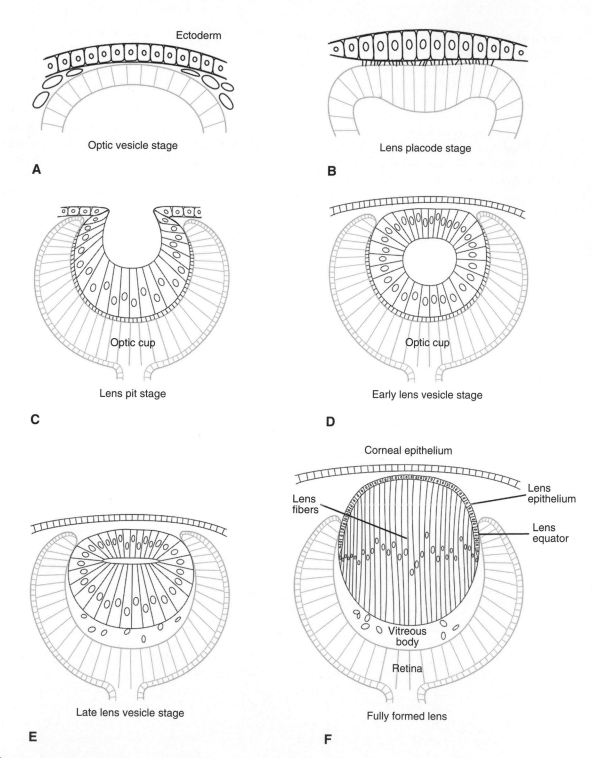

FIGURE 5-4   The early stages of lens formation. **A,** The lens vesicle contacts the surface ectoderm. **B,** The optic vesicle adheres to the surface ectoderm and the prospective lens cells elongate to form the lens placode. **C,** The lens placode and the outer surface of the optic vesicle invaginate to form the lens pit and the optic cup, respectively. **D,** The lens vesicle separates from the surface ectoderm. **E,** The primary lens fibers elongate and begin to occlude the lumen of the vesicle. The posterior of the lens vesicle separates from the inner surface of the optic cup. Capillaries from the hyaloid artery invade the primary vitreous body. **F,** The configuration of the lens as it begins to grow. Secondary fiber cells have not yet developed and organelles are still present in all fiber cells. (Modified from McAvoy J: Developmental biology of the lens. In Duncan G [ed]: *Mechanism of cataract formation,* London, 1981, Academic Press.)

which eventually contact the surface ectoderm cells (Figure 5-4, *A*). The cells of the lens vesicles also express *Pax-6*, a characteristic that is essential for eye formation.[148,391] Some of the genes that regulate and are regulated by *Pax-6* at early stages of eye formation are now known, although the number of genes involved and the knowledge about their interactions are likely to increase.[278,393,412]

After they make contact, the optic vesicles and the prospective lens cells secrete an extracellular matrix that causes them to adhere tightly to each other[144] (Figure 5-4, *B*) The surface epithelial cells that adhere to the optic vesicle then elongate, forming the thickened lens placode[143] (see Figure 5-4, *B*). Soon after, the lens placode and the adjacent cells of the optic vesicle buckle inward[328] (Figure 5-4, *C*). This morphologic transformation results in the formation of the optic cup from the optic vesicle. The invaginated lens placode soon separates from the surface ectoderm by a process involving the death of the cells in the connecting stalk between the cells of the surface ectoderm and the lens[109] (Figure 5-4, *D*). The *Pax-6*–expressing ectodermal cells adjacent to the lens placode that remain on the surface of the eye become corneal and conjunctival epithelial cells.[198]

Shortly after lens invagination, the extracellular matrix between the optic vesicle and the lens begins to dissolve and the two tissues separate[144,289] (Figure 5-4, *E*). The space that is formed between them is rapidly filled with a loose extracellular matrix, the *primary vitreous body,* that is secreted by the cells of the inner layer of the optic cup[343] (see Figure 5-4, *E*).

The epithelial cells that give rise to the lens vesicle originally lay on a thin basal lamina. In the process of invagination, this basal lamina comes to surround the lens vesicle. It gradually thickens by the deposition of successive layers of basal lamina material to form the lens capsule.[290,340]

Soon after the lens vesicle separates from the surface ectoderm, the cells in the posterior portion of the vesicle closest to the retina begin to elongate. The elongation of these primary fiber cells soon obliterates the lumen of the vesicle as their apical ends contact the apical ends of the anterior epithelial cells (Figure 5-4, *E* and *F*). Primary fiber cell formation establishes the fundamental structure of the lens, with epithelial cells covering the anterior surface and elongated fiber cells filling the bulk of the lens.

At this stage, most of the lens epithelial cells are actively proliferating. Cells at the margin of the epithelium are pushed toward the equator and are

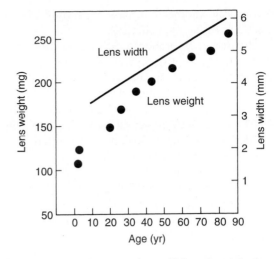

FIGURE 5-5 Changes in lens width and weight from birth to 90 years of age. (Data from Scammon RE, Hesdorfer MB: *Arch Ophthalmol* 17:104, 1937; and Brown N: *Med Biol Illus* 23:192, 1973.)

stimulated to differentiate into secondary fiber cells by factors present in the vitreous body.[20,68,69,329] As the secondary fibers elongate and their basal and apical ends curve toward the center of the lens, they displace the central primary fibers from their attachments with the capsule and the lens epithelium. The primary fiber cells are buried in the center of the lens during this process (see Figure 5-1). In the adult lens these cells form the embryonic nucleus. Deposition of successive layers of secondary fiber cells continues throughout life. The rate of fiber cell formation and therefore lens growth is rapid in the embryo and slows greatly after birth[326] (Figure 5-5).

In addition to *Pax-6*, several transcription factors have been shown to be essential for lens formation.[278] In chicken embryos, prospective lens cells express *L-maf,* a member of the *maf* family of *bZIP* transcription factors, soon after they contact the optic vesicle.[277] When modified forms of this protein that bind to deoxyribonucleic acid (DNA) but do not activate transcription are expressed in the prospective lens-forming region, the formation of the lens placode and lens vesicle is suppressed. Expression of *L-maf* in regions of the head ectoderm outside of the lens placode (but within the area expressing *Pax-6*) leads to the formation of extra lenses.[277] Although members of the *maf* family of transcription factors are expressed during lens formation in mammals, there is no factor comparable in sequence and expression pattern to *L-maf.*

Presumably, another molecule has subsumed the function of *L-maf* in mammals.

The proper separation of lens vesicle from the overlying presumptive corneal epithelium is defective in the mouse mutant, *dysgenetic lens (dyl)*. Recently, a mutation was identified in the "forkhead" transcription factor, *FoxE3*, in the *dyl* strain. *FoxE3* is selectively expressed in the lens placode and developing lens epithelium.[32,43] Therefore it is likely that *FoxE3* plays an early and important role in lens development.

Targeted disruption of the genes encoding three additional transcription factors that are normally expressed during primary fiber cell differentiation, *c-maf, sox1,* and *prox1*, leads to failure of elongation of primary lens fiber cells.[179,182,271,312] In mice lacking any one of these genes, lens fiber cells do not elongate or express the high level of lens crystallins that are characteristic of primary fiber cells. The factors that regulate the expression of *prox1, sox1,* and *c-maf* in lens fiber cells have not yet been identified. The diffusible factors that trigger fiber cell formation and the mechanisms responsible for fiber cell elongation and the regulation of crystallin synthesis are subsequently discussed.

Mice homozygous for the *aphakia* mutation form lens vesicles, but the lens cells degenerate soon after.[383] Recently, the *aphakia* mutation was mapped close to the gene encoding a homeodomain transcription factor, *Pitx3*.[332] *Pitx3* is expressed early in lens development and is not detected in any other cells in the embryo.[330] Two families have been described in which affected individuals have hereditary congenital cataracts and point mutations in *Pitx3*.[331] Semina et al.[332] identified a deletion of 652-bp in the region upstream of the *Pitx3* coding sequence in the *aphakia* strain. This deletion probably removes part of the promoter sequence required for the expression of Pitx3 and therefore could be the cause of the *aphakia* phenotype. Another group mapped and sequenced the *aphakia* locus and found the deletion in the promoter regions and a second deletion that removes part of the coding sequence of *Pitx3*.[311] This group showed that *Pitx3* was expressed at low levels in the *aphakia* strain and that the genes flanking *Pitx3* are normally expressed only either after lens formation or at similar levels in wild-type and *aphakia* mice. These results indicate that the deletions are likely to affect the expression of only *Pitx3*.[311] Therefore *Pitx3* is another transcription factor that is essential for normal lens development.

LENS FIBER CELL DIFFERENTIATION

Lens fiber cells are highly specialized, terminally differentiated cells. During their differentiation, fiber cells withdraw from the cell cycle; elongate greatly; express large amounts of proteins, the *crystallins;* acquire several specializations of their plasma membranes; and degrade all membrane-bound organelles.

The first evidence of fiber cell differentiation is withdrawal from the cell cycle. After their last mitosis, epithelial cells leave the germinative zone and move in a posterior direction into the transitional zone (Figure 5-6). Cells in the transitional zone are postmitotic but have not yet begun to elongate. Studies in chicken embryos and newborn mice in which the lens was rotated so that the epithelial cell faced the vitreous body demonstrated that a factor (or factors) in the vitreous humor stimulates fiber cell differentiation.[68,413] Epithelial cells exposed to vitreous humor in this manner elongated like primary fiber cells. Furthermore, chicken embryo lens epithelial cells stopped progressing through the cell cycle within 9 hours after lens rotation, indicating that control of cell proliferation depends on factors from outside the lens.[422]

Several proteins that are known to be involved in regulating the cell cycle in many cell types appear to play an essential role in the cessation of lens fiber cell proliferation. Included in this group are the cyclin-dependent kinase inhibitor protein p57 (KIP2) and the retinoblastoma protein (pRb). Progression through the cell cycle requires the phosphorylation of regulatory proteins, called *cyclins,* by cyclin-dependent kinases. The cyclin-dependent kinase inhibitor protein p57, an inhibitor of cell cycle progression, is expressed in the early stage of lens fiber cell differentiation, where it is found bound to cyclins.[106,231] In lenses that lack the gene for the retinoblastoma protein pRb, a well-known regulator of the cell cycle, p57 levels are low and lens fiber cells do not withdraw from the cell cycle.[104,263] This finding suggests that pRb is required for the expression of p57 and that at least one function of p57 is to maintain lens fiber cells in the nonproliferating state by complexing with cyclins. Absence of both cyclin-dependent kinase inhibitors expressed in the lens, p27 and p57, leads to extensive lens fiber cell proliferation, even in the presence of pRb, confirming that these molecules play an important role in the withdrawal of fiber cells from the cell cycle.[417] Lenses lacking both p27 and p57 also do not make detectable levels of crystallins, suggesting that the func-

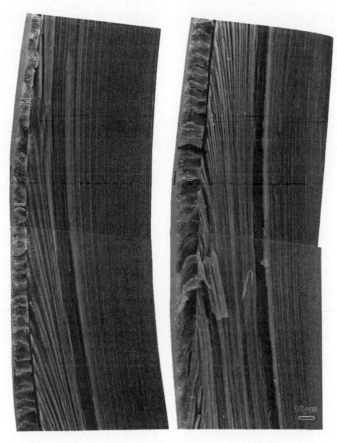

FIGURE 5-6 A montage of photomicrographs showing the organization of cells in the pregerminative zone (*curly brackets*), germinative zone (*square brackets*), and transitional zone (*curved brackets*) of the equatorial lens epithelium. The image on the right is a continuation of the one on the left showing the change in cell morphology as the cells of the transitional zone elongate (*asterisk*) to form lens fiber cells. The images were obtained with a scanning electron microscope (×780). (Courtesy Dr. J. Kuszak.)

tion of these molecules is essential for normal gene expression during fiber cell differentiation.[417] Other than the requirement for pRb, the mechanisms responsible for increasing the expression of p27 and p57 in lens fiber cells have not been determined.

Some of the basic mechanisms responsible for the extensive cell elongation that characterizes lens fiber cell differentiation have been described, but this process is not understood in detail. Early studies suggested that the microtubules of the lens fiber cytoskeleton are required for fiber cell elongation.[292,296] However, later experiments showed that fiber cells could elongate in culture in the absence of microtubules.[21] Whether other components of the cytoskeleton play an essential role in fiber cell elongation has not been demonstrated.

Evidence suggests that lens fiber cell elongation is driven by an increase in cell volume.[22] Initiation of fiber cell elongation is accompanied by changes in the ionic permeability of the plasma membrane. The resulting accumulation of potassium and chloride ions in the cytoplasm leads to an osmotically driven increase in cell volume.[288] Continued cell elongation depends on sustained protein synthesis.[262,297] The mechanism by which fiber cell elongation is regulated at different stages of differentiation, especially when fiber cells reach the sutures and stop elongating, has not been studied.

Several growth factors are capable of initiating lens fiber cell differentiation when added to cultured lens epithelia or, in some cases, when overexpressed in the lens in vivo. Among these are members of the fibroblast growth factor (FGF) and insulin-like growth factor (IGF) families. Studies in chicken embryos identified IGF-1 as a potent activator of fiber cell differentiation.[23] However, experiments in rats and mice showed that, although IGFs may play some role in fiber cell differentiation, members of the FGF family appear to be more important in mammals.* It is possible that different growth factors stimulate fiber cell differentiation in birds and mammals. Although FGFs are strong candidates for the fiber differentiation factors in mammals, it is not yet certain that they are essential for this process.[213] It remains a possibility that the authentic factor or factors responsible for fiber cell differentiation in vivo have not yet been found.

Lens Crystallins

The synthesis and accumulation of large amounts of crystallins characterize lens fiber cell differentiation. As much as 40% of the wet weight of the lens fiber cell can be accounted for by crystallins, a protein concentration that is approximately three times higher than that in the cytoplasm of typical cells.[96] Crystallin proteins can be classified as either *classical* or *taxon specific*. The classical crystallins include members of the α-crystallin family and the β/γ-crystallin superfamily. All vertebrate lenses accumulate large amounts of classical crystallins in their fiber cells. In many species, fiber cells also produce large amounts of taxon-specific crystallins.[298,406] As the name implies, different taxon-specific crystallins are found in the lenses of different species. Taxon-specific crystallins are functional enzymes or proteins that are structurally similar to enzymes but that lack enzymatic activity. The levels of taxon-specific crystallins sometimes exceed those of the classical crystallins. Adult human lenses do not produce taxon-specific crystallins, although the enzyme betaine-homocysteine methyltransferase is present at high levels in the embryonic nucleus, indicating that this enzyme serves as a taxon-specific crystallin during the early development of the human lens.[306]

Many of the transcription factors responsible for the high lens-specific expression of the crystallin genes have been identified. The details of these studies are described in comprehensive reviews and are not considered further here.†

Human lenses express two α-crystallin genes: αA and αB. Examination of the protein structure of the α-crystallins showed that they are members of the family of small heat shock proteins.[162,193,293] An important function of small heat shock proteins is to stabilize proteins that are partially unfolded and prevent them from aggregating (chaperone activity).

The role of the α-crystallins in preventing protein aggregation and precipitation has been demonstrated in experiments performed in vitro.[158] A similar in vivo role for αA-crystallin has been inferred in mice in which the αA-crystallin gene was disrupted.[38] The function of the α-crystallins in preventing protein aggregation has obvious importance for the lens because the proteins in lens fiber cells must persist for the life of the individual and excessive protein aggregation could lead to light scattering and cataract formation (see following discussion).

α-Crystallins are also enzymes because they possess serine-threonine autokinase activity.[173] It is not yet clear whether the α-crystallins phosphorylate other proteins in lens fiber cells to regulate lens metabolic activity. The α-crystallins are, themselves, normally phosphorylated in vivo and can be phosphorylated in vitro in a cyclic adenosine monophosphate–dependent manner.[53,348] The kinases responsible for the phosphorylation of α-crystallin in the lens and the importance of this phosphorylation, if any, for the function of lens cells have not been determined.[392]

α-Crystallin proteins normally associate in the lens cell cytoplasm to make high-molecular-weight complexes containing approximately 30 subunits. The structure of these complexes has been revealed by cryoelectron microscopy.[159] These observations show that native α-crystallin complexes can be assembled in a number of configurations, indicating that there is substantial flexibility in the way the subunits associate. α-Crystallin monomers also readily exchange between high-molecular-weight complexes, further supporting the view that α-crystallin complexes are plastic.[36]

The phenotype of αA-crystallin knockout mice provides insight into the function of α-crystallins in vivo.[38] The lenses of these animals are slightly smaller than normal but structurally similar to the normal lens. Mature fiber cells contain aggregates of proteins that lead to the formation of cataracts in the first few weeks after birth. Analysis of these aggregates shows that they contain large amounts of αB-crystallin and smaller amounts of other proteins. These results suggest that, in the fiber cell cytoplasm, αA-crystallin is partly responsible for preventing αB from aggregating. In addition, when lens epithelial cells from these animals were cultured in vitro, they grew more slowly than normal cells, were more sensitive to stress, and appeared to undergo a higher rate of apoptosis.[8] Therefore αA-crystallin appears to be important for the normal function of lens epithelial cells and fiber cells.

---

*References 49, 50, 54, 213, 217, 226, 246, 315, 316, 329, 353.
†References 76, 77, 196, 248, 278, 294, 295.

In addition to being expressed at high levels in the lens, αB-crystallin is present in a variety of cells throughout the body, especially in heart and skeletal muscle.[92] The protein is also found in damaged areas of the central nervous system in a variety of neurodegenerative diseases.[122,381] A naturally occurring mutation in the αB-crystallin gene leads to the formation of cataracts and myopathy.[386] In vitro tests showed that the mutant form of the protein had no chaperone activity and even enhanced the aggregation of test proteins.[37] These studies suggest that αB-crystallin has important chaperone functions in the lens and in other cells of the body. However, the fact that the mutant protein accelerated the denaturation of test proteins leaves open the possibility that the mutant is a gain-of-function. In this case, the cataracts and myopathy seen in individuals harboring this mutation could be a result of the destabilizing function of the protein rather than loss of its putative function as a chaperone.

The β/γ-crystallin superfamily is more diverse than the α-crystallins, and the function of its members in the lens is less evident. The β- and γ-crystallins were originally thought to be two distinct protein families. However, once the protein sequences of representative members of these families were available, it was clear that they were closely related.[91] The major difference in these proteins is the tendency for most of the β-crystallins to form multimers, whereas the γ-crystallins exist as monomers. Solving the three-dimensional structure of these molecules confirmed their close structural relationship and provided a structural rationale for why the β-crystallins form higher-order aggregates.[18,200] Six β-crystallin polypeptides (βA1, βA3, βA4, βB1, βB2, βB3) and three γ-crystallins (γS, γC, γD) are expressed in the human lens, although the βA1 and βA3 polypeptides are derived from the same gene (βA3/A1).[212,249] The only enzymatic activity identified to date in a member of the β/γ-crystallin superfamily is the detergent-activated proteolytic activity of βA3/A1.[350] This enzymatic activity has not yet been found in vivo.

Lens Fiber Cell Cytoskeleton

Microtubules are abundant beneath the plasma membranes of lens fiber cells, where they probably play an important role in stabilizing the fiber cell membrane.[208] Microtubules may also be important for transporting vesicles to the apical and basal ends of elongating fiber cells, although neither of these functions has been demonstrated in vivo. In addition to microtubules, there is an abundant network of actin-containing microfilaments beneath the plasma membrane of lens fiber cells. These microfilaments associate with the cytoplasmic surfaces of the adhesive junctions between lens fibers and are also likely to interact with the spectrin-containing submembrane meshwork.[214,228] This submembrane scaffold also contains tropomyosin and tropomodulin, proteins that may alter the structure of the microfilaments.[99]

Lens fiber cells also contain an unusual complement of intermediate filaments, including those composed of vimentin.[101] This is unusual because vimentin intermediate filaments are usually restricted to cells of mesodermal, not epithelial, origin. The function of vimentin-containing intermediate filaments in the lens is not evident because mice lacking vimentin appear to have normal lenses.[65] Overexpression of vimentin in the lens leads to cataract formation and abnormal fiber cell maturation.[47] Whether this is a specific effect of excessive vimentin levels in the lens or the response of the lens to protein overexpression in general has not been demonstrated.

In addition to vimentin, the lens contains intermediate filaments consisting of the proteins filensin and phakinin.[114,302] These filaments have an unusual "knobby" structure, leading to the name *beaded filaments*.[165] Beaded filament proteins have been found only in lens fiber cells, suggesting that they have a specialized role in these cells.[165] Mutations in the phakinin gene appear to be the cause of cataracts in two separate pedigrees.[66,168] Despite this useful information, the cataracts in these individuals could be caused by gain-of-function mutations (e.g., excessive protein aggregation resulting from misfolding of the abnormal phakinin protein). The normal function of beaded filaments in the lens is unknown.

Other Cellular and Biochemical Specializations Found in Lens Fiber Cells

In fiber cells at early stages of elongation, the lateral plasma membranes are smooth. However, as fiber cells reach the sutures, the membranes become progressively more interdigitated, forming interlocking "ball-and-socket" junctions[202,401] (Figure 5-7). Ball-and-socket junctions may stabilize the lateral membranes of the fiber cells and ensure that the cells remain tightly connected during accommodation. The mechanisms responsible for the formation of these unusual membrane specializations have not been identified.

The membranes of mature fiber cells have an unusual lipid composition. Human lens fiber cells

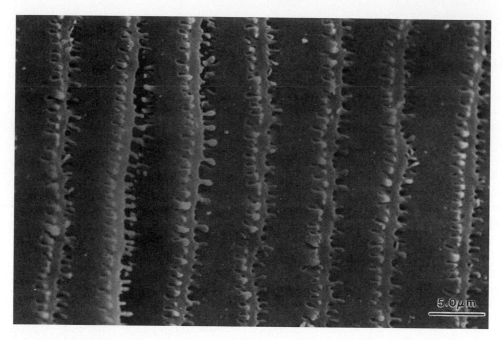

FIGURE 5-7   Visualization of the ball-and-socket interdigitations at the lateral surfaces of lens fiber cells. The tissue was fractured to show the surface morphology of the cells and viewed with a scanning electron microscope. (Courtesy Dr. J. Kuszak.)

have the highest proportion of cholesterol of any plasma membrane in the body, and the amount of cholesterol increases as the fiber cells mature.[33,34] The cholesterol/phospholipid ratio is nearly three-fold greater in nuclear than in cortical fiber cells. Partially purified fiber cell membranes have a substantially lower cholesterol/phospholipid ratio than that found in the whole tissue, although membranes from nuclear fibers still have proportionally higher cholesterol content than membranes from the cortex.[34] This finding suggests that some of the cholesterol in mature lens fiber cells may be associated with a complex that is not an integral component of the plasma membrane. There is also a high percentage of sphingomyelin in lens membrane phospholipids.[33] The presence of high concentrations of cholesterol and sphingomyelin is likely to cause lens fiber cell membranes to be rigid.[34] The functional significance of these biochemical specializations is unknown.

In addition to its unusual lipid content, lens fiber cell plasma membranes contain several unique proteins. The most abundant of these is the *major intrinsic polypeptide* (MIP). MIP accounts for as much as 50% of the total protein of the lens fiber cell membrane and has not been detected in any other cells in the body. When the MIP complementary

DNA was first cloned and sequenced, it encoded a protein sequence that was unrelated to any known protein.[127] Later, when the aquaporin family of water channel proteins was identified, MIP was recognized to be its "founding" member.[2] Despite its strong structural resemblance to the other aquaporins, MIP is a relatively inefficient water channel.[51] The reason for its abundance in the lens and its function there are not well understood, although MIP plays a prominent role in a theoretical model of fluid and ion flow in the lens.[242] Mutations in the MIP gene lead to cataracts in mice and humans.[28,336] These mutations could cause cataracts because they reduce MIP function or because they interfere with the normal function of the lens by generating large amounts of abnormal membrane protein.[336]

The gap junctions of the lens are assembled from a unique set of subunits, or *connexins*. The cell-to-cell transport of small molecules mediated by these gap junctions is likely to be important for the function of the lens because most of the fiber cells are far from the nutrients supplied by the aqueous and vitreous humors.[125] Not surprisingly, lens fiber cells have the highest concentration of gap junction plaques of any cells in the body (Figure 5-8).

Three connexins are found in lens cells: α1, α3, and α8. Connexin α1 (also known as *Cx43*) is

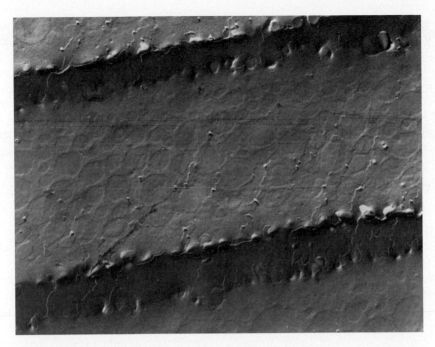

FIGURE 5-8   Scanning electron micrograph showing the abundant gap junction plaques on the surface of young lens fiber cells (×270,000). (From FitzGerald PG, Bok D, Horwitz J: *Curr Eye Res* 4:1204, 1985.)

found in many tissues in the body. In the lens, it is present only in the epithelial cells.[264] Connexins α3 (Cx46) and α8 (Cx50) are abundant in fiber cells but are also expressed at lower levels in the lens epithelial cells of some species.[78,123] Whether connexins α3 and α8 are found in human lens epithelial cells is not yet known. Gap junction plaques containing both connexins α3 and α8 are present along the lateral membranes of lens fiber cells.[187]

Although the presence of a large number of gap junctions seems to be essential for the normal function of the lens, recent studies have shown that the lenses of mice lacking either the connexin α3 or α8 gene are only mildly affected. In the case of the α3 knockout mice, fiber cell differentiation proceeds normally, although nuclear cataracts appear shortly after birth.[123] However, no cataracts form when the disrupted α3 connexin gene is bred onto a different genetic background, indicating that genetic modifiers can compensate for the absence of this connexin in maintaining lens transparency.[124] The lenses of the α8 knockouts grow more slowly than the lenses of the wild-type mice in the first 2 weeks after birth and develop diffuse nuclear cataracts.[400] Considering the abundance of specialized connexins in the lens, these phenotypes seem surprisingly mild. Unpublished reports indicate that animals

lacking both fiber-specific connexins have more severe cataracts, suggesting that the functions of these proteins may partially overlap.

A possible alternative pathway for nutrient diffusion from more superficial to deeper fiber cells has been described recently. In chicken embryos, fiber cells fuse with their neighbors late in their differentiation, just before they degrade their organelles.[335] This event links the cytoplasm of cells containing organelles with the cytoplasm of cells that have already degraded their organelles. Fiber cell fusions have been described previously in the lenses of several species, although it is not yet evident whether these fusions are as abundant as those described in chicken embryos.[204,205] If fiber cell fusions occur frequently in human lenses, newly formed proteins and essential metabolites could diffuse from metabolically active, superficial cells to older, less metabolically active fibers. The question of whether the extensive cytoplasmic continuity present in chicken embryo lenses is a common feature of the lens fiber cells of other species should be answered in the near future.

The second most abundant protein in the lens fiber cell membrane is MP20. The sequence of MP20 gives little clue to its function because it is unlike that of known proteins. However, mutations in the MP20 gene in mice lead to the formation of congenital cataracts.[351] As with the mutations in MIP, it is not clear whether these mutations cause cataracts by loss of an essential function or by gain of a deleterious one.

Lens fiber cells are linked to their neighbors all along their lateral membranes by N-cadherin, a calcium-dependent, homophilic cell adhesion molecule.[24,211] N-cadherin is typically linked to the actin cytoskeleton by a complex of proteins that includes α- and β-catenin. Therefore, as the lens changes shape during accommodation, the lateral membranes of the fiber cells are held together tightly by interlocking ball-and-socket junctions and N-cadherin–containing cell-to-cell adhesion complexes. These adhesion complexes may also contribute to the close association between the lateral membranes of lens fiber cells, thereby minimizing the extracellular space and reducing light scattering.

In addition to the lateral cell adhesion complexes, lens fiber cells are joined tightly to each other at their apical and basal ends.[16,24,229] These complexes contain abundant N-cadherin and vinculin, a protein that plays an important role in regulating the interaction between adhesion molecules and the actin cytoskeleton. Membrane complexes at the basal ends of the lens fiber cells, along the posterior capsule, probably attach the fiber cells to the capsule because they contain a rich actin cytoskeleton, the contractile protein myosin, and integrin extracellular-matrix receptors.[16,390] It is possible that the basal membrane complex also plays a role in the migration of the basal ends of the lens fiber cells toward the sutures.[16]

The lens grows by progressively adding new layers of fiber cells to its outer surface. These new fiber cells elongate, gradually extending their apical and basal ends toward the sutures. Once the tips of an elongating fiber cell reach the sutures, they meet a fiber cell coming from the opposite side of the lens. The cells then form new junctions at the apical and basal ends and detach from the posterior capsule (see Figure 5-1). They are gradually buried deeper within the lens by successive layers of fiber cells.

Soon after they detach from the posterior capsule, fiber cells suddenly degrade all of their membrane-bound organelles, including their mitochondria, endoplasmic reticulum, and nuclei.[12,15,209] Organelle degradation is complete within a few hours.[12] The mechanism responsible for organelle degradation in lens fiber cells is not known, although it has been suggested that the enzyme 15-lipoxygenase mediates organelle loss in the lens, as it does during the maturation of erythrocytes.[380]

In primates, the outer shell of fiber cells that contain organelles is only about 100 microns wide. For the most part, these organelle-containing cells are located outside of the optical axis of the lens[11] (see Figure 5-1). The absence of organelles in most lens fibers increases transparency by reducing light scattering. However, organelle loss also makes the fiber cells in the center of the lens dependent on the superficial fiber cells, an arrangement that may contribute to age-related cataract formation (see subsequent discussion).

Control of Growth

The human lens grows rapidly in the embryo and during the first postnatal year. The rate of lens growth slows between ages 1 and 10 years, then continues at a much slower, nearly linear rate throughout life[326,349] (see Figure 5-5). The factors that regulate lens growth in humans are not known. Many growth factors have been shown to stimulate lens epithelial cell proliferation in vitro, and the receptors for several families of growth factors have been identified in the human lens and in the lenses of other species. These include the FGF family, the IGF family, the epidermal growth factor (EGF) family, platelet-derived growth factor (PDGF), hepatocyte growth factor, and vascular endothelial cell growth factor (Shui et al., unpublished results from the author's laboratory).[29,103,395] In addition to these growth factor receptors, there are many other kinds of receptors, including muscarinic acetylcholine receptors and purinergic receptors.[310,402] However, it is unknown whether any of these signaling systems is essential for lens growth in vivo. In mice, absence of signaling through EGF, PDGF, or IGF receptors has not been associated with any defects in lens growth or development.[300]

Communication between Lens Epithelial and Fiber Cells

The apical ends of the lens epithelial cells abut the apical ends of elongating fiber cells. It has been suggested that nutrients are provided to the underlying fiber cells through gap junctions that link the apposed ends of these cells.[125,303,400] Other studies have questioned this interpretation because gap junctions are rarely detected at the apical ends of central epithelial cells.[17,78] Because the peripheral fiber cells contain a full complement of organelles, it is unclear whether transport from the epithelium is necessary for lens viability. However, damage to lens epithelial cells compromises the viability of underlying lens fibers.[147] Whether this is caused by the absence of metabolites provided by the epithelium or by some other role of the epithelium has not been determined.

Vascular Support during Development

Soon after the lens is formed, it becomes invested with a meshwork of capillaries. In the posterior of the lens, this network, the *tunica vasculosa lentis,* arises from the hyaloid artery. The capillaries at the anterior of the lens arise from blood vessels of the developing iris stroma to form the *anterior pupillary membrane.* These capillary networks join with each other near the lens equator. The importance of the fetal vasculature to normal lens development is unknown. In nonmammalian species there are no vessels around the lens during its development.

During the second trimester of human development, the capillaries of the tunica vasculosa lentis and the anterior pupillary membrane regress.[418] Decreasing levels of plasma-derived vascular endothelial cell growth factor may be one of the factors involved in the normal regression of these vessels.[256] Macrophages in the vitreous body also appear to play an essential role in regression.[87,418]

A number of hereditary and acquired ocular diseases are accompanied by persistence of the fetal vasculature.[121] At present, it is unclear why the fetal vasculature fails to regress in so many different syndromes and hereditary diseases. Better understanding of the factors that regulate vascular regression in normal ocular development is needed to address this question.

The Lens as the Organizer of the Anterior Segment

Studies performed in the 1960s and extended in the last few years suggest that the lens plays an important role in the development of the other tissues of the anterior segment.[19,112,113,332,358] Absence of the lens at an early stage of embryogenesis leads to the absence of the corneal endothelium; abnormal differentiation of the corneal stroma; and absence of the iris, ciliary body, and anterior chamber.[19,113,332,358,370] Therefore the lens not only receives signals from its environment but also sends signals to nearby tissues that are essential for their normal development.

SPECIAL PROBLEMS OF LENS CELL METABOLISM

Overview

The lens, like all biologic systems, is subjected to oxidative stress. Oxidation can be caused by molecular oxygen or free radicals. Free radicals are generated by the normal activity of mitochondria, by other normal metabolic processes, and by the absorption of light.[375] To counteract the effects of oxidation, all cells maintain a reducing environment in their cytoplasm. The generation of reducing equivalents requires the expenditure of energy and therefore presents an especially difficult problem for the deeper lens fiber cells that lack mitochondria. Enzyme systems in these deeper cells are also less active because they may have been synthesized decades earlier. For this reason, central fiber cells maintain a precarious balance between the catastrophic damage that would be caused by the unchecked oxidation of membrane lipids and cytoplasmic proteins and the diffusion from the more superficial cells in the lens of molecules that protect against oxidative damage.[371]

The unique structure of the lens creates special problems for the majority of fiber cells that do not contact the lens epithelium or capsule. Nutrients must reach these cells by diffusion, either through the space between cells, through specialized cell-to-cell junctions, or through cell fusions. To reduce light scattering and maintain transparency, lens fiber cells must maintain a small extracellular space. Therefore nutrient and metabolite transport is more likely to occur through cells rather than between them. This predicts that metabolites will accumulate in the center of the lens and that diffusion will limit the availability of nutrients and essential metabolites to cells deeper in the lens. Most fiber cells do not synthesize proteins and must deal with the consequences of molecular senescence without the capacity for repair.

The lens derives much of its energy from glycolysis. The end product of glycolysis is lactic acid. As a result of lactate accumulation, intracellular pH drops significantly from peripheral to deeper fiber cells.[14,243] As a result, pH-sensitive processes are differentially affected in different regions of the lens.[13] Gap junction conductance is one of the systems in the lens that should be affected because gap junction permeability is generally decreased at low pH. Interestingly, connexin α8 (Cx50) is cleaved by proteolysis in the deeper fiber cells, a process that abolishes its pH sensitivity.[222] Other structural and metabolic adaptations to the standing pH gradient in the lens are likely to exist.

Another problem that the lens faces is the need to maintain protein stability for many decades. Once the lens is formed, proteins are synthesized only in the superficial fiber cells. Therefore proteins made during embryogenesis in humans may have to last for more than 100 years. Accumulated damage leads to loss of enzymatic activity. Altering the structure of the crystallins, cytoskeletal proteins, and enzymes also increases their propensity for aggregation, a process that can lead to cataract formation.

Oxidants within and around the Lens

All of the cells of the body exist in an oxidizing environment. Molecular oxygen is, directly or indirectly, the source of most oxidative damage. If cells could survive in an atmosphere free of oxygen, most oxidative damage could be avoided. For most cells this is not possible. However, human lenses can be maintained in an atmosphere of pure nitrogen for some time, as long as adequate amounts of glucose are provided.[185] This is possible because the lens obtains much of its energy from glycolysis.[55,405]

The oxygen tension around the lens in the living eye is low, approximately 15 mm Hg (approximately 2% O_2).[142,210,253] The low oxygen tension around and within the lens probably protects lens proteins and lipids from oxidative damage. Even with this low level of oxygen, the lens normally derives a substantial proportion of its adenosine triphosphate (ATP) from oxidative phosphorylation, a process that, of necessity, generates free radicals.[375,405]

Hydrogen peroxide is another molecule that may be responsible for oxidative stress in the lens. Hydrogen peroxide is produced in mitochondria by superoxide dismutase from a by-product of oxidative phosphorylation, the superoxide anion. Hydrogen peroxide can also be produced by the oxidation of ascorbic acid. Because ascorbic acid levels in the aqueous humor are high (approximately 1 mM), both processes may contribute to the hydrogen peroxide that has been detected within the lens.[85,345] Although hydrogen peroxide by itself is not a particularly strong oxidant, it readily produces damaging free radicals in the presence of ferrous ions by means of the Fenton reaction. One of the mechanisms that protects against this form of damage is the presence of high concentrations of the protein transferrin in the aqueous humor.[252] Transferrin binds iron and may inhibit it from reacting with hydrogen peroxide to produce free radicals.

The level of hydrogen peroxide in the aqueous humor has been reported to average more than 30 μM and to exceed 200 μM in approximately one third of cataract patients.[344,345] However, recent studies suggest that, for methodologic reasons, the level of hydrogen peroxide in aqueous humor was overestimated in these earlier studies.[31,108,347] Reexamination of the levels of hydrogen peroxide around the human lens using methods not subject to these errors is needed.

The lens is exposed to solar irradiation throughout its life. Although much of the most energetic and potentially harmful ultraviolet light that reaches the eye is absorbed by the cornea, the remaining solar radiation could have harmful effects, especially on the metabolically vulnerable fiber cells.[89] If light is not absorbed, it produces no damage. However, ultraviolet light is readily absorbed by a number of cellular constituents, including DNA, proteins, nucleoside-containing metabolites, flavonoids, and pigments. Flavonoids and pigments also absorb visible light, especially the shorter wavelengths of visible light. All of these interactions are potential sources of free radicals. Free radicals oxidize DNA, lipids, and proteins. Whether free radicals are produced by the absorption of light depends on the chemical nature of the molecule that is interacting with light and the molecular environment.

Despite its exposure to light throughout life and the presence of abundant targets for light damage, there is no evidence for the photo-oxidation of proteins in the central region of the lens, even in lenses from older individuals.[137,138] It is likely that lens constituents are protected against the harmful effects of light-generated free radicals by the high intracellular concentration of reducing substances (see following discussion) and by the low concentration of oxygen around and within the lens.[142]

Protection against Oxidative Damage

Glutathione, a tripeptide of the amino acids glutamine, cysteine, and glycine, provides most of the protection against oxidative damage in the lens. It can prevent the oxidation of components of the lens cytoplasm because its concentration in the lens is high, approximately 4 to 6 mM, and its sulfhydryl group is readily oxidized. When glutathione levels have been lowered in lens epithelial cells or whole lenses, cell damage and cataract formation follow rapidly.[45,308,309]

Lens epithelial and superficial fiber cells can synthesize glutathione, and glutathione can be transported into lens from the aqueous humor.[170,171,309] Reduced glutathione is regenerated from oxidized glutathione (GSSG) by glutathione reductase and NADPH[309] (Figure 5-9). Much of the NADPH in the lens is produced by the hexose monophosphate shunt, the activity of which is important for the continued production of reduced glutathione.[55]

However, fiber cells deeper in the lens have minimal capacity for the synthesis or reduction of glutathione. They must obtain most of their reduced glutathione by diffusion from more superficial fiber cells.[309,359] Glutathione can form disulfide bonds with the oxidized sulfhydryl groups of proteins. These glutathione-protein mixed disulfides can then be reduced by a second molecule of glutathione, a process

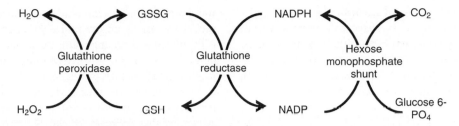

FIGURE 5-9   Diagram showing the major reactions responsible for the reduction of glutathione (*right side*) and the use of glutathione to reduce hydrogen peroxide (*left side*).

that is facilitated by the enzyme thioltransferase.[230] This regenerates the protein sulfhydryl and forms disulfide-linked glutathione (GSSG). The GSSG that results from this process must then diffuse to more superficial layers of the lens, where it can be reduced to form two molecules of glutathione (Figure 5-10). It is likely that this two-way diffusion is the rate-limiting step in maintaining a reducing environment in the center of the lens.[371] Recent studies show that the rate of diffusion between the superficial and deeper layers of the lens diminishes with age.[359] Therefore proteins and lipids in the nuclei of older lenses must be less able to withstand oxidative stress than those in younger lenses.

Ascorbic acid is also likely to protect the lens against oxidative damage. Ascorbic acid is actively transported from the blood to the aqueous humor by a sodium dependent transporter located in the ciliary epithelium, and it reaches concentrations in the aqueous humor that are up to 20 times higher than levels in the blood.[317,374] The ascorbate levels in the lens and other intraocular tissues are also substantial, although the prevailing evidence is that the lens does not contain a sodium-dependent ascorbate transporter.[180] Dehydroascorbate, the oxidized form of ascorbic acid, can enter the lens by way of the glucose transporter, where it can be reduced by glutathione-dependent processes.[317,404] Like glutathione, ascorbate is readily oxidized, forming dehydroascorbic acid in the process. Therefore ascorbate can react with free radicals and other oxidants in the aqueous humor and the lens, preventing these molecules from damaging lens lipids, proteins, and nucleic acids.

In addition to high levels of transferrin in the aqueous humor, which may minimize the harmful effects of hydrogen peroxide, the lens has two enzyme systems to detoxify this metabolite. Lens epithelial cells have abundant levels of catalase, which converts hydrogen peroxide to water, and glu-

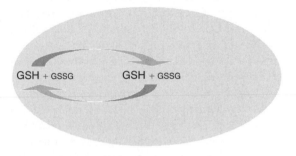

FIGURE 5-10   Diagrammatic representation of the distribution of reduced glutathione (*GSH*) and oxidized glutathione disulfide (*GSSG*) in the adult human lens. An increased fraction of glutathione is in the oxidized form in the center of the lens, a situation that is often increased in the aging lens.

tathione peroxidase, an enzyme that couples the reduction of hydrogen peroxide to the oxidation of glutathione.[307] Studies on cultured lenses and lens epithelial cells suggest that glutathione peroxidase provides most of the protection against the potential damaging effects of physiologic levels of hydrogen peroxide. Catalase is effective only against relatively high concentrations of peroxide.[116]

ENERGY PRODUCTION

As a result of the lack of blood supply, the oxygen concentration within and around the lens is much lower than that in most other parts of the body.[142,253] Therefore the lens depends on glycolytic metabolism to produce much of the ATP and the reducing equivalents required for its metabolic activities.[185,405] The glucose required for glycolytic metabolism is derived from the aqueous humor. Aqueous humor glucose levels are maintained by facilitated diffusion across the ciliary epithelium.

However, lens epithelial cells and superficial fiber cells also contain numerous mitochondria. Therefore cells near the surface of the lens may use both gly-colytic and oxidative pathways to derive energy from glucose. Approximately 50% of the ATP produced by rabbit lens epithelial cells is derived from oxidative metabolism, whereas glycolysis accounts for nearly all the ATP produced in lens fiber cells.[405]

Water and Electrolyte Balance

Because of the lens' high protein concentration and lack of a blood supply, it faces special problems in regulating its water content and in transporting nutrients to cells deeper in the lens. A gradient of increasing protein concentration is found as the lens is inspected from the more superficial fiber cells to fiber cells deeper in the lens.[96] However, this protein gradient is not associated with a reciprocal gradient in the osmotic activity of water because water does not have a tendency to flow into the cells of lens nucleus. The mechanism by which this large potential osmotic gradient is neutralized is unknown. The simplest explanation is that there is a decreasing gradient of protein osmotic activity deeper in the lens. Decreased protein osmotic activity might result from the increase in the short-range interactions between protein molecules, which contributes to lens transparency.[83] The mechanism by which proteins can be concentrated in an osmotically neutral manner remains an important unsolved question in the biophysics of the lens.

Recently, investigators have suggested that there is a fluid circulation within the lens. It has been suggested that these hypothetic water currents are driven by ionic gradients generated by the transport activities of lens epithelial and superficial fiber cells.

Vibrating electrodes have detected gradients of electrical potential around the lens.[287,314] Positive charges flow into the lens near the anterior and posterior sutures and out at the equator. Like most cells, the membranes of lens epithelial and superficial fiber cells contain sodium-potassium–activated ATPase (Na^+-K^+-ATPase) activity. The Na^+-K^+-ATPase generates an electrochemical gradient across the surface membranes of the lens, with the interior of the lens more negative than the extracellular space. This electrochemical potential tends to drive positive charges, largely sodium ions, into lens cells. This appears to be the origin of the inward positive current at the sutures.[287,314,403] The positive current flowing out at the lens equator is likely to be carried by potassium ions.[403]

A model that takes into account the electrical and biophysical properties of the lens predicts that water will follow the flow of ions into and out of the lens, creating an internal circulation system.[242] Although this is an appealing construct, direct evidence for water flow through the lens fiber cell cytoplasm has not been provided.

In support of the idea that water flows into the lens, lens epithelial cells contain the water channel aquaporin-1 (previously known as *CHIP28*), and as mentioned earlier, lens fiber cell membranes have high levels of aquaporin-0, or MIP.[268] Recent studies show that the lens epithelium actively moves water from the aqueous humor into the lens fiber mass.[98] Water flow across the lens epithelial cells can be blocked by agents that prevent the function of aquaporin-1. It has not been determined whether this water percolates between lens fiber cells or whether it enters the lens fiber cell cytoplasm, perhaps through channels formed by aquaporin-0. In either case, if this observation is confirmed, it indicates that a substantial flow of water enters and leaves the lens. This can be one way that the lens transports metabolites to and from the deeper lens fiber cells.[98,242]

The transmembrane potential of the human lens decreases steadily with age.[94] This decrease is caused by an increase in the permeability of the fiber cell membranes to sodium and calcium ions through nonselective cation channels. It is unclear whether the increased cation permeability is caused by increased numbers of these channels, by the appearance of the new type of channel, or by an increase in the activity (open probability) of preexisting channels. The increase in cation permeability is balanced by an increase in the activity of membrane ATPases, which remove sodium and calcium from lens cells. Despite the increased pump activity, free sodium and calcium levels increase in the cytoplasm of older lenses.[94] Because the transmembrane potential of all cells indirectly provides the driving force for the transport of many metabolites and nutrients, the age-related decrease in the transmembrane potential of the lens may have important consequences for lens metabolism and ionic homeostasis. Elevated calcium levels can also lead to metabolic disturbances and destruction of cell components through the activation of calcium-sensitive proteases.

Like all cells, lens epithelial and fiber cells maintain a much lower concentration of free calcium ions in their cytoplasm than is found in the extracellular space. However, free calcium levels measured in fiber cell cytoplasm are substantially higher than the levels in epithelial cells.[94,166] In addition, there appears to be a gradient of free calcium that decreases from the posterior to the anterior ends of lens fiber cells.[166] These observations are consistent with the view that calcium slowly leaks into lens fiber cells and is removed by membrane pumps at the lens surface. The activity of these pumps in maintaining low cytoplasm calcium concentrations is important because treatments that abruptly raise free calcium levels lead to rapid degradation of the lens fiber cell cytoskeleton, uncontrolled proteolysis, cell swelling, and opacification.[61,95,167,237,373]

Lens epithelial cells transport nutrients into their cytoplasm from the aqueous humor. Although the transport of small molecules from epithelial cells to fiber cells has been demonstrated, the relative importance of this pathway in providing nutrients to the fiber cells, compared with transport directly across the surface membranes of superficial fiber cells, has not been measured.[303,400] When metabolite transporters have been examined in lens fiber cells, these molecules have usually been found. The distribution of glucose transporters in the lens illustrates this issue. Lens epithelial cells express abundant levels of the glucose transporter glut1, which is presumably used for the uptake of glucose from the aqueous humor.[260] Although fiber cells express little glut1, they express large amounts of the higher-affinity glucose transporter glut3. Therefore fiber cells can transport glucose into their cytoplasm from the extracellular milieu, a finding that raises questions about the relative importance of the epithelial cells in providing glucose to the fiber cells.

TRANSPARENCY AND REFRACTION

Vertebrate lenses are remarkably effective optical devices. An efficient lens must be transparent to the wavelengths of light that can be detected by the photoreceptors, must have a focal point that is appropriate for the optical system in which it functions, and must have a minimum of spherical and chromatic aberration. Lens transparency depends on the organization of the cells of the lens and of the distribution of the proteins within. The precise organization of the fiber cells, their high protein concentration, and the absence of organelles from the fiber cells that lie in the optical axis ensure that a minimum of scattering occurs as light passes through the lens.

The cellular and molecular interactions responsible for establishing and maintaining the curvature of the lens surfaces are unknown. Studies in chicken embryos demonstrated that influences from outside the lens normally regulate its shape and rate of growth.[69] Lenses in different species range from nearly spherical (rodents) to an axial ratio of more than 2:1 (humans). As the human lens grows, the radii of curvature of its anterior and posterior surfaces decrease significantly.[40] Despite this, the focal point of the lens remains remarkably constant, suggesting that the refractive power of the lens cytoplasm is altered to compensate for the change in curvature of the refractive surfaces. Control of lens shape is one of the most fascinating unanswered aspects of lens biology.

The high protein concentration of the lens fiber cells causes the refractive index of the lens to be higher than that of the fluid around it. Fiber cells close to the surface of the lens have a lower protein concentration than fiber cells deeper in the lens, creating a gradient of refractive index that at least partially corrects for spherical aberration.[199,341,342]

Although the human lens is transparent to most wavelengths of visible light, it produces and accumulates chromophores that absorb the shortest wavelengths of the visible spectrum. At birth, the human lens is pale yellow. With increasing age, the amount of yellow pigmentation in the lens increases. This pigmentation absorbs the shorter, more energetic wavelengths of light, preventing them from reaching the retina. The predominant yellow chromophores in the young human lens are metabolites of tryptophan, especially *N*-formyl kynurenine glucoside.[157] With aging, an increasing variety of soluble and protein-bound chromophores are found in the lens fiber cells.[105,299] When especially high concentrations of these chromophores accumulate, they can reduce visual acuity by increasing light absorbance, leading to the formation of what is termed a *brunescent* or *nigrescent cataract*. The factors responsible for the excessive accumulation of chromophores in some lenses are not known, although recent studies suggest that the oxidative modification of proteins may play a significant role.[105] Brunescent cataract is more common in developing countries, which suggests that environmental or nutritional factors may be important.

CHANGES WITH AGING

Fiber cells in the center of an adult lens are produced during early embryonic life, whereas those at the surface of the lens may be weeks or months old. It has been widely assumed that, by studying the composition of fiber cells at different depths within the lens, one can determine the changes that occur as a result of aging. For this reason, many authors have touted the lens as a valuable model system for studying aging. However, unique properties of the lens, especially the lens fibers, probably make it an inappropriate model for aging in most cell types.

Protein synthesis ceases at about the time that fiber cells degrade their organelles.[334] It has therefore been assumed that any changes in protein structure in deeper layers of the lens fibers result solely from the effects of age. However, in chicken embryo lenses, fiber cells fuse with their neighbors just before they degrade their organelles, and some degree of fiber cell fusion is a common property of the lenses of many species.[204,205,335] It seems possible that newly synthesized proteins might diffuse slowly from more superficial, younger fiber cells into older fiber cells deeper in the lens through these membrane fusions. Therefore protein modifications found with increasing depth in the lens may not be strictly proportional to increasing age.

One way to have increased confidence that changes in the composition of the lens are related to age is to correlate changes in fiber cells from lenses of different ages and from different layers of the same lens. With use of this approach it was shown that, in the human lens, many of the soluble crystallins are sequentially truncated by proteolysis over months to years.[110] Some of the β-crystallins showed a relatively rapid rate of degradation, whereas other crystallins were degraded much more slowly. However, by the end of the first 20 years of life, most of the crystallins appeared to reach a steady state after which little additional degradation occurred. Therefore, in older lenses, crystallins in the center of the lens and crystallins a short distance from the surface of the lens showed similar degrees of proteolysis.[110] These studies examined only changes in soluble crystallins. Further studies may show that crystallins in the insoluble fraction are more extensively degraded.

The proteins of the lens are often characterized by their relative solubility, typically being separated into fractions that are water soluble, urea soluble, and insoluble. As one goes from the more superficial to the deeper fiber cells, an increasing percentage of the crystallins are found in the insoluble fraction. In addition, when the water-soluble crystallins are separated by size, an increasing proportion is found in high molecular aggregates. Therefore there is a tendency for proteins to become aggregated and less soluble in the older fiber cells.[313,346] α-Crystallin is a good example. In the lens nucleus from individuals of increasing age, decreasing amounts of soluble α-crystallin are found. By age 45 years, no α-crystallin is detectable in the water-soluble fraction from the lens nucleus.[251,322]

The gradual insolubilization of α-crystallin is likely to be related to its function as a molecular chaperone.[158] When lens proteins are unfolded, hydrophobic domains are exposed. α-Crystallin binds to these hydrophobic regions, presumably preventing further unfolding and protein aggregation. It seems likely that accumulated damage to the crystallins leads to increased association with α-crystallin. Interestingly, despite the loss of soluble α-crystallin, a precipitous increase in the rate of protein aggregation in the lens nucleus is not seen after age 45 years.

Another age-related change seen in crystallin structure is the increasing racemization of aspartic acid, methionine, and tyrosine, and the deamidation of glutamine and asparagine.[111,154,241] Although racemization and deamidation alter protein structure, these changes correlate well with age but do not differ significantly in clear and cataractous lenses of the same age.

Some components of the lens fiber cell cytoskeleton are disassembled in older fiber cells. Vimentin intermediate filaments are degraded in the deeper lens cortex, well after the loss of membrane-bound organelles.[301] Beaded filaments made up of phakinin and filensin persist into the lens nucleus and may last for the life of the lens.[302] Actin microfilaments also appear to survive in the oldest fiber cells, although the persistence and continued association of these filaments with the plasma membrane has been questioned.[63,181,236] Proteolysis and insolubilization of the components of the cytoskeleton appear to contribute to their disassembly.[63,301,302]

STRUCTURE AND DEVELOPMENT OF SUTURES

Sutures form at the anterior and posterior poles of the lens, where fiber cells growing from opposite sides of the lens abut at their apical and basal ends. In some species, all fiber cells meet near the midline of the lens, forming an "umbilical" suture.[203] However, in most species the sutures form along planes. In human embryos, elongated lens fiber cells meet at three planes, forming an upright Y at their anterior ends (with respect to the superior-inferior axis of the eye) and an inverted Y posteriorly (Figure 5-11, *A*). As the human lens grows, the suture planes formed by more superficial shells of fibers become increasingly complex. The first evidence of this typically occurs soon after birth, when two new suture planes form at the ends of each of the three branches of the Y sutures (Figure 5-11, *B*). As new fibers are added during lens growth, the branch points gradually migrate toward the center, eventually forming a six-pointed "star" suture[203] (Figure 5-11, *C*). Branching again occurs at the tips of each of these six planes, eventually forming a total of 12 suture planes at the anterior and posterior surfaces of the lens[203] (Figure 5-11, *D* and *E*). The increasing geometric complexity of the suture patterns in older human lenses results in lenses with better optical proper-

ties than in species that maintain a simple Y-suture pattern throughout life.[206]

The structure and orientation of the sutures result in a challenging problem for developmental and structural biologists. The lens appears to be radially symmetric about the optical axis, yet the sutures form in a pattern that breaks this symmetry. The spatial cues that lead to the precise alignment of the suture planes with respect to the axes of the body are unknown.

LENS CAPSULE

When the lens placode invaginates from the surface ectoderm early in embryonic life, it is already

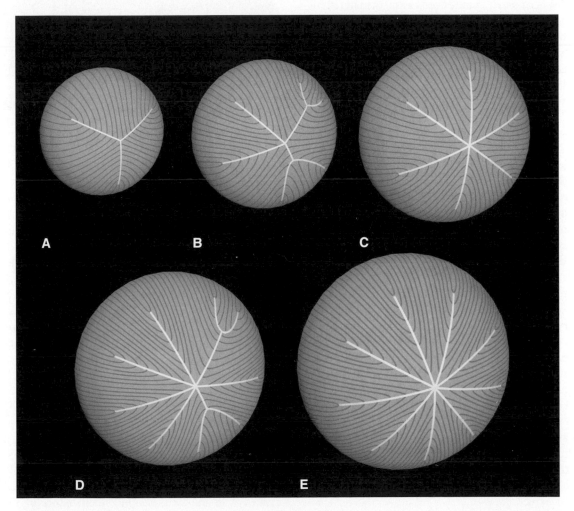

FIGURE 5-11 Diagram illustrating the increasing complexity of the sutures as the lens grows. The sizes of the lenses depicted are to scale. **A–C,** The tripartite Y suture that forms during embryogenesis as a result of secondary fiber cell formation is converted into a six-pointed star suture by the continued deposition of new fiber cells. If the fibers from the lens depicted in **C** were peeled away, the initial tripartite suture pattern would be revealed. **D** and **E,** Further growth results in the formation of additional suture planes.

supported by a thin basal lamina.[340] This extracellular matrix surrounds the lens vesicle after it detaches from the surface ectoderm. The lens epithelial and superficial fiber cells continue to secrete the components of the basal lamina, which thickens to become the lens capsule.[290,340] Structural examination of the lens capsule in the electron microscope shows that it is composed of multiple laminae, as if the basal lamina had been reduplicated many times.[46] Studies of the synthesis of the lens capsule in experimental animals showed that newly synthesized capsular materials are originally deposited close to the basal ends of epithelial and fiber cells.[415] With time, the labeled components of the capsule move farther away from the surface of the cells because they are displaced by successive layers of newly synthesized capsular material.

Clinical observations have supported the view that the human lens capsule is also synthesized from the inside out. In certain cases, foreign materials can be deposited in the capsule during its synthesis. These deposits can be viewed in slit-lamp or Scheimpflug images.[276] Eventually, these deposits disappear from the lens. One interpretation of this observation is that, as new layers are laid down on the inner surface of the capsule, capsular material is lost from the surface of the lens. If this interpretation is correct, the rate of synthesis of components of the capsule at its inner surface and the rate of degradation at its outer surface regulate its thickness. The capsule also must be remodeled during embryonic life, when the surface area of the lens is increasing rapidly.[169] It is not known which enzymes may be responsible for the degradation or remodeling of the capsule.

In keeping with its similarity to typical basal laminae, the capsule is predominantly composed of type IV collagen, laminin, entactin (nidogen), and heparan sulfate proteoglycans.[46,281,289] However, studies have shown that some components of the capsule differ in the anterior, posterior, and equatorial regions of the lens.[100,169,415] In the adult lens, the capsule is significantly thicker over the epithelium and thinner over the basal ends of the superficial fiber cells. The factors that regulate the differential distribution and accumulation of the components of the lens capsule remain to be identified.

ZONULES

The zonules (suspensory ligament, zonules of Zinn) are composed of thin fibrils that suspend the lens in the anterior of the eye. Zonular fibers insert

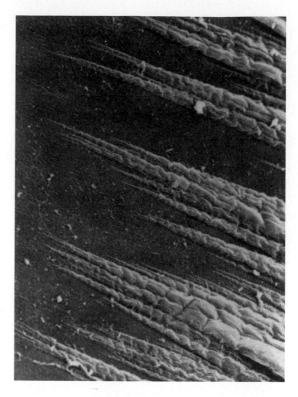

FIGURE 5-12 Scanning electron micrograph showing tapering bundles of zonular fibers inserting into the lens capsule (×780). (From Streeten BW: *Invest Ophthalmol Vis Sci* 16:364, 1977.)

into the lens capsule near the equator and into the basal lamina of the nonpigmented layer of the ciliary epithelium[355] (Figure 5-12). It is likely that the ciliary epithelial cells synthesize the components of these fibrils.[399] The primary structural protein in zonular fibers is fibrillin.[254,357,399] Mutations in the fibrillin gene are responsible for Marfan syndrome, in which dislocation of the lens is a common clinical finding.[86,215]

Examination of the insertion of zonular fibers into the lens capsule shows that these fibers are intimately interwoven with the components of the capsule.[97,355,399] If, as suggested previously, the capsule is continuously degraded at its outer surface, it is unclear how the zonular fibers and capsular fibers maintain their connections.

This is only one of the topologic paradoxes associated with the synthesis and maintenance of the zonules. For example, it is also unclear how the components of the fibrils are originally inserted into the lens capsule, especially when they are under tension, or how the zonular fibers are physically attached to the basal lamina of the ciliary epithelial cells while

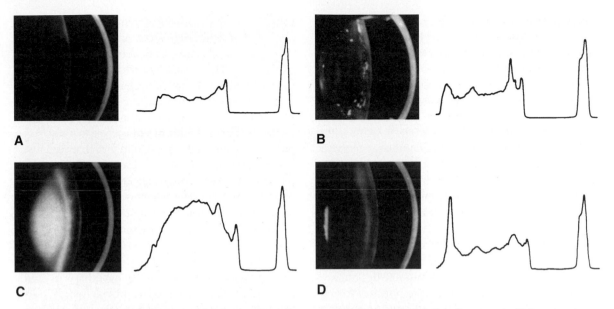

FIGURE 5-13 Photographs of the anterior portion of human eyes taken using a Scheimpflug camera. Light scattering from the cornea, the lens capsule epithelium, and any opacity in the lens can be seen in the photographs. Scattering intensity is shown in scans of the photographs made with a densitometer. **A,** Normal lens. **B,** Cortical cataract. **C,** Nuclear cataract. **D,** Posterior subcapsular cataract.

being synthesized by these same cells. Presumably, the zonular fibers establish their attachment between the lens capsule and ciliary epithelium early in development, when these basal laminae are in direct contact. If this assumption is correct, it predicts that the number of zonular fibers should not change throughout life. If it is not correct, a mechanism must exist for these fibrils to be assembled across the space between the ciliary epithelium and the lens capsule, a remarkable feat of bioengineering.

As the lens grows, the position of insertion of the zonules shifts anteriorly.[97] Because the zonules are believed to maintain a fixed point of insertion into the lens capsule, this shift has been interpreted as evidence for a relative increase in capsule synthesis at the lens equator.[97] It is possible that the age-related anterior shift in the zonular insertion point alters the forces applied on the lens during accommodation and may contribute to presbyopia.[97]

CATARACT

A *cataract* is any opacification of the lens. Cataracts are considered clinically significant when opacification interferes with visual function. Loss of lens transparency can be caused by an increase in light scattering or light absorption. Increased light scattering can be caused by disruption of the structure

of lens fiber cells, increases in protein aggregation, phase separation in the lens cell cytoplasm, or a combination of these processes.

Age-related cataracts are classified on the basis of the region of the lens that is affected (Figure 5-13). The most common types of age-related cataracts are nuclear, cortical, and posterior subcapsular. Nuclear cataracts occur in the oldest fiber cells, those formed during embryonic and fetal life. Cortical cataracts occur in cells formed later in life. These cataracts typically occur in a sector of the lens and affect mature cells that have already degraded their organelles. Posterior subcapsular cataracts (PSCs) result from light scattering by a plaque of swollen cells at the posterior pole of the lens.

In addition to age-related cataracts, a variety of less common cataracts are usually classified on the basis of their cause. These cataracts include the opacification of the posterior lens capsule that sometimes occurs after cataract surgery, referred to as *secondary cataracts, after cataracts,* or *posterior capsular opacification (PCO)*. Age-related cataracts are discussed first, followed by each of the several types of cataracts for which specific causes are known.

Age-Related Nuclear Cataracts

In the United States and most Western countries, nuclear cataracts are most often associated with increased light scattering in the nuclear fiber cells. In many developing countries, brunescent nuclear cataracts are more common. These opacities are associated with increased lens color and consequent light absorption. Whether a result of light scattering or absorption, nuclear cataract is the most common type, typically accounting for more than 60% of cataract surgery.

Abundant evidence shows that nuclear cataracts are associated with increased oxidative damage to lens proteins and lipids.[90,309,344,361,372] The formation of disulfide bonds between protein subunits can lead to aggregation and increased light scattering, although other forms of protein-to-protein interactions may occur.[309] Evidence also suggests that crystallins may associate with lens fiber cell membranes in an increased amount in nuclear cataracts.[160,161,197,360] The factors responsible for increased oxidation in nuclear cataracts are not fully understood. However, the marked age dependence of nuclear cataracts and the concurrent increase in oxidized glutathione in the lens nucleus suggests that disturbances in the balance between protein and lipid oxidation and glutathione-dependent reduction may be involved.[35,309,359]

Persuasive evidence for an association between oxidation, age, and cataract formation was provided by studies of patients treated with hyperbaric oxygen to alleviate the complications of peripheral vascular disease.[284] These individuals were exposed to 2.0 to 2.5 atmospheres of pure oxygen for 1 hour each day for up to 3 years. Of the 25 patients treated in this study, all but one had increased light scatter in the lens nucleus and seven developed frank nuclear cataracts. All of the individuals who showed increased light scattering or opacification in the nucleus were older than 50 years of age. The individual who did not show increased light scatter was 24 years old. Patients of slightly older average age with the same presenting symptoms, but not treated with hyperbaric oxygen, served as the control group. None of the individuals in the control group developed cataracts over the study period. After the termination of treatment, some of the patients who had been treated with hyperbaric oxygen and had developed increased light scatter showed improvements in their visual acuity and decreases in the amount of light scattering in their lenses. This result suggests that, even in older individuals, the lens has the capacity to reverse oxidative damage to the components of the nucleus.[284]

The onset of nuclear cataract formation is often associated with an increase in the refractive power of the lens.[41] For patients with hyperopia, this myopic shift temporarily causes an improvement in their near visual acuity, a phenomenon often called *second sight*. This increase in refractive power is associated with hardening of the lens nucleus. It is not surprising that the term *nuclear sclerotic cataract* is used to describe the opacities that soon follow.

Patients treated with hyperbaric oxygen also experienced significant myopic shift, like that seen just before the formation of a nuclear sclerotic cataract. As with the light scattering described previously, these increases in lens refractive power usually reversed during treatment or soon thereafter.[234,284,318]

Isolated lenses and experimental animals have also been treated with hyperbaric oxygen. The results of these studies are in general agreement with the findings in patients receiving hyperbaric oxygen therapy. These animal models provide useful tools to study the effects of oxidative stress on cataract formation.[115,117,282]

Studies of patients treated with hyperbaric oxygen suggest that molecular oxygen or a metabolite derived from molecular oxygen contributes to nuclear sclerosis and nuclear cataract formation. Studies of the effect of hyperbaric oxygen on the lens also provide some of the strongest evidence that the cells of the lens nucleus are in a delicate balance between their ability to prevent or reverse oxidative damage and the tendency for oxidation to occur. The fact that hyperbaric oxygen leads to opacification of the lens nucleus, but not the more superficial lens fiber cells, shows that the central fibers are more susceptible to oxidative damage. Age-associated changes in the level and rate of diffusion of glutathione in the lens nucleus are likely to be part of the reason for this increased susceptibility.[35,309,359,371]

Nuclear cataracts commonly occur in older patients within 6 months to 3 years after vitrectomy. Several studies have reported that the incidence of cataracts is as high as 80% after the removal of the vitreous body.* The incidence of postvitrectomy cataracts is significantly higher in patients older than 50 years than in younger patients.[257] To date, there have been no studies of the mechanism of postvitrectomy cataracts in humans and only one published study in experimental animals.[207]

Because there have been no studies of the changes in the human lens after vitrectomy, we do not know whether the same oxidative changes seen in typical age-related nuclear cataract also occur in postvitrectomy nuclear cataracts. However, the appearance of

---

*References 52, 80, 81, 257, 274, 279, 369, 378.

the lens in postvitrectomy nuclear cataracts is similar to typical age-related nuclear cataracts, the only difference being the rapidity of onset of cataracts after vitrectomy. If it is assumed that the cause of the cataracts in both cases is the same, there is likely to be an increase in oxidative damage in the lens after vitrectomy. The lens is usually not touched during vitrectomy, and the time between surgery and cataract formation is at least several months. Therefore the high incidence of nuclear cataracts after this procedure is probably a result of changes in the environment around the lens, rather than a direct effect of the procedure on the lens.

One potential source of increased oxidative stress to the lens after vitrectomy is an increase in the oxygen tension around the lens. The oxygen tension in the anterior vitreous is normally low, approximately 16 mm Hg (approximately 2%).[324] However, the oxygen tension in the posterior vitreous near the retinal vessels is high, decreasing in a sharp gradient within the first 1 mm of the vitreous body.[3] It is possible that when the vitreous is removed and the fluid in the eye can circulate freely, the lens is exposed to increased oxygen from the retina. This can tip the balance between reduction and oxidation in the lens nucleus, leading to rapid cataract formation. The details of this hypothesis remain to be tested.

The increased light scattering associated with nuclear cataract formation can be caused by protein aggregation or by separation of the lens cell cytoplasm into protein-rich and protein-poor liquid phases.[82,362,363] Evidence suggests that phase separation accounts for some of the opacification that occurs in several experimental models of cataract formation.[25,57-60,62,150,333] Phase separation can be caused by modifications to the soluble proteins in the lens nucleus or by alterations in the ionic composition of the solvent phase in this region.

Electron microscopic examination of the fiber cells in the lens nucleus suggests that nuclear cataract formation is usually not associated with a gross disruption of cell membranes, obvious protein aggregation, or phase separation[4,5,367] (Figure 5-14). Techniques aimed at detecting subtle alterations in the organization of the fiber cell cytoplasm have not found significant differences between clear lenses and lenses with nuclear cataracts in most cases.[367] Changes in cytoplasmic organization are easily demonstrated in experimental models in which cataracts are caused by reversible phase separation.[58,59,376,377] These observations suggest that extensive phase separation is not likely to play a major role in nuclear cataract formation. More subtle changes in the organization of the cytoplasm, whether caused by protein aggregation or microscopic phase separation, cannot be ruled out.

Therefore, despite the dramatic change in the hardness of the lens nucleus that typically occurs during nuclear cataract formation, the changes in

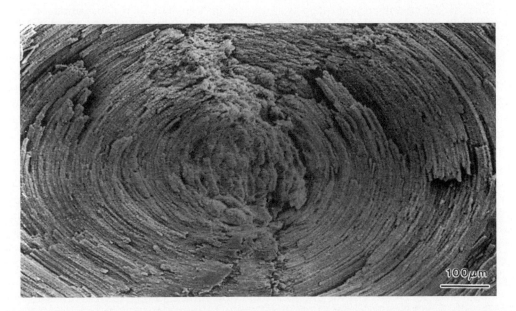

FIGURE 5-14 Scanning electron micrograph of the lens fiber cells in the embryonic nucleus of a lens from an 80-year-old. The fiber cells are still well organized and intact. (Courtesy Dr. J. Kuszak.)

the organization of proteins that lead to cataract formation appear to be subtle. It may be useful to remember that the protein concentration in the normal lens nucleus is much higher than that in typical cells and that there is, as yet, no obvious biophysical explanation for this high protein concentration. The increase in lens protein concentration that accompanies nuclear sclerosis may be a pathologic exaggeration of the mechanism responsible for protein concentration in the normal nucleus. If the mechanism responsible for the high protein concentration seen in the normal lens was understood, insight into the mechanism of nuclear sclerosis and nuclear cataract formation might be obtained.

It is also important to recognize that only a small fraction of the protein in the lens fiber cell cytoplasm needs be aggregated to increase light scattering dramatically.[384] This makes it difficult to identify the changes that lead to opacification among the many alterations of lens proteins that occur with aging.

In summary, it is likely that the aging lens is susceptible to oxidative damage as a result of the increased difficulty in maintaining the cytoplasm of the lens nucleus in the reduced state.[371] Any increase in oxidative load or further decrease in the ability of the lens nucleus to cope with the normal level of oxidation is likely to lead to nuclear cataract formation.

Age-Related Cortical Cataracts

The cells that are affected in cortical cataracts are mature fiber cells that lie close to the surface of the lens. Cortical cataracts most often occur in the inferior half of the lens, with a tendency for these cataracts to occur in the inferior nasal quadrant.[73,259] Cortical opacities usually begin in small regions of the lens periphery and, over years, may spread around the circumference of the lens. Early-stage cortical cataracts are usually not clinically significant because the opacity is limited to the lens periphery and does not impinge on the visual axis. As the cataract progresses, the opacity may spread toward the visual axis, eventually interfering with vision. However, an individual may have a cortical opacity for years without experiencing a diminution of visual function.

Like all mature lens fiber cells, the superficial lens fiber cells that are involved in cortical cataracts span from the posterior suture near the midline to the anterior suture. Therefore the peripheral opacities characteristic of early-stage cortical cataracts occur only in the central part of the affected fiber cells, with the apical and basal ends of these cells remaining transparent.[42,388] The spread of the cortical cataract around the lens circumference involves progressive damage to an increasing number of lens fiber cells of similar age, whereas the extension of a cortical cataract into the visual axis involves progressive opacification of the extremities of the same cohort of lens fiber cells. It is remarkable that the central region of a group of fiber cells can be completely opaque while the tips of the same cells remain transparent. Extension of the opacity along the lengths of a small cluster of fiber cells leads to the formation of the "cortical spokes" that are often described in these cataracts.

In contrast to the subtle morphologic changes that occur during nuclear cataract formation, cellular the damage found in cortical cataracts is catastrophic. Examination of the affected regions of lens fiber cells in a cortical cataract reveals almost complete disruption of cell structure.[93,387,388] Plasma membranes are ruptured, and many whorls and vesicles of membranelike material can be found in the cytoplasm. Cytoplasmic proteins are typically aggregated to such an extent that the cytoplasm takes on a chalky appearance when the cataractous region of the lens is disrupted during cataract surgery or during dissection. Therefore cortical cataract formation involves damage to all components of the cell.

Only a small group of cells is affected in the early stages of cortical cataract formation. Several mechanisms can lead to the formation of this initial opacity, including damage to the fiber cell plasma membrane, inhibition of the ion pumps or transporters in these membranes, damage to the system responsible for calcium homeostasis, excessive proteolysis, or the local loss of protective molecules such as glutathione. The occurrence of any one of these essential factors is likely to lead to all the others. This makes it particularly difficult to identify the initiating event in cortical cataract formation.

No matter what the initiating event, the loss of calcium homeostasis can underlie the radial and circumferential spread of opacification. Cytoplasmic calcium levels are abnormally high in the damaged cells of cortical cataracts.[93,238,389] As mentioned previously, lens fiber cells typically maintain their intracellular calcium concentration in the low micromolar range. Experimental elevation of lens cytoplasmic calcium levels leads to widespread proteolysis.[238] Gap junction communication is usually blocked by high levels of cytoplasmic calcium, presumably helping prevent the spread of calcium-induced damage to neighboring cells. However, if adjacent fiber cells are joined by membrane fusions, it may be difficult to prevent the eventual spread of high levels of calcium into adjacent cells.

The mechanism that initially prevents the spread of damage from the central portion of the lens fiber cell toward its basal and apical ends must involve the creation of a barrier between the central, cataractous region of the cell and the transparent, distal regions. Numerous membrane blebs and vesicles are seen in the opaque regions of cortical cataracts, a phenomenon that has been termed *globular degeneration.*[70] If the cytoplasm were to fragment into such vesicles during cataract formation, it is likely that the proximal ends of the fiber cells, adjacent to the damage, would be sealed by fusion of the plasma membrane. This could "wall off" the damaged region of the cell, thereby slowing the spread of damage.[93] Because fiber cells are connected to their neighbors by gap junctions all along their lateral membranes, walling off the central region of the cell does not isolate the tips of the cell from the rest of the lens.

The presence of a protective mechanism to prevent the spread of damage along the length of a fiber cell in typical age-related cortical cataracts is also seen in traumatic cataracts. Local physical damage to the lens, caused by traumatic injury to the eye or by touching the lens during surgery, usually leads to the formation of a local opacity. Such opacities may be restricted to the affected cells for many years, becoming buried deeper in the lens as new fiber cells are added, or the opacity may slowly spread to adjacent fiber cells in a manner that appears similar to the progression of nontraumatic cortical cataracts.[304]

Posterior Subcapsular Cataracts. PSCs are caused by light scattering in a cluster of swollen cells at the posterior pole of the lens, just beneath the capsule. Because the opacity produced by these cells is in the optical axis, PSCs are particularly disabling. Careful examination has shown that, in lenses with PSCs, the most superficial fiber cells are disorganized in localized regions at the lens equator. A "stream" of epithelial-like cells leads from the affected region of the equator to the opacity at the posterior pole.[356] This suggests that PSCs result from the abnormal migration of lens epithelial cells or the aberrant differentiation of lens fiber cells.

Opacities can also occur at the posterior pole as a result of swelling of the posterior ends of the fibers along the suture planes. These "sutural"

cataracts can sometimes resemble PSCs. However, sutural opacities are typically associated with inherited cataracts and are not common in age-related cataract.

"Pure" PSCs (PSCs not associated with another kind of cataract) are less common than either age-related nuclear or cortical cataracts, typically accounting for less than 10% of cataracts in humans. However, PSCs commonly occur in conjunction with nuclear or cortical opacities. Although specific risk factors are associated with PSCs (described in a later section), little information about the cellular or molecular defects associated with the formation of these cataracts is available.

One potentially valuable model system for the study of the cell biology of PSCs is experimentally induced radiation cataracts. Both amphibians and rodents have been used to study the cortical and posterior subcapsular opacities that develop over weeks to months after exposure to sufficient levels of ionizing radiation.[258,285,339,411] These models are relevant to PSCs in humans because patients whose lenses are exposed to ionizing radiation during interventional radiotherapy also develop PSCs. Some of the characteristics of radiation cataracts are described subsequently.

Mixed Cataracts. Patients with cataracts often have a combination of nuclear, cortical, and/or posterior subcapsular cataracts. It is not clear whether having one kind of cataract predisposes a person to developing an additional kind of cataract, although it seems likely that such an association would have been noticed. This is particularly likely in the case of a preexisting cortical cataract, which may be detectable but clinically insignificant for many years. However, I am not aware of studies showing that the presence of a cortical cataract is a risk factor for the later formation of a nuclear cataract or PSC. In the case of mixed cataracts, it is possible that the factors that led to the formation of one kind of cataract also contributed to the formation of the second or third type.

In most developed countries, cataracts are removed as soon as they become visually disabling. However, if a cataract is not removed, it may progress to a total or "morgagnian" cataract. There is no specific cause for total cataracts. They are simply the result of the progression of a more localized cataract to the point at which it affects the entire lens.

Secondary Cataracts. There are two general strategies for the removal of cataracts. The most common approach taken in developed countries is to remove a portion of the anterior lens epithelium and capsule to expose the underlying fiber mass; extract the nuclear and cortical fiber cells, often using instruments for "phacoemulsification"; and implant a plastic intraocular lens (IOL) in the capsular bag. This method of cataract removal is a form of *extracapsular cataract extraction.* Before IOLs were available, the entire lens was removed to remove the cataract. This is called *intracapsular cataract extraction* and is still the most common type of cataract surgery performed in developing countries.

A common complication of extracapsular cataract extraction is the formation of secondary cataracts, also called *after cataracts* or *PCO.* Removal of the cataractous fiber mass leaves the posterior capsule free of cells. Lens epithelial cells near the lens equator persist after cataract surgery and can migrate beneath the IOL onto the denuded posterior capsule. Epithelial cells that remain close to the equator may differentiate into a mass of fiberlike cells, forming a band called *Soemmering's ring,* around the equator.[177] If the epithelial cells migrate further onto the posterior capsule, they may differentiate into small "lentoid bodies," also called *Elschnig's pearls,* or they may form fibrotic plaques. Both Elschnig's pearls and fibrotic plaques scatter light, degrade the visual image, and result in secondary cataract formation.

The cells found in Elschnig's pearls resemble the large, swollen cells seen in PSCs.[176] They are likely to result from lens epithelial cells that were stimulated to undergo aberrant fiber cell differentiation. Instead of forming precisely organized, elongated lens fibers, they form small, rounded clumps of cells that act as miniature lenses, thereby degrading the image produced by the implanted IOL.

Fibrotic plaques contain contractile, myofibroblast-like cells in an abundant extracellular matrix, thereby resembling in many ways the fibrosis seen in anterior polar cataracts (see following discussion).[239,250,275,327] Myofibroblasts are contractile cells found during wound healing in many parts of the body. They express the contractile protein, α–smooth muscle actin, and secrete an abundant collagenous extracellular matrix, properties that may be important in wound healing. In addition to the light scattered by the cells and matrix in these plaques, the contractile cells wrinkle the posterior capsule, further contributing to light scattering.

The cytokine transforming growth factor-β (TGF-β) has been implicated as a stimulant of the capsular fibrosis seen in secondary cataracts.[131,227] Lenses and lens epithelial cells treated with activated TGF-β form plaques of myofibroblast-like cells similar to those seen in secondary cataracts.[130,133,201]

Other studies have suggested that the migration or spreading of lens epithelial cells on the posterior capsule may, by itself, contribute to myofibroblast differentiation.[266] Because active TGF-β is likely to be found in the eye after cataract surgery and cataract surgery always provides a surface on the posterior capsule for the migration of lens epithelial cells, it is possible that both of these conditions contribute to the formation of myofibroblasts after cataract surgery.

Less Common Types of Cataract. *Congenital cataracts* are cataracts that are present at birth or that appear soon after birth. They can include early-onset hereditary cataracts or cataracts caused by infectious agents. Most congenital cataracts are total, although some may affect specific regions of the lens. In most cases the cause of congenital cataracts is unknown, although the presence of a family history of congenital cataracts suggests a genetic component.

One infectious cause of congenital cataracts is rubella infection in early pregnancy.[394] The rubella virus has been isolated from the lenses of affected individuals, and experimental infection of early-stage human lens tissue with the rubella virus has been demonstrated. It is likely that the lens is susceptible to infection only early in gestation, before the separation of the lens vesicle from the overlying ectoderm. After this stage of lens development, the capsule appears to prevent the entry of the virus into the lens tissue.[178] Immunization against rubella in industrialized countries has reduced the incidence of rubella cataracts and other types of birth defects associated with this disease. However, rubella cataracts are still common in nonimmunized populations.

One of the cytologic characteristics of lenses infected with the rubella virus is the failure of organelle degradation in lens fiber cells.[420] The mechanism by which the rubella virus prevents organelle loss is not understood. However, several genetic and transgenic mouse models of cataract also show a failure of organelle degradation, suggesting that inhibition of organelle loss may be a nonspecific side effect of a variety of factors that perturb lens fiber cell differentiation.[47,195]

Anterior polar cataract is another type of congenital or early-onset cataract. Anterior polar cataracts typically involve the formation of an opaque plaque near the center of the lens epithelium. Microscopic examination of these plaques shows spindle-shaped lens epithelial cells embedded in a large amount of extracellular matrix, the plaque taking on the appearance of a connective tissue. The fiber cells that lie beneath these plaques are often disrupted, a factor that may contribute to the opacity. The spindle-shaped lens cells in these plaques express several of the proteins characteristic of myofibroblast cells, including α–smooth muscle actin, fibronectin, type I collagen, TGF-β, and connective tissue growth factor.[131,216,227] Experimental studies have shown that exposing lenses to TGF-β in vivo or in vitro can trigger the formation of myofibroblast-like cells and plaques that resemble those seen in anterior polar cataracts, although it has not yet been shown that anterior polar cataracts in humans are associated with exposure of the lens to high levels of TGF-β.[130,133]

Mutations in several lens-specific genes have been implicated in hereditary cataracts in humans. These include genes encoding αA- and αB-crystallin, members of the β/γ-crystallin superfamily, the lens-specific connexins α3 and α8, and the lens-specific intermediate filament protein phakinin.* To date, all mutations identified in these genes are dominant, resulting in a phenotype when only one allele is mutated.

The association of cataract and mutations in these genes does not necessarily demonstrate that the proteins they encode are essential to the function of the lens. For example, deletion of one copy of the genes encoding either of the two lens-specific connexins in mice does not result in cataract formation.[123,400] However, if one allele of these genes is mutated in humans, cataract can result.[235,337] Similarly, one mutant allele of any of several of the genes encoding members of the β/γ superfamily of crystallins is sufficient to cause cataracts.[129,146,195,352] In these cases the mutant allele may lead to the production of a protein that interferes with the function of the normal protein, thereby disrupting its function and leading to cataract formation. However, this kind of "dominant interference" has not yet been conclusively demonstrated as the cause of these cataracts.

Numerous hereditary syndromes include cataracts as one of their characteristic features. The genes responsible for these syndromes are known in several cases, including the oculocerebrorenal syndrome of Lowe (a protein similar to inositol polyphosphate-5-phosphatase),[10] neurofibromatosis type 2 (a member of the ezrin/radixin/moesin [ERM] family of cell membrane–associated proteins),[321] galactokinase deficiency (galactokinase 1),[120] galactosemia (galactose-1-phosphate uridyltransferase),[126] hyperferritinemia (ferritin light chain),[119] Werner syndrome (*recQ*-related helicase),[416] myotonic dystrophy (*SIX5* homeobox gene),[194,325] and several others. For most of these diseases, knowing the gene responsible has not provided an obvious explanation for why cataracts are part of the phenotype. Understanding the molecular and biochemical mechanisms underlying cataract formation in these syndromes may provide information about the mechanisms of age-related cataract formation.

Exceptions to this generalization include galactosemia and galactokinase deficiency, in which the sugar galactose accumulates to high levels in the body. High levels of galactose lead to the accumulation of the polyol galactitol in the lens fiber cell cytoplasm. This is caused by the activity of the enzyme aldose reductase, which converts galactose to galactitol. Accumulation of galactitol leads to osmotic swelling of lens fiber cells, damage to fiber cell membranes, and cataract formation. The possible role of aldose reductase in the formation of cataracts seen in diabetic patients is discussed further in a following section.

Exposure of the eye to several kinds of electromagnetic radiation can lead to cataract formation. The best studied of these are cataracts caused by ionizing radiation.[64] In experimental animals, x- or γ-irradiation causes characteristic changes in the cells of the lens, leading to PSCs and cortical cataracts. The initial insult in the cataractogenic process may be damage to the proliferating cells in the germinative zone of the lens epithelium, which leads to extensive cell death in this region.[285,408-410,421] Exposure of only the central epithelial cells and mature fibers to high levels of x-irradiation does not lead to cataract formation, as long as the germinative zone is protected from irradiation.[6] Furthermore, animals in which cell division in the lens can be stopped by environmental or experimental means are resistant to radiation cataracts.[218,320] Cell death in the germinative zone is followed by a delay in cell division and a wave of compensatory mitosis. When the epithelial cells that resulted from this increased proliferation begin to differentiate, the usually precise organization of the fiber cells is disrupted.[409] As they elongate, these fiber cells become distorted and may appear swollen, although their average cell volume is unchanged.[421] The appearance of fiber cell swelling may be a result of the presence of distended and attenuated regions along

---

*References 66, 146, 168, 224, 225, 235, 337, 352, 386.

the length of a fiber instead of the uniform geometry of normal fiber cells. Instead of remaining in a compact arc (the "lens bow"), the nuclei of these elongating fibers move posteriorly. This posterior movement of the nuclei probably reflects the flow of the entire cytoplasm of these cells. Eventually, these abnormal fibers form "balloon cells" or "Wedl cells" at the posterior pole, resulting in the formation of a PSC. During the later stages of this process, there is evidence of increased membrane permeability in the affected lens fibers. Glutathione levels decrease, the potassium concentration in the cytoplasm declines, the sodium concentration increases, and the synthesis of proteins slows.[107,244]

Exposure to x-rays or γ-radiation is a risk factor for cortical cataract and PSC formation in humans. Radiologists routinely seek to minimize the exposure of the lens to ionizing radiation. In cases in which this is impossible, cataracts often follow and must be dealt with surgically.

Nonionizing radiation can also contribute to cataract formation. The effects of ultraviolet (UV) light on the eye have been intensively studied. Epidemiologic studies have linked high lifetime exposure to UV light with the formation of cortical cataracts in humans.[72,73,247,365,397] The effects of UV light have been clearly demonstrated in individuals who are exposed to high levels of UV as a consequence of their occupation.[365,366] The risk of developing cortical cataracts is increased only slightly in individuals who receive higher-than-normal levels of UV but whose occupation does not routinely expose them to high levels of UV light.[397] The same studies have suggested that the shorter wavelengths of UV light (UV-B) reaching the eye, and not the longer, less energetic UV-A, is likely to be responsible for increased risk of cortical cataract.[366] However, studies in diurnal animals exposed to UV-A suggest that these longer wavelengths can also contribute to cataract formation (see subsequent discussion).

The mechanism by which UV exposure leads to cataract formation in humans has not been identified. Studies in experimental animals, on lenses cultured in vitro, and on isolated lens proteins have been used to examine the potential damaging effects of UV light on the lens or lens components. Although these studies have suggested that UV-generated free radicals can damage components of the lens in a similar manner to that seen in cataract formation, these studies often do not fully take into account the biology of the human lens. For example, most studies of the effects of UV light on the

lens in experimental animals have been performed in rodents or rabbits. These are nocturnal animals that are not adapted to high levels of light exposure. Many potential protective mechanisms found in the human eye, like the high ascorbic acid content of the aqueous humor, are not present in these species. Furthermore, treatment of the isolated lenses or lens proteins with UV light has usually been performed at ambient oxygen concentrations (21%), not at the low levels of oxygen typically found around the lens in vivo (2% or less).[142] Experiments performed under these conditions may yield results that are substantially different from what is found as the result of light exposure in the eye. Finally, UV exposure in experimental animals is often acute; high levels of UV light are used. This differs significantly from the chronic, lower level of exposure over a lifetime that is typical in humans.

In a few cases the effects of UV light on the lens were tested in diurnal species chronically exposed to more physiologic levels of light over a substantial proportion of their lifetime. In contrast to epidemiologic studies of human populations, these experiments indicated that UV-A light might also be a risk for cataract formation.[419] UV-A light can be absorbed by several chromophores in the lens, a process that may lead to the generation of free radicals.[88,105] These studies suggest that protection against free radical generation or the effects of free radicals might help reduce the incidence of cataracts. They also suggest that the role of UV-A light in human cataract formation is worthy of further study.

One of the paradoxic findings concerning the role of UV light in cataract formation is that the cells that are affected are those best protected from light exposure. As indicated previously, epidemiologic studies have associated UV light with the formation of cortical, not nuclear, cataracts. Cortical cataracts form in superficial fiber cells. Because they lie behind the densely pigmented iris epithelium, superficial fiber cells and the peripheral epithelial cells that give rise to them are better protected from light exposure than any other part of the lens. This is especially true in bright light, when the iris is maximally constricted and the size of the pupil is small. Conversely, epidemiologic and experimental studies indicate that the fiber cells in the center of the lens, those directly exposed to light entering the eye through the pupil, are usually not damaged by exposure to light.[138,365,397]

Studies using model eyes have suggested that light entering the eye from the temporal side of the head may be focused by the curvature of the cornea onto the cortical fiber cells on the opposite (nasal) side of the lens.[67,259] Although this hypothesis might provide an explanation for the higher frequency of cortical cataract formation on the nasoinferior side of the lens, it would not appear to account for the higher frequency of cortical cataracts in the remainder of the inferior half of the lens.[190] Studies are needed to explain the selective effects of light exposure on cortical fiber cells and to better understand the proposed role of ocular sunlight exposure in cortical cataract formation.

Long-term exposure to infrared light and focused, high-energy microwaves can also cause cataracts. Evidence that infrared light can cause cataracts comes mostly from epidemiologic studies in individuals exposed as a result of their occupation.[232,233] This type of cataract is also called *glassblowers cataract.* High-energy microwaves appear to cause cataracts by directly damaging lens fiber cell membranes.[9,71,261] It seems unlikely that either kind of cataract will provide significant insight into the cause of more common types of cataracts.

Long-term exposure to high-dose steroids is a significant risk factor for PSC formation in humans.[56,223] There are few animal models with which to study the effect of chronic steroid administration on the biology of the lens, and those that are available have not yet been used for biochemical or cellular biologic studies.[338,339] Consequently, little is known about the alterations in lens cells caused by steroids. This is unfortunate because knowledge of the cellular and molecular alterations leading to the formation of steroid-induced PSCs might provide information about the cause of PSCs not associated with steroid use. The extensive knowledge about the effects of steroids in other biologic systems has not yet provided insight about the mechanism of steroid-induced PSC formation.

People with diabetes are at increased risk for early-onset cataracts, and the lens has provided a useful system with which to study diabetic complications. Like other organ systems affected in diabetes, damage to the lens seems to entirely result from high levels of glucose. It is the mechanism by which elevated glucose leads to cellular damage that is the question. Investigators studying diabetic cataracts have been leaders in illustrating the potential importance of the enzyme aldose reductase in diabetic complications.[184,186] Aldose reductase catalyzes the reduction of a variety of aldehydes, including glucose and galactose. These sugars are relatively poor substrates for the enzyme, but their

metabolism by aldose reductase becomes significant when concentrations exceed normal levels. Species that have high levels of aldose reductase in the lens seem to be particularly susceptible to diabetic cataract formation.[79] Inhibitors of aldose reductase protect these animals against diabetic cataracts.[79,184,382] Mice, which have low levels of aldose reductase in the lens, are not particularly susceptible to diabetic cataracts. However, when aldose reductase is overexpressed in the lenses of transgenic mice, these animals become susceptible to hexose-induced cataract formation.[414] These studies convincingly show that a high level of aldose reductase in the lens is sufficient to cause diabetic cataracts in this species. Humans have relatively low levels of aldose reductase in the lens, a situation that has led to controversy about the relative role of aldose reductase in human diabetic cataracts.

It has been suggested that aldose reductase causes cataracts in people with diabetes because of the accumulation of the polyol sorbitol in lens fiber cells. Sorbitol accumulation can lead to osmotic damage. However, because aldose reductase uses reducing equivalents from NADH to produce polyols, it is possible that the high glucose flux through the polyol pathway could also create oxidative stress in lens fiber cells.

Three hypotheses are currently favored to explain diabetic complications in affected organs: (1) increased flux through the polyol pathway mediated by aldose reductase, (2) glucose-mediated activation of a specific isoform of protein kinase C, and (3) generation of increased amounts of advanced glycation end products (AGEs).[44,183] AGEs are produced by the nonenzymatic reaction of aldehydes, such as glucose, with a variety of chemical species. People with diabetes and animals with experimental diabetes accumulate increased levels of AGEs in connective tissues and within cells. Treatments that block each of these three biochemical pathways have been shown to reduce or prevent diabetic complications in one or more experimental systems. A recent study suggests that the three major pathways thought to be responsible for diabetic complications might be explained by a single mechanism: the effect of high glucose on mitochondrial oxidative phosphorylation.[272] High levels of glucose cause increased flux of reducing equivalents through the mitochondrial electron transport system, overwhelming the capacity of the mitochondria to generate ATP from adenosine diphosphate (ADP). This leads to increased production of superoxide anion, which is converted to hydrogen peroxide by the enzyme superoxide dismutase. This study showed that excess production of superoxide anion leads to the activation of aldose reductase, increased protein kinase C activity, and increased production of an early metabolite that is involved in the formation of AGEs.[272] When several approaches were used to prevent the production of excessive amounts of superoxide anion, the activation of aldose reductase and protein kinase C and the production of increased amounts of AGEs were prevented. If the results of this study are confirmed for the lens, it may be possible to intervene in the process that leads to diabetic cataracts, not to mention enable us to reduce diabetic complications in other tissues.

Epidemiology

A few of the risk factors for the formation of specific kinds of cataracts have already been discussed, including diabetes for cortical and posterior subcapsular cataracts, long-term sunlight exposure for cortical cataracts, and prolonged steroid therapy for PSCs. Epidemiologic studies have identified several other general and specific risk factors for cataract formation. Not surprisingly, age is the primary risk factor for the most common kinds of cataract. There is an exponentially increasing incidence of cataract after age 50 years. One risk factor common to most kinds of cataract is lower socioeconomic status or lower education level. Because lower socioeconomic status may predispose patients to nutritional deficiencies, increased exposure to diseases, poor general health status, and increased occupational exposure to cataractogenic agents, it is difficult to determine the specific aspects that are important for cataract formation.

Sex is also an important influence on the incidence of cataract. Women are at increased risk for most kinds of cataract.* Conversely, studies suggest that estrogen protects against cataract formation in humans and animals and that cataracts may be delayed by late menopause.† Lowering estrogen function with the antiestrogen tamoxifen increased the risk of cataracts when used for a long duration.[128,283] The protective effect of estrogen demonstrated by these studies makes the increased overall levels of cataract in women more difficult to understand. If estrogen is protective, other factors, as yet unknown, must strongly predispose women to cataract formation.

---

*References 48, 84, 149, 189, 191, 219, 220.
†References 26, 30, 74, 132, 188, 192.

When the influences of age, sex, and socioeconomic status are removed, specific risks for different types of cataracts are revealed. Smoking and high alcohol consumption have been identified in several studies as dose-dependent risk factors for nuclear and, in some cases, cortical cataracts.[84,153,291,396] Dark iris color is associated with a higher incidence of all types of lens opacities,[75,84,134] a finding that may also be related to higher levels of cortical cataract in African-Americans than in Caucasians.[220] Other than steroid exposure, fewer risk factors have been consistently identified for PSCs. However, this could be the statistical consequence of the relatively lower frequency of PSCs than of other types of cataract. Numerous epidemiologic studies have identified additional risk factors for specific kinds of cataracts. These are not detailed here, either because their association with cataract was not particularly strong or because they have not been seen in most epidemiologic studies of cataract.

Several studies have found an interesting and potentially important association between cataracts and increased mortality. When confounding variables, including smoking, age, race, and gender, are removed, the presence of clinically significant cataracts remains as a strong, independent predictor of mortality.[151,255,354,398] These findings suggest a significant connection between cataracts and systemic phenomena influencing survival. Considered in another way, behavioral, nutritional, and biochemical factors that prevent age-related cataract formation may lengthen life span.

Overview of Age-Related Cataract Formation. The previously presented data that describe different types of cataracts, the basics of lens physiology, and the risk factors for cataract formation provide suggestions about the mechanism of human cataract formation. However, testing hypotheses about the mechanism of cataract formation are complicated because cataracts typically occur late in life. The lifetime experience and genetic characteristics of an individual are likely to have a significant influence on whether he or she develops cataracts. Experimental studies have shown that individual insults that, by themselves, do not cause cataracts may lead to cataract formation when combined.[152,339] These considerations make it particularly difficult to identify the mechanisms of age-related cataract formation.

As described previously, excessive oxidative damage to lens crystallins and fiber cell membranes remains an attractive explanation for nuclear cataract formation. Increased oxidative damage in the lens nucleus must result from an imbalance between the factors that protect lens proteins from oxidative damage and the tendency for such damage to occur in a general environment that has abundant oxygen and free radicals. The age-related decrease in the diffusion of glutathione to the center of the lens is likely to be of central importance in this balance.[359,371] Whether there are also age-related changes that increase the delivery of oxidants to the lens remains to be determined. If oxidative damage is the common denominator in the formation of nuclear cataracts, the firm association between cataract and early mortality suggests that strategies that decrease systemic oxidative imbalance may have benefit throughout the body.

Cortical cataracts are associated with gross disorganization and disruption of fiber cells. This makes it even more difficult to identify the initiating insult for this type of cataract because the wreckage that ensues obscures the early damage. Although many possible inciting factors have been suggested, a comprehensive hypothesis that explains the subcellular and anatomic location of the damage in cortical cataracts (initial involvement of the center of affected fiber cells only, preferential location in inferior half of the lens) is lacking. Although epidemiologic studies suggest that light exposure contributes to cortical cataract formation, no evidence indicates whether the damage to the lens results from the interaction of light with the affected cells or with other parts of the eye. For example, light could cause the release of substances from the iris that contribute to cortical cataract formation,[7] a possibility that seems consistent with the increase in cataract in persons with dark iris color.[75,84,134] It is even possible that physical forces acting on the aging lens, such as those generated during accommodation, could rupture fiber cell membranes, initiating cataract formation or contributing to the gradual progression of cortical cataracts.

PERSPECTIVES FOR THE FUTURE

One of the most unusual aspects of the lens is its continued growth throughout life. Because fiber cells are not replaced once they differentiate and epithelial cells continue to divide to produce new lens fibers, the number of fiber cells in the lens increases steadily with age, approximately doubling between ages 1 and 90 years. Although the rate of addition of new fiber cells is slow after age 10 years, most of the cells in the outer part of the lens, in-

cluding the fiber cells involved in cortical cataract formation, are produced after childhood. It is worth asking whether the age-related increase in the number of lens fiber cells plays a role in cataract formation. Can cortical cataract formation be prevented or slowed by reducing the rate of lens cell proliferation? Is it possible that the age-related decline in metabolite diffusion to and from the lens nucleus could be prevented if lenses contained fewer fiber cells? Does slowing lens growth delay the onset of presbyopia? These questions could be approached if there were an experimental means to slow or stop the formation of new lens fiber cells in mammals.

At present, it is not possible to block lens growth in most mammals. However, in amphibians, removing the pituitary gland stops lens cell division. This approach was used to show that x-ray–induced cataracts could be avoided if cell division were halted, even if the pituitary gland were removed after the lens had been irradiated.[139,156,320] Restoration of lens cell growth by hormone supplementation led to cataract formation if the lenses had been irradiated before hypophysectomy.[156,319] These studies provide tantalizing support for the possibility that reducing the rate of lens growth could slow or prevent cataract formation.

Another area that is likely to provide important information about cataract formation is the study the genetics of human cataracts. Some of the genes responsible for congenital cataracts were described in a previous section. It is not surprising that the known genes that cause cataracts without affecting other parts of the body encode proteins that are expressed selectively and at high levels in the lens. Once a hereditary cataract is mapped close to one of these "lens-specific" genes, it is relatively easy to connect the disease to a change in the sequence of that gene. However, several loci responsible for hereditary cataracts do not map closely to the genes encoding known lens-specific proteins.[27,163,164] Identifying these genes and studying their function in the lens may give important clues about the factors required to maintain lens transparency.

Equally important will be the identification of genes that predispose the lens to cataracts in middle life. Some of these adult-onset hereditary cataracts are likely to be caused by mutations in genes that protect the lens from cataract-causing damage over a lifetime. Studies of twins suggest that heredity accounts for approximately 50% of the factors responsible for nuclear and cortical cataracts.[135,136] Other statistical analyses of epidemiologic data support these conclusions and suggest that a relatively small number of genes determine the probability of developing nuclear and cortical cataracts.[140,141] The identification of these genes is likely to suggest therapeutic approaches to delay cataractogenesis.

Additional clues to the genes responsible for counteracting cataract formation may come from novel molecular approaches that have recently been applied to the lens. Several genes that are expressed at higher or lower levels in the epithelial cells of age-matched normal and cataractous lenses have been identified.[174] One of the genes whose transcripts are selectively increased in cataracts is osteonectin (also known as *SPARC* or *BM-40*), a secreted glycoprotein that associates with basal laminae in many parts of the body.[155,172,175,368] Interestingly, mice in which the osteonectin gene has been disrupted develop cataracts.[118,273] These results show that osteonectin is important for normal lens function, but they do not explain why osteonectin messenger ribonucleic acid (mRNA) levels are elevated in cataracts. The identification of additional genes whose expression is altered in cataracts may provide candidates for further study.

Cataract blindness is a serious and growing problem in developing countries. The early onset and higher incidence of cataracts in these populations suggests that basic nutritional, environmental, and hygienic factors contribute to cataract formation. Elimination of these predisposing conditions could preserve the vision of millions of individuals who would otherwise be deprived of their sight and productivity for a substantial proportion of their lifetime. The World Health Organization, through its program, "Vision 2020: The Right to Sight," has developed plans to eliminate preventable blindness by the year 2020. Cataract blindness will be addressed in this program by providing increased access to affordable cataract surgery (www.who.int/inf-fs/en/fact213.html).[286] Although greatly increased numbers of cataract surgeries are essential to the goals of this project, concomitant improvement of basic living conditions should reduce the rate of cataract formation, and along with it, a host of other diseases.

Cataract is one of a number of diseases whose prevalence increases greatly with age. There is good reason to believe that the factors responsible for age-related cataract formation are similar to the factors that contribute to other diseases of aging. For example, moderate caloric restriction, which reduces cataract incidence and slows cataract progression in animals, also slows or prevents a variety of other age-related conditions.[240,267,364,407] Conversely, Werner syndrome, a hereditary disease that causes systemic changes that resemble many of the features of aging, is associated with early-onset cataract formation.[323] There is also the strong statistical association between cataract surgery and mortality. Therefore understanding the causes of cataract may provide insight into the causes of other age-related diseases and vice versa.

Numerous epidemiologic studies suggest that nutrition plays an important role in cataract formation. However, there are few interventional studies to test whether supplementation with specific nutrients can protect against cataract formation or progression, probably because such studies are expensive and difficult to conduct. However, clinical trials are one of the few reliable sources of information about the specific dietary factors that influence cataractogenesis in a given population. Information from the Age-Related Eye Disease Study, a large-scale clinical trial of the effects of selected vitamin and nutrient supplementation on the progression of eye diseases, may provide useful guidelines for the effects of a few components of the diet on cataract formation.[1] Other studies will probably be required in the future to better delineate the relationship between diet and cataract.

Alternatively, studying the importance of individual components of the diet on cataract incidence and progression may obscure a larger picture. The message that seems to underlie most studies of the relationship between nutrition and cataract is one that is echoed in many studies of nutrition and disease: A moderate diet with abundant fruits and vegetables is likely to provide an effective foundation for good visual health.

Secondary cataracts remain an important clinical problem. These opacities are routinely treated by ablating the posterior capsule with a laser, a procedure that is costly, depends on advanced technology, and is associated with increased risk of serious complications.[280] The frequency with which secondary cataracts develop depends on the patient's age and the type of IOL that is implanted. Children have a high incidence of secondary cataract formation, a fact that complicates and limits the options for treating congenital cataracts. In older patients the composition and design of the IOL can significantly influence the need for laser surgery after cataract extraction.[265,269,270] Further studies of the factors responsible for secondary cataract and its prevention are needed to simplify pediatric cataract surgery and reduce the need to treat secondary cataracts in adults.

New technologies are likely to provide valuable advances in cataract surgery, IOL design, and cataract prevention. It should not be long before IOLs that preserve accomodation are available, offering the possibility of substantially improving visual function in elderly individuals. Such improvements could increase the demand for replacement of the lens even before cataract formation. Although cataract surgery is now a relatively simple surgery, new technologies are likely to further simplify and expedite this most common procedure. Drugs to prevent or delay cataract formation have not been widely sought by the pharmaceutical industry. This may be because of the relatively low cost of cataract surgery coupled with the cost and potential risk of anticataract medications that may need to be taken for many years. Better understanding of the cause of cataracts may point to therapies that are effective, minimally invasive, and inexpensive.

Cataract is now thought to be inevitable if one is fortunate enough to live a long life. However, better understanding of cellular biology, biophysics, and physiology of the lens, along with greater insight into the aging process, should provide strategies to prevent or significantly delay cataract formation in most individuals.

ACKNOWLEDGMENTS
Many thanks to the colleagues, students, residents, and fellows whose stimulating discussions and healthy skepticism helped me formulate some of the ideas expressed in this chapter. I especially thank Drs. Steven Bassnett, Ying-Bo Shui, Toshiyuki Nagamoto, Carmelann Zintz, Joram Piatigorsky, and Leo Chylack. Cheryl Armbrecht provided expert assistance with graphics, and Dr. Jer Kuszak generously contributed figures. Support for preparing this manuscript was derived from Research to Prevent Blindness, National Institutes of Health (NIH) Grants EY04853 and EY07528, and a Core Grant from the National Eye Institute to the Department of Ophthalmology and Visual Sciences at Washington University.

REFERENCES

1. The Age-Related Eye Disease Study (AREDS): Design implications, AREDS report no. 1. The Age-Related Eye Diseases Study Group, *Control Clin Trials* 20:573, 1999.
2. Agre P et al: Aquaporin CHIP: the archetypal molecular water channel, *Am J Physiol* 265:F463, 1993.
3. Alder VA, Cringle SJ: The effect of the retinal circulation on vitreal oxygen tension, *Curr Eye Res* 4:121, 1985.
4. al-Ghoul KJ, Costello MJ: Fiber cell morphology and cytoplasmic texture in cataractous and normal human lens nuclei, *Curr Eye Res* 15:533, 1996.
5. al-Ghoul KJ et al: Distribution and type of morphological damage in human nuclear age-related cataracts, *Exp Eye Res* 62:237, 1996.
6. Alter AJ, Leinfelder PJ: Roentgen-ray cataract: effects of shielding the lens and ciliary body, *Arch Ophthalmol* 49:257, 1953.
7. Andley UP et al: The role of prostaglandins E2 and F2 alpha in ultraviolet radiation-induced cortical cataracts in vivo, *Invest Ophthalmol Vis Sci* 37:1539, 1996.
8. Andley UP et al: The molecular chaperone alphaA-crystallin enhances lens epithelial cell growth and resistance to UVA stress, *J Biol Chem* 273:31252, 1998.
9. Appleton B, McCrossan GC: Microwave lens effects in humans, *Arch Ophthalmol* 88:259, 1972.
10. Attree O et al: The Lowe's oculocerebrorenal syndrome gene encodes a protein highly homologous to inositol polyphosphate-5-phosphatase, *Nature* 358:239, 1992.
11. Bassnett S: Mitochondrial dynamics in differentiating fiber cells of the mammalian lens, *Curr Eye Res* 11:1227, 1992.
12. Bassnett S, Beebe DC: Coincident loss of mitochondria and nuclei during lens fiber cell differentiation, *Dev Dyn* 194:85, 1992.
13. Bassnett S, Croghan P, Duncan G: Diffusion of lactate and its role in determining intracellular pH, *Exp Eye Res* 44:143, 1987.
14. Bassnett S, Duncan G: Direct measurement of pH in the rat lens by ion-sensitive microelectrodes, *Exp Eye Res* 40:585, 1985.
15. Bassnett S, Mataic D: Chromatin degradation in differentiating fiber cells of the eye lens, *J Cell Biol* 137:37, 1997.
16. Bassnett S, Missey H, Vucemilo I: Molecular architecture of the lens fiber cell basal membrane complex, *J Cell Sci* 112:2155, 1999.
17. Bassnett S et al: Intercellular communication between epithelial and fiber cells of the eye lens, *J Cell Sci* 107:799, 1994.
18. Bax B et al: X-ray analysis of beta B2-crystallin and evolution of oligomeric lens proteins, *Nature* 347:776, 1990.
19. Beebe DC, Coats JM: The lens organizes the anterior segment: specification of neural crest cell differentiation in the avian eye, *Dev Biol* 220:424, 2000.
20. Beebe DC, Feagans DE, Jebens HA: Lentropin: a factor in vitreous humor which promotes lens fiber cell differentiation, *Proc Natl Acad Sci USA* 77:490, 1980.
21. Beebe DC et al: Lens epithelial cell elongation in the absence of microtubules: evidence for a new effect of colchicine, *Science* 206:836, 1979.
22. Beebe DC et al: The mechanism of cell elongation during lens fiber cell differentiation, *Dev Biol* 92:54, 1982.
23. Beebe DC et al: Lentropin, a protein that controls lens fiber formation, is related functionally and immunologically to the insulin-like growth factors, *Proc Natl Acad Sci USA* 84:2327, 1987.
24. Beebe DC et al: Changes in adhesion complexes define stages in the differentiation of lens fiber cells, *Invest Ophthalmol Vis Sci* 42:727, 2001.
25. Benedek GB et al: Theoretical and experimental basis for the inhibition of cataract, *Prog Retin Eye Res* 18:391, 1999.
26. Benitez del Castillo JM, del Rio T, Garcia-Sanchez J: Effects of estrogen use on lens transmittance in postmenopausal women, *Ophthalmology* 104:970, 1997.
27. Berry V et al: A locus for autosomal-dominant anterior polar cataract on chromosome 17p, *Hum Mol Genet* 5:415, 1996.
28. Berry V et al: Missense mutations in MIP underlie autosomal-dominant 'polymorphic' and lamellar cataracts linked to 12q, *Nat Genet* 25:15, 2000.

29. Bhuyan DK, Reddy PG, Bhuyan KC: Growth factor receptor gene and protein expressions in the human lens, *Mech Ageing Dev* 113:205, 2000.

30. Bigsby RM et al: Protective effects of estrogen in a rat model of age-related cataracts, *Proc Natl Acad Sci USA* 96:9328, 1999.

31. Bleau G, Giasson C, Brunette I: Measurement of hydrogen peroxide in biological samples containing high levels of ascorbic acid, *Anal Biochem* 263:13, 1998.

32. Blixt A et al: A forkhead gene, FoxE3, is essential for lens epithelial proliferation and closure of the lens vesicle, *Genes Dev* 14:245, 2000.

33. Bloemendal H et al: The plasma membranes of eye lens fibres: biochemical and structural characterization, *Cell Differ* 1:91, 1972.

34. Borchman D et al: Studies on the distribution of cholesterol, phospholipid, and protein in the human and bovine lens, *Lens Eye Toxic Res* 6:703, 1989.

35. Bova LM et al: Major changes in human ocular UV protection with age, *Invest Ophthalmol Vis Sci* 42:200, 2001.

36. Bova MP et al: Subunit exchange of alphaA-crystallin, *J Biol Chem* 272:29511, 1997.

37. Bova MP et al: Mutation R120G in alphaB-crystallin, which is linked to a desmin-related myopathy, results in an irregular structure and defective chaperone-like function, *Proc Natl Acad Sci USA* 96:6137, 1999.

38. Brady JP et al: Targeted disruption of the mouse alpha A-crystallin gene induces cataract and cytoplasmic inclusion bodies containing the small heat shock protein alpha B-crystallin, *Proc Natl Acad Sci USA* 94:884, 1997.

39. Brown N: Slit-image photography and measurement of the eye, *Med Biol Illus* 23:192, 1973.

40. Brown N: The change in lens curvature with age, *Exp Eye Res* 19:175, 1974.

41. Brown NA, Hill AR: Cataract: the relation between myopia and cataract morphology, *Br J Ophthalmol* 71:405, 1987.

42. Brown NP et al: Is cortical spoke cataract due to lens fibre breaks? The relationship between fibre folds, fibre breaks, waterclefts and spoke cataract, *Eye* 7:672, 1993.

43. Brownell I, Dirksen M, Jamrich M: Forkhead FoxE3 maps to the dysgenetic lens locus and is critical in lens development and differentiation, *Genesis* 27:81, 2000.

44. Brownlee M: Negative consequences of glycation, *Metabolism* 49:9, 2000.

45. Calvin H et al: Rapid deterioration of lens fibers in GSH-depleted mouse pups, *Invest Ophthalmol Vis Sci* 32:1916, 1991.

46. Cammarata PR et al: Macromolecular organization of bovine lens capsule, *Tissue Cell* 18:83, 1986.

47. Capetanaki Y, Smith S, Heath J: Overexpression of the vimentin gene in transgenic mice inhibits normal lens cell differentiation, *J Cell Biol* 109:1653, 1989.

48. Carlsson B, Sjostrand J: Increased incidence of cataract extractions in women above 70 years of age: a population based study, *Acta Ophthalmol Scand* 74:64, 1996.

49. Chamberlain CG, McAvoy JW: Evidence that fibroblast growth factor promotes lens fibre differentiation, *Curr Eye Res* 6:1165, 1987.

50. Chamberlain CG, McAvoy JW, Richardson NA: The effects of insulin and basic fibroblast growth factor on fibre differentiation in rat lens epithelial explants, *Growth Factors* 4:183, 1991.

51. Chandy G et al: Comparison of the water transporting properties of MIP and AQP1, *J Membr Biol* 159:29, 1997.

52. Cherfan GM et al: Nuclear sclerotic cataract after vitrectomy for idiopathic epiretinal membranes causing macular pucker, *Am J Ophthalmol* 111:434, 1991.

53. Chiesa R et al: Definition and comparison of the phosphorylation sites of the A and B chains of bovine alpha-crystallin, *Exp Eye Res* 46:199, 1988.

54. Chow RL et al: FGF suppresses apoptosis and induces differentiation of fibre cells in the mouse lens, *Development* 121:4383, 1995.

55. Chylack LT Jr, Friend J: Intermediary metabolism of the lens: a historical perspective 1928-1989, *Exp Eye Res* 50:575, 1990.

56. Chylack LT Jr et al: Ocular manifestations of juvenile rheumatoid arthritis, *Am J Ophthalmol* 79:1026, 1975.

57. Clark JI, Carper D: Phase separation in lens cytoplasm is genetically linked to cataract formation in the Philly mouse, *Proc Natl Acad Sci USA* 84:122, 1987.

58. Clark JI, Clark JM: Lens cytoplasmic phase separation, *Int Rev Cytol* 192:171, 2000.

59. Clark JI, Livesey JC, Steele JE: Phase separation inhibitors and lens transparency, *Optom Vis Sci* 70:873, 1993.

60. Clark JI, Osgood TB, Trask SJ: Inhibition of phase separation by reagents that prevent X-irradiation cataract in vivo, *Exp Eye Res* 45:961, 1987.

61. Clark JI et al: Cortical opacity, calcium concentration and fiber membrane structure in the calf lens, *Exp Eye Res* 31:399, 1980.

62. Clark JI et al: Phase separation of X-irradiated lenses of rabbit, *Invest Ophthalmol Vis Sci* 22:186, 1982.

63. Clark JI et al: Lens cytoskeleton and transparency: a model, *Eye* 13:417, 1999.

64. Cogan DG, Donaldson DD, Reese AB: Clinical and pathological characteristics of radiation cataract, *AMA Arch Ophthalmol* 47:55, 1952.

65. Colucci-Guyon E et al: Mice lacking vimentin develop and reproduce without an obvious phenotype, *Cell* 79:679, 1994.

66. Conley YP et al: A juvenile-onset, progressive cataract locus on chromosome 3q21-q22 is associated with a missense mutation in the beaded filament structural protein-2, *Am J Hum Genet* 66:1426, 2000.

67. Coroneo MT, Muller-Stolzenburg NW, Ho A: Peripheral light focusing by the anterior eye and the ophthalmohelioses, *Ophthalmic Surg* 22:705, 1991.

68. Coulombre JL, Coulombre AJ: Lens development: fiber elongation and lens orientation, *Science* 142:1489, 1963.

69. Coulombre JL, Coulombre AJ: Lens development: IV. Size, shape, and orientation, *Invest Ophthalmol* 8:251, 1969.

70. Creighton MO et al: Globular bodies: a primary cause of the opacity in senile and diabetic posterior cortical subcapsular cataracts? *Can J Ophthalmol* 13:166, 1978.

71. Creighton MO et al: In vitro studies of microwave-induced cataract: II. Comparison of damage observed for continuous wave and pulsed microwaves, *Exp Eye Res* 45:357, 1987.

72. Cruickshanks KJ: Sunlight exposure and risk of lens opacities in a population-based study, *Arch Ophthalmol* 116:1666, 1998.

73. Cruickshanks KJ, Klein BE, Klein R: Ultraviolet light exposure and lens opacities: the Beaver Dam Eye Study, *Am J Public Health* 82:1658, 1992.

74. Cumming RG, Mitchell P: Hormone replacement therapy, reproductive factors, and cataract: the Blue Mountains Eye Study, *Am J Epidemiol* 145:242, 1997.

75. Cumming RG, Mitchell P, Lim R: Iris color and cataract: the Blue Mountains Eye Study, *Am J Ophthalmol* 130:237, 2000.

76. Cvekl A, Piatigorsky J: Lens development and crystallin gene expression: many roles for Pax-6, *Bioessays* 18:621, 1996.

77. Cvekl A et al: A complex array of positive and negative elements regulates the chicken alpha A-crystallin gene: involvement of Pax-6, USF, CREB and/or CREM, and AP-1 proteins, *Mol Cell Biol* 14:7363, 1994.

78. Dahm R et al: Gap junctions containing alpha8-connexin (MP70) in the adult mammalian lens epithelium suggests a re-evaluation of its role in the lens, *Exp Eye Res* 69:45, 1999.

79. Datiles MB, Fukui H: Cataract prevention in diabetic Octodon degus with Pfizer's sorbinil, *Curr Eye Res* 8:233, 1989.

80. de Bustros S et al: Nuclear sclerosis after vitrectomy for idiopathic epiretinal membranes, *Am J Ophthalmol* 105:160, 1988.

81. de Bustros S et al: Vitrectomy for idiopathic epiretinal membranes causing macular pucker, *Br J Ophthalmol* 72:692, 1988.

82. Delaye M, Clark JI, Benedek GB: Coexistence curves for the phase separation in the calf lens cytoplasm, *Biochem Biophys Res Commun* 100:908, 1981.

83. Delaye M, Tardieu A: Short-range order of crystallin proteins accounts for eye lens transparency, *Nature* 302:415, 1983.

84. Delcourt C et al: Risk factors for cortical, nuclear, and posterior subcapsular cataracts: the POLA study. Pathologies Oculaires Liees a l'Age, *Am J Epidemiol* 151:497, 2000.

85. Devamanoharan P, Ramachandran S, Varma S: Hydrogen peroxide in the eye lens: radioisotopic determination, *Curr Eye Res* 10:831, 1991.

86. Dietz HC et al: Marfan syndrome caused by a recurrent de novo missense mutation in the fibrillin gene, *Nature* 352:337, 1991.

87. Diez-Roux G et al: Macrophages kill capillary cells in G1 phase of the cell cycle during programmed vascular regression, *Development* 126:2141, 1999.

88. Dillon J et al: Electron paramagnetic resonance and spin trapping investigations of the photoreactivity of human lens proteins, *Photochem Photobiol* 69:259, 1999.

89. Dillon J et al: The optical properties of the anterior segment of the eye: implications for cortical cataract, *Exp Eye Res* 68:785, 1999.

90. Dische Z, Zil HA: Studies on the oxidation of cysteine to cystine in lens proteins during cataract formation, *Am J Ophthalmol* 34:104, 1951.

91. Driessen HP et al: Primary structure of the bovine beta-crystallin Bp chain: internal duplication and homology with gamma-crystallin, *Eur J Biochem* 121:83, 1981.

92. Dubin RA, Wawrousek EF, Piatigorsky J: Expression of the murine alpha B-crystallin gene is not restricted to the lens, *Mol Cell Biol* 9:1083, 1989.

93. Duindam JJ et al: Cholesterol, phospholipid, and protein changes in focal opacities in the human eye lens, *Invest Ophthalmol Vis Sci* 39:94, 1998.

94. Duncan G et al: Human lens membrane cation permeability increases with age, *Invest Ophthalmol Vis Sci* 30:1855, 1989.

95. Fagerholm PP: The influence of calcium on lens fibers, *Exp Eye Res* 28:211, 1979.

96. Fagerholm PP, Philipson BT, Lindstrom B: Normal human lens: the distribution of protein, *Exp Eye Res* 33:615, 1981.

97. Farnsworth TN et al: Surface ultrastructure of the human lens capsule and zonular attachments, *Invest Ophthalmol* 15:36, 1976.

98. Fischbarg J et al: Transport of fluid by lens epithelium, *Am J Physiol* 276:C548, 1999.

99. Fischer RS, Lee A, Fowler VM: Tropomodulin and tropomyosin mediate lens cell actin cytoskeleton reorganization in vitro, *Invest Ophthalmol Vis Sci* 41:166, 2000.

100. Fitch JM, Linsenmayer TF: Monoclonal antibody analysis of ocular basement membranes during development, *Dev Biol* 95:137, 1983.

101. FitzGerald P: Methods for the circumvention of problems associated with the study of the ocular lens plasma membrane-cytoskeleton complex, *Curr Eye Res* 9:1083, 1990.

102. FitzGerald PG, Bok D, Horwitz J: The distribution of the main intrinsic membrane polypeptide in ocular lens, *Curr Eye Res* 4:1203, 1985.

103. Fleming TP, Song Z, Andley UP: Expression of growth control and differentiation genes in human lens epithelial cells with extended life span, *Invest Ophthalmol Vis Sci* 39:1387, 1998.

104. Fromm L, Overbeek PA: Regulation of cyclin and cyclin-dependent kinase gene expression during lens differentiation requires the retinoblastoma protein, *Oncogene* 12:69, 1996.

105. Fu S et al: The hydroxyl radical in lens nuclear cataractogenesis, *J Biol Chem* 273:28603, 1998.

106. Gao CY et al: Changes in cyclin dependent kinase expression and activity accompanying lens fiber cell differentiation, *Exp Eye Res* 69:695, 1999.

107. Garadi R et al: Protein synthesis in x-irradiated rabbit lens, *Invest Ophthalmol Vis Sci* 25:147, 1984.

108. Garcia-Castineiras S et al: Aqueous humor hydrogen peroxide analysis with dichlorophenol-indophenol, *Exp Eye Res* 55:9, 1992.

109. Garcia-Porrero JA, Colvee E, Ojeda JL: The mechanisms of cell death and phagocytosis in the early chick lens morphogenesis: a scanning electron microscopy and cytochemical approach, *Anat Rec* 208:123, 1984.

110. Garland DL et al: The nucleus of the human lens: demonstration of a highly characteristic protein pattern by two-dimensional electrophoresis and introduction of a new method of lens dissection, *Exp Eye Res* 62:285, 1996.

111. Garner WH, Spector A: Racemization in human lens: evidence of rapid insolubilization of specific polypeptides in cataract formation, *Proc Natl Acad Sci USA* 75:3618, 1978.

112. Genis-Galvez JM: Role of the lens in the morphogenesis of the iris and cornea, *Nature* 210:209, 1966.

113. Genis-Galvez JM, Santos-Gutierrez L, Rios-Gonzalez A: Causal factors in corneal development: an experimental analysis in the chick embryo, *Exp Eye Res* 6:48, 1967.

114. Georgatos SD et al: To bead or not to bead? Lens-specific intermediate filaments revisited, *J Cell Sci* 110:2629, 1997.

115. Giblin FJ et al: Exposure of rabbit lens to hyperbaric oxygen in vitro: regional effects on GSH level, *Invest Ophthalmol Vis Sci* 29:1312, 1988.

116. Giblin FJ et al: The relative roles of the glutathione redox cycle and catalase in the detoxification of H_2O_2 by cultured rabbit lens epithelial cells, *Exp Eye Res* 50:795, 1990.

117. Giblin FJ et al: Nuclear light scattering, disulfide formation and membrane damage in lenses of older guinea pigs treated with hyperbaric oxygen, *Exp Eye Res* 60:219, 1995.

118. Gilmour DT et al: Mice deficient for the secreted glycoprotein SPARC/osteonectin/BM40 develop normally but show severe age-onset cataract formation and disruption of the lens, *EMBO J* 17:1860, 1998.

119. Girelli D et al: A linkage between hereditary hyperferritinaemia not related to iron overload and autosomal-dominant congenital cataract, *Br J Haematol* 90:931, 1995.

120. Gitzelmann R: Deficiency of erythrocyte galactokinase in a patient with galactose diabetes, *Lancet* 2:670, 1965.

121. Goldberg MF: Persistent fetal vasculature (PFV): an integrated interpretation of signs and symptoms associated with persistent hyperplastic primary vitreous (PHPV). LIV Edward Jackson Memorial Lecture, *Am J Ophthalmol* 124:587, 1997.

122. Goldman JE, Corbin E: Rosenthal fibers contain ubiquitinated alpha B-crystallin, *Am J Pathol* 139:933, 1991.

123. Gong X et al: Disruption of alpha3 connexin gene leads to proteolysis and cataractogenesis in mice, *Cell* 91:833, 1997.

124. Gong X et al: Genetic factors influence cataract formation in alpha 3 connexin knockout mice, *Dev Genet* 24:27, 1999.

125. Goodenough DA, Dick JS 2nd, Lyons JE: Lens metabolic cooperation: a study of mouse lens transport and permeability visualized with freeze-substitution autoradiography and electron microscopy, *J Cell Biol* 86:576, 1980.

126. Goppert F: Galaktosurie nach Milchzuckergabe bei angeborenem, familiaerem chronischem Leberleiden, *Klin Wschr* 54:473, 1917.

127. Gorin MB et al: The major intrinsic protein (MIP) of the bovine lens fiber membrane: characterization and structure based on cDNA cloning, *Cell* 39:49, 1984.

128. Gorin MB et al: Long-term tamoxifen citrate use and potential ocular toxicity, *Am J Ophthalmol* 125:493, 1998.

129. Graw J: Mouse models of congenital cataract, *Eye* 13:438, 1999.

130. Hales AM, Chamberlain CG, McAvoy JW: Cataract induction in lenses cultured with transforming growth factor-beta, *Invest Ophthalmol Vis Sci* 36:1709, 1995.

131. Hales AM et al: TGF-beta 1 induces lens cells to accumulate alpha-smooth muscle actin, a marker for subcapsular cataracts, *Curr Eye Res* 13:885, 1994.

132. Hales AM et al: Estrogen protects lenses against cataract induced by transforming growth factor-beta (TGF-beta), *J Exp Med* 185:273, 1997.

133. Hales AM et al: Intravitreal injection of TGF-beta induces cataract in rats, *Invest Ophthalmol Vis Sci* 40:3231, 1999.

134. Hammond BR Jr et al: Iris color and age-related changes in lens optical density, *Ophthalmic Physiol Opt* 20:381, 2000.

135. Hammond CJ et al: Genetic and environmental factors in age-related nuclear cataracts in monozygotic and dizygotic twins, *N Engl J Med* 342:1786, 2000.

136. Hammond CJ et al: The heritability of age-related cortical cataract: the twin eye study, *Invest Ophthalmol Vis Sci* 42:601, 2001.

137. Harding J: *Cataract: biochemistry, epidemiology and pharmacology,* London, 1991, Chapman & Hall.

138. Harding JJ: The untenability of the sunlight hypothesis of cataractogenesis, *Doc Ophthalmol* 88:345, 1994.

139. Hayden JH et al: Hypophysectomy exerts a radioprotective effect on frog lens, *Experientia* 36:116, 1980.

140. Heiba IM et al: Genetic etiology of nuclear cataract: evidence for a major gene, *Am J Med Genet* 47:1208, 1993.

141. Heiba IM et al: Evidence for a major gene for cortical cataract, *Invest Ophthalmol Vis Sci* 36:227, 1995.

142. Helbig H et al: Oxygen in the anterior chamber of the human eye, *Ger J Ophthalmol* 2:161, 1993.

143. Hendrix RW, Zwaan J: Cell shape regulation and cell cycle in embryonic lens cells, *Nature* 247:145, 1974.

144. Hendrix RW, Zwaan J: The matrix of the optic vesicle-presumptive lens interface during induction of the lens in the chicken embryo, *J Embryol Exp Morphol* 33:1023, 1975.

145. Henry J, Grainger R: Early tissue interactions leading to embryonic lens formation, *Dev Biol* 141:149, 1990.

146. Heon E et al: The gamma-crystallins and human cataracts: a puzzle made clearer, *Am J Hum Genet* 65:1261, 1999.

147. Hightower KR et al: Lens epithelium: a primary target of UVB irradiation, *Exp Eye Res* 59:557, 1994.

148. Hill RE et al: Mouse small eye results from mutations in a paired-like homeobox-containing gene, *Nature* 355:750, 1992.

149. Hiller R, Sperduto RD, Ederer F: Epidemiologic associations with nuclear, cortical, and posterior subcapsular cataracts, *Am J Epidemiol* 124:916, 1986.

150. Hiraoka T et al: Effect of selected anti-cataract agents on opacification in the selenite cataract model, *Exp Eye Res* 62:11, 1996.

151. Hirsch RP, Schwartz B: Increased mortality among elderly patients undergoing cataract extraction, *Arch Ophthalmol* 101:1034, 1983.

152. Hockwin O: Clinical significance of the production of experimental cataract by means of addition of subliminal injuries, *Ophthalmologica* 158:481, 1969.

153. Hodge WG, Whitcher JP, Satariano W: Risk factors for age-related cataracts, *Epidemiol Rev* 17:336, 1995.

154. Hoenders HJ, Bloemendal H: Lens proteins and aging, *J Gerontol* 38:278, 1983.

155. Holland PW et al: In vivo expression of mRNA for the Ca^{++}-binding protein SPARC (osteonectin) revealed by in situ hybridization, *J Cell Biol* 105:473, 1987.

156. Holsclaw DS et al: Modulating radiation cataractogenesis by hormonally manipulating lenticular growth kinetics, *Exp Eye Res* 59:291, 1994.

157. Hood BD, Garner B, Truscott RJ: Human lens coloration and aging: evidence for crystallin modification by the major ultraviolet filter, 3-hydroxy-kynurenine O-beta-D-glucoside, *J Biol Chem* 274:32547, 1999.

158. Horwitz J: Alpha-crystallin can function as a molecular chaperone, *Proc Natl Acad Sci USA* 89:10449, 1992.

159. Horwitz J: The function of alpha-crystallin in vision, *Semin Cell Dev Biol* 11:53, 2000.

160. Ifeanyi F, Takemoto L: Differential binding of alpha-crystallins to bovine lens membrane, *Exp Eye Res* 49:143, 1989.

161. Ifeanyi F, Takemoto L: Specificity of alpha crystallin binding to the lens membrane, *Curr Eye Res* 9:259, 1990.

162. Ingolia TD, Craig EA: Four small Drosophila heat shock proteins are related to each other and to mammalian alpha-crystallin, *Proc Natl Acad Sci USA* 79:2360, 1982.

163. Ionides A et al: The clinical and genetic heterogeneity of autosomal dominant cataract, *Acta Ophthalmol Scand* 219(suppl):40, 1996.

164. Ionides A et al: Clinical and genetic heterogeneity in autosomal dominant cataract, *Br J Ophthalmol* 83:802, 1999.

165. Ireland M, Maisel H: A cytoskeletal protein unique to lens fiber cell differentiation, *Exp Eye Res* 38:637, 1984.

166. Jacob TJ: A direct measurement of intracellular free calcium within the lens, *Exp Eye Res* 36:451, 1983.

167. Jacob TJ: Raised intracellular free calcium within the lens causes opacification and cellular uncoupling in the frog, *J Physiol (Lond)* 341:595, 1983.

168. Jakobs PM et al: Autosomal-dominant congenital cataract associated with a deletion mutation in the human beaded filament protein gene BFSP2, *Am J Hum Genet* 66:1432, 2000.

169. Johnson MC, Beebe DC: Growth, synthesis and regional specialization of the embryonic chicken lens capsule, *Exp Eye Res* 38:579, 1984.

170. Kannan R et al: Molecular characterization of a reduced glutathione transporter in the lens, *Invest Ophthalmol Vis Sci* 36:1785, 1995.

171. Kannan R et al: Identification of a novel, sodium-dependent, reduced glutathione transporter in the rat lens epithelium, *Invest Ophthalmol Vis Sci* 37:2269, 1996.

172. Kantorow M, Horwitz J, Carper D: Up-regulation of osteonectin/SPARC in age-related cataractous human lens epithelia, *Mol Vis* 4:17, 1998.

173. Kantorow M, Piatigorsky J: Alpha-crystallin/small heat shock protein has autokinase activity, *Proc Natl Acad Sci USA* 91:3112, 1994.

174. Kantorow M et al: Differential display detects altered gene expression between cataractous and normal human lenses, *Invest Ophthalmol Vis Sci* 39:2344, 1998.

175. Kantorow M et al: Increased expression of osteonectin/SPARC mRNA and protein in age-related human cataracts and spatial expression in the normal human lens, *Mol Vis* 6:24, 2000.

176. Kappelhof JP, Vrensen GF: The pathology of after-cataract: a minireview, *Acta Ophthalmol* 205(suppl):13, 1992.

177. Kappelhof JP et al: The ring of Soemmerring in the rabbit: a scanning electron microscopic study, *Graefes Arch Clin Exp Ophthalmol* 223:111, 1985.

178. Karkinen-Jaaskelainen M et al: Rubella cataract in vitro: sensitive period of the developing human lens, *J Exp Med* 141:1238, 1975.

179. Kawauchi S et al: Regulation of lens fiber cell differentiation by transcription factor c-maf, *J Biol Chem* 274:19254, 1999.

180. Kern HL, Zolot SL: Transport of vitamin C in the lens, *Curr Eye Res* 6:885, 1987.

181. Kibbelaar MA et al: Is actin in eye lens a possible factor in visual accommodation? *Nature* 285:506, 1980.

182. Kim JI et al: Requirement for the c-maf transcription factor in crystallin gene regulation and lens development, *Proc Natl Acad Sci USA* 96:3781, 1999.

183. King GL et al: Biochemical and molecular mechanisms in the development of diabetic vascular complications, *Diabetes* 45(suppl 3):S105, 1996.

184. Kinoshita JH: A thirty-year journey in the polyol pathway, *Exp Eye Res* 50:567, 1990.

185. Kinoshita JH, Kern HL, Merola OH: Factors affecting the cation transport of calf lens, *Biochim Biophys Acta* 47:458, 1961.

186. Kinoshita JH, Nishimura C: The involvement of aldose reductase in diabetic complications, *Diabetes Metab Rev* 4:323, 1988.

187. Kistler J et al: Ocular lens gap junctions: protein expression, assembly, and structure-function analysis, *Microsc Res Tech* 31:347, 1995.

188. Klein BE: Lens opacities in women in Beaver Dam, Wisconsin: is there evidence of an effect of sex hormones? *Trans Am Ophthalmol Soc* 91:517, 1993.

189. Klein BE, Klein R, Lee KE: Incidence of age-related cataract: the Beaver Dam Eye Study, *Arch Ophthalmol* 116:219, 1998.

190. Klein BE, Klein R, Linton KL: Prevalence of age-related lens opacities in a population: the Beaver Dam Eye Study, *Ophthalmology* 99:546, 1992.

191. Klein BE, Klein R, Moss SE: Incident cataract surgery: the Beaver Dam eye study, *Ophthalmology* 104:573, 1997.

192. Klein BE, Klein R, Ritter LL: Is there evidence of an estrogen effect on age-related lens opacities? The Beaver Dam Eye Study, *Arch Ophthalmol* 112:85, 1994.

193. Klemenz R et al: Alpha B-crystallin is a small heat shock protein, *Proc Natl Acad Sci USA* 88:3652, 1991.

194. Klesert TR et al: Mice deficient in Six5 develop cataracts: implications for myotonic dystrophy, *Nat Genet* 25:105, 2000.

195. Klopp N et al: Three murine cataract mutants (Cat2) are defective in different gamma-crystallin genes, *Genomics* 52:152, 1998.

196. Kodama R, Eguchi G: Gene regulation and differentiation in vertebrate ocular tissues, *Curr Opin Genet Dev* 4:703, 1994.

197. Kodama T, Takemoto L: Characterization of disulfide-linked crystallins associated with human cataractous lens membranes, *Invest Ophthalmol Vis Sci* 29:145, 1988.

198. Koroma BM, Yang JM, Sundin OH: The Pax-6 homeobox gene is expressed throughout the corneal and conjunctival epithelia, *Invest Ophthalmol Vis Sci* 38:108, 1997.

199. Kroger RH et al: Refractive index distribution and spherical aberration in the crystalline lens of the African cichlid fish *Haplochromis burtoni*, *Vision Res* 34:1815, 1994.

200. Kroone RC et al: The role of the sequence extensions in beta-crystallin assembly, *Protein Eng* 7:1395, 1994.

201. Kurosaka D et al: Growth factors influence contractility and alpha-smooth muscle actin expression in bovine lens epithelial cells, *Invest Ophthalmol Vis Sci* 36.1701, 1995.

202. Kuszak J, Alcala J, Maisel H: The surface morphology of embryonic adult chick lens-fiber cells, *Am J Anat* 159:395, 1980.

203. Kuszak JR: The development of lens sutures, *Prog Retin Eye Res* 14:567, 1995.

204. Kuszak JR et al: Cell-to-cell fusion of lens fiber cells in situ: correlative light, scanning electron microscopic, and freeze-fracture studies, *J Ultrastruct Res* 93:144, 1985.

205. Kuszak JR et al: The contribution of cell-to-cell fusion to the ordered structure of the crystalline lens, *Lens Eye Toxic Res* 6:639, 1989.

206. Kuszak JR et al: The interrelationship of lens anatomy and optical quality: II. Primate lenses, *Exp Eye Res* 59:521, 1994.

207. Kuszak JR et al: The relationship between rabbit lens optical quality and sutural anatomy after vitrectomy, *Exp Eye Res* 71:267, 2000.

208. Kuwabara T: Microtubules in the lens, *Arch Ophthalmol* 79:189, 1968.

209. Kuwabara T: The maturation of the lens cell: a morphologic study, *Exp Eye Res* 20:427, 1975.

210. Kwan M, Niinikoski J, Hunt TK: In vivo measurements of oxygen tension in the cornea, aqueous humor, and anterior lens of the open eye, *Invest Ophthalmol* 11:108, 1972.

211. Lagunowich LA, Grunwald GB: Expression of calcium-dependent cell adhesion during ocular development: a biochemical, histochemical and functional analysis, *Dev Biol* 135:158, 1989.

212. Lampi KJ et al: Sequence analysis of betaA3, betaB3, and betaA4 crystallins completes the identification of the major proteins in young human lens, *J Biol Chem* 272:2268, 1997.

213. Lang RA: Which factors stimulate lens fiber cell differentiation in vivo? *Invest Ophthalmol Vis Sci* 40:3075, 1999.

214. Lee A, Fischer RS, Fowler VM: Stabilization and remodeling of the membrane skeleton during lens fiber cell differentiation and maturation, *Dev Dyn* 217:257, 2000.

215. Lee B et al: Linkage of Marfan syndrome and a phenotypically related disorder to two different fibrillin genes, *Nature* 352:330, 1991.

216. Lee EH, Joo CK: Role of transforming growth factor-beta in transdifferentiation and fibrosis of lens epithelial cells, *Invest Ophthalmol Vis Sci* 40:2025, 1999.

217. Leenders WP et al: Synergism between temporally distinct growth factors: bFGF, insulin and lens cell differentiation, *Mech Dev* 67:193, 1997.

218. Leinfelder PJ, Dickerson J: Species variation of the lens epithelium to ionizing radiation, *Am J Ophthalmol* 50:175, 1960.

219. Leske MC et al: Prevalence of lens opacities in the Barbados Eye Study, *Arch Ophthalmol* 115:105, 1997.

220. Leske MC et al: Incidence and progression of lens opacities in the Barbados Eye Studies, *Ophthalmology* 107:1267, 2000.

221. Li HS et al: Pax-6 is first expressed in a region of ectoderm anterior to the early neural plate: implications for stepwise determination of the lens, *Dev Biol* 162:181, 1994.

222. Lin JS et al: Spatial differences in gap junction gating in the lens are a consequence of connexin cleavage, *Eur J Cell Biol* 76:246, 1998.

223. Lipworth BJ: Systemic adverse effects of inhaled corticosteroid therapy: a systematic review and meta-analysis, *Arch Intern Med* 159:941, 1999.

224. Litt M et al: Autosomal-dominant cerulean cataract is associated with a chain termination mutation in the human beta-crystallin gene CRYBB2, *Hum Mol Genet* 6:665, 1997.

225. Litt M et al: Autosomal-dominant congenital cataract associated with a missense mutation in the human alpha crystallin gene CRYAA, *Hum Mol Genet* 7:471, 1998.

226. Liu J, Chamberlain CG, McAvoy JW: IGF enhancement of FGF-induced fibre differentiation and DNA synthesis in lens explants, *Exp Eye Res* 63:621, 1996.

227. Liu J et al: Induction of cataract-like changes in rat lens epithelial explants by transforming growth factor beta, *Invest Ophthalmol Vis Sci* 35:388, 1994.

228. Lo WK: Adherens junctions in the ocular lens of various species: ultrastructural analysis with an improved fixation, *Cell Tissue Res* 254:31, 1988.

229. Lo WK et al: Spatiotemporal distribution of zonulae adherens and associated actin bundles in both epithelium and fiber cells during chicken lens development, *Exp Eye Res* 71:45, 2000.

230. Lou MF: Thiol regulation in the lens, *J Ocul Pharmacol Ther* 16:137, 2000.

231. Lovicu FJ, McAvoy JW: Spatial and temporal expression of p57(KIP2) during murine lens development, *Mech Dev* 86:165, 1999.

232. Lydahl E: Infrared radiation and cataract, *Acta Ophthalmol* 166(suppl):1, 1984.

233. Lydahl E, Philipson B: Infrared radiation and cataract: II. Epidemiologic investigation of glass workers, *Acta Ophthalmol (Copenh)* 62:976, 1984.

234. Lyne AJ: Ocular effects of hyperbaric oxygen, *Trans Ophthalmol Soc UK* 98:66, 1978.

235. Mackay D et al: Connexin46 mutations in autosomal-dominant congenital cataract, *Am J Hum Genet* 64:1357, 1999.

236. Maisel H, Ellis M: Cytoskeletal proteins of the aging human lens, *Current Eye Res* 3:369, 1984.

237. Marcantonio JM, Duncan G: Calcium-induced degradation of the lens cytoskeleton, *Biochem Soc Trans* 19:1148, 1991.

238. Marcantonio JM, Duncan G, Rink H: Calcium-induced opacification and loss of protein in the organ-cultured bovine lens, *Exp Eye Res* 42:617, 1986.

239. Marcantonio JM, Vrensen GF: Cell biology of posterior capsular opacification, *Eye* 13:484, 1999.

240. Masoro EJ: Caloric restriction and aging: an update, *Exp Gerontol* 35:299, 2000.

241. Masters PM, Bada JL, Zigler JS Jr: Aspartic acid racemization in heavy molecular weight crystallins and water insoluble protein from normal human lenses and cataracts, *Proc Natl Acad Sci USA* 75:1204, 1978.

242. Mathias RT, Rae JL, Baldo GJ: Physiological properties of the normal lens, *Physiol Rev* 77:21, 1997.

243. Mathias RT, Riquelme G, Rae JL: Cell to cell communication and pH in the frog lens, *J Gen Physiol* 98:1085, 1991.

244. Matsuda H, Giblin FJ, Reddy VN: The effect of x-irradiation on cation transport in rabbit lens, *Exp Eye Res* 33:253, 1981.

245. McAvoy J: Developmental biology of the lens. In Duncan G (ed): *Mechanism of cataract formation,* London, 1981, Academic Press.

246. McAvoy JW, Chamberlain CG: Fibroblast growth factor (FGF) induces different responses in lens epithelial cells depending on its concentration, *Development* 107:221, 1989.

247. McCarty CA, Taylor HR: Recent developments in vision research: light damage in cataract, *Invest Ophthalmol Vis Sci* 37:1720, 1996.

248. McDermott JB, Cvekl A, Piatigorsky J: A complex enhancer of the chicken beta A3/A1-crystallin gene depends on an AP-1-CRE element for activity, *Invest Ophthalmol Vis Sci* 38:951, 1997.

249. McDermott JB, Peterson CA, Piatigorsky J: Structure and lens expression of the gene encoding chicken beta A3/A1-crystallin, *Gene* 117:193, 1992.

250. McDonnell PJ, Stark WJ, Green WR: Posterior capsule opacification: a specular microscopic study, *Ophthalmology* 91:853, 1984.

251. McFall-Ngai MJ et al: Spatial and temporal mapping of the age-related changes in human lens crystallins, *Exp Eye Res* 41:745, 1985.

252. McGahan MC, Fleisher LN: Inflammation-induced changes in the iron concentration and total iron-binding capacity of the intraocular fluids of rabbits, *Graefes Arch Clin Exp Ophthalmol* 226:27, 1988.

253. McLaren JW et al: Measuring oxygen tension in the anterior chamber of rabbits, *Invest Ophthalmol Vis Sci* 39:1899, 1998.

254. Mecham RP et al: Development of immunoreagents to ciliary zonules that react with protein components of elastic fiber microfibrils and with elastin-producing cells, *Biochem Biophys Res Commun* 151:822, 1988.

255. Meddings DR et al: Mortality rates after cataract extraction, *Epidemiology* 10:288, 1999.

256. Meeson AP et al: VEGF deprivation–induced apoptosis is a component of programmed capillary regression, *Development* 126:1407, 1999.

257. Melberg NS, Thomas MA: Nuclear sclerotic cataract after vitrectomy in patients younger than 50 years of age, *Ophthalmology* 102:1466, 1995.

258. Merriam GR Jr, Worgul BV: Experimental radiation cataract-its clinical relevance, *Bull NY Acad Med* 59:372, 1983.

259. Merriam JC: The concentration of light in the human lens, *Trans Am Ophthalmol Soc* 94:803, 1996.

260. Merriman-Smith R, Donaldson P, Kistler J: Differential expression of facilitative glucose transporters GLUT1 and GLUT3 in the lens, *Invest Ophthalmol Vis Sci* 40:3224, 1999.

261. Milroy WC, Michaelson SM: Microwave cataractogenesis: a critical review of the literature, *Aerosp Med* 43:67, 1972.

262. Milstone LM, Piatigorsky J: Rates of protein synthesis in explanted embryonic chick lens epithelia: differential stimulation of crystallin synthesis, *Dev Biol* 43:91, 1975.

263. Morgenbesser SD et al: p53-dependent apoptosis produced by Rb-deficiency in the developing mouse lens, *Nature* 371:72, 1994.

264. Musil L, Beyer E, Goodenough D: Expression of the gap junction protein connexin43 in embryonic chick lens: molecular cloning, ultrastructural localization, and post-translational phosphorylation, *J Membr Biol* 116:163, 1990.

265. Nagamoto T, Eguchi G: Effect of intraocular lens design on migration of lens epithelial cells onto the posterior capsule, *J Cataract Refract Surg* 23:866, 1997.

266. Nagamoto T, Eguchi G, Beebe DC: Alpha-smooth muscle actin expression in cultured lens epithelial cells, *Invest Ophthalmol Vis Sci* 41:1122, 2000.

267. Nicolas AS, Lanzmann-Petithory D, Vellas B: Caloric restriction and aging, *J Nutr Health Aging* 3:77, 1999.

268. Nielsen S et al: Distribution of the aquaporin CHIP in secretory and resorptive epithelia and capillary endothelia, *Proc Natl Acad Sci USA* 90:7275, 1993.

269. Nishi O, Nishi K, Sakanishi K: Inhibition of migrating lens epithelial cells at the capsular bend created by the rectangular optic edge of a posterior chamber intraocular lens, *Ophthalmic Surg Lasers* 29:587, 1998.

270. Nishi O, Nishi K, Wickstrom K: Preventing lens epithelial cell migration using intraocular lenses with sharp rectangular edges, *J Cataract Refract Surg* 26:1543, 2000.

271. Nishiguchi S et al: Sox1 directly regulates the gamma-crystallin genes and is essential for lens development in mice, *Genes Dev* 12:776, 1998.

272. Nishikawa T et al: Normalizing mitochondrial superoxide production blocks three pathways of hyperglycaemic damage, *Nature* 404:787, 2000.

273. Norose K et al: SPARC deficiency leads to early-onset cataractogenesis, *Invest Ophthalmol Vis Sci* 39:2674, 1998.

274. Novak MA et al: The crystalline lens after vitrectomy for diabetic retinopathy, *Ophthalmology* 91:1480, 1984.

275. Novotny GE, Pau H: Myofibroblast-like cells in human anterior capsular cataract, *Virchows Arch A Pathol Anat Histopathol* 404:393, 1984.

276. Obara H et al: Usefulness of Scheimpflug photography to follow up Wilson's disease, *Ophthalmic Res* 27:100, 1995.

277. Ogino H, Yasuda K: Induction of lens differentiation by activation of a bZIP transcription factor, L-maf, *Science* 280:115, 1998.

278. Ogino H, Yasuda K: Sequential activation of transcription factors in lens induction, *Dev Growth Differ* 42:437, 2000.

279. Ogura Y, Kitagawa K, Ogino N: Prospective longitudinal studies on lens changes after vitrectomy: quantitative assessment by fluorophotometry and refractometry, *Nippon Ganka Gakkai Zasshi* 97:627, 1993.

280. Olsen G, Olson RJ: Update on a long-term, prospective study of capsulotomy and retinal detachment rates after cataract surgery, *J Cataract Refract Surg* 26:1017, 2000.

281. Onodera S: Presence of the basement membrane component—heparan sulfate proteoglycan—in bovine lens capsules, *Chem Pharm Bull (Tokyo)* 39:1059, 1991.

282. Padgaonkar VA et al: Hyperbaric oxygen in vivo accelerates the loss of cytoskeletal proteins and MIP26 in guinea pig lens nucleus, *Exp Eye Res* 68:493, 1999.

283. Paganini-Hill A, Clark LJ: Eye problems in breast cancer patients treated with tamoxifen, *Breast Cancer Res Treat* 60:167, 2000.

284. Palmquist BM, Philipson B, Barr PO: Nuclear cataract and myopia during hyperbaric oxygen therapy, *Br J Ophthalmol* 68:113, 1984.

285. Palva M, Palkama A: Ultrastructural lens changes in x-ray induced cataract of the rat, *Acta Ophthalmol* 56:587, 1978.

286. Pararajasegaram R: Vision 2020: the right to sight—from strategies to action, *Am J Ophthalmol* 128:359, 1999.

287. Parmelee JT: Measurement of steady currents around the frog lens, *Exp Eye Res* 42:433, 1986.

288. Parmelee JT, Beebe DC: Decreased membrane permeability to potassium is responsible for the cell volume increase that drives lens fiber cell elongation, *J Cell Physiol* 134:491, 1988.

289. Parmigiani C, McAvoy J: Localisation of laminin and fibronectin during rat lens morphogenesis, *Differentiation* 28:53, 1984.

290. Parmigiani CM, McAvoy JW: The roles of laminin and fibronectin in the development of the lens capsule, *Curr Eye Res* 10:501, 1991.

291. Phillips CI et al: Human cataract risk factors: significance of abstention from, and high consumption of, ethanol (U-curve) and non-significance of smoking, *Ophthalmic Res* 28:237, 1996.

292. Piatigorsky J: Lens cell elongation in vitro and microtubules, *Ann NY Acad Sci* 253:333, 1975.

293. Piatigorsky J: Molecular biology: recent studies on enzyme/crystallins and alpha-crystallin gene expression, *Exp Eye Res* 50:725, 1990.

294. Piatigorsky J: Puzzle of crystallin diversity in eye lenses, *Dev Dyn* 196:267, 1993.

295. Piatigorsky J: Multifunctional lens crystallins and corneal enzymes: more than meets the eye, *Ann NY Acad Sci* 842:7, 1998.

296. Piatigorsky J, Rothschild SS, Wollberg M: Stimulation by insulin of cell elongation and microtubule assembly in embryonic chick-lens epithelia, *Proc Natl Acad Sci USA* 70:1195, 1973.

297. Piatigorsky J, Webster H, Wollberg M: Cell elongation in the cultured embryonic chick lens epithelium with and without protein synthesis, *J Cell Biol* 55:82, 1972.

298. Piatigorsky J, Wistow GJ: Enzyme/crystallins: gene sharing as an evolutionary strategy, *Cell* 57:197, 1989.

299. Pirie A: Color and solubility of the proteins of human cataracts, *Invest Ophthalmol* 7:634, 1968.

300. Potts JD, Kornacker S, Beebe DC: Activation of the Jak-STAT-signaling pathway in embryonic lens cells, *Dev Biol* 204:277, 1998.

301. Prescott AR et al: The intermediate filament cytoskeleton of the lens: an ever changing network through development and differentiation—a minireview, *Ophthalmic Res* 28:58, 1996.

302. Quinlan RA et al: The eye lens cytoskeleton, *Eye* 13:409, 1999.

303. Rae JL et al: Dye transfer between cells of the lens, *J Membr Biol* 150:89, 1996.

304. Rafferty NS, Goossens W, March WF: Ultrastructure of human traumatic cataract, *Am J Ophthalmol* 78:985, 1974.

305. Rafferty NS, Rafferty KA: Cell population kinetics of the mouse lens epithelium, *J Cell Physiol* 107:309, 1981.

306. Rao PV et al: Betaine-homocysteine methyltransferase is a developmentally regulated enzyme crystallin in rhesus monkey lens, *J Biol Chem* 273:30669, 1998.

307. Reddan JR et al: Regional differences in the distribution of catalase in the epithelium of the ocular lens, *Cell Mol Biol* 42:209, 1996.

308. Reddan JR et al: Protection from oxidative insult in glutathione depleted lens epithelial cells, *Exp Eye Res* 68:117, 1999.

309. Reddy V: Glutathione and its function in the lens: an overview, *Exp Eye Res* 50:771, 1990.

310. Riach RA et al: Histamine and ATP mobilize calcium by activation of H1 and P2u receptors in human lens epithelial cells, *J Physiol (Lond)* 486:273, 1995.

311. Rieger DK et al: A double-deletion mutation in the Pitx3 gene causes arrested lens development in aphakia mice, *Genomics* 72:61, 2001.

312. Ring BZ et al: Regulation of mouse lens fiber cell development and differentiation by the *maf* gene, *Development* 127:307, 2000.

313. Ringens PJ, Hoenders HJ, Bloemendal H: Effect of aging on the water-soluble and water-insoluble protein pattern in normal human lens, *Exp Eye Res* 34:201, 1982.

314. Robinson KR, Patterson JW: Localization of steady currents in the lens, *Curr Eye Res* 2:843, 1982.

315. Robinson M et al: Extracellular FGF-1 acts as a lens differentiation factor in transgenic mice, *Development* 121:505, 1995.

316. Robinson ML et al: Dysregulation of ocular morphogenesis by lens-specific expression of FGF-3/int-2 in transgenic mice, *Dev Biol* 198:13, 1998.

317. Rose RC, Bode AM: Ocular ascorbate transport and metabolism, *Comp Biochem Physiol* 100A:273, 1991.

318. Ross ME et al: Myopia associated with hyperbaric oxygen therapy, *Optom Vis Sci* 73:487, 1996.

319. Rothstein H et al: Somatomedin C: restoration in vivo of cycle traverse in G0/G1 blocked cells of hypophysectomized animals, *Science* 208:410, 1980.

320. Rothstein H et al: G0/G1 arrest of cell proliferation in the ocular lens prevents development of radiation cataract, *Ophthalmic Res* 14:215, 1982.

321. Rouleau GA et al: Alteration in a new gene encoding a putative membrane-organizing protein causes neuro-fibromatosis type 2, *Nature* 363:515, 1993.

322. Roy D, Spector A: Absence of low-molecular-weight alpha crystallin in nuclear region of old human lenses, *Proc Natl Acad Sci USA* 73:3484, 1976.

323. Ruprecht KW: Ophthalmological aspects in patients with Werner's syndrome, *Arch Gerontol Geriatr* 9:263, 1989.

324. Sakaue H, Negi A, Honda Y: Comparative study of vitreous oxygen tension in human and rabbit eyes, *Invest Ophthalmol Vis Sci* 30:1933, 1989.

325. Sarkar PS et al: Heterozygous loss of Six5 in mice is sufficient to cause ocular cataracts, *Nat Genet* 25:110, 2000.

326. Scammon RE, Hesdorfer MB: Growth in mass and volume of the human lens in postnatal life, *Arch Ophthalmol* 17:104, 1937.

327. Schmitt-Graff A et al: Appearance of alpha-smooth muscle actin in human eye lens cells of anterior capsular cataract and in cultured bovine lens-forming cells, *Differentiation* 43:115, 1990.

328. Schook P: A review of data on cell actions and cell interaction during the morphogenesis of the embryonic eye, *Acta Morphol Neerl Scand* 16:267, 1978.

329. Schulz MW et al: Acidic and basic FGF in ocular media and lens: implications for lens polarity and growth patterns, *Development* 118:117, 1993.

330. Semina EV, Reiter RS, Murray JC: Isolation of a new homeobox gene belonging to the Pitx/Rieg family: expression during lens development and mapping to the aphakia region on mouse chromosome 19, *Hum Mol Genet* 6:2109, 1997.

331. Semina EV et al: A novel homeobox gene PITX3 is mutated in families with autosomal-dominant cataracts and ASMD, *Nat Genet* 19:167, 1998.

332. Semina EV et al: Deletion in the promoter region and altered expression of Pitx3 homeobox gene in aphakia mice, *Hum Mol Genet* 9:1575, 2000.

333. Shearer TR, David LL, Anderson RS: Selenite decreases phase separation temperature in rat lens, *Exp Eye Res* 42:503, 1986.

334. Shestopalov VI, Bassnett S: Exogenous gene expression and protein targeting in lens fiber cells, *Invest Ophthalmol Vis Sci* 40:1435, 1999.

335. Shestopalov VI, Bassnett S: Expression of autofluorescent proteins reveals a novel protein permeable pathway between cells in the lens core, *J Cell Sci* 113:1913, 2000.

336. Shiels A, Bassnett S: Mutations in the founder of the MIP gene family underlie cataract development in the mouse, *Nat Genet* 12:212, 1996.

337. Shiels A et al: A missense mutation in the human connexin50 gene (GJA8) underlies autosomal-dominant "zonular pulverulent" cataract, on chromosome 1q, *Am J Hum Genet* 62:526, 1998.

338. Shui YB, Kojima M, Sasaki K: A new steroid-induced cataract model in the rat: long-term prednisolone applications with a minimum of x-irradiation, *Ophthalmic Res* 28:92, 1996.

339. Shui YB et al: In vivo morphological changes in rat lenses induced by the administration of prednisolone after subliminal x-irradiation: a preliminary report, *Ophthalmic Res* 27:178, 1995.

340. Silver PH, Wakely J: The initial stage in the development of the lens capsule in chick and mouse embryos, *Exp Eye Res* 19:73, 1974.

341. Sivak JG, Kreuzer RO: Spherical aberration of the crystalline lens, *Vision Res* 23:59, 1983.

342. Sivak JG, Luer CA: Optical development of the ocular lens of an elasmobranch, *Raja eglanteria, Vision Res* 31:373, 1991.

343. Smith GN Jr, Linsenmayer TF, Newsome DA: Synthesis of type II collagen in vitro by embryonic chick neural retina tissue, *Proc Natl Acad Sci USA* 73:4420, 1976.

344. Spector A: Oxidative stress-induced cataract: mechanism of action, *FASEB J* 9:1173, 1995.

345. Spector A, Garner WH: Hydrogen peroxide and human cataract, *Exp Eye Res* 33:673, 1981.

346. Spector A, Li S, Sigelman J: Age-dependent changes in the molecular size of human lens proteins and their relationship to light scatter, *Invest Ophthalmol* 13:795, 1974.

347. Spector A, Ma W, Wang RR: The aqueous humor is capable of generating and degrading H_2O_2, *Invest Ophthalmol Vis Sci* 39:1188, 1998.

348. Spector A et al: cAMP-dependent phosphorylation of bovine lens alpha-crystallin, *Proc Natl Acad Sci USA* 82:4712, 1985.

349. Spencer RP: Change in weight of the human lens with age, *Ann Ophthalmol* 8:440, 1976.

350. Srivastava OP, Srivastava K: Characterization of a sodium deoxycholate-activatable proteinase activity associated with betaA3/A1-crystallin of human lenses, *Biochim Biophys Acta* 1434:331, 1999.

351. Steele EC Jr et al: Identification of a mutation in the MP19 gene, Lim2, in the cataractous mouse mutant To3, *Mol Vis* 3:5, 1997.

352. Stephan DA et al: Progressive juvenile-onset punctate cataracts caused by mutation of the gammaD-crystallin gene, *Proc Natl Acad Sci USA* 96:1008, 1999.

353. Stolen CM, Griep AE: Disruption of lens fiber cell differentiation and survival at multiple stages by region-specific expression of truncated FGF receptors, *Dev Biol* 217:205, 2000.

354. Street DA, Javitt JC: National five-year mortality after inpatient cataract extraction, *Am J Ophthalmol* 113:263, 1992.

355. Streeten BW: The zonular insertion: a scanning electron microscopic study, *Invest Ophthalmol Vis Sci* 16:364, 1977.

356. Streeten BW, Eshaghian J: Human posterior subcapsular cataract: a gross and flat preparation study, *Arch Ophthalmol* 96:1653, 1978.

357. Streeten BW, Licari PA: The zonules and the elastic microfibrillar system in the ciliary body, *Invest Ophthalmol Vis Sci* 24:667, 1983.

358. Stroeva OG: Relation of proliferative and determinative processes in the morphogenesis of the iris and ciliary body of mammals, *Zh Obshch Biol* 28:684, 1967.

359. Sweeney MH, Truscott RJ: An impediment to glutathione diffusion in older normal human lenses: a possible precondition for nuclear cataract, *Exp Eye Res* 67:587, 1998.

360. Takehana M, Takemoto L: Quantitation of membrane-associated crystallins from aging and cataractous human lenses, *Invest Ophthalmol Vis Sci* 28:780, 1987.

361. Takemoto LJ, Azari P: Isolation and characterization of covalently linked, high molecular weight proteins from human cataractous lens, *Exp Eye Res* 24:63, 1977.

362. Tanaka T, Benedek GB: Observation of protein diffusivity in intact human and bovine lenses with application to cataract, *Invest Ophthalmol* 14:449, 1975.

363. Tanaka T, Ishimoto C, Chylack LT Jr: Phase separation of a protein-water mixture in cold cataract in the young rat lens, *Science* 197:1010, 1977.

364. Taylor A et al: Moderate caloric restriction delays cataract formation in the Emory mouse, *FASEB J* 3:1741, 1989.

365. Taylor HR: Ultraviolet radiation and the eye: an epidemiologic study, *Trans Am Ophthalmol Soc* 87:802, 1989.

366. Taylor HR et al: Effect of ultraviolet radiation on cataract formation, *N Engl J Med* 319:1429, 1988.

367. Taylor VL, Costello MJ: Fourier analysis of textural variations in human normal and cataractous lens nuclear fiber cell cytoplasm, *Exp Eye Res* 69:163, 1999.

368. Termine JD et al: Osteonectin, a bone-specific protein linking mineral to collagen, *Cell* 26:99, 1981.

369. Thompson JT et al: Progression of nuclear sclerosis and long-term visual results of vitrectomy with transforming growth factor beta-2 for macular holes, *Am J Ophthalmol* 119:48, 1995.

370. Thut CJ et al: A large-scale in situ screen provides molecular evidence for the induction of eye anterior segment structures by the developing lens, *Dev Biol* 231:63, 2001.

371. Truscott RJ: Age-related nuclear cataract: a lens transport problem, *Ophthalmic Res* 32:185, 2000.

372. Truscott RJ, Augusteyn RC: Oxidative changes in human lens proteins during senile nuclear cataract formation, *Biochim Biophys Acta* 492:43, 1977.

373. Truscott RJ et al: Calcium-induced opacification and proteolysis in the intact rat lens, *Invest Ophthalmol Vis Sci* 31:2405, 1990.

374. Tsukaguchi H et al: A family of mammalian Na+-dependent L-ascorbic acid transporters, *Nature* 399:70, 1999.

375. Turrens JF, Alexandre A, Lehninger AL: Ubisemiquinone is the electron donor for superoxide formation by complex III of heart mitochondria, *Arch Biochem Biophys* 237:408, 1985.

376. Vaezy S, Clark JI: Characterization of the cellular microstructure of ocular lens using 2D power law analysis, *Ann Biomed Eng* 23:482, 1995.

377. Vaezy S, Clark JI, Clark JM: Quantitative analysis of the lens cell microstructure in selenite cataract using a two-dimensional Fourier analysis, *Exp Eye Res* 60:245, 1995.

378. Van Effenterre G et al: Is vitrectomy cataractogenic? Study of changes of the crystalline lens after surgery of retinal detachment, *J Fr Ophtalmol* 15:449, 1992.

379. Van Heyningen R: Fluorescent glucoside in the human lens, *Nature* 230:393, 1971.

380. van Leyen K et al: A function for lipoxygenase in programmed organelle degradation, *Nature* 395:392, 1998.

381. van Rijk AF, Bloemendal H: Alpha-B-crystallin in neuropathology, *Ophthalmologica* 214:7, 2000.

382. Varma SD, Mizuno A, Kinoshita JH: Diabetic cataracts and flavonoids, *Science* 195:205, 1977.

383. Varnum DS, Stevens LC: Aphakia, a new mutation in the mouse, *J Hered* 59:147, 1968.

384. Velasco PT et al: Hierarchy of lens proteins requiring protection against heat-induced precipitation by the alpha crystallin chaperone, *Exp Eye Res* 65:497, 1997.

385. Veretout F, Delaye M, Tardieu A: Molecular basis of eye lens transparency: osmotic pressure and x-ray analysis of alpha-crystallin solutions, *J Mol Biol* 205:713, 1989.

386. Vicart P et al: A missense mutation in the alphaB-crystallin chaperone gene causes a desmin-related myopathy, *Nat Genet* 20:92, 1998.

387. Vrensen GF: Aging of the human eye lens: a morphological point of view, *Comp Biochem Physiol A Physiol* 111:519, 1995.

388. Vrensen GF, Willekens B: Biomicroscopy and scanning electron microscopy of early opacities in the aging human lens, *Invest Ophthalmol Vis Sci* 31:1582, 1990.

389. Vrensen GF et al: Heterogeneity in ultrastructure and elemental composition of perinuclear lens retrodots, *Invest Ophthalmol Vis Sci* 35:199, 1994.

390. Walker JL, Menko AS: Alpha6 integrin is regulated with lens cell differentiation by linkage to the cytoskeleton and isoform switching, *Dev Biol* 210:497, 1999.

391. Walther C, Gruss P: Pax-6, a murine paired box gene, is expressed in the developing CNS, *Development* 113:1435, 1991.

392. Wang K, Gawinowicz MA, Spector A: The effect of stress on the pattern of phosphorylation of alphaA and alphaB crystallin in the rat lens, *Exp Eye Res* 71:385, 2000.

393. Wawersik S et al: BMP7 acts in murine lens placode development, *Dev Biol* 207:176, 1999.

394. Webster WS: Teratogen update: congenital rubella, *Teratology* 58:13, 1998.

395. Weng J et al: Hepatocyte growth factor, keratinocyte growth factor, and other growth factor-receptor systems in the lens, *Invest Ophthalmol Vis Sci* 38:1543, 1997.

396. West SK, Valmadrid CT: Epidemiology of risk factors for age-related cataract, *Surv Ophthalmol* 39:323, 1995.

397. West SK et al: Sunlight exposure and risk of lens opacities in a population-based study: the Salisbury Eye Evaluation project, *JAMA* 280:714, 1998.

398. West SK et al: Mixed lens opacities and subsequent mortality, *Arch Ophthalmol* 118:393, 2000.

399. Wheatley HM et al: Immunohistochemical localization of fibrillin in human ocular tissues: relevance to the Marfan syndrome, *Arch Ophthalmol* 113:103, 1995.

400. White TW, Goodenough DA, Paul DL: Targeted ablation of connexin50 in mice results in microphthalmia and zonular pulverulent cataracts, *J Cell Biol* 143:815, 1998.

401. Willekens B, Vrensen G: The three-dimensional organization of lens fibers in the rhesus monkey, *Graefe Arch Clin Exp Ophthalmol* 219:112, 1982.

402. Williams MR et al: Acetylcholine receptors are coupled to mobilization of intracellular calcium cultured human lens cells, *Exp Eye Res* 57:381, 1993 (letter).

403. Wind BE, Walsh S, Patterson JW: Equatorial potassium currents in lenses, *Exp Eye Res* 46:117, 1988.

404. Winkler BS, Orselli SM, Rex TS: The redox couple between glutathione and ascorbic acid: a chemical and physiological perspective, *Free Radic Biol Med* 17:333, 1994.

405. Winkler BS, Riley MV: Relative contributions of epithelial cells and fibers to rabbit lens ATP content and glycolysis, *Invest Ophthalmol Vis Sci* 32:2593, 1991.

406. Wistow G, Piatigorsky J: Recruitment of enzymes as lens structural proteins, *Science* 236:1554, 1987.

407. Wolf NS et al: Normal mouse and rat strains as models for age-related cataract and the effect of caloric restriction on its development, *Exp Eye Res* 70:683, 2000.

408. Worgul BV, Rothstein H: Radiation cataract and mitosis, *Ophthal Res* 7:21, 1975.

409. Worgul BV, Rothstein H: On the mechanism of radio-cataractogenesis, *Medikon* I:5, 1977.

410. Worgul BV et al: Lens epithelium and radiation cataract, *Arch Ophthalmol* 94:996, 1976.

411. Worgul BV et al: Radiation cataractogenesis in the amphibian lens, *Ophthalmic Res* 14:73, 1982.

412. Xu PX et al: Mouse eye homologues of the Drosophila eyes absent gene require Pax-6 for expression in lens and nasal placode, *Development* 124:219, 1997.

413. Yamamoto Y: Growth or lens and ocular environment: role of the neural retina in the growth of mouse lens as revealed by an implantation experiment, *Dev Growth Diff* 18:273, 1976.

414. Yamaoka T et al: Acute onset of diabetic pathological changes in transgenic mice with human aldose reductase cDNA, *Diabetologia* 38:255, 1995.

415. Young RW, Ocumpaugh DE: Autoradiographic studies on the growth and development of the lens capsule in the rat, *Invest Ophthal* 5:583, 1966.

416. Yu CE et al: Positional cloning of the Werner's syndrome gene, *Science* 272:258, 1996.

417. Zhang P et al: Cooperation between the Cdk inhibitors p27(KIP1) and p57(KIP2) in the control of tissue growth and development, *Genes Dev* 12:3162, 1998.

418. Zhu M et al: The human hyaloid system: cell death and vascular regression, *Exp Eye Res* 70:767, 2000.

419. Zigman S et al: Effect of chronic near-ultraviolet radiation on the gray squirrel lens in vivo, *Invest Ophthalmol Vis Sci* 32:1723, 1991.

420. Zimmerman LE: Histopathologic basis for ocular manifestations of congenital rubella syndrome, *Am J Ophthalmol* 65:837, 1968.

421. Zintz C, Beebe DC: Morphological and cell volume changes in the rat lens during the formation of radiation cataracts, *Exp Eye Res* 42:43, 1986.

422. Zwaan J, Kenyon RE: Cell replication and terminal differentiation in the embryonic chicken lens: normal and forced initiation of lens fibre formation, *J Embryol Exp Morph* 84:331, 1984.

SECTION 4

OPTICS AND REFRACTION

DAVID MILLER

CHAPTER 6

◆

PHYSIOLOGIC OPTICS AND REFRACTION

DAVID MILLER

THE YOUNG EYE

Primate and human infants must normally pass head first through their mother's pelvis to accommodate the limited opening determined by the bony configuration. Therefore the size of the mother's pelvis limits the head and brain size of the infant. Specifically, the brain of an infant ape is 55% of its full size, and the brain of a present-day human infant is only 23% of the adult size.[11] The result is a human infant who is neurologically immature.[19] Notice that the baby monkey can immediately cling tightly to the fur on its mother's stomach, whereas the human infant has poor muscle strength, has little motor control, and is completely dependent on his or her mother for survival. While immature, the human infant lives in a restricted and artificial reality, interacting primarily with his or her mother. The human infant interacts little with the forces of life in the outside world.

It is possible that this early immaturity and restricted world contact are naturally beneficial. The infant's restricted curriculum concentrates on a few priorities necessary for survival. Without words, the infant must be able to announce all his or her needs and encourage a high level of motherly devotion. To communicate with his or her mother, the infant must be able to read facial expressions and respond with a nonverbal vocabulary. If this speculation is correct, what vision equipment does the infant have to perform these functions?

Relevant Anatomy

Axial Length. Larsen[52] noted that the axial length of the neonate's eye was 17 mm and that it increases 25% by the time the child reaches adolescence. The size of the normal infant's eye is about three fourths

that of the adult size. Geometric optics teaches us that the retinal image of the normal infant eye is therefore be about three fourths the size of the adult's image.* A smaller image also means that much less fine detail is recorded. The small retinal image may be but one reason why an infant's visual acuity is poorer than that of the adult. In fact, experiments have shown that the neonate's visual appreciation for fine detail at birth is one thirtieth, or approximately 3%, of the development of the adult,† yet the neonate appreciates large objects (e.g., nose, mouth, eyes of close faces) as does the adult. Figure 6-1 shows that visual acuity swiftly improves, and by the age of 12 months, the infant's level of visual acuity is 25% (20/80) of optimal adult visual acuity. This improvement in acuity seems to parallel eyeball growth. By the age of 5 years, the child usually has 20/20 vision.[11,29,32,82,102] What other factors beyond eye size account for the young child's lowered visual acuity? As the eye grows, the optical power of the eye lens and cornea must weaken in a tightly coordinated fashion so that the world stays in sharp focus on the retina. If this tight coordination of growth fails, the infant may become nearsighted or farsighted. Because the coordination of eye length growth and the focusing power of the cornea and eye lens may be imperfect, is there some compensation provided, early in life, guaranteeing that almost every child can process a sharply focused retinal image of the world?

---

*Specifically, the size of the retinal image depends on an entity known as the *nodal distance,* which averages 11.7 mm in the newborn and 16.7 mm in the adult emmetropic schematic eye, giving a ratio of adult to infant retinal images of 1.43.[6]
†The infant's visual acuity is about 20/600 versus the normal visual acuity of an adult, which is 20/20.

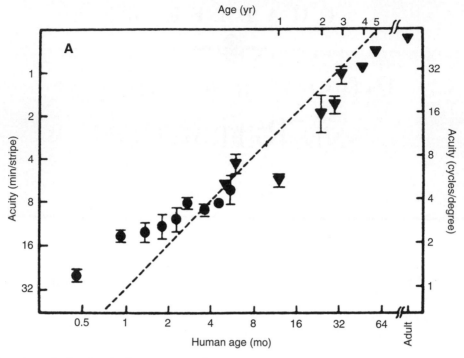

FIGURE 6-1   A graph showing the improvement of visual acuity in the baby as it ages. The method of preferential viewing was used to achieve these results. (From Teller DG: The development of visual function in infants. In Cohen B, Bodis-Wollner I [eds]: *Vision and brain,* New York, 1990, Raven Press.)

Accommodation is the safety valve that can help provide a sharp image, even if all the ocular components are not perfectly matched. In the young child the range of accommodation is greater than 20 diopters. This range, in addition to the farsightedness of almost all infants, means that most young eyes can focus almost any object by using part or all of this enormous focusing capacity.

Because of the infant's smaller pupil, a second factor that helps the infant achieve a sharper retinal image is an increased depth of focus.[32] Photographers use this device when they use larger F-stops (F 32, F 64) to keep objects at different distances all in focus.

Figure 6-2 shows the importance of the nodal point in determining the size of the retinal image in a typical human eye. To help us appreciate the basic optical principles operating within the human eye and avoid being confused by their many details (e.g., the many different radii of curvature, the different indices of refraction), an all-purpose, simplified eye was developed. Such model eyes have many names (e.g., reduced, schematic, simplified eye)

and were developed by some of the true giants of physiologic optics.*

Figure 6-2 depicts such an eye with its cardinal points (the principal points, focal points, and nodal points). Knowing the location of the cardinal points of a lens system, the optical designer can calculate all of the relationships between an object and an image. For example, to determine the image size of the reduced eye, one simply traces the ray, starting from the top of the object, which goes undeviated through the nodal point and lands on the top of the inverted retinal image. As the distance between the nodal point and the retina increases, the image size increases. The addition of a plus spectacle lens to the eye's optic system moves the nodal point of the new system forward (increasing the nodal point to retina distance), thus magnifying the retinal image. The re-

---

*A partial list of giants of physiologic optics who have created schematic or reduced eyes include Listing, Helmholtz, Wüllner, Tserning, Matthiessen, Gullstrand, Legrand, Ivanoff, and Emsley.

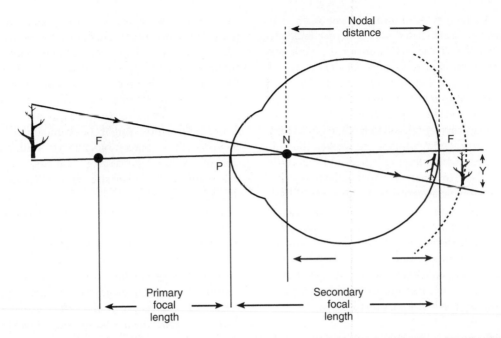

Figure 6-2 A diagram of a reduced human eye. *F,* Focal points; *N,* nodal point; *P,* principle point. The *dotted line* represents the retina of an enlarged eye.

verse is true with a negative spectacle lens. Therefore a contact lens or a refractive cornea on which surgery has been performed enlarges the image size for a person with myopia who previously wore spectacles.

Emmetropization. The coordination of the power of the cornea, crystalline lens, and axial length to process a sharp retinal image of a distant object is known as *emmetropization.* In the United States, more than 70% of the population is either emmetropic or mildly hyperopic (easily corrected with a small accommodative effort).

With age, the cornea, lens, and axial length undergo coordinated changes. Essentially, the optical components (cornea and lens) must lose refractive power as the axial length increases so that a sharp image remains focused on the retina.

The cornea, which averages 48 diopters of power at birth and has an increased elasticity, loses about 4 diopters by the time the child is 2 years of age.[41,42] One may assume that the spurt in growth of the sagittal diameter of the globe during this period pulls the cornea into a flatter curvature. The fact that the average corneal diameter is 8.5 mm at 34 weeks of gestation, 9 mm at 36 weeks, 9.5 mm at

term, and about 11 mm in the adult eye supports this "pulling, flattening" hypothesis.[108]

On the other hand, other coordinated events also occur, such as the change of lens power and the coordinated increase in eye size (most important, an increase in axial length). The crystalline lens, which averages 45 diopters during infancy, loses about 20 diopters of power by age 6.[71,118] To compensate for this loss of lens power, the axial length increases by 5 to 6 mm in that same time frame.[52] (In general, 1 mm of change in axial length correlates with a 3-diopter change in refractive power of the eye.)

Now let us examine a possible mechanism that could account for most of the data.[38,71] As the cross-sectional area of the eye expands, there is an increased pull on the lens zonules and a subsequent flattening of the lens (the anterior lens surface is affected a bit more and the posterior lens surface a bit less), thus decreasing the overall lens power. There also may be a related decrease in the refractive index of the lens, which also contributes to the reduction in lens power. Because the incidence of myopia starts to accelerate significantly around the age of 10,[71] one may question whether there could be a decoupling of the previously described coordinated drop in lens power and increase in axial length. An increased amount of near work (e.g., schoolwork) is associated with a higher incidence of myopia.[120] It is also well known that genetic predisposition influences myopia incidence, as evidenced by the fact that more Oriental children than Caucasian children are myopic.[120] Thus one might hypothesize that the long periods of accommodation that accompany schoolwork (ciliary body contraction) may tend to stretch and weaken the linkage between the enlarging scleral shell and the ciliary body. If this were to happen, the lens would flatten less during eye growth. Another way of looking at this phenomenon is to theorize that with the linkage weakened, the restraining effect of the lens-zonule combination on eye growth is also weakened, which results in an increase in axial length in the myopic student. Many studies demonstrating that the myopic eye has a greater axial length than the emmetropic eye support this idea.[31]

Retinal Receptors. The cone photoreceptors of the retina are responsible for sharp vision under daylight conditions. The denser the cones are packed, the more acute the vision.[11,82] To use a photographic analogy, film with the highest resolution has smaller photosensitive grains, packed tightly, whereas a film with large grains of silver halide yields a coarser picture.

The most sensitive part of the retina is the fovea.* Here the cones are even finer and are packed together even tighter. The fovea of the infant eye is packed less than one fourth the density of that of the adult. Furthermore, the synapse density in the neural portion of the retina, as well as the visual brain, is low at birth. The combination of these two anatomic configurations means that fewer fine details of the retinal image are recorded and sent to the brain.

Neural Processing. Finally, the nerves that transmit the visual information to the brain, as well as the nerve fibers at the various levels within the brain, are poorly myelinated in the infant. Myelin is the insulating wrap around each nerve fiber. A normally myelinated nerve can transmit nerve impulses swiftly and without static or "cross talk" from adjacent nerves. To use a computer analogy, one might

think of the infant brain as being connected with poorly insulated wires. Therefore sparks, short circuits, and static all slow or interfere with perfect transmission, and only the strongest messages get through. Figure 6-3 represents an appropriate analogy. The face of Albert Einstein is shown on a computer screen with larger and larger pixels. The infant's early vision might be comparable to the picture with the biggest block pixels. With maturation of the brain processing elements, the neurologic equivalent of pixel size gets smaller and more details can be registered. Thus the equivalent of the photographic film grain size in the retina and the equivalent of pixel size in the brain processor both get smaller as the child grows. Lakshiminarayanan, who created Figure 6-3, speculated that the immaturity of the infant's memory capacity may be one reason why its visual images have less detail. In other words, the coarseness of the infant visual system does not overtax the immature memory system.

Relevant Early Physiology
Experiments with infants reveal that good color vision does not appear for about 3 months. The infant also takes longer to "make sense" of the retinal image. Specifically, the infant must stare for relatively long periods (1 to 3 minutes), blinking rarely during this period.[11,82]

Recognizing Faces. The remarkable thing about the infant's eyesight is that the relatively poor level of resolution just described still allows the infant to recognize different faces and different facial expressions. We know this to be true in some newborn infants, who can accurately imitate the expressions of an adult, as seen in Figure 6-4. You might think of the baby using his or her own face as a canvas to reproduce the facial expression of the onlooker.

Experiments with infants demonstrate that infants prefer to look at faces or pictures of faces rather than to look at other objects. By the age of 6 weeks, infants can discern specific features of the face. For example, they can lock in on their mother's gaze. By age 6 months, they can also recognize the same face in different poses. In fact, they are experts at recognizing a face, be it upside down or right side up, till the age of 6 years. After age 6, infants actually lose their skill at quickly recognizing upside-down faces.[82]

A closer examination of the eye at 6 months of age is worthwhile because an unusual change has started to take place in the optics of the eye at this

---

*F.W. Campbell[14] quotes Stuart Ansti's clear analogy of how the fovea functions: "A retina with a fovea surrounded by a lower acuity periphery can be compared to a low magnification finder telescope with a large field of view which will find any interesting target and then steer on to it a high powered main telescope, with a very small field which could examine the target in detail."

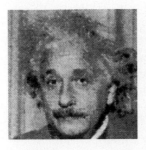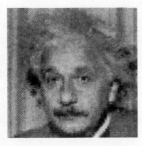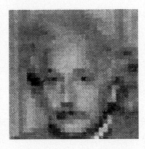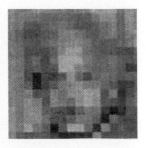

FIGURE 6-3 A computer display of the face of Albert Einstein, with pixels of different size. (From Lakshiminarayanan V et al: Human face recognition using wavelengths In *Vision science and its application,* Santa Fe, 1995, Optical Society of America.)

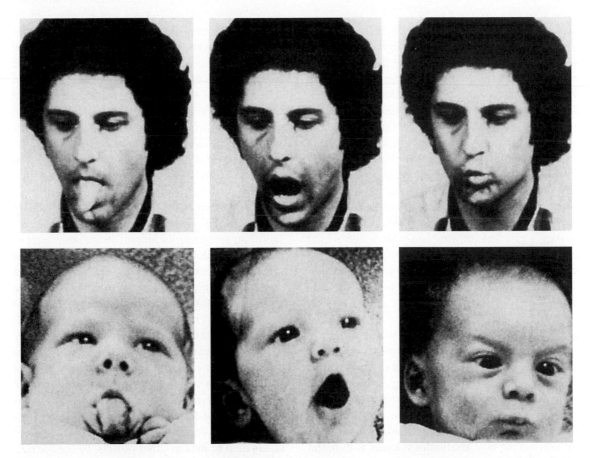

FIGURE 6-4 This photo shows a recently born infant mimicking the expression of psychologist Dr. A Meltzoff. The baby is obviously able to perceive the different expressions in order to mimic them. (From Klaus MH, Klaus PH: *The amazing newborn,* Reading, Mass, 1985, Addison Wesley.)

time. Gwiazda et al.[33] found that a significant amount of astigmatism develops in 56% of the infants studied. This condition remains for only 1 to 2 years.[31,33,69,120]

The transient astigmatism just described tends to elongate tiny dots of the retinal image into lines.

In essence, these create the equivalent of a line drawing of the retinal image. For example, think of a mime (i.e., a painted face with a few dark lines and spots for eyes and nose) as creating different line drawings of the face. What is astonishing is that, although made of only a few dark lines, the

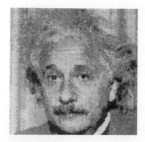 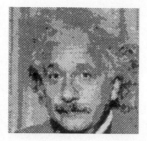 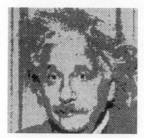 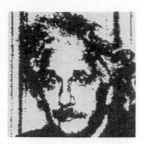

FIGURE 6-5   A series of computer simulations of the face of Albert Einstein with an extensive gray scale on the left (16 gray scale) and only a 2 gray scale on the right, the latter being similar to a line drawing. (From Lakshiminarayanan V et al: Human face recognition using wavelength. In *Vision science and its applications,* Santa Fe, 1995, Optical Society of America.)

mime can recreate most human expressions. It seems reasonable to imagine that the mime presents faces similar to those seen by the young child or found in a child's drawing. The faces have no texture, no shadowing, and no creases—only a line for a mouth, circle for eyes, and occasionally, a dot for a nose. Is it not then possible that infant astigmatism helps represent faces as line drawings to the infant visual system? Line drawings also save memory storage space, which would be an advantage for the small infant brain.* Figure 6-5 illustrates this point in a different way. The face of Albert Einstein is shown with a complete gray scale on the left and is shown as a line drawing (only black and white) on the right. The line drawing requires much less computing power than a face with texture and would be more compatible with the child's immature processing system.

Line Orientation Receptors. As noted earlier, in many infants the amount of astigmatism can rise to a level of greater than 2 diopters in the first year of life. The orientation of the distortion is usually horizontal (180 degrees) initially. In the course of the next 2 years, the meridian of distortion rotates to the vertical and the amount of the astigmatism diminishes. This slow rotation of the axis of exaggeration can help activate different groups of brain cells, which become sensitive to features in the retinal image with different tilts. In fact, the discovery of these brain cells with orientation selectively leads to a ground-breaking understanding of the functional architecture in the higher brain. Torsten Wiesel and David Hubel, working in their labora-

tory at the Harvard Medical School, late one night, in 1958, implanted electrodes in the visual cortex of an anesthetized cat to record cortical cell responses to patterns of light, which they projected onto a screen in front of the cat. After 4 hours of intense work, the two scientists put the dark spot slide into the projector, where it jammed. As the edge of the glass slide cast an angled shadow on the retina, the implanted cell in the visual cortex fired a burst of action potentials. Torsten Wiesel described that moment as the "door to all secrets." The pair went on to prove that cells in the cortex responded only to stimuli of a particular orientation. Similar responding cells were all located in the same part of the cortex. This work opened up the area of how and where the brain encodes specific features of the retinal image. Fittingly, Drs. Hubel and Wiesel were awarded the Nobel Prize for Medicine in 1981.[98]

Monitoring Other's Eye Movements. Another function of great survival value to the infant is the ability to follow the eye movements of his or her caretakers. Consider this a near task involving the contrast discrimination of a 12-mm dark iris against a white sclera framed by the palpebral fissure; such a task can be accomplished with a visual acuity of 20/200.

The British psychologist Simon Baron-Cohen, in his book *Mindblindness,** suggests that a major evolutionary advance has been the human's ability to understand and then interact with others in a social group (e.g., playing social chess). He further suggests that we accomplish this social intelligence

---

*This idea was suggested by David Marr in "Early Processing of Visual Information," published in *Transactions of the Royal Society of London,* Series B, 275:483, 1976.

*In his book *Mindblindness: An Essay on Autism and Theory of Mind,* published by MIT Press in 1995, Baron-Cohen ferrets out the key features of "eye following" in the normal child by comparing them with those of the autistic child.

primarily by following the eye movements of others, which begins at a young age. For example, an infant of 2 months begins to concentrate on the eyes of adults. Infants have been shown to spend as much time on the eyes as all other features of an observer's face.

By 6 months of age, infants look at the face of an adult who is looking at them two to three times longer than an adult who is looking away. We also know that when infants achieve eye contact, a positive emotion is achieved (i.e., infants smile). By age 14 months, infants start to read the direction that an adult is looking. Infants turn in that direction and then continue to look back at the adult to check that both are looking at the same thing. By age 2, infants typically can read fear and joy from eye and facial expression.

Recognizing Movement. Infants are capable of putting up their arms to block a threatening movement. This act tells us that infants appreciate both movement and the implied threat of this particular movement.[12,29] Admittedly, infants cannot respond if the threat moves too quickly, probably because the immature myelinization of the nerves slows the neural circuits. Nevertheless, a definite appreciation of movement and threat exists.

For movement to be registered accurately, the infant retina probably records an object at point A. That image is then physiologically erased (in the brain and/or retina), and the object is now seen at point B. This physiologic erasure is important because, without it, movement would produce a smeared retinal image. Researchers think that the infant probably sees movement as a smoothed series of sharp images, not smears.[106] This hypothesis is supported by other experiments demonstrating that the infant can appreciate the on/off quality of a rapidly flickering light at an early age. It seems logical that the movement of an image across the retina (with the inherent erasures) is physiologically related to the rapid on/off registration of a flickering light.

A related reflex, the foveal reflex, is triggered by stimulation of the peripheral retina, activating the eye movement system so that the fovea is directed to the visual stimulus.

Summary
Social Seeing. Although the visual system of the infant is immature, some infants can recognize and respond to adult facial expressions on the first day of life and follow their mother's glances by 6 weeks

of age. Clearly, the infant's top priority is to maintain a social relationship with his or her mother or other caring adults. This idea was described succinctly by the "language expert" Pinker[77]: "Most normally developing babies like to schmooze." As infants grow, they learn to see people and objects in the way that their culture demands and communicate in the expected manner; that is, "We don't see things as they are but as we are." Is it possible that the immature eye and visual system actually facilitate socially biased seeing? Perhaps the smaller, simpler retinal images, along with the less sophisticated brain processing, prevent the many other details of life from confusing the key message; that is, social interaction takes top priority.

THE IMAGE OF THE HUMAN ADULT EYE

The image quality of the human adult eye is far superior to that of the human infant, although probably inferior to certain predator birds. Its wide focusing range is smaller than that of certain diving birds, and its fine sensitivity to low light levels is weaker than spiders or animals with a tapetum lucidum. Its ability to repair itself if probably not as efficient as some animals (e.g., newts, which can form a new lens if the original is damaged). Finally, the human eye has the ability to transmit emotional information[49] (e.g., excitement by means of pupil dilation, sadness by means of weeping), but with less forcefulness than some fish, who uncover a pigmented bar next to the eye when they are about to attack,[26] or the horned lizard, which squirts a jet of blood from its eye when it is threatened.[87] Thus, in reading this chapter, one must appreciate the eye's level of performance in light of its large spectrum of functions.

Tuned to Visible Light Waves
When our retinas receive an image of a spotted puppy in a room, what is really happening in terms of information transfer? Light waves from the ceiling light are cast onto the puppy. The puppy's body reflects and scatters the light waves into our eyes. In a sense, information about the puppy has been encoded into visible light waves. The optical elements of the eye focus the encoded light waves onto our retina as a map of bright and dim colored dots, known as the *retinal image*. Nerve signals report the retinal image to the brain. In the brain the nerve signals are recreated into the impression that a real puppy is in the room.

One might liken the function of the eye to that of a radio, which receives radio waves carrying a Beethoven symphony. The specific station broadcasting the symphony beams it out on a specific radio wavelength. The radio then receives the radio waves, and the speaker reconverts the waves to musical sounds. If the eye is to receive and process visible light, it must be constructed with the ability to be tuned to the wavelengths of visible light. The physicist would substitute the term *resonate* for *tune*. Literally, *resonate* means to resound another time. A simple example of resonance is an opera singer who can make a wine glass hum when the frequency (or wavelength) of the note is the same as the natural frequency of the glass. What is the natural frequency of anything? The answer has to do with composition and size. Organ pipes of different lengths resonate at different frequencies and wavelengths. Changing the length of the antenna on a car radio allows the frequencies of different stations to be received. The best receiver for a specific wavelength (frequency is the reciprocal of wavelengths) is physically the same size as the wavelength, a precise number of wavelengths, or a precise faction (one fourth, one half) of the size of the wavelength. Therefore optical theory demands that the size of the key components of the eye be the size of a wavelength of visible light or some number (n) times the size of, or a fraction of the size of, the wavelengths of visible light; in addition, the key components must be made of a resonating material.

Role of the Cornea. The human cornea is a unique tissue. First, it is the most powerful focusing element of the eye, roughly twice as powerful as the lens within the eye. It is mechanically strong and transparent. Its strength comes from its collagen fiber layers. Some 200 fiber layers crisscross the cornea in different directions. These fibers are set in a thick, watery jelly called *glycosaminoglycan*. The jelly gives the cornea pliability. For a long time, no one could explain convincingly the transparency of the cornea. No one could understand how nature combined tough, transparent collagen fibers (with their unique index of refraction) with the transparent glycosaminoglycan matrix, which had a different index of refraction, and still maintain clarity. Perhaps an everyday example of this phenomenon will help. When a glass is filled from the hot water tap, the solution looks cloudy. Looking closely, one can see many fine, clear expanded air bubbles (which have a unique index of refraction) within the water (which has different refractive properties). Conversely, cold water appears clear because

its air bubbles are tiny. The normal corneal structure might be considered optically similar to the structure of the cold water (i.e., tiny components with different indices of refraction).

Miller and Benedek[63] were ultimately able to prove that if the spaces consisting of glycosaminoglycan and the size of the collagen fibers were smaller than one half a wavelength of visible light, the cornea is clear, even if the fibers were arranged randomly. An orderly arrangement of the fibers also helps maintain corneal transparency.

Another way to explain it is to say that the cornea is basically transparent to visible light because its internal structures are tuned to the size of a fraction of the wavelengths of visible light. Figure 6-6 is an electron micrograph showing the fibers of the human cornea. The black dots are cross sections of collagen fibers imbedded in the glycosaminoglycan matrix. Note that in this specimen, the fibers are spaced closer than half a wavelength of visible light apart, and the fibers in each of the major layers are arranged in an orderly manner.

This arrangement of corneal fibers serves a number of important functions. First, the arrangement offers maximal strength and resistance to injury from any direction.* Second, the arrangement produces a transparent, stable optical element. Third, the spaces between the major layers act as potential highways for white blood cell migration if any injury or infection occurs.

Role of the Crystalline Lens. Have you ever noticed that you see things much better underwater if you wear goggles?† Without goggles, the water practically cancels the focusing power of the cornea,‡ leaving objects blurred. The goggles ensure an envelope of air in front of the cornea, restoring its optical power. If water cancels optic power, how can we explain the focusing ability of the crystalline lens, which lies inside the eye and is

---

*A fiber-matrix structure like the cornea has a number of mechanical advantages. For example, fibers separated by a softer matrix cannot transfer stress cracks and tears to neighboring fibers. During bending, the separating matrix prevents fibers from abrading each other. Upon loading, the matrix can transmit forces around torn fibers.

†Because the index of refraction of water is greater than air, objects underwater appear about one third closer and thus one third larger than they would in air (i.e., magnification = $1.33\times$).[61]

‡The cornea is a focusing element for two reasons. First, it has a convex surface. Second, it has a refractive index greater than air. Actually, its refractive index is close to that of water. Thus, when one is underwater, the surrounding water on the outside and the aqueous humor inside the eye combine to neutralize the cornea's focusing power.

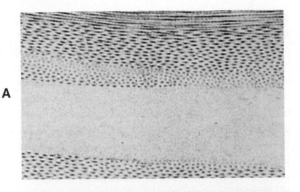

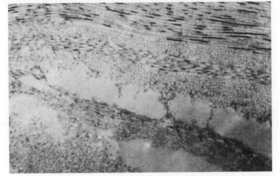

A

B

FIGURE 6-6 **A,** Electron micrograph showing the neat pattern of corneal collagen fibers. The black dots are the fibers cut on end. In this photo the spacing between fibers is less than a wavelength of light apart. **B,** Large spaces between collagen fibers, as seen in a waterlogged, hazy cornea. (From Miller D, Benedek G: *Intraocular light scattering,* Springfield, Ill, 1973, Charles C Thomas.)

surrounded by a fluid known as *aqueous humor?* The answer is that the focusing power resides in the unusually high protein content of the lens. The protein concentration may reach 50% or more in certain parts of the lens.* Such a high concentration increases the refractive index above that of water and allows the focusing of light. Now we are ready to appreciate the real secret of the lens.[62,63]

Normally, a 50% protein solution is cloudy, with precipitates floating about like curdled lumps of milk in a cup of coffee. However, the protein molecules of the normal lens do not precipitate. In a manner not fully understood, the large protein molecules known as *crystallins*† seem to repel each other, or at least prevent aggregation, to maintain tiny spaces between each other. The protein size and the spaces between them are equivalent to a

small fraction of a light wavelength. Spaced as they are, one might say that they are tuned to visible light and allow the rays to pass through unimpeded. On the other hand, if some pathologic process occurs, the protein molecules clump together and the lens loses its clarity. When this happens, light is scattered about as it passes through the lens. The result is a cataract.

Accommodation. If the emmetropic eye is in sharp focus for the distant world, it must refocus (accommodate) to see closer objects.* For example, the child's range of accommodation is large, as noted earlier. This allows the child to continue to keep objects in sharp focus from an infinite distance away to objects brought to the tip of the nose. The act of accommodation is fast, taking only about one third of a second. Our range of accommodation decreases with each passing year, so by the age of 45, most of us are left with about 20% of the amplitude of accommodation we started with.

With age, the lens enlarges and becomes denser and more rigid. In so doing, it progressively loses the ability to accommodate. Parenthetically, the cornea of many birds, from pigeons to hawks, can change shape to accommodate.[76] The avian cornea does not change flexibility with age; therefore these birds do not become presbyopic. However, there is no "free lunch" in nature. The human lens, sitting within the eye surrounded by protective fluid is far less vulnerable to injury than the cornea.

Role of the Retina. After light passes through the cornea, the aqueous humor, the lens, and the vitreous humor, it is focused onto the retinal photoreceptors. The light must pass through a number of retinal layers of nerve fibers, nerve cells, and blood vessels before striking the receptors. These retinal layers (aside from blood vessels) are transparent because of the small size of the elements and the tight packing arrangement.

The bird retina does not have blood vessels. The human retina has retinal blood vessels that cover some of the retinal receptors and produce fine angioscotomas. A bird's retina obtains much of its oxygen and nutritive supply from a tangle of blood vessels (the pectin), which is covered with black pigment and sits in the vitreous in front of the retina and above the macula (so as to function as a

---

*The chemical composition of a focusing element such as the crystalline lens determines the refractive index. Water has a refractive index of 1.33. As the protein concentration of the lens rises, the index of refraction approaches 1.42.
†*Crystallins* are large protein molecules ranging in size from 45 to 2000 kD.

---

*The question "How does accommodation 'know' it has achieved the sharpest focus?" seems to be best answered by a sensing system in the brain. However, some have suggested that the system takes advantage of the naturally occurring chromatic aberration of the primate eye to fine-tune focusing.[1]

visor). The negative aspect of such a vascular system is vulnerability to a direct blunt or penetrating injury that can lead to a vitreous hemorrhage and sudden blindness. Obviously, this is less probable in the bird because of its lifestyle.

Rhodopsin. The rods and cones are made up of a biologic molecule that absorbs visible light and then traduces that event into an electrical nerve signal. The rhodopsin molecule is an example of Einstein's photoelectric effect.* In fact, only one quanta (the smallest possible amount of light) of visible light† is needed to trigger the molecule, that is, snap the molecule into a new shape.‡

The internal structure of the molecule allows the wavelengths of visible light to resonate within its electron cloud and within 20 million millionths of a second, inducing the change in the molecule that starts the reaction.

Probably the earliest chemical relative of rhodopsin is to be found in a primitive purple-colored bacteria called *Holobacterium halobium.* Koji Nakanishi, a biochemist at Columbia University, in an article titled "Why 11-cis-Retinal?"[72] (a type of rhodopsin) notes that this bacteria has been on the planet for the last 1.3 billion years.[73,93] Its preference for low oxygen and a salty environment places its origin at a time on earth where there was little or no oxygen in the atmosphere and a high salt concentration in the sea. Although found in primeval bacteria, bacteriorhodopsin is a rather complicated molecule, containing 248 amino acids. It is thought that this bacteria probably used rhodopsin for photosynthesis, rather than light sensing. Time-resolved spectroscopic measurements have determined that this molecule changes shape within one trillionth of a second after light stimulation.[3] This early form of rhodopsin absorbs light most efficiently in the blue-green part of the spectrum, although it does respond to all colors.[119]

To function as the transducer for vision, the photopigment must capture light and then signal the organism's brain that the light has registered. As noted earlier, one molecule needs only one quanta to start the reaction. Even more amazing is the molecule's stability. Although only one quanta of visible light is necessary to trigger it, the molecule will not trigger accidentally. In fact, it has been estimated that spontaneous isomerization of retinal (the light-sensing chromophore portion of rhodopsin) occurs once in a thousand years.[3] If this were not so, we would see light flashes every time there is a rise in body temperature (a fever). To better understand the rhodopsin mechanism, one may picture a hair trigger on a pistol that takes only the slightest vibration (but only a special type of vibration) to be activated. As noted, the activating quanta must be of the proper energy level to "kick in" the reaction. That is, the quanta of light must be made of wavelengths of visible light.

Receptor Size and Spacing. Retinal receptor factors that influence the optical limits of visual acuity occur in the foveal macular area. The fovea itself subtends an arc of about 0.3 degree. It is an elliptical area with a horizontal diameter of 100 μm. The area contains more than 2000 tightly packed cones. The distance between the centers of these tightly packed cones is about 2 μm. The cone diameters themselves measure about 1.5 μm (a dimension comparable to three wavelengths of green light) and are separated by about 0.5 μm.[16,25,89,90] Therefore the fine details of the retinal image occupy an elliptical area only about 0.1 mm in maximum width.

A discussion of the diffraction limits of resolution, in a theoretical emmetropic human eye, must involve the anatomic size of the photoreceptors and the pupil. A point on an object is focused on the retina as an Airy disc because of diffraction. The angular size of the Airy disc is determined as follows:

Equation 6-1

$$\text{Angular size} = \frac{1.22 \text{ (wavelength)}}{\text{Pupil diameter}}$$

Let the pupil diameter be 2.4 mm (optimal balance between diffraction and spherical aberration in the human eye), and let the wavelength be 0.00056 mm (yellow green/light):

Equation 6-2

$$\text{Angular size} = \frac{1.22 \ (0.00056)}{2.4} = 0.0003$$

$$= \text{Tangent of 1 minute of arc*}$$

---

*Some wavelengths of light are powerful enough to knock electrons of certain molecules out of their orbits, thereby producing an electric current. Einstein was awarded the Nobel Prize for explaining the "photoelectric effect."

†In 1942, Selig Hecht and his co-workers in New York first proved that only one quanta of visible light could trigger rhodopsin to start a cascade of biochemical events eventuating in the sensing of light.

‡Photoactivation of one molecule of rhodopsin starts an impressive example of biologic amplification, in which hundreds of molecules of the protein transducer each activate a like number of phosphodiesterase molecules, which in turn, hydrolyze a similar number of cyclic guanine monophosphate (cGMP) molecules, which then trigger a neural signal to the brain.[100]

---

*One minute of arc is the spacing between the bars of a 20/20 symbol. Interestingly, the sizing of the symbol was originally determined empirically.

Given this angle of 1 minute, the actual size of the Airy disc can be calculated if the distance from the nodal point to the retina is known. The optimal distance depends on the diameter of the photoreceptors. Because these act as light guides, the theoretical limit is 1 to 2 μm. To obtain the maximum visual information available, Kirschfield calculated that more than five receptors are required to scan the Airy disc.[62] Assume that each foveal cone is 1.5 μm in diameter and that there is an optimal space of 0.5 μm between receptors. The following equation describes the situation for three cones and two spaces (5.5 μm).

EQUATION 6-3

$$\text{Tan 1 minute} = \frac{5.5 \ \mu m}{\text{Nodal point to retina distance}}$$

Substituting 0.0003 from equation 2 into equation 3 gives equation 4:

EQUATION 6-4

$$0.0003 = \frac{5.5 \ \mu m}{\text{Nodal point to retina distance}}$$

From equation 4 the distance from the nodal point to the retina can be rounded off to 18.00 mm, which is close to the distance between the secondary nodal point and the retina in the schematic human eye.

How closely does optical theory agree with reality? The average visual acuity for healthy eyes in the age group younger than 50 was better than 20/16. In the distribution within the group younger than 40, the top 5% had an acuity of close to 20/10.[23]

Another related factor must be kept in mind. The fixating eye is in constant motion, as opposed to a camera on a tripod. Presumably, these movements prevent bleaching or fading within individual photoreceptors. These small movements, called either *tremors, drifts,* or *microsaccades,* range in amplitude from seconds to minutes of angular arc. Such movements tend to smear rather than enhance our traditional concept visual resolution. It can only be presumed that to maintain high resolution within the context of this physiologic nystagmus, the visual system takes quick, short samples of the retinal image during these potentially smearing movements and then recreates an image of higher resolution.[80,83,84]

The unique essence of the vertebrate retina is that the structure of the transparent optical components, the rhodopsin molecule, and the size of the foveal cones are all tuned to interact optimally with wavelengths of visible light.[22,113] It is earth's unique atmosphere and its unique relationship to the sun that have allowed primarily visible light, a tiny band from the enormous electromagnetic spectrum of the sun, to rain down upon us at safe energy levels. Our eyes are a product of an evolutionary process that has tuned to these unique wavelengths at these levels of intensity.[109,121]

With this basic science background, we can discuss how functions such as visual acuity and contrast sensitivity are monitored in a clinical setting.

Visual Acuity Testing. The idea that the minimum separation between two point sources of light was a measure of vision dates back to Hooke in 1679, when he noted "tis hardly possible for any animal eye well to distinguish an angle much smaller than that of a minute: and where two objects are not farther distant than a minute, if they are bright objects, they coalesce and appear as one."[56] In the early nineteenth century, Purkinje and Young used letters of various sizes for judging the extent of the power of distinguishing objects. Finally, in 1863, Professor Hermann Snellen of Utrecht developed his classic test letters. He quantitated the lines by comparison of the visual acuity of a patient with that of his assistant, who had good vision. Thus 20/200 (6/60) vision meant that the patient could see at 20 feet (6 m) what Snellen's assistant could see at 200 feet (60 m).[56]

The essence of correct identification of the letters on the Snellen chart is to see the clear spaces between the black elements of the letter. The spacing between the bars of the "E" should be 1 minute for the 20/20 (6/6) letter. The entire letter is 5 minutes high. To calculate the height of "x" (i.e., a 20/20 or 6/6 letter), use the following equation:

EQUATION 6-5

$$\text{Tan 5 minutes} = \frac{\text{x feet}}{20}$$

$$0.0015 = \frac{x}{20 \text{ feet}}$$

$$x = 0.36 \text{ inches (9.14 mm)}$$

The 20/200 (6/6) letter is 10 times larger, or 3.6 inches (9.14 cm).

Chart Luminance. In clinical visual acuity testing, the chart luminance should (1) represent typical real work photopic conditions and (2) be set at a level where variation produced by dust accumulation in the projector system, bulb decline, or normal variation in electrical current levels minimally affect visual performance. Thus chart luminance between 80 and 320 cd/m² meet such criteria (160 cd/m² is a favorite level of illumination).

Visual Acuity As Log MAR. If one looks at a standard Snellen acuity chart, the lines of symbols progress as follows: 20/400, 20/200, 20/150, 20/120, 20/100, 20/80, 20/70, 20/60. 20/50, 20/40, 20/30, 20/25, 20/20, 20/15, and 20/10. Thus the line-to-line decrease in symbol size varies from 25% (20/20 to 20/150) to 20% (20/120 to 20/100) to 16.7% (20/30 to 20/25).

Would it not be more logical to create a chart of uniform decrements, that is, a chart in which the line-to-line diminution in resolution angle were 0.1 steps? To create such a chart, one must first describe the spaces within a symbol (i.e., spaces between the bars of "E") in terms of "minutes of arc" (MAR) at 20 feet (6 m). Thus the 20/20 line represents a resolution of 1 MAR. If we take the log to the base of 10 of 1 (minute), we get 0. A spacing of 1.25 MAR (the equivalent of 20/30) yields a log value of 0.2, whereas a spacing of 1.99 MAR (the equivalent of 20/40) yields a log MAR of 0.3.

The Bailey-Lovie acuity chart (Figure 6-7) uses the log MAR sizing system.

Visual Acuity Chart Contrast. Clean printed charts using black characters on a white background usually have a character-to-background luminance contrast ratio between 1/20 and 1/33. For projected charts, the contrast ratio drops to a range of 1/5 to 1/10. Such a decrease in contrast is probably the result of the light scattering produced within the projector and the ambient light falling on the screen. Therefore the test should be performed in a dark room to ensure the highest contrast levels.

Contrast Sensitivity Testing. Visual acuity testing is relatively inexpensive, takes little time to perform, and describes visual function with one notation, that is, 20/40 (6/12). Best of all, for more than 150 years it has provided an end point for the correction of a patient's refractive error. However, contrast sensitivity testing, a time-consuming test born in the laboratory of the visual physiologist and described by a graph rather than a simple notation, has recently become a popular clinical test. It describes a number of subtle levels of vision, not accounted for by the visual acuity test; thus it more accurately quantifies the loss of vision in cataracts, corneal edema, neuroophthalmic diseases, and certain retinal diseases. These assets have been known for a long time, but the recent enhanced popularity has arisen because of cataract patients. As life span increases, more patients who have

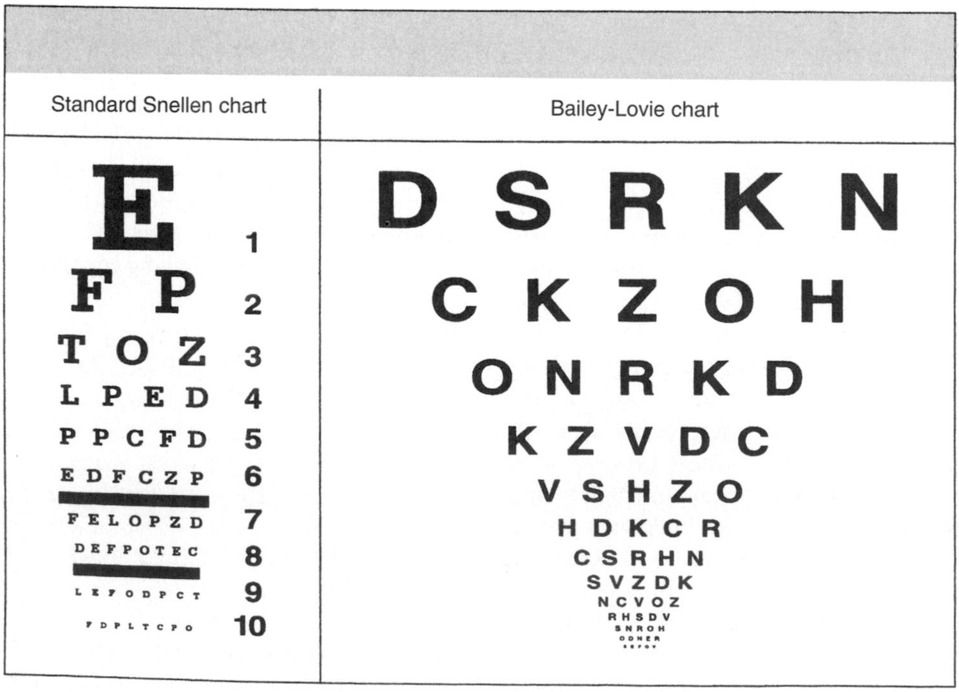

FIGURE 6-7   The standard Snellen chart and the Bailey-Lovie chart are examples of visual acuity charts.

cataracts request medical help. Often, their complaints of objects that appear faded or objects that are more difficult to see in bright light are not described accurately by their Snellen acuity scores. Contrast sensitivity tests and glare sensitivity tests can quantitate these complaints.

Contrast sensitivity testing is related to visual acuity testing. Contrast sensitivity tests the equivalent of four to eight differently sized Snellen letters in six or more shades of gray.

Definition and Units

Contrast. Whereas a black letter on a white background is a scene of high contrast, a child crossing the road at dusk and a car looming up in a fog are scenes of low contrast. Thus contrast may be considered as the difference in the luminance of a target against the background.

EQUATION 6-6

$$\text{Contrast} = \frac{\text{Target luminance} - \text{Background luminance}}{\text{Target luminance} + \text{Background luminance}}$$

To compute contrast, one uses a photometer to measure the luminance of a target against the background. For example, a background of 100 units of light and a target of 50 units of light yields the following:

EQUATION 6-7

$$\text{Contrast} = \frac{50 - 100}{50 + 100} = \frac{-50}{150} = 33\%$$

Contrast Sensitivity. Suppose the contrast of a scene is 33%, or one third, which also represents the patient's threshold (i.e., the patient cannot identify targets of lower contrast). The patient's contrast sensitivity is the reciprocal of the fraction (i.e., 3). A young, healthy subject may have a contrast threshold of 1%, or 1/100 (i.e., a contrast sensitivity of 100). Occasionally, subjects have even better contrast thresholds. A subject could have a threshold of 0.003 (0.03%, or 1/1000), which converts into a contrast sensitivity of 3000. In the visual psychology literature, the contrast threshold is described in logarithmic terms. Therefore a contrast sensitivity of 10 is 1, a contrast sensitivity of 100 is 2, and a contrast sensitivity of 1000 is 3.

However, the video engineer describes contrast by using a gray scale that may contain more than 100 different levels of gray. A newspaper printer may use the term *halftones* in place of gray scale and may need more than 100 different halftones

(densities of black dots) to describe the contrast of a scene.

Targets

Both the visual scientist and the optical engineer use a series of alternating black and white bars as targets. The optical engineer describes the fineness of a target by the number of line pairs per millimeter (a line pair is a dark bar and the white space next to it); the higher the number of line pairs per millimeter, the finer the target. For example, about 100 line pairs per millimeter is equivalent to a space of 1 minute between two black lines, which is almost equivalent to the spacing of the 20/20 (6/6) letter (in experimental testing, 109 line pairs per millimeter is equivalent to 20/15 [6/4.5]).

The vision scientist describes the alternating bar pattern in terms of spatial frequency; the units are cycles per degree (cpd). A cycle is a black bar and a white space. To convert Snellen units into cycles per degree, one must divide the Snellen denominator into 600, or 180 if meters are used, for example, 20/20 (6/6) converts to 30 cpd (600/20, or 180/6), and 20/200 (6/60) converts into 3 cpd (600/200, or 180/60).

Sine Waves

So far, targets have been described as dark bars of different spatial frequency against a white background. These are also known as *square waves* or *Foucalt gratings*. However, in optics, few images can be described as perfect square waves with perfectly sharp edges. Diffraction tends to make most edges slightly fuzzy, as do spherical aberration and oblique astigmatism. If the light intensity is plotted across a black bar with fuzzy edges against a light background, a sine wave pattern results. Sine wave patterns have great appeal because they can be considered the essential element from which any pattern can be constructed. The mathematician can break down any alternating pattern (be it an electrocardiogram or a trumpet's sound wave) into a unique sum of sine waves, known as a *Fourier transformation*. Joseph Fourier, a French mathematician, initially developed this waveform language to describe heat waves. Fourier's theorem states that a wave may be written as a sum of sine waves that have various spatial frequencies, amplitudes, and phases.

It also is thought that the visual system of the brain may operate by breaking down observed patterns and scenes into sine waves of different frequencies. The brain then adds them again to produce the mental impression of a complete picture.

Fourier transformations may be the method the visual system uses to encode and record retinal images. In fact, it has been shown that different cells or "channels" occur in the retina, lateral geniculate body, and cortex and selectively carry different spatial frequencies. So far, six to eight channels have been identified. It also has been shown that all channels respond to contrast. Interestingly, the cortex shows a linear relationship between the amplitude of the neuronal discharge and the logarithm of the grating contrast.[58] As a result of the preceding reasoning, most contrast sensitivity tests are based on sine wave patterns rather than square wave patterns of different frequency.

Recording Contrast Sensitivity

Figure 6-8 shows a number of functions, including the contrast sensitivity testing function for a normal subject. The shape of the human contrast function is different from that of almost all good optical systems, which have a high contrast sensitivity for low spatial frequency. The contrast sensitivity gradually diminishes at the higher spatial frequencies, as diffraction and other aberrations make discrimination of finer details more difficult. The contrast sensitivity function for the purely optical portion of the visual system (cornea and lens) is the modulation transfer function. The human contrast sensitivity function is different from the sum of its components because the retina-brain processing system is programmed to enhance the spatial frequencies in the range of 2 to 6 Hz. Receptor fields, on/off systems, and lateral inhibition are the well-known physiologic mechanisms that influence the different spatial frequency channels and are responsible for such enhancement.

In Figure 6-8, the wave labeled "retinal testing function" represents the retinal neural system performance.[15,17,59]

Normal variations are found in the contrast sensitivity function. For example, contrast sensitivity decreases with age. Two factors appear to be responsible: First, the normal crystalline lens scatters more light with increasing age, which thus blurs the edges of targets and degrades the contrast. Second, the retina-brain processing system itself loses some ability to enhance contrast with increasing age.

The contrast sensitivity also decreases as the illumination decreases. Thus contrast sensitivity for a spatial frequency of 3 cpd drops from 300 to 150 to 10 as the retinal luminance drops from 9 to 0.09

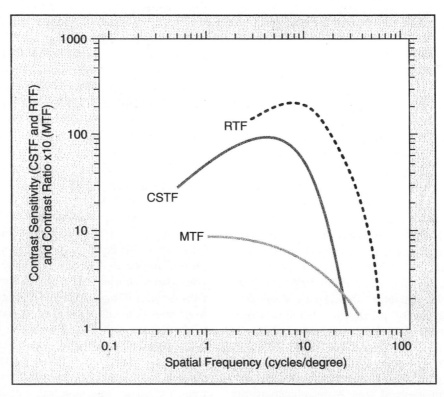

FIGURE 6-8   The normal human contrast sensitivity function (*CSTF*) is the sum of the contrast sensitivity of the purely optical contribution (*MTF*), and the neuroretinal enhancement system (*RTF*). (Modified from Mainster M: *Surv Ophthalmol* 23:135, 1978.)

to 0.0009 trolands. (The *troland* is a psychophysical unit; 1 troland is the retinal luminance produced by the image of an object, the luminance of which is 1 lux, for an area of the entrance pupil of 1 mm².)

The contrast sensitivity function also is an accurate method by which to follow certain disease states. For example, the contrast sensitivity of a patient who has a cataract is diminished, as it is in another light-scattering lesion, corneal edema. Because the contrast sensitivity function depends on central nervous system processing, it is not surprising that conditions such as optic neuritis and pituitary tumors also characteristically have diminished contrast sensitivity functions.

GLARE, TISSUE LIGHT SCATTERING, AND CONTRAST SENSITIVITY

When a transparent structure loses its clarity, the physicist describes it as a light *scatterer* rather than a light *transmitter*. This concept is foreign to the clinician whose textbooks talk about opaque lenses and corneas. The word *opaqueness* conjures up the image of a cement wall that stops light. Of all the experiments demonstrating that most cataracts scatter light rather than stop light, the most graphic involves the science of holography. If it is true that a cataract splashes or scatters oncoming light, resulting in a poor image focused on the retina, it should theoretically be possible to collect all the scattered light with a special optical element and recreate a sharp image. The essence of such an optical element, one that would take the scattered light of the cataract and rescatter it so that a proper image could be formed, would be a special inverse hologram of the cataract itself. Figure 6-9 shows how such a filter would work. Miller et al.[67] were able to demonstrate how an extracted cataract (the patient's visual acuity was worse than 20/200) would be made relatively transparent by registering a special inverse hologram of that specific cataract in front of the cataract.

To follow the progress of conditions such as cataracts or corneal edema, one should use a measure of tissue transparency or tissue backscattering. Although photoelectric devices can be used to quantitate the amount of light scattered by various ocular tissues, a subjective discrimination system is needed to evaluate patient complaints. The Snellen visual acuity test was the traditional index, but it is not sensitive enough. In Figure 6-10, LeClaire et al.[51] illustrate that many patients with cataracts showed good visual acuity but had poor contrast sensitivity in the face of a

glare source. In fact, this should not come as a surprise because the essence of vision is the discrimination of the light intensity of one object as opposed to another, often with a natural glare source present. Thus a plane is seen against the sky because the retinal image of the plane does not stimulate the photoreceptors to the same degree that the sky does. Terms such as *contrast luminance* and *intensity discrimination* are used to describe differences in brightness between an object and its background.

How then can ocular light scattering, glare, and contrast sensitivity be linked together to give the clinician a useful index? An industrialist scientist named Holliday set the stage to solve this puzzle.[39] In 1926, Holliday developed the concept of glare and glare testing to measure the degrading effect of stray light. In the 1960s, Wolfe, a visual physiologist working in Boston, realized that glare testing could

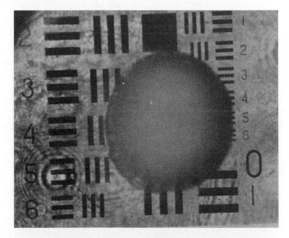

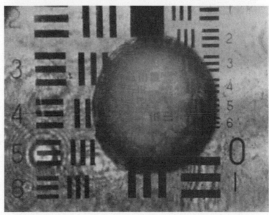

FIGURE 6-9   Note how the addition of the inverse conjugate hologram in registration with the cataract allows you to see the resolution chart. (From Miller D, Benedek G: *Intraocular light scattering,* Springfield, Ill, 1973, Charles C Thomas.)

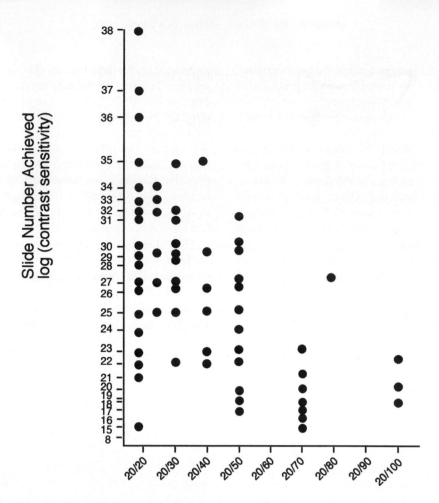

FIGURE 6-10   A study of visual acuity versus glare sensitivity (arbitrary units) in 144 cataract patients showed that many with 20/40 or better visual acuity had low glare scores. (From LeClaire J et al: *Arch Ophthalmol* 100:153; 1982.)

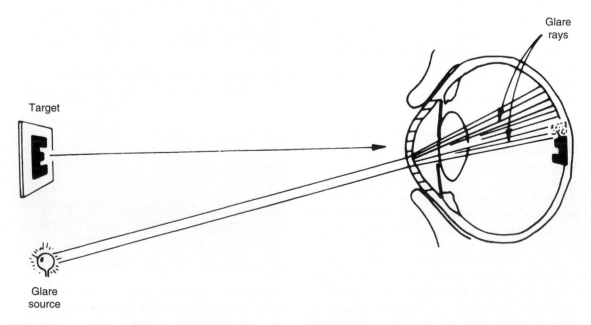

FIGURE 6-11   Corneal edema scatters the light from the peripheral light source onto the fovea, decreasing the contrast of the foveal image. (From Miller D, Benedek GB: *Intraocular light scattering,* Springfield, Ill, 1973, Charles C Thomas.)

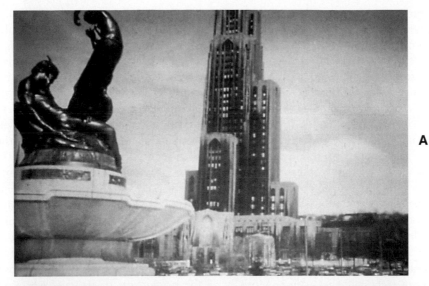

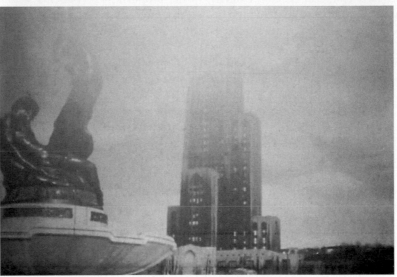

FIGURE 6-12 Photograph of the way the scene would appear to a normal patient (**A**) and a patient with corneal edema (**B**) in the face of glare. (From Miller D, Benedek GB: *Intraocular light scattering*, Springfield, Ill, 1973, Charles C Thomas.)

be a useful way to describe the increase in light scattering seen in different clinical conditions.[116,117] How does increased light scattering produce a decrease in the contrast of the retinal image in the presence of a glare source? Figure 6-11 shows how corneal edema splashes light from a naked light bulb onto the foveal image, reducing the contrast of the image of the target. Figure 6-12 illustrates the way a patient with a cataract or corneal edema would see a scene in the presence of a glare source. In the mid-1970s, Nadler observed that many of his cataract patients complained of annoying glare. His observations rekindled interest in glare testing and

led to the first clinical glare tester—the Miller-Nadler glare tester.[65]

CLINICAL CONDITIONS AFFECTING GLARE AND CONTRAST SENSITIVITY
Optical Conditions
This section describes how contact lenses, cataracts, opacified posterior capsules, displaced intraocular lenses (IOLs), and multifocal IOLs affect glare sensitivity and contrast. With the exception of IOLs, these conditions primarily diminish contrast sensitivity because of increased light scattering.

Corneal Conditions

Corneal Edema. Studies tracing the progression of corneal decompensation have shown that the stroma increases in thickness before the epithelium changes.[64] The stroma may increase in thickness by up to 30% before the epithelium becomes edematous. Studies have shown that an increase in stromal thickness above 30% need not influence Snellen visual acuity results if there is no epithelial edema.[51] Unlike Snellen visual acuity, both contrast sensitivity and glare sensitivity are compromised as soon as the stroma thickens. Mild edema affects only the middle and high frequencies of a contrast sensitivity test, sparing the low frequencies. With further edema, the sparing of the low frequencies disappears and contrast sensitivity is decreased throughout the spatial frequency spectrum.[65] Glare sensitivity measurements also detect early epithelial edema. A mildly edematous epithelium is roughly equivalent to an increase of 10% in stromal thickness, whereas moderate to significant epithelial edema has a profound effect on glare and contrast sensitivity.

Contact Lens Wear. The wearing of contact lenses may reduce contrast sensitivity in a number of subtle ways. Patients with significant corneal astigmatism who wear thin soft contact lenses experience blur that affects their contrast sensitivity. Aging of the plastic material itself or surface-deposit accumulations can affect soft lens hydration and ultimately influence acuity, glare, and contrast sensitivity. Most important, contact lens–induced epithelial edema produces increased glare disability and reduced contrast sensitivity.[65]

Keratoconus. Patients with keratoconus demonstrate attenuation of contrast sensitivity with relative sparing of low spatial frequencies despite normal Snellen visual acuity. However, once scarring develops in the keratoconic cornea, all frequencies become attenuated. In addition, glare sensitivity acutely increases as soon as scarring develops. Thus contrast sensitivity testing at a number of spatial frequencies, with or without a glare source, may be an excellent way of following the progression of keratoconus.[65]

Nephrotic Cystinosis. In a study of patients with infantile-onset cystinosis, contrast sensitivities were reduced at all frequencies, although the loss at high frequencies was the greatest. Of 12 subjects, 10 showed glare disability, compared with a control population.[45]

Penetrating Keratoplasty. Contrast sensitivity or glare testing may also be useful in detecting the earliest signs of graft rejection. In such cases, the earliest corneal damage is corneal edema. Although visual acuity may remain normal, contrast and glare performance start to slip. As the edema progresses to involve the epithelium, the degradation of these visual functions is accentuated. Similarly, reversal of graft rejection may be followed by an improvement in the contrast sensitivity function.[65]

Refractive Surgery. Some patients who have undergone radial keratotomy or photorefractive keratoplasty with postoperative corneal haze have been reported to experience increased glare sensitivity.[85,111] The extent of the problem and the number of patients complaining of heightened glare sensitivity varies from study to study and depends on the time elapsed since the surgery and the method by which the glare was assessed. Nevertheless, it can be concluded that glare is a postoperative complication of radial keratotomy and that the proportion of patients who complain about glare and the severity of the problem decrease as the time after surgery increases.

Harper and Halliday[34] reported on four unilaterally aphakic patients and found significant contrast sensitivity losses in the eyes with epikeratoplasty when compared with the normal fellow eye.

Cataracts and Opacified Posterior Capsules. Figure 6-11 demonstrates the way that an edematous cornea or cataract scatters stray light onto the fovea and degrades contrast sensitivity, thereby heightening glare disability. Thus measurements of contrast sensitivity are usually better correlated with patient complaints than with a visual acuity measurement. The addition of a glare source to a contrast sensitivity test causes a dramatic decrease in the contrast function. Of the various cataract types, the posterior subcapsular cataract degrades the glare and contrast function the most. It should be noted that the presence of a glare light diminishes both visual acuity and contrast sensitivity in cataract patients. In the presence of a glare light, the contrast sensitivity function gradually diminishes as a simulated cataract increases in severity, whereas the visual acuity function holds steady until an 80% simulated cataract produces a dramatic drop in visual acuity.

Progressive opacification of the posterior capsule after an extracapsular cataract extraction produces a progressive increase in glare disability.[48] A neodymium:yttrium-aluminum-garnet (Nd:YAG) laser capsulotomy in such cases improves the visual function. The improvement of contrast and glare sensitivity after Nd:YAG laser treatment depends on the ratio of the area of the clear opening to the area of the remaining opaque capsule. Thus a photopic pupil of 4 mm would require a 4-mm capsulotomy for best results in daylight. However, if the pupil dilates to 6 mm at night, an oncoming headlight would induce an annoying glare unless the capsulotomy were enlarged to 6 mm in diameter. Thus the smallest capsulotomy is not necessarily the best from an optical point of view.

Modulation Transfer Function. Optical engineers generally evaluate optical systems by means of a system similar to contrast sensitivity, called the *modulation transfer function* (MTF). The MTF is the ratio of image-to-object contrast as a function of spatial frequency, where the object is either a bar graph or a sinusoidal grating. It gives more information than the parameter of resolving power. For example, two systems may have the same resolving power, but one might be unable to form useful images of low-contrast objects, which the other could readily form. A smaller pupillary aperture introduces diffraction interference, which makes it difficult to resolve fine detail (higher spatial frequencies). Thus the spatial frequency cutoff occurs sooner with the small aperture system. In an MTF plot, the vertical axis is akin to contrast sensitivity (see Figure 6-8). Because it represents the ratio of contrast of image against contrast of object, its values decrease from 1.0 to 0. The MTF is conceptually similar to the manner in which electronic engineers evaluate an amplifier. The performance of an amplifier is described by the output/input ratio, or the gain, for different sound frequencies. The MTF concept also may be useful in the comparison of the performance of the eye with that of optical and electronic instruments. Campbell and Green[15] plotted the MTF of the human eye for various pupillary diameters and found that a smaller pupil system has a better contrast ratio than a larger pupil system. This probably reflects the opposing factors of a somewhat better performance with greater illumination and the degrading effect of spherical aberration with a larger pupil. As noted earlier, a pupil size in the range 2.0 to 2.8 mm gives the maximum MTF for high spatial frequencies.

Depth of Focus. How can an insect or a small animal like a rat see objects clearly from 10 m to 10 cm without an accommodating mechanism? How does a pinhole allow a patient with presbyopia to read the newspaper without a reading correction? The answer is that both situations rely on an optical system with an increased depth of focus.

Recall that an image can be thought of as being made up of an array of points. Thus the finite size of the pixels, the photographic grains, or the photoreceptor clusters ultimately determine the fineness of details of the recorded image. This means that a blur of a focused point is tolerated if it is no bigger than the size of the receptor. Because a point of light is focused as an Airy disc, a cluster or two to five cones is considered the "limiting grain size." Let us review two important definitions:

Depth of focus: the amount of blur in diopters or millimeters from the retina that will be tolerated or go unnoticed

Depth of field: the distance range, in object space, that an object can move toward or away from a fixed focus optical system and still be considered in focus

Figure 6-13 is a schematic of the eye. For simplicity, we used a reduced eye, with a biconvex lens representing the cornea and lens.

Let $()$ = the object that can move from infinity to a near point N

ρ = pupillary diameter

f = focal length of the model eye

x = distance from the retina that near point remains in focus

c = limiting photoreceptor cluster size (i.e., limiting grain size or pixel size)

N = refractive index of the model eye

$D_1 = \dfrac{n}{f}$ (i.e., dioptric power of eye when viewing a finite object)

$D_2 = \dfrac{n}{f}$ (i.e., dioptric power of eye when near object at N)

(In this case, the eye can be considered to have lengthened [theoretically] by a distance x.)

Depth of focus is as follows:

EQUATION 6-8

$$D_1 - D_2 = \frac{n}{f} - \frac{n}{f+x} = \frac{n\,x(f+x) - nf}{f(f+x)} = \frac{nx}{f(f+x)}$$

(but by similar triangles)
Thus

EQUATION 6-9

$$D_1 - D_2 = \frac{nc}{f\rho}$$

This equation tells us that the depth of focus in diopters ($D_1 - D_2$) is proportional to the index of refraction (n) and the limiting photoreceptor of grain size *c*. The depth of focus is also inversely proportional to the pupil size (ρ) or the focal length of the system (f).

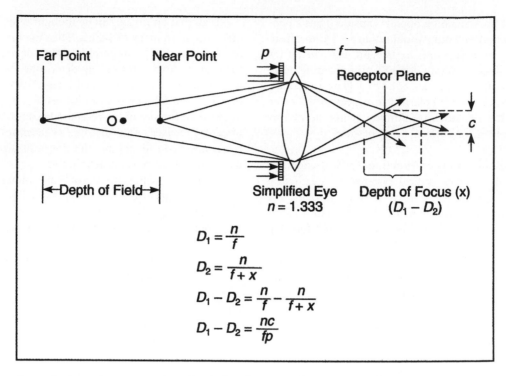

FIGURE 6-13   A schematic representation of a single refracting surface model eye where ρ = pupillary diameter, f = focal length distance from the retina where image of near object falls, c = limiting photoreceptor cluster size (i.e., similar to grain or pixel size), n = refractive index, D_1 = n/f dioptric power of eye when viewing infinite object, D_2 = n/(f + x) (i.e., dioptric power of an eye when viewing near object). Thus depth of focus = $D_1 - D_2$ = n/f − n/(f + x). Ultimately, we find $D_1 - D_2$ = nc/fρ.

For example, determine the depth of focus for a reduced human eye under the following conditions:

Let pupil (ρ) = 3 mm, or 0.003 m

Focal length (f) = 22.2 mm, or 0.0222 m

Limiting cone cluster (c) = 5 cones (Assume each cone is 1.5 μ in diameter and spacing between cones is 0.5 μ. The total cluster of 5 cones + 4 spaces = 9.5 μ, or 0.0000095 m.)

Index of refraction (n) = 1.333

$$\text{Depth of focus } (D_1 - D_2) = \frac{1.33 \times 0.0000095}{0.0222 \times 0.003} = 0.189$$

Our calculation of 0.189 for the reduced (hypothetical) eye with a pupil of 3 mm is about half of the 0.40 diopter (Figure 6-14, *A*), which is the average value from four (real) human studies.[13,18,74,107] Thus we may conclude that the normal eye has a modest depth of focus.

Interestingly, Figure 6-14, *B*, represents a study in which artificial pupils (placed in front of the cornea) between 1 and 2 mm were used. Within this range of apertures, a depth of focus between 2 and 4 diopters was obtained.[62]

Do we ever see the equivalent of pupillary apertures of between 1 and 2 mm in human patients? Yes, we do in cases of trauma, disease, or use of strong miotics. Figure 6-15 demonstrates four examples of 1- to 2-mm clear areas within a corneal opacity. Actually, the patient shown in the upper left had an acuity of 20/20. Figure 6-16 shows four examples of 1- to 2-mm clear areas within traumatic cataracts or 1- to 2-mm spaces between traumatic cataracts and iris tears. In Figure 6-17, we can see the equivalent of a reduced pupillary aperture produced by a ptosis or a conscious reduction of the palpebral fissure as a result of squinting. It is comforting to know that in cases of trauma, disease, or significant refractive error, the human eye can call on a 2- to 3-diopter depth of focus mechanism.

Optical Aberrations

The famous nineteenth century German physiologist Herman von Helmholtz, in Volume 1 of his "Treatise on Physiologic Optics,"[36] wrote that the optical aberrations of the human eye are "of a kind

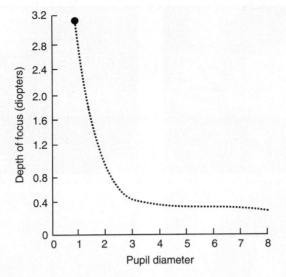

A

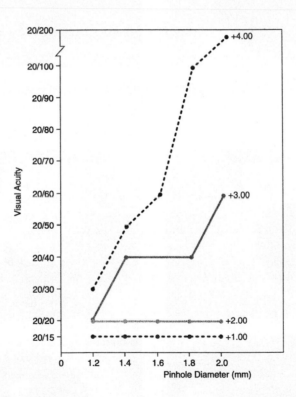

B

FIGURE 6-14 **A,** An averaged depth of focus versus pupil size function representing four different studies.[13,18,71,99] **B,** Plot of visual acuity versus pinhole diameters (between 1 and 2 mm) using different blurring lenses (i.e., +1 diopter, +2 diopters, +3 diopters, and +4 diopters). Thus, for example, the subject could achieve a visual acuity of 20/40 through a 1.8-mm pinhole, but vision would be blurred by a 3-diopter lens. (Modified from Miller D: *Optics and refraction: a user friendly guide,* St Louis, 1991, Gower Medical.)

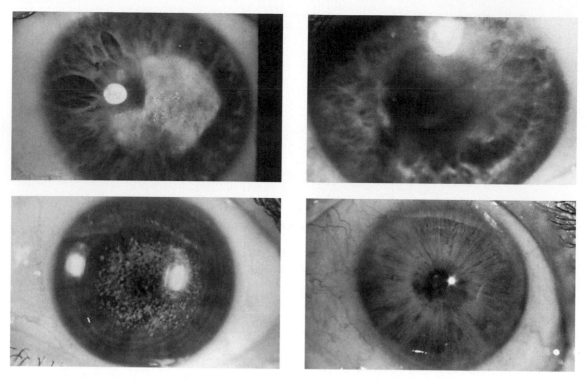

FIGURE 6-15   Four examples of small clear areas within corneal opacities that operated as pinholes.

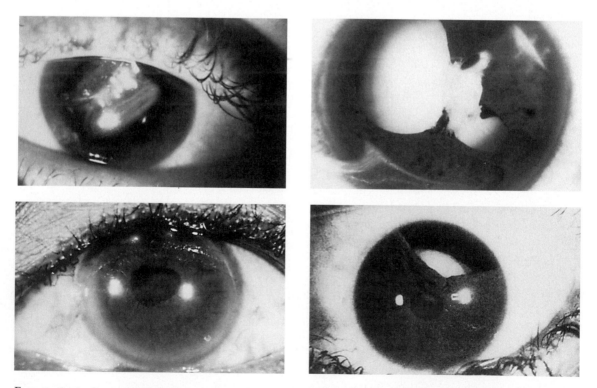

FIGURE 6-16   Four examples of 1- to 2-mm clear area within traumatic cataracts or 1- to 2-mm spaces between traumatic cataracts and iris tears.

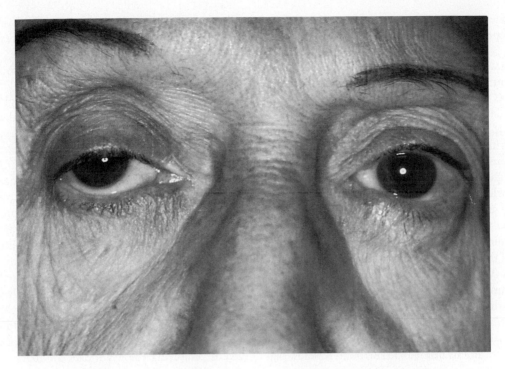

FIGURE 6-17   The equivalent of a reduced aperture produced by a ptosis.

that is not permissible in well constructed instruments." The implication is that the optical design of the human eye would receive low marks if evaluated by someone from the optical industry. If we are to simply compare the optical quality of the living human eye with that of our best cameras and telescopes under ordinary static daylight conditions, then Helmholtz was correct. The optical imperfections noted by Helmholtz are discussed in the following sections.

Light Scattering. Fingerprints on spectacle lenses scatter light, making small letters difficult to read. Raindrops or windshield wiper smears on the car windshield make the reading of street signs difficult. In a similar way, small bubbles from the warm water tap give a haze to a glass of water and make it difficult to see the details at the bottom of the glass. These are all examples of light scattering, which can obscure the details of any object.

As noted earlier, the cornea is clear, but technically speaking, it is not perfectly transparent. Its composition of fine collagen fibers, loaded into a watery matrix of glycosaminoglycans and populated by fine cells that swim in the matrix, scatter a small percentage (10% of incident light) and create a slight haze. This is unquestionably a flaw, as opposed to the glass optical systems of cameras and telescopes. However, the "imperfect" corneal structure allows for healing. Thus we can appreciate that a 10% level of light scatter is a fair price to pay for a self-healing system.

The lens of the eye is made up of tens of thousands of fine fibers (each a bag of clear protein solution) packed closely together. The living lens continually adds outside fibers and packs old cells in its nucleus throughout life, ultimately increasing its volume by a factor of 3 in the older eye. The refractive index of the fibers differs from that of the thin spaces between the fibers. Thus the young lens scatters about 20% of the incident light. Is there a practical advantage to the fiber structure of the lens? There are many ways that the lens may be injured, including inflammation from diseases inside the eye, blunt blows from fists or rocks, periods of malnutrition, poisoning, and osmotic upset from systemic disease. In all of these situations, the part of the lens being laid down at the time of the injury or disease loses transparency. This hazy section may also be lumpy in thickness. However, in a short time, new transparent layers cover and compress the hazy ones, smoothing and reducing the blurring effect of the injury. Again, we now understand that a small level of light scattering resulting from this fiber layering system is a fair price to pay for a self-repairing lens system.

Natural Defenses against Light Scattering. The reader may have been led astray in thinking that the eye has no defense against normal light scattering. In fact, it does. For example, the birefringent capacity of the collagen fibers in the cornea, in combination with the birefringence of the fovea, may cancel out some annoying glare caused by light scattering through a process known as *destructive interference,* somewhat akin to the way polarizing sunglasses cancel annoying glare.

The retina has three defenses against the image-degrading effects of scattered light. To appreciate one of the defenses, one first must know that not all colors (wavelengths) are scattered equally. The fine components of eye tissue scatter blue light 16 times more than red light. Therefore a defense that can reduce blue scattered light would be disproportionately helpful. Sprinkled throughout the ultrasensitive fovea and its immediate surround is yellow pigment. The yellow pigment is efficient at absorbing the scattered blue light, thus preventing much of it from degrading the retinal image.[62]

The second defense used by the retina involves the positioning of the rods and cones. Each rod or cone functions as a light guide. To enter the guide, light must enter at a specific angle. Interestingly, normally focused light enters a photoreceptor at a different angle than does scattered light.[24] The photoreceptors of the retina are so directed that they primarily receive focused light, but not scattered light (Figure 6-18).

The dark brown pigment of the retinal pigment epithelium and the choroid absorbs any stray light

that has passed through the retina and prevents such light from backscatter, which would reverberate among the neighboring photoreceptors. None of these defenses is perfect, but all work to reduce the annoyance of scattered light.

The brow and eyelid may also be thought of as blocking annoying glare sources such as the overhead sun. Interestingly, the Oriental lid has a double fold and serves as a more effective thicker visor than the Caucasian lid, thereby more effectively blocking the glaring effect of the sun overhead.

Chromatic Aberrations. The rainbow is produced by millions of tiny round droplets of water vapor that hover over the earth during or after a rain. Each water droplet functions as a tiny, powerful round lens. Such a powerful lens bends each wavelength of color differently. A rainbow is caused by the chromatic aberration of the water droplets. Thus, like Newton's prism, the tiny droplets break up white light into the colors of the rainbow. The phenomenon of strong lenses producing colored fringes around a focused image is known as *chromatic aberration.*[103,110] The optical components of the eye (cornea and lens), like the fine water droplets, also produce chromatic aberration. The total chromatic aberration of the photopic human eye is about 3 diopters. However, we do not see colored fringes around objects because significant colored fringes of red and blue are less likely to be seen as a result of the cones' relative insensitivity to the colors at the ends of the spectrum. Also, the visual processing in the retina and brain can sharpen the edges of the retinal image and "erase" the colored blur. Although we rarely consciously sense the chromatic aberration of the eye, some researchers believe that the retina may make use of the faint colored fringes around images to help accommodation reach a precise end point.[1,105]

Spherical Aberration. A major distortion produced by many high-powered optical systems such

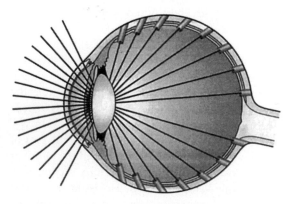

FIGURE 6-18   The orientation of the retinal photoreceptors in the normal human eye. Note that they are directed to the second nodal point of the eye.

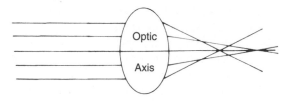

FIGURE 6-19   An illustration of the smearing of sharp focus created by spherical aberration. Note that the peripheral rays are bent more than the paraxial rays of light.

as the cornea or lens is called *spherical aberration.* Figure 6-19 shows the results of this aberration. The rays at the edge of the lens are bent more than those going through the center of the lens, creating a smeared focus. The cornea (a strong optical element) is subject to spherical aberration. Figure 6-20 shows that the cornea sits at the front of the eye like a small, strongly curved dome. The steeper the dome (shorter its radius of curvature), the more spherical aberration created. We have known since the time of the French mathematician Descartes that spherical aberration can be controlled by flattening the curvature of the edge of a lens, thereby weakening the focusing power of the lens periphery. Descartes described such a surface as *aspheric.* Most cameras today use lenses with aspheric surfaces. The average cornea is somewhat aspheric as well. It gets a bit flatter at its periphery, allowing it to more smoothly merge with the sclera. However, there are some real-world considerations that make it advantageous to keep the cornea steeply curved. This is only supposition, of course, but in the event of a direct blow to the eye by a blunt object, the steep protruding cornea can absorb the blow, much like a spring. The steeper the cornea, the more it vaults over the rest of the eye and the greater the spring effect. Such a spring-dampening effect protects the deeper eye structures. How then does the eye satisfy both needs? In daylight, with the pupil being constricted, the iris tissue essentially blocks many of the light rays coming through the corneal periphery and effectively cancels most of the spherical aberration. Thus spherical aberration from the cornea has an important degrading effect only when illumination is dim and the pupil is large. Happily, in dim light, the human eye switches to the rod retinal system in which seeing fine details takes a lower priority than simply seeing large shapes.

The crystalline lens is also a powerful optical element and therefore is also vulnerable to spherical aberration. Although an aspheric surface corrects the aberration in cameras and telescopes, nature has chosen a different approach for the crystalline lens. Recall that refraction, or the bending of light, can be controlled by either the curvature of the lens surface or the index of refraction of the composition of the lens. The high index of refraction of the crystalline lens is the result of a high concentration of protein. The lens has a lower refractive index near its edge than at its center. Therefore the lens periphery has a weaker focusing action and self-corrects spherical aberration, much as an aspheric surface.[26]

However, even with the aforementioned correction factors, the total spherical aberration of the human eye varies from 0.25 to 2.00 diopters. The corneal shape is the most important factor in the induction of spherical aberration.[9]

Abolition of spherical aberration not only sharpens focus but can be thought of as concentrating the light at the focus. Concentrating light energy at a focus makes it easier to see a dimly lit

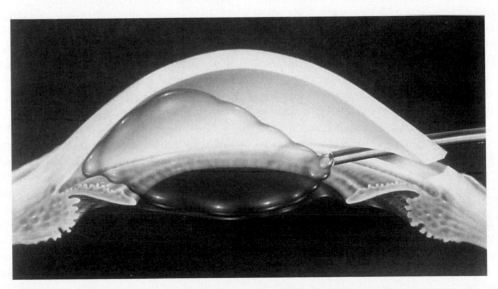

FIGURE 6-20   Three-dimensional drawing of the cornea sitting atop the eye as a small dome, vaulting over the internal structures. The viscoelastic material injected into the anterior chamber should remind the reader that the vitreous humor (similar properties) serves as a second damping element in the event of blunt trauma.

object. Therefore cameras, or creatures with an optical system of minimal spherical aberration, function well in low illumination.

Light Absorption. The lens of a typical 20-year-old absorbs about 30% of incident blue light. At age 60, the typical lens absorbs about 60% of incident blue light.[86] This increase in lens absorption of blue light results in both a decrease in subtle color discrimination and a decrease in chromatic aberration.

Summary

A Compromise of Eye Function. The human eye (which is similar to the monkey eye) is a fairly good resolving optical instrument.[7,14,46] Admittedly, the eyes of certain birds are even better optical instruments, reaching the outer limits of the constraints of the laws of physics. One must appreciate that the evolution of better and better optics had to be balanced against other useful functions, such as glare prevention, injury prevention, injury repair, and use of the eyes for nonverbal communication.

THE AGING EYE

The components of human eyes usually last a lifetime. This was reinforced to me years ago when our eye team did a visual screening of residents in a housing project for older adults. On average, most residents were older than 80 years. The number of residents with 20/40 vision in at least one eye was more than 90%.[66] This finding should not minimize the disability of people with cataracts (which affect 9.4 million people older than age 65 in the United States).[78] However, it is important to recognize that a high percentage of people live their entire lives with good vision—thanks to a number of positive compensations that help the aging eye. For example, the human macula is particularly vulnerable to damage from ultraviolet and blue light. Fortunately, a yellow pigment effectively absorbs or scatters away most of these harmful wavelengths, thus diminishing the potential damage to the macula.[112]

One of the more remarkable aspects of the aging eye is that the eye lens continually acquires new layers of fibers, becoming both progressively thicker and steeper. These changes would normally lead to an increase in lens focusing power and a tendency toward nearsightedness in older eyes. In fact, this does not happen universally because the index of refraction of the cortex of the lens decreases in a perfectly compensatory fashion,[37] so the lens power often stays constant.

Evolution of Ocular Components

Human eyes are fascinating examples of a potpourri of components seen all along the evolutionary trail. Indeed, human eyes contain components previously developed for other uses. For example, our retinal rhodopsin may have come from an ancient bacterium, which may have used the rhodopsin for photosynthesis. Our rounded corneal curvature originally comes from primitive fish. As noted earlier, when a person is under water, the corneal refractive power is canceled by the surrounding water. However, rounded shape helps decrease water resistance because the eye is then more streamlined. Finally, and most difficult to explain, many of the special crystalline proteins that have been identified in animal eye lenses are similar to metabolic enzymes found elsewhere in the body. For example, lactic dehydrogenase-β is similar to E-crystalline found in the lens: arginosuccinate lyase is similar to γ-crystalline found in the lens.[114] Nonlenticular enzymes have been adapted to also function as special lens proteins, a process known as *gene sharing*. The term *gene sharing* simply names the phenomenon without giving us an idea of which function came first or what evolutionary pressures forced the new use of the molecules. In summary, one might think of this entire process of nature as reaching into its dusty attic to find new uses for old creations as the ultimate in recycling efficiency.

Nonoptical Brain Mechanisms That Enhance the Retinal Image

There is a group of visual phenomena in which the retinal image is enhanced or made complete by the brain.[30] They represent ways of improving the retinal image in nonoptical ways. One might think of these brain-processing effects as an example of method of going beyond the limits of the laws of optics to bring out visual information.[55]

Filling in Information. Figure 6-21 is an example of the "completing the picture" illusion. Because of our previous visual experience, we assume that the partially covered words represent "THE EYE." Wrong!

If there is a discontinuity in an object, we almost always assume that the object is partially covered. We simple create a full impression of the covered object in our mind. In Figure 6-22, we are made to think that one geographic form covers the other, although the artist simply fitted the outline of one triangle next to the other.

These illusions illustrate the ability of our visual processing system to fill in all sorts of blanks and

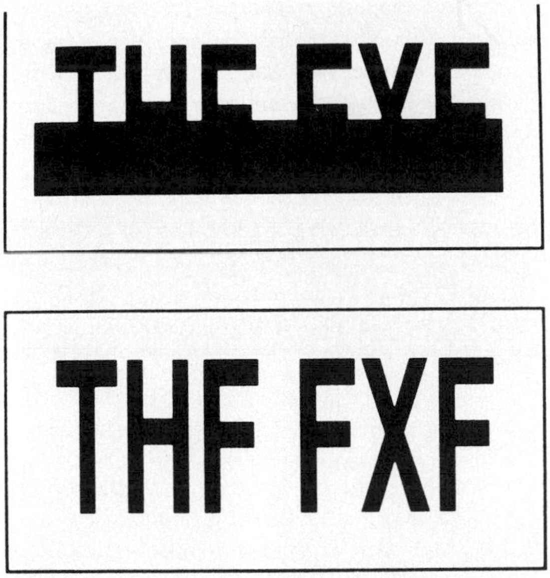

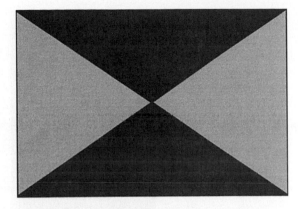

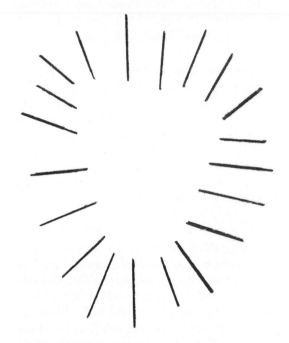

FIGURE 6-21 Because of our previous visual experience, we assume the line covered words will spell "THE EYE." On removal of the cover, we see we were wrong.

FIGURE 6-22 A group of triangles with some seeming to cover the others. In fact, the edges of the shapes simply abut each other.

incongruities within the retinal image to create a coherent story.

Suppose that the object of regard is not covered but that the observer has a brain lesion that has produced a small scotoma in the visual field. When such a patient is presented with a circle or square in which part of the figure resides inside the scotoma, after a brief period, the patient reports that the gap has filled in and the figure looks whole. The same phenomenon takes place if part of an image falls on the physiologic blind spot. It suggests that the visual system, faced with a gap in the information, hypothesizes (gambles) that the region surrounding the scotoma has the needed data and places that data within the scotoma to produce a complete scene.[79]

There is another series of illusions known as *gap figures.*[44] Figure 6-23 shows an example of a gap illusion. The defect (gap) is strongly highlighted by the radiating lines as a footprint might appear highlighted to a skilled guide.

A related phenomenon is presented in Conan Doyle's story *The Adventure of Silver Blaze,* in which Sherlock Holmes identifies the murderer when he concludes that the watchdog must have known the murderer because no barking was heard on the night of the murder. As in the gap figure, the gap in the expected pattern of the dog's behavior takes on a heightened importance. Hearst appropriately called this phenomenon "getting something for nothing."[35]

FIGURE 6-23 A gap figure (modified from an Ehrenstein illusion). Note that the radiating lines seem to create the outline of a foot.

Finally, mention should be made of a related temporal blocking of a visual scene, that is, our failure to notice the fleeting disappearance of an image during a blink, a twitch, a flicker, or a saccade.

Contrast Enhancement. Interestingly, the visual brain has the ability to sharpen the contrast of elements in the retinal image. Figure 6-24 presents

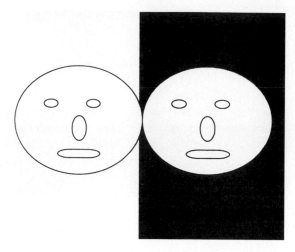

FIGURE 6-24 *Right,* Gray face is seen against a black background. *Left,* Same gray face is seen against a white background. A contrast enhancement function makes the gray face look lighter on the black and darker on the white side. (Illusion created by R. Miller, F. Miller, and D. Miller.)

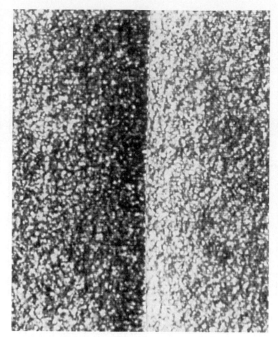

FIGURE 6-25 The Craik-Cornsweet-O'Brien illusion. The perceived difference in the darkness of the vertical panels disappears if you place a pencil or your finger along the border between panels. The effect persists even if the panel details are blurred.

two faces of the same grayness. In the right figure, the face is seen against a black background, whereas in the left figure, it is seen against a white background. The gray face on the black background looks lighter (enhancing its contrast), whereas the gray face looks darker on the white background. This effect is reduced when the edges of the faces are fuzzy. One might speculate that a sharper edge on an object brings out a stronger contrast enhancement response.

Edge Sharpening. If you wear glasses for myopia or hyperopia, take them off for a moment and look across the room at a framed picture. True, you cannot see any of the details within the picture. However, notice the edges of the frame. There is a distinct boundary against the wall. The visual system places a priority on sharpening the edge of the retinal image, even though the details within remain hazy. One might suppose that in the case of the picture on the wall, recognizing the edges of the frame tells you that the fuzzy blob on the wall is a picture rather than a swarm of insects.

There is a second way that the brain works on the edge of a retinal image. If two objects of similar brightness are placed next to each other, they should appear to merge into one object. However, if the connecting edge of one of these similar objects is a bit darker than the connecting edge of the other, the entire side with the darker edge appears

darker than the lighter one. The greater contrast at the edge has spread across the whole panel.

This phenomenon, known as the *Craik-Cornsweet-O'Brien illusion,* is seen in Figure 6-25. If you put your finger or a pencil between the two vertical rectangles (occluding the boundary), you will see that they are actually the same brightness.

Vernier Acuity. Earlier in this chapter, it was noted that a normal-sighted human being (with 20/20 visual acuity) can detect a separation between two objects as small as 1 minute of angular subtense. Interestingly, it was said that Ted Williams, the great outfielder of the Boston Red Sox, had a visual acuity of 20/10 (could detect a ½ minute of angular separation). However, there is a visual task (Vernier acuity), which has a threshold of about 5 seconds of arc ($\frac{1}{12}$ of a minute of arc). Indeed, most normal-sighted people can line up dots or notice a discrepancy in the alignment of dots or lines as small as 5 seconds of arc or less. Figure 6-26 demonstrates two typical alignment tasks presented to experimental subjects. We know that the brain is involved in the processing because the experiment can be re-

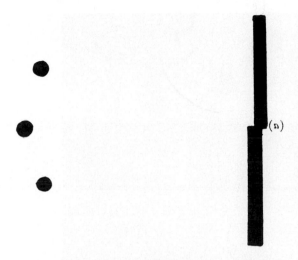

FIGURE 6-26 Two typical targets for measuring vernier acuity. The subject either notes misalignment of the vertical lines or of the three dots.

designed so that one eye is presented with the top and bottom dot (which are in alignment), while the other eye is allowed to see only the middle dot. Subjects show similar thresholds whether the experiment is done this way or done monocularly. Clearly, the brain must be where the ultimate processing occurs in these experiments. Because a threshold of less than 5 seconds is well beyond the optical diffraction limit of the eye, Vernier acuity represents a special example of sophisticated brain processing. The challenge is to try to conceptualize some important task necessary for the survival of our *Homo sapien* ancestors that required such precision. Incidentally, we also know that the macaque monkey demonstrates a high level of Vernier acuity. In fact, the adult monkey averages a threshold of about 13 seconds of arc.[101] Thus it is possible that monkeys and early humans used Vernier acuity to detect the presence of an animal or an enemy hiding behind a stalk or a tree by noting a misalignment between the edge of the tree or stalk and the protruding body of the enemy. If that possible scenario was true, normal Vernier acuity might save a life. Once again, brain enhancement of the retinal image brings out details well beyond the limits of the best optical resolution.

Removing Distractions. In Figure 6-27, a deer is hidden in the high grass. Almost completely closing the eyes creates a blurring of the overlying fine grass, making the animal more vividly seen. A similar effect

can be achieved through a heavy rain. Again, almost closing the eyes allows figures to be seen more easily through the rain. This is an example of erasing the distractions that have a high spatial frequency.

Refractive Errors

Thus far, when pertinent, this chapter has covered the physiologic optics of the average, emmetropic eye. However, the average refractive error in certain populations is not emmetropia. For example, in many Asian groups the incidence of myopia may between 80% and 90%.

Therefore, for a broader perspective for a review of physiologic optics, this last section covers some of the essential epidemiologic aspects of the refractive errors other than emmetropia.

Prevalence. Studies that tabulate the distribution of refractive errors often are taken from data on young army recruits,[91,99] which show the incidence of myopia to be about 10%. However, this group of healthy young men is not representative of the general population. Stenstrom's study in Uppsala, Sweden, consisted of the clinic patients, colleagues, nurses, and cadet officers, which is a group more reflective of the general population.[94] His study showed that about 20% of the population has lower myopia (less than 2 diopters), 7% has moderate myopia (2 to 6 diopters), and another 2.5% has high myopia (greater than 6 diopters). The great majority of this population (just less than 70%) clustered between emmetropia and 2 diopters of hyperopia; the rest were high hyperopes and aphakes.

The spectacle-wearing population of a typical Western country provides a different focus on emmetropes. Bennett[8] surveyed the distribution of spectacles dispensed in England. His study indicates the distribution of refractions carried out by the average eye clinician showed that about 20% are myopic refractions and 75% of all refractions require prescriptions from −0.5 to +8.00 diopters. Subtraction of Stenstrom's estimate of the percentage of high hyperopes shows that about 65% of all refraction prescriptions are for presbyope.

Myopia
Pathologic Myopia. Curtin[21] estimates that 2% to 3% of the population has pathologic myopia (a condition in which there is a significant enlargement of the eyeball with a lengthening of the posterior segment). This group falls into Stenstom's group of patients with myopia of greater than 6 diopters. The

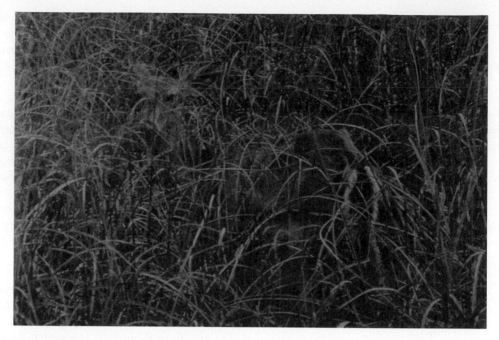

FIGURE 6-27   Note the deer hidden in the bush. By almost closing your eyes, the distraction of the high grass is canceled and the animal is easier to see. (From Osborne C (ed), Tanner O: *Animal defenses,* New York, 1978, Time-Life Films.)

term *pathologic* is used because these patients show significant choroidal and retinal degenerative changes, a high incidence of retinal detachment, glaucoma, and increased occurrence of staphyloma development. At present, high myopia (greater than 6 diopters) is considered a sex-linked, recessive inherited disorder.[2,115]

Physiologic, or School, Myopia. As noted by Stenstom,[94] most patients have myopia that is less than 2 diopters; this type of myopia is called *physiologic,* or *school, myopia.* The word *physiologic* implies that this form of myopia is a normal, physiologic response to a stress. In fact, substantial evidence exists that increased time spent reading from early teenage to the midtwenties is that stress.[2,5]

However, near work is not the sole cause of physiologic myopia. Racial and ethnicity studies show that myopia is more prevalent among Orientals and Jewish persons and less prevalent among African-Americans.[85] (The results of a study in Taiwan showed the incidence of myopia to be about 12% in children 6 years of age or younger, 55% in children 12 years of age or younger, 75% in children 15 years of age or younger, and 84% in those older than 18 years of age.[57]) Thus it appears

that an inherited predisposition, linked with excessive close work during the student years, results in most of the cases of physiologic myopia.

Astigmatism

About 50% of term infants in their first years of life show astigmatism of more than 2 diopters.[10,40,70] This may arise from the influence of the recti muscles that pull on the delicate infant sclera, because the astigmatism seems to change in different gaze directions. Howland et al.[40] suggested that the high astigmatism helps the infant bracket the position of best focus while learning to accommodate. By adulthood, this high incidence of astigmatism has disappeared. Studies show that about 15% of the adult population has astigmatism greater than 1 diopter and only 2% have astigmatism greater than 3 diopters. It is possible that much of the high astigmatism in this last group is related to some form of intraocular surgery (e.g., corneal transplants, cataract surgery, repair of corneal lacerations).

Presbyopia

Although presbyopia is age related, its age of onset varies around the world. For example, presbyopia develops earlier in people who live closer to the

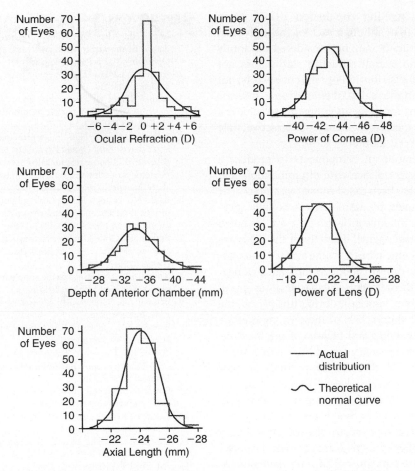

FIGURE 6-28 Curves of distribution of refraction and its components in 194 eyes. (Adapted from Sorsby A, Sheridan M, Leary GA: *BMJ* 1394, 1960; and Sorsby A et al: *Med Res Counc Special Rep Serv Rep* 293, 1959.)

equator.[47,68] Specifically, the age of onset of presbyopia was noted to be 37 years in India, 39 years in Puerto Rico, 41 years in Israel, 42 years in Japan, 45 years in England, and 46 years in Norway. Further studies show the important variable to be ambient temperature rather than latitude. Thus the higher the ambient temperature, the earlier the onset of presbyopia.

On the other hand, life expectancy is lower in developing countries where the ambient temperatures are usually high. Thus, although presbyopia starts at a young age in the developing world, fewer persons with presbyopia are found in the general population. For example, in Haiti the prevalence rate of presbyopia is about 16% for the normal population, whereas in the United States it is 31%.[88] The lower rate of presbyopia in Haiti is paradoxical. The reason is probably that the average life span in Haiti is much shorter than in Western countries. Seen in perspective, presbyopia constitutes about 65% of all those who wear glasses in developed Western countries. Thus it is of little surprise that the first spectacles produced sometime in the fourteenth century were created for persons with presbyopia.

Components of Ametropia

The overall refractive state of the eye is determined by four components:

- Corneal power (mean, 43 diopters)
- Anterior chamber depth (mean, 3.4 mm)
- Crystalline lens power (mean, 21 diopters)
- Axial length (mean, 24 mm)

Figure 6-28 shows the distribution of total refraction and the four components just mentioned for 194 eyes.[92]

The most striking conclusion drawn from Figure 6-28 is that, although each of the individual optical components may be considered randomly distributed, the overall refractive status does not show a normal distribution of refractive errors, but rather a skew in the region of emmetropia. It seems that the various components cooperate to achieve a higher-than-expected incidence of refractive state between 0 and +2 diopters.

This cooperation of components to produce a higher-than-expected incidence of emmetropia and low hyperopia has been called *emmetropization*.[92] The process of emmetropization seems to be fully effective during the infantile growth of the eye. As noted earlier, the average sagittal diameter of the eye is approximately 18 mm at birth. By the age of 3 years, the axial length increases to about 23 mm. Such elongation of the eye theoretically yields a state of myopia of about 15 diopters. However, during this period, the data show that almost 75% of these young eyes are hyperopic.[20] Between 3 and 14 years of age, the elongation increases, on average, an additional millimeter. Again, this should theoretically produce another 3 diopters of myopia. However, at 14 years of age, the average refractive state shows a strong clustering in the emmetropic neighborhood. Because the cornea and anterior chamber depth change little during these periods of eye growth, it appears that the power of the crystalline lens must change to maintain emmetropia. It seems possible that the process is coordinated by the retina-brain complex, which might tune each component to ensure a sharp image. However, studies of infant monkeys who were raised in the dark or who have had their optic nerve sectioned suggest that emmetropization is largely programmed on a genetic basis.[81] The experiments further showed that procedures that result in significant degradation of the retinal image, such as the suturing of the lids together or induction of a corneal opacity during the early growth period, influence the axial growth process. Surprisingly, these types of opacification significantly increase the axial length and produce states of myopia of up to 12 diopters. Such excessive image degradation seems to override the emmetropization process and result in high levels of axial myopia.

In conclusion, it appears that a genetic bias underscores the refractive state of the eye. However, this genetic program can be tuned by environmental and intrinsic (i.e., intraocular) factors. Koretz et al.,[50] and Laties and Stone,[52] and Stone et al.[43,50,75,95-97,104] have provided further insights into the biophysical and chemical controls of emmetropization and their failure.

REFERENCES

1. Aggurwala KR, Nowbotsing S, Kruger PB: Accommodation to monochromatic and white-light targets, *Invest Ophthalmol Vis Sci* 36:2695, 1995.
2. Angle J, Wissman DA: The epidemiology of myopia, *Am J Epidemol* 111:220, 1980.
3. Atkins GH et al: Picosecond time resoled fluorescence spectroscopy of K-590 in the bacteriorhodopsin photocycle, *Biophys J* 55:263, 1989.
4. Bailey H, Lovie JE: New design principles for visual acuity letter charts, *Am J Optom Physiol Opt* 53:740, 1976.
5. Baldwin WR: Some relationships between ocular, anthropometric and refractive variables in myopia, doctoral thesis, Indianapolis, 1964, Indiana University.
6. Banks MS, Bennett PG: Optical and photoreceptor immaturity's limit the spatial and chromatic vision of human neonates, *J Opt Soc Am* 5A:2059, 1988.
7. Barlow HB: Critical limiting factors in the design of the eye and visual cortex: the Ferrier lecture, 1980, *Proc R Soc (Lond)* 212B:1, 1981.
8. Bennett AG: Lens usage in the supplementary ophthalmic service, *Optician* 149:131, 1965.
9. Bennett AG, Rabbetts RB: *Clinical visual optics,* London, 1984, Butterworths.
10. Bennett AG, Rabbetts RB: *Clinical visual optics,* ed 2, London, 1989, Butterworths.
11. Boothe RG, Dobson V, Teller DY: Post natal development of vision in human and nonhuman primates, *Ann Rev Neurosci* 8:495, 1985.
12. Bower TG: The perceptual world of the child, Cambridge, 1977, Harvard University Press.
13. Campbell FW: The depth of field of the human eye, *Optica Acta* 4:157, 1957.
14. Campbell FW: The physics of visual perception, *Philos Trans R Soc Lond B Biol Sci* 290:5, 1980.
15. Campbell FW, Green DG: Optical and retinal factors affecting visual resolution, *J Physiol* 181:576, 1965.
16. Campbell FW, Gubisch RW: Optical quality of the human eye, *J Physiol* 186:558, 1966.
17. Campbell FW, Robson JG: Application of Fourier analysis to the visibility of gratings, *J Physiol* 186:558, 1966.
18. Charman WN, Whitefoot H: Pupil diameter and the depth of field of the human eye as measured by laser speckle, *Optica Acta* 24:1211, 1977.
19. Collins D: *The human revolution: from ape to artist,* London, 1976, Phaidon.
20. Cook RC, Glasscock RE: Refractive and ocular findings in the newborn, *Am J Ophthalmol* 34:1407, 1951.
21. Curtin BJ: *The myopias: basic science and clinical management,* Philadelphia, 1985, Harper and Row.
22. Eakin RM: Evolution of photoreceptors. In Robzhansky T, Hetch MK, Steere WC (eds): *Evolutionary biology,* vol 2, New York, 1968, Appleton-Century-Crofts.
23. Elliott DB, Yang KGH, Whitaker D: Visual acuity changes throughout adulthood in normal healthy eyes seeing beyond 6/6, *Optom Vis Sci* 72:186, 1995.
24. Enoch JM: Retinal receptor orientation and the role of fiber optics in vision, *Am J Optometry* 49:455, 1972.
25. Fein A, Szutz EZ: *Photoreceptors: their role in vision,* Cambridge, 1982, Cambridge University Press.
26. Fernald RD: Vision and behavior in an African cichild fish, *Am Sci* 72:58, 1984.
27. Ferris FL et al: New visual acuity charts for clinical research, *Am J Ophthalmol* 94:91, 1982.

28. Findlay JBC: The biosynthetic, functional and evolutionary implications of the structure of rhodopsin. In Stieve H (ed): *The molecular mechanism of photoreception: report on the Dahlem Workshop on the Molecular Mechanism of Photoreception,* Berlin, 1986, Springer-Verlag.

29. Frantz RL: Visual perception from birth as shown by pattern selectivity, *Ann NY Acad Sci* 118:793, 1965.

30. Frisby JP: *Illusion, brain and mind,* Oxford, 1980, Oxford University Press.

31. Goss DA: Development of the ametropias. In Benjamin WJ (ed): *Borish's clinical refraction,* Philadelphia, 1998, WB Saunders.

32. Green DG, Powers MK, Banks MS: Depth of focus, eye size, visual acuity, *Vis Res* 20:827, 1980.

33. Gwiazda J et al: Astigmatism in children: changes in axis and amount from birth to six years, *Invest Ophthalmol Vis Sci* 25:99, 1984.

34. Harper RA, Halliday BL: Glare and contrast sensitivity in contact lens corrected aphakia, epikeratophakia and pseudophakia, *Eye* 3:562, 1989.

35. Hearst E: Psychology of nothing, *Am Sci* 79:432, 1991.

36. Helmholtz H: *Handbuch der Physiologische Optik,* Leipzig, 1909, Hamburg University.

37. Hemenger RP, Garner LF, Ooi CS: Change with age of the refractive index gradient of the human ocular lens, *Invest Ophthalmol Vis Sci* 36:703, 1995.

38. Hofstetter HW: Emmetropization-biological process or mathematical artifact? *Am J Optom Arch Am Acad Optom* 46:447, 1969.

39. Holliday LL: The fundamentals of glare and visibility, *J Opt Soc Am* 12A:492, 1926.

40. Howland HC et al: Astigmatism measured by photorefraction, *Science* 202:331, 1978.

41. Inagaki Y: The rapid change of corneal curvature in the neonatal period and infancy, *Arch Ophthalmol* 104:1026, 1986.

42. Insler MS et al: Analysis of corneal thickness and corneal curvature in infants, *CLAO J* 3:192, 1987.

43. Iuvone PM et al: Effects of apomorphine, a dopamine receptor agonist, on ocular refraction and axial elongation in a primate model of myopia, *Invest Ophthalmol Vis Sci* 32:1674, 1991.

44. Kanizsa G: Subjective contours, *Sci Am* 234:48, 1976.

45. Katz B, Melles RB, Schneider JA: Glare disability in nephrotic cystinosis, *Arch Ophthalmol* 105:1670, 1987.

46. Katz M: the human eye as an optical system. In Duane TD (ed): *Clinical ophthalmology,* New York, 1990, Harper and Row.

47. Klemstein RN: Epidemiology of presbyopia. In Start L, Obrecht G (eds): *Presbyopia,* New York, 1987, Professional Press.

48. Koch D et al: Glare following posterior chamber lens implantation, *J Cataract Refract Surg* 12:480, 1986.

49. Kohda Y, Watanabe M: The aggression releasing effect of the eye-like spot of the Oyanirami Coreopera Kawamebari, a fresh water serranid fish, *Ethology* 84:162, 1990.

50. Koretz JF, Rogot A, Kaufman PL: Physiological strategies for emmetropia, *Trans Am Ophthalmol Soc* 93:105, 1995.

51. Lancon M, Miller D: Corneal hydration, visual acuity and glare sensitivity, *Arch Ophthalmol* 90:227, 1973.

52. Larsen JS: The sagittal growth of the eye: ultrasonic measurements of axial length of the eye from birth to puberty, *Acta Ophthalmol* 49:872, 1971.

53. Laties AM, Stone RA: Some visual and neurochemical correlates of refractive development, *Vis Neurosci* 7:125, 1991.

54. LeClaire J et al: A new glare tester for clinical testing, *Arch Ophthalmol* 100:153, 1982.

55. Lee DN: The optic flow field: the foundation of vision, *Philos Trans R Soc London B Biol Sci* 290:169, 1980.

56. Levene JR: *Clinical refraction and visual science,* London, 1977, Butterworths.

57. Luke LK et al: Epidemiological study of ocular refraction amount school children in Taiwan, *Invest Ophthalmol Vis Sci* 6:1002, 1996.

58. Maffei L, Fiorentin A: The visual cortex as a spatial frequency analyzer, *Vis Res* 3:1255, 1973.

59. Mainster MD: Contemporary optics and ocular pathology, *Surv Ophthalmol* 23:135, 1978.

60. Marsh P (ed): *Eye to eye,* Salem, 1988, Salem Press.

61. Miles S: Underwater medicine, Philadelphia, 1966, Heppesen Sandreson.

62. Miller D: Optics and refraction: a user friendly guide, St Louis, 1991, Gower Medical.

63. Miller D, Benedek G: Intraocular light scattering, Springfield, Ill, 1973, Charles C Thomas.

64. Miller D, Dohlman CH: The effect of cataract surgery on the cornea, *Trans Am Acad Ophthalmol Otolaryngol* 74:369, 1970.

65. Miller D, Sanghvi S: Contrast sensitivity and glare testing in corneal disease. In Nadler M, Miller D, Nadler DJ (eds): *Glare and contrast sensitivity for clinicians,* New York, 1990, Springer-Verlag.

66. Miller D, Stern R: Vision and hearing screening for the elderly, *EENT Monthly* 13:128, 1974.

67. Miller D, Zuckerman JL, Reynolds GO: Holographic filter to negate the effect of cataract, *Arch Ophthalmol* 90:323, 1973.

68. Miranda MH: The environmental factor in the onset of presbyopia. In Stark L, Obrecht G (eds): *Presbyopia,* New York, 1987, Professional Press.

69. Mohindra I, Held R, Gwiazda J: Astigmatism in infants, *Science* 202:329, 1978.

70. Mohundra I et al: Astigmatism in infants, *Science* 202:329, 1978.

71. Mutti DO et al: Optical and structural development of the crystalline lens in childhood, *Invest Ophthalmol Vis Sci* 39:120, 1997.

72. Nakanishi K: Why 11-cis-retinal, *Am Zool* 31:479, 1991.

73. Oesterhelt D, Stoekenius W: Rhodopsin-like protein from the membrane of *Holobacterium halobium. Nature New Biol* 233:149, 1971.

74. Ogle KN, Schwartz JT: Depth of focus of the human eye, *J Opt Soc Am* 49:273, 1959.

75. Papastergiou GI et al: Induction of axial eye elongation and myopic refractive shift in one-year old chickens, *Vis Res* 38:1883, 1998.

76. Pardue MT, Anderson ME, Sivak J: Accommodation in raptors, *Invest Ophthalmol Vis Sci* 37:725, 1996.

77. Pinker S: *The language instinct,* New York, 1994, Penguin Books.

78. Pizzarellio LD: The dimensions of the problems of eye disease among the elderly, *Ophthalmology* 94:1191, 1987.

79. Ramachandran VS: 2-D or not 2-D, that is the question. In Gregory R et al (eds): *The artful eye,* Oxford, 1995, Oxford University Press.

80. Ratliff F: The role of physiologic nystagmus in monocular acuity, *J Exp Psychol* 43:163, 1952.

81. Raviola E, Wiesel TN: Animal model for myopia, *N Engl J Med* 312:1609, 1985.

82. Reynolds CR, Fletcher F, Janzen E: *Handbook of clinical child neurophysiology,* New York, 1989, Plenum Press.

83. Riggs LA: Visual acuity. In Graham CH (ed): *Vision and visual perception,* New York, 1965, John Wiley & Sons.

84. Riggs LA et al: The disappearance of steadily fixated visual test objects, *J Opt Soc Am* 43:495, 1953.

85. Rowsey JJ, Balyeat HD: Preliminary results and complications of radial keratotomy, *Am J Ophthalmol* 93:347, 1983.

86. Said FS, Weale RA: The variation with age of the human spectral transmissivity of the living human crystalline lens, *Gerontologia* 3:213, 1959.

87. Sherbrooke W: Personal communication, Santa Fe, 1995.

88. Stark L, Obrecht G: *Presbyopia: recent research and reviews from the Third International symposium,* New York, 1987, Professional Press.

89. Snyder AW, Bossomaier JR, Hughes A: Optical image quality and the cone mosaic, *Science* 231:499, 1986.

90. Snyder AW, Menzal R: *Photoreceptor optics,* Berlin, 1975, Springer-Verlag.

91. Sorsby A, Sheridan M, Leary GA: Vision, visual acuity and ocular refraction in young men, *BMJ* 1394, 1960.

92. Sorsby A et al: Emmetropia and its aberrations, *Med Res Counc Special Rep Serv Rep* 293, 1959.

93. Spudich JL, Bogomolni RD: Sensory rhodopsins of *Halobacteria, Annu Rev Biophys Biophys Chem* 17:183, 1988.

94. Stenstom S: Untersuchungen uber die variation fon ko-variation des optishen elements des menschlichen auges, *Acta Ophthalmol* 26(suppl), 1946.

95. Stone RA, Lin T, Laties AM: Muscarinic antagonist effects on experimental chick myopia, *Exp Eye Res* 52:755, 1991.

96. Stone RA et al: Retinal dopamine and form-deprivation myopia, *Proceedings of the National Academy of Sciences of the United States of America* 86:704, 1989.

97. Stone RA et al: Postnatal control of ocular growth: dopaminergic mechanisms, *Ciba Foundation Symposium* 155:45, 1990.

98. Strickland C: *Torsten Wiesel, winner of 1981 Nobel Prize for Vision Research,* San Francisco, 1995, American Academy of Ophthalmology.

99. Stromberg E: Uber refraktion und Achsenlange des menchlicken Auges, *Acta Ophthalmol* 14:281, 1936.

100. Stryer L: Mini review: visual excitation and recovery, *J Biol Chem* 266:1071, 1991.

101. Tang C, Kiorpes L, Morshon JA: Stereo acuity and vernier acuity in Macaque monkeys, *Invest Ophthal* 36:5365, 1995 (abstract).

102. Teller DY: First glances: the vision of infants, *Invest Ophthalmol Vis Sci* 38:2183, 1997.

103. Thisbos LN, Zhang X, Ming Y: The chromatic eye: a new model of ocular chromatic aberration, *Appl Opt* 31:3594, 1992.

104. Tigges M et al: Effects of muscarinic cholinergic receptor antagonists on postnatal eye growth of rhesus monkeys, *Opt Vis Sci* 76:397, 1999.

105. Troelsta Z et al: Accommodative tracking: a trial and error function, *Vis Res* 4:585, 1964.

106. Tronick E: Simultaneous control and growth of the infant's effective visual field, *Perception Psychophysics* 11:373, 1972.

107. Tucker J, Charman WN: The depth of focus of the human eye for Snellen letters, *Am J Optom Physiol Opt* 52:3, 1975.

108. Tucker SM et al: Corneal diameter, axial length and intraocular pressure in premature infants, *Ophthalmology* 99:1296, 1992.

109. Von Ditfurther H: *Children of the universe,* New York, 1976, Athenaeum Press.

110. Wald G, Griffin DR: The change in refractive power of the human eye in dim and bright light, *J Opt Soc Am* 37:321, 1947.

111. Waring GO et al: Results of the progressive evaluation of radial keratotomy (PERK) study one year after surgery, *Ophthalmology* 92:177, 1985.

112. Weiter JJ: Phototoxic changes in the retina. In Miler D (ed): *Clinical light damage to the eye,* New York, 1987, Springer-Verlag.

113. Williams DR: Topography of the foveal cone mosaic in the living human eye, *Vis Res* 28:433, 1988.

114. Wistow GJ, Piatigorsky J: Recruitment of enzymes as lens structural proteins, *Science* 236:1554, 1987.

115. Wold KC: Hereditary myopia, *Arch Ophthalmol* 42:225, 1949.

116. Wolfe E: Glare and age, *Arch Ophthalmol* 64:502, 1960.

117. Wolfe E, Gardiner JS: Studies on the scatter of light in the dioptric median of the eye as a basis for visual glare, *Arch Ophthalmol* 37:450, 1963.

118. Wood ICJ, Mutti DO, Zadnik K: Crystalline lens parameters in infancy, *Ophthalmol Physiol Opt* 6:310, 1996.

119. Yokoyama S, Yokoyama R: Molecular evolution of human visual pigment genes, *Mol Biol Evol* 6:186, 1989.

120. Zadnik K, Mutti DO: Development of ametropias. In Benjamin WJ (ed): *Borish's clinical refraction,* Philadelphia, 1998, WB Saunders.

121. Zeilik M: *Astronomy: the evolving universe,* ed 3, New York, 1982, Harper and Row.

SECTION 5

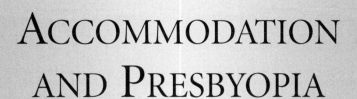

ACCOMMODATION AND PRESBYOPIA

ADRIAN GLASSER AND PAUL L. KAUFMAN

C H A P T E R   7

ACCOMMODATION AND PRESBYOPIA

ADRIAN GLASSER AND PAUL L. KAUFMAN

"There is no other portion of physiological optics where one finds so many differing and contradictory ideas as concerns the accommodation of the eye where only recently in the most recent time have we actually made observations where previously everything was left to the play of hypotheses."

H. VON HELMHOLTZ (1909)

It is primarily to Helmholtz[51] that we owe our current understanding of the accommodative mechanism of the human eye. His insight came from his own work and from pioneers before him. Thomas Young[124] was instrumental in demonstrating that accommodation occurs, not through changes in corneal curvature or axial length as those before him believed, but through changes in the curvature of the lens.[55] Young's painstaking anatomic investigations[124] were insufficient for him to rule out the possibility that the crystalline lens received direct innervation from a branch of the ciliary nerves to allow it to contract as a muscle. It was only after the work of Crampton,[17] who first described the ciliary muscle from his investigation of bird eyes, that a mechanistic description of how the ciliary muscle might alter lens curvatures was proposed by Müller.[72] The understanding of human accommodation was hindered by numerous investigations of the eyes of birds and other vertebrates (studied for their comparatively large size to gain insight into the human accommodative mechanism) now known to effect accommodation through mechanisms quite different from the human eye.[44,46,47]

Our current understanding of accommodation stems from the work of many, including Brücke,[11] Cramer,[16] Hess,[53] Müller,[79] and Helmholtz and Gullstrand.[51] This path was made tortuous by the diversity of accommodative mechanisms of the various vertebrates studied. Possibly the most an-cient of accommodative mechanisms is that of the Sauropsida (lizards, birds, and turtles). Although these eyes differ from the primate eye, these species all share many unusual ocular characteristics, including striated intraocular muscles, bony plates or ossicles in the sclera, attachment of the ciliary processes to the lens equator, the absence of a circumlental space, a lens annular pad, and in some species, corneal accommodation and iris-mediated lenticular accommodation. The diversity of avian visual habitats (aerial, aquatic, and terrestrial), eye shapes (tubular, globose, and flattened), and feeding behaviors in all likelihood dictates their accommodative needs. Corneal accommodation, of considerable value to terrestrial birds, is of no value to aquatic birds, for whom the corneal optical power is neutralized by water. The evolutionarily divergent accommodative mechanisms, or the absence of accommodation in other vertebrates, is, by reasonable conjecture, determined by feeding behaviors. Herbivorous animals (e.g., sheep, horses, cows), those that forage and dig for food primarily using olfactory cues (e.g., pigs), or those with relatively poor visual abilities (e.g., mice, rats, rabbits) do not appear to accommodate. Carnivores have better developed ciliary muscles than these other species, but they still have relatively little accommodative ability; the raccoon is the only nonprimate terrestrial mammal with substantial accommodative amplitude.[91] Cats are suggested, and raccoons and fish are shown to translate the lens forward without lenticular thickening.[2-4,83,91,102,116] Other adaptations in the lens, iris, or retina allow other lower vertebrates functional near and distance vision, although these cannot be classified as true accommodation because they rely on static optical adaptations.

Among the vertebrates that do accommodate, the amplitude varies considerably. Diving birds have among the largest amplitudes, with cormorants having approximately 50 diopters and diving ducks suggested to have 70 to 80 diopters.[53,103] Among the mammals, vervet and cynomolgus monkeys have approximately 20 diopters, young rhesus as much as 40 diopters, and raccoons about 20 diopters.[8,57,91,112,113] We humans, for only a few short childhood years, may have a maximum of about 15 diopters but find much less accommodation adequate for most visual tasks. Although accommodative amplitude gradually declines until about age 50 years, at which time it is almost com-

pletely lost, the deficit in most individuals appears to be of sudden onset when the accommodative amplitude is diminished to a few diopters as presbyopia develops. Although persons with presbyopia may read at intermediate distances, the reason is almost certainly due to the depth of focus (see later discussion) resulting from pupillary constriction rather than active accommodation. The word *presbyopia* (Greek *presbys* meaning an aged person and *opsis* meaning vision) possibly derives from Aristotle's use of the term *presbytas* to describe "those who see well at distance, but poorly at near."[52] Historically, the term was used to describe the condition in which the near point has receded too far from the eye as a result of a diminution in the range of accommodation.[25] Despite the wealth of studies of accommodation on vertebrates, only primates are shown to systematically lose the ability to accommodate with increasing age. It may be no coincidence that although absolute life spans differ considerably, the relative age course of the

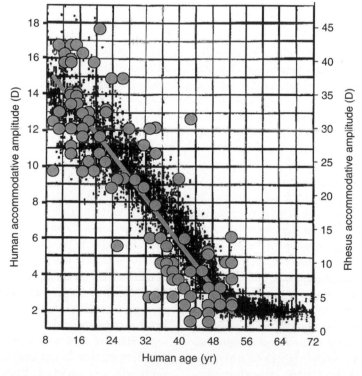

FIGURE 7-1   Progression of presbyopia in humans (Duane,[27] *small solid black symbols*) as measured subjectively with a push-up test and in rhesus monkeys (Bito et al.,[8] *larger gray symbols* and *solid line*) as measured objectively with a Hartinger coincidence refractometer after topical application of the cholinergic agonist pilocarpine. The horizontal axis is in human years and the rhesus monkey data are scaled to human years such that 25 rhesus monkey years are equivalent to 52 human years. The vertical axis is scaled such that the mean amplitude of 14 diopters in humans is equivalent to 35 diopters in rhesus monkeys. In humans and rhesus monkeys, presbyopia progresses at the same rate relative to the absolute age span of each species. (From Bito LZ et al: *Invest Ophthalmol Vis Sci* 23:23, 1982; and Duane, *JAMA* 59:1010, 1912. Reproduced with permission from the Association for Research in Vision and Ophthalmology and the author.)

progression of presbyopia is similar in humans and monkeys (Figure 7-1).

ACCOMMODATION

Accommodation is a dynamic, optical change in the dioptric power of the eye. It provides the ability to change the point of focus of the eye from distant to near objects. In the primate this is mediated through a contraction of the ciliary muscle, release of resting zonular tension at the lens equator, and a "rounding up" of the crystalline lens through the force exerted on it by the lens capsule. The increased optical power is achieved through increased anterior and posterior lens surface curvatures and increased thickness of the lens (Figure 7-2). In an emmetropic eye (an eye without refractive error), distant objects at or beyond what is considered optical infinity for the eye (6 m or 20 feet) are focused on the retina when accommodation is relaxed. When objects are brought closer to the eye, the eye must accommodate to maintain a clearly focused image on the retina. Myopic eyes, typically too long for the optical power of the lens and cornea combined, are unable to attain a sharply focused image for objects at optical infinity unless optical compensation is provided such as through negatively powered spectacle lenses. Persons with myopia can focus clearly on objects closer than optical infinity without accommodation (i.e., objects at their far point; see Chapter 6). Persons with hyperopia are able to focus clearly on objects at optical infinity only through an accommodative increase in the optical power of the eye or with the use of positively powered spectacle lenses.

Optics of the Eye

Light from an object enters the eye at the cornea and is brought to a focus on the retina through the combined optical power of the cornea and the lens. When light is focused on the retina of an emmetropic eye, a clear, well-focused image is per-

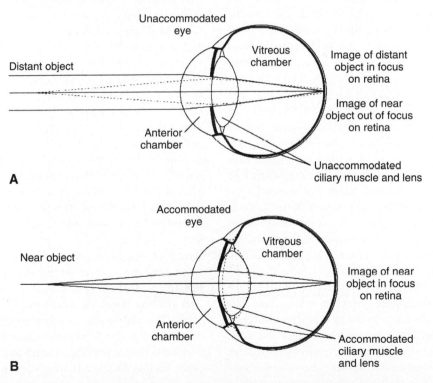

FIGURE 7-2 The accommodative optical changes in the eye occur through an increase in optical power of the crystalline lens. Unaccommodated eye focused on distant object (**A**) and accommodated eye focused on near object (**B**). In the unaccommodated eye (**A**), the image of a distant object is focused on the retina *(solid rays)*, while the image of a near object forms an out-of-focus blur circle on the retina *(dashed rays)*. In **B** the anterior and posterior lens surface curvatures and the lens thickness increase with accommodation. The anterior chamber depth and, to a lesser extent, the vitreous chamber depth decrease. These physical movements result in the optical changes that allow the eye to focus the image of a near object on the retina.

ceived. This enables the performance of everyday visual tasks such as reading, writing, sewing, and driving. If the image is not focused on the retina, these tasks become difficult or impossible to perform without optical correction to bring the image to focus on the retina.

The optical elements of the eye—the cornea, aqueous humor, crystalline lens, and vitreous humor—all contribute to the optical power of the eye. Specific details for schematic eyes are given in Bennett and Rabbetts.[6] In the adult human eye the cornea has a radius of curvature of about +7.8 mm, a thickness of about 0.25 mm near the optical axis, and provides approximately 70% of the optical power of the eye. Light passes from an air environment, with a refractive index of approximately 1.00, into the cornea. The cornea is composed largely of fluid and proteins and therefore has a higher refractive index of about 1.376. The optical power of the cornea is attributable to a combination of the positive radius of curvature and the higher refractive index than the surrounding air. Light then passes through the cornea and into the aqueous humor. Because the refractive index of the aqueous humor is close to that of the cornea (about 1.336), the optical effect at the posterior cornea/aqueous interface is relatively little. Light then enters the anterior surface of the crystalline lens. The surface of the crystalline lens has a refractive index slightly higher than that of the aqueous humor (about 1.386). The lens anterior surface has a radius of curvature of about +10.00 mm, which adds to the optical power of the eye. The crystalline lens has a gradient refractive index that gradually increases from the surface to a value of about 1.406 at the center and then decreases toward the posterior lens surface. The posterior surface of the crystalline lens has a radius of curvature of about −6.00 mm. Although this is a concave surface relative to the direction of propagation of light, because the light passes from the higher refractive index of the lens to the lower refractive index of the vitreous humor (about 1.336), the posterior lens surface also adds to the optical power of the eye, relatively more than the anterior lens surface because the posterior surface curvature is steeper than the anterior surface curvature. The lens anterior and posterior surface curvatures are important to the optical power of the eye, and it is these surface curvatures that steepen when accommodation occurs. Historically, it has been suggested that the posterior lens surface did not move with accommodation and that the posterior surface curvature did not change appre-

ciably.[51,63] However, the posterior lens surface does undergo an increase in curvature and moves backward with accommodation.[32,41,63] High-resolution partial coherence interferometric studies in human subjects 25 to 39 years of age show an average of 185 μm of forward movement of the anterior lens surface and 69 μm of posterior movement of the posterior lens surface.[26] The possibility also exists that the gradient refractive index of the lens changes with accommodation.[40] Presbyopia, the age-related loss of accommodation, occurs in conjunction with a gradual decline in the change in the lens optical power with accommodative effort.

The Optical Requirements for Accommodation

The optical power of the crystalline lens increases (i.e., the lens focal length decreases) with accommodation. As a consequence, the eye is able to change its point of focus from distance to near so that near objects are brought to focus on the retina. This dioptric change in power of the eye is called *accommodation*. Accommodation is measured in units of diopters. A diopter is a reciprocal meter and is a measure of the vergence of light. *Positive vergence* denotes rays converging toward a point image, and *negative vergence* denotes rays diverging from a point object. When an emmetropic eye is focused for distant objects, the eye is unaccommodated. If the eye accommodates from an object at optical infinity so that, for example, an object 1.0 m in front of the eye is focused on the retina, this represents 1.0 diopter of accommodation. If the eye accommodates from an object at infinity to an object 0.5 m from the eye, this is 2 diopters; from infinity to 0.1 m is 10 diopters, and so on.

Depth of Focus. Accommodation is often measured subjectively by moving a near reading target toward the eye. The subject then reports when the near reading target can no longer be held in clear focus. The amplitude of accommodation is then determined as the difference in dioptric power between the closest reading distance and the most remote reading distance at which text is in sharp focus. Because accommodation is most easily and most commonly (although not most accurately) measured this way, depth of focus of the eye is an important consideration in determining the accommodative amplitude.

Depth of field is the range over which a target can be moved toward or away from the eye without a perceptible change in the blur or focus of the image. Depth of focus is the focusing error that can be tolerated without an appreciable decrease in acuity or change in blur or focus of the image on the retina. For any given accommodative state, there is a range of distances over which an object is perceived to be in focus. This is the depth of focus and is dependent on pupil size. A small pupil results in a relatively larger depth of focus, and a larger pupil size results in a relatively smaller depth of focus. The depth of focus of an eye is also dependent on the level of illumination. For a brightly illuminated object, pupil size decreases and depth of focus increases. With accommodation and with increasing age, the pupil size decreases. These two factors result in a greater depth of focus of the aging eye during accommodation. When accommodation is measured with subjective methods, such as the push-up approach, the depth of focus of the eye results in an overestimation of true accommodative amplitude. It is for this reason that when accommodation is measured with a push-up method, about 1 diopter of "accommodation" is still seen even in the most elderly of patients.[27,66]

Visual Acuity. In addition to the depth of focus of the eye, acuity or contrast sensitivity of the eye also affects the subjective measurement of accommodative amplitude. The subjective push-up measurement of accommodation relies heavily on the subject perceiving when the object can no longer be seen in sharp focus. As a near reading target is brought closer to the eye, the subject must decide at what point the letters are no longer in acceptable focus. As mentioned, the level of illumination of the target can affect the depth of focus of the eye, but it also affects the contrast and the brightness of the image. If the target is viewed in dim illumination, it is more difficult to detect when it is in clear and sharp focus. A brightly illuminated reading target is seen more clearly. Because the increased illumination provides higher contrast on the target, smaller changes in focus or blur of the target is more easily detected (although increased illumination also causes decreased pupil size and increased depth of focus).

Similarly, in cases of cataract or other opacities of the ocular optical media, the near target is not seen clearly; therefore small changes in the focus of the object cannot be detected. With increasing age the optical clarity of the lens decreases and the prevalence of cataract increases. Elderly patients often have reduced visual acuity or reduced contrast

sensitivity, although not solely because of decreased optical performance.[12] For this reason, if the accommodative amplitude is measured in a presbyope with cataracts by means of a subjective push-up measurement, the true accommodative amplitude is likely overestimated. Although increasing the level of illumination helps improve the contrast sensitivity and acuity, it also decreases the pupil size and thereby increases the depth of focus of the eye; thus it also increases subjectively measured apparent accommodative amplitude.

The Anatomy of the Accommodative Apparatus

The accommodative apparatus of the eye consists of the ciliary body, the ciliary muscle, the choroid, the anterior and posterior zonular fibers, the lens capsule, and the crystalline lens (Figure 7-3). Support for and against a role for the vitreous in accommodation exists.[14,38,59] The ciliary muscle is located within the ciliary body beneath the anterior sclera. The ciliary muscle is composed of three muscle fiber groups oriented longitudinally, radially (obliquely), and circularly. The anterior zonular fibers span the circumlental space extending between the ciliary processes and the lens equator. Equatorial zonular fibers constitute the suspensory elements of the crystalline lens. Posterior zonular fibers extend between the tips of the ciliary processes and the pars plana of the posterior ciliary body near the ora serrata. The crystalline lens consists of a central nucleus and a surrounding cortex. This lens is surrounded by the collagenous elastic lens capsule.

The Ciliary Body. The ciliary body is a triangular-shaped region bounded on its outer surface by the anterior sclera and on its inner surface by the pigmented epithelium. It lies between the scleral spur anteriorly and the retina posteriorly. The anterior ciliary body begins at the scleral spur at the angle of the anterior chamber. The peripheral iris inserts into the anterior ciliary body. Posterior to the iris, the ciliary processes are found at the anterior innermost point of the ciliary body and form the corrugated pars plicata of the ciliary body. Posterior to the pars plicata, the smooth inner surface of the ciliary body is called the *pars plana*. The inner surface of the pars plana is spanned by longitudinally oriented posterior zonular fibers.[48] The most posterior aspect of the ciliary body joins the ora serrata of the retina. The outer surface of the ciliary body beneath the anterior sclera is the suprachoroidal lamina or *supraciliaris,* formed by a

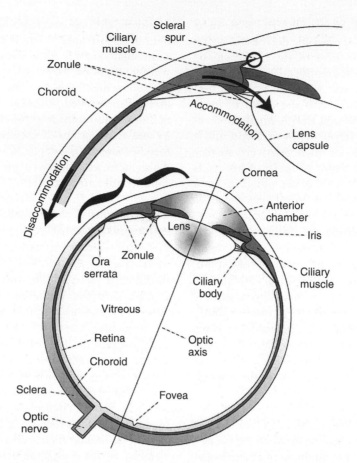

FIGURE 7-3   Schematic representation of a sagittal section of the anatomy of the accommodative apparatus at the ciliary region of the eye (**A**) in relation to a midsagittal section of the eye as a whole (**B**). The schematic shows that the lens capsule, zonule, ciliary muscle, and choroid constitute a single elastic "sling" anchored at the posterior scleral canal where the optic nerve leaves the globe, and anteriorly at the scleral spur. The action of accommodation results in a movement of the ciliary body forward and toward the axis of the eye against the elasticity of the posterior attachment of the ciliary muscle and the posterior zonular fibers. With a cessation of an accommodative effort, the ciliary muscle is returned to its unaccommodated configuration through the elasticity of choroid and posterior zonular fibers.

---

thin layer of collagen fibers, fibroblasts, and melanocytes.[110] Ultrastructural differences exist between the ciliary nonpigmented epithelial cells at the tips of the processes and those in the valleys, the former being adapted for fluid secretion and the latter for mechanical anchoring of the zonule.[49] The ciliary body from the tips of the ciliary processes to the ora serrata is longest temporally and shortest nasally.[54]

The Ciliary Muscle.   The ciliary muscle occupies a triangular-shaped region within the ciliary body beneath the anterior sclera (see Figure 7-3). It has an anterior origin at the scleral spur in proximity to Schlemm's canal.[54,71] Anterior ciliary muscle tendons insert into the scleral spur and the trabecular meshwork, which serve as a fixed anterior anchor against which the ciliary muscle contracts.[110]

Posterior to the scleral spur, the outer surface of the ciliary muscle is attached only loosely to the inner surface of the anterior sclera. The posterior attachment of the ciliary muscle is to the stroma of the choroid. The anterior and inner surfaces of the ciliary muscle are bounded anteriorly by the stroma of the pars plicata and posteriorly by the pars plana of the ciliary body. The ciliary muscle fiber bundles beneath the sclera are oriented such that a contraction of the ciliary muscle results in a forward and inward redistribution of the mass of the ciliary body and a narrowing of the ciliary ring as a result of ciliary muscle movement along the inner surface of the sphere formed by the anterior sclera. This causes the anterior choroid to be pulled forward.

The ciliary muscle is a smooth muscle, with a dominant parasympathetic innervation causing contraction mediated by M_3 muscarinic receptors and a sympathetic innervation causing relaxation mediated by β_2-adrenergic receptors. These apparently antagonistic functions may serve to smooth accommodative tracking, with the muscle in effect acting as its own antagonist, in contrast to the skeletal muscle system in which this smoothing function is served by separate antagonistic muscles (e.g., biceps and triceps during flexion or extension of the forearm). The ciliary muscle is atypical for smooth muscles in its speed of contraction; the large size of its motor neurons; the distance between the muscle and the motor neurons (unlike the gut, for instance, where the cell bodies are actually within the muscle); and the unusual ultrastructure of the ciliary muscle cells, which in some ways resemble skeletal muscle (indeed, in birds it is a striated skeletal muscle). There are also regional differences in ultrastructure and histochemistry among different regions of the primate ciliary muscle, suggesting that the longitudinal portion may be acting like a fast skeletal muscle to "set" or "brace" the system rapidly, for the slightly slower contraction of the inner portion to be most effective.[39]

The ciliary muscle is composed of three muscle fiber groups identified by their relative positions and orientations, forming a morphologically and functionally integrated three-dimensional syncytium or reticulum[110] (Figure 7-4). The major group of muscle fibers is the peripheral meridional or longitudinal fibers, or Brücke's muscle.[11] They extend longitudinally between the scleral spur and the choroid adjacent to the sclera. Located inward to the longitudinal fibers are the reticular, or radial, fibers, which constitute a relatively smaller proportion of the ciliary muscle. The radial fibers are branching V- or Y-shaped fibers. They attach anteriorly to the scleral spur and the peripheral wall of the anterior ciliary body at the insertion of the iris and posteriorly to the elastic tendons of the choroid. Beneath the radial fibers and positioned more anteriorly in the ciliary body and closest to the lens are the equatorial or circular fibers, or Müller's muscle.[79] These constitute the smallest proportion of the ciliary muscle. The division of the ciliary muscle into three muscle fiber groups is somewhat artificial. In reality, there is a gradual transition from the outermost longitudinal muscle fibers to the radial fibers to the innermost circular muscle fibers, with some intermingling of the different fiber types. A contraction of the ciliary muscle results in a contraction of all three muscle fiber groups together.

With a contraction of the ciliary muscle, there is a gradual rearrangement of fibers, with an increase in the proportion of circular fibers at the expense of the proportion of radial and longitudinal fibers.[110] A contraction of the entire ciliary muscle as a whole pulls the anterior choroid forward and serves the primary function of releasing resting zonular tension at the lens equator to allow accommodation to occur.

The Zonule. The zonular tissue has alternatively been called *zonular fibers, zonular apparatus, zonule,* or *zonules.* The zonular fibers are a complex meshwork of fibrils. Fibrils 70 to 80 nm in diameter are grouped into fiber bundles estimated to be between 4 to 50 μm in diameter.[24,29] The zonule is composed of the noncollagenous carbohydrate-protein mucopolysaccharide and glycoprotein complexes secreted by the ciliary epithelium. The zonular fibers are elastin-based elastic fibers and are thought to be much more elastic than the lens capsule. Their primary function is to stabilize the lens and allow accommodation to occur. Because the zonule is not a continuous tissue but is composed of fibers, it also allows fluid flow from the posterior chamber behind the iris through to the vitreous chamber (see Chapter 8).

Because of difficulty in visualizing the zonular fibers, the different techniques used to study it and the different terminology used to describe it, descriptions vary (Figure 7-5). The zonule arises from its posterior insertion at the posterior pars plana region of the ciliary body near the ora serrata. There the zonular fibers attach to the ciliary epithelium by the internal limiting membrane but do not enter the cytoplasm of the underlying cells.[62,90] The zonular fibers extend longitudinally toward the pars plicata of the ciliary body as a mat or flat meshwork of interlacing fibers. A few coronally oriented fibers run across the main fiber direction and are attached to the surface of the mat or more anteriorly to the crests of the ciliary processes.[24,90] Although scanning electron microscopy studies of fixed specimens suggest that this mat lies flat against the pars plana of the ciliary body, ultrasound biomicroscopy of living human and monkey eyes shows that the posterior zonule in fact follows a "straight line" path through the vitreous toward the tips of the ciliary processes.[48,70] This arrangement of the posterior zonule shows a pronounced nasal/temporal asymmetry in rhesus monkey eyes, with the zonule closer to the ciliary body nasally than temporally[48] (see Figure 7-5).

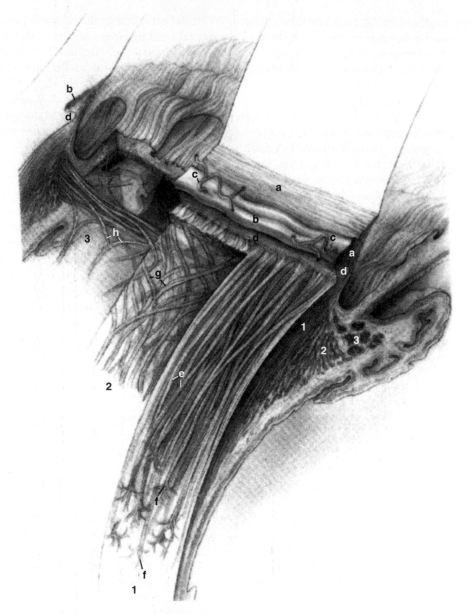

FIGURE 7-4   Drawing of the ciliary muscle showing a sequential dissection following removal of the outer layers of the globe to reveal the orientation of the underlying ciliary muscle fibers. After removal of the overlying sclera (*right*), first the meridional, or longitudinal, fibers; then the reticular, or radial, fibers; and finally the equatorial, or circular, fibers (*left*) of the ciliary muscle are revealed. (From Hogan MJ, Alvarado JA, Weddell JE: *Histology of the human eye*, Philadelphia, 1971, WB Saunders.)

A branching of the posterior zonule as it courses forward to the pars plicata is also observed. Most posterior zonular fibers course forward to the pars plicata and enter the valleys between the ciliary processes, inserting into the ciliary epithelium of the valleys and the walls of the ciliary processes.[29] This region is generally considered to separate the posterior zonule from the anterior zonule.[29] These zonu-

lar regions are alternatively called the *pars plana zonular fibers* and the *anterior zonule*, or *zonulelike strands* and the *true zonule*, respectively.[24,90]

The description of the zonule as it passes through the pars plicata and ciliary processes to the lens varies. Although scanning electron microscopic images clearly show zonular fibers passing from the pars plana zonule through the valleys be-

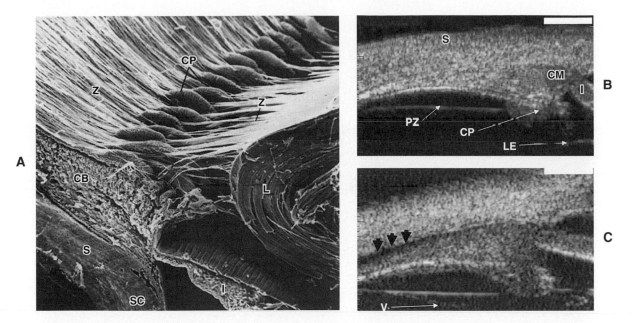

FIGURE 7-5   A, Scanning electron micrograph (SEM) of the accommodative apparatus of a cynomolgus monkey eye. Note that in the SEM the anterior zonular fibers appear to insert at the lens (*L*) equator in discreet bundles (see Figure 7-8) and that the posterior zonular (*Z*) fibers appear as a flat mat or meshwork of fibers against the ciliary body (*CB*). These features of the anterior and posterior zonule may be caused by artifact associated with the tissue processing required of SEM. When the zonule is viewed in unfixed tissues either directly or with ultrasound biomicroscopy (*UBM*) in the intact primate eye (**B** and **C**), these features of the zonular apparatus are not observed. **B,** UBM image of the temporal quadrant of a living, atropinized rhesus monkey eye. A bundle of posterior zonular fibers extends as a straight line between the ciliary processes (*CP*) and the posterior attachment of the ciliary muscle (*CM*). (Scale bar = 1 mm.) **C,** UBM image of an intact, enucleated human donor eye. Here too, a posterior zonular fiber bundle appears as a straight line (when carefully oriented such that the bundle is orthogonal to the plane of oscillation of the UBM transducer), extending between the ciliary processes and the posterior attachment of the ciliary muscle. The vitreous face (*V*) appears as a diffuse line coursing away from the PZ bundle. The ciliary muscle has become detached from the sclera (*S*) (*arrowheads*), an artifact commonly observed in postmortem, enucleated eyes. (Scale bar = 1 mm.) *I,* Iris; *L,* lens; *SC,* Schlemm's canal. (**A** from Rohen JW: *Invest Ophthalmol Vis Sci* 18:137, 1979, with permission from the Association for Research in Vision and Ophthalmology and the author. **B** from Glasser A et al: *Optom Vis Sci* 78:417, 2001.)

tween the ciliary processes and on to the anterior zonule (Figure 7-6), others suggest that this is not the case and that these anterior zonular fibers originate from the ciliary epithelium along the ridges of the ciliary processes without passing through the processes.[24,29,90] Tissue-processing techniques, specimen age, comparisons between healthy and pathologic tissues, and comparisions between humans and monkeys may account for these differences. Rohen[90] differentiates between two functionally different sets of zonular fibers: the *main fiber* and the *spanning, or tension, fiber system.* The tension fiber system consists of many finer strands that join each other to form the zonular plexus; the plexus attaches the zonule to the ciliary epithelium in the ciliary process valleys. This anchors the anterior and pars plana zonule to the ciliary epithelium of the ciliary body and serves as a fulcrum. Anteriorly,

the zonule splits to form the *zonular fork* of two main fiber groups extending to the anterior and posterior lens surfaces (Figure 7-7). Finally, the anterior zonule inserts onto the capsule at the lens equatorial region and terminates within zonular lamella of the lens capsule.[90] On the lens anterior surface the zonule is a broad and flattened ramification or band inserting approximately the same distance from the lens equator along a circular line.[24,75,90] The insertion of the zonule onto the posterior capsular surface is at a variety of levels and is not as evenly distributed as the circular line visible on the anterior lens surface.[29,75]

The attachment of the zonular fibers to the lens capsule is superficial, with few fibers penetrating into the capsule with a mechanical (possibly similar to Velcro) or chemical union.[31] On the basis of scanning electron microscopy, this anterior zonule

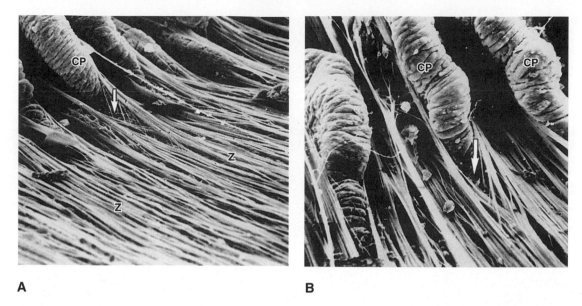

A   **B**

FIGURE 7-6   Posterior zonular fibers entering into the valleys between the ciliary processes at the transition zone between the pars plana and the pars plicata. The zonular fibers cross in a regular pattern at the posterior end of the ciliary processes (*arrows*). *CP,* Ciliary process; *Z,* zonule. (Scanning electron micrograph, cynomolgus monkey; **A,** ×200, **B,** ×240). (From Rohen JW: *Invest Ophthalmol Vis Sci* 18:1136, 1979, with permission from the Association for Research in Vision and Ophthalmology and the author.)

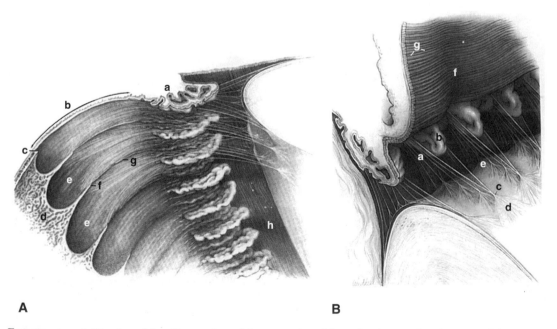

A   **B**

FIGURE 7-7   **A,** Drawing of the ciliary region of the eye as viewed from the vitreous chamber. From left to right, anterior to the ora serrata of the retina is the ciliary body consisting of the pars plana, the pars plicata, and ciliary processes. The mat of posterior zonular fibers on the pars plana extend toward the valleys between the ciliary processes. The anterior zonular fibers extend across the circumlental space and insert into the capsule at the lens equator. **B,** Drawing of the circumlental space and anterior zonules as viewed from the anterior chamber after the iris is raised up. The anterior zonule extends from the valleys between the ciliary processes, across the circumlental space to the capsule at the lens equator. (From Hogan MJ, Alvarado JA, Weddell JE: *Histology of the human eye,* Philadelphia, 1971, WB Saunders.)

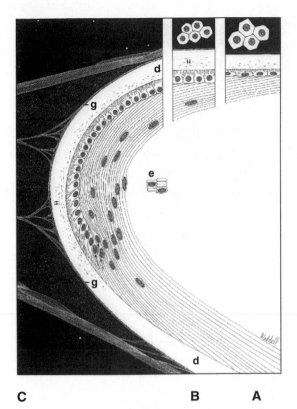

C   **B**   **A**

Figure 7-8 A composite drawing of the lens cortex, epithelium, capsule, and zonular attachments. At **A** is the anterior central lens epithelium, seen in flat and cross section. The size and shape of these cells can be compared with those in **B**, the intermediate zone, and **C**, the equatorial zone. At the lens equator the dividing cells are elongated to form lens cortical cells. As they elongate, they send processes anteriorly and posteriorly toward the sutures, and their nuclei migrate somewhat anterior to the equator to form the lens bow. At the same time the nuclei become more and more displaced into the lens as new cells are formed at the equator. The lens capsule (*d*) is thicker anterior and posterior to the equator than it is at the equator itself. The anterior and equatorial capsule contains fine filamentous inclusions (*b* and *c; double arrows*); these are not present posteriorly. Zonular fibers (*f*) are depicted to attach to the anterior, posterior, and equatorial capsule, forming the pericapsular or zonular lamella of the lens (*g*). This depiction, not observed in fresh unfixed tissues (see Figure 7-5), may be an artifact of tissue-processing techniques. (From Hogan MJ, Alvarado JA, Weddell JE: *Histology of the human eye,* Philadelphia, 1971, WB Saunders.)

crossing the circumlental space and extending to the lens is alternatively described as (1) consisting of three fiber strands running to the anterior, equatorial, and posterior lens surfaces; (2) fibers that insert along a circular line on the anterior and posterior surface of the lens with some fibers inserting di-

rectly on the equator; (3) a zonular fork with two main fiber groups extending to the lens anterior and posterior surfaces with finer bundles seemingly of relatively unimportance running to the lens equator; or (4) successive sagittal lines of insertion from lens anterior to posterior surface and two coronal lines of insertion, one where the fibers insert onto the capsule around the anterior surface and another where the fibers insert onto the capsule around the posterior surface[24,29,75,77,90] (Figure 7-8).

Although no systematic crossing of anterior zonular fibers was described by McCulloch,[77] crossing has been seen by others in both the human and monkey.[24,29,42] From histologic preparations, when an appropriate plane of section is obtained, a continuous line of zonular insertion into the entire lens equator is seen.[77] Unfixed specimens show a continuous meshwork of fibers uniformly covering the entire lens equator and crossing of zonular fibers[42] (Figure 7-9).

Observations of the ciliary region during accommodation show that the posterior ciliary body slides forward against the curvature of the anterior sclera, moving the posterior insertion of the posterior zonule forward. However, contraction of the ciliary muscle stretches the posterior zonule as a result of a greater forward movement of the tips of the ciliary processes. This suggests that the stretched posterior zonule may assist in pulling the ciliary muscle back to its unaccommodated position after an accommodative effort ceases.

The Crystalline Lens. The crystalline lens is surrounded by the lens capsule (Figures 7-8 and 7-9). The human capsule is not of uniform thickness. Fincham[33] studied the capsule in histologic section and found it to be of relatively uniform thickness in nonaccommodating mammals; however, in primates, Fincham determined that the capsule is thickest at the peripheral anterior surface and thins again toward the lens equatorial region. On the posterior surface the capsule shows a peripheral thickening, but it is thinnest at the region of the posterior pole of the lens.[32] The lens itself consists of a nucleus and a cortex (Figure 7-10). The embryonic nucleus, present at birth, remains present at the center of the lens throughout life as the cortex, by the addition of an increasing number of layers of lens fiber cells, grows progressively around it. The lens consists of layers of lens fiber cells laid down in a radial pattern. The lens grows throughout life by adding lens fibers at its outer edge and shows a linear increase in mass with increasing age. The lens thickness increases

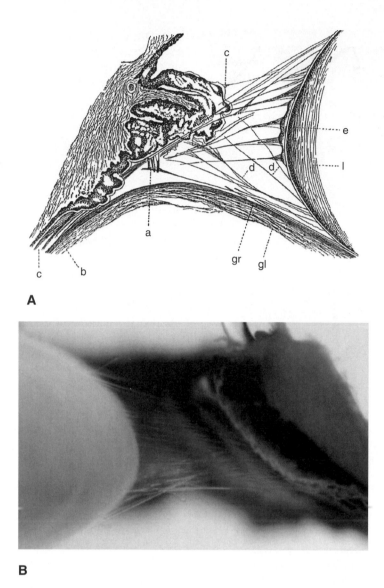

A

B

FIGURE 7-9   Because of the delicate nature of the zonule and the difficulties in observing it, descriptions of the insertion of the anterior zonule onto the lens equator differ. **A,** Early anatomists with relatively crude methods produced remarkably accurate diagrams of the structure of the anterior zonule showing crossing of zonular fibers, fiber bundles of varying thickness, and insertion into a thickened region of the capsule at the lens equator. **B,** Photograph of a partially dissected 42-year-old human eye showing uniform insertion of the zonule around the lens equator, crossing of zonular fibers and the insertion of these anterior zonular fibers all along the length of the ciliary process. (**A** from Helmholtz von HH: *Handbuch der Physiologishen Optik,* New York, 1909, Dover. [Translated by JPC Southall, 1962.]) **B** from Glasser A, Campbell MCW: *Vision Res* 38:209, 1998, with permission from Elsevier Science Ltd.)

---

with a resulting increase in the anterior surface and posterior surface curvatures with increasing age. It has also been suggested that the lens equatorial diameter increases throughout life, although recent measurements disprove this and show that the adult lens diameter is age independent.[106]

The crystalline lens has a gradient refractive index, with a refractive index of 1.385 near the poles and a higher refractive index of 1.406 at the center of the nucleus. The lens is not optically homogeneous, and when viewed through a slit lamp, several optical zones of discontinuity are observed, which allow visual differentiation of the lens nucleus from the surrounding lens cortex. The unaccommodated young adult human lens is roughly 9.0 mm in diameter and 3.6 mm thick. The lens thickness increases by approximately 0.5 mm with 8 diopters of accommodation.

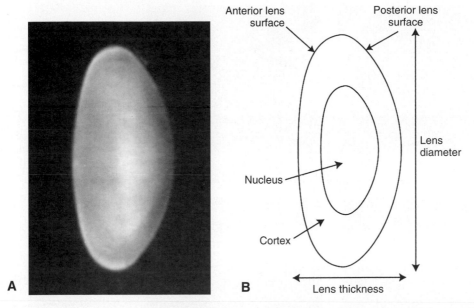

FIGURE 7-10 Photograph of the profile of an isolated 75-year-old human lens (**A**) and outline of the same lens showing the relative arrangements of the lens nucleus and cortex (**B**). The lens anterior surface curvature is flatter than the posterior surface curvature.

The Mechanism of Accommodation

Our current understanding of the accommodative mechanism stems primarily from the early writings of Helmholtz and Gullstrand[51] and Fincham[33] (Figure 7-11). At rest, when the eye is focused for distance, resting tension on the zonular fibers spanning the circumlental space (collectively called the *anterior zonule*) applies an outward directed tension on the lens equator through the lens capsule. This holds the lens in a relatively flattened and unaccommodated state. When the ciliary muscle contracts, the inner apex of the ciliary body moves forward and toward the axis of the eye (Figure 7-12). This results in a stretching of the posterior attachment of the ciliary muscle to the choroid and the posterior zonular fibers. The movement of the apex of the ciliary muscle releases the resting tension on all the zonular fibers inserting on the lens. On release of the outward-directed force at the lens equator, the lens capsule molds the lens substance into a more spherical, accommodated form.[33] The lens diameter decreases, and the anterior surface curvature and, to a lesser extent, the lens posterior surface curvature increase and the lens thickness increases (Figure 7-13). This results in an increase in the optical power of the crystalline lens. In addition, the anterior chamber depth is decreased as a result of the forward movement of the lens anterior surface. There is also a small decrease in vitreous chamber depth because of posterior movement of

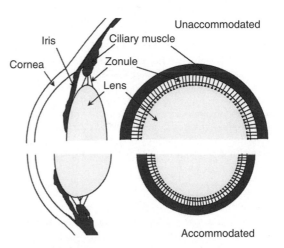

FIGURE 7-11 Diagram showing the Helmholtz accommodative mechanism. In the upper half of the diagram, the eye is in the unaccommodated state. In the lower half, the eye is in the accommodated state. The *left side* shows a sagittal section and the *right side* a frontal section through the anterior segment of the eye. In the unaccommodated state, resting tension on the zonule at the lens equator holds the lens in a relatively flattened and unaccommodated state. When the ciliary muscle contracts, this resting zonular tension is released and the lens is allowed to round up through the force exerted on the lens substance by the lens capsule. Lens axial thickness increases, lens equatorial diameter decreases, anterior chamber depth decreases, and vitreous chamber depth decreases with accommodation The lens anterior and posterior surface curvatures increase to increase the optical power of the lens. (Redrawn from Koretz JF, Handelman GH: *Sci Am* 259:92, 1988, with permission from the artist.)

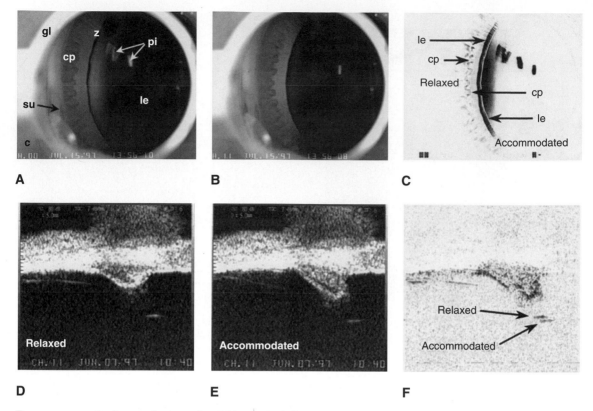

FIGURE 7-12   Gonioscopy images of an iridectomized rhesus monkey eye in the unaccommodated (**A**) and accommodated (**B**) state. **C,** The subtracted difference image shows the accommodative movements of the lens equator and ciliary processes and the relative stability of the eye. The lens equator and the ciliary processes move away from the sclera, with accommodation to roughly the same extent. Ultrasound biomicroscopy images of an iridectomized rhesus monkey eye in the unaccommodated (**D**) and accommodated (**E**) states. **F,** The subtracted difference image shows the accommodative movements of the ciliary muscle and the lens equator. The apex of the ciliary muscle and the lens equator (*short horizontal line* and identified with *arrows*) move away from the sclera with accommodation. *c,* Cornea; *cp,* ciliary processes; *gl,* gonioscopy lens; *le,* lens; *pi,* lens Purkinje images; *su,* suture; *z,* zonule. (From Glasser A, Kaufman PL: *Ophthalmology* 106:863, 1999, with permission from Elsevier Science Ltd.)

the lens posterior surface. This too contributes to an overall increase in the refractive power of the eye. When the accommodative effort ceases, the elasticity of the posterior attachment of the choroid and the posterior zonular fibers pulls the ciliary muscle back toward its flattened and unaccommodated configuration. This once again increases the resting tension on the anterior zonular fibers at the lens equator to pull the lens into its flattened and unaccommodated configuration.

Modifications to the classical description of the accommodative mechanism have been provided by Gullstrand[51] and now also include a well-accepted role for the lens capsule.[33] Clearly, the capsule provides the major force, if not all of the force, to accommodate the lens, and the lens substance in fact retards the extent and rate of capsule movement. When the lens substance is removed in monkeys, leaving the empty cap-

sular bag still suspended by the zonule, the elasticity of the empty capsular bag actively pulls the ciliary processes inward faster and to a greater extent during an accommodative effort than when the lens substance is present.[22] Variants on this generalized accommodative mechanism have been described to include a prominent role for the vitreous, which is questioned.[13,14,38] Revisionist accommodative theories have been presented but are not supported by experimental evidence in primates.[45,95,99]

Tscherning[115] suggested that accommodation occurs through a flattening of the peripheral lens surface curvature and an increase in the curvature of the central lens surface. Tscherning in part erroneously reached this conclusion from studying the behavior of lenses from ungulate eyes, which almost certainly do not accommodate. Pig lenses, for example, have spherical surface curvatures and are firmer and dis-

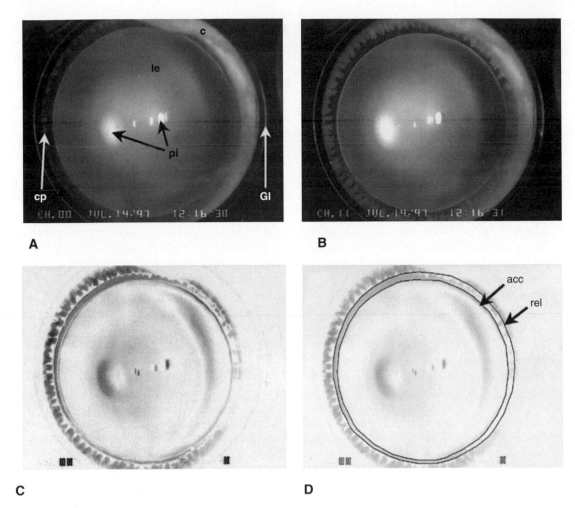

FIGURE 7-13 Goldmann lens images of an iridectomized rhesus monkey eye in the unaccommodated (**A**) and accommodated (**B**) states. **C,** Subtracted difference image to show the accommodative movements of the lens. The lens undergoes a concentric decrease in diameter and the ciliary processes move concentrically inward with accommodation. There is a virtual absence of eye movements, as evident form the absence of additional detail in the difference image. **D,** The outlines of the accommodated and unaccommodated lens diameter are shown superimposed on the difference image demonstrating a concentric decrease in lens diameter with accommodation in accordance with the Helmholtz accommodative mechanism. *acc,* Accommodated; *c,* conjunctiva; *cp,* ciliary process; *Gl,* Goldmann lens; *le,* lens; *pi,* lens Purkinje images; *rel,* relaxed. (From Glasser A, Kaufman PL: *Ophthalmology* 106:863, 1999, with permission from Elsevier Science Ltd.)

---

similar to accommodative lenses.[120] Tscherning[115] describes squeezing the equator of ox and horse lenses and observing a flattening of the lens surfaces, or pulling on the zonules and observing an increase in curvature. Tscherning's theory has again been proposed, but without a role for the vitreous, as Tscherning originally suggested.[95] Ironically, the behavior of nonaccommodating bovine lenses is, once again, offered as proof of this theory.[98] Acceptance of this alternative theory requires significant modification of thinking on the anatomy of the accommodative apparatus and its action. It is suggested that the zonule at the lens equator is composed of three distinct groups of fibers, which originate at the anterior, equatorial, and posterior lens equatorial surfaces; that the equatorial zonular fibers insert not to the base of the ciliary body, but to the anterior face of the ciliary muscle beneath the iris; and that the anterior and posterior fibers course through the ciliary processes to the ciliary body. It is suggested that a contraction of the ciliary muscle selectively moves the anterior face of the ciliary muscle posteriorly to increase tension on the equatorial zonular group while releasing tension on the anterior and posterior zonular groups.[95] It is postulated that this increases lens diameter during accommodation, to flatten the peripheral lens surface curvature and increases the central lens surface curvature. Although small movements of the lens equator toward the sclera have been described during accommodation in humans, other studies show a more pronounced movement of the lens equator away from the sclera.[100,122] Experimental investigations in live monkeys show no evidence to support this revisionist accommodative mechanism.[45]

The Stimulus to Accommodate

At rest, the eyes have some residual or resting level of accommodation amounting to approximately 1.5 diopters. This is called *tonic accommodation.* The act of accommodation causes three physiologic responses: The pupil constricts, the eyes converge, and the eyes accommodate. Together these are referred to as the *accommodative triad,* or the *near reflex.* These three actions are neuronally coupled through the preganglionic parasympathetic innervation extending from the Edinger-Westphal (EW) nucleus in the brain. The intraocular muscles are innervated by the postganglionic parasympathetic innervation. The extraocular muscles of the eyes are innervated by the oculomotor (III), trochlear (IV), and abducent (VI) nerves, the axons of which originate from motor nerve nuclei in the brainstem, which receive impulses from the EW nucleus. Accommodation and convergence are coupled in both eyes. An accommodative stimulus presented monocularly results in a binocular accommodation and convergence response. Similarly, a convergence stimulus in one eye results in pupil constriction, convergence, and accommodation in both eyes.

Accommodation can be stimulated in various ways. Accommodation is blur driven. If a myopic blur is presented to one or both eyes by placing a negative-powered lens in front of the eye, the eyes will accommodate in an attempt to overcome the imposed defocus. If the vergence of the eyes is increased, for instance by placing base-out prisms in front of the eyes, pupil constriction, convergence, and accommodation occur. These two stimulus conditions result in coupled binocular accommodation. Blur- and vergence-driven accommodation can be induced simultaneously through a proximal stimulus. If a near object is presented, coupled accommodation and convergence occur.

Studies aimed at addressing how the eye detects defocus have shown that the longitudinal chromatic aberration (LCA) of the eye is an important factor. The optics of the eye cause considerable LCA, with the result that short wavelengths of light are focused further forward in the eye than the long wavelengths. Removing the LCA by testing under monochromatic light or optically neutralizing or reversing the LCA disrupts the normal reflex accommodative response.[69] In addition, the eye focuses more accurately when broader spectral bandwidths are available than in monochromatic light.[1]

Accommodation can also be induced through pharmacologic stimulation. Topical application of muscarinic cholinergic agonists (e.g., pilocarpine) to the human eye results in direct pharmacologic stimulation of the ciliary muscle.[20] In rhesus monkeys, pharmacologically stimulated accommodation is found to be of higher amplitude than centrally stimulated accommodation attributable to a supramaximal pharmacologic response of the ciliary muscle and iris, which is unlikely to occur naturally.[18,19,65] Pupil constriction also occurs with pharmacologic stimulation, but convergence does not. When applied topically, anticholinesterases such as echothiophate iodide produce a resting tonus of accommodation.[57] This results from the spontaneous release of acetylcholine at the neuromuscular junction, normally broken down by cholinesterases. Accommodative esotropia, often occurring in uncorrected persons with hyperopia as a consequence of a need to accommodate even to see distant objects in focus, can be treated with topical echothiophate. With an increased production of accommodative tonus without an increased neuronal input, the stimulus for convergence is lessened, and the reduced accommodation convergence/accommodation (AC/A) ratio is lessened, helping alleviate the accommodative esotropia.[84] Certain anticholinesterases produce a long response to a single administration and so are more therapeutically useful than shorter-acting cholinomimetics such as pilocarpine (see Chapter 36).

The Pharmacology of Accommodation

Accommodation occurs when the postganglionic parasympathetic innervation to the ciliary muscle releases the neurotransmitter acetylcholine at the neuromuscular junctions. Acetylcholine is a muscarinic agonist that binds with the muscarinic receptors in the ciliary muscle to cause the muscle to contract. Topically applied muscarinic agonists, such as pilocarpine, also bind to the muscarinic receptors and cause ciliary muscle contraction. This results in an involuntary monocular accommodative response, which in some individuals can be of higher amplitude than voluntary accommodation and is greater in eyes with lighter colored irises.[123] The sensitivity of an individual to topically applied autonomic drugs depends on iris pigmentation, with individuals having light-colored irides (blue) being more sensitive. Individuals with dark irides (brown) are less sensitive because of increased pigment in the iris pigment epithelium and the ciliary muscle itself, which binds topically applied agents and decreases their bioavailability for stimulating the ciliary muscle. The dependence of ocular pigmentation on the ocular hypotensive response to pilocarpine, also through the action of the drug on the ciliary muscle, is well known.[50] Just as accommodation can be stimulated pharmacologically, so too can accommodation be pharmacologically blocked. This is called *cycloplegia.* Cycloplegia can be induced by topical application of muscarinic antagonists such as atropine, cyclopentolate, or tropicamide. These agents competitively bind to the same muscarinic receptors as the agonists but do not activate the receptor, thereby preventing the agonist binding and so blocking accommodation.

Measurement of Accommodation

Although good objective methods are available for measurement of accommodation, unfortunately, clinically subjective methods are used most often. The push-up method requires the patient to report when a near letter chart can no longer be maintained in sharp focus as the chart is gradually brought closer to the eye. This requires a subjective evaluation of best image focus, which can be influenced by depth of focus, visual acuity, contrast sensitivity of the eye, and contrast of the image, for example. A dimly illuminated reading chart may provide a poor stimulus to accommodate or may not allow an accurate detection of defocus. Different levels of illumination alter pupil diameter and depth of focus of the eye, thus influencing the apparent accommodative amplitude. Push-up measurements are also confounded by increasing image size as a reading chart is brought closer to the eye unless carefully controlled by maintaining the image angular magnification with scaled letter sizes. An alternative subjective measurement of accommodative amplitude can also be obtained with negatively powered trial lenses placed in front of one or both eyes to blur a distant letter chart and stimulate accommodation. Lens power can be increased until the smallest legible letter line of a distance Snellen letter chart can no longer be maintained in sharp focus. Accommodative amplitude is determined by the strongest powered negative lens through which

the smallest legible Snellen letter line can still be read clearly.

Subjective methods traditionally used for evaluating accommodative amplitude are inherently inaccurate and tend to overestimate true accommodative amplitude. Near vision can be and is improved through nonaccommodative optical compensation. Multifocal intraocular lenses or multifocal contact lenses, for example, allow some functional near vision to persons with presbyopia, but without accommodation. Similarly, astigmatism or ocular aberrations provide some degree of multifocality to the eye. The ability to read near text does not imply that accommodation occurs, and subjective methods to measure accommodation cannot differentiate between true accommodation and optical compensation such as occurs with multifocal contact lenses.

Because accommodation results in a change in refractive power of the eye, it can readily be measured objectively. Objective methods should be used to get a true measure of accommodative amplitude. Accurate objective measurement of accommodation requires the use of either static or dynamic refractometers.[66,76,101] Only when objective methods are used is a complete loss of accommodation demonstrated at the end point of presbyopia, as is the absence of accommodation after scleral expansion surgery to restore accommodation.[66,76] The success of objective instruments to measure maximal accommodation relies on the accuracy and measurement range of the instrument and on the elicitation of the maximal accommodative response from the subject. Objective instruments differ in whether they measure static refraction or dynamic accommodation. If a single static measurement is made, this may miss the point of maximum accommodation. Dynamic optometers sometimes provide a real-time graphic display of the accommodative response and provide a reliable method to ascertain true accommodative amplitude. The success of these instruments at measuring maximal accommodation also depends on how well distant and near targets can be presented and whether monocular or binocular measurements can be made.

Accommodation can be stimulated in a number of ways. If a negative-powered trial lens is placed in front of one eye while viewing a distant letter chart, the consensual accommodative response can be measured in the contralateral eye. Accommodation can also be stimulated by topically applied muscarinic agonists (e.g., pilocarpine); the resulting accommodative response can be measured periodically over 30 to 45 minutes until the maximal response is attained (Figure 7-14). The accommodative amplitude measured in this way is independent of a visible accommodative stimulus and of patient subjectivity. However, the response does depend on dose, intraocular pharmacokinetics, iris pigmentation, and other factors that influence how much or how quickly the drug reaches the ciliary muscle.

PRESBYOPIA

Presbyopia is the age-related loss in accommodative ability and results in a nearly complete loss in accommodative ability by about 50 years of age. Duane[27] measured the subjective push-up amplitude of accommodation in approximately 1500 subjects as a function of age (see Figure 7-1). He found that the gradual age-related loss of accommodation starts early in life and that about 1 diopter of accommodation still remains after 50 years of age. Objective measurement of accommodation shows a linear decline of about 2.3 diopters per decade, culminating in a complete loss of accommodation by about age 50.8 years.[66] Subjective measurement in the same subjects shows a 2-diopter higher accommodative amplitude in youth and a slightly faster decline of 2.4 diopters per decade, with a residual accommodative amplitude of about 2 diopters after age 50.[66]

Presbyopia may be unique in that it results in the complete loss of a physiologic function roughly two thirds of the way through the human life span. Few other physiologic functions undergo such a profound and systematic deterioration so soon and with such certainty in so many individuals. Presbyopia must be a consequence of age changes in the accommodative apparatus that begin early in life and continue beyond the point at which accommodation is lost, possibly until death. Because two thirds of our accommodative amplitude is lost between ages 15 and 35, this is the age group of most interest in trying to understand the progression of the "disease." However, although what happens after the age of 45 to 50 may not be of particular relevance as far as causes of presbyopia, these age changes may represent a part of the continuum that earlier in life leads to presbyopia. Understanding the causes of presbyopia may be best achieved by studying how and why accommodation is lost, but understanding the age changes that continue beyond the age of presbyopia may also provide important insights.

Factors Contributing to Presbyopia

Because the accommodative apparatus is composed of many different tissues and systems and accommodation is a complex interaction of these components, the factors potentially contributing to presbyopia are

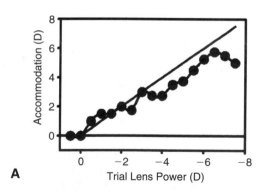

A Trial Lens Power (D)

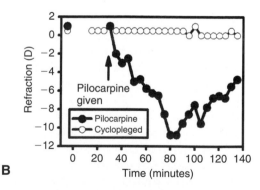

B Time (minutes)

FIGURE 7-14   Two techniques for objective measurement of accommodation in humans. **A,** The accommodative response of the right eye is measured with a Hartinger coincidence refractometer as increasingly powered negative trial lenses are placed in front of the left eye of a 35-year-old subject viewing a distant letter chart. As the letter chart is viewed through increasing powered negative trial lenses, the accommodative response increases toward the maximal accommodative amplitude of 6 diopters. A further increase in trial lens power results in no further increase in accommodation. **B,** The right eye is dilated with one drop of phenylephrine, and the baseline resting refraction is measured four times in both eyes. The left eye (*open symbols*) is then cyclopleged with 1% cyclopentolate, and accommodation is stimulated in the right eye (*solid symbols*) with one drop of 6% pilocarpine. Refraction is measured in each eye three times at the end of each 5-minute interval with a Hartinger coincidence refractometer. The pilocarpine stimulated accommodative response in the right eye of the same 35-year-old subject as in **A** reaches a maximum of 11 diopters approximately 30 minutes after instillation of pilocarpine. The pilocarpine-stimulated accommodative response is greater than the voluntary accommodative response elicited from negative lens–induced defocus.

numerous. Aging affects many of these tissues and systems to different extents; therefore the reasons accommodation is lost as a consequence of aging are potentially many and complex. Although several fundamental changes that occur, such as loss of compliance of the posterior attachment of the ciliary muscle or hardening of the lens, must necessarily have a profound effect on the ability of the eye to accommodate, consideration must be given to each aspect of ocular aging and how it may affect accommodative amplitude. Furthermore, many studies of the aging eye show age changes that progress beyond that age at which accommodation is lost. Most fundamental to understanding the causes of presbyopia are the age changes that occur between the ages of 15 and 45, the period during which most of the accommodative amplitude is lost. In the following sections, age changes in the ciliary muscle, lens, lens capsule, zonule, and associated tissues are considered in terms of their possible roles in presbyopia.

Age Changes in Rhesus Ciliary Muscle. Histologic investigations show that the rhesus monkey ciliary muscle undergoes chanes with increasing age.[70] However, because accommodation is lost with increasing age and is mediated by the ciliary muscle, the question arises whether presbyopia results from a loss in ability of the ciliary muscle to contract. Because pupillary constriction and convergence are part of the near reflex but do not decrease with increasing age, this suggests that loss of muscle contractility is not a normal part of presbyopia.[7] Accommodative excursion of the ciliary muscle is reduced in presbyopic rhesus monkeys, as seen from both direct observation in surgically aniridic animals in which accommodation is stimulated by an electrode placed in the EW nucleus and from histologic study of ciliary muscle topography in eyes fixed in the presence of pilocarpine or atropine[73,81] (Figure 7-15). The posterior attachment of the rhesus ciliary muscle, which is composed of elastic tendons continuous with Bruch's membrane, show pronounced structural changes with increasing age.[108] Whereas the elastic tendons of the young monkey eye stain strongly for actin and desmin, in the aging eye, this region exhibits increased collagen fibers that adhere to the elastic fibers, thickening of the elastic tendons, and increased microfibrils[109] (Figure 7-16). These anatomic changes may lead to decreased compliance of the posterior attachment of the ciliary muscle and the choroid. This is supported by the observation that in aged rhesus monkey eyes in which the posterior attachment of the

ciliary muscle is severed before pilocarpine stimulation, a configurational change occurs that is otherwise absent[109] (Figure 7-17). The contractile force of isolated rhesus ciliary muscle strips to pilocarpine stimulation is not reduced with increasing age[88] (Figure 7-18). Although there is some loss of ciliary muscle mass, there is no loss of muscarinic receptor number or binding affinity, nor is there any change in cholineacetyltransferase or acetylcholinesterase activity.[114] These histologic, histochemical, and ultrastructural studies show that the reduced ciliary muscle accommodative movement in presbyopic monkey eyes is caused by a loss of elasticity of the posterior attachment of the ciliary muscle and choroid to the sclera. This tissue is normally elastic and is stretched during accommodation in the young eye. If the tissue becomes less extensible with advancing age, the ciliary muscle must work harder to move forward during accommodation. At the extreme, ciliary muscle contraction becomes essentially isometric with no forward movement. Together these findings suggest that decreased compliance of the posterior attachment of the ciliary muscle must be considered as a factor in presbyopia in rhesus monkeys.

Age Changes in Human Ciliary Muscle. With increasing age, the human ciliary muscle shows a loss of muscle fibers and an increase in connective tissue.[82,85,111] Despite this, studies using impedance cyclography to indirectly measure force of contraction of the ciliary muscle, or mechanical stretching of ocular tissues to infer force of contraction of the human ciliary muscle, suggest that human ciliary muscle contractile force does not decrease but indeed may increase and reach a maximum at the age at which presbyopia is manifest.[37,93,107] These findings are consistent with the maintenance of ciliary muscle contractile responses to cholinomimetic drugs throughout the life span in monkeys, but unfortunately, they do not provide information about configurational changes in the muscle upon accommodative effort. Histologic study of the atropinized human ciliary muscle shows that total area, area of longitudinal and reticular portion, and length of the muscle decrease with age. In addition, the inner apex of the unaccommodated ciliary muscle resides further forward and inward toward the anteroposterior axis in the aging eye, so the configuration of the older unaccommodated ciliary muscle appears more like that of the young accommodated ciliary muscle[111] (Figure 7-19). Whether this is causal or a consequence of the anterior zonule gradually

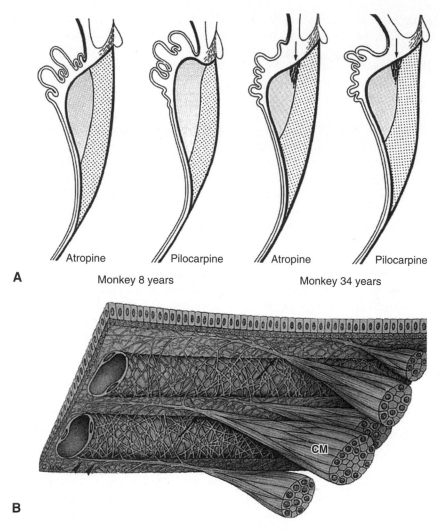

FIGURE 7-15   A, Diagrams of the configuration of the ciliary muscle (*CM*) from an 8-year-old (*left pair of images*) and a 34-year-old (*right pair of images*) enucleated rhesus monkey eye after each globe was bisected and one half (*left*) was placed in an atropine solution and the other half (*right*) was placed in a pilocarpine solution. Representative sections, based on histologic specimens, are shown. In the young, but not the old, eye, the pilocarpine-treated CM showed a configurational change similar to that which occurs with accommodation. The CM from the older eye fails to undergo an accommodative configurational change because of the loss of elasticity of the posterior attachment of the CM to the choroid. The 8-year-old rhesus monkey exhibits essentially no intramuscular connective tissue, whereas the 34-year-old rhesus monkey exhibits connective tissue (*arrows*) only anteriorly between longitudinal and reticular zones of the CM. **B,** Diagram of the posterior attachment of the CM in rhesus monkeys. The meridional muscle fiber bundles (*arrows*) are attached to the elastic layer of Bruch's membrane by means of the elastic tendons. Smaller elastic fibers connect (*arrowheads*) the tendons of different bundles to the elastic network that surrounds the vessels of the pars plana. (**A** from Lütjen-Drecoll E et al: *Arch Ophthalmol* 106:1591, 1988, with permission from the American Medical Association. **B** from Tamm E et al: *Invest Ophthalmol Vis Sci* 32:1680, 1991, with permission from the Association for Research in Vision and Ophthalmology and the author.)

---

pulling the ciliary muscle inward is unclear. On the basis of this result, it has been suggested that, at rest, the aged human ciliary muscle may be less able to hold or pull the crystalline lens into its flattened and unaccommodated configuration.[7]

Age Changes in the Zonule. The attachment of the anterior zonular fibers onto the equatorial region of the lens serves a fundamental role in the accommodative process. It is the outward force directed through these zonular fibers and the resulting ten-

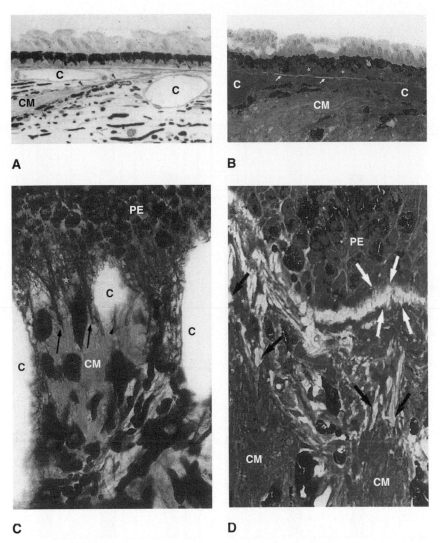

FIGURE 7-16   Histologic sections of the posterior attachment of the ciliary muscle (*CM*) in young and old rhesus monkeys. **A,** Young monkey meridional section. The posterior attachment of the CM is attached to Bruch's membrane (*arrows*) by the elastic tendon (*arrowheads*). *C,* Capillaries in the loose connective tissue. **B,** Young monkey, oblique-tangential section. The asterisk denotes the network of elastic fibers surrounding the vessels of the posterior ciliary body (see Figure 7-15, *B*) that connect the elastic tendons (*arrows*) to the CM bundles. This elastic network is continuous with the elastic layer of Bruch's membrane next to the pigment epithelium (*PE*). *C,* Capillaries. **C,** Old (31 years) monkey, meridional section. The elastic lamina of Bruch's membrane (*arrows*) is thickened, and a marked hyalinization is seen (*asterisks*) between the elastic lamina and the PE associated with the posterior ends of the meridional muscle bundles (*CM*). *C,* Capillary. **D,** Old (34 years) monkey, oblique-tangential section. Thickened and irregularly shaped elastic tendons (*arrows*) are seen originating from the muscle bundles (*CM*) in older eyes. Thickened and hyalinized connective tissue is observed between the elastic tendons and the ciliary PE. (From Tamm E et al: *Invest Ophthalmol Vis Sci* 32:1678, 1991, with permission from the Association for Research in Vision and Ophthalmology and the author.)

---

sion on the lens capsule that maintain the unaccommodated lens in its flattened state. The release of this resting tension during the act of accommodation allows the capsule to mold the lens into its more spherical and accommodated form.[33] Thus any age changes that may affect this zonular attachment are likely to affect the accommodative process

and may therefore contribute to presbyopia. The zonule is a fine, delicate network of fibers and is especially difficult to study; thus relatively few studies have been done. Zonular spring constants determined indirectly by stretching human tissues show no correlation with age.[117] Scanning electron microscopic studies of human eyes over a range of ages

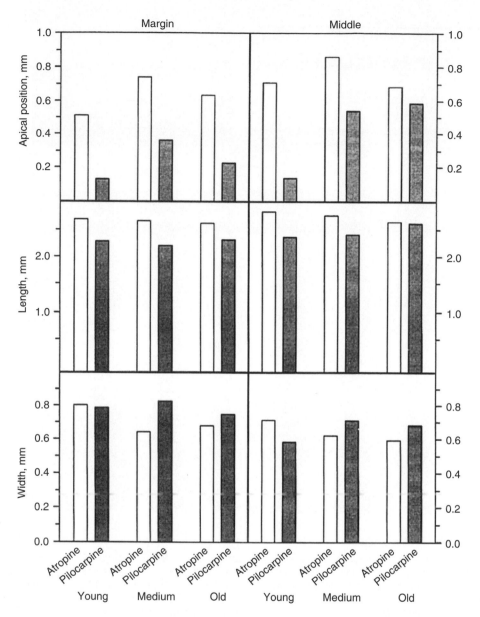

FIGURE 7-17   Bar graphs showing the results from morphometric tracings of the ciliary muscle from young, middle-aged, and old rhesus monkey eyes placed in fixative with atropine (*open bars*) or pilocarpine (*shaded bars*). The left column shows tracings from the ciliary muscle adjacent to the cut margin of bisected eyes. The right column shows data from tracings of the ciliary muscle in the middle of the bisected globe farthest from the cut margin. The top panel shows the anteroposterior position of the ciliary muscle apex in relation to the scleral spur; the middle panel, the length of the ciliary muscle; and the lower panel, the width of the ciliary muscle. Although an age-dependent configurational change in the ciliary muscle to pilocarpine stimulation is observed at the middle region of the globe (e.g., apical position and length), this age dependence is not observed in the ciliary muscle adjacent to the cut margin. The disruption of the posterior muscle tendons from sections adjacent to the cut margin allow configurational changes in the old monkey ciliary muscle while the configurational changes are prevented from occurring in those regions in which the posterior muscle tendons remain intact near the middle regions of the globe. (From Tamm E et al: *Arch Ophthalmol* 110:871, 1992, with permission from the American Medical Association.)

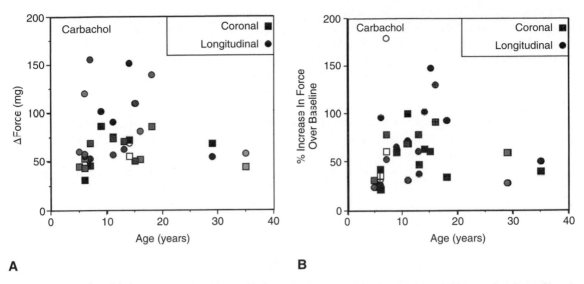

A   **B**

FIGURE 7-18   Force of contraction (**A**) and percentage of increase in force of contraction (**B**) over baseline of longitudinal (*circles*) and coronal (*squares*) strips of isolated rhesus monkey ciliary muscle stimulated with muscarinic agonists aceclidine (50 μM) or carbachol (1 μM). No age dependence in force of contraction of the isolated ciliary muscle was observed. (Adapted with new data from Poyer JF, Kaufman PL, Flügel C: *Curr Eye Res* 12:413, 1993, with permission from Swetz & Zeitlinger Publishers.)

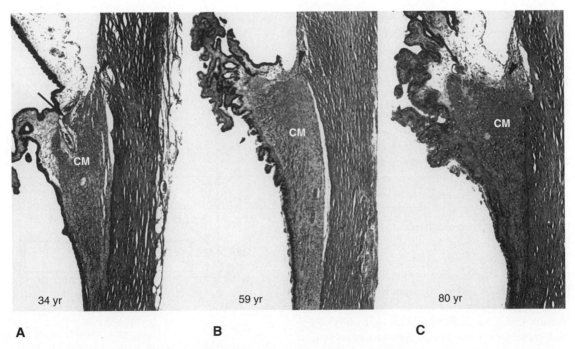

A   **B**   **C**

FIGURE 7-19   Age changes in the configuration of the atropinized human ciliary muscle. Histologic sections from a 34-year-old (**A**), a 59-year-old (**B**), and an 80-year-old (**C**) human donor eye. The aging, atropinized human ciliary muscle looks more like a young accommodated ciliary muscle with the inner apex of the ciliary muscle moving forward and toward the axis of the eye. (From Tamm S, Tamm E, Rohen JW: *Mech Ageing Dev* 62:209, 1992, with permission from Elsevier Science Ltd.)

have shown that an anterior zonular/capsular shift on the lens occurs with increasing age.[30] The distance from the zonular/capsule insertion to the lens equator increases, the distance from the zonular/capsule insertion to the ciliary processes is unchanged, the circumlental space decreases with age (see following discussion), and the rate of increase in distance from zonular/capsular insertion to lens equator remains relatively constant until the fifth decade and then increases dramatically.[30] On the basis of the constancy of the distance between the zonular/capsular insertion and the ciliary body, it is suggested that there would be no change in zonular length or zonular tension with increasing age provided zonular elasticity remains unchanged.

It is therefore possible that the decreased circumlental space previously described is either caused by centripetal pulling of the ciliary body by the zonule as the zonule/capsular shift occurs with increasing lens thickness or caused by the inward expansion of the ciliary muscle, rather than an increase in the equatorial diameter of the lens (see following discussion).[111] Farnsworth and Shyne[30] theorized that the anterior zonular shift occurs because the capsule is thinner on the posterior lens surface and is therefore stretched more than the anterior capsule as the lens continues to grow equatorially within the capsule. This anterior zonular/capsular shift may occur not through an increase in equatorial diameter of the lens but through the well-established increase in lens thickness, which can reliably be measured in vivo with A-scan ultrasonography. A zonular/capsular shift could reasonably occur because the posterior capsule is thinner and therefore likely to stretch more than the anterior capsule as lens thickness increases.[33] As a consequence of this zonular/capsular shift, in older eyes the attachment of the anterior zonular fiber to the lens is anterior to the equator, the fine zonular fibers that reside at the lens equator in the young eye are found anterior to the equator, and fewer zonular fibers are found at the equator.[30] This would result in diminution of the outward directed force on the lens equator by the anterior zonular fibers as a whole and is suggested as a contributing factor in the age-related loss of accommodation.[30] Measurements on unfixed human eyes from which the lens substance was removed by phacoemulsification also show an age-dependent increase in the distance from the anterior zonular/capsular insertion to the equatorial edge of the capsular bag, a decrease in circumlental space, and an age-dependent increase in the distance from the anterior zonular/capsular insertion to the ciliary body.[92] However, absence of the lens substance from the capsular bag complicates interpretation of these measurements.

Age Changes in the Capsule. The thickness of the anterior lens capsule increases from about 11 μm at birth to approximately 20 μm at 60 years and then decreases slightly thereafter.[34,94] Krag[67] found an increase from 11 to 33 μm up to age 75 and then a slight decrease thereafter. Fisher[34] measured the extensibility of the human lens capsule by applying a fluid pressure behind the central part of the anterior lens capsule clamped between two rings and found it to be 29% and age independent. Despite the increased capsular thickness with increasing age, Fisher[34] showed a decrease in Young's modulus of elasticity of the capsule from 6×10^7 dyn/cm^2 in infancy to 2×10^7 dyn/cm^2 in old age. Fisher suggests that the force that can be transmitted per unit thickness of the capsule decreases by half by age 60 but that the increased thickness offers some compensation for the loss of elasticity. Salzman[94] suggests that a loss of capsular thickness occurs with increasing age, especially at the lens equator, and that variations of capsular thickness are directly related to presence or absence of the zonular insertions. Age change in lens volume may account for the variations in thickness of the capsule at a specified region

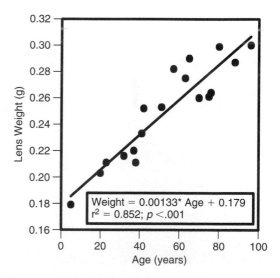

FIGURE 7-20 The human lens continues to grow throughout life, as evident from an increase in mass of the isolated human lens. The wet weight of 18 human lenses was measured after isolating the lenses from human eye-bank eyes ranging in age from 5 to 96 years of age. (From Glasser A, Campbell MCW: *Vis Res* 39:1991, 1999, with permission from Elsevier Science Ltd.)

on the lens. Krag, Olsen, and Andreasson's[67] measurements of extensibility of a ring cut from the anterior capsule show that although the young capsule can be stretched to 108% of its unstretched length, there is a linear decline in strain to 40% at age 98. The force required to break the capsular ring remained constant until age 35 and decreased linearly thereafter. With increasing age, the capsule gets thicker, less extensible, and more brittle.[67]

Growth of the Crystalline Lens. The crystalline lens continues to grow throughout life. In humans, this is reflected by the linear increase in mass of more than 1.5 times over the human life span[43] (Figure 7-20). The human lens also continues to increase in thickness as a consequence of the addition of lens fiber cells to the anterior and posterior cortex[66] (Figure 7-21). Scheimpflug slit-lamp measure-

ments show that both the anterior and posterior lens surface curvatures increase with increasing age.[10,28] This change in mass and volume of the lens results in a forward movement of the center of the lens and a decrease in anterior chamber depth, but without a change in the position of the posterior surface of the lens[66] (Figure 7-22). Qualitatively similar age changes have been identified in the anterior segment of the rhesus monkey eye.[64] Because the thickness and anterior and posterior surface curvatures of the lens increase with increasing age, the external shape of the aged lens resembles that of the young accommodated lens. However, the increased polar thickness with age is caused by an increase of the anterior and posterior cortical thickness, whereas accommodation in a young lens is caused by an increase in thickness of the nucleus.[9,10,63] In addition, the adult lens nuclear thickness does not

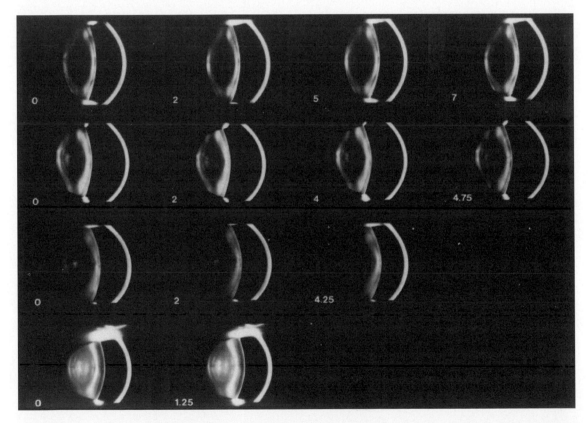

FIGURE 7-21 Composite of axial slit-lamp Scheimpflug photographs of human eyes. The corneal section is at the right of each panel. *First row,* 21-year-old subject; *left to right,* unaccommodated, 2, 5, and 7 diopters of accommodation. *Second row,* 28-year-old subject; unaccommodated, 2, 4, and 4.75 diopters of accommodation. *Third row,* 39-year-old subject; unaccommodated, 2, and 4.25 diopters of accommodation. *Forth row,* 57-year-old subject; unaccommodated and 1.25 diopters of accommodation. In each row the final panel is the maximum accommodation for that subject. Diopters of accommodation are given in the lower left corner of each panel. Lens thickness and curvature increase with increasing age and accommodation. Zones of discontinuity increase in number and prominence with age; after approximately 45 years the zones tend to merge. (From Hart WM Jr [ed]: *Adler's physiology of the eye,* St Louis, 1992, Mosby.)

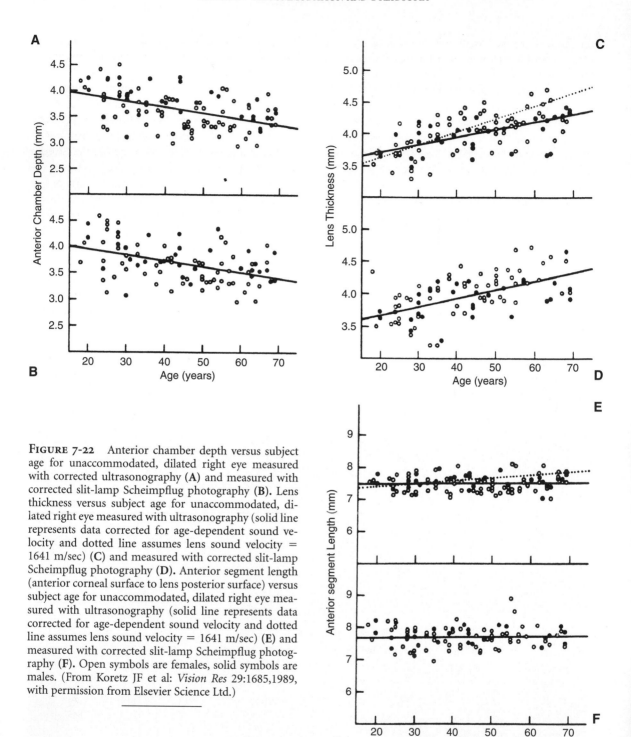

FIGURE 7-22 Anterior chamber depth versus subject age for unaccommodated, dilated right eye measured with corrected ultrasonography (**A**) and measured with corrected slit-lamp Scheimpflug photography (**B**). Lens thickness versus subject age for unaccommodated, dilated right eye measured with ultrasonography (solid line represents data corrected for age-dependent sound velocity and dotted line assumes lens sound velocity = 1641 m/sec) (**C**) and measured with corrected slit-lamp Scheimpflug photography (**D**). Anterior segment length (anterior corneal surface to lens posterior surface) versus subject age for unaccommodated, dilated right eye measured with ultrasonography (solid line represents data corrected for age-dependent sound velocity and dotted line assumes lens sound velocity = 1641 m/sec) (**E**) and measured with corrected slit-lamp Scheimpflug photography (**F**). Open symbols are females, solid symbols are males. (From Koretz JF et al: *Vision Res* 29:1685,1989, with permission from Elsevier Science Ltd.)

increase with growth. The optical changes that occur in the lens with accommodation and aging differ in several respects. Although accommodation results in an increase in the extent of the negative spherical aberration of young lenses, aging results in a systematic change in sign of spherical aberration from negative to positive.[42,43] Despite the external

similarity between the old lens and the young accommodated lens, the presbyopic eye clearly is not focused for near distance because presbyopia results in a loss of near vision. The incongruity between the increasing lens surface curvatures and the gradual loss of near vision has been termed the *lens paradox.*[60] It has been suggested that an age-related change in the gradient refractive index of the lens prevents the presbyopic eye from becoming nearsighted, despite the increasing lens surface curvatures.[86,104] If the increased power of the lens resulting from increasing surface curvatures is exactly compensated for by a decrease in the refractive index of the lens, overall lens power could be maintained. The increased thickness of the lens would also serve to reduce its refractive power in the face of increasing surface curvatures. Although age changes in the refractive index distribution of the lens are theoretically feasible, the practical difficulties in accurately measuring the lens gradient refractive index have precluded experimental verification.

In addition to the increased thickness and increased surface curvatures of the human lens, the equatorial diameter of the lens has been suggested to increase with age.[89,95,121] These works all directly or indirectly cite an original study in which lens equatorial diameter was measured in isolated human lenses.[105] Smith,[105] Fincham,[33] and Glasser and Campbell[42,43] recognized that when removed from the eye and isolated from external zonular forces, younger lenses tend to become accommodated while older presbyopic lenses do not undergo a change in shape. Until recently, it has been impossible to measure the diameter of the lens in the living eye. Therefore information on the change in diameter of the lens has relied on these measurements from human cadaver eyes. Because the lens becomes accommodated on removal from the eye, relatively more so for young accommodating lenses than for older presbyopic lenses, lens diameter is reduced relatively more in young than in older isolated lenses.[33,42] Studies of isolated lenses, therefore, compare young accommodated lenses with older unaccommodated lenses. Although such studies have found an age-dependent increase in lens diameter, this trend is almost certainly not caused by age but by the accommodative state of the isolated lens.[105] Therefore measurements from isolated adult lenses do not reflect the equatorial diameter of the lens in vivo. Recent studies have used magnetic resonance imaging (MRI) to measure the thickness and diameter of the lens in the living eye[106] (Figure 7-23). These results show, in accordance with A-scan ultrasonographic measurements, that unaccommodated lens thickness increases with increasing age and that, contrary to measurements on isolated human lenses, no change in equatorial lens diameter occurs as a function of age.[66,106] This result has important implications for presbyopia because the lens is held suspended by the zonule, which is attached at the lens equator. If lens diameter were to increase with

increasing age, this could significantly alter the forces on the lens at rest. On the basis of these recent findings, however, this appears not to occur.

Loss of Ability of the Human Lens to Accommodate. The accommodative performance of the human crystalline lens in vitro changes with increasing age. Human lenses subjected to high-speed rotational forces designed to simulate the forces that act on the lens during accommodation show an age-dependent decline in deformability.[35] For a given rotational stress, the equatorial and polar strain (change in lens diameter and thickness) decrease by about one third between the ages of 15 and 65. Calculated Young's modulus of polar and equatorial elasticity undergoes a more than threefold increase over the same age range.[35] Fisher[36] also calculates that a decrease in elastic modulus of the capsule, an increase in elastic modulus of the lens substance, and a flattening of the lens are sufficient to account for the loss of accommodation by the age of 61 years. However, Fisher's[36] assumptions of no age change in lens shape or zonular insertion onto the lens, refuted in subsequent studies, render his conclusions equivocal.[10,23]

Young lenses undergo substantial changes in power from stretching forces applied through the intact zonular apparatus. These changes in power correspond well with the accommodative dioptric change in power of the eye. The change in optical power that the human lens can undergo with mechanical stretching gradually decreases with increasing age.[37,42] By the age of 55 years, human lenses are unable to undergo any change in power with the same degree of stretching that produces 14 diopters of change in power of young lenses[42] (Figure 7-24). These experiments show that regardless of what other age changes may occur in the human eye, the human lens ultimately completely loses the ability to be accommodated through the capsular forces. Neither increasing nor completely releasing zonular tension results in any alteration of the optical power of these presbyopic lenses.[42]

After the zonule is cut, the young isolated lens is in a maximally accommodated form as a result of the forces of the lens capsule.[33,43,105] Removing the capsule tends to unaccommodate the lens.[33,43] In actuality, removing the capsule produces optical changes that differ from the optical changes that occur with physiologic disaccommodation.[35,43] Despite these differences, removing the capsule results in systematic optical changes in young lenses, which cause a decrease in optical power; however, it produces no

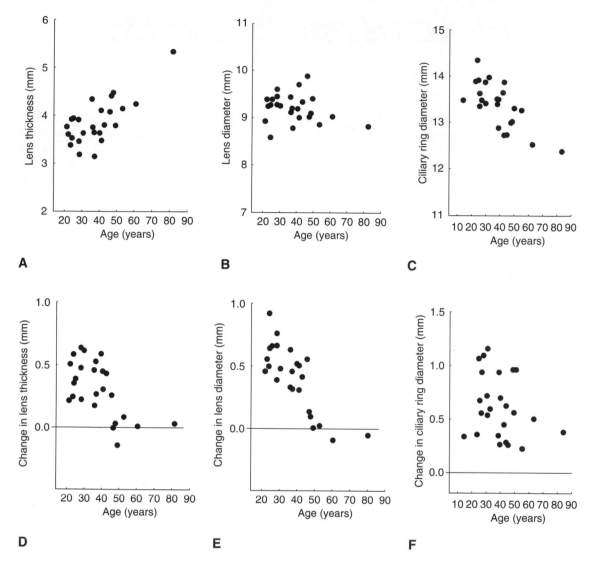

FIGURE 7-23 Magnetic resonance imaging measurements of resting, unaccommodated lens thickness (**A**), lens diameter (**B**), and ciliary ring diameter (**C**) in human eyes as a function of age. Subjects viewed a near target (8 diopters of accommodative demand) and magnetic resonance imaging measurements were repeated to determine the change in lens thickness (**D**), the change in lens diameter (**E**), and the change in ciliary ring diameter (**F**) with accommodation. The accommodative change in lens thickness and lens diameter reach zero (*horizontal lines*) by approximately 50 years of age, whereas the accommodative change in ciliary ring diameter, although reduced with increasing age, does not. (From Strenk SA: *Invest Ophthalmol Vis Sci* 40:1162, 1999, with permission from the Association for Research in Vision and Ophthalmology and the author.)

systematic change in power of lenses over 50 years.[43] This, together with data from mechanical stretching experiments, suggests that the lens substance of older human lenses is incapable of undergoing the capsule-induced optical alterations required for accommodation and disaccommodation.[42]

Through in vitro experiments, Fisher[37] indirectly calculated the force of contraction of the human ciliary muscle required to produce the maximal accommodative amplitude at each age. His calculations suggest that the force of contraction of the ciliary muscle increases up to age 45 and thereafter decreases, and that for a constant ciliary muscle contractile force, a lens from a 15-year-old will undergo a fourfold higher dioptric change than that from a 55-year-old. These calculations were made by comparing changes in lens thickness from spinning experiments, in which the forces on the lens

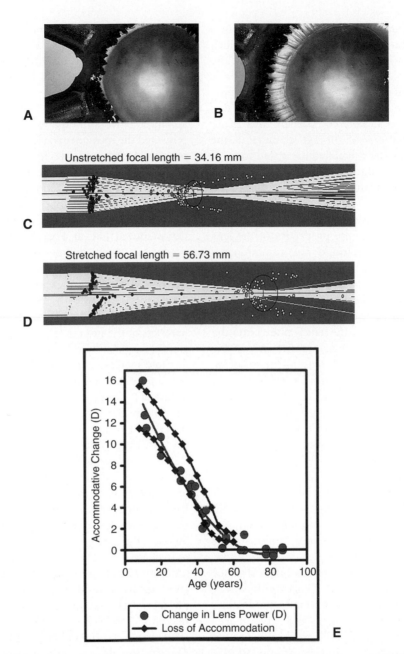

FIGURE 7-24   **A,** The anterior segment of a partially dissected 54-year-old human donor eye glued to the arms of a mechanical stretching apparatus. The zonule can be completely relaxed to allow the lens to become maximally accommodated (**A**) or the zonule stretched to disaccommodate the lens (**B**). Scanning laser measurements of the focal length of a 10-year-old human lens measured in the unstretched, accommodated state (focal length = 34.16 mm) (**C**) and in the maximally stretched and unaccommodated state (focal length = 57.73 mm) (**D**). Parallel laser beams enter the lens, are refracted by the lens (*at dark symbols, left*), and cross the optical axis (*dark horizontal line*) at the position identified (*light symbols, right*). The distance from the lens (*dark symbols, left*) to the average focus of all rays (*+ sign* and *large circle*) represents the lens focal length. **E,** The change in focal length converted to diopters (*solid line* and *circles*) as a function of the applied stretch shows that young lenses undergo 12 to 16 diopters of change in power with stretching, but that by age 60, the same extent of applied stretch results in no change in lens power. The data from the human lenses are plotted together with Duane's[27] data (*solid lines, diamonds*), showing the range of accommodative amplitudes from approximately 1500 subjects as measured with a push-up technique. (From Glasser A, Campbell MCW: *Vision Res* 38:209, 1998, with permission from Elsevier Science Ltd.)

could be computed, with changes in lens thickness from mechanical stretching experiments for which the dioptric power changes could be measured. By relating the forces on the lens to the lens dioptric changes, the ciliary muscle force required to produce maximum accommodation at any age was indirectly deduced. This comparison was made from determinations of the age changes in the lens, and despite the calculated increased force of contraction, accommodation still declines because the lens is becoming ever more resistant to deformation.[37]

The maximum rate of far-to-near (FN) accommodation is limited by the properties of the lens alone because the lens could not accommodate faster than the ciliary processes allow it to. However, the maximum rate of near-to-far (NF) disaccommodation relies on the properties of the lens and the choroid because it is through the elasticity of the choroid that the lens is pulled into the unaccommodated state. Dynamic measures of the time constants for changes in lens thickness during FN accommodation and NF disaccommodation in humans show that both time constants increase with age at an approximately equal rate.[5] Similarly, the velocity of changes in lens thickness with accommodation and disaccommodation also decrease with age in rhesus monkeys.[21] An analysis of the human time constant age changes with a biomechanical model suggests that because the lens is the only common rate-limiting factor in both NF disaccommodation and FN accommodation, the time constants for both are primarily dominated by the properties of the lens.[5] Active disaccommodation of the lens by the choroid has little influence on the time constant for NF disaccommodation, suggesting a lenticular contribution to presbyopia. The rhesus monkey experiments also show an age-dependent decrease in ciliary muscle velocity for both accommodation and disaccommodation.[21] Caution should be used in interpreting age change in velocity of movements with progression of presbyopia because, of course, in conjunction with aging, accommodative amplitude also declines. Findings of a change in rate of accommodation with age may simply reflect the declining accommodative response, rather than a change in absolute rate. Indeed, rate of accommodation and disaccommodation in rhesus monkeys shows a linear dependence on amplitude.[119] The disaccommodative response is systematically faster than the accommodative response.[21,119] When accommodative rates as a function of age are compared, this should be done for the same accommodative amplitude in all subjects.

Recent high-resolution MRI studies have shown important new insights on aging of the accommodative apparatus from direct measurements in aging human eyes.[106] Strenk et al.[106] presented an 8-diopter accommodative stimulus to all their subjects and measured the movements of the accommodative apparatus. Accommodative lens thickening and accommodative decrease in lens equatorial diameter both decline to zero by about age 50, whereas accommodative change in ciliary ring diameter, although reduced in the elderly, still occurs. This evidence shows that, at least in these persons with presbyopia, the crystalline lens fails to undergo accommodative changes while at least some ciliary muscle contraction is present.

Increased Hardness of the Human Lens. The hardness of the human lens increases exponentially from early childhood, undergoing more than a fourfold increase over the life span[43] (Figure 7-25). It is a fundamental requirement that if accommodation is to occur, the lens substance must remain sufficiently pliable so that capsular forces can act on it to flatten and unaccommodate it and to increase the curvatures into a more accommodated state. Because accommodation relies on the capsular forces, a small change in the ratio of capsular and lens elastic forces would negatively affect the accommodative process. Although presbyopia results in a complete loss of accommodation by the age of 50 years, the hardness of the human lens continues to increase beyond this age throughout the human life span. The predominant increase in hardness occurs after accommodation is lost, and this may simply represent a continuation of the aging process that ultimately leads to cataract. The progressive increase in lens hardness from birth concurs with the characteristic decline in accommodative amplitude that begins at a young age. If no other age-related changes were to occur in the eye, an increased hardness of the lens alone could account for the loss of accommodation with advancing age. In the young eye the lens is a highly viscous elastic material, which, in the absence of the capsule, has a tendency to take on a relatively flattened and unaccommodated state.[33,43] The capsule provides the molding forces to shape the lens substance into an accommodated form. An increase in the viscosity of the lens, a loss of elasticity (i.e., becoming firmer), or both could provide sufficient resistive force against which the lens capsule could no longer act.

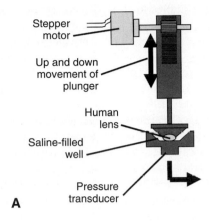

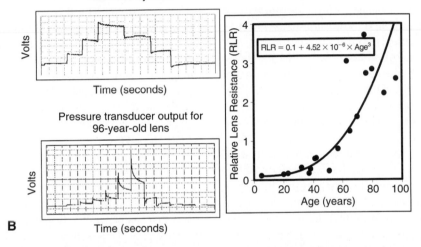

FIGURE 7-25 The method and results of measurement of the hardness of isolated human lenses. **A,** Human lenses from donor eyes were placed on a pressure transducer in a saline-filled well, and a plunger was driven down onto the lenses in six discrete steps and then off again in six discrete steps. The pressure transducer calibrated previously with a closed fluid-filled system (*upper trace*) showed a stepwise response to increasing pressure. The response of the pressure transducer to a 96-year-old human lens (*lower trace*), in contrast, shows a response suggesting viscous and elastic material properties of the human lens. **B,** Nineteen human lenses ranging in age from 5 to 96 years show an exponential increase in hardness with a more than fourfold increase in hardness over the human life span, which continues well after the age at which accommodation is completely lost. (Adapted from Glasser A, Campbell MCW: *Vision Res* 39:1991, 1999, with permission from Elsevier Science Ltd.)

Presbyopia has classically been attributed to the hardening, or "sclerosis," of the lens. Some confusion exists as to the meaning of the term *lenticular sclerosis*. This should be thought of as a gradual but progressive hardening throughout life that at some point leads to an inability of the lens to undergo the optical changes required for accommodation.

Ciliary Muscle Immobility. In addition to the age changes in the rhesus monkey ciliary muscle previously mentioned, in vivo studies of accommoda-tion in aging rhesus monkeys have allowed both qualitative and quantitative assessments of the age-dependent changes in the dynamic movements of the accommodative apparatus. Accommodation can be stimulated with an electrode surgically implanted in the EW nucleus of the monkey brain.[18] Prior surgical removal of the iris allows the anterior ciliary processes and lens equator to be visualized through the cornea during accommodation.[58,81] Although surgical iridectomy reduces supramaximal pharmacologically induced accommodative amplitude, it is unlikely to alter the submaximal pharmacologic or centrally stimulated accommodative amplitude or mechanism.[19] This technique has served not only to identify age-dependent changes related to presbyopia but also to verify the accommodative mechanism.[45,81] In monkeys centrally stimulated, accommodative amplitude declined significantly with increasing age.[81] Furthermore, Scheimpflug imaging shows an age-dependent decrease in lens axial thickening in addition to decreased lens transparency and increased prominence of lenticular zones of discontinuity. Gonioscopic examination shows that the extent of accommodative movement of the ciliary processes and the lens equator are reduced with increasing age and that movement of the ciliary processes in the oldest monkeys is barely perceptible.[81] Thus ciliary muscle mobility is *present* even in the oldest animals, as indicated by both in vivo videographic measurements and histologic measurements, but it is significantly *reduced.*[109] This, in conjunction with MRI measurements showing reduced accommodative excursion of the human ciliary muscle, provides evidence for extralenticular factors contributing to the progression of presbyopia.[106] The reduced responsiveness of the ciliary processes does not imply loss of ciliary muscle contractility but rather is consistent with anatomic evidence showing loss of elasticity of the posterior attachment of the ciliary muscle.[81] The human ciliary muscle and choroid have also been shown to become significantly stiffer with increasing age, as assessed by mechanical stretching experiments.[117] These results provide a clear indication that significant age changes in the accommodative function outside of the lens must be considered in the etiology of presbyopia. Dynamic analysis of the accommodative movements of aging rhesus monkey eyes shows a decline in accommodative amplitude, velocity of ciliary body movement, and velocity of lens thickening, as well as an increase in the latency of these movements.[21] Whether these age changes in the monkey eye are a cause or a consequence of the reduced lens accommodative movements with increasing age is unclear, but it is certainly clear that ciliary body dysfunction must be considered as a factor in presbyopia in rhesus monkeys.[21]

Theories of Presbyopia

Because of the multitude of age-related changes that have been identified in the eye, many theories of presbyopia have been proposed. Many of these theories are based on specific age changes in the eye, but others consider a combination of factors. Although it is relatively easier to identify specific age changes, it is more difficult to show how they cause presbyopia. Nevertheless, many of these individual factors, at one time or another, have been (or continue to be) proposed as the leading or sole cause of presbyopia. The findings of hardening, or sclerosis, of the lens have led to the lenticular hardening theory of presbyopia. Age changes in the thickness of the lens and consequent changes in the geometry of the zonular attachment to the lens have led to the geometric theory of presbyopia. Increased growth of the lens throughout life has led to the suggestion that a gradual reduction in zonular tension occurs with increasing age, thus allowing the lens to assume an accommodated configuration and leading to the disaccommodation theory of presbyopia. Continued growth of the lens, together with a controversial and uncorroborated revisionist theory of accommodation proposed by Schachar, has led to Schachar's theory of presbyopia.[95] Because so many age-related changes have been found in the eye, some investigators suggest that all of these age-related changes in part contribute to the gradual reduction in accommodation. Such multifactorial theories of presbyopia do not consider any one specific age change as being the sole, or even the major contributor to presbyopia.

Lenticular Sclerosis. The classical theory of presbyopia, recognized for as long as the accommodative mechanism and its gradual decline have been studied, is that the crystalline lens becomes harder with increasing age. This is often referred to as *lenticular sclerosis* and is the most commonly articulated explanation for presbyopia. In light of what is known about the accommodative mechanism, it is easy to understand how hardening of the lens can result in a loss of accommodation. If the lens substance becomes hardened, the lens could no longer be molded into an accommodated state by the lens capsule when the resting zonular tension is released.[33] In addition, the hardened lens substance would also be incapable of being pulled into a flattened and unaccommodated state by the zonular tension. Thus a hardened lens would be in a fixed state and could not undergo accommodative optical changes. Because presbyopia is a loss of near vision, the emmetropic presbyopic eye has a fixed focus for distant objects. The presbyopic lens should therefore be considered to be in an unaccommodated state in the presbyopic eye and incapable of accommodating. Past and recent experimental evidence lends credence to hardening of the lens as a major contributor to presbyopia. Most recently, experiments show not only that appropriate age-dependent dioptric changes can be induced in the lens with mechanical stretching but also that by the age of 50 years, mechanical stretching can induce no optical changes in the lens. This together with a direct demonstration of exponential increase in hardness of the lens dictates that lens hardening could be a major factor in the progression of presbyopia.

Geometric Theory of Presbyopia. Because with increasing age the crystalline lens gets thicker and an anterior zonular shift occurs, it has been proposed that presbyopia is a consequence of the altered geometry of the lens/zonular relationships with increasing age.[30,61,62,66] In the young lens the anterior zonular connections are relatively near the lens equator and so can exert considerable influence on the anterior curvature of the lens through alterations in tension with accommodation. The geometric theory argues that in the aged lens, where the point of attachment of the anterior zonule to the lens is further forward on the lens anterior surface and the angle between the zonular fibers and the lens anterior surface is altered, there is no effective relaxation of the anterior zonular/capsular force with an accommodative ciliary muscle contraction.[61] This theory argues that as a result of this altered geometry, the zonular fibers in presbyopic eyes exert a force that is nearly tangential to the surface of the lens, so relaxation of the zonule would have little effect on the capsule and on the shape of the lens.[62] The theory is said to provide a plausible explanation for presbyopia in the absence of changes in lens elasticity or ciliary muscle degeneration, but the presbyopic lens is suggested not to be accommodated.[15,61] The theory does not address how the aged lens/zonular geometry can provide the necessary force to maintain the lens in an unaccommodated form but fail to allow accommodation to occur. Although presbyopia is said to be predominantly a geometric disorder and is plausibly based on the independent observations of changes in lens thickness and zonular connections, systematic age-dependent zonular geometric alterations have not been demonstrated. Furthermore, the inability of the aged human crystalline lens to undergo optical changes with stretching or relaxation of the zonule mitigates against the geometric theory providing a sole explanation for presbyopia.[42]

Disaccommodation Theory of Presbyopia. The disaccommodation theory suggests that presbyopia is not caused by a failure of the lens to accommo-date, but rather by a gradual failure of the lens to be held in an unaccommodated form at rest.[7,87] Support for this theory comes from evidence suggesting that the lens anterior and posterior surface curvatures increase with increasing age.[10] This theory holds that because of increased growth and equatorial diameter of the lens, altered zonular/lens geometric relationships, altered configuration of the aging ciliary muscle, and loss of compliance of the choroid, the accommodative apparatus is no longer able to apply resting zonular tension to hold the lens in its unaccommodated state.[61,111] As a consequence, the lens progressively assumes a more accommodated configuration, and in the final stages of presbyopia, the lack of accommodation is then caused not by inherent failure in accommodation, but rather by the lens already being in a fully accommodated state. The eye is said to remain emmetropic in the face of the increased lens surface curvatures (i.e., the "lens paradox"[60]) through an active compensation of the lens gradient refractive index to maintain a constant lens power with increasing age.[28,62,86] Although the theoretic feasibility of an age-dependent alteration in the lens gradient refractive index has been shown, it has not been empirically verified to occur.[104] This theory contravenes the observations that neither increasing nor releasing zonular tension can alter the elderly crystalline lens focal length, that no paradox is found between lens surface curvatures and lens focal length, that there is no age constancy of the presbyopic lens focal length, and that the shape of the nucleus of the presbyopic lens is unlike that of the young accommodated lens.[15,42,43]

Schachar's Theory of Presbyopia. Continued lens equatorial growth has been suggested as a theory of presbyopia.[95] This is based on the revisionist theory of accommodation, which suggests that accommodation occurs through an increase in zonular tension to pull the lens equator toward the sclera.[96-98] The age-dependent increase in lens diameter with so-called crowding of the posterior chamber is suggested to result in a gradual slackening of the zonular tension at the lens equator such that the accommodative effort fails to increase the older slackened zonule sufficiently to actively pull on the lens equator.[99]

This theory of presbyopia fails on many grounds. Certainly, the lens continues to grow throughout life as reflected by an increase in mass, but this occurs through an increase in axial thickness but without an increase in diameter.[43] As previously mentioned, it is only when the diameter of isolated human lenses are measured that an apparent age-related increase in diameter is observed because the isolated lens tends to be in an accommodated state, relatively more so for the younger than the older lenses.[89,105] When lens diameter is measured in vivo in living human eyes, it is shown to be age independent.[106] Furthermore, were this theory of presbyopia correct, the speculated increase in lens diameter and resulting loss of zonular tension would predict more pronounced accommodative microfluctuations in older eyes as a result of reduced stability of the lens. However, the accommodative microfluctuations are more pronounced in young eyes and are all but absent in persons with presbyopia.[76,118] No independent conformation of this revisionist accommodative mechanism exists, and attempts to verify it found no evidence to support it.[45] This novel theory of accommodation serves as the basis for performing scleral expansion as a surgical procedure to restore accommodation in persons with presbyopia.[95] The only objective assessment of accommodation in postoperative scleral expansion patients found no evidence that accommodation is restored.[76] The possibility exists that scleral expansion surgery may alter the normal aberrations of the eye to induce some degree of multifocality. This could provide some degree of near vision, but without restoration of accommodation.

Multifactorial Theory of Presbyopia. Given the preponderance of evidence for age changes in the various aspects of the accommodative structures of the eye, it has been proposed that presbyopia results not from any single causal factor but through a global deterioration of accommodative function of several or many aspects of the accommodative apparatus.[87] Such multifactorial theories of presbyopia argue against any one factor such as lenticular sclerosis or hardening or loss of ciliary muscle contractility, for example, as representing any more significant causal factor to the loss of accommodation than any other age-related change. For example, if the force of contraction of the ciliary muscle diminishes and the lens hardness and size increases, it is clear that at some point along this continuum of age changes an accommodative effort is no longer able to induce optical changes in the lens. Presbyopia then is not an end point in itself, but is simply one time point in a gradual and progressive continuum of deterioration in the accommodative structures, which ultimately culminates in the loss of a physiologic function.

Correcting Presbyopia

Because the prevalence of presbyopia is 100% in individuals older than 50 years of age, presbyopia represents a source of inconvenience and annoyance and an economic burden for many. Spectacle lenses alone result in considerable health care costs, compounded by lost workdays attributable to headache, migraine, and other asthenopic symptoms associated with the strain of near work. As a consequence of this considerable economic impact, much is being done to improve optical compensation for persons with presbyopia. No known preventions or cures exist for presbyopia, but many old and new methods are being used to provide persons with presbyopia with some degree of functional near vision. These range from the use of traditional low-cost reading addition lenses, to improved bifocal or multifocal spectacle, contact, or intraocular lenses, to experimental and controversial surgical procedures aimed at restoring dynamic accommodation in persons with presbyopia.

Optical Compensation for Presbyopia. Optical compensation for persons with presbyopoa is achieved with spectacle lenses, contact lenses, corneal refractive surgical procedures, or artificial intraocular lenses (IOLs). Although all offer functional near vision with different approaches, costs, and degrees of success, they are all aimed at providing near vision while still affording functional distance vision.

Given the ease with which presbyopia is and has traditionally been optically compensated with spectacle lenses, the vast array of options now available to persons with presbyopia is a testament to the level of inconvenience or disability that losing accommodation imposes. Spectacle lens compensation for presbyopia includes bifocal, trifocal, or multifocal (progressive) addition lenses. Bifocal or multifocal contact lenses also provide optical compensation, although at the corneal vertex. Contact lenses are also offered for monovision compensation for persons with presbyopia for whom different powered contact lenses afford distance vision for one eye and intermediate or near vision for the other eye corrected for near.

Surgical Compensation for Presbyopia. Surgical options for persons with presbyopia included corneal refractive surgery, cataract surgery, accommodative IOLs, and new surgical options claim to actually restore the natural accommodative ability. The frequency and success with which cataract surgery is performed provide the motivation for surgical intervention to correct for presbyopia with an accommodative IOL. When the cataractous crystalline lens is replaced with an artificial IOL, best corrected distance acuity typically is restored, but the patient is left unable to accommodate for near vision tasks. A number of different IOL designs are available, such as bifocal, multifocal, diffractive, or so-called accommodative IOLs. In addition several corneal refractive surgery approaches are offered to persons with presbyopia, including monovision, bifocal, multifocal, or astigmatic corneal corrections. Controversial surgical interventions claimed to actually restore natural accommodation, such as scleral expansion surgery, started phase I U.S. Food and Drug Administration (FDA)–approved clinical trials in the year 2000. Independent attempts to restore accommodation with scleral expansion show only limited and transient benefits.[56,74] Any short-term benefits of such surgical procedures are limited by the high incidence of age-related cataract and an almost inevitable need to replace the crystalline lens with an IOL. Future surgical prospects for reintroducing accommodation in persons with presbyopia may include deformable polymer (e.g., silicone, hydrogel) IOLs or lenses with hinged or spring haptics permitting movement of one or more solid optics or through intralenticular laser photodisruption of the hardened presbyopic crystalline lens.[23,69,80] Prospects for achieving some level of functional near vision with accommodative IOLs are good because considerable benefit would be conferred to persons with presbyopia through the introduction of as little as 2 to 3 diopters of accommodation. With designs that most effectively use the accommodative function, it may be possible, albeit not necessary, to restore accommodation to a magnitude comparable to that available in youth. The success and longevity of these approaches ultimately depend on the extent to which the aging accommodative apparatus is able to continue to exert an accommodative effort.

REFERENCES

1. Aggarwala KR et al: Spectral bandwidth and ocular accommodation, *J Opt Soc Am A* 12:450, 1995.
2. Andison ME, Sivak JG: The naturally occurring accommodative response of the oscar, *Astronotus ocellatus,* to visual stimuli, *Vision Res* 36:3021, 1996.
3. Armaly MF: Studies on intraocular effects of the orbital parasympathetic pathway. I. Techniques and effects on morphology, *Arch Ophthalmol* 61:14, 1959.
4. Beer T: Die Accommodation des Fischauges, *Archiv Gesamte Physiolgie Mens Tiere (Pfluegers)* 58:523, 1894.
5. Beers APA, Van der Heijde GL: Presbyopia and velocity of sound in the lens, *Optom Vis Sci* 71:250, 1994.
6. Bennett A, Rabbetts RB: *Clinical visual optics,* ed 3, Boston, 1998, Butterworth-Heinemann.
7. Bito LZ, Miranda OC: Accommodation and presbyopia. In Reinecke RD (ed): *Ophthalmology annual,* New York, 1989, Raven Press.
8. Bito LZ et al: Age-dependent loss of accommodative amplitude in rhesus monkeys: an animal model for presbyopia, *Invest Ophthalmol Vis Sci* 23:23, 1982.
9. Brown N: The change in shape and internal form of the lens of the eye on accommodation, *Exp Eye Res* 15:441, 1973.
10. Brown N: The change in lens curvature with age, *Exp Eye Res* 19:175, 1974.
11. Brücke E: Über den musculus Cramptonianus und den Spannmuskel der Choroidea, *Archiv für Anatomie, Physiologie und Wissenschaftliche Medicine* 1:370, 1846.
12. Calver RI, Cox MJ, Elliott DB: Effect of aging on the monochromatic aberrations of the human eye, *J Opt Soc Am A Opt Image Sci Vis* 16:2069, 1999.
13. Coleman DJ: Unified model for accommodative mechanism, *Am J Ophthalmol* 69:1063, 1970.
14. Coleman DJ: On the hydraulic suspension theory of accommodation, *Tr Am Ophth Soc* 84:846, 1986.
15. Cook CA et al: Aging of the human crystalline lens and anterior segment, *Vision Res* 34:2945, 1994.
16. Cramer A: Het accommodatievermogen der oogen, physiologisch toegelicht, *Hollandsche Maatschappij der Wetenschappen te Haarlem* 1:139, 1853.
17. Crampton P: The description of an organ by which the eyes of birds are accommodated to the different distances of objects, *Thompson's Annals of Philosophy* 1:170, 1813.
18. Crawford K, Terasawa E, Kaufman PL: Reproducible stimulation of ciliary muscle contraction in the cynomolgus monkey via permanent indwelling midbrain electrode, *Brain Res* 503:265, 1989.
19. Crawford KS, Kaufman PL, Bito LZ: The role of the iris in accommodation of rhesus monkeys, *Invest Ophthalmol Vis Sci* 31:2185, 1990.
20. Croft MA et al: Aging effects on accommodation and outflow facility responses to pilocarpine in humans, *Arch Ophthalmol* 114:586, 1996.
21. Croft MA et al: Accommodation dynamics in aging rhesus monkeys, *Am J Physiol* 275:R1885, 1998.
22. Croft MA et al: Lens and ciliary muscle function in young and old rhesus monkeys, *Invest Ophthalmol Vis Sci* 40(suppl):S361, 1999 (ARVO abstract).
23. Cumming JS, Slade SG, Chayet A: Clinical evaluation of the model AT-45 silicone accommodating intraocular lens: results of feasibility and the initial phase of a Food and Drug Administration clinical trial, *Ophthalmology* 108:2122, 2001.
24. Davanger M: The suspensory apparatus of the lens. The surface of the ciliary body. A scanning electron microscopic study, *Acta Ophthalmol* 53:19, 1975.
25. Donders FC: *On the anomalies of accommodation and refraction of the eye with preliminary essay on physiological dioptrics,* London, 1864, The New Sydenham Society.
26. Drexler W et al: Biometric investigation of changes in the anterior eye segment during accommodation, *Vision Res* 37:2789, 1997.

27. Duane A: Normal values of the accommodation at all ages, *JAMA* 59:1010, 1912.
28. Dubbelman M, Van der Heijde GL: The shape of the aging human lens: curvature, equivalent refractive index and the lens paradox, *Vis Res* 41:1867, 2001.
29. Farnsworth PN, Burke P: Three-dimensional architecture of the suspensory apparatus of the lens of the rhesus monkey, *Exp Eye Res* 25:563, 1977.
30. Farnsworth PN, Shyne SE: Anterior zonular shifts with age, *Exp Eye Res* 28:291, 1979.
31. Farnsworth PN et al: Surface ultrastructure of the human lens capsule and zonular attachments, *Invest Ophthalmol Vis Sci* 15:36, 1976.
32. Fincham EF: The changes in the form of the crystalline lens in accommodation, *Trans Optical Soc* 26:240, 1925.
33. Fincham EF: The mechanism of accommodation, *Br J Ophthalmol Monograph*, No. VIII, 1:1937.
34. Fisher RF: Elastic constants of the human lens capsule, *J Physiol* 201:1, 1969.
35. Fisher RF: The elastic constants of the human lens, *J Physiol* 212:147, 1971.
36. Fisher RF: Presbyopia and the changes with age in the human crystalline lens, *J Physiol* 228:765, 1973.
37. Fisher RF: The force of contraction of the human ciliary muscle during accommodation, *J Physiol* 270:51, 1977.
38. Fisher RF: Is the vitreous necessary for accommodation in man, *Br J Ophthalmol* 67:206, 1983.
39. Flügel C, Barany EH, Lutjen-Drecoll E: Histochemical differences within the ciliary muscle and its function in accommodation, *Exp Eye Res* 50:219, 1990.
40. Garner LF, Smith G: Changes in equivalent and gradient refractive index of the crystalline lens with accommodation, *Optom Vis Sci* 74:114, 1997.
41. Garner LF, Yap MKH: Changes in ocular dimensions and refraction with accommodation, *Ophthal Physiol Opt* 17:12, 1997.
42. Glasser A, Campbell MCW: Presbyopia and the optical changes in the human crystalline lens with age, *Vision Res* 38:209, 1998.
43. Glasser A, Campbell MCW: Biometric, optical and physical changes in the isolated human crystalline lens with age in relation to presbyopia, *Vision Res* 39:1991, 1999.
44. Glasser A, Howland HC: A history of studies of visual accommodation in birds, *Quart Rev Biol* 71:475, 1996.
45. Glasser A, Kaufman PL: The mechanism of accommodation in primates, *Ophthalmology* 106:863, 1999.
46. Glasser A, Troilo D, Howland HC: The mechanism of corneal accommodation in chicks, *Vision Res* 34:1549, 1994.
47. Glasser A et al: The mechanism of lenticular accommodation in the chick eye, *Vision Res* 35:1525, 1995.
48. Glasser A et al: Ultrasound biomicroscopy of the aging rhesus monkey ciliary region, *Optom Vision Sci* 78:417, 2001.
49. Hara K et al: Structural differences between regions of the ciliary body in primates, *Invest Ophthalmol Vis Sci* 16:912, 1977.
50. Harris LS, Galin MA. Effect of ocular pigmentation on hypotensive response to pilocarpine, *Am J Ophthalmol* 72:923, 1971.
51. Helmholtz von HH: *Handbuch der Physiologishen Optik*, New York, 1909, Dover. (Translated by JPC Southall, 1962.)
52. Herschberg J: *The history of ophthalmology*, vol 1, Bonn, 1889, Antiquity. (Translated by CF Blodi, 1982.)
53. Hess C: Vergleichende Untersuchungen über den Einfluss der Accommodation auf den Augendruck in der Wirbelthierreihe, *Archiv für Augenheilkunde* 63:88, 1909.
54. Hogan MJ, Alvarado JA, Wedell JE: *Histology of the human eye*, Philadelphia, 1971, WB Saunders.
55. Homes E: The Croonian lecture on muscular motion, *Phil Trans Royal Soc Lond* 85:1, 1795.
56. Kaufman PL: Scleral expansion surgery for presbyopia, *Ophthalmology* 108:2161, 2001.
57. Kaufman PL, Bárány EH: Subsensitivity to pilocarpine in primate ciliary muscle following topical anticholinesterase treatment, *Invest Ophthalmol Vis Sci* 14:302, 1975.
58. Kaufman PL, Lütjen-Drecoll E: Total iridectomy in the primate in vivo: surgical technique and postoperative anatomy, *Invest Ophthalmol Vis Sci* 14:766, 1975.
59. Koretz JF, Handelman GH: A model for accommodation in the young human eye: the effects of lens elastic anisotropy on the mechanism, *Vision Res* 23:1679, 1983.
60. Koretz JF, Handelman GH: The "lens paradox" and image formation in accommodating human eyes, *Top Aging Res Eur* 6:57, 1986.
61. Koretz JF, Handelman GH: Modeling age-related accommodative loss in the human eye, *Mathematical Modeling* 7:1003, 1986.
62. Koretz JF, Handelman GH: How the human eye focuses, *Sci Am* 259:92, 1988.
63. Koretz JF, Handelman GH, Brown NP: Analysis of human crystalline lens curvature as a function of accommodative state and age, *Vision Res* 24:1141, 1984.
64. Koretz JF et al: Slit-lamp studies of the rhesus monkey eye. I. Survey of the anterior segment, *Exp Eye Res* 44:307, 1987.
65. Koretz JF et al: Slit-lamp studies of the rhesus monkey eye. II. Changes in crystalline lens shape, thickness and position during accommodation and aging, *Exp Eye Res* 45: 317, 1987.
66. Koretz JF et al: Accommodation and presbyopia in the human eye: aging of the anterior segment, *Vision Res* 29:1685, 1989.
67. Krag S, Olsen T, Andreassen T: Biomechanical characteristics of the human anterior lens capsule in relation to age, *Invest Ophthalmol Vis Sci* 38:357, 1999.
68. Krueger RR et al: Experimental increase in accommodative potential after neodymium: yttrium-aluminum-garnet laser photodisruption of paired cadaver lenses, *Ophthalmology* 108:2122, 2001.
69. Kruger PB et al: Chromatic aberration and ocular focus: Fincham revisited, *Vision Res* 33:1397, 1993.
70. Ludwig K et al: In vivo imaging of the human zonular apparatus with high-resolution ultrasound biomicroscopy, *Graefe's Arch Clin Exp Ophthalmol* 237:361, 1999.
71. Lütjen-Drecoll E: Functional morphology of the trabecular meshwork in primate eyes, *Prog Retinal Res* 18:91, 1998.
72. Lütjen-Drecoll E, Tamm E, Kaufman PL: Age changes in rhesus monkey ciliary muscle: light and electron microscopy, *Exp Eye Res* 47:885, 1988.
73. Lütjen-Drecoll E, Tamm E, Kaufman PL: Age-related loss of morphologic responses to pilocarpine in rhesus monkey ciliary muscle, *Arch Ophthalmol* 106:1591, 1988.
74. Malecaze FJ et al: Scleral expansion bands for presbyopia, *Ophthalmology* 108:2165, 2001.
75. Marshall J, Beaconsfield M, Rothery S: The anatomy and development of the human lens and zonules, *Trans Ophthal Soc UK* 102:433, 1982.
76. Mathews S: Scleral expansion surgery does not restore accommodation in human presbyopia, *Ophthalmology* 106:873, 1999.
77. McCulloch C: The zonule of Zinn: its origin, course, and insertion, and its relation to neighboring structures, *Trans Am Ophthal Soc* 52:525, 1954.
78. Müller H: Über den Accommodations-apparat im Auge der Vogel, besonders der Falken, *Archiv für Ophthalmologie* 3:25, 1857.

79. Müller H: Über einen ringförmigen Muskel am Ciliarmuskel des Menschen und über den Mechanismus der Akkommodation. Albrecht v. Graefes, *Arch Ophthalmol* 3:1, 1858.

80. Murthy SK, Ravi N: Hydrogels as potential probes for investigating the mechanism of lenticular presbyopia, *Curr Eye Res* 22:384, 2001.

81. Neider MW et al: In vivo videography of the rhesus monkey accommodative apparatus: age-related loss of ciliary muscle response to central stimulation, *Arch Ophthalmol* 108:69, 1990.

82. Nishida S, Mizutani S: Quantitative and morphometric studies of age-related changes in human ciliary muscle, *Jpn J Ophthalmol* 36:380, 1992.

83. O'Neill WD, Brodkey JS: A nonlinear analysis of the mechanics of accommodation, *Vision Res* 10:375, 1970.

84. Owens PL, Amos DM: Pharmacologic management of strabismus. In Bartlett JF, Jaanus SD (eds): *Clinical ocular pharmacology,* ed 3, Boston, 1995, Butterworth-Heinemann.

85. Pardue MT, Sivak JG: Age-related changes in human ciliary muscle, *Optom Vis Sci* 77:204, 2000.

86. Pierscionek BK: What we know and understand about presbyopia, *Clin Exp Optom* 76:83, 1993.

87. Pierscionek BK, Weale RA: Presbyopia: a maverick of human aging, *Arch Gerontol Geriat* 20:229, 1995.

88. Poyer JF, Kaufman PL, Flugel C: Age does not affect contractile responses of the isolated rhesus monkey ciliary muscle to muscarinic agonists, *Curr Eye Res* 12:413, 1993.

89. Rafferty NS: Lens morphology. In Maisel H (ed): *The ocular lens: structure, function, and pathology,* New York, 1985, Marcel Dekker.

90. Rohen JW: Scanning electron microscopic studies of the zonular apparatus in human and monkey eyes, *Invest Ophthalmol Vis Sci* 18:133, 1979.

91. Rohen JW et al: Functional morphology of accommodation in raccoon, *Exp Eye Res* 48:523, 1989.

92. Sakabe I et al: Anterior shift of zonular insertion onto the anterior surface of human crystalline lens with age, *Ophthalmology* 105:295, 1998.

93. Saladin JJ, Stark L: Presbyopia: new evidence from impedance cyclography supporting the Hess-Gullstrand theory, *Vision Res* 15:537, 1975.

94. Salzman M: *The anatomy and histology of the human eyeball in the normal state, its development and senescence,* Chicago, 1912, Lithographed Photopress.

95. Schachar RA: Cause and treatment of presbyopia with a method for increasing the amplitude of accommodation, *Ann Ophthalmol* 24:445, 1992.

96. Schachar RA: Zonular function: a new hypothesis with clinical implications, *Arch Ophthalmol* 26:36, 1994.

97. Schachar RA, Anderson D: The mechanism of ciliary muscle function, *Ann Ophthalmol* 27:126, 1995.

98. Schachar RA, Cudmore DP, Black TD: Experimental support for Schachar's hypothesis of accommodation, *Arch Ophthalmol* 25:404, 1993.

99. Schachar RA et al: The mechanism of accommodation and presbyopia in the primate, *Ann Ophthalmol* 27:58, 1995.

100. Schachar RA et al: In vivo increase of the human lens equatorial diameter during accommodation, *Am J Physiol* 271:670, 1996.

101. Schaeffel F, Wilhelm H, Zrenner E: Inter-individual variability in the dynamics of natural accommodation in humans: relation to age and refractive errors, *J Physiol* 461:301, 1993.

102. Sivak J, Howland HC. Accommodation in the northern rock bass *(Ambloplites rupestris)* in response to natural stimuli, *Vision Res* 13:2059,1973.

103. Sivak JG, Hildebrand T, Lebert C: Magnitude and rate of accommodation in diving and nondiving birds, *Vision Res* 25:925, 1985.

104. Smith G, Atchison DA, Pierscionek BK: Modeling the power of the aging human eye, *J Opt Soc Am A* 9:2111, 1992.

105. Smith P: Diseases of the crystalline lens and capsule: on the growth of the crystalline lens, *Trans Ophthalmol Soc UK* 3:79, 1883.

106. Strenk SA et al: Age-related changes in human ciliary muscle and lens: a magnetic resonance imaging study, *Invest Ophthalmol Vis Sci* 40:1162, 1999.

107. Swegmark G: Studies with impedance cyclography on human ocular accommodation at different ages, *Acta Ophthalmol* 46:1186, 1969.

108. Tamm E et al: Posterior attachment of ciliary muscle in young, accommodating old, presbyopic monkeys, *Invest Ophthalmol Vis Sci* 32:1678, 1991.

109. Tamm E et al: Age-related loss of ciliary muscle mobility in the rhesus: role of the choroid, *Arch Ophthalmol* 110:871, 1992.

110. Tamm ER, Lütjen-Drecoll E: Ciliary body, *Micros Res Tech* 33:390, 1996.

111. Tamm S, Tamm E, Rohen JW: Age-related changes of the human ciliary muscle: a quantitative morphometric study, *Mech Age Dev* 62:209, 1992.

112. Tornqvist G: Effect on refraction of intramuscular pilocarpine in two species of monkey *(Cercopithecus aethiops* and *Macaca irus)*, *Invest Ophthalmol Vis Sci* 4:211, 1965.

113. Tornqvist G: Effect of topical carbachol on the pupil and refraction in young and presbyopic monkeys, *Invest Ophthalmol Vis Sci* 5:186, 1966.

114. True-Gabelt B, Kaufman PL, Polansky JR: Ciliary muscle muscarinic binding sites, choline acetyltransferase, and acetylcholinesterase in aging rhesus monkeys, *Invest Ophthalmol Vis Sci* 31:2431, 1990.

115. Tscherning M: Accommodation. In *Physiologic optics,* ed 2, Philadelphia, 1904, The Keystone.

116. Vakkur GJ, Bishop PO: The schematic eye in the cat, *Vision Res* 3:357, 1963.

117. Van Alphen GWHM, Graebel WP: Elasticity of tissues involved in accommodation, *Vision Res* 31:1417, 1991.

118. Van der Heijde GL, Beers APA, Dubbelman M: Microfluctuations of steady-state accommodation measured with ultrasonography, *Ophthal Physiol Opt* 16:216, 1996.

119. Vilupuru AS, Glasser A: Dynamic accommodation in rhesus monkeys, *Vis Res* 42:125, 2002.

120. Vilupuru AS, Glasser A: Optical and biometric relationships of the isolated pig crystalline lens, *Ophthalmic Physiol Opt* 21:296, 2001.

121. Weale RA: *A biography of the eye: development, growth, age,* London, 1982, HK Lewis.

122. Wilson RS: Does the lens diameter increase or decrease during accommodation? Human accommodation studies: a new technique using infrared retro-illumination video photography and pixel unit measurements, *Trans Am Ophthalmol Soc* 95:261, 1997.

123. Wold J et al: Measurement of human accommodative amplitude, *Optom Vis Sci* 77(suppl):185, 2000.

124. Young T: On the mechanisms of the eye, *Phil Trans Lond* 91:23, 1801.

SECTION 6

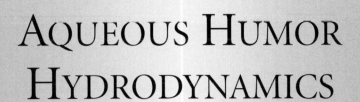

AQUEOUS HUMOR HYDRODYNAMICS

B'ANN TRUE GABELT AND PAUL L. KAUFMAN

CHAPTER 8

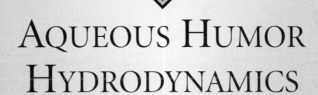

AQUEOUS HUMOR HYDRODYNAMICS

B'ANN TRUE GABELT AND PAUL L. KAUFMAN

In the healthy eye, flow of aqueous humor against resistance generates an intraocular pressure (IOP) of approximately 15 mm Hg, which is necessary for the proper shape and optical properties of the globe.[462] The circulating aqueous humor nourishes the cornea and lens, structures that must be transparent and therefore devoid of blood vessels and the trabecular meshwork (TM).[462] The aqueous humor also provides a transparent and colorless medium of refractive index 1.33332 between the cornea and lens, thus constituting an important component of the eye's optical system.[462] The basic anatomy of the primate anterior ocular segment and the normal pathways of aqueous humor flow (AHF) are illustrated schematically in Figures 8-1 and 8-2. Aqueous humor is secreted by the ciliary epithelium lining the ciliary processes (CPs) (as a consequence of active ionic transport across the ciliary epithelium and hydrostatic and osmotic gradients between the posterior chamber and the CP vasculature and stroma) and enters the posterior chamber. The humor then flows around the lens and through the pupil into the anterior chamber (AC). Convection flow of aqueous humor exists in the AC—downward close to the cornea, where the temperature is cooler, and upward near the lens, where the temperature is warmer (seen clinically when there is particulate matter in the AC, e.g., cells). Aqueous humor leaves the eye by passive bulk flow via two pathways at the AC angle: (1) through the TM, across the inner wall (IW) of Schlemm's canal (SC) into its lumen, and from there into collector channels, aqueous veins, and the episcleral venous circulation—the trabecular or conventional route—and (2) across the iris root,

the uveal meshwork, and the anterior face of the ciliary muscle (CM), through the connective tissue between the muscle bundles, through the suprachoroidal space, and from there out through the sclera—the uveoscleral, posterior, or unconventional route. Whether there is net osmotic resorption of some of the aqueous humor passing through the uvea by the uveal venous circulation is still under debate.[332,516] In young individuals of various monkey species, total aqueous drainage is relatively evenly divided between the two pathways.* In the healthy human eye, the importance of the uveoscleral pathway has not been well quantified. In elderly eyes with posterior segment tumors, the uveoscleral pathway accounts for 10% of total aqueous humor drainage, whereas in young individuals it may account for more than 30%.[104,682,684] More recently, Toris et al.[682] have shown that in healthy subjects 60 years of age or older, uveoscleral outflow (F_u) is significantly reduced compared with that of 20- to 30-year-olds (mean ± standard deviation = 1.10 ± 0.81 versus 1.52 ± 0.81 μl/min; p .009). Similarly, in rhesus monkeys older than 25 years of age (human equivalent, older than 62 years of age), F_u was even more dramatically reduced (0.02 ± 0.06 versus 0.42 ± 0.08 μl/min).[259] The historic human/monkey disparity may represent age differences rather than species differences. There is no significant net fluid movement across the cornea, iris vasculature, or vitreoretinal interface, although ion fluxes exist.[95,97]

Because of the autonomic innervation and receptors of the relevant structures, adrenergic and

---

*References 81, 259, 354, 494, 637.

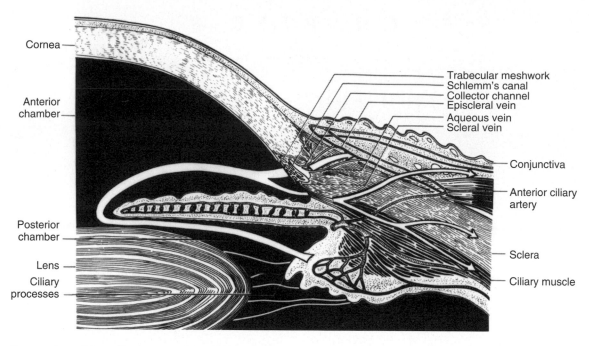

Figure 8-1   Schematic representation of the primate anterior ocular segment. *Arrows* indicate aqueous humor flow pathways. Aqueous humor is formed by the ciliary processes, enters the posterior chamber, flows through the pupil into the anterior chamber, and exits at the chamber angle via the trabecular and uveoscleral routes. (From Kaufman PL, Wiedman T, Robinson JR: Cholinergics. In Sears ML [ed]: *Pharmacology of the eye: handbook of experimental pharmacology,* Berlin, 1984, Springer-Verlag.)

cholinergic mechanisms play major roles in aqueous humor formation and drainage in terms of both normal physiology and glaucoma therapeutics, although evidence for other mechanisms, including serotonergic, dopaminergic, adenosinergic, and especially, prostaglandinergic, is amassing.*

AQUEOUS HUMOR FORMATION AND COMPOSITION

Physiology of Aqueous Humor Formation

Until the early twentieth century, aqueous humor was regarded as a stagnant fluid.[604] However, since then, it has been shown to be continuously formed and drained, and the associated anatomic drainage portals (e.g., SC, collector channels, aqueous veins, CM interstices) have been described.†

Three physiologic processes contribute to the formation and chemical composition of the aqueous humor: diffusion, ultrafiltration (and the related dialysis), and active secretion.[462] The first two

processes are passive and hence require no active cellular participation. *Diffusion* of solutes across cell membranes occurs down a concentration gradient; substances with high lipid-solubility coefficients that can easily penetrate biologic membranes move readily in this way. *Ultrafiltration* is the term used to describe the bulk flow of blood plasma across the fenestrated ciliary capillary endothelia into the ciliary stroma; it can be increased by augmentation of the hydrostatic driving force (see Figure 8-2). The processes of diffusion and ultrafiltration are responsible for the formation of the "reservoir" of the plasma ultrafiltrate in the stroma, from which the posterior chamber aqueous humor is derived (by means of active secretion across the ciliary epithelium). *Active secretion* requires energy, normally provided by the hydrolysis of adenosine triphosphate (ATP). The energy is used to secrete substances against a concentration gradient. Energy-dependent active transport of sodium into the posterior chamber by the nonpigmented ciliary epithelium (Figure 8-3) results in water movement from the stromal pool into the posterior chamber. Although controversy has surrounded the relative quantitative roles of ultrafiltration and active secretion, it seems fairly

*References 10, 18, 19, 42, 55, 89, 91, 115, 117, 140, 145, 149, 150, 160, 168, 177, 178, 180, 184, 191, 255, 266, 301, 349, 386, 405, 417, 435, 458, 461, 482, 494, 498, 590, 601, 641, 664, 681, 765, 766.
†References 27, 28, 97, 276, 374, 603.

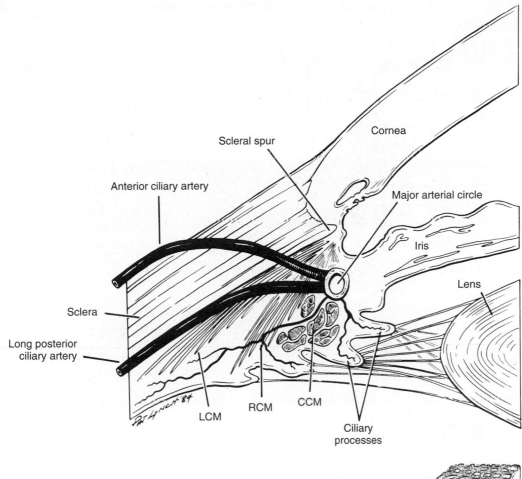

A

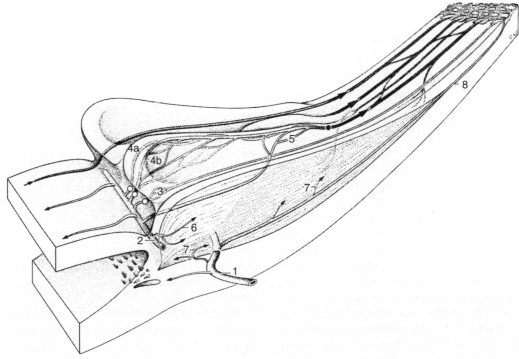

B

FIGURE 8-2 **A,** Blood supply to the ciliary processes. *CCM,* Circular ciliary muscle; *LCM,* longitudinal ciliary muscle; *RCM,* radial ciliary muscle. **B,** Vascular architecture in the human ciliary body. *1,* Perforating branches of the anterior ciliary arteries; *2,* major arterial circle of iris; *3,* first vascular territory. The second vascular territory is depicted in *4a,* marginal route, and *4b,* capillary network in the center of this territory. *5,* Third vascular territory; *6* and *7,* arterioles to the ciliary muscle; *8,* recurrent choroidal arteries. *Light circles,* terminal arterioles; *dark circle,* efferent venous segment. (From Caprioli J: The ciliary epithelia and aqueous humor. In Hart WM [ed]: *Adler's physiology of the eye: clinical application,* ed 9, St Louis, 1992, Mosby; and Funk R, Rohen JW: *Exp Eye Res* 51:651, 1990.)

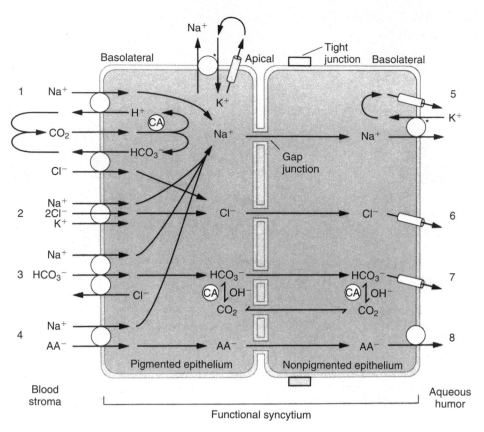

FIGURE 8-3   Diagram of possible secretory pathways in the ciliary processes. *AA,* Ascorbic acid; *CA,* carbonic anhydrase. (From Wiederholt M, Helbig H, Korbmacher C: Ion transport across the ciliary epithelium: lessons from cultured cells and proposed role of the carbonic anhydrase. In Botrè F, Gross G [eds]: *Carbonic anhydrase,* Cambridge, 1991, Verlag-Chemie.)

certain that under normal conditions active secretion accounts for perhaps 80% to 90% of total aqueous humor formation.[*] The observation that moderate alterations in systemic blood pressure and CP blood flow have little effect on aqueous humor formation rate supports this notion.[94,95,743] Furthermore, Bill[94] noted that the hydrostatic and oncotic forces that exist across the ciliary epithelium–posterior aqueous interface would favor resorption, not secretion, of aqueous humor. Active secretion is essentially pressure insensitive at near-physiologic IOP. However, the ultrafiltration component of aqueous humor formation is sensitive to changes in IOP, decreasing with increasing IOP. This phenomenon is quantifiable and is termed *facility of inflow,* or pseudofacility (C_{ps}), the latter because a pressure-induced decrease in inflow appears as an increase in outflow when techniques such as tonography and constant-pressure perfusion are used to measure outflow facility (OF).[*] Although measurements vary, C_{ps} in the noninflamed monkey and human eye constitutes a small percentage of total facility.[†]

In most mammalian species the turnover constant of the AC aqueous humor is approximately 0.01 to 0.015 × min^{-1}, that is, the rate of aqueous humor formation and drainage is approximately 1.0% to 1.5% of the AC volume per minute.[‡] This is true also in the healthy human eye, in which the aqueous humor formation rate is approximately 2.5 μl × min^{-1}.[§]

More comprehensive theoretical analyses of the fluid mechanics of aqueous humor production can be found elsewhere.[||]

[*]References 94, 95, 126, 141, 165, 166, 281, 447, 462, 515.

[*]References 36, 40, 86, 93, 99, 277, 353, 462.
[†]References 69, 93, 128, 129, 252, 353, 395, 443, 473.
[‡]References 92, 141, 164, 216, 331, 517.
[§]References 187, 267, 388, 462, 673, 684, 753.
[||]References 36, 299, 388, 463, 492, 518.

BIOCHEMISTRY OF AQUEOUS HUMOR FORMATION

The active process of aqueous humor secretion is mediated by selective transport of certain ions and substances across the basolateral membrane of the nonpigmented epithelium (NPE) against a concentration gradient. Two enzymes abundantly present in the NPE are intimately involved in this process: sodium-potassium–activated adenosine triphosphatase (Na$^+$-K$^+$-ATPase) and carbonic anhydrase (CA).* Na$^+$-K$^+$-ATPase is found predominantly bound to the plasma membrane of the basolateral infoldings of the NPE.† The enzyme provides the energy for the metabolic pump, which transports sodium into the posterior chamber by catalyzing the following reaction:

$$ATP \rightarrow ADP + Pi + energy$$

where

ATP = Adenosine triphosphate
ADP = Adenosine diphosphate
 Pi = Inorganic phosphate

As a result of active transport, aqueous humor in humans exhibits increased levels of ascorbate, some amino acids, and certain ions such as Cl$^-$.[187,388] There is also passive transport for HCO$_3^-$.[449,462] A summary of the biochemistry of aqueous humor secretion is shown in Figure 8-3.

Inhibition of the CP Na$^+$-K$^+$-ATPase by cardiac glycosides (e.g., ouabain) or vanadate (VO$_3^-$,VO$_4^{3-}$) significantly reduces the rate of aqueous humor formation and IOP in experimental animals and in humans.‡ Cardiac glycosides appear to act at the extracellular aspect of the membrane-bound enzyme, whereas vanadate acts at the cytoplasmic surface.[377,625] Cardiac glycosides given topically are ineffective as ocular hypotensives and may cause corneal edema by interfering with the Na$^+$-K$^+$-ATPase–dependent sodium pump in the corneal endothelium.[65] Intravitreal and systemic administration are effective but carry unacceptable ocular and cardiovascular risks, respectively.[65,626] Vanadate is effective topically in both rabbits and monkeys, apparently without producing corneal edema acutely.[66,387,534] However, the minimal IOP reduction (8%) after multiple dosing in patients with ocular hypertension precluded vanadate from being pursued further as an antiglaucoma agent (T. Krupin, personal communication, 2001).

CA is abundantly present in erythrocytes, renal tubules, and the basal and lateral membranes and cytoplasm of the pigmented epithelium (PE) and NPE of the CP.* Two isoenzymes of CA (II and IV) are present in the CPs.[124] CA catalyzes reaction I of the following sequence:

$$CO_2 + H_2O \rightarrow H_2CO_3 \rightarrow H^+ + HCO_3^-$$
$$\quad\quad\quad I \quad\quad\quad\quad II$$

Reaction II is a spontaneous, virtually instantaneous ionic dissociation.[475,733] The actual sequence may be far more complex, involving energy-dependent separation of H$^+$ and OH$^-$ at membrane boundaries within the NPE cell and formation of HCO$_3^-$ by CA-catalyzed association of OH$^-$ with CO$_2$.[246,447] The reaction sequence presented previously provides the HCO$_3^-$, which is essential for the active secretion of aqueous humor. Although the exact roles of CA and HCO$_3^-$ are still debated, it has been demonstrated that inhibition of the production of HCO$_3^-$ also leads to an inhibition of the active transport of Na$^+$ across the NPE into the first-formed aqueous humor, thereby reducing active aqueous humor formation.† The following hypotheses attempt to explain the relationship between reduction in NPE intracellular HCO$_3^-$ and inhibition of Na$^+$ transport: (1) inhibition of CA causing a decrease in HCO$_3^-$ available for transport with Na$^+$ from the cytosol of the NPE to the aqueous, required to maintain electroneutrality; (2) reduction in intracellular pH inhibiting Na$^+$-K$^+$-ATPase; and (3) decreased availability of H$^+$ produced by reaction II decreasing H$^+$-Na$^+$ exchange and reducing the availability of intracellular Na$^+$ for transport into the intercellular channel.[462] In addition, inhibition of renal and erythrocyte CA leads to a systemic acidosis, which promotes inhibition of AHF.[362]

CA inhibitors (e.g., acetazolamide, methazolamide, ethoxzolamide, dichlorphenamide, aminozolamide, trifluormethazolamide) given systemically can reduce secretion by up to 50% and have been in use for clinical glaucoma therapy for more than 40 years.‡ With low dosages of certain CA inhibitors (e.g., methazolamide), it is possible to inhibit the ocular enzyme without affecting the renal and erythrocyte enzymes, thus producing submaximal secretory suppression without systemic

---

*References 32, 75, 118, 119, 163 165, 236, 466, 562, 563, 691, 696, 746.
†References 118, 119, 163, 166, 236, 562, 563, 696.
‡References 65, 66, 118, 387, 403, 404, 532, 534, 562, 625.

*References 432, 433, 445-447, 475, 477.
†References 60, 141, 166, 246-248, 447, 449.
‡References 59, 199, 247, 248, 312, 315, 362, 432, 433, 445, 448, 451, 452, 477, 528, 593, 648, 649, 747.

acidosis.[340,445,447,448,450] It was once thought that the drug concentration at the ciliary epithelium required to produce the almost continuous, total ciliary CA inhibition necessary to achieve adequate and sustained reduction in AHF (more than 99% of the ciliary enzyme must be inhibited to achieve significant secretory suppression) might never be attainable via the eyedrop route.[445,447,448,450] However, the topically effective CA inhibitors dorzolamide and brinzolamide are now available; these CA inhibitors may achieve a reduction in IOP nearly as substantial as the earlier oral CA inhibitors but without their systemic side effects.*

AQUEOUS HUMOR COMPOSITION

The composition of aqueous humor differs from that of plasma as a result of two important physiologic characteristics of the anterior segment: a mechanical epithelial/endothelial blood-aqueous barrier (BAB) and active transport of various organic and inorganic substances by the ciliary epithelium. The greatest differences are the low protein and high ascorbate concentrations in the aqueous humor relative to plasma (200 times less and 20 times greater, respectively).† The high ascorbate concentration may help protect the anterior ocular structures from ultraviolet light–induced oxidative damage. When the aqueous humor protein concentration rises much above its normal 20 mg/100 ml, as in uveitis, the resultant light scattering (Tyndall effect) makes visible the slit-lamp beam as it traverses the AC (a phenomenon known as *flare*).[141] Lactate is also normally in excess in the aqueous humor, presumably as a result of glycolytic activity of the lens, cornea, and other ocular structures.[141,312] Other compounds or ions in excess in the aqueous humor relative to plasma are Cl^- and certain amino acids.[187]

BLOOD-AQUEOUS BARRIER

The BAB is a functional concept, rather than a discrete structure, invoked to explain the degree to which various solutes are relatively restricted in travel from the ocular vasculature into the aqueous humor. The capillaries of the CP and choroid are fenestrated, but the interdigitating surfaces of the retinal PE and the CP NPE, respectively, are joined to each other by tight junctions (zonulae occludens) and constitute an effective barrier to intermediate- and high-molecular-weight substances, such as proteins.* The endothelia of the IW of SC are similarly joined, preventing retrograde movement of solutes and fluid from the canal lumen into the TM and AC.[309,554] The iris and retina have no similar epithelium between their vasculature and the ocular fluids, but their capillaries are of the nonfenestrated, impermeable type.[6,95,141,187] For present purposes, one may say that the BAB consists of the tight junctions of the CP NPE, the IW endothelium of SC, the iris vasculature, and the outward-directed active transport systems of the CP (see following discussion). A more universal concept of the BAB must deal with the movement of smaller molecules, lipid-soluble substances, and water into the eye.[141]

With trauma-, disease-, or drug-induced breakdown of the BAB (Table 8-1), plasma components enter the aqueous humor. Net fluid movement from blood to aqueous increases, but so does its IOP dependence (pseudofacility [C_{ps}]).[455] Total facility, as measured by IOP-altering techniques, cannot distinguish C_{ps} from total OF (C_{tot}); therefore the C_{ps} component is erroneously recorded as increased C_{tot} (hence the term C_{ps}) and the extent to which the outflow pathways have been compromised by the insult is underestimated. Under these circumstances, increased C_{ps} provides some protection against a precipitous rise in IOP; as IOP rises, aqueous humor inflow by ultrafiltration is partly suppressed, blunting (but not completely suppressing) further IOP elevation.[88,93] In addition, the inflammatory process that occurs during BAB breakdown leads to a reduction in active secretion of aqueous humor, possibly by means of interference with active transport mechanisms.[677] This in turn may actually produce ocular hypotony, despite compromised outflow pathways (as a result of plasma protein blockage of the TM). Prostaglandin (PG) release during inflammation may contribute to the hypotony by increasing aqueous humor outflow via the uveoscleral route.[355,359] When the noxious stimulus is removed, however, the ciliary body may recover before the TM and the resulting normalization of AHF rate in

---

*References 292, 320, 362, 418, 533, 624, 648, 649, 707, 721, 724, 741.
†References 194, 232, 269, 380, 470, 606, 643.

*References 6, 80, 87, 141, 309, 570, 621, 630, 699, 700, 709.

Table 8-1

Factors Interrupting the Blood-Aqueous Barrier

I. Traumatic
  A. Mechanical
    1. Paracentesis
    2. Corneal abrasion
    3. Blunt trauma
    4. Intraocular surgery
    5. Stroking of the iris
  B. Physical
    1. Radiotherapy
    2. Nuclear radiation
  C. Chemical
    1. Alkali
    2. Irritants (e.g., nitrogen mustard)
II. Pathophysiologic
  A. Vasodilation
    1. Histamine
    2. Sympathectomy

  B. Corneal and intraocular infections
  C. Intraocular inflammation
  D. Prostaglandins (varies with dose, type, and species)
  E. Anterior segment ischemia
III. Pharmacologic
  A. Melanocyte-stimulating hormone
  B. Nitrogen mustard
  C. Cholinergic drugs, especially cholinesterase inhibitors
  D. Plasma hyperosmolality

Modified from Stamper RL: Aqueous humor: secretion and dynamics. In Tasman W, Jaeger EA (eds): *Clinical ophthalmology*, vol 2, Philadelphia, 1979, Lippincott.

---

the face of still compromised outflow pathways leads to elevated IOP, as seen from the modified Goldmann equation:

$$IOP = [(AHF - F_u)/C_{trab}] + P_e$$

where

AHF = Aqueous humor formation
C_{trab} = Facility of outflow from the AC via the TM and SC
IOP = Intraocular pressure
P_e = Episcleral venous pressure (the pressure against which fluid leaving the AC via the trabecular-canalicular route must drain)
F_u = uveoscleral outflow[343]

Active Transport

The CP possesses the ability to actively transport a variety of organic and inorganic compounds and ions out of, or to exclude them from, the eye; that is, the CP can move them from the aqueous or vitreous humor to the blood against a concentration gradient. *para*-Aminohippurate, Diodrast, and penicillin are examples of large anions that are actively transported out of the eye. These systems are similar to those in the renal tubules and satisfy all the criteria for active transport: saturability, energy and temperature dependence, Michaelis Menten kinetics, inhibition by ouabain and probenecid,

and so forth.* In addition, another system can actively excrete injected iodide from the aqueous humor, resembling iodide transport in the thyroid and salivary glands.[63] The physiologic role of these outward-directed systems is unknown. With the discovery that PGs may be actively transported out of the eye, some workers have suggested that such outward-directed mechanisms may rid the eye of biologically active substances that are no longer needed or that may even be detrimental.[62,108-112,114] Other outwardly directed ion-uptake mechanisms are present in the eye. For example, the anterior uvea of the rabbit eye accumulates the anions cholate, glycocholate, deoxycholate, chenodeoxycholate, iodipamide, and o-iodohippurate.[43,47] At least one outwardly directed cationic pump has also been reported; iris/ciliary body (ICB) preparations accumulate the cation emperonium, although a later report questioned whether any other cations are actively eliminated from the eye.[48,49]

Bárány,[44] making an analogy to the ion pump located at the renal peritubular cell border adjacent to the blood, which pumps simple cations from the blood to the kidney tubule, investigated whether there are any inwardly directed complex cation pump systems from blood to aqueous but concluded that such mechanisms probably do not ex-

---

*References 43-47, 62, 63, 114, 187, 195, 239, 645, 646.

ist, at least in the rabbit. All of these transport systems (inwardly and outwardly directed) are thought to be located in the NPE.[141]

Pharmacology and Regulation of Aqueous Humor Formation and Composition

Sympathetic and parasympathetic nerve terminals are present in the ciliary body arising from branches of the long and short posterior ciliary nerves.[197,198,399,487,582] These nerve fibers are of both the myelinated and nonmyelinated varieties. Parasympathetic fibers originate in the Edinger-Westphal nucleus of the third cranial nerve, run with the inferior division of this nerve in the orbit, and synapse in the ciliary ganglion.[131] Nerve fibers originating in the pterygopalatine ganglion release nitric oxide and vasoactive intestinal peptide (VIP) to increase choroidal blood flow in the rat.[755] Isotope injection of the pterygopalatine ganglion in rats anterogradely labels fibers passing through the ciliary ganglion that innervate the conjunctiva, limbus, and parts of the choroid.[660] Nerves displaying VIP immunoreactivity were also detected in the CP, in the posterior third of the CM, and around small to medium blood vessels in the posterior uvea of the cat.[692] In the cat eye, nerve fibers containing pituitary adenylate cyclase–activating polypeptide (PACAP) were detected in the iris, ciliary body, and conjunctiva. PACAP immunoreactivity colocalized with VIP in the sphenopalatine ganglion and with calcitonin gene-related peptide in the trigeminal ganglion.[202] Human eyes specifically have an intrinsic nerve cell plexus in the temporocentral portion of the choroid, indicating a functional significance of the nitrergic choroidal innervation for the fovea.[238] Stimulation of the facial nerve causes vasodilation in the uvea.[103] Sympathetic fibers synapse in the superior cervical ganglion and are distributed to the muscles and blood vessels of the ciliary body. Stimulation of the cervical sympathetic nerves in vervet monkeys significantly increased the rate of aqueous humor formation.[91] Numerous unmyelinated nerve fibers surround the stromal vessels of the CP; these are most likely noradrenergic and subserve vasomotion.[141] Sensory fibers arise from the ophthalmic division of the trigeminal nerve and enter the ciliary body, but their distribution and function have not been well studied. No innervation of the ciliary epithelium has been found anatomically, but stimulation of the ciliary ganglion leads to an increase in AHF in the enucleated arterially perfused cat eye, suggesting that neurotransmitters released in the ciliary stroma might diffuse toward the epithelia.[309,442]

Sympathetic denervation in monkeys does not alter resting AHF and marginally affects the AHF response to timolol or epinephrine (EPI).[260] In humans with unilateral Horner syndrome, IOP, daytime AHF, tonographic OF, and the flow and IOP response to timolol were similar in both eyes.[730] However, eyes of patients with Horner syndrome showed a decrease in AHF in response to EPI instead of the normal increase. Conversely, isoproterenol increased flow during sleep in eyes both of healthy subjects and those with Horner syndrome, no significant effect on flow was noted in either group during the day.[398] Chemical sympathectomy with guanethidine sulfate in glaucomatous humans lowered IOP, presumably by reducing aqueous humor production measured indirectly by tonography.[116] VIP-stimulated aqueous humor formation after intravenous (IV) administration in monkeys results from activation of the sympathetic nervous system, whereas intracameral administration of VIP directly effects the ciliary epithelium.[495] The role of sympathetic innervation in mediating aqueous humor inflow and outflow responses to pharmacologic agents remains largely uncertain.

Cholinergic Mechanisms

The effects of cholinergic drugs on AHF, aqueous humor composition, and the BAB are unclear. Overall, cholinomimetics have little effect on the volumetric rate of AHF. In general, cholinergic drugs cause vasodilation in the anterior segment, resulting in increased blood flow to the choroid, iris, CP, and CM.* However, cholinergic drugs may also promote vasoconstriction, for example, in rat coronary arteries and rat outer descending vasa recta, perfused in vitro, and in the rabbit eye.[105,132] These responses are mediated by muscarinic receptors (M_3) in the anterior uveal arterioles, perhaps associated with facial parasympathetic nerve terminals.[7,493,580] Congestion in the iris and ciliary body is a well-recognized clinical side effect of topical cholinomimetics, especially the anticholinesterases.[314] The presence of flare and cells in the aqueous humor, detected by biomicroscopy, indicates that these agents can also cause breakdown of the BAB and perhaps frank inflammation.[314] Pilocarpine (PILO) increases BAB permeability to iodide and in-

---

*References 7, 54, 79, 132, 264, 324, 587, 740.

ulin.[64,653] Cholinergic drug–induced vasodilation might cause a weakening of tight junctions in anterior uveal blood vessels, perhaps contributing to breakdown of the BAB.[609] Cholinergic drugs may alter the aqueous humor concentration of inorganic ions and the movement of certain amino acids from the blood into the aqueous humor and may also influence the outward-directed transport systems of the CP.[113,717,718] Cholinergic agents can disrupt the coupling and Na^+ currents between PE and NPE cells in vitro, suggesting a possible inhibitory effect on aqueous humor secretion.[618,640]

Under certain conditions, PILO may increase C_{ps}.[36,252] Using a variety of species, conditions, and experimental techniques, researchers have reported that cholinergic agents or parasympathetic nerve stimulation increases, decreases, or does not alter the AHF rate and increases slightly the episcleral venous pressure.* These apparently confusing results may indicate that cholinergic drug effects on these parameters are extremely dependent on species and technique-related factors and on the ambient neurovascular milieu. In any event, the effects on the rate of AHF and episcleral venous pressure are minor in most instances and are not responsible for the drug-induced decrease in IOP that forms the basis of PILO's therapeutic efficacy in chronic glaucoma. PILO's efficacy is in its ability to decrease outflow resistance through its effect on the CM, and perhaps to a much lesser extent, directly on the TM[214] (see section Aqueous Humor Drainage).

Adrenergic Mechanisms

The precise role and receptor specificity of adrenergic mechanisms in regulating the rate of AHF are unclear. At one time it was generally believed that long-term topical administration of EPI, a combined $\alpha_1,\alpha_2,\beta_1,\beta_2$-adrenergic agonist, would decrease the rate of AHF.[311] This effect was thought to be mediated by β-adrenergic receptors in the NPE, through activation of a membrane adenylate cyclase, although the consequent biochemical events were (and still are) unknown.[282,489,691,716] In support of these observations, activation of ocular adenylate cyclase by means of its G_s protein by close arterial infusion of cholera toxin decreases AHF and lowers IOP in the rabbit.[282] Furthermore, in some studies forskolin, a naturally occurring diterpene

derivative of the coleus plant (*Coleus forskohlii*), which directly and irreversibly activates intracellular adenylate cyclase, decreased the rate of AHF when given topically or intravitreally.[613,620,629] Although vascular phenomena could theoretically be involved in the secretion and pressure responses, these observations are consistent with primary epithelial action of these drugs. The relationship between ocular vascular events and IOP modulation, if any, has yet to be established.*

Fluorophotometric studies have shown that short-term topical administration of EPI increases AHF[18,260,590,684]; studies with other adrenergic agonists, including salbutamol, isoproterenol (isoprenaline), and terbutaline, have supported this finding and are consistent with many studies showing that β-adrenergic antagonists unequivocally decrease AHF.†

The ocular hypotensive action of β-antagonists has led to their becoming mainstays of clinical glaucoma therapy: the nonselective β_1,β_2-antagonists timolol, levobunolol, and metipranolol; the nonselective β_1,β_2-partial agonist carteolol; and the relatively selective β_1-selective antagonist betaxolol.‡ Adrenergic receptors in the ciliary epithelium are of the β_2-subtype, but antagonists that are relatively selective for β_1-receptors (e.g., betaxolol) are effective (although less potent and efficacious) in suppressing AHF.§ However, the apparent β_1-efficacy may be related to a sufficiently high concentration reaching the ciliary epithelium so that nonselective blockade of β_2-receptors may occur.[714]

It has been questioned whether β-adrenergic antagonists suppress AHF through their effect on ciliary epithelial β-adrenergic receptors.‖ Evidence suggests that classical β-adrenergic blockade may not be involved and that other receptor types, such as 5-HT_{1A}, may be relevant (see subsequent discussion).[55,386,461,505] Furthermore, $Na^+\text{-}K^+\text{-}2Cl^-$ cotransport stimulated by EPI and isoproterenol can be inhibited by β_2-adrenergic–receptor antagonists in human fetal nonpigmented ciliary epithelial cells, although timolol had no effect on Na^+ entry into the rabbit posterior chamber after IV injection of ^{22}Na.[175,176,453]

---

*References 71, 72, 107, 151, 252, 280, 392, 419, 440-442, 478, 642, 697, 698, 717.

*References 58, 152, 303, 463, 471, 529, 722.
†References 19, 117, 121, 160, 161, 184, 267, 398, 444, 465, 482, 498, 590, 641, 753, 766.
‡References 19, 160, 184, 465, 590, 641, 752, 753.
§References 4, 5, 73, 74, 130, 135, 412, 426, 480, 481, 600, 641.
‖References 57, 66, 142, 143, 153, 282, 366, 419, 420, 460, 464, 559, 560, 592, 613, 614, 620, 629, 708, 730.

AHF is reduced by nearly 50% during sleep as a result of the β-Arrestin–cyclic adenosine monophosphate (cAMP) cascade regulation of signal transduction from the β-adrenergic receptor to the ciliary epithelium.[130,141,187,557] This results in a circadian fluctuation of IOP.[720] However, there is some question about whether IOP actually decreases in humans at night. Liu et al.[422,423] suggest that IOP may actually increase in humans at night and that technical limitations may be responsible for previously reported IOP decreases. β-Antagonists produce little additional decrease in AHF during sleep or in pentobarbital-anesthetized monkeys.[568,673] Because sympathetic tone is reduced during both sleep and barbiturate anesthesia, these findings provide further indirect evidence that β-adrenergic tone/stimulation enhances AHF, whereas β-adrenergic blockade decreases it.[227] Sympathetic fibers synapse in the superior cervical ganglion and are distributed to the muscles and blood vessels of the ciliary body regulating blood flow to the CP vasculature. Catecholaminergic and neuropeptide Y (NPY)-ergic nerve fibers preferentially supply vasculature and epithelium of the monkey anterior CP, suggesting a crucial function of these structures for the precise regulation of aqueous humor formation.[565] Adrenergic drugs may exert their effect by causing localized constriction in the arterioles that supply the CP.[704,705] Stimulation of the cervical sympathetic nerves in vervet monkeys significantly increases the rate of aqueous humor formation.[91] However, adrenergic tone to the ciliary epithelium may be humoral catecholaminergic rather than sympathetic innervational. AHF in human subjects was correlated with circulating catecholamine levels during sleep and wakefulness.[439] Two major hormones of the adrenal gland, EPI and cortisol, can regulate aqueous formation.[322]

Topically applied α_1-adrenergic agonists and antagonists appear to have little effect on fluorophotometrically determined AHF in the normal intact human eye, although these compounds do reduce AHF in the rabbit.* However, in eyes under β-adrenergic blockade, topical EPI acutely produces a small decrease, rather than increase, in AHF, perhaps indicating a weak α-adrenergic influence, possibly mediated by local vasoconstriction.[307,662] Clonidine, which has both α_1-antagonist and α_2-agonist properties, decreases AHF and ocular blood flow.[100,268,381,402] Therefore EPI may have a dual effect on AHF: stimulation by means of β-adrenoceptors and inhibition by means of α_2-adrenoceptors.[325,421,479,594] α_2-Adrenergic agonists, such as apraclonidine and brimonidine, are powerful ocular hypotensive agents when applied topically and are believed to lower IOP primarily by decreasing AHF.[358,456] Other mechanisms such as increased OF (e.g., with apraclonidine use) and increased F_u (e.g., with brimonidine use) have been suggested but remain controversial.[679,680] The results of one study in humans conclude that brimonidine and apraclonidine are similar in their effects on the aqueous system and reduce IOP primarily, if not exclusively, by suppressing AHF.[456] However, the results of another study in humans suggest that brimonidine suppresses AHF early on, but after 8 to 29 days of treatment the predominant effect is on F_u.[675]

OTHER AGENTS

AHF can be reduced pharmacologically in many other ways (Table 8-2). Effective compounds include the guanylate cyclase activators; atrial natriuretic factor (ANF); and the nitrovasodilators sodium nitroprusside, sodium azide, and nitroglycerin.* In contrast, Krupin et al.[391] proposed that the IOP rise in rabbits after topical application of sodium azide or sodium nitroprusside was a result of an increase in AHF because blood pressure was not elevated, tonographic OF was unchanged, and posterior chamber ascorbate levels were decreased. 8-Bromocyclic guanosine monophosphate also reduces the AHF rate by 15% to 20% in the monkey.[367] ANF injected intravitreally reduced IOP and AHF in rabbits and monkeys.[378,585] The calcium channel antagonists verapamil, nifedipine, and diltiazem have been reported to reduce AHF in rabbits, although no apparent change in IOP, visual fields, or optic discs were found in patients with open-angle glaucoma who were using calcium channel blockers for nonophthalmic diseases.[424,586]

The serotonergic antagonist ketanserin reduces the AHF rate in rabbits, cats, and monkeys.[145] The endogenous agonist serotonin (5-HT) may also reduce AHF; topical application results in decreased IOP in the rabbit, but intracameral injection in the same species increases IOP.[386] Serotonergic receptors of a 5-HT_{1A}–like subtype have been reported to exist in the ICB of rabbits and humans.[55,147,461,505] It has been suggested that these receptors may be antagonized by timolol and other β-blockers.[505] The 5-HT_{1A} agonist 8-OH-DPAT dose-dependently decreased IOP in normotensive rabbits during light

---

*References 302, 389, 400, 401, 467, 468, 607.

*References 378, 469, 483, 484, 585, 612.

Table 8-2
Factors Causing Reduced Aqueous Humor Secretion

I. General
- A. Age
- B. Diurnal cycle
- C. Exercise

II. Systemic
- A. Reduction in blood pressure
- B. Artificial reduction in internal carotid arterial blood flow
- C. Diencephalic stimulation
- D. Hypothermia
- E. Acidosis
- F. General anesthesia

III. Local
- A. Increased IOP (pseudofacility)
- B. Uveitis (especially iridocyclitis)
- C. Retinal detachment
- D. Retrobulbar anesthesia
- E. Choroidal detachment

IV. Pharmacologic
- A. β-Adrenoceptor antagonists (e.g., timolol, betaxolol, levobunolol, carteolol, metipranolol)
- B. Carbonic anhydrase inhibitors
- C. Nitrovasodilators; atrial natriuretic factor
- D. Calcium channel antagonists
- E. 5-HT$_{1A}$ antagonists (e.g., ketanserin)
- F. DA$_2$ agonists (e.g., pergolide, lergotrile, bromocriptine)
- G. α$_2$-Adrenoceptor agonists (e.g., apraclonidine, brimonidine)
- H. ACE inhibitors
- I. H$_1$-receptor antagonists (e.g., antazoline, pyrilamine)
- J. Δ9-Tetrahydrocannabinol (Δ9-THC)
- K. Metabolic inhibitors (e.g., DNP, fluoroacetamide)
- L. Cardiac glycosides (e.g., ouabain, digoxin)
- M. Spironolactone
- N. Plasma hyperosmolality
- O. cGMP

V. Surgical
- A. Cyclodialysis
- B. Cyclocryothermy
- C. Cyclodiathermy
- D. Cyclophotocoagulation

Modified from Stamper RL: Aqueous humor: secretion and dynamics. In Tasman W, Jaeger EA (eds): *Clinical ophthalmology,* vol 2, Philadelphia, 1979, Lippincott.
ACE, Angiotensin-converting enzyme; *cGMP,* cyclic guanosine monophosphate; *DA$_2$,* dopamine; *DNP,* dinitrophenol; *IOP,* intraocular pressure.

and dark cycles.[148,156] However, the precise nature of the putative 5-HT$_{1A}$–like receptor subtype in the ciliary epithelium is still in question. In addition, IOP and AHF suppression of 5HT$_{1A}$–receptor agonists in nonhuman primates is variable.[262] Components of the renin-angiotensin system have been measured in the ocular tissues of several species, including humans.* Several angiotensin-converting

enzyme inhibitors, when topically applied to rabbit eyes, reduce secretion.[712] However, there was no reduction in IOP in healthy humans, hypertensive humans, or monkeys after topical application of a renin inhibitor.[497,520] H$_1$-antihistamines, such as antazoline and pyrilamine, decrease AHF in rabbits, although the effect may be unrelated to histamine-receptor binding.[390] Metabolic inhibitors such as 2,4-dinitrophenol (DNP) decrease AHF, as do the cardiac glycosides ouabain and digoxin, which in-

*References 123, 231, 323, 396, 506, 552, 622, 638, 712, 715, 719, 732.

hibit the ciliary epithelial Na^+-K^+-ATPase enzyme.[308,375] None of these has yet been shown to have any clinical relevance for the human.

Other local, systemic, and surgical factors can reduce AHF rate, as can age and exercise (see Table 8-2). In a study of 300 normal volunteers ages 5 to 83 years, there was an average decline in aqueous flow of 25% between the ages of 10 and 80 years.[130] A smaller decline was observed by Toris et al.[682] in humans older than 65 years of age. No age-related decline in AHF was seen in rhesus monkeys up to 25 to 29 years of age (human equivalent, 62 to 73 years).[259]

Aqueous Humor Drainage

Fluid Mechanics

The tissues of the AC angle normally offer a certain resistance to fluid outflow. IOP builds up in response to the inflow of aqueous humor to the level that is sufficient to drive fluid across that resistance at the same rate it is produced by the ciliary body; this is the *steady-state IOP*. In the glaucomatous eye, this resistance is often unusually high, resulting in elevated IOP. IOP is thought to be one of the causal risk factors in the development and progression of glaucoma.[1,631,632] Understanding the factors governing normal and abnormal AHF, aqueous humor outflow, IOP, and their interrelationships and manipulations is vital in understanding and treating glaucoma.

Briefly, let:

F = Flow (μl/min)

F_{in} = Total aqueous humor inflow (human = approximately $2.5\ \mu l \times min^{-1}$)*

F_S = Inflow from active secretion

F_f = Inflow from ultrafiltration

F_{out} = Total aqueous humor outflow

F_{trab} = Outflow via trabecular pathway

F_u = Outflow via uveoscleral pathway (0.3 μl/min, measured invasively by radioactive tracer, in primarily elderly human eyes with malignant melanoma, tumor, or glaucoma[104]; 1.64 μl/min in healthy subjects ages 20 to 30 years; and 1.16 ± 0.82 μl/min in subjects older than 60 years, measured by noninvasive fluorophotometry[682])

P = Pressure (mm Hg)

P_i = IOP (humans = 16 mm Hg)[23,61]

P_e = Episcleral venous pressure (human = 9 mm Hg)[313,679]

R = Resistance to flow (mm Hg × min/μl)

C = Facility or conductance of flow (μl/min/mm Hg) = $1/R$

C_{tot} = Total aqueous humor OF (humans ages 20 to 30 years, 0.25 ± 0.12 μl/min/mm Hg; older than 60 years, 0.19 ± 0.11 μl/min/mm Hg[682]; OF = 0.54 − (0.0042 × age in years) μl/min/mm Hg[173]; 0.243 μl/min/mm Hg[278]; younger than 40 years, 0.331 ± 0.067 μl/min/mm Hg; older than 60 years, 0.233 ± 0.046 μl/min/mm Hg[61]; 0.28 ± 0.01 μl/min/mm Hg[394] all measured by indentation tonography)

C_{trab} = Facility of outflow via trabecular pathway (humans 20 to 30 years, 0.21 ± 0.10 μl/min/mm Hg; older than 60 years, 0.25 ± 0.10 μl/min/mm Hg [fluorophotometry][678]; 0.22 ± 0.01 μl/min/ mm Hg [tonography])[394]

C_u = Facility of outflow via uveoscleral pathway (humans = 0.02 μl/min/mm Hg[299]; probably based on reported monkey values[93,353])

C_{ps} = Facility of inflow (human = 0.06 μl/min/mm Hg[393,394]; 0.08 μl/min/mm Hg[69]; these values for C_{ps} are most likely overestimates: under normal circumstance, in a noninflamed eye the phenomenon is negligible[473]; values for the normal monkey measured by a more precise tracer technique are less than 0.02 μl/min/mm Hg[93,353])

Then:

$$F_{in} = F_S + F_f$$
$$F_{out} = F_{trab} + F_u$$
$$C_{tot} = C_{trab} + C_u + C_{ps}$$

At steady state:

$$F = F_{in} = F_{out}$$

The simplest hydraulic model, represented by the classic Goldmann equation, views aqueous flow as passive, non–energy-dependent bulk fluid movement down a pressure gradient, with aqueous humor leaving the eye only via the trabecular route, where $\Delta P = P_i - P_e$, so that $F = C_{trab}(P_i - P_e)$. This relationship is correct, but it is vastly oversimplified. Because there is no complete endothelial layer covering the anterior surface of the ciliary body and no delimitation of the spaces between the trabecular beams and the spaces between the CM bundles, fluid can pass from the chamber angle into the tissue spaces within the CM.[309] These spaces, in turn, open into the suprachoroid, from which fluid can pass through the scleral substance or the perivascular/perineural scleral spaces into the episcleral tissues. Some investigators believe that some fluid may also be drawn osmotically into the vortex veins by the high protein content in the blood of these vessels.[332] Along these uveal routes, the fluid mixes with

---

*References 187, 267, 337, 388, 462, 673, 682, 684, 753.

tissue fluid from the CM, CP, and choroid. Thus this flow pathway may be analogous to lymphatic drainage of tissue fluid in other organs (there are no ocular lymphatics) and provide an important means of ridding the eye of potentially toxic tissue metabolites.* Flow from the AC across the TM into SC is pressure dependent, but drainage via the uveoscleral pathway is virtually independent of pressure at IOP levels greater than 7 to 10 mm Hg.[83,86,95] Although the actual drainage rates (μl/min) via the trabecular and uveoscleral routes in the monkey may be approximately equal, measured facility of F_u (C_u, determined by measuring F_u at two different IOP levels) is only approximately 0.02 μl/min/mm Hg, or less than one twentieth the facility of trabecular outflow.[83] The reasons for the pressure independence of the uveoscleral pathway are not entirely clear but might be consequent to the complex nature of the pressure and resistance relationships between the various fluid compartments within the soft intraocular tissues along the route.[95] For instance, pressure in the potential suprachoroidal space (P_s) is directly dependent on IOP, such that at any IOP level, P_s is considerably but constantly less than IOP.[95] Because the pressure gradient between the AC and suprachoroid is thus independent of IOP, bulk fluid flow between these compartments is also IOP independent. Intraorbital pressure is such that under normal circumstances there is always a positive-pressure gradient between the suprachoroidal and intraorbital spaces.[95] Fluid and solutes, including large protein molecules, can thus easily exit the eye by passing through the spaces surrounding the neural or vascular scleral emissaria or through the scleral substance itself.[81,84,92] At low IOP levels, the net pressure gradient across the uveoscleral pathways is apparently so low that uveoscleral drainage decreases.[86] The absence of an outflow gradient from the suprachoroid may contribute to the development of choroidal detachments seen during the ocular hypotony that sometimes follows intraocular surgery.[95]

However, other investigators[370,516,676] have found unconventional flow to be more pressure sensitive than did Bill, and F_u may become more sensitive to pressure following PG treatment.[255,681] There is no need for fluid flow to carry tracer across the sclera because it can diffuse across on its own, based on calculations of diffusional transport porperties.[332] Direct evidence for a uveovortex pathway was pro-

vided by Pederson et al.,[516] who demonstrated that after perfusion of the AC with fluorescein, the fluorescein concentration in the vortex veins was higher than that in the general circulation. In addition, flow across the sclera is pressure dependent.[370] Uveovortex flow explains the relative insensitivity of the flow to pressure because most of the driving force would then be that of osmotic pressure of the blood that draws the fluid into these vessels.[332] Clearly, more needs to be learned about this flow pathway.

Because, under normal steady-state conditions, C_{ps} and C_u are so low compared with C_{trab}, the hydraulics of aqueous dynamics may be reasonably approximated for clinical purposes by the following equation:

$$F_{in} = F_{out} = C_{trab}(P_i - P_e) + F_u$$

Clinically significant increases in inflow occur only in situations involving breakdown of the BAB. The pressure sensitivity of the ultrafiltration component of aqueous secretion blunts the tendency for IOP to rise under such conditions; that is, C_{ps} is increased. Elevated episcleral venous pressure, such as may occur with arteriovenous communications resulting from congenital malformations or trauma, causes a nearly mm Hg–for–mm Hg increase in IOP.[316] Pharmacologic agents may exert small and probably clinically insignificant effects on C_{ps}, C_u, or P_e.* Major, clinically relevant alterations in outflow physiology are achieved by iatrogenic manipulation of C_{trab} or F_u.

PHARMACOLOGY AND REGULATION

Most aqueous humor leaves the eye through the TM and SC. This outflow is pressure dependent. SC and the TM lie within the internal scleral groove between the scleral spur and the ring of Schwalbe's line at the termination of Descemet's membrane. The TM extends from the level of the scleral spur to Schwalbe's line. An anterior nonfiltering portion can be distinguished from a posterior filtering portion of the meshwork. The TM itself consists of three functionally and structurally different parts: the iridic and uveal part, which represents the innermost portion of the meshwork; the corneoscleral part, which extends between the scleral spur and the cornea; and the juxtacanalicular (JXT) part or cribriform layer, which lies adjacent to the IW of SC (Figure 8-4). In the primate eye, approximately 60% to 80% of the

---

*References 81-83, 85, 86, 92, 95, 97, 101, 104, 106, 107, 309, 355, 677.

---

*References 36, 42, 85, 90, 91, 107, 251, 252, 392, 393, 740.

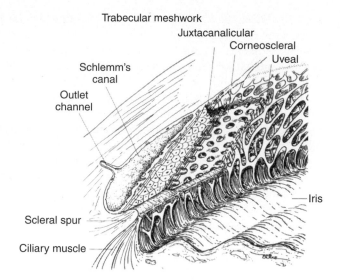

FIGURE 8-4   Three layers of trabecular meshwork (shown in cutaway view): uveal, corneoscleral, and juxtacanalicular. (From Shields
MB: Aqueous humor dynamics: I. Anatomy and
physiology. In Shields MB [ed]: *Textbook of
glaucoma*, Baltimore, 1998, Williams &
Wilkins.)

resistance to aqueous humor outflow resides in the
tissues between the AC and the lumen of SC.*

The iridic, uveal, and corneoscleral portions of
the TM consist of connective tissue plates or lamellas, which are completely covered by endothelial
cells resting on a basement membrane. The iridic
and uveal meshwork is posteriorly contiguous with
the ciliary body and the iris root. The iridic portion
consists mainly of intermeshed, radially oriented,
more or less round tissue strands that originate in
the stroma of the iris root or in the connective tissue in front of the CM. They become fixed anteriorly in the corneal stroma or in the nonfiltering
portion of the TM. Between the radial strands are
large spaces or openings.

In the uveal meshwork, as in the corneoscleral
part of the meshwork, the trabecular lamellas form
netlike sheets oriented mainly in an equatorial direction. The endothelial cells completely covering
these sheets or beams connect the sheets also in the
radial, outward-inward direction so that a three-
dimensional spongelike mesh is formed. The intertrabecular spaces and openings are relatively large
in the inner parts of the meshwork but become
smaller toward the cribriform layer. Each trabecular lamella has a central core containing ground
substance rich in glycoproteins and hyaluronic acid
and collagenous and elastic-like fibers. The collagenous and elastic-like fibers form a regular network
of interlacing bundles, their main course following
an equatorial direction.[429,430]

The major resistance site within the trabecular
structures has still not been identified, but most investigators believe that it resides in the cribriform
portion of the meshwork (CAI tissue), the outermost part of the mesh consisting of several layers of
endothelial cells embedded in a ground substance
consisting of a wide variety of macromolecules, including hyaluronic acid, other glycosaminoglycans
(GAGs), collagen, fibronectin, and other glycoproteins.* These macromolecules are presumably produced by meshwork endothelial cells, and their synthesis and turnover may be one means by which
outflow resistance is modulated.[242,539] However, if
this is the case, the control mechanisms are largely
unknown, despite new evidence suggesting that
modulation of TM-inducible glucocorticoid response (TIGR)/myocilin gene expression and protein production may play an important role.[541,644]
However, some investigators consider the main resistance to lie slightly proximal to the CAI tissue.[14,476] In
contrast to the corneoscleral meshwork, the cribriform layer is not organized into cell-covered lamellas, so aqueous humor directly penetrates this tissue
layer, thereby coming into contact with the extracellular substances and fibrous material. The cribriform
layer is supported by an elastic-like fiber network
and fine collagen fiber bundles (Figure 8-5) that have
the same orientation as the elastic-like network in
the central core of the trabecular lamellas.[573] This
network is connected to the IW endothelium of SC
by fine, bent, connecting fibrils.

*References 95, 106, 201, 279, 321, 428, 526, 650, 701, 702.

*References 95, 106, 200, 201, 279, 300, 321, 428, 429, 561, 576,
588, 589, 650.

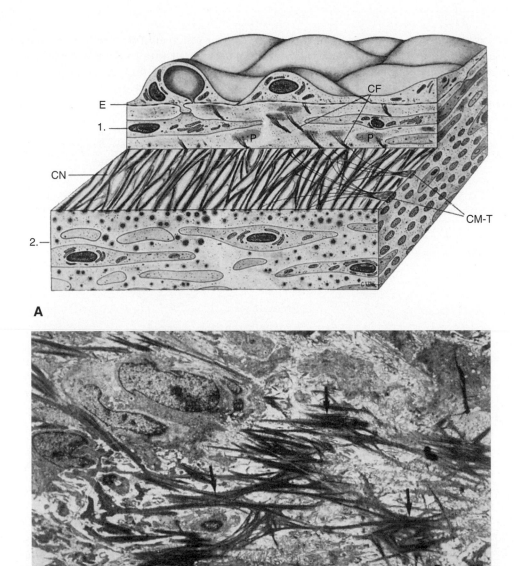

FIGURE 8-5 A, Schematic drawing of the cribriform meshwork and the endothelial lining of Schlemm's canal (*E*). Note the connection between the ciliary muscle tendons (*CM-T*) and the elastic-like fiber plexus, or "cribriform plexus" (*CN*), located mainly in the region between the first and second subendothelial cell layers (*1.* and *2.*). The cribriform plexus is connected to the inner wall endothelium and the plaque material (*P*) by a system of fine fibrils or "connecting fibrils" (*CF*). **B,** Electron micrograph of a tangential section through the cribriform region almost at the level between the second subendothelial cell layer and the first corneoscleral trabecular lamellas (normal eye). The cells seen in the *upper left* are subendothelial. The elastic-like fibers of the cribriform region (*arrows*) form a plexus that shows the same equatorial orientation as the network of the elastic-like fibers of the trabecular lamellas. (From Rohen JW, Futa R, Lütjen-Drecoll E: *Invest Ophthalmol Vis Sci* 21:574, 1981.)

SC itself possesses a complete endothelial lining, which does not rest on a continuous basement membrane. A subendothelial cell layer is oriented predominantly in a radial direction, whereas the endothelial cells of the canal run mostly in an equa-

torial direction.[571] The two cell layers are closely related to each other by interdigitating cell processes. The extracellular material (ECM) between the cells, rich in glycoproteins and fine collagenous fibrils, might serve for fixation of the two cell layers. A small percentage of the resistance, perhaps 10% to 25%, resides in the IW of SC.[106,650,651] The basement membrane and apparently empty spaces between it, and the IW may also play a role. The basement membrane and subendothelial matrix are known to be discontinuous.[572] Other factors involved in creating resistance in these gaps include proteogly-

cans or other substances within the gaps that are not visualized with conventional fixation and processing, the AHF through nongap regions of the basement membrane, resistance offered by the IW endothelial cells, or proteoglycans within the optically empty spaces of the entire TM.[223,454] Calculations show that gaps make the basement

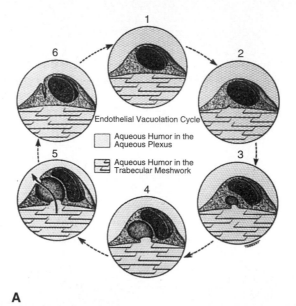

A

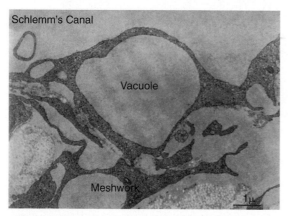

B

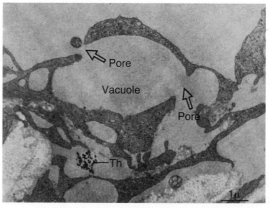

C

FIGURE 8-6   **A,** Resting state before initiation of transcellular transport *(1)*. Theory of transcellular aqueous transport in which a series of pores and giant vacuoles open (probably in response to transendothelial hydrostatic pressure) on the connective tissue side of the juxtacanalicular meshwork *(2 to 4)*. Fusion of basal and apical cell plasmalemma creates a temporary transcellular channel *(5)* that allows bulk flow of aqueous humor into Schlemm's canal. **B,** Transmission electron micrograph of the inner wall of Schlemm's canal and the adjacent subendothelial tissue showing empty spaces or "giant vacuoles" within the endothelial cells. **C,** Serial sections of the inner wall of Schlemm's canal indicate that the "giant vacuoles" of the endothelial cells have openings toward the trabecular side, indicating that they are invaginations from the trabecular side. Some of the invaginations also have openings (pores) into Schlemm's canal. Aqueous humor can pass through the cells via the invaginations and the pores. Arrows indicate possible routes for aqueous humor outflow through the pores. *Th,* Thorotrast. (From Inomata H, Bill A, Smelser GK: *Am J Ophthalmol* 73:760, 1972; and Tripathi RC: *Exp Eye Res* 11:116, 1971.)

membrane of the IW leakier than basement membranes in other tissues.[327] Digestion of heparan sulfate, a component of basement membranes, by heparinase treatment of human anterior segments in organ culture increases OF by 55%.[329]

Fluid movement across the inner canal wall endothelium itself appears to be predominantly via passive pressure-dependent transcellular pathways, including giant vacuole formation (Figure 8-6), especially near collector channels and pore formation, often associated with the giant vacuoles, but also found in thin, flat regions in the IW.* Three-dimensional analysis of the TM reveals large fluid spaces with numerous interconnections randomly arranged.[136] With serial sectioning, it can be shown that some "vacuoles" have openings on the inner and outer sides, so they can be considered transcellular microchannels.[106,321] When the IOP is experimentally elevated, the number and size of these giant vacuoles are increased, whereas vacuolization decreases at lower pressure gradients.[288,336] Because the openings of these microchannels at the abluminal (meshwork) side are often larger than those at the luminal side and because their apical pores are usually located not directly opposite the basal openings, some authors have assumed that these structures provide a valvular function.[233,688] Calculations of the number and size of pores and openings in the IW endothelium of SC are too large to account for most of the outflow resistance. These and other findings lead to the assumption that the main resistance to aqueous humor outflow is located internal to the endothelial lining (i.e., within the subendothelial or cribriform layer).

Although the pores themselves contribute negligible flow resistance, because they force the fluid to funnel through those regions of the CAI tissue nearest the pores, their number and size can greatly increase the effective outflow resistance of the CAI tissue.[333] However, two studies[224,627] failed to find a correlation between OF and IW pore density, as would be expected if the funneling effect contributed to aqueous humor outflow resistance.[332] Studies with gold particles suggest that exclusion of large segments of the trabecular outflow pathway may help maintain high resistance to flow. Expanding the areas available for fluid drainage by relaxation of the IW cells and the adjacent CAI region may be a possible approach to glaucoma therapy[583] (Figure 8-7).

Experimental studies of the transendothelial passage of ferritin particles in monkeys have indicated that ferritin also traverses tortuous paracellular routes that lie between the endothelial cells of SC.[210] The functional significance of these paracellular routes for aqueous humor outflow are unknown. Tight junctions between endothelial cells of SC become less complex with increasing pressure, suggesting that the paracellular pathway into SC in the healthy eye may be sensitive to modulation within a range of physiologically relevant pressures.[758] However, gold tracer does not cross junctions between the cells at a pressure of 25 mm Hg; perhaps a higher pressure gradient is required to disrupt normal cellular junctions.[583]

Obstruction of these cribriform pathways or a collapse of the cribriform layer as a whole results in increased outflow resistance and, if compensatory mechanisms fail, increased IOP. In glaucomatous eyes there is an increase in ECM beneath the IW of SC and in the cribriform region of the TM and thickening of the trabecular lamellas compared with age-matched healthy controls.[434,437] In advanced cases of primary open-angle glaucoma (POAG), there is additional loss of trabecular cells beyond that associated with normal aging.[11,291] In addition, in POAG the inner uveal and corneoscleral lamellas can be "glued" together and SC can be partly obliterated.[291] Areas with more ECM are less perfused, presumably because of the higher resistance of the area.[188] The origin of the increased amounts of ECM in glaucomatous eyes is still unknown. In addition, most specimens of glaucomatous eyes investigated morphologically are derived from patients who have been treated for many years with antiglaucoma drugs, which can themselves induce changes in the biology of the trabecular cells.[431]

Cholinergic Mechanisms

Conventional (Trabecular) Outflow. In primates the iris root inserts into the CM and the uveal meshwork just posterior to the scleral spur, whereas the CM inserts at the scleral spur and the posterior inner aspect of the TM.[6,575,654] The influence of these two contractile, cholinergically innervated structures on resistance to aqueous humor outflow has long been a source of speculation. The anterior tendons of the longitudinal portion of the CM insert into the outer lamellated portion of the TM and into the cribriform meshwork (Figure 8-8). Electron microscopy shows that the elastic tendons of the CM insert into the elastic fiber network of the cribriform layer of the TM, which is connected

---

*References 284, 285, 287, 321, 336, 509.

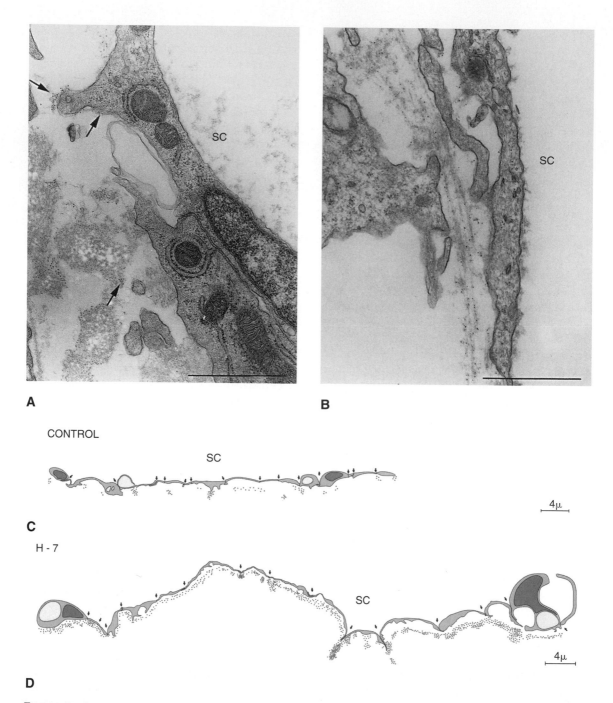

FIGURE 8-7   Distribution of perfused gold particles in the juxtacanalicular area of eyes treated with H-7 (1-[5-isoquinoline sulfonyl]-2-methyl piperazine) and in control eyes. **A** and **B,** Electron micrographs showing gold particle distribution under inner wall endothelial cells. There is focal distribution of gold particles in control eyes (*arrows* in **A**) compared with wide distribution following H-7 treatment **(B).** (Bars = 1 μm.) Schematic drawings depicting 15-cell stretches (cell-cell junctions marked by *arrows*) along the Schlemm's canal (*SC*) of control **(C)** and H-7–treated **(D)** eyes. The location of individual gold particles is represented by *red dots*. (Bars = 4 μm.) (From Sabany I et al: *Arch Ophthalmol* 118:955, 2000.)

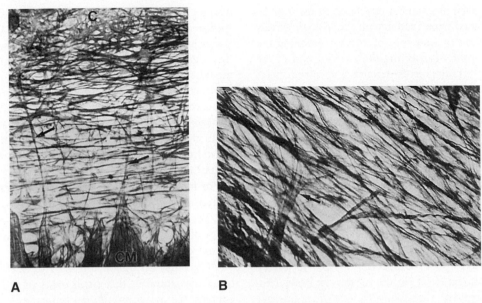

FIGURE 8-8 Light micrographs of tangential sections through the trabecular meshwork of a normal human eye showing different types of ciliary muscle tendons (Gomori's silver-impregnation method). **A,** Type B tendons (*arrows*) penetrate the corneoscleral trabecula and enter the cornea (*C*). (Magnification ×160.) **B,** Tangential section through the fiber network of the corneoscleral trabecula. Note the anterior ciliary muscle tendons (type C) entering the net while bending to 90 degrees (*arrows*). (Magnification ×320.) *CM,* Anterior ciliary muscle tips. (From Rohen JW, Futa R, Lütjen-Drecoll E: *Invest Ophthalmol Vis Sci* 21:574, 1981.)

to the IW endothelium by bent connecting fibrils.[573] During contraction the CM moves anterior inwardly, forming an inner edge of circularly arranged fibers.[427] This contraction results not only in spreading of the lamellated portion of the meshwork but also in an inward pulling of the cribriform elastic fiber plexus and straightening of the connecting fibrils and, perhaps, dilation of SC. Movement of the IW region might affect the area and configuration of the outflow pathways and thereby outflow resistance.[429]

Voluntary accommodation (human); electrical stimulation of the third cranial nerve (cat); topical, intracameral, or systemic administration of cholinergic agonists (monkey and human); and in enucleated eyes (monkey and human), pushing of the lens posteriorly with a plunger through a corneal fitting all decrease outflow resistance, whereas ganglionic blocking agents and cholinergic antagonists increase resistance.* Furthermore, the resistance-decreasing effect of IV PILO in monkeys is virtually instantaneous, implying that the effect is mediated by an arterially perfused structure or structures.[41] These findings collectively suggest that iris sphincter and/or CM contraction physically alters mesh-

work configuration so as to decrease resistance, whereas muscle relaxation deforms it so as to increase resistance.[41] However, not all of the experimental evidence supported this strictly mechanical view of cholinergic and anticholinergic effects on meshwork function. For example, in monkeys, IV atropine rapidly reverses some of the PILO-induced resistance decrease and topical PILO causes a much greater resistance decrease per diopter of induced accommodation than does systemic PILO (monkey) or voluntary accommodation (human).[35,39,611] The inability of atropine to rapidly and completely reverse the PILO-induced facility increase in healthy eyes could be a result of mechanical hysteresis of the meshwork; CM contraction forces a rapid structural change on the meshwork, but muscle relaxation itself cannot reverse this change; elasticity of the meshwork is involved and its effect may be slow.[346] The variation in the relative magnitude of PILO-induced accommodation and resistance decrease when the drug is administered by different routes might reflect differences in bioavailability of the drug to different regions of the muscle. The possible existence of slowly developing (weeks or longer) primary cholinomimetic effects directly on the endothelium of the TM or SC was especially intriguing.[35,39]

---

*References 20-22, 25, 51, 52, 263, 298, 342, 591, 706.

Secondary mechanical effects of drugs may be distinguished from primary pharmacologic effects in the living monkey eye by totally removing the iris at its root, disinserting the anterior end of the CM over its entire circumference, and retrodisplacing it to a more posterior position on the inner scleral wall.[345,361] Total removal of the iris has no effect on IOP, resting outflow resistance, or resistance responses to IV or intracameral PILO.[339] However, after CM disinsertion and total iris removal, there is virtually no acute resistance response to IV or intracameral PILO and no response to topical PILO given at 6-hour intervals for 18 to 24 hours.[345,346] Thus it seems virtually certain that the acute resistance-decreasing action of PILO, and presumably other cholinomimetics, is mediated entirely by drug-induced CM contraction, with no direct pharmacologic effect on the meshwork itself. This is consistent with the relative paucity of cholinergic nerve endings in the meshwork, most of which are located posteriorly in proximity to the CM insertion and are probably of no significance.[346,496,581,582]

Cholinergic and nitrergic nerve terminals that could induce contraction and relaxation of TM and scleral spur cells have been observed in primate TM and scleral spur. Terminals contacting the elastic-like network of the TM and containing substance P immunoreactive fibers resemble afferent mechanoreceptor-like terminals.[605] Afferent mechanoreceptors that measure stress or strain in the connective tissue elements of the scleral spur have also been identified.[656] These findings raise the possibility that the TM may have some ability to self-regulate aqueous humor outflow.

Muscarinic receptors and contractile elements are present in the TM (Figure 8-9). The M_3 messenger ribonucleic acid (mRNA) muscarinic receptor transcript was detected in human TM (HTM) of cadaver eyes.[293] Carbachol (CARB)–induced mobilization of Ca^{2+} and phosphoinositide production in HTM cells in culture has been associated with the M_3 muscarinic receptor.[610] Pharmacologically, the functional muscarinic receptors in isolated bovine TM strips were also shown to be of the M_3 subtype.[737] Smooth muscle–specific contractile proteins have been discovered in cells within the HTM and adjacent to the outer wall of SC and the collector channels.[167,189,190,237] Transformed TM cells from a patient with glaucoma also demonstrated vimentin, tubulin, and smooth muscle–specific α-actin.[508] Cultured HTM cells showed electrophysiologic responses typical for smooth muscle cells in response to endothelin-1 and cholinergic agonists.[408] Isolated bovine TM strips contracted isometrically in response to CARB, PILO, aceclidine (ACEC), and acetylcholine and endothelin-1.[406,407,737] However, in the organ-cultured perfused bovine anterior segment, endothelin-1–induced and CARB-induced contractions resulted in an increase in resistance and a reduction of the outflow rate.[736] In addition, low (10^{-8} to 10^{-6} M), but not high (10^{-4} to 10^{-2} M), doses of PILO, ACEC, or CARB induce increased OF in human perfused anterior ocular segments devoid of CM.[214] Small doses of PILO had no effect on OF in living monkeys eyes[369]; facility increases occurred only at doses, which also produced miosis and accommodation. However, responses to small doses of PILO still remain to be examined in CM disinserted monkey eyes.[345]

ACEC may act directly on the TM, as evidenced by studies showing that small doses of ACEC can enhance OF in organ-cultured human eyes in vitro and in monkey eyes in vivo where the CM has been disinserted from the scleral spur.[214,318] The presence of adenylate cyclase II, IV, and V in normal human outflow tissue supports the hypothesis that cholinergics may exert an effect on OF mediated by cAMP.[763,764] CARB, ACEC, PILO, and oxotremorine-M increased intracellular calcium and phospholipase C activity in a dose-dependent manner in HTM cells by means of M_3-receptor stimulation.[610] These findings raise the possibility of an OF-relevant direct cholinergic effect on the TM and/or that OF and accommodative functions subserved by the CM may be regionalized anatomically and pharmacologically within the muscle. Because receptor subtype specificity is concentration dependent, it is important to stay within the appropriate dosage range and/or to span the dose-response curve. Small PILO doses theoretically could stimulate M_2-receptor–mediated cAMP elevation in the TM and consequent relaxation of the meshwork.[214] These potential direct actions of cholinomimetics notwithstanding, the major effect of cholinomimetics on facility is almost surely related to CM contraction.

Recently, noncholinergic agents, such as certain protein kinase inhibitors (e.g., H-7), have been shown to relax the TM, leading to an increase in facility.[583,661,669] PILO-induced CM contraction actually spreads the TM, perhaps with the same physiologic consequences as direct relaxation of the meshwork—decreased tissue density and thus decreased flow resistance resulting from opening of new flow pathways.

Light and electron microscopic studies of the TM and SC have demonstrated PILO-induced al-

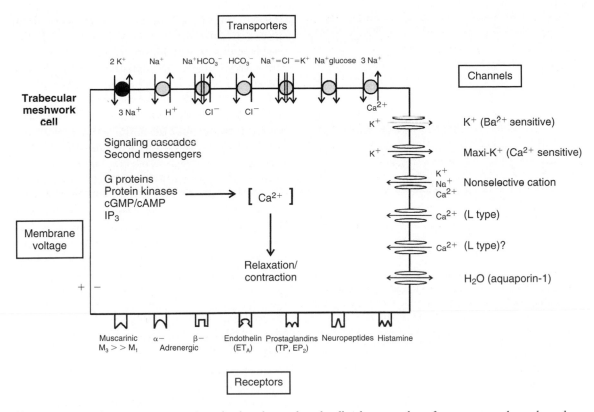

FIGURE 8-9 Schematic representation of trabecular meshwork cell. A large number of transporters, channels, and receptors have been identified in these cells, many of which are involved in regulating smooth muscle contractility. *cAMP*, Cyclic adenosine monophosphate; *cGMP*, cyclic guanosine monophosphate; *EP₂*, prostaglandin E₂; *TP*, thromboxane A₂. (From Wiederholt M, Stumpff F: The trabecular meshwork and aqueous humor reabsorption. In Civan MM: *Current topics in membranes,* San Diego, 1998, Academic Press.)

terations in the size and shape of the intertrabecular spaces and in various characteristics, including vacuolization of the endothelium of the inner canal wall.* The area of empty spaces beneath the IW endothelium in monkeys may represent flow pathways through the meshwork and is positively correlated with OF under PILO or hexamethonium.[428] However, these alterations are all considered the result of PILO-induced CM contraction and augmented transtrabecular outflow.[289] Furthermore, it is unknown what anatomic alteration in the meshwork accounts for the CM contraction-induced decrease in resistance to passive bulk fluid outflow. It is also unknown whether opening entirely new channels, decreasing the resistance of some or all existing channels, widening SC, or some other alteration is critical, as is any understanding of how CM traction on the meshwork brings about the

critical change. In short, we are rather ignorant of the physics behind the physiology.

At least two different subtypes of muscarinic receptors, M_2 and M_3, are present in the CM.[293,294,762] The M_3 subtype appears to mediate the OF and accommodative responses to PILO and ACEC in monkeys.[256,257] The M_2 receptor shows preferential localization to the longitudinal, putatively more facility-relevant portion of the CM, but to date no functional role for this subtype has been elucidated.[294] In monkeys the outer longitudinal region of the CM differs ultrastructurally and histochemically from the inner reticular and circular portions.[235] ACEC increases OF with little accommodative response (Figure 8-10) after intracameral administration in monkey eyes or topical administration in humans.* No differences were found between the contraction response to ACEC in the lon-

---

*References 26, 240, 241, 310, 436, 474.

*References 192, 219, 225, 257, 357, 414, 578.

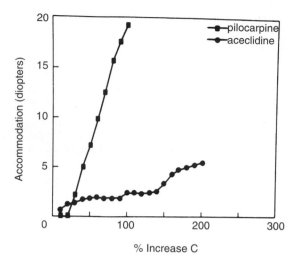

FIGURE 8-10 Comparison of accommodative amplitude versus increased facility of outflow induced by pilocarpine or aceclidine. Data points represent the mean calculated diopters of accommodation in $n = 5$ eyes occurring at calculated mean drug concentrations necessary to induce 10% to 200% increases on facility of outflow in pilocarpine-treated ($n = 6$) and aceclidine-treated ($n = 5$) eyes. (From Erickson-Lamy K, Schroeder A: *Exp Eye Res* 50:143, 1990.)

gitudinal and circular vectors of the isolated rhesus monkey CM.[543] Differences in muscarinic receptor subtypes also do not appear to play a role in the dissociation of the accommodative and OF responses.[257] Similarly, in cultured human CM cells, the M_3 receptor mediates the contractile response to CARB.[507] mRNA from the m_2, m_3, and m_5 subtypes was strongly expressed in the longitudinal and circular portions of human CM cells and tissue.[762] The M_3 subtype is also the predominant receptor in the human ocular anterior segment.[270] Although differential distribution of muscarinic subtypes is probably not responsible for the OF accommodation dissociation occurring under certain conditions, functional dissociation might be produced by combinations of drugs from different classes.

Unconventional (Uveoscleral) Outflow. When the CM contracts in response to exogenous PILO (Figure 8-11), the spaces between the muscle bundles are essentially obliterated.[52,431,575] Conversely, during atropine-induced muscle relaxation, the spaces are widened.[52] If mock aqueous humor containing albumin labeled with iodine-125 or iodine-131 (which under resting conditions leave the AC essentially by bulk flow via the trabecular and uveoscleral drainage routes) is perfused through the AC, autoradiographs may be made to show qualitatively the distribution of the flow.[85,104] In the eye being treated with PILO, radioactivity is present in the iris stroma, the iris root, the region of SC and the surrounding sclera, and the most anterior portion of the CM. In the eye being treated with atropine, radioactivity is found in all of these tissues, as well as throughout the entire CM and even further posteriorly in the suprachoroid/sclera.[85,104] In other perfusion experiments quantifying uveoscleral drainage, eyes treated with PILO demonstrate only a fraction of the uveoscleral flow in eyes treated with atropine.[85,90,107] Thus, to generalize in the primate eye, PILO (and presumably all cholinergic agonists) augments aqueous humor drainage via the trabecular route and diminishes drainage via the uveoscleral route.

ALTERATIONS IN CHOLINERGIC SENSITIVITY OF THE OUTFLOW APPARATUS

Given the long-term use of cholinergic agonists in glaucoma therapy and the vital role of CM tone in regulating outflow resistance, it is important to note that in the monkey, topical administration of the cholinesterase inhibitor echothiophate or the direct-acting agonist PILO can induce subsensitivity of the OF and accommodative responses to PILO, accompanied by decreased numbers of muscarinic receptors in the CM.* Even a single dose of PILO or CARB reduces the number of receptors.[34]

The molecular mechanisms involved may bear on potentially important clinical questions. Will patients receiving long-term cholinergic drug treatment for glaucoma eventually become refractory to therapy? How can drug-induced refractoriness be distinguished clinically from progression of the disease? Will certain agonists be more likely to induce profound refractoriness than others? Can the problem be alleviated by periodically switching from one cholinomimetic to another or by alternating periods of cholinomimetic therapy and abstinence? Will the obvious clinical advantages of low-dose, sustained-release systems over pulsed topical eye drop delivery be offset by a greater tendency to induce subsensitivity?[33] Will the induced subsensitivity be as reversible in the diseased human eye as it apparently is in the healthy animal eye?[172,222] Can noniatrogenic abnormalities in cholinergic systems be causally related to glaucoma? These questions

---

*References 33, 34, 50, 172, 338, 344, 347, 360.

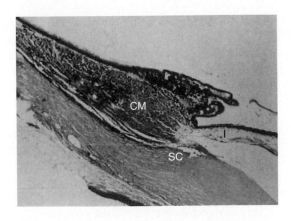
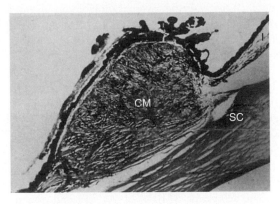

A   **B**

FIGURE 8-11   Histologic sagittal sections through the chamber angle region of monkey eyes treated acutely with atropine (**A**) or pilocarpine (**B**) topically. After treatment with pilocarpine, the muscle moves anteriorly and inwardly, thereby expanding the trabecular lamellas and widening Schlemm's canal. This contraction also obliterates the spaces between the ciliary muscle bundles, obstructing uveoscleral outflow. Conversely, atropine relaxes the ciliary muscle bundles. *CM*, Ciliary muscle; *I*, iris; *SC*, Schlemm's canal. (Vervet monkey, Azan stain; original magnification ×25.) (From Lütjen-Drecoll E, Kaufman PL: *J Glaucoma* 2:316, 1993.)

will be difficult to answer, especially because the parameter of greatest clinical interest, IOP, is influenced by so many anatomic structures and physiologic processes. Clinical experience to date with sustained-release PILO delivery systems does not appear to consistently demonstrate a progressive loss of IOP-lowering efficacy analogous to the experimental results in the monkey, although some late therapeutic failures certainly occur.[550,750]

Adrenergic Mechanisms

Conventional (Trabecular) Outflow. Topical and intracameral EPI increase OF in rabbit and primate eyes.* Much work has been done attempting to define the time course, type of receptors (e.g., α, β, adenosine), and biochemical pathways (e.g., PGs, cAMP) involved in these responses.[136] Adrenergic agonists affect smooth muscle tone in the iris and ciliary body.[683,701,702] CM receptors are of the β_2-subtype.[425] Adrenergic-receptor stimulation could alter intraocular, intrascleral, and extrascleral vascular tone, as well as having possible direct effects on the endothelium lining the outflow pathways, all of which might alter facility. These potential sites of action are not mutually exclusive, and indeed that might account for much of the variability and confusion in the literature.

The facility increases and dose-response relationships for EPI and norepinephrine are virtually identi-

cal in surgically untouched and totally iridectomized monkey eyes and in eyes with the CM disinserted from the TM and scleral spur, indicating that neither the iris nor the CM is involved in the responses.[350,363]

It was proposed that the facility-increasing action of adrenergic agonists is related primarily to the agonists' effects on intrascleral and extrascleral vasculature.[397] However, intracameral infusion of the noncatecholamine vasoconstrictors ergotamine and angiotensin II and the vasoactive agents histamine, serotonin, and bradykinin, which may have either vasoconstricting or vasodilating effects depending on the particular vascular bed, decreased facility in surgically untouched, aniridic, and CM disinserted eyes.[350,351,363] Although various vascular beds may react differently to any given vasoconstrictor or vasodilator, these results did not support the contention that the facility-increasing effects of catecholamines such as EPI (vasoconstrictor/vasodilator, depending on ambient condition of vascular tone) and norepinephrine (vasoconstrictor) are a result of their vascular actions.

In surgically untouched, aniridic, and CM disinserted monkey eyes with widely varying starting facilities, EPI and norepinephrine increased facility by a constant percentage of the starting facility, indicating that the drugs exert their effects on whatever is responsible for the major part of the variation in starting facility. Attributing entirely to C_{ps} or facility of uveoscleral routes, the constant percentage increase in facility observed in eyes with start-

---

*References 18, 31, 42, 68, 89, 91, 169, 382-385, 490, 545, 599, 601, 725.

ing facilities varying over a fourfold to fivefold range requires that virtually all of the starting facility be C_{ps} or uveoscleral facility, which of course is not so.[42,83,350,353,363]

Similarly, because PILO exerts its resistance-decreasing effect by way of CM traction on the TM and because, in the healthy monkey eye, PILO greatly decreases and ganglionic blockade with hexamethonium significantly increases both outflow resistance and its interindividual variability, most of the variability in starting resistance must reside at sites other than the sclera.[38,345,350,363]

This leaves the TM/IW of SC. EPI and norepinephrine exert their action on whatever characteristic of the meshwork/canal that accounts for interindividual variability in starting facility. One possibility is an increase in the hydraulic conductivity per unit filtering area.[350,363] HTM or SC endothelial cells grown on porous filter supports separated and shrank when exposed to isoproterenol or EPI, resulting in increased transendothelial fluid flow.[15] Biochemical evidence also points to the meshwork as the target tissue. It appears that the facility-increasing effect of EPI and norepinephrine is mediated by β_2-adrenergic receptors on the trabecular endothelial cells and the subsequent G protein adenylate cyclase–cAMP cascade.[492] The evidence for this is as follows: Trabecular cells in culture express β-adrenergic receptors (as measured by ^{125}I-hydroxybenzylpindolol [HYP] binding), which have been characterized by competition studies as being of the β_2-subtype.[723] Trabecular OF increases in response to β-adrenergic agonists.[12,18,91,684] Trabecular cells synthesize cAMP in response to stimulation with β-adrenoceptor–selective agonists.[489,599,601] The increase in cAMP synthesis by TM cells in response to EPI can be blocked by timolol, although not by betaxolol (a β_1-receptor antagonist), which is consistent with the hypothesis that only β_2-receptors are present in the TM.[601] Topically applied adrenergic agonists elevate aqueous humor cAMP levels, and intracameral injection of cAMP or its analogs (but not the inactive metabolite 5′AMP) lowers IOP and increases OF.[133,341,488-490] The cAMP-induced facility increase is not additive to that induced by adrenergic agonists or vice versa.[486] EPI increases facility and perfusate cAMP levels in the organ-cultured perfused human anterior segment, effects that are blocked by timolol and the selective β_2-antagonist ICI118,551.[220] Thus the adrenergic agonist–induced facility increase seems to be mediated via the adenylate cyclase cAMP pathway. However, cycloheximide blocked the effect on OF of both EPI and forskolin, but it did not block the rise in

cAMP, suggesting that protein synthesis may play a role in the EPI-induced facility increase at some point beyond the second messenger level.[212] The facility-increasing effect of EPI is blocked by timolol,[182,662] but not betaxolol, in both humans and monkeys, which is consistent with the hypothesis that there are no β_1-receptors present in the primate TM.[4,5,182,566,662] Topical pretreatment of rabbits with an adenosine A_1 antagonist inhibited the EPI-induced hypotensive and increased OF responses, suggesting activation of ocular adenosine receptors as part of the ocular hypotensive action of EPI.[179]

Adrenergic innervation of the primate TM is sparse and concentrated mainly in the region of the meshwork near the CM tendons. No functional significance can as yet be ascribed to these terminals.[198,496,581] However, even noninnervated cells may express autonomic receptors.[29,77,78,411]

The nature of the physiologic change in the meshwork responsible for the decreased flow resistance remains uncertain. Studies suggest an EPI-induced disruption of actin filaments within the TM cells, with consequent alteration in cell shape and cell-to-cell and cell-to-extracellular matrix (C-ECM) adhesions within the meshwork, resulting in altered meshwork geometry and increased hydraulic conductivity across the meshwork. Thus cytochalasin B (a disruptor of actin filament formation) potentiates the facility-increasing effect of EPI, whereas phalloidin (a stabilizer of actin filaments) inhibits it.[567,569] Continuous exposure to EPI at a concentration of 10 μM produced arrest of normal cytokinetic cell movements, inhibition of mitotic and phagocytic activity, significant cell retraction, and separation from the substrate and cellular degeneration after 4 to 5 days in cultured human trabecular cells.[686] Similarly, the hydraulic conductivity of trabecular cell monolayer cultures grown on filters was increased by EPI and associated with changes in cell shape and with separation between cells.[12] These actions of EPI were all partially blocked by pretreatment with timolol. EPI is known to alter cell adhesion and the actin cytoskeleton in other cell systems. EPI costimulates tyrosine phosphorylation of pp[125]FAK (focal adhesion kinase, a tyrosine kinase involved in the formation of C-ECM adherens junctions) in human platelets; induces a dose-dependent decrease in macrophage spreading, associated with changes in the distribution of F-actin; and promotes detachment of natural killer cells from umbilical cord vein endothelial cells.[70,527,615] These effects are all likely mediated by β_2-adrenergic receptors acting through a cAMP-dependent mechanism. cAMP itself promotes F-actin disassembly and inhibits actin polymerization in macrophages under certain conditions.[297] β-Adrenergic agonists (EPI or isoproterenol) and analogs of cAMP increased phosphorylation of the intermediate-size filament vimentin in human or rabbit CP or cultured ciliary epithelial-derived cells. Phosphorylation of vimentin increased by β-adrenergic agonists could be blocked by the β-adrenergic antagonist timolol.[162]

It is hoped that in the coming years we will see the integration of physiologic, pharmacologic, biochemical, morphologic, and cell biologic data into a comprehensive scheme of adrenergic modulation of aqueous humor outflow.

Unconventional (Uveoscleral) Outflow. β-Adrenergic receptors are present in the primate CM and their physiologic or pharmacologic stimulation relaxes the muscle.[144,683,701,702] In addition to increasing trabecular outflow, EPI also increases F_u in monkeys and in humans.[89,590,684] The mechanism is unknown but may, in part, be caused by the mildly relaxant effect of EPI on the CM, presumably acting by means of its β-adrenergic receptors.[197,683,701,702] However, adrenergic agonists also stimulate PG biosynthesis in several tissues, including rabbit and bovine iris.[204,759] Pretreatment with the cyclooxygenase inhibitor indomethacin inhibits the ocular hypotensive effect of topically applied EPI in rabbits and in humans, suggesting that the IOP-lowering action of EPI may be mediated at least in part by PGs or other cyclooxygenase products.[18,76,761]

Numerous clinical studies in humans claim that topical application of timolol, a nonselective $β_1,β_2$-adrenergic–receptor antagonist, induces no change in the distance refraction.[311] However, a single topical application of 0.5% timolol may increase myopia by nearly 1 diopter, presumably by blocking the effect of endogenous CM-relaxing sympathetic neuronal tone.[271] Indirect fluorophotometric estimates have failed to demonstrate any effect of timolol on F_u per se.[590] However, timolol may reduce EPI-induced increases in F_u when the two drugs are applied concurrently.[590] These findings are consistent with the data concerning adrenergic influences on CM contractile tone and also illustrate the importance of the ambient neuronal and pharmacologic adrenergic tone in determining the response of a target tissue to an exogenous adrenergic agent.

In addition to suppressing aqueous humor formation (see previous discussion), $α_2$-adrenergic agonists may enhance F_u. Brimonidine apparently increased F_u in rabbits in the treated eye and lowered IOP in both the treated and contralateral eyes, although measurements of uveoscleral flow in the rabbit are difficult to interpret because of the substantially different anatomy of the rabbit's outflow apparatus compared with the monkey's.[542] In humans, apraclonidine- and brimonidine-induced IOP reductions are associated with decreased AHF and decreased (apraclonidine) or increased (brimonidine) F_u.[679,680] Treatment of patients with ocular hypertension with brimonidine for 1 month resulted in a suppression of aqueous humor formation early on with a later increase in F_u.[675] A single topical application of either brimonidine or apraclonidine decreased IOP and AHF by similar amounts in timolol-treated healthy human eyes, suggesting that both $α_2$-agonists act by a similar mechanism.[456] The human F_u methodology has some variability, because calculations are based on the results of several indirect measurements, each with its own assumptions and uncertainties.[258,751]

PROSTAGLANDIN MECHANISMS

Nilsson et al.[494] reported a 60% increase in aqueous humor outflow via the uveoscleral pathway in monkeys after a single submaximal dose of PGF$_{2α}$-1-isopropyl ester (PGF$_{2α}$-IE). Following multiple submaximal doses (Table 8-3), there was a greater than 100% increase.[255] In both instances, aqueous humor outflow was substantially redirected from the trabecular to the uveoscleral pathway. The effect is likely consequent to an initial PGF$_{2α}$-induced relaxation of the CM (probably consequent to PGF$_{2α}$ action at specific prostanoid receptors). In vitro, PGF$_{2α}$ produces a weak dose-dependent relaxation of CARB-precontracted rhesus monkey CM strips and in CM strips from cats, rabbits, monkeys, and humans precontracted with eserine and acetylcholine, PILO, or KCl.[544,703] Such relaxation may contribute to widening the intermuscular spaces in vivo.[655] ECM remodeling in the anterior segment resulting from PGF$_{2α}$ treatment is characterized by an increase in matrix metalloproteinase (MMP)-1, MMP-2, and MMP-3 and reduction in collagen types I, II, and IV within the CM, iris root, and periciliary body sclera, and may be associated with activation of the protooncogene *c-fos*.[415-417,584] PGF$_{2α}$ and latanoprost (13,14-dihydro-17-phenyl-18,19,20-trinor-PGF$_{2α}$-isopropyl ester) caused reductions in collagen types I, III, and IV; fibronectin; and laminin and hyaluronan immunoreactivity in the CM and adjacent sclera, whereas MMP-2 and

Table 8-3
Uveoscleral Outflow on Day 5 of Twice-Daily Unilateral Treatment with PGF$_{2\alpha}$

	Treated	Control	Treated/Control
(a) Spontaneous IOP; Approximately 235-325 min (n = 6)			
Albumin	$0.78 \pm 0.12^*$	0.46 ± 0.03	$1.66 \pm 0.20^\dagger$
Dextran	$0.89 \pm 0.13^*$	0.48 ± 0.11	$1.99 \pm 0.22^\ddagger$
(b) IOP = 17-18 mm Hg; Approximately 240-335 min (n = 2)			
Albumin	$1.45 \pm 0.01^\S$	0.62 ± 0.11	2.41 ± 0.42
Dextran	$1.42 \pm 0.15^*$	0.52 ± 0.07	$2.75 \pm 0.08^\dagger$
(c) IOP = 17-18 mm Hg; Approximately 135-195 min (n = 1)			
Albumin	2.03	0.63	3.21
Dextran	1.74	0.49	3.53
(d) All IOP Time Groups Combined (n = 9)			
Albumin	$1.07 \pm 0.17^\S$	0.52 ± 0.04	$2.00 \pm 0.24^\ddagger$
Dextran	$1.10 \pm 0.14^\S$	0.49 ± 0.07	$2.33 \pm 0.24^\|$

From Gabelt BT, Kaufman PL: *Exp Eye Res* 49:389, 1989.
FITC, Fluorescein isothiocyanate; *IOP,* intraocular pressure; *MW,* molecular weight; *PGF$_{2\alpha}$,* prostaglandin F$_{2\alpha}$.
On day 5, anterior chambers were exchanged with 2 ml of a mixture of FITC-dextran (46,600 MW) and either ^{125}I- or ^{131}I-albumin. Infusion was continued at a lower rate for the balance of the indicated times. Pressures other than spontaneous were maintained by tracer flow from an elevated reservoir. Animals were then sacrificed and the equivalent anterior chamber fluid recovered in the ocular and periocular tissues was determined. Overall, PGF$_{2\alpha}$ increased uveoscleral outflow approximately twofold compared with control eyes with either tracer. Data are mean $\pm$ standard error of mean uveoscleral outflow (μl/min) for *n* animals, each contributing one treated and one control eye, following the ninth unilateral dose of PGF$_{2\alpha}$ on day 5; *min* indicates time window following PGF$_{2\alpha}$ encompassed by the measurement. Significantly different from 1.0 by the two-tailed paired t-test: $^\dagger p < .05$; $^\ddagger p < .01$; $^\| p < .001$. Significantly different from contralateral control by the two-tailed two sample t-test: $^* p < .05$; $^\S p < .01$.

MMP-3 were increased. Generation of plasmin (an activator of MMPs) was enhanced.[504,584]

This system likely evolved to protect the eye in several ways during inflammation. The TM may become compromised by inflammation or obstructed by inflammatory debris, and the choroid may be overloaded with debris and extravasated proteins that must be removed from the eye.[355] In this situation, PGs would be released and, as autocoids or hormones that are synthesized, released, and locally acting, would induce the changes described. Because the eye has no lymphatics, F$_u$ may serve as an analog to an intraocular lymphatic drainage system.[95] The normal low flow rate that is sufficient to remove normal levels of extravascular protein may be inadequate when protein levels are increased, as in uveitis. Redirection of aqueous humor outflow from the trabecular to the uveoscleral pathway would both rid the eye of excess proteins and maintain physiologic IOP. This could also explain the low IOP that often accompanies uveitis; during experimental iridocyclitis in monkeys, F$_u$ is increased approximately fourfold[677] (Table 8-4).

The increase in F$_u$ in response to these compounds is so great that a larger reduction in IOP is possible than with any other known substance. It has yet to be established whether endogenous PGs have a physiologic or only a pathophysiologic role in regulating uveoscleral flow. Nonetheless, PGF$_{2\alpha}$ analogs and metabolites are clinically useful ocular hypotensive agents, despite some undesirable side effects (e.g., conjunctival foreign body sensation, conjunctival hyperemia, stinging pain, photophobia, increased iris pigmentation in some instances).*

Corticosteroid Mechanisms

Topical or systemic glucocorticoids may induce elevation of IOP in susceptible persons as a result of decreased OF.[24,67,376,596] Glucocorticoids may play a major role in the normal physiologic regulation of OF and IOP. Although glucocorticoid receptors have been identified in the cells of the outflow pathways, the biochemical and consequent physical processes causing the facility decrease are unclear.[305,658,726] However, the mechanism may be caused by modulation of macromolecular metabolism or PG-adrenergic interactions involving the outflow system. For example, the elevated IOP of albino

---

*References 8, 9, 30, 115, 249, 273, 317, 674, 710, 711, 756, 761.

TABLE 8-4

DISTRIBUTION OF DEXTRAN TRACER, UVEOSCLERAL OUTFLOW, PROTEIN, AND INTRAOCULAR PRESSURE IN CONTROL AND INFLAMED CYNOMOLGUS MONKEY EYES

	CONTROL EYE (μl)	INFLAMED EYE (μl)	PROBABILITY*
Iris	$1.2 \perp 0.3$	$2.4 \perp 0.3$	0.07
Anterior uvea	8.5 ± 2.4	18.6 ± 4.3	0.43
Posterior uvea	0.3 ± 0.2	4.2 ± 0.8	0.006
Anterior sclera	8.4 ± 1.6	28.4 ± 4.4	0.01
Posterior sclera	1.9 ± 0.9	21.5 ± 3.9	0.006
Retina	0.1 ± 0.1	2.1 ± 0.9	0.08
Fluid†	0.7 ± 0.4	11.2 ± 3.4	0.03
TOTAL	21.0 ± 4.7	88.4 ± 14.7	0.009
Uveoscleral outflow (μl/min)	0.7 ± 0.2	2.9 ± 0.5	0.009
AC protein (mg/ml)	0.20 ± 0.02	7.8 ± 4.0	0.006
Pre-IOP	16.7 ± 0.8	15.2 ± 1.3	0.43
Post-IOP	14.2 ± 1.6	3.0 ± 1.1	<0.001

From Toris CB, Pederson JE: *Invest Ophthalmol Vis Sci* 28:477, 1987.
AC, Anterior chamber; *IOP,* intraocular pressure.
Inflammation was induced by intravitreal injection of bovine serum albumin. Two days later, tracers were perfused through the anterior chamber and F_u was determined after 30 minutes at 15 mm Hg. Uveoscleral outflow was increased in inflamed eyes up to fourfold with the 70,000 molecular weight (MW) fluoresceinated dextran. Values are mean standard error of mean; $n = 6$.
*Paired t-test analysis value.
†Includes vitreous, posterior chamber fluid, suprachoroidal fluid.

rabbits, caused by the administration of either dexamethasone (DEX) or DEX plus 5β-dihydrocortisol, is reduced after 3 to 7 days of dosing with 0.1% 3α, 5β-tetrahydrocortisol, a cortisol metabolite. This metabolite has no effect on the IOP of untreated, normotensive rabbits or on the IOP or OF of normotensive monkeys.[602,635] The oral administration of the glucocorticoid biosynthesis inhibitor metyrapone in patients with glaucoma has been observed to elicit a small, transient decline in IOP.[410] A generalized cellular hypersensitivity to glucocorticoids is not intrinsic to POAG.[538] Patients with glaucoma have increased plasma levels of cortisol compared with healthy individuals.[597,598]

The glucocorticoid effect on the physiology of the outflow pathways may be more rapid than previously believed, certainly less than the 3 to 6 weeks classically described following topical administration of eye drops, and perhaps in a matter of hours.[727] DEX alters complex carbohydrate, hyaluronic acid, protein, and collagen synthesis and distribution in cells and tissues of rabbit and human aqueous humor outflow systems.* In TM cells, DEX inhibits PG synthesis (90%), reduces phagocytic and extracellular protease activity, changes gene expression, and increases nuclear deoxyribonucleic acid (DNA) content.* Cortisol metabolism may be altered in cultured TM cells obtained from patients with POAG. These cells accumulate 5β-dihydrocortisol and, to a lesser extent, 5α-dihydrocortisol, metabolites that potentiate the facility-decreasing and IOP-increasing effects of DEX; these cells produce only relatively little 3′,5′-tetrahydrocortisol from cortisol.[636] Normal HTM cells show no accumulation of active dihydrocortisol intermediates; all cortisol is rapidly metabolized to the inactive tetrahydrocortisols. Peripheral lymphocytes from patients with glaucoma do not show these abnormalities, indicating that the defects are not found in all cortisol-metabolizing cells.[634,728] 3′,5′-Tetrahydrocortisol applied topically decreases IOP and increases OF in glaucomatous human eyes and antagonizes DEX-induced cytoskeletal reorganization in normal HTM cells.[159,636] However, it has no effect on OF in normotensive monkeys after intracameral injection or 10 days of topical administration.[602] Identification of the mRNAs for these or other relevant steroid-induced effects on TM cell biology is needed.[540,687,760]

A stress and glucocorticoid-inducible response gene product (TIGR protein; myocilin), whose progressive induction over time matches the time course

---

*References 304, 306, 371, 539, 633, 639, 685, 690, 727.

*References 514, 537, 540, 623, 658, 760.

of clinical steroid effects on IOP and OF, has been associated with a role in outflow obstruction and glaucoma pathogenesis.[541,644] Recombinant TIGR increases outflow resistance in the organ-cultured human anterior segment.[229] This molecule appears to be a secreted glycoprotein with aggregation and extracellular matrix–binding groups.[491,540] The regulation of human trabecular cell TIGR/myocilin mRNA appears to be distinct in HTM cells compared with other cell types.[536] Alteration in TIGR/myocilin expression affects TM cell adhesion, proliferation, and phagocytosis.[731] The TIGR gene has been directly linked to patients with POAG.[644] Three mutations in the gene for myocilin lie within the interval on chromosome 1 that was originally associated with juvenile open-angle glaucoma.[558,617,738] In contrast to juvenile glaucoma, mutations in the myocilin/TIGR gene are present in only a minor percentage (approximately 4.6%) of patients with adult forms of POAG.[16] The TIGR gene product has been identified as a novel protein-glycoprotein induction, which became prominent at 55 kD in human TM cells after 1 to 3 weeks of DEX treatment.[228,491,535] In addition to the 55-kD form of TIGR, a large DEX induction of a glycosylated form of TIGR was found extracellularly in the 66-kD region. Maintaining elevated pressure in human anterior segment organ culture for 7 days caused a sharp increase in TIGR/myocilin mRNA, with a narrowing of intertrabecular spaces, increased fine fibrillar material, and increased plaque material in the CAI region.[579]

However, TIGR may play a role in maintaining normal outflow pathways (Figure 8-12). It may serve a structural function within the cytoplasm, or it may associate with other molecules within the cell, perhaps as a molecular chaperone. Extracellularly, it may be involved in creating resistance to aqueous humor outflow by binding to other extracellular molecules or to the cell membrane of trabecular cells.[328] Dynamic mechanical stimuli maintain myocilin/TIGR expression in TM in situ.[657] Blocking TIGR gene expression was associated with a reduction in intercellular space and a decrease in hydraulic conductivity of TM cells.[695] Overexpression of the amino terminal domain or full-length TIGR/myocilin protein after injection of recombinant plasmid cyclic DNA in the human anterior segment organ culture produced an increase in OF.[120,134]

Combined with recent work on changes in laminin and fibronectin and alterations in phagocytosis and surface binding properties, studies of DEX effects in cultured human TM cells may provide clues to the changes in pressure-dependent outflow seen with corticosteroid use.[193] Prolonged treatment of HTM cells with DEX decreased hyaluronan synthesis. Hyaluronan is an inert molecule that may be necessary to prevent adherence of larger molecules to the cribriform meshwork.[203] Cultured HTM cells exposed to DEX also exhibit increased cell and nuclear size, an unusual stacked arrangement of smooth and rough endoplasmic reticulum, proliferation of the Golgi apparatus, pleomorphic nuclei, and perhaps most intriguing in terms of outflow resistance, increased amounts of extracellular matrix material and unusual geodesic, domelike, cross-linked actin networks[157,203,742] (Figure 8-13). Greater strength of cell-to-cell and cell-to-substrate attachment is found in DEX-treated HTM cells.[499] Cell volume may be altered by an early DEX-induced enhancement of Na^+-K^+-Cl^- cotransport.[547] Eyes with glucocorticoid glaucoma and those with POAG both exhibit increased amounts of ECM in the meshwork.[574] However, the ECM that accumulates in eyes with corticosteroid-induced glaucoma differs from that seen in eyes with POAG.[326] The human anterior segment in organ culture exposed to DEX exhibits morphologic changes similar to those reported for corticosteroid glaucoma and a resulting increase in IOP and decrease in OF.[158]

Precisely how steroids affect aqueous humor outflow remains controversial. HTM and human SC cell monolayers grown on filters exhibit enhanced tight junction formation and decreased hydraulic conductivity in the presence of DEX.[694] The number of tight junctions increased twofold, the mean area occupied by interendothelial "gaps" or preferential flow channels was reduced tenfold to thirtyfold, and the expression of the junction-associated protein ZO-1 increased threefold to fivefold. Inhibition of ZO-1 expression abolished the DEX-induced increase in resistance and the accompanying alteration in cell junctions and gaps. These results support the hypothesis that intercellular junctions are necessary for the development and maintenance of transendothelial flow resistance in cultured TM and SC cells and may be involved in the mechanism of increased resistance associated with glucocorticoid exposure.

OTHER MECHANISMS

Na^+-K^+-Cl^- cotransporter is a plasma membrane protein that participates in vectorial transport of Na^+ and Cl^- across epithelia and also regulates

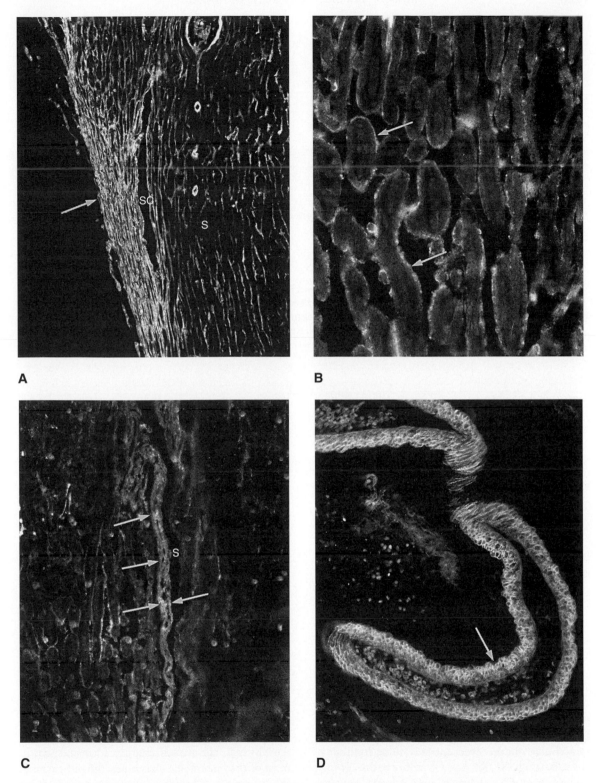

A

B

C

D

Figure 8-12 Immunoreactivity for myocilin–trabecular meshwork–inducible glucocorticoid response (TIGR) in trabecular meshwork and sclera. **A,** Intense staining for myocilin-TIGR is seen in the trabecular meshwork (*arrow*) and between the collagen bundles of the adjacent sclera. (Magnification ×280.) **B,** Trabecular meshwork cells covering the lamellas of the corneoscleral and uveal meshwork are positively labeled (*arrows*). No immunoreactivity is observed in the connective tissue core of the lamellas. (Magnification ×1550.) **C,** Positive immunoreactivity is seen in large areas of the cribriform or juxtacanalicular meshwork (*arrows*) close to Schlemm's canal. (Magnification ×710.) **D,** Vascular smooth muscle cells of arteries and arterioles passing through the sclera into the uvea are labeled for myocilin-TIGR (*arrow*). *S,* Sclera; *SC,* Schlemm's canal. (From Karali A et al: *Invest Ophthalmol Vis Sci* 41:729, 2000.)

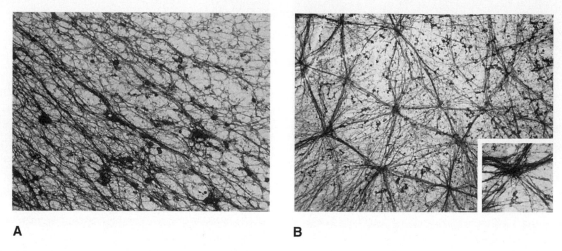

A   **B**

FIGURE 8-13   Whole mount transmission electron micrographs of the cytoskeleton of control trabecular meshwork cells (**A**) and trabecular meshwork cells exposed to $10-7$ M dexamethasone for 14 days (**B**). The stress fibers in the control cells are arranged in normal linear arrays, whereas dexamethasone-treated microfilaments are grouped into 90- to 120-nm bundles radiating from electron-dense vertices. (From Clark AF et al: *Invest Ophthalmol Vis Sci* 35:281, 1994.)

intracellular volume in a variety of cell types, both epithelial and nonepithelial.[295,501,503] The transporter is an obligate symporter, requiring the presence of all three ion species—Na^+, K^+, and Cl^-—to operate and is specifically inhibited by loop diuretics, such as bumetanide. Cultured TM cells exhibit a high level of Na^+-K^+-Cl^- cotransporter protein expression and cotransport activity. The cotransporter regulates the volume of these cells by contributing to the maintenance of steady-state volume under basal, isotonic conditions and mediates volume recovery after hypertonicity-induced cell shrinkage.[502] When TM cells are shrunk by exposure to hypertonic media, the Na^+-K^+-Cl^- cotransporter is activated to bring Na^+, K^+, and Cl^- into the cell. As osmotically obligated water follows the ions, intracellular volume is increased to normal levels and cotransporter activity then decreases to normal levels as well.[502] When TM cells are exposed to bumetanide to inhibit Na^+-K^+-Cl^- cotransport activity, the cells shrink.[502] This indicates that cotransporter activity is required to maintain TM intracellular volume, even under isotonic conditions, by offsetting Na^+, K^+, and Cl^- efflux pathways such as K^+ and Cl^- channels and K^+-Cl^- cotransport.[226,510,729] Na^+-K^+-Cl^- cotransport function and regulation are altered in glaucomatous TM cells compared with that of normal TM cells. However, the cell volume of glaucomatous TM cells is greater than that of normal TM cells, despite reduced Na^+-K^+-Cl^- cotransport activity, suggesting that other

volume-regulatory ion flux pathways may be involved.[548] The elevated intracellular volume could be caused by altered function of other ionic influx pathways such as Na^+-H^+ exchange and Cl^--HCO_3^- exchange or altered function of ionic efflux pathways, or both.[510,511] Changes in TM cell volume by agents that modulate Na^+-K^+-Cl^- cotransport activity affect OF in human and calf eyes in vitro.[2] However, no change in OF was observed in monkeys in vivo after administration of the Na^+-K^+-Cl^- inhibitor bumetanide.[261]

In eyes with POAG, there appears to be deposition of an as yet only partially characterized complex electron-dense substance (possibly incorporating GAG material within its structure) in the JXT, although the incidence of the confounding variables of age and prior medical therapy needs to be assessed.[430,573] How important this substance is in increasing resistance to aqueous humor outflow (and thus increasing IOP) in open-angle glaucoma is uncertain. The endothelial cells of the TM have phagocytic capabilities.[283,539,577] It has been proposed that the TM is in effect a self-cleaning filter and that in most of the open-angle glaucomas, the self-cleaning (i.e., phagocytic) function is deficient or at least inadequate to cope with the amount of material present.[13,96] Phagocytosis, especially of particulate matter and red blood cells, is also carried out by trabecular macrophages. Although this process may be important in clearing the AC of some inflammatory and other debris, it is probably not significant for bulk outflow of aqueous humor. Interestingly, however, artificial perfusion (even with pooled homologous aqueous humor or an artificial solution closely resembling it) of the AC in primates is associated with a progressive time-dependent decrease in outflow resistance.* This occurs even when the CM has been detached from the scleral spur.[350] Although the precise mechanism responsible for this phenomenon is unknown, washout of resistance-contributing ECM from the TM has been a leading theory.[253,254] However, although such washout occurs in enucleated or organ-cultured calf eyes and in enucleated and live monkey eyes, it is not seen in enucleated or organ-cultured human eyes or in bovine eyes if the pressure is less than 7 mm Hg.[217,218]

Combining the clogged-filter concept of glaucoma and the washout concept of perfusion-induced resistance decrease inevitably led to interest in compounds (e.g., cytochalasins B and D, calcium chelators, ethacrynic acid, H-7, staurosporine, latrunculin A) that might disrupt or remodel the structure of the meshwork and canal IW so as to enhance flow through the tissue and/or to promote washout of normal and pathologic resistance-producing ECM (see following discussion). Such compounds might provide insights into cellular and extracellular mechanisms governing outflow resistance in normal and glaucomatous states.† In addition, if normal or pathologic ECM required many years to accumulate to the extent that IOP became elevated, perhaps a one-time washout would provide years of normalized outflow resistance and IOP.[97,205,364]

IOP is decreased and OF is increased in monkeys after topical application of adenosine A_1 agonists.[664] The addition of adenosine A_1 agonists to HTM cells produces a dramatic increase in the secretion of matrix metalloproteinases.[616] Aqueous adenosine levels were positively correlated with IOP in individuals with ocular hypertension and could possibly serve as an endogenous modulator of IOP.[181]

HYALURONIDASE AND PROTEASE-INDUCED FACILITY INCREASES

GAGs contribute to the filtration barrier of aqueous humor outflow through the TM. A quantitative biochemical profile of GAGs from normal and POAG TM suggests that there is a depletion of hyaluronic

acid and an accumulation of chondroitin sulfates in the POAG TM.[372,373] Substantial hyaluronan is present in the nonglaucomatous outflow pathway associated with the endothelial cells lining the trabecular beams. This finding supports potential roles for this GAG in the regulation of the physiologic aqueous humor outflow resistance or in the maintenance of the outflow channels, or both.[409]

Intracameral infusion of hyaluronidase greatly increases facility in the bovine eye, presumably as the result of washout of acid mucopolysaccharide–rich ECM in the chamber angle tissues.[53] Effects in primates are much more variable.[243,279,319,519,526] The variations have been attributed to interspecies differences, the type and source of hyaluronidase, and the conditions used for the enzymatic digestion that may have contributed to a variable and incomplete degradation of hyaluronic acid. In the enucleated human eye perfused at room temperature, α-chymotrypsin has little effect on facility.[279] However, effects of trypsin may be masked at low temperatures, and a combination of trypsin and ethylenediaminetetraacetate (EDTA) may have a substantial effect in dissociating cultured cells not easily dissociated by either agent alone.[556,672] Perfusion of the AC of living monkeys with 50 U/ml α-chymotrypsin gives a large facility increase that persists for several hours even after the enzyme is removed from the infusate.[98] The facility increase induced by intracameral 0.5 mM Na_2EDTA is augmented and prolonged by α-chymotrypsin.[98] Exposure of porcine TM cells to growth factors, such as transforming growth factor–β, induced increases in MMPs such as stromelysin, gelatinase B, and collagenase, suggesting a role in the regulation of ECM turnover by TM cells.[3] Purified MMPs increased OF in organ-cultured human anterior segments by 160% for at least 125 hours.[122]

CYTOSKELETAL AND CELL JUNCTIONAL MECHANISMS

The adhesion of cells to their neighbors or to the extracellular matrix has multiple effects on cell shape and dynamics. Cell-to-cell and cell-to-extracellular matrix adherens junctions are complex and dynamic, comprising numerous proteins, and are modulated by the ambient physical (e.g., pressure, shear stress) and chemical (e.g., endogenous hormonal and biochemical, exogenous pharmacologic) milieu. They play a role in signaling to the cell the state of its external environment. Actin filaments play a central role as the "backbone" of the

---

*References 35, 37, 90, 91, 213, 253, 254, 348, 350, 363.
†References 102, 170, 171, 348, 352, 356, 364, 413, 523, 524, 567, 663, 665, 666, 669.

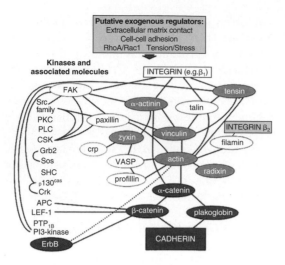

Figure 8-14 Schematic diagram of protein-protein interactions between cell adhesion receptors, cytoskeletal proteins, and signal transduction molecules. *Dotted line* indicates a possible indirect interaction. *Open ovals* indicate intracellular molecules associated with integrin-type receptors, *dark gray ovals* indicate molecules associated with cadherins, and *light gray ovals* indicate molecules associated with both types of adhesion systems. Several proposed exogenous regulators of these binding interactions are listed at the top. The kinases and associated molecules shown *at the left* are involved in adhesion complexes, but their specific binding interactions with other components of cell adhesions are not yet clear. *CSK,* Carboxy-terminal Src kinase; *LEF-1,* lymphoid enhancer factor-1; *PI3-kinase,* phosphatidylinositol 3′-kinase; *PKC,* protein kinase C; *PLC,* phospholipase C; *PTP_{1B},* protein tyrosine phosphatase_{1B}; *VASP,* vasodilator-stimulated phosphoprotein. (From Yamada KM, Geiger B: *Curr Opin Cell Biol* 9:75, 1997.)

submembrane plaque in both types of junctions (Figure 8-14), with the coupling of actin and myosin being essential for cell contractility.[265,754]

Monkey and human trabecular and SC endothelial cells are no exception to the previous discussion and contain an abundant actin filament network.* Cytochalasin B is a fungal metabolite that interferes with polymerization of cytoplasmic actin to form actin microfilaments, causing changes in cell shape and motility properties, and also inhibits hexose transport across the cell membrane.[127,186,274,531] Cytochalasin D, a structural analog of cytochalasin B, is many times more potent in interfering with the formation of actin microfilaments but has virtually no effect on hexose transport. Cytochalasin D thus permits distinction between actin filament dis-

ruption and hexose transport inhibition as a possible basis for cytochalasin effects on a given biologic system.[125,186,274,531]

AC infusion of microgram doses of cytochalasin B and D in cynomolgus and rhesus monkeys sharply increases total OF within minutes.[335,348,567] A similar response to cytochalasin D is observed in the human anterior segment organ culture system.[327] Tracer studies demonstrate that the increase in total facility represents increased facility across the meshwork and inner canal wall and is not related to contraction of the CM because the effect is similar in eyes with and without surgically disinserted CMs.[348,352] Rather, it is because of distention of the cribriform meshwork and separation of its cells, ruptures of the IW endothelium of SC, and washout of ECM.[335,364,652] Cytochalasin D is approximately 25 times more potent than cytochalasin B, although the maximal response, an approximate doubling of starting facility, is almost the same for the two analogs, indicating an effect on actin filaments.[356]

AC perfusion with other cytoskeletal agents, such as ethacrynic and tienilic acids (phenoxyacetic acids that induce shape changes in cultured TM cells), H-7 and staurosporine (inhibitors of various protein kinases), and latrunculins A and B (marine sponge macrolides that bind monomeric G-actin and inhibit actin polymerization), also increase OF more than twofold.* The main targets of H-7 are JXT and SC cells, which undergo an apparent "relaxation" accompanied by an increase in extracellular spaces in the JXT region; loss of ECM deposits, which are usually present in that region; and expansion of new fluid flow pathways (see Figure 8-7). A potentially important effect of H-7 treatment is the clearance of ECM from the JXT area. Numerous vesicles containing ECM inside the IW cells of SC in eyes treated with H-7 support the view that the primary effect of H-7 is an extension of the outflow pathways rather than a direct effect on the ECM.[583] Relaxation of the cells and the entire TM appears important for facility-increasing action of these cytoskeletal agents. Relaxation of CARB-precontracted TM strips in vitro by cytochalasin D and by protein kinase C inhibitors, including H-7, has been demonstrated.[647,661,735] In the case of H-7, no relaxation was demonstrated in CARB-precontracted bovine CM strips.[661] Conversely, H-7 inhibited PILO-induced contraction of monkey CM in vitro in both the facility-relevant longitudinal vector

---

*References 272, 285, 286, 290, 564, 689.

*References 170, 174, 209, 221, 330, 413, 522, 524, 525, 663, 666-668.

and the accommodation-relevant circular vector, but it had no effect on PILO-stimulated accommodation in vivo.[665] Compared with CM, TM has a higher expression of the protein kinase C–e isoform that is known to be both Ca^{2+} independent and associated with smooth muscle contraction under Ca^{2+}-free conditions.[661] H-7 also inhibits myosin light-chain kinase and rho kinase.[155,713] Studies suggest that the major effect of H-7 relevant to cellular relaxation is blocking cellular actomyosin-driven contractility through inhibition of myosin light-chain kinase, rho kinase, or both.[155,553,693] Such a decrease in contractility is followed by a rapid deterioration of actin-containing stress fibers and focal contacts.

Microtubules contain 25-nm-diameter hollow polar fibers, densely packed near the nucleus and extending toward the cell periphery. They are not intrinsically contractile but are important for directional cell motility and, driven by specific microtubule motor proteins such as kinesins and dyneins, for cytoplasmic traffic of vesicles and organelles. Associated proteins bind to microtubules and can affect their stability and potentially attach them to other cellular structures, including other cytoskeletal filaments. Microtubule function could affect outflow pathway events through direct cellular mechanical effects, influences on extracellular or cell membrane turnover, or secondary signaling leading to activation of the actin cytoskeleton.[670] Microtubule disrupting agents such as ethacrynic acid, colchicine, and vinblastine, which have been shown to increase OF, cause cellular contraction in HTM cells if the actin cytoskeleton is intact.[221,530] Ethacrynic acid reduces outflow resistance in enucleated calf and human eyes and in living monkey eyes and concomitantly reduces IOP in live rabbit, monkey, and human eyes.[170,211,459] In enucleated human eyes, lower resistance-effective ethacrynic acid doses do not produce morphologic changes in the TM, whereas higher dosages induce separations between TM and SC cells.[330,413] However, more recently, the effects of ethacrynic acid are postulated to be more directly related to its dephosphorylation of focal adhesion kinase or paxillin, two proteins prevalent in focal adhesions, which regulate cellular attachments to the extracellular matrix, rather to an effect directly on microtubules.[500]

Perfusion of the monkey AC with calcium- and magnesium-free mock aqueous humor containing 4 to 6 mM Na_2EDTA or with calcium-free mock aqueous humor containing 4 mM ethylene glycol bis (aminoethylether) tetraacetate (EGTA) also causes large facility increases and ultrastructural changes in which the junctions are clearly fractured, which is not the case with H-7 (see previous discussion).[102] Because EDTA chelates both calcium and magnesium, whereas EGTA is much more specific for calcium, calcium appears to be a critical cation in maintaining the structural and functional integrity of the conventional outflow pathway.[102] The calcium channel antagonist verapamil increased OF in organ-cultured human eyes.[215]

Although neither the precise subcellular events nor the exact pathophysiologic sequence responsible for the chamber angle alterations produced by these agents has yet been elucidated, it seems that agents that alter the cytoskeleton, cell junctions, contractile proteins, or ECM are, in effect, capable of producing a "pharmacologic trabeculotomy." Much work remains before clinical use of such agents can be considered, but the prospect is enormously exciting.

CELL AND OTHER PARTICULATE-INDUCED FACILITY DECREASES

Normal erythrocytes are deformable and pass easily from the AC through the tortuous pathways of the TM and the IW of SC.[321] However, nondeformable erythrocytes such as sickled or clastic (ghost) cells may become trapped within and obstruct the TM, elevating outflow resistance and IOP.[137,138,275] Similarly, macrophages that have swollen after having ingested lens proteins leaking from a hypermature cataract or breakdown products from intraocular erythrocytes or pigmented tumors (or the tumor cells themselves) may produce meshwork obstruction.[230,234,757] Pigment liberated from the iris spontaneously (i.e., pigmentary dispersion syndrome) or iatrogenically (i.e., following argon-laser iridotomy) may clog or otherwise alter the meshwork function, presumably without prior ingestion by wandering macrophages, as may zonular fragments after iatrogenic enzymatic zonulolysis or lens capsular fragments after neodymium:yttrium-aluminum-garnet laser posterior capsulotomy.* Perfusion of the anterior segment with cross-linked polyacrylamide microgels, similar to those contained in flawed batches of the viscoelastic Orcolon (which produced severe glaucoma in some patients), produced persistent elevated IOP in monkeys and decreased OF in both monkeys and in organ-cultured human and calf anterior segments resulting from obstruction of trabecular drainage.[365] Ocular amyloidosis can lead to

---

*References 17, 146, 279, 521, 549, 748.

elevated IOP as a result of blockage of the TM with amyloid particles.[485]

PROTEIN AND OTHER MACROMOLECULE-INDUCED FACILITY DECREASES

Glaucoma resulting from hypermature cataract (i.e., phacolytic glaucoma) or uveitis has long been ascribed to trabecular obstruction. In the former entity the presence of protein-laden macrophages lining the chamber angle seemed adequate to account for the increased outflow resistance.[234] The uveitis-related glaucomas comprise many different entities, and the cause of the increased outflow resistance seems less clear; postulated mechanisms include trabecular involvement by the primary inflammatory process, trabecular obstruction by inflammatory cells, or secondary alteration of trabecular cellular physiology by inflammatory mediators or by-products released elsewhere in the eye.

Small amounts of purified high-molecular-weight, soluble lens proteins or serum itself, when perfused through the AC of freshly enucleated human eyes, causes an acute and significant increase in outflow resistance.[206-208] Thus it may be that specific proteins, protein subfragments, or other macromolecules are themselves capable of obstructing or altering the meshwork so as to increase outflow resistance, perhaps contributing to the elevated IOP in entities such as the phacolytic, uveitic, exfoliation, and hemolytic glaucomas.[185,230] The protein concentration in the peripheral portion of the AC, close to the meshwork, may be much higher than that in the more central region because of protein entry from the ciliary stroma through the peripheral iris.[56,244,245,555] Experimental perfusion of the enucleated calf eye or monkey eye in vivo with medium containing higher protein concentrations than found in normal aqueous humor has indeed reduced or eliminated resistance washout.[334,368,628] Perhaps protein in the TM is essential for maintenance of normal resistance either by providing resistance itself or by signaling or modifying some property of the meshwork such as stimulation of focal adhesion and stress fiber formation, which would enhance adhesion of TM cells to the extracellular matrix.[154,368,608]

In human eyes, hyaluronate-based and chondroitin sulfate–based agents used as tissue spacers during intraocular surgery (i.e., viscoelastic agents) may raise IOP, presumably by obstructing trabecular outflow, if not completely removed

from the eye by irrigation/aspiration at the conclusion of a procedure.[183,196,546,551,619]

OUTFLOW BIOMECHANICS

Aqueous humor outflow via the conventional drainage pathway is a physical process that can be altered pharmacologically. In every instance an alteration of some physical characteristic of the meshwork/canal must account for the altered outflow. Understanding the physics of pharmacologically induced alterations in outflow is crucial in developing new pharmacologic approaches to manipulating meshwork physics to improve aqueous humor outflow in glaucomatous states.

A nonpharmacologic approach to altering physical characteristics of the meshwork/canal has been the application of laser energy to the TM. Initial efforts were directed at punching holes in the meshwork and inner canal wall. Such holes could be produced with resultant increases in OF and decreases in IOP, but patency was nearly always transient; the openings scarred over, and facility and IOP usually returned to their former levels.* Indeed, in monkeys, intensive circumferential treatment of the meshwork with argon-laser energy can produce sufficient scarring to significantly decrease facility and increase IOP long term.[250]

However, spacing approximately 50 to 100 small (50 μm), less intensive argon-, krypton-, or diode-laser burns evenly around the circumference of the meshwork of the glaucomatous human eye can result in a significant and long-term increase in OF and decrease in IOP, apparently without actually producing a "hole" in the meshwork or inner canal wall.† Indeed, histologic studies demonstrate the expected scar formation at the lasered sites.[745] Although the presence of an undetected puncture leading from the AC into the canal lumen cannot be unequivocally excluded, it may be that contracture of the laser-produced scars tightens and narrows the trabecular ring and the distortion somehow expands the meshwork, opens aqueous channels, and improves hydraulic conductance.[734,744,745] This may be somewhat analogous to the effect of CM contraction. Other data suggest that laser energy–induced alterations in trabecular cell biosynthetic, biodegradative, or phagocytic functions result in less hydraulic resistance. Increases in MMPs, gelatinase B, and stromelysin,

---

*References 296, 379, 659, 671, 734, 749.
†References 438, 457, 472, 595, 739, 744, 745.

which can degrade trabecular proteoglycans, has been demonstrated in human anterior segment organ cultures following argon-laser trabeculoplasty.[512,513] Definitive proof of the facility-increasing mechanism of laser trabeculoplasty remains to be established.

REFERENCES

1. The advanced glaucoma intervention study (AGIS): 7: The relationship between control of intraocular pressure and visual field deterioration, *Am J Ophthalmol* 130:429, 2000.
2. Al-Aswad LA et al: Effects of Na-K-2Cl cotransport regulators on outflow facility in calf and human eyes in vitro, *Invest Ophthalmol Vis Sci* 40:1695, 1999.
3. Alexander JP, Samples JR, Acott TS: Growth factors and cytokine modulation of trabecular meshwork matrix metalloproteinase and TIMP expression, *Curr Eye Res* 17:276, 1998.
4. Allen RC, Epstein DL: Additive effects of betaxolol and epinephrine in primary open angle glaucoma, *Arch Ophthalmol* 104:1178, 1986.
5. Allen RC et al: A double-masked comparison of betaxolol vs timolol in the treatment of open-angle glaucoma, *Am J Ophthalmol* 101:535, 1986.
6. Alm A: Ocular circulation. In Hart WMJ (ed): *Adler's physiology of the eye,* ed 9, St Louis, 1992, Mosby.
7. Alm A, Bill A, Young FA: The effects of pilocarpine and neostigmine on the blood flow through the anterior uvea in monkeys: a study with radioactively labelled microspheres, *Exp Eye Res* 15:31, 1973.
8. Alm A, Villumsen J: PhXA34, a new potent ocular hypotensive drug: a study on dose-response relationship and on aqueous humor dynamics in healthy volunteers, *Arch Ophthalmol* 109:1564, 1991.
9. Alm A et al: Intraocular-pressure-reducing effect of PhXA41 in patients with increased eye pressure: a one-month study, *Ophthalmology* 100:1312, 1993.
10. Alm A et al: Latanoprost administered once daily caused a maintained reduction of intraocular pressure in glaucoma patients treated concomitantly with timolol, *Br J Ophthalmol* 79:12, 1995.
11. Alvarado J, Murphy C, Juster R: Trabecular meshwork cellularity in primary open-angle glaucoma and nonglaucomatous normals, *Ophthalmology* 91:564, 1984.
12. Alvarado JA: Epinephrine effects on major cell types of the aqueous outflow pathway: in vitro studies/clinical implications, *Trans Am Ophthalmol Soc* 88:267, 1990.
13. Alvarado JA, Murphy CG: Outflow obstruction in pigmentary and primary open angle glaucoma, *Arch Ophthalmol* 110:1769, 1992.
14. Alvarado JA, Yun AJ, Murphy CG: Juxtacanalicular tissue in primary open-angle glaucoma and in nonglaucomatous normals, *Arch Ophthalmol* 104:1517, 1986.
15. Alvarado JA et al: Effect of β-adrenergic agonists on paracellular width and fluid flow across outflow pathway cells, *Invest Ophthalmol Vis Sci* 39:1813, 1998.
16. Alward WL et al: Clinical features associated with mutations in the chromosome 1 open-angle glaucoma gene, *N Engl J Med* 338:1022, 1998.
17. Anderson DR: Experimental alpha chymotrypsin glaucoma studied by scanning electron microscopy, *Am J Ophthalmol* 71:470, 1971.
18. Anderson L, Wilson WS: Inhibition by indomethacin of the increased facility of outflow induced by adrenaline, *Exp Eye Res* 50:119, 1990.
19. Araie M, Takase M: Effects of S-596 and carteolol, new β-adrenergic blockers, and flurbiprofen on the human eye: a fluorometric study, *Graefes Arch Clin Exp Ophthalmol* 222:259, 1985.
20. Armaly MF: Studies on intraocular effects of the orbital parasympathetic pathway: I. Technique and effects on morphology, *Arch Ophthalmol* 61:14, 1959.
21. Armaly MF: Studies on intraocular effects of the orbital parasympathetic pathway: II. Effects on intraocular pressure, *Arch Ophthalmol* 62:117, 1959.
22. Armaly MF: Studies on intraocular effects of the orbital parasympathetic pathway: III. Effect on steady state dynamics, *Arch Ophthalmol* 62:817, 1959.
23. Armaly MF: On the distribution of applanation pressure, *Arch Ophthalmol* 73:11, 1965.
24. Armaly MF: Steroids and glaucoma. In Samson CLM et al (eds): *Symposium on glaucoma: transactions of the New Orleans Academy of Ophthalmology,* St Louis, 1967, Mosby.
25. Armaly MF, Burian HM: Changes in the tonogram during accommodation, *Arch Ophthalmol* 60:60, 1958.
26. Asayama J: Zur anatomie des ligamentum pectinatum, *Graefes Arch Clin Exp Ophthalmol* 53:113, 1902.
27. Ascher KW: Aqueous veins: preliminary note, *Am J Ophthalmol* 25:31, 1942.
28. Ashton N: Anatomical study of Schlemm's canal and aqueous veins by means of neoprene casts: part I. Aqueous veins, *Br J Ophthalmol* 35:291, 1951.
29. Aurbach GD, Spiegel AM, Gardner JD: Beta-adrenergic receptors, cyclic AMP, and ion transport in the avian erythrocyte, *Adv Cyclic Nucleotide Res* 5:117, 1975.
30. Azuma I et al: Double-masked comparative study of UF-021 and timolol ophthalmic solutions in patients with primary open-angle glaucoma or ocular hypertension, *Jpn J Ophthalmol* 37:514, 1993.
31. Ballintine EJ, Garner LL: Improvement of the coefficient of outflow in glaucomatous eyes: prolonged local treatment with epinephrine, *Arch Ophthalmol* 66:314, 1961.
32. Ballintine EJ, Maren TH: Carbonic anhydrase activity and the distribution of Diamox in the rabbit eye, *Am J Ophthalmol* 40:148, 1955.
33. Bárány E: Pilocarpine-induced subsensitivity to carbachol and pilocarpine of ciliary muscle in vervet and cynomolgus monkeys, *Acta Ophthalmol* 55:141, 1977.
34. Bárány E et al: The binding properties of the muscarinic receptors of the cynomolgus monkey ciliary body and the response to the induction of agonist subsensitivity, *Br J Pharmacol* 77:731, 1982.
35. Bárány EH: The mode of action of pilocarpine on outflow resistance in the eye of a primate (*Cercopithecus ethiops*), *Invest Ophthalmol* 1:712, 1962.
36. Bárány EH: A mathematical formulation of intraocular pressure as dependent on secretion, ultrafiltration, bulk outflow, and osmotic reabsorption of fluid, *Invest Ophthalmol* 2:584, 1963.
37. Bárány EH: Simultaneous measurements of changing intraocular pressure and outflow facility in the vervet monkey by constant pressure infusion, *Invest Ophthalmol* 3:135, 1964.
38. Bárány EH: Relative importance of autonomic nervous tone and structure as determinants of outflow resistance in normal monkey eyes (*Cercopithecus ethiops* and *Macaca irus*). In Rohen JW (ed): *The structure of the eye,* 2nd symposium, Stuttgart, 1965, Schattauer.

39. Bárány EH: The mode of action of miotics on outflow resistance: a study of pilocarpine in the vervet monkey (*Cercopithecus ethiops*), *Trans Ophthalmol Soc UK* 86:539, 1966.

40. Bárány EH: Pseudofacility and uveoscleral outflow routes: some nontechnical difficulties in the determination of outflow facility rate and rate of formation of aqueous humor. In Leydhecker W (ed): *Glaucoma symposium, Tutzing Castle,* Basel, 1966, Karger.

41. Bárány EH: The immediate effect on outflow resistance of intravenous pilocarpine in the vervet monkey, *Invest Ophthalmol* 6:373, 1967.

42. Bárány EH: Topical epinephrine effects on true outflow resistance and pseudofacility in vervet monkeys studied by a new anterior chamber perfusion technique, *Invest Ophthalmol* 7:88, 1968.

43. Bárány EH: Inhibition by hippurate and probenecid of in vitro uptake of iodipamide and o-iodohippurate-composite uptake system for iodipamide in choroid plexus, kidney cortex, and anterior uvea of several species, *Acta Physiol Scand* 86:12, 1972.

44. Bárány EH: The liver-like anion transport system in rabbit kidney, uvea, and choroid plexus: I. Selectivity of some inhibitors, direction of transport, possible physiological substrates, *Acta Physiol Scand* 88:412, 1973.

45. Bárány EH: The liver-like anion transport system in rabbit kidney, uvea, and choroid plexus: II. Efficiency of acidic drugs and other anions as inhibitors, *Acta Physiol Scand* 88:491, 1973.

46. Bárány EH: Bile acids as inhibitors of the liver-like anion transport system in the rabbit kidney, uvea, and choroid plexus, *Acta Physiol Scand* 92:195, 1974.

47. Bárány EH: In vitro uptake of bile acids by choroid plexus, kidney cortex, and anterior uvea: I. The iodipamide sensitive transport systems in the rabbit, *Acta Physiol Scand* 93:250, 1975.

48. Bárány EH: Organic cation uptake in vitro by the rabbit iris-ciliary body, renal cortex, and choroid plexus, *Invest Ophthalmol* 15:341, 1976.

49. Bárány EH: Elimination of organic cations from the eye, *Klin Monatsbl Augenheilkd* 184:290, 1984.

50. Bárány EH: Muscarinic subsensitivity without receptor change in monkey ciliary muscle, *Br J Pharmacol* 84:193, 1985.

51. Bárány EH, Christensen RE: Cycloplegia and outflow resistance, *Arch Ophthalmol* 77:757, 1967.

52. Bárány EH, Rohen JW: Localized contraction and relaxation within the ciliary muscle of the vervet monkey (*Cercopithecus ethiops*). In Rohen JW (ed): *The structure of the eye,* 2nd symposium, Stuttgart, 1965, Schattauer.

53. Bárány EH, Scotchbrook S: Influence of testicular hyaluronidase on the resistance to flow through the angle of the anterior chamber, *Acta Physiol Scand* 30:240, 1954.

54. Barbelivian A, MacKenzie ET, Dauphin F: Regional cerebral blood flow responses to neurochemical stimulation of the substantia innominata in the anesthetized rat, *Neurosci Lett* 190:81, 1995.

55. Barnett NL, Osborne NN: The presence of serotonin (5-HT1) receptors negatively coupled to adenylate cyclase in rabbit and human ciliary processes, *Exp Eye Res* 57:209, 1993.

56. Barsotti M et al: The source of proteins in the aqueous humor of the normal monkey eye, *Invest Ophthalmol Vis Sci* 33:581, 1992.

57. Bartels SP, Lee SR, Neufeld AH: The effects of forskolin on cyclic AMP, intraocular pressure and aqueous humor formation in rabbits, *Curr Eye Res* 6:307, 1987.

58. Baxter GM et al: Color Doppler ultrasound of orbital and optic nerve blood flow: effects of posture and timolol 0.5%, *Invest Ophthalmol Vis Sci* 33:604, 1992.

59. Becker B: Decrease in intraocular pressure in man by a carbonic anhydrase inhibitor, Diamox, *Am J Ophthalmol* 37:13, 1954.

60. Becker B: The mechanism of the fall in intraocular pressure induced by the carbonic anhydrase inhibitor Diamox, *Am J Ophthalmol* 39:177, 1955.

61. Becker B: The decline in aqueous secretion and outflow facility with age, *Am J Ophthalmol* 46:731, 1958.

62. Becker B: The transport of organic anions by the rabbit eye: I. In vitro iodopyracet (Diodrast) accumulation by ciliary body-iris preparations, *Am J Ophthalmol* 50:862, 1960.

63. Becker B: Iodide transport by the rabbit eye, *Am J Physiol* 200:804, 1961.

64. Becker B: The measurement of rate of aqueous flow with iodide, *Invest Ophthalmol* 1:52, 1962.

65. Becker B: Ouabain and aqueous humor dynamics in the rabbit eye, *Invest Ophthalmol* 2:325, 1963.

66. Becker B: Vanadate and aqueous humor dynamics: Proctor lecture, *Invest Ophthalmol Vis Sci* 19:1156, 1980.

67. Becker B, Hahn K: Topical corticosteroids and heredity in primary open-angle glaucoma, *Am J Ophthalmol* 57:543, 1964.

68. Becker B, Pettit TH, Gay AJ: Topical epinephrine therapy of open-angle glaucoma, *Arch Ophthalmol* 66:219, 1961.

69. Beneyto MP, Fernandez-Vila PC, Perez TM: Determination of the pseudofacility by fluorophotometry in the human eye, *Int Ophthalmol* 19:219, 1995-1996.

70. Benschop RJ et al: β2-Adrenergic stimulation causes detachment of natural killer cells from cultured endothelium, *Eur J Immunol* 23:3242, 1993.

71. Berggren L: Effect of parasympathomimetic and sympathomimetic drugs on secretion in vitro by the ciliary processes of the rabbit eye, *Invest Ophthalmol* 4:91, 1965.

72. Berggren L: Further studies on the effect of autonomic drugs on in vivo secretory activity of the rabbit eye ciliary processes. A: Inhibition of the pilocarpine effect by isopilocarpine, arecoline, and atropine. B: Influence of isoproterenol and norepinephrine, *Acta Ophthalmol* 48:293, 1970.

73. Berrospi AR, Leibowitz HM: Betaxolol: a new β-adrenergic blocking agent for the treatment of glaucoma, *Arch Ophthalmol* 100:943, 1982.

74. Berry DPJ, van Buskirk EM, Shields MB: Betaxolol and timolol: a comparison of efficacy and side-effects, *Arch Ophthalmol* 102:42, 1984.

75. Bhattacherjee P: Distribution of carbonic anhydrase in the rabbit eye as demonstrated histochemically, *Exp Eye Res* 1971;12:356, 1971.

76. Bhattacherjee P, Hammond BR: Effect of indomethacin on the ocular hypotensive action of adrenaline in the rabbit, *Exp Eye Res* 24:307, 1977.

77. Bilezikian JP: A beta-adrenergic receptor of the turkey erythrocyte: I. Binding of catecholamine and relationship to adenylate cyclase activity, *J Biol Chem* 248:5577, 1973.

78. Bilezikian JP, Aurbach GD: A beta-adrenergic receptor of the turkey erythrocyte: II. Characterization and solubilization of the receptor, *J Biol Chem* 248:5584, 1973.

79. Bill A: Autonomic control of uveal blood flow, *Acta Physiol Scand* 56:70, 1962.

80. Bill A: The drainage of albumin from the uvea, *Exp Eye Res* 3:179, 1964.

81. Bill A: The aqueous humor drainage mechanism in the cynomolgus monkey (*Macaca irus*) with evidence for unconventional routes, *Invest Ophthalmol* 4:911, 1965.

82. Bill A: The protein exchange in the eye with aspects on conventional and uveoscleral bulk drainage of aqueous humor in primates. In Rohen JW (ed): *The structure of the eye,* 2nd symposium, Stuttgart, 1965, Schattauer.

83. Bill A: Conventional and uveoscleral drainage of aqueous humor in the cynomolgus monkey (*Macaca irus*) at normal and high intraocular pressures, *Exp Eye Res* 5:45, 1966.

84. Bill A: The routes for bulk drainage of aqueous humor in rabbits with and without cyclodialysis, *Doc Ophthalmol* 20:157, 1966.

85. Bill A: Effects of atropine and pilocarpine on aqueous humour dynamics in cynomolgus monkeys (*Macaca irus*), *Exp Eye Res* 6:120, 1967.

86. Bill A: Further studies on the influence of the intraocular pressure on aqueous humor dynamics in cynomolgus monkeys, *Invest Ophthalmol* 6:364, 1967.

87. Bill A: Capillary permeability to and extravascular dynamics of myoglobin, albumin, and gammaglobulin in the uvea, *Acta Physiol Scand* 73:204, 1968.

88. Bill A: The effect of ocular hypertension caused by red cells on the rate of formation of aqueous humor, *Invest Ophthalmol* 7:162, 1968.

89. Bill A: Early effects of epinephrine on aqueous humor dynamics in vervet monkeys (*Cercopithecus ethiops*), *Exp Eye Res* 8:35, 1969.

90. Bill A: Effects of atropine on aqueous humor dynamics in the vervet monkey (*Cercopithecus ethiops*), *Exp Eye Res* 8:284, 1969.

91. Bill A: Effects of norepinephrine, isoproterenol and sympathetic stimulation on aqueous humour dynamics in vervet monkeys, *Exp Eye Res* 1970;10:31, 1970.

92. Bill A: Aqueous humor dynamics in monkeys (*Macaca irus* and *Cercopithecus ethiops*), *Exp Eye Res* 11:195, 1971.

93. Bill A: Effects of longstanding stepwise increments in eye pressure on the rate of aqueous humor formation in a primate (*Cercopithecus ethiops*), *Exp Eye Res* 12:184, 1971.

94. Bill A: The role of ciliary blood flow and ultrafiltration in aqueous humor formation, *Exp Eye Res* 16:287, 1973.

95. Bill A: Blood circulation and fluid dynamics in the eye, *Physiol Rev* 55:383, 1975.

96. Bill A: Editorial: the drainage of aqueous humor, *Invest Ophthalmol* 14:1, 1975.

97. Bill A: Basic physiology of the drainage of aqueous humor. In Bito LZ, Davson H, Fenstermacher JD (eds): *The ocular and cerebrospinal fluids: Fogarty International Center Symposium,* London, 1977, Academic Press.

98. Bill A: Effects of Na2EDTA and alpha-chymotrypsin on aqueous humor outflow conductance in monkey eyes, *Uppsala J Med Sci* 85:311, 1980.

99. Bill A, Bárány EH: Gross facility, facility of conventional routes, and pseudofacility of aqueous humor outflow in the cynomolgus monkey, *Arch Ophthalmol* 75:665, 1966.

100. Bill A, Heilmann K: Ocular effects of clonidine in cats and monkeys (*Macaca irus*), *Exp Eye Res* 21:481, 1975.

101. Bill A, Hellsing K: Production and drainage of aqueous humor in the cynomolgus monkey (*Macaca irus*), *Invest Ophthalmol* 4:920, 1965.

102. Bill A, Lutjen-Drecoll E, Svedbergh B: Effects of intracameral Na2EDTA and EGTA on aqueous outflow routes in the monkey eye, *Invest Ophthalmol Vis Sci* 19:492, 1980.

103. Bill A, Nilsson SF: Control of ocular blood flow, *J Cardiovasc Pharmacol* 7(suppl 3):S96, 1985.

104. Bill A, Phillips I: Uveoscleral drainage of aqueous humor in human eyes, *Exp Eye Res* 21:275, 1971.

105. Bill A, Stjernschantz J: Cholinergic vasoconstrictor effects in the rabbit eye: vasomotor effects of pentobarbital anesthesia, *Acta Physiol Scand* 108:419, 1980.

106. Bill A, Svedbergh B: Scanning electron microscopic studies of the trabecular meshwork and the canal of Schlemm: an attempt to localize the main resistance to outflow of aqueous humor in man, *Acta Ophthalmol* 50:295, 1972.

107. Bill A, Walinder P-E: The effects of pilocarpine on the dynamics of aqueous humor in a primate (*Macaca irus*), *Invest Ophthalmol* 5:170, 1966.

108. Bito LZ: Accumulation and apparent active transport of prostaglandins by some rabbit tissues in vitro, *J Physiol* 221:371, 1972.

109. Bito LZ: Comparative study of concentrative prostaglandin accumulation by various tissues of mammals and marine vertebrates and invertebrates, *Comp Biochem Physiol* 43:65, 1972.

110. Bito LZ: Species differences in the response of the eye to irritation and trauma: a hypothesis of divergence in ocular defense mechanisms, and the choice of experimental animals for eye research, *Exp Eye Res* 39:807, 1984.

111. Bito LZ: Prostaglandins: old concepts and new perspectives, *Arch Ophthalmol* 105:1036, 1987.

112. Bito LZ, Davson H, Salvador EV: Inhibition of in vitro concentrative prostaglandin accumulation by prostaglandins, prostaglandin analogues, and by some inhibitors of organic anion transport, *J Physiol* 256:257, 1976.

113. Bito LZ, Davson H, Snider N: The effects of autonomic drugs on mitosis and DNA synthesis in the lens epithelium and on the composition of the aqueous humor, *Exp Eye Res* 4:54, 1965.

114. Bito LZ, Salvador EV: Intraocular fluid dynamics: 3. The site and mechanism of prostaglandin transfer across the blood intraocular fluid barriers, *Exp Eye Res* 14:233, 1972.

115. Bito LZ et al: The ocular effects of prostaglandins and the therapeutic potential of a new PGF2α analog, PhXA41 (latanoprost), for glaucoma management, *J Lipid Mediators* 6:535, 1993.

116. Bonomi L, Di Comite P: Outflow facility after guanethidine sulfate administration, *Arch Ophthalmol* 78:337, 1967.

117. Bonomi L, Steindler P: Effect of pindolol on intraocular pressure, *Br J Ophthalmol* 59:301, 1975.

118. Bonting SL, Becker B: Studies on sodium-potassium activated adenosine triphosphatase: XIV. Inhibition of enzyme activity and aqueous humor flow in the rabbit eye after intravitreal injection of ouabain, *Invest Ophthalmol* 3:523, 1964.

119. Bonting SL, Simon KA, Hawkins NM: Studies on sodium-potassium-activated adenosine triphosphatase: I. Quantitative distribution in several tissues of the cat, *Arch Biochem* 95:416, 1961.

120. Borrás T et al: Trabecular meshwork gene transfer: its effects on intraocular pressure (IOP), *Exp Eye Res* 71 (suppl 1):S3, 2000 (abstract 8).

121. Bouzoubaa M et al: Synthesis and β-adrenergic blocking activity of new aliphatic and alicyclic oxime ethers, *J Med Chem* 27:1291, 1984.

122. Bradley JM et al: Effect of matrix metalloproteinases activity on outflow in perfused human organ culture, *Invest Ophthalmol Vis Sci* 39:2649, 1998.

123. Brandt CR et al: Renin mRNA is synthesized locally in rat ocular tissues, *Curr Eye Res* 13:755, 1994.

124. Brechue WF, Maren TH: A comparison between the effect of topical and systemic carbonic anhydrase inhibitors on aqueous humor secretion, *Exp Eye Res* 57:67, 1993.

125. Brenner SL, Korn ED: Substoichiometric concentrations of cytochalasin D inhibit actin polymerization: additional evidence for an F-actin treadmill, *J Biol Chem* 254:9982, 1979.

126. Brodwell J, Fischbarg J: The hydraulic conductivity of rabbit ciliary epithelium in vitro, *Exp Eye Res* 34:121, 1982.

127. Brown SS, Spudich JA: Mechanism of action of cytochalasin: evidence that it binds to actin filament ends, *J Cell Biol* 88:487, 1981.

128. Brubaker RF: The measurement of pseudofacility and true facility by constant pressure perfusion in the normal rhesus monkey eye, *Invest Ophthalmol* 9:42, 1970.

129. Brubaker RF: Physiology of aqueous humor formation. In Drance S, Neufeld A (eds): *Applied pharmacology in the medical treatment of glaucoma*, New York, 1984, Grune & Stratton.

130. Brubaker RF: Flow of aqueous humor in humans, *Invest Ophthalmol Vis Sci* 32:3145, 1991.

131. Bryson JM, Wolter JR, O'Keefe NT: Ganglion cells in the human ciliary body, *Arch Ophthalmol* 75:57, 1966.

132. Burlington RF, Milsom WK: Differential effects of acetylcholine on coronary flow in isolated hypothermic hearts from rats and ground squirrels, *J Exp Biol* 185:17, 1993.

133. Busch MJ, van Oosterhout EJ, Hoyng PF: Effects of cyclic nucleotide analogs on intraocular pressure and trauma-induced inflammation in the rabbit eye, *Curr Eye Res* 11:5, 1992.

134. Caballero M, Rowlette LL, Borrás T: Altered secretion of a TIGR/MYOC mutant lacking the olfactomedin domain, *Biochem Biophys Acta* 1502:447, 2000.

135. Caldwell DR, Salisbury CR, Guzek JP: Effects of topical betaxolol in ocular hypertensive patients, *Arch Ophthalmol* 102:539, 1984.

136. Camp JJ et al: Three-dimensional reconstruction of aqueous channels in human trabecular meshwork using light microscopy and confocal microscopy, *Scanning* 19:258, 1997.

137. Campbell DG, Essingman EM: Hemolytic ghost cell glaucoma: further studies, *Arch Ophthalmol* 97:2141, 1979.

138. Campbell DG, Simmons RJ, Grant WM: Ghost cells as a cause of glaucoma, *Am J Ophthalmol* 81:441, 1976.

139. Camras CB et al: Inhibition of the epinephrine-induced reduction of intraocular pressure by systemic indomethacin in humans, *Am J Ophthalmol* 100:169, 1985.

140. Camras CB et al: Latanoprost, a prostaglandin analog, for glaucoma therapy, *Ophthalmology* 103:1916, 1996.

141. Caprioli J: The ciliary epithelia and aqueous humor. In Hart WM (ed): *Adler's physiology of the eye: clinical application*, ed 9, St Louis, 1992, Mosby.

142. Caprioli J, Sears M: Forskolin lowers intraocular pressure in rabbits, monkeys, and man, *Lancet* 1:958, 1983.

143. Caprioli J, Sears M, Bausher L: Forskolin lowers intraocular pressure by reducing aqueous inflow, *Invest Ophthalmol Vis Sci* 25:268, 1984.

144. Casey WJ: Cervical sympathetic stimulation in monkeys and the effects on outflow facility and intraocular volume: a study in the East African vervet (*Cercopithecus aethiops*), *Invest Ophthalmol* 5:33, 1966.

145. Chang FW, Burke JA, Potter DE: Mechanism of the ocular hypotensive action of ketanserin, *J Ocular Pharmacol* 1:137, 1985.

146. Channell MM, Beckman H: Intraocular pressure changes after neodynium-YAG laser posterior capsulotomy, *Arch Ophthalmol* 102:1024, 1984.

147. Chidlow G, Le Corre S, Osborne NN: Localization of 5-hydroxytryptamine1A and 5-hydroxytryptamine7 receptors in rabbit ocular and brain tissues, *Neuroscience* 87:675, 1998.

148. Chidlow G et al: The 5-HT1A receptor agonist 8-OH-DPAT lowers intraocular pressure in normotensive NZW rabbits, *Exp Eye Res* 69:587, 1999.

149. Chiou GCY: Ocular hypotensive actions of haloperidol, a dopaminergic antagonist, *Arch Ophthalmol* 102:143, 1984.

150. Chiou GCY: Treatment of ocular hypertension and glaucoma with dopamine antagonists, *Ophthalmic Res* 16:129, 1984.

151. Chiou GCY, Liu HK, Trzeciakowski J: Studies of action mechanism of antiglaucoma drugs with a newly developed cat model, *Life Sci* 27:2445, 1980.

152. Chiou GCY, Yan HY: Effects of antiglaucoma drugs on the blood flow in rabbit eyes, *Ophthalmic Res* 18:265, 1986.

153. Chiou GCY et al: Are β-adrenergic mechanisms involved in ocular hypotensive actions of adrenergic drugs? *Ophthalmic Res* 17:49, 1985.

154. Chrzanowska-Wodnicka M, Burridge K: Tyrosine phosphorylation is involved in reorganization of the actin cytoskeleton in response to serum or LPA stimulation, *J Cell Sci* 107:3643, 1994.

155. Chrzanowska-Wodnicka M, Burridge K: Rho-stimulated contractility drives the formation of stress fibers and focal adhesions, *J Cell Biol* 133:1403, 1996.

156. Chu T-C, Ogidigben MJ, Potter DE: 8OH-DPAT-induced ocular hypotension: sites and mechanisms of action, *Exp Eye Res* 69:227, 1999.

157. Clark AF et al: Glucocorticoid-induced formation of cross-linked actin networks in cultured human trabecular meshwork cells, *Invest Ophthalmol Vis Sci* 35:281, 1994.

158. Clark AF et al: Dexamethasone-induced ocular hypertension in perfusion-cultured human eyes, *Invest Ophthalmol Vis Sci* 36:478, 1995.

159. Clark AF et al: Inhibition of dexamethasone-induced cytoskeletal changes in cultured human trabecular meshwork cells by tetrahydrocortisol, *Invest Ophthalmol Vis Sci* 37:805, 1996.

160. Coakes RL, Brubaker RF: The mechanism of timolol in lowering intraocular pressure, *Arch Ophthalmol* 96:2045, 1978.

161. Coakes RL, Siah PB: Effects of adrenergic drugs on aqueous humor dynamics in the normal human eye: I. Salbutamol, *Br J Ophthalmol* 68:393, 1984.

162. Coca-Prados M: Regulation of protein phosphorylation of the intermediate-sized filament vimentin in the ciliary epithelium of the mammalian eye, *J Biol Chem* 260:10332, 1985.

163. Coca-Prados M, Lopez-Briones LG: Evidence that the a and the a(+) isoforms of the catalytic subunit of (Na+, K+)-ATPase reside in distinct ciliary epithelial cells of the mammalian eye, *Biochem Biophys Res Commun* 145:460, 1987.

164. Colasanti BK: Aqueous humor dynamics in the enucleated deer eye, *Comp Biochem* 78:755, 1985.

165. Cole DF: Effects of some metabolic inhibitors upon the formation of the aqueous humor in rabbits, *Br J Ophthalmol* 44:739, 1960.

166. Cole DF: Secretion of the aqueous humor, *Exp Eye Res* 25(suppl):161, 1977.

167. Coroneo MT et al: Electrical and morphological evidence for heterogeneous populations of cultured bovine trabecular meshwork cells, *Exp Eye Res* 52:375, 1991.

168. Crawford K, Kaufman PL, True Gabelt B: Prostaglandins and aqueous humor dynamics. In Shields MB, Pollack IP, Kolker AE (eds): *Perspectives in glaucoma: transactions of the First Scientific Meeting of the American Glaucoma Society*, Thorofare, NJ, 1988, Slack.

169. Criswick VG, Drance SM: Comparative study of four different epinephrine salts on intraocular pressure, *Arch Ophthalmol* 75:768, 1966.

170. Croft MA, Hubbard WC, Kaufman PL: Effect of ethacrynic acid on aqueous outflow dynamics in monkeys, *Invest Ophthalmol Vis Sci* 35:1167, 1994.

171. Croft MA, Kaufman PL: Effect of daily topical ethacrynic acid on aqueous humor dynamics in monkeys, *Curr Eye Res* 14:777, 1995.

172. Croft MA et al: Accommodation and ciliary muscle muscarinic receptors after echothiophate, *Invest Ophthalmol Vis Sci* 32:3288, 1991.

173. Croft MA et al: Aging effects on accommodation and outflow facility responses to pilocarpine in humans, *Arch Ophthalmol* 114:586, 1996.

174. Croft MA et al: Effect of ticrynafen on aqueous humor dynamics in monkeys, *Arch Ophthalmol* 116:1481, 1998.

175. Crook RB, Polansky JR: Stimulation of Na+, K+, Cl- cotransport by forskolin-activated adenylyl cyclase in fetal human nonpigmented epithelial cells, *Invest Ophthalmol Vis Sci* 35:3374, 1994.

176. Crook RB, Riese K: Beta-adrenergic stimulation of Na+, K+, Cl- cotransport in fetal nonpigmented ciliary epithelial cells, *Invest Ophthalmol Vis Sci* 37:1047, 1996.

177. Crosson CE, Gray T: Modulation of intraocular pressure by adenosine agonists, *J Ocular Pharmacol* 10:379, 1994.

178. Crosson CE, Gray T: Characterization of ocular hypertension induced by adenosine agonists, *Invest Ophthalmol Vis Sci* 37:1833, 1996.

179. Crosson CE, Petrovich M: Contributions of adenosine receptor activation to the ocular actions of epinephrine, *Invest Ophthalmol Vis Sci* 40:2054, 1999.

180. Crosson CE et al: Pharmacological evidence for heterogeneity of ocular α2 adrenoceptors, *Curr Eye Res* 11:963, 1992.

181. Crosson CE et al: Elevated adenosine levels in the aqueous humor of ocular hypertensive individuals, *Invest Ophthalmol Vis Sci* 41:S576, 2000 (ARVO abstract 3061).

182. Cyrlin MN, Thomas JV, Epstein DL: Additive effect of epinephrine to timolol therapy in primary open-angle glaucoma, *Arch Ophthalmol* 100:414, 1982.

183. Dada VK, Sindhu N, Sachdev MS: Postoperative intraocular pressure changes with use of different viscoelastics, *Ophthal Surg* 25:540, 1994.

184. Dailey RA, Brubaker RF, Bourne WM: The effects of timolol maleate and acetazolamide on the rate of aqueous formation in normal human subjects, *Am J Ophthalmol* 93:232, 1982.

185. Davanger M: On the molecular composition and physiochemical properties of the pseudoexfoliation material, *Acta Ophthalmol* 1977;55:621, 1977.

186. Davies P, Allison AC: Effects of cytochalasin B on endocytosis and exocytosis. In Tannenbaum SW (ed): *Cytochalasins: biochemical and cell biological aspects,* Amsterdam, 1978, North-Holland.

187. Davson H: The aqueous humor and the intraocular pressure. In Davson H (ed): *Physiology of the eye,* New York, 1990, Pergamon Press.

188. de Kater AW, Melamed S, Epstein DL: Patterns of aqueous humor outflow in glaucomatous and nonglaucomatous human eyes, *Arch Ophthalmol* 107:572, 1989.

189. de Kater AW, Shahsafaei A, Epstein DL: Localization of smooth muscle and nonmuscle actin isoforms in the human aqueous outflow pathway, *Invest Ophthalmol Vis Sci* 33:424, 1992.

190. de Kater AW, Spurr-Michaud SJ, Gipson IK: Localization of smooth muscle myosin-containing cells in the aqueous outflow pathway, *Invest Ophthalmol Vis Sci* 31:347, 1990.

191. De Vries GW, Mobasser A, Wheeler LA: Stimulation of endogenous cyclic AMP levels in ciliary body by SK&F28526, a novel dopamine receptor agonist, *Curr Eye Res* 5:449, 1986.

192. Demailly PH: Place de l'acéclidine dans le traitement du glaucome chronique simple à angle ouvert, *Arch Ophthalmol* 28:735, 1968.

193. Dickerson JE et al: The effect of dexamethasone on integrin and laminin expression in cultured human trabecular meshwork cells, *Exp Eye Res* 66:731, 1998.

194. DiMatteo J: Active transport of ascorbic acid into lens epithelium of the rat, *Exp Eye Res* 49:873, 1989.

195. Duke-Elder S: The aqueous humor. In Duke-Elder S (ed): *The physiology of the eye and of vision: system of ophthalmology,* vol 4, St Louis, 1968, Mosby.

196. Duperre J et al: Effect of timolol vs acetazolamide on sodium hyaluronate-induced rise in intraocular pressure after cataract surgery, *Can J Ophthalmol* 29:182, 1994.

197. Ehinger B: Adrenergic nerves to the eye and to related structures in man and in the cynomolgus monkey (*Macaca irus*), *Invest Ophthalmol* 5:42, 1966.

198. Ehinger B: A comparative study of the adrenergic nerves to the anterior segment of some primates, *Zeitschr Zellforschung* 116:157, 1971.

199. Eller MG, Schoenwald RD, Dixson JA: Topical carbonic anhydrase inhibitors: III. Optimization model for corneal penetration of ethoxzolamide analogues, *J Pharm Sci* 74:155, 1985.

200. Ellingsen BA, Grant WM: Influence of intraocular pressure and trabeculotomy on aqueous outflow in enucleated monkey eyes, *Invest Ophthalmol* 10:705, 1971.

201. Ellingsen BA, Grant WM: Trabeculotomy and sinusotomy in enucleated human eyes, *Invest Ophthalmol* 11:21, 1972.

202. Elsas T, Uddman R, Sundler F: Pituitary adenylate cyclase-activating peptide-immunoreactive nerve fibers in the cat eye, *Graefes Arch Clin Exp Ophthalmol* 234:573, 1996.

203. Engelbrecht-Schnur S et al: Dexamethasone treatment decreases hyaluronan formation by primate trabecular meshwork cells in vitro, *Exp Eye Res* 64:539, 1997.

204. Engstrom P, Dunham EW: Alpha-adrenergic stimulation of prostaglandin release from rabbit iris-ciliary body in vitro, *Invest Ophthalmol Vis Sci* 22:757, 1982.

205. Epstein DL: Open angle glaucoma: why not a cure? *Arch Ophthalmol* 105:1187, 1987 (editorial).

206. Epstein DL, Hashimoto JM, Grant WM: Serum obstruction of aqueous outflow in enucleated eyes, *Am J Ophthalmol* 86:101, 1978.

207. Epstein DL, Jedziniak JA, Grant WM: Identification of heavy molecular weight soluble lens protein in aqueous humor in phakolytic glaucoma, *Invest Ophthalmol Vis Sci* 17:398, 1978.

208. Epstein DL, Jedziniak JA, Grant WM: Obstruction of aqueous outflow by lens particles and by heavy-molecular weight soluble lens proteins, *Invest Ophthalmol Vis Sci* 17:272, 1978.

209. Epstein DL, Roberts BC, Skinner LL: Nonsulfhydryl-reactive phenoxyacetic acids increase aqueous humor outflow facility, *Invest Ophthalmol Vis Sci* 38:1526, 1997.

210. Epstein DL, Rohen JW: Morphology of the trabecular meshwork and inner wall endothelium after cationized ferritin perfusion in the monkey eye, *Invest Ophthalmol Vis Sci* 32:160, 1991.

211. Epstein DL et al: Influence of ethacrynic acid on outflow facility in the monkey and calf eye, *Invest Ophthalmol Vis Sci* 28:2067, 1987.

212. Erickson K et al: Adrenergic regulation of aqueous outflow, *J Ocular Pharmacol* 10:241, 1994.

213. Erickson KA, Kaufman PL: Comparative effects of three ocular perfusates on outflow facility in the cynomolgus monkey, *Curr Eye Res* 1:211, 1981.

214. Erickson KA, Schroeder A: Direct effects of muscarinic agents on the outflow pathways in human eyes, *Invest Ophthalmol Vis Sci* 41:1743, 2000.

215. Erickson KA, Schroeder A, Netland PA: Verapamil increases outflow facility in the human eye, *Exp Eye Res* 61:565, 1995.

216. Erickson KA et al: The cynomolgus monkey as a model for orbital research: III. Effects on ocular physiology of lateral orbitotomy and isolation of the ciliary ganglion, *Curr Eye Res* 3:557, 1984.

217. Erickson-Lamy K, Rohen JW, Grant WM: Outflow facility studies in the perfused bovine aqueous outflow pathways, *Curr Eye Res* 7:799, 1988.

218. Erickson-Lamy K et al: Absence of time-dependent facility increase ("wash-out") in the perfused enucleated human eye, *Invest Ophthalmol Vis Sci* 31:2384, 1990.

219. Erickson-Lamy KA, Kaufman PL, Polansky JR: Dissociation of cholinergic supersensitivity from receptor number in ciliary muscle, *Invest Ophthalmol Vis Sci* 29:600, 1988.

220. Erickson-Lamy KA, Nathanson JA: Epinephrine increases facility of outflow and cyclic AMP content in the human eye in vitro, *Invest Ophthalmol Vis Sci* 33:2672, 1992.

221. Erickson-Lamy KA, Schroeder A, Epstein DL: Ethacrynic acid induces reversible shape and cytoskeletal changes in cultured cells, *Invest Ophthalmol Vis Sci* 33:2631, 1992.

222. Erickson-Lamy KA et al: Cholinergic drugs alter ciliary muscle response and receptor content, *Invest Ophthalmol Vis Sci* 28:375, 1987.

223. Ethier CR et al: Calculations of flow resistance in the juxtacanalicular meshwork, *Invest Ophthalmol Vis Sci* 27:1741, 1986.

224. Ethier CR et al: Two pore types in the inner-wall endothelium of Schlemm's canal, *Invest Ophthalmol Vis Sci* 39:2041, 1998.

225. Étienne R, Barut C, Gonzalès-Bouchon J: Un nouvel hypotenseur oculaire: l'acéclidine, *Ann Oculist* 200:287, 1967.

226. Eveloff J, Warnock D: Activation of ion transport systems during cell volume regulation, *Am J Physiol* 252:F1, 1987.

227. Exley KA: Depression of autonomic ganglia by barbiturates, *Br J Pharmacol Chemother* 9:170, 1954.

228. Fauss DJ et al: Glucocorticoid (GC) effects on HTM cells: biochemical approaches and growth factor responses. In Lütjen-Drecoll E (ed): *Basic aspects of glaucoma research III.* International symposium held at the Department of Anatomy, University of Erlangen-Nürnberg, FRG, September 23-25, 1991, Stuttgart; New York, 1993, Schattauer.

229. Fautsch MP et al: Recombinant TIGR/MYOC increases outflow resistance in the human anterior segment, *Invest Ophthalmol Vis Sci* 41:4163, 2000.

230. Fenton RH, Zimmerman LE: Hemolytic glaucoma: an unusual cause of acute open-angle secondary glaucoma, *Arch Ophthalmol* 70:236, 1963.

231. Ferrari-Dileo G et al: Angiotensin-converting enzyme in bovine, feline, and human ocular tissues, *Invest Ophthalmol Vis Sci* 29:876, 1988.

232. Fielder AR, Rahi AHS: Immunoglobulins of normal aqueous humor, *Trans Ophthalmol Soc UK* 99:120, 1979.

233. Fink AI, Gelix MD, Fletcher RC: Schlemm's canal and adjacent structures in glaucomatous patients, *Am J Ophthalmol* 74:893, 1972.

234. Flocks M, Littwin CS, Zimmerman LE: Phacolytic glaucoma: clinicopathologic study of 138 cases of glaucoma associated with hypermature cataract, *Arch Ophthalmol* 54:37, 1955.

235. Flügel C, Bárány EH, Lütjen-Drecoll E: Histochemical differences within the ciliary muscle and its function in accommodation, *Exp Eye Res* 50:219, 1990.

236. Flügel C, Lütjen-Drecoll E: Presence and distribution of Na+/K+-ATPase in the ciliary epithelium of the rabbit, *Histochemistry* 88:613, 1988.

237. Flügel C et al: Age-related loss of α-smooth muscle actin in normal and glaucomatous human trabecular meshwork of different age groups, *J Glaucoma* 1:165, 1992.

238. Flügel C et al: Species differences in choroidal vasodilative innervation: evidence for specific intrinsic nitrergic and VIP-positive neurons in the human eye, *Invest Ophthalmol Vis Sci* 35:592, 1994.

239. Forbes M, Becker B: The transport of organic anions by the rabbit eye: II. In vivo transport of iodopyracet (Diodrast), *Am J Ophthalmol* 50:867, 1960.

240. Fortin EP: Canal de Schlemm y ligamento pectineo, *Arch Ophthalmol* 4:454, 1925.

241. Fortin EP: Action du muscle ciliare sur la circulation de l'oeil: insertion du muscle ciliare sur la paroi du canal de Schlemm—signification physiologique et pathologique, *CR Soc Biol* 102:432, 1929.

242. Francois J: The importance of the mucopolysaccharides in intraocular pressure regulation, *Invest Ophthalmol Vis Sci* 14:173, 1975.

243. Francois J, Rabaey M, Neetens A: Perfusion studies on the outflow of aqueous humor in human eyes, *Arch Ophthalmol* 55:193, 1956.

244. Freddo TF: The Glenn A. Fry award lecture 1992: aqueous humor proteins—a key for unlocking glaucoma? *Optom Vis Sci* 70:263, 1993.

245. Freddo TF et al: The source of proteins in the aqueous humor of the normal rabbit, *Invest Ophthalmol Vis Sci* 31:125, 1990.

246. Friedenwald JS: The formation of the intraocular fluid: Proctor award lecture of the Association for Research in Ophthalmology, *Am J Ophthalmol* 32:9, 1949.

247. Friedenwald JS: Carbonic anhydrase inhibition and aqueous flow, *Am J Ophthalmol* 39:59, 1955.

248. Friedenwald JS: Current studies on acetazolamide (Diamox) and aqueous humor flow, *Am J Ophthalmol* 40:139, 1955.

249. Fujimori C et al: The clinical evaluation of UF-021, a new prostaglandin related compound, in low tension glaucoma patients (Japanese), *Nippon Ganka Gakkai Zasshi* 97:1231, 1993.

250. Gaasterland D, Kupfer C: Experimental glaucoma in the rhesus monkey, *Invest Ophthalmol* 13:455, 1974.

251. Gaasterland D, Kupfer C, Ross K: Studies of aqueous humor dynamics in man: III. Measurements in young normal subjects using norepinephrine and isoproterenol, *Invest Ophthalmol Vis Sci* 12:267, 1973.

252. Gaasterland D, Kupfer C, Ross K: Studies of aqueous humor dynamics in man: IV. Effects of pilocarpine upon measurements in young normal volunteers, *Invest Ophthalmol* 14:848, 1975.

253. Gaasterland DE, Pederson JE, MacLellan HM: Perfusate effects upon resistance to aqueous humor outflow in the rhesus monkey eye, *Invest Ophthalmol Vis Sci* 17:391, 1978.

254. Gaasterland DE et al: Rhesus monkey aqueous humor composition and a primate ocular perfusate, *Invest Ophthalmol Vis Sci* 18:1139, 1979.

255. Gabelt BT, Kaufman PL: Prostaglandin $F_{2\alpha}$ increases uveoscleral outflow in the cynomolgus monkey, *Exp Eye Res* 49:389, 1989.

256. Gabelt BT, Kaufman PL: Inhibition of outflow facility, accommodative, and miotic responses to pilocarpine in rhesus monkeys by muscarinic receptor subtype antagonists, *J Pharmacol Exp Ther* 263:1133, 1992.

257. Gabelt BT, Kaufman PL: Inhibition of aceclidine-stimulated outflow facility, accommodation and miosis by muscarinic receptor subtype antagonists in rhesus monkeys, *Exp Eye Res* 58:623, 1994.

258. Gabelt BT, Kaufman PL: Normal physiology. In Alm A, Weinreb RN (eds): *Uveoscleral outflow: biology and clinical aspects,* London, 1998, Mosby-Wolfe.

259. Gabelt BT, Kaufman PL: Uveoscleral outflow decreases in old rhesus monkeys, *Invest Ophthalmol Vis Sci* 40:S253, 2000 (ARVO abstract 1328).

260. Gabelt BT et al: Superior cervical ganglionectomy in monkeys: aqueous humor dynamics and their responses to drugs. *Exp Eye Res* 1995;60:575-84.

261. Gabelt BT et al: Anterior segment physiology following bumetanide inhibition of Na-K-Cl cotransport, *Invest Ophthalmol Vis Sci* 38:1700, 1997.

262. Gabelt BT et al: Effect of serotonergic compounds on aqueous humor dynamics in monkeys, *Curr Eye Res,* 2002 (in press).

263. Galin MA: Mydriasis provocative test, *Arch Ophthalmol* 66:353, 1961.

264. Gartner S: Blood vessels of the conjunctiva, *Arch Ophthalmol* 32:464, 1944.

265. Geiger B, Yehuda-Levenberg S, Bershadsky AD: Molecular interactions in the submembrane plaque of cell-cell and cell-matrix adhesions, *Acta Anat* 154:46, 1995.

266. Geyer O, Robinson D, Lazar M: Hypotensive effect of bromocriptine in normal eyes, *J Ocul Pharmacol* 3:291, 1987.

267. Gharagozloo NZ, Larson RS, Kullerstrand W: Terbutaline stimulates aqueous humor flow in humans during sleep, *Arch Ophthalmol* 106:1218, 1988.

268. Gharagozloo NZ, Relf SJ, Brubaker RF: Aqueous flow is reduced by the alpha-adrenergic agonist, apraclonidine hydrochloride (ALO 2145), *Ophthalmology* 95:1217, 1988.

269. Ghose T et al: Immunoglobulins in aqueous humor and iris from patients with endogenous uveitis and patients with cataract, *Br J Ophthalmol* 57:897, 1973.

270. Gil DW et al: Muscarinic receptor subtypes in human iris-ciliary body measured by immunoprecipitation, *Invest Ophthalmol Vis Sci* 38:1434, 1997.

271. Gilmartin B, Hogan RE, Thompson SM: The effect of timolol maleate on tonic accommodation, tonic vergence, and pupil diameter, *Invest Ophthalmol Vis Sci* 25:763, 1984.

272. Gipson IK, Anderson RA: Actin filaments in cells of human trabecular meshwork and Schlemm's canal, *Invest Ophthalmol Vis Sci* 18:547, 1979.

273. Giuffré G: The effects of prostaglandin F$_{2\alpha}$ in the human eye, *Graefes Arch Clin Exp Ophthalmol* 222:139, 1985.

274. Godman GC, Miranda AF: Cellular contractility and the visible effects of cytochalasin. In Tannenbaum SW (ed): *Cytochalasins: biochemical and cell biological aspects,* Amsterdam, 1978, North-Holland.

275. Goldberg MF: The diagnosis and treatment of sickled erythrocytes in human hyphemias, *Trans Am Ophthalmol Soc* 76:481, 1978.

276. Goldmann H: Enhalten die kammervasservener kammervasser? *Ophthalmologica* 117:240, 1949.

277. Goldmann H: On pseudofacility, *Bibl Ophthalmol* 76:1, 1968.

278. Grant WM: Tonographic method for measuring the facility and rate of aqueous flow in human eyes, *Arch Ophthalmol* 44:204, 1950.

279. Grant WM: Experimental aqueous perfusion in enucleated human eyes, *Arch Ophthalmol* 69:783, 1963.

280. Green K, Padgett D: Effects of various drugs on pseudofacility and aqueous humor formation in rabbit eye, *Exp Eye Res* 28:239, 1979.

281. Green K, Pederson JE: Contribution of secretion and filtration to aqueous humor formation, *Am J Physiol* 222:1218, 1972.

282. Gregory D, Sears M, Bausher L: Intraocular pressure and aqueous flow are decreased by cholera toxin, *Invest Ophthalmol Vis Sci* 20:371, 1981.

283. Grierson I, Lee WR: Erythrocyte phagocytosis in the human trabecular meshwork, *Br J Ophthalmol* 57:400, 1973.

284. Grierson I, Lee WR: The fine structure of the trabecular meshwork at graded levels of intraocular pressure: 1. Pressure effects within the near physiological range (8-30mmHg), *Exp Eye Res* 20:505, 1975.

285. Grierson I, Lee WR: The fine structure of the trabecular meshwork at graded levels of intraocular pressure: 2. Pressures outside the physiological range (0 and 50 mmHg), *Exp Eye Res* 20:523, 1975.

286. Grierson I, Lee WR: Pressure-induced changes in the ultrastructure of the endothelium lining of Schlemm's canal, *Am J Ophthalmol* 80:863, 1975.

287. Grierson I, Lee WR: Light microscopic quantitation of the endothelial vacuoles in Schlemm's canal, *Am J Ophthalmol* 84:234, 1977.

288. Grierson I, Lee WR: Pressure effects on flow channels in the lining endothelium of Schlemm's canal, *Acta Ophthalmol* 56:935, 1978.

289. Grierson I, Lee WR, Abraham S: Effects of pilocarpine on the morphology of the human outflow apparatus, *Br J Ophthalmol* 62:302, 1978.

290. Grierson I, Rahi AH: Microfilaments in the cells of the human trabecular meshwork, *Br J Ophthalmol* 63:3, 1979.

291. Grierson I et al: The effects of age and antiglaucoma drugs on the meshwork cell population, *Res Clin Forum* 4:69, 1982.

292. Gunning FP et al: Two topical carbonic anhydrase inhibitors sezolamide and dorzolamide in Gelrite vehicle: a multiple-dose efficacy study, *Graefes Arch Clin Exp Ophthalmol* 231:384, 1993.

293. Gupta N et al: Localization of M3 muscarinic receptor subtype and mRNA in the human eye, *Ophthalmic Res* 26:207, 1994.

294. Gupta N et al: Muscarinic receptor M1 and M2 subtypes in the human eye: QNB, pirenzepine, oxotremorine, and AFDX-116 in vitro autoradiography, *Br J Ophthalmol* 78:555, 1994.

295. Haas M: The Na-K-Cl cotransporters, *Am J Physiol* 267:C869, 1994.

296. Hager H: Besondere mickrochirurgische eingraffe: II. Erste erfahrugen mid dem argon laser gerät 800, *Klin Monatsbl Augenheilkd* 162:437, 1973.

297. Hamachi T, Hirata M, Koga T: Effect of cAMP-elevating drugs on Ca2+ efflux and actin polymerization in peritoneal macrophages stimulated with N-formyl chemotactic peptide, *Biochim Biophys Acta* 804:230, 1984.

298. Harris LS: Cycloplegic-induced intraocular pressure elevations, *Arch Ophthalmol* 79:242, 1968.

299. Hart WM: Intraocular pressure. In Hart WM (ed): *Adler's physiology of the eye,* ed 9, St Louis, 1992, Mosby.

300. Hassel JR, Newsome DA, Martin GR: Isolation and characterization of the proteoglycans and collagens synthesized by cells in culture, *Vision Res* 21:49, 1981.

301. Hayashi M, Yablonski ME, Bito LZ: Eicosanoids as a new class of ocular hypotensive agents: 2. Comparison of the apparent mechanism of the ocular hypotensive effects of A and F type prostaglandins, *Invest Ophthalmol Vis Sci* 28:1639, 1987.

302. Hedler L et al: Functional characterization of central α-adrenoceptors by yohimbine diastereoisomers, *Eur J Pharmacol* 70:43, 1981.

303. Henkind P: Ocular circulation. In Records RE (ed): *Physiology of the human eye and visual system,* New York, 1979, Harper & Row.

304. Hernandez MR et al: The effect of dexamethasone on the in vitro incorporation of precursors of extracellular matrix components in the outflow pathway region of the rabbit eye, *Invest Ophthalmol Vis Sci* 24:704, 1983.

305. Hernandez MR et al: Glucocorticoid target cells in human outflow pathway: autopsy and surgical specimens, *Invest Ophthalmol Vis Sci* 24:1612, 1983.

306. Hernandez MR et al: The effect of dexamethasone on the synthesis of collagen in normal human trabecular meshwork explants, *Invest Ophthalmol Vis Sci* 26:1784, 1985.

307. Higgins RG, Brubaker RF: Acute effect of epinephrine on aqueous humor formation in the timolol-treated normal eye as measured by fluorophotometry, *Invest Ophthalmol Vis Sci* 19:420, 1980.

308. Hoffman BF, Bigger JTJ: Digitalis and allied cardiac glycosides. In Gilman AG et al (eds): *Goodman and Gilman's the pharmacological basis of therapeutics,* New York, 1990, McGraw-Hill.

309. Hogan MJ, Alvarado JA, Weddell JE: Ciliary body and posterior chamber. In Hogan MJ, Alvarado JA, Weddell JE (eds): *Histology of the human eye,* Philadelphia, 1971, WB Saunders.

310. Holmberg Å, Bárány EH: The effect of pilocarpine on the endothelium forming the inner wall of Schlemm's canal: an electron microscopic study in the monkey *Cercopithecus ethiops, Invest Ophthalmol* 5:53, 1966.

311. Hoskins HD, Kass MA: Adrenergic agonists. In Hoskins HD, Kass MA (eds): *Becker-Shaffer's diagnosis and therapy of the glaucomas,* St Louis, 1989, Mosby.

312. Hoskins HD, Kass MA: Aqueous humor formation. In Klein EA (ed): *Becker-Shaffer's diagnosis and therapy of the glaucomas,* ed 6, St Louis, 1989, Mosby.

313. Hoskins HD, Kass MA: Aqueous humor outflow. In Hoskins HD, Kass MA (eds): *Becker-Shaffer's diagnosis and therapy of the glaucomas,* St Louis, 1989, Mosby.

314. Hoskins HD, Kass MA: Cholinergic drugs. In Hoskins HD, Kass MA (eds): *Becker-Shaffer's diagnosis and therapy of the glaucomas,* ed 6, St Louis, 1989, Mosby.

315. Hoskins HD, Kass MA: Medical treatment. In Hoskins HD, Kass MA (eds): *Becker-Shaffer's diagnosis and therapy of the glaucomas,* ed 6, St Louis, 1989, Mosby.

316. Hoskins HD, Kass MA: Secondary open-angle glaucoma. In Hoskins HD, Kass MA (eds): *Becker-Shaffer's diagnosis and therapy of the glaucomas,* ed 6, St Louis, 1989, Mosby.

317. Hotehama Y et al: Ocular hypotensive effect of PhXA41 in patients with ocular hypotension or primary open-angle glaucoma, *Jpn J Ophthalmol* 37:270, 1993.

318. Hubbard WC, Kee C, Kaufman PL: Aceclidine effects on outflow facility after ciliary muscle disinsertion, *Ophthalmologica* 210:303, 1996.

319. Hubbard WC et al: Intraocular pressure and outflow facility are unchanged following acute and chronic intracameral Chondroitinase ABC and hyaluronidase in monkeys, *Exp Eye Res* 65:177, 1997.

320. Ingram CJ, Brubaker RF: Effect of brinzolamide and dorzolamide on aqueous humor flow in human eyes, *Am J Ophthalmol* 128:292, 1999.

321. Inomata H, Bill A, Smelser GK: Aqueous humor pathways through the trabecular meshwork and into Schlemm's canal in the cynomolgus monkey (*Macaca irus*): an electron microscopic study, *Am J Ophthalmol* 73:760, 1972.

322. Jacob E, FitzSimon JS, Brubaker RF: Combined corticosteroid and catecholamine stimulation of aqueous humor flow, *Ophthalmology* 103:1303, 1996.

323. Jan Danser AH et al: Angiotensin levels in the eye, *Invest Ophthalmol Vis Sci* 35:1008, 1994.

324. Janes RG, Calkins JP: Effect of certain drugs on iris vessels, *Arch Ophthalmol* 57:414, 1957.

325. Jin Y, Verstappen A, Yorio T: Characterization of alpha 2-adrenoceptor binding sites in rabbit ciliary body membranes, *Invest Ophthalmol Vis Sci* 35:2500, 1994.

326. Johnson D et al: Ultrastructural changes in the trabecular meshwork of human eyes treated with corticosteroids, *Arch Ophthalmol* 115:375, 1997.

327. Johnson DH: The effect of cytochalasin D on outflow facility and the trabecular meshwork of the human eye in perfusion organ culture, *Invest Ophthalmol Vis Sci* 38:2790, 1997.

328. Johnson DH: Myocilin and glaucoma: a TIGR by the tail, *Arch Ophthalmol* 118:974, 2000.

329. Johnson DH, Bahler CK: Heparintinase increases outflow facility in the human eye, *Invest Ophthalmol Vis Sci* 40:S504, 1999 (ARVO abstract 2657).

330. Johnson DH, Tschumper RC: Ethacrynic acid: outflow effects and toxicity in human trabecular meshwork in perfusion organ culture, *Curr Eye Res* 12:385, 1993.

331. Johnson F, Maurice D: A simple method of measuring aqueous humor flow with intravitreal fluoresceinated dextrans, *Exp Eye Res* 39:791, 1984.

332. Johnson M, Erickson K: Mechanisms and routes of aqueous humor drainage. In Albert DM, Jakobiec FA (eds): *Principles and practice of ophthalmology,* Philadelphia, 2000, WB Saunders.

333. Johnson M et al: Modulation of outflow resistance by the pores of the inner wall endothelium, *Invest Ophthalmol Vis Sci* 33:1670, 1992.

334. Johnson M et al: Serum proteins and aqueous outflow resistance in bovine eyes, *Invest Ophthalmol Vis Sci* 34:3549, 1993.

335. Johnstone M et al: Concentration-dependent morphologic effects of cytochalasin B in the aqueous outflow system, *Invest Ophthalmol Vis Sci* 19:835, 1980.

336. Johnstone MA, Grant WM: Pressure-dependent changes in structure of the aqueous outflow system of human and monkey eye, *Am J Ophthalmol* 75:365, 1973.

337. Jones RF, Maurice DM: New methods of measuring the rate of aqueous flow in man with fluorescein, *Exp Eye Res* 5:208, 1966.

338. Kaufman PL: Anticholinesterase-induced cholinergic subsensitivity in primate accommodative mechanism, *Am J Ophthalmol* 85:622, 1978.

339. Kaufman PL: Aqueous humor dynamics following total iridectomy in the cynomolgus monkey, *Invest Ophthalmol Vis Sci* 18:870, 1979.

340. Kaufman PL: Aqueous humor dynamics. In Duane TD (ed): *Clinical ophthalmology,* New York, 1985, Harper & Row.

341. Kaufman PL: Adenosine 3',5' cyclic monophosphate and outflow facility in monkey eyes with intact and retrodisplaced ciliary muscle, *Exp Eye Res* 44:415, 1987.

342. Kaufman PL: Accommodation and presbyopia: neuromuscular and biophysical aspects. In Hart WM (ed): *Adler's physiology of the eye,* ed 9, St Louis, 1992, Mosby.

343. Kaufman PL: Pressure-dependent outflow. In Ritch R, Shields MB, Krupin T (eds): *The glaucomas*, ed 2, St Louis, 1996, Mosby.

344. Kaufman PL, Bárány EH: Subsensitivity to pilocarpine in primate ciliary muscle following topical anticholinesterase treatment, *Invest Ophthalmol* 14:302, 1975.

345. Kaufman PL, Bárány EH: Loss of acute pilocarpine effect on outflow facility following surgical disinsertion and retrodisplacement of the ciliary muscle from the scleral spur in the cynomolgus monkey, *Invest Ophthalmol* 15:793, 1976.

346. Kaufman PL, Bárány EH: Residual pilocarpine effects on outflow facility after ciliary muscle disinsertion in the cynomolgus monkey, *Invest Ophthalmol* 15:558, 1976.

347. Kaufman PL, Bárány EH: Subsensitivity to pilocarpine of the aqueous outflow system in monkey eyes after topical anticholinesterase treatment, *Am J Ophthalmol* 82:883, 1976.

348. Kaufman PL, Bárány EH: Cytochalasin B reversibly increases outflow facility in the eye of the cynomolgus monkey, *Invest Ophthalmol Vis Sci* 16:47, 1977.

349. Kaufman PL, Bárány EH: Recent observations concerning the effects of cholinergic drugs on outflow facility in monkeys. In Bito LZ, Davson H, Fenstermacher JD (eds): *The ocular and cerebrospinal fluids*: Fogarty International Center Symposium, *Exp Eye Res* 25(suppl): 415, 1977.

350. Kaufman PL, Bárány EH: Adrenergic drug effects on aqueous outflow facility following ciliary muscle retrodisplacement in the cynomolgus monkey, *Invest Ophthalmol Vis Sci* 20:644, 1981.

351. Kaufman PL, Bárány EH, Erickson KA: Effect of serotonin, histamine, and bradykinin on outflow facility following ciliary muscle retrodisplacement in the cynomolgus monkey, *Exp Eye Res* 35:191, 1982.

352. Kaufman PL, Bill A, Bárány EH: Effect of cytochalasin B on conventional drainage of aqueous humor in the cynomolgus monkey. In Bito LZ, Davson H, Fenstermacher JD (eds): *The ocular and cerebrospinal fluids*: Fogarty International Center Symposium, *Exp Eye Res* 25(suppl): 411, 1977.

353. Kaufman PL, Bill A, Bárány EH: Formation and drainage of aqueous humor following total iris removal and ciliary muscle disinsertion in the cynomolgus monkey, *Invest Ophthalmol Vis Sci* 16:226, 1977.

354. Kaufman PL, Crawford K: *Aqueous humor dynamics: how $PGF_{2\alpha}$ lowers intraocular pressure.* In Bito LZ, Stjernschantz J (eds): *The ocular effects of prostaglandins and other eicosanoids*, New York, 1989, Alan R. Liss.

355. Kaufman PL, Crawford K, Gabelt BT: The effects of prostaglandins on aqueous humor dynamics. In Kooner KS, Zimmerman TJ (eds): *New ophthalmic drugs*, Philadelphia, 1989, WB Saunders.

356. Kaufman PL, Erickson KA: Cytochalasin B and D dose-outflow facility response relationships in the cynomolgus monkey, *Invest Ophthalmol Vis Sci* 23:646, 1982.

357. Kaufman PL, Gabelt BT: Cholinergic mechanisms and aqueous humor dynamics. In Drance SM, Van Buskirk EM, Neufeld AH (eds): *Pharmacology of glaucoma*, Baltimore, 1992, Williams & Wilkins.

358. Kaufman PL, Gabelt BT: α2-Adrenergic agonist effects on aqueous humor dynamics, *J Glaucoma* 4(suppl 1):S8, 1995.

359. Kaufman PL, Gabelt BT: Presbyopia, prostaglandins and primary open angle glaucoma. In Krieglstein GK (ed): *Glaucoma update: V.* Proceedings of the Symposium of the Glaucoma Society of the International Congress of Ophthalmology in Quebec City, June 1994, New York; Berlin, 1995, Springer-Verlag.

360. Kaufman PL, Gabelt BT: Direct, indirect and dual acting parasympathetic drugs. In Zimmerman TJ (ed): *Textbook of ocular pharmacology*, Philadelphia, 1997, Lippincott-Raven.

361. Kaufman PL, Lütjen-Drecoll E: Total iridectomy in the primate in vivo: surgical technique and postoperative anatomy, *Invest Ophthalmol* 14:766, 1975.

362. Kaufman PL, Mittag TW: Medical therapy of glaucoma. In Kaufman PL, Mittag TW (eds): *Glaucoma*, London, 1994, Mosby-Year Book Europe, Ltd.

363. Kaufman PL, Rentzhog L: Effect of total iridectomy on outflow facility responses to adrenergic drugs in cynomolgus monkeys, *Exp Eye Res* 33:65, 1981.

364. Kaufman PL, Svedbergh B, Lütjen-Drecoll E: Medical trabeculocanalotomy in monkeys with cytochalasin B or EDTA, *Ann Ophthalmol* 11:795, 1979.

365. Kaufman PL et al: Obstruction of aqueous humor outflow by cross-linked polyacrylamide microgels in bovine, monkey and human eyes, *Ophthalmology* 101:1672, 1994.

366. Keates EU, Stone R: The effect of d-timolol on intraocular pressure in patients with ocular hypertension, *Am J Ophthalmol* 98:73, 1984.

367. Kee C, Kaufman PL, Gabelt BT: Effect of 8-Br cGMP on aqueous humor dynamics in monkeys, *Invest Ophthalmol Vis Sci* 35:2769, 1994.

368. Kee C et al: Serum effects on aqueous outflow during anterior chamber perfusion in monkeys, *Invest Ophthalmol Vis Sci* 37:1840, 1996.

369. Kiland JA, Hubbard WC, Kaufman PL: Low doses of pilocarpine do not significantly increase outflow facility in the cynomolgus monkey, *Exp Eye Res* 70:603, 2000.

370. Kleinstein RN, Fatt I: Pressure dependency of trans-scleral flow, *Exp Eye Res* 24:335, 1977.

371. Knepper PA, Collins JA, Frederick R: Effects of dexamethasone, progesterone, and testosterone on IOP and GAGS in the rabbit eye, *Invest Ophthalmol Vis Sci* 26:1093, 1985.

372. Knepper PA, Goossens W, Palmberg PF: Glycosaminoglycan stratification of the juxtacanalicular tissue in normal and primary open-angle glaucoma, *Invest Ophthalmol Vis Sci* 37:2414, 1996.

373. Knepper PA et al: Glycosaminoglycans of the human trabecular meshwork in primary open-angle glaucoma, *Invest Ophthalmol Vis Sci* 37:1360, 1996.

374. Knutson SL, Sears ML: Herman Boerhaave and the history of vessels carrying aqueous humor from the eye, *Am J Ophthalmol* 76:648, 1973.

375. Kodama T, Reddy VN, Macri FJ: Pharmacological study on the effects of some ocular hypotensive drugs on aqueous humor formation in the arterially perfused enucleated rabbit eye, *Ophthalmic Res* 17:120, 1985.

376. Kolker AE, Becker B: Topical corticosteroids and glaucoma: current status. In Bellows JG (ed): *Contemporary ophthalmology*, Baltimore, 1972, Williams & Wilkins.

377. Korenbrot JI: Ion incorporation in membranes: incorporation of biological ion-translocating proteins in model membrane systems, *Annu Rev Physiol* 39:19, 1977.

378. Korenfeld MS, Becker B: Atrial natriuretic peptides: effects on intraocular pressure, cGMP, and aqueous flow, *Invest Ophthalmol Vis Sci* 30:2385, 1989.

379. Krasnov MM: Laser puncture of anterior chamber angle in glaucoma, *Am J Ophthalmol* 75:674, 1973.

380. Krause U, Raunio V: Proteins of the normal human aqueous humor, *Ophthalmologica* 159:178, 1969.

381. Krieglstein GK, Langham ME, Leydhecker W: The peripheral and central neural actions of clonidine in normal and glaucomatous eyes, *Invest Ophthalmol Vis Sci* 17:149, 1978.

382. Krill AE, Newell FW, Novak KM: Early and long-term effects of levo-epinephrine on ocular tension and outflow, *Am J Ophthalmol* 59:833, 1965.

383. Kronfeld PC: Dose-effect relationships as an aid in the evaluation of ocular hypotensive drugs, *Invest Ophthalmol* 3:258, 1964.

384. Kronfeld PC: The efficacy of combinations of ocular hypotensive drugs: a tonographic approach, *Arch Ophthalmol* 78:140, 1967.

385. Kronfeld PC: Early effect of single and repeated doses of l-epinephrine in man, *Am J Ophthalmol* 72:1058, 1971.

386. Krootila K, Palkama A, Uusitalo H: Effect of serotonin and its antagonist (ketanserin) on intraocular pressure in the rabbit, *J Ocular Pharmacol* 3:279, 1987.

387. Krupin T, Becker B, Podos SM: Topical vanadate lowers intraocular pressure in rabbits, *Invest Ophthalmol Vis Sci* 19:1360, 1980.

388. Krupin T, Civan MM: Physiologic basis of aqueous humor formation. In Ritch R, Shields MB, Krupin T (eds): *The glaucomas*, ed 2, St Louis, 1996, Mosby.

389. Krupin T, Feitl M, Becker B: Effect of prazosin on aqueous humor dynamics in rabbits, *Arch Ophthalmol* 98:1639, 1980.

390. Krupin T, Siverstein B, Feitl M: The effect of H1-blocking antihistamines on intraocular pressure in rabbits, *Ophthalmology* 87:1167, 1980.

391. Krupin T et al: Increased intraocular pressure following topical azide or nitroprusside, *Invest Ophthalmol Vis Sci* 16:1002, 1977.

392. Kupfer C: Clinical significance of pseudofacility: Sanford R. Gifford memorial lecture, *Am J Ophthalmol* 75:193, 1973.

393. Kupfer C, Gaasterland D, Ross K: Studies of aqueous humor dynamics in man: II. Measurements in young normal subjects using acetazolamide and l-epinephrine, *Invest Ophthalmol* 10:523, 1971.

394. Kupfer C, Ross K: Studies of aqueous humour dynamics in man: I. Measurements in young normal subjects, *Invest Ophthalmol* 10:518, 1971.

395. Kupfer C, Sanderson P: Determination of pseudofacility in the eye of man, *Arch Ophthalmol* 80:194, 1968.

396. Laliberte MF et al: Immunohistochemistry of angiotensin-I converting enzyme in rat eye structures involved in aqueous humor regulation, *Lab Invest* 59:263, 1988.

397. Langham ME: The aqueous outflow system and its response to autonomic receptor agonists, *Exp Eye Res* 25(suppl):311, 1977.

398. Larson RS, Brubaker RF: Isoproterenol stimulates aqueous flow in humans with Horner's syndrome, *Invest Ophthalmol Vis Sci* 29:621, 1988.

399. Laties AMD, Jacobowitz D: A comparative study of the autonomic innervation of the eye in monkey, cat and rabbit, *Anat Record* 156:383, 1966.

400. Lee DA, Brubaker RF: Effect of phenylephrine on aqueous humor flow, *Curr Eye Res* 83:89, 1982.

401. Lee DA, Brubaker RF, Nagataki S: Acute effect of thymoxamine on aqueous humor formation in the epinephrine-treated normal eye as measured by fluorophotometry, *Invest Ophthalmol Vis Sci* 24:165, 1983.

402. Lee DA, Topper JE, Brubaker RF: Effect of clonidine on aqueous humor flow in normal human eyes, *Exp Eye Res* 38:239, 1984.

403. Lee P-Y et al: Pharmacological testing in the laser-induced monkey glaucoma model, *Curr Eye Res* 4:775, 1985.

404. Lee P-Y et al: Intraocular pressure effects of multiple doses of drugs applied to glaucomatous monkey eyes, *Arch Ophthalmol* 105:249, 1987.

405. Lee P-Y et al: The effect of prostaglandin $F_{2\alpha}$ on intraocular pressure in normotensive human subjects, *Invest Ophthalmol Vis Sci* 29:1474, 1988.

406. Lepple-Wienhues A, Stahl F, Wiederholt M: Differential smooth muscle-like contractile properties of trabecular meshwork and ciliary muscle, *Exp Eye Res* 53:33, 1991.

407. Lepple-Wienhues A et al: Endothelin-evoked contractions in bovine ciliary muscle and trabecular meshwork: interaction with calcium, nifedipine and nickel, *Curr Eye Res* 10:983, 1991.

408. Lepple-Wienhues A et al: Electrophysiological properties of cultured human trabecular meshwork cells, *Exp Eye Res* 59:305, 1994.

409. Lerner LE et al: Hyaluronan in the human trabecular meshwork, *Invest Ophthalmol Vis Sci* 38:1222, 1997.

410. Levi L, Schwartz B: Decrease of ocular pressure with oral metyrapone: a double masked crossover trial, *Arch Ophthalmol* 105:777, 1987.

411. Levitzki A: The binding characteristics and number of beta-adrenergic receptors in the turkey erythrocyte, *Proc Natl Acad Sci USA* 71:2773, 1974.

412. Levy NS, Boone L, Ellis E: A controlled comparison of betaxolol and timolol with long-term evaluation of safety and efficacy, *Glaucoma* 7:54, 1985.

413. Liang L-L et al: Ethacrynic acid increases facility of outflow in the human eye in vitro, *Arch Ophthalmol* 110:106, 1992.

414. Lieberman TW, Leopold IH: The use of aceclidine in the treatment of glaucoma: its effect on intraocular pressure and facility of aqueous humor outflow as compared to that of pilocarpine, *Am J Ophthalmol* 64:405, 1967.

415. Lindsey JD, To HD, Weinreb RN: Induction of c-fos by prostaglandin F2 alpha in human ciliary smooth muscle cells, *Invest Ophthalmol Vis Sci* 35:242, 1994.

416. Lindsey JD et al: Prostaglandins increase proMMP-1 and proMMP-3 secretion by human ciliary smooth muscle cells, *Curr Eye Res* 15:869, 1996.

417. Lindsey JD et al: Prostaglandin action on ciliary smooth muscle extracellular matrix metabolism: implications for uveoscleral outflow, *Surv Ophthalmol* 41(suppl 2):S53, 1997.

418. Lippa EA et al: Dose response and duration of action of dorzolamide, a topical carbonic anhydrase inhibitor: *Arch Ophthalmol* 110:495, 1992.

419. Liu HK, Chiou GCY: Continuous, simultaneous, and instant display of aqueous humor dynamics with a microspectrophotometer and a sensitive drop counter, *Exp Eye Res* 32:583, 1981.

420. Liu JH, Bartels SP, Neufeld AH: Effects of l- and d-timolol on cyclic AMP synthesis and intraocular pressure in water-loaded, albino and pigmented rabbits, *Invest Ophthalmol Vis Sci* 24:1276, 1983.

421. Liu JH, Gallar J: In vivo cAMP level in rabbit iris-ciliary body after topical epinephrine treatment, *Curr Eye Res* 15:1025, 1996.

422. Liu JH et al: Elevation of human intraocular pressure at night under moderate illumination. *Invest Ophthalmol Vis Sci* 40:2439, 1999.

423. Liu JH et al: Twenty-four-hour pattern of intraocular pressure in the aging population, *Invest Ophthalmol Vis Sci* 40:2912, 1999.

424. Liu S et al: Lack of effect of calcium channel blockers on open-angle glaucoma, *J Glaucoma* 5:187, 1996.

425. Lograno MD, Reibaldi A: Receptor-responses in fresh human ciliary muscle, *Br J Pharmacol* 87:379, 1986.

426. Lotti VJ, LeDouarec JC, Stone CA: Autonomic nervous system: adrenergic antagonists. In Sears ML (ed): *Pharmacology of the eye: handbook of experimental pharmacology*, Berlin, 1984, Springer-Verlag.

427. Lütjen E: Histometrische untersuchungen über den ziliarmuskel der primaten, *Graefes Arch Clin Exp Ophthalmol* 171:121, 1966.

428. Lütjen-Drecoll E: Structural factors influencing outflow facility and its changeability under drugs: a study of Macaca arctoides, *Invest Ophthalmol* 12:280, 1973.

429. Lütjen-Drecoll E: Functional morphology of the trabecular meshwork in primate eyes, *Prog Retin Eye Res* 18:91, 1998.

430. Lütjen-Drecoll E, Futa R, Rohen JW: Ultrahistochemical studies on tangential sections of the trabecular meshwork in normal and glaucomatous eyes, *Invest Ophthalmol Vis Sci* 21:563, 1981.

431. Lütjen-Drecoll E, Kaufman PL: Morphological changes in primate aqueous humor formation and drainage tissues after long-term treatment with antiglaucomatous drugs, *J Glaucoma* 2:316, 1993.

432. Lütjen-Drecoll E, Lonnerholm G: Carbonic anhydrase distribution in the rabbit eye by light and electron microscopy, *Invest Ophthalmol Vis Sci* 21:782, 1981.

433. Lütjen-Drecoll E, Lonnerholm G, Eichhorn M: Carbonic anhydrase distribution in the human and monkey eye by light and electron microscopy, *Graefes Arch Clin Exp Ophthalmol* 220:285, 1983.

434. Lütjen-Drecoll E, Rohen JW: Morphology of aqueous outflow pathways in normal and glaucomatous eyes. In Ritch R, Shields MB, Krupin T (eds): *The glaucomas,* St Louis, 1989, Mosby.

435. Lütjen-Drecoll E, Tamm E: Morphological study of the anterior segments of cynomolgus monkey eyes following treatment with prostaglandin $F_{2\alpha}$, *Exp Eye Res* 47:761, 1988.

436. Lütjen-Drecoll E, Weindl H, Kaufman PL: Acute and chronic structural effects of pilocarpine on monkey outflow tissues, *Trans Am Ophthalmol Soc* 96:171, 1998.

437. Lütjen-Drecoll E et al: Quantitative analysis of "plaque material" in the inner and outer wall of Schlemm's canal in normal and glaucomatous eyes, *Exp Eye Res* 42:443, 1986.

438. Lyle WM, Cullen AP, Charman WN: Role of lasers in eye care, *Optom Vis Sci* 70:136, 1993.

439. MacCumber MW et al: Endothelin mRNAs visualized by in situ hybridization provides evidence for local action, *Proc Natl Acad Sci USA* 86:7285, 1989.

440. Macri FJ, Cevario SJ: The induction of aqueous humor formation by the use of Ach + eserine, *Invest Ophthalmol* 12:910, 1973.

441. Macri FJ, Cevario SJ: The dual nature of pilocarpine to stimulate or inhibit the formation of aqueous humor, *Invest Ophthalmol* 13:617, 1974.

442. Macri FJ, Cevario SJ: A possible vascular mechanism for the inhibition of aqueous humor formation by ouabain and acetazolamide, *Exp Eye Res* 20:563, 1975.

443. Mäepea O, Nilsson SF: Suppression of VIP- and terbutaline-stimulated aqueous humor flow by increased intraocular pressure in the cynomolgus monkey, *Curr Eye Res* 10:703, 1991.

444. Main BG, Tucker H: Recent advances in beta-adrenergic blocking agents. In Ellis GP, West GB (eds): *Progress in medicinal chemistry,* Amsterdam, 1985, Elsevier.

445. Maren TH: Carbonic anhydrase: chemistry, physiology, and inhibition, *Physiol Rev* 47:595, 1967.

446. Maren TH: Bicarbonate formation in cerebrospinal fluid: role in sodium transport and pH regulation, *Am J Physiol* 222:885, 1972.

447. Maren TH: HCO_3^- formation in aqueous humor: mechanism and relation to the treatment of glaucoma, *Invest Ophthalmol* 13:479, 1974.

448. Maren TH: The development of ideas concerning the role of carbonic anhydrase in the secretion of aqueous humor: relations to the treatment of glaucoma. In Drance SM, Neufeld AH (eds): *Glaucoma: applied pharmacology in medical treatment,* Orlando, 1984, Grune & Stratton.

449. Maren TH: Biochemistry of aqueous humor inflow. In Kaufman PL, Mittag TW (eds): *Glaucoma,* London, 1994, Mosby-Year Book Europe, Ltd.

450. Maren TH, Haywood JR, Chapman SK: The pharmacology of methazolamide in relation to the treatment of glaucoma, *Invest Ophthalmol Vis Sci* 16:730, 1977.

451. Maren TH, Mayer E, Wadsworth BC: Carbonic anhydrase inhibition: I. The pharmacology of Diamox (1-acetylamino 1,3,4-thiadiazole-5-sulfonamide), *Johns Hopkins Med J* 95:199, 1954.

452. Maren TH et al: The transcorneal permeability of sulfonamide carbonic anhydrase inhibitors and their effect on aqueous humor secretion, *Exp Eye Res* 36:457, 1983.

453. Maren TH et al: Timolol decreases aqueous humor flow but not Na+ movement from plasma to aqueous, *Invest Ophthalmol Vis Sci* 38:1274, 1997.

454. Marshall GE, Konstas AG, Lee WR: Immunogold localization of type IV collagen and laminin in the aging human outflow system, *Exp Eye Res* 51:691, 1990.

455. Masuda M: Effects of prostaglandins on inflow and outflow of the aqueous humor in rabbits, *Jpn J Ophthalmol* 17:300, 1973.

456. Maus TL, Nau C, Brubaker RF: Comparison of the early effects of brimonidine and apraclonidine as topical ocular hypotensive agents, *Arch Ophthalmol* 117:586, 1999.

457. McMillan TA et al: Comparison of diode and argon laser trabeculoplasty in cadaver eyes, *Invest Ophthalmol Vis Sci* 35:706, 1994.

458. Mekki QA, Hassan SM, Turner P: Bromocriptine lowers intraocular pressure without affecting blood pressure, *Lancet* 1:1250, 1983.

459. Melamed S et al: The effect of intracamerally injected ethacrynic acid on intraocular pressure in patients with glaucoma, *Am J Ophthalmol* 113:508, 1992.

460. Merte HJ, Stryz J: Present day possibilities of glaucoma therapy. In Merte HJ (ed): *Metipranolol: pharmacology of beta-blocking agents and use of metipranolol in ophthalmology—contributions to the first metipranolol symposium,* Vienna, 1983, Springer-Verlag.

461. Meyer-Bothling U, Bron AJ, Osborne NN: Topical application of serotonin or the 5-HT1a-agonist 5-CT increases intraocular pressure in rabbits, *Invest Ophthalmol Vis Sci* 34:3035, 1993.

462. Millar C, Kaufman PL: Aqueous humor: secretion and dynamics. In Tasman W, Jaeger EA (eds): *Duane's foundations of clinical ophthalmology,* Philadelphia, 1995, Lippincott-Raven.

463. Millar JC et al: Drug effects on intraocular pressure and vascular flow in the bovine perfused eye using radiolabelled microspheres, *J Ocular Pharmacol Ther* 11:11, 1995.

464. Mills KB, Jacobs NJ, Vogel R: A study of the effects of four concentrations of d-timolol, 0.25% l-timolol, and placebo on intraocular pressure in patients with raised intraocular pressure, *Br J Ophthalmol* 72:469, 1988.

465. Mills KB, Wright G: A blind randomized cross-over trial comparing metipranolol 0.3% with timolol 0.25% in open-angle glaucoma: a pilot study, *Br J Ophthalmol* 70:39, 1986.

466. Mishima H et al: Ultracytochemistry of cholera toxin binding sites in ciliary processes, *Cell Tissue Res* 223:241, 1982.

467. Mittag TW: Ocular effects of selective alpha-adrenergic agents: a new drug paradox? *Ann Ophthalmol* 15:201, 1983.

468. Mittag TW et al: Alpha-adrenergic antagonists: correlation of the effect on intraocular pressure and on $\alpha 2$-adrenergic receptor binding specificity in the rabbit eye, *Exp Eye Res* 40:591, 1985.

469. Mittag TW et al: Atrial natriuretic peptide (ANP), guanylate cyclase, and intraocular pressure in the rabbit eye, *Curr Eye Res* 6:1189, 1987.

470. Mondino BJ, Rao H: Complement levels in normal and inflamed aqueous humor, *Invest Ophthalmol Vis Sci* 24:380, 1983.

471. Morgan TR, Green K, Bowman K: Effects of adrenergic agonists upon regional ocular blood flow in normal and ganglionectomized rabbits, *Exp Eye Res* 32:691, 1981.

472. Moriarty AP: Diode lasers in ophthalmology, *Int Ophthalmol* 17:297, 1993-1994.

473. Moses RA, Grodzki WJ Jr, Carras PL: Pseudofacility, *Arch Ophthalmol* 103:1653, 1985.

474. Moses RA, Grodzki WJ Jr, Etheridge EL: Schlemm's canal: the effect of intraocular pressure, *Invest Ophthalmol Vis Sci* 20:61, 1981.

475. Mudge GH, Weiner IM: Agents affecting volume and composition of body fluids. In Goodman LS, Gilman AG (eds): *Goodman and Gilman's the pharmacological basis of therapeutics,* ed 8, New York, 1990, Pergamon Press.

476. Murphy CG, Johnson M, Alvarado JA: Juxtacanalicular tissue in pigmentary and primary open-angle glaucoma: the hydrodynamic role of pigment and other constituents, *Arch Ophthalmol* 110:1779, 1992.

477. Muther TF, Friedland BR: Autoradiographic localization of carbonic anhydrase in the rabbit ciliary body, *J Histochem Cytochem* 28:1119, 1980.

478. Nagataki S, Brubaker RF: The effect of pilocarpine on aqueous humor formation in human beings, *Arch Ophthalmol* 100:818, 1982.

479. Nakamura T et al: Signal transduction system in epinephrine stimulated platelets: comparison between epinephrine sensitive and insensitive platelets, *Thromb Res* 85:83, 1997.

480. Nathanson JA: Adrenergic regulation of intraocular pressure: identification of beta 2-adrenergic-stimulated adenylate cyclase in the ciliary process epithelium, *Proc Natl Acad Sci USA* 77:7420, 1980.

481. Nathanson JA: Human ciliary process adrenergic receptor: pharmacological characterization, *Invest Ophthalmol Vis Sci* 21:798, 1981.

482. Nathanson JA: Biochemical and physiological effects of S-32-468, a beta adrenoceptor antagonist with possible oculoselectivity, *Curr Eye Res* 4:191, 1985.

483. Nathanson JA: Nitrovasodilators as a new class of ocular hypotensive agents, *J Pharmacol Exp Ther* 260:956, 1992.

484. Nathanson JA: Nitric oxide and nitrovasodilators in the eye: implications for ocular physiology and glaucoma, *J Glaucoma* 2:206, 1993.

485. Nelson GA, Edward DP, Wilensky JT: Ocular amyloidosis and secondary glaucoma, *Ophthalmology* 106:1363, 1999.

486. Neufeld AH: Influences of cyclic nucleotides on outflow facility in the vervet monkey, *Exp Eye Res* 27:387, 1978.

487. Neufeld AH, Bartels SP: Receptor mechanisms for epinephrine and timolol. In Lütjen-Drecoll E (ed): *Basic aspects of glaucoma research.* International symposium held at the Department of Anatomy, University Erlangen-Nürnberg, September 17 and 18, 1981, Stuttgart; New York, 1982, Schattauer.

488. Neufeld AH, Jampol LM, Sears ML: Cyclic-AMP in the aqueous humor: the effects of adrenergic agonists, *Exp Eye Res* 14:242, 1972.

489. Neufeld AH, Sears ML: Cyclic-AMP in ocular tissues of the rabbit, monkey, and human, *Invest Ophthalmol* 13:475, 1974.

490. Neufeld AH, Sears ML: Adenosine $3',5'$-monophosphate analogue increases the outflow facility of the primate eye, *Invest Ophthalmol* 14:688, 1975.

491. Nguyen TD et al: Glucocorticoid (GC) effects on HTM cells: molecular biology approaches. In Lütjen-Drecoll E (ed): *Basic aspects of glaucoma research III.* International symposium held at the Department of Anatomy, University of Erlangen-Nürnberg, FRG, September 23-25, 1991, Stuttgart; New York, 1993, Schattauer.

492. Nilsson SF, Bill A: Physiology and neurophysiology of aqueous humor inflow and outflow. In Kaufman PL, Mittag TW (eds): *Glaucoma,* London, 1994, Mosby-Year Book Europe, Ltd.

493. Nilsson SF, Sperber GO, Bill A: Effects of vasoactive intestinal polypeptide (VIP) on intraocular pressure, facility of outflow and formation of aqueous humor in the monkey, *Exp Eye Res* 43:849, 1986.

494. Nilsson SF et al: Increased uveoscleral outflow as a possible mechanism of ocular hypotension caused by prostaglandin $F_{2\alpha}$-1-isopropylester in the cynomolgus monkey, *Exp Eye Res* 48:707, 1989.

495. Nilsson SF et al: Effects of timolol on terbutaline- and VIP-stimulated aqueous humor flow in the cynomolgus monkey, *Curr Eye Res* 9:863, 1990.

496. Nomura T, Smelser GK: The identification of adrenergic and cholinergic nerve endings in the trabecular meshwork, *Invest Ophthalmol* 13:525, 1974.

497. Nordmann JP et al: Evaluation of safety and efficacy of CGP 38560, a renin inhibitor, in healthy volunteers and glaucoma subjects, *Invest Ophthalmol Vis Sci* 36:S719, 1995 (ARVO abstract 3317).

498. Novack GD: Ophthalmic β-blockers since timolol, *Surv Ophthalmol* 31:307, 1987.

499. O'Brien ET et al: Dexamethasone inhibits trabecular cell retraction, *Exp Eye Res* 62:675, 1996.

500. O'Brien ET et al: A mechanism for trabecular meshwork cell retraction: ethacrynic acid initiates the dephosphorylation of focal adhesion proteins, *Exp Eye Res* 65:471, 1997.

501. O'Donnell ME: Role of Na-K-Cl cotransport in vascular endothelial cell volume regulation, *Am J Physiol* 264:C1316, 1993.

502. O'Donnell ME, Brandt JD, Curry FR: Na-K-Cl cotransport regulates intracellular volume and monolayer permeability of trabecular meshwork cells, *Am J Physiol* 268:C1067, 1995.

503. O'Grady SM, Palfrey HC, Field M: Characteristics and functions of Na-K-Cl cotransport in epithelial tissues, *Am J Physiol* 253:C177, 1987.

504. Ocklind A: Effect of latanoprost on the extracellular matrix of the ciliary muscle: a study on cultured cells and tissue sections, *Exp Eye Res* 67:179, 1998.

505. Osborne NN, Chidlow G: Do beta-adrenoceptors and serotonin 5-HT1A receptors have similar functions in the control of intraocular pressure (IOP) in the rabbit? *Ophthalmologica* 210:308, 1996.

506. Osusky R et al: Individual measurements of angiotensin II concentrations in aqueous humor of the eye, *Eur J Ophthalmol* 4:228, 1994.

507. Pang IH et al: Characterization of muscarinic receptor involvement in human ciliary muscle cell function, *J Ocular Pharmacol* 10:125, 1994.

508. Pang IH et al: Preliminary characterization of a transformed cell strain derived from human trabecular meshwork, *Curr Eye Res* 13:51, 1994.

509. Parc C, Johnson DH, Vrilakis H: Giant vacuoles are found preferentially near collector channels, *Invest Ophthalmol Vis Sci* 41:2924, 2000.

510. Parker J: Coordinated regulation of volume-activated transport pathways. In Strange K (ed): *Cellular and molecular physiology of cell volume regulation,* Boca Raton, Fla, 1994, CRC Press.

511. Parker J, Colclasure G, McManus T: Coordinated regulation of shrinkage-induced Na/H exchange and swelling induced KCl cotransport in dog red cells, *J Gen Physiol* 98:869, 1991.

512. Parshley DE et al: Early changes in matrix metalloproteinases and inhibitors after in vitro laser treatment to the trabecular meshwork, *Curr Eye Res* 14:537, 1995.

513. Parshley DE et al: Laser trabeculoplasty induces stromelysin expression by trabecular juxtacanalicular cells, *Invest Ophthalmol Vis Sci* 37:795, 1996.

514. Patridge CA et al: Dexamethasone induces specific proteins in human trabecular meshwork cells, *Invest Ophthalmol Vis Sci* 30:1843, 1989.

515. Pederson JE: Fluid permeability of monkey ciliary epithelium in vivo, *Invest Ophthalmol Vis Sci* 23:176, 1982.

516. Pederson JE, Gaasterland DE, MacLellan HM: Uveoscleral aqueous outflow in the rhesus monkey: importance of uveal reabsorption, *Invest Ophthalmol Vis Sci* 16:1008, 1977.

517. Pederson JE, Gaasterland DE, MacLellan HM: Anterior chamber volume determination in the rhesus monkey, *Invest Ophthalmol Vis Sci* 17:784, 1978.

518. Pederson JE, Green K: Aqueous humor dynamics: a mathematical approach to measurement of facility, pseudofacility, capillary pressure, active secretion and Xc, *Exp Eye Res* 15:265, 1973.

519. Pedler WS: The relationship of hyaluronidase to aqueous outflow resistance, *Trans Ophthalmol Soc UK* 76:51, 1956.

520. Percicot CL, Mauget M, Pages C: Effects of topical renin inhibitor, CGP 38560 versus timolol on intraocular pressure in normal and ocular hypertensive animal models, *Invest Ophthalmol Vis Sci* 36:S719, 1995 (ARVO abstract 3318).

521. Peterson HP: Can pigmentary deposits on the trabecular meshwork increase the resistance of the aqueous outflow? *Acta Ophthalmol* 47:743, 1969.

522. Peterson JA et al: Latrunculin's effects on intraocular pressure, aqueous humor flow and corneal endothelium, *Invest Ophthalmol Vis Sci* 41:1749, 2000.

523. Peterson JA et al: Latrunculin-A causes mydriasis and cycloplegia in the cynomolgus monkey, *Invest Ophthalmol Vis Sci* 40:631, 1999.

524. Peterson JA et al: Latrunculin-A increases outflow facility in the monkey, *Invest Ophthalmol Vis Sci* 40:931, 1999.

525. Peterson JA et al: Effect of latrunculin-B on outflow facility in monkeys, *Exp Eye Res* 70:307, 2000.

526. Peterson WS, Jocson VL: Hyaluronidase effects on aqueous outflow resistance: quantitative and localizing studies in the rhesus monkey eye, *Am J Ophthalmol* 77:573, 1974.

527. Petty HR, Martin SM: Combinative ligand-receptor interactions: effects of cAMP, epinephrine, and met-enkephalin on RAW264 macrophage morphology, spreading, adherence, and microfilaments, *J Cell Physiol* 138:247, 1989.

528. Pierce WMJ, Sharir M, Waite KJ: Topically active ocular carbonic anhydrase inhibitors: novel biscarbonylamidothiadiazole sulfonamides as ocular hypotensive agents, *Proc Soc Exp Biol Med* 203:360, 1993.

529. Pillunat L, Stodtmeister R: Effect of different antiglaucomatous drugs on ocular perfusion pressures, *J Ocular Pharmacol* 4:231, 1988.

530. Pitzer Gills J, Roberts BC, Epstein DL: Microtubule disruption leads to cellular contraction in human trabecular meshwork cells, *Invest Ophthalmol Vis Sci* 39:653, 1998.

531. Plagemann PGW et al: Inhibition of carrier mediated and non-mediated permeation processes by cytochalasin B. In Tannenbaum SW (ed): *Cytochalasins: biochemical and cell biological aspects,* Amsterdam, 1978, North-Holland.

532. Podos SM, Camras CB, Serle JB: Experimental compounds to lower intraocular pressure, *Aust NZ J Ophthalmol* 17:129, 1989.

533. Podos SM, Serle JB: Topically active carbonic anhydrase inhibitors for glaucoma, *Arch Ophthalmol* 109:38, 1982.

534. Podos SM et al: The effect of vanadate on aqueous humor dynamics in cynomolgus monkeys, *Invest Ophthalmol Vis Sci* 25:359, 1984.

535. Polansky JR: HTM cell culture model for steroid effects on intraocular pressure: overview. In Lütjen-Drecoll E (ed): *Basic aspects of glaucoma research III.* International symposium held at the Department of Anatomy, University of Erlangen-Nürnberg, FRG, September 23-25, 1991, Stuttgart; New York, 1993, Schattauer.

536. Polansky JR, Fauss D, Zimmerman CC: Regulation of TIGR/MYOC gene expression in human trabecular meshwork cells, *Eye* 14:503, 2000.

537. Polansky JR, Kurtz RM, Fauss DJ: In vitro correlates of glucocorticoid effects on intraocular pressure. In Krieglestein GK, International Congress of Ophthalmology, Glaucoma Society (eds): *Glaucoma update IV,* Berlin; New York, 1991, Springer-Verlag.

538. Polansky JR, Palmberg P, Matulich D: Cellular sensitivity to glucocorticoids in patients with POAG: steroid receptors and responses in cultured skin fibroblasts, *Invest Ophthalmol Vis Sci* 26:805, 1985.

539. Polansky JR, Wood IS, Alvarado JA: Trabecular meshwork cell culture in glaucoma research: evaluation of biological activity and structural properties of human trabecular cells in vitro, *Ophthalmology* 91:580, 1984.

540. Polansky JR et al: Eicosanoid production and glucocorticoid regulatory mechanisms in cultured human trabecular meshwork cells, *Prog Clin Biol Res* 312:113, 1989.

541. Polansky JR et al: Cellular pharmacology and molecular biology of the trabecular meshwork inducible glucocorticoid response gene product, *Ophthalmologica* 211:126, 1997.

542. Poyer JF, Gabelt BT, Kaufman PL: The effect of topical $PGF_{2\alpha}$ on uveoscleral outflow and outflow facility in the rabbit eye, *Exp Eye Res* 54:277, 1992.

543. Poyer JF, Gabelt BT, Kaufman PL: The effect of muscarinic agonists and selective receptor subtype antagonists on the contractile response of the isolated rhesus monkeys' ciliary muscle, *Exp Eye Res* 59:729, 1994.

544. Poyer JF, Millar C, Kaufman PL: Prostaglandin $F_{2\alpha}$ effects on isolated rhesus monkey ciliary muscle, *Invest Ophthalmol Vis Sci* 36:2461, 1995.

545. Prijot E: Contribution to the study of tonometry and tonography in ophthalmology, *Doc Ophthalmol* 15:1, 1961.

546. Probst LE, Hakim OJ, Nichols BD: Phacoemulsification with aspirated or retained Viscoat, *J Cataract Refract Surg* 20:145, 1994.

547. Putney LK, Brandt JD, O'Donnell ME: Effects of dexamethasone on sodium-potassium-chloride cotransport in trabecular meshwork cells, *Invest Ophthalmol Vis Sci* 38:1229, 1997.

548. Putney LK, Brandt JD, O'Donnell ME: Na-K-Cl cotransport in normal and glaucomatous human trabecular meshwork cells, *Invest Ophthalmol Vis Sci* 40:425, 1999.

549. Quigley HA: Long-term follow-up of laser iridotomy, *Ophthalmology* 88:218, 1981.

550. Quigley HA, Pollack IP, Harbin TS Jr: Pilocarpine Ocuserts: long-term clinical trials and selected pharmacodynamics, *Arch Ophthalmol* 93:771, 1975.

551. Raitta C et al: A randomized, prospective study on the use of sodium hyaluronate (Healon) in trabeculectomy, *Ophthalmol Surg* 25:536, 1994.

552. Ramirez M et al: The renin-angiotensin system in the rabbit eye, *J Ocular Pharmacol* 12:299, 1996.

553. Rao PV et al: Modulation of aqueous humor outflow facility by the Rho kinase-specific inhibitor Y-27632, *Invest Ophthalmol Vis Sci* 42:1029, 2001.

554. Raviola G: Effects of paracentesis on the blood-aqueous barrier: an electron microscopic study on *Macaca mulatta* using horseradish peroxidase as a tracer, *Invest Ophthalmol* 13:828, 1974.

555. Raviola G: The structural basis of the blood-ocular barriers, *Exp Eye Res* 25:27, 1977.

556. Rees D, Lloyd CW, Thom D: Control of grip and stick in cell adhesion through lateral relationships of membrane glycoproteins, *Nature* 267:124, 1977.

557. Reiss GR et al: Aqueous humor flow during sleep, *Invest Ophthalmol Vis Sci* 25:776, 1984.

558. Richards JE et al: Mapping of a gene for autosomal dominant juvenile-onset open-angle glaucoma to chromosome 1q, *Am J Hum Genet* 54:62, 1994.

559. Richards R, Tattersfield AE: Bronchial β-adrenoceptor blockade following eyedrops of timolol and its isomer L-714,465 in asthmatic subjects, *Br J Clin Pharmacol* 24:459, 1985.

560. Richards R, Tattersfield AE: Comparison of the airway response to eye drops of timolol and its isomer L-714,465 in asthmatic subjects, *Br J Clin Pharmacol* 24:485, 1987.

561. Richardson TM: Distribution of glycosaminoglycans in the aqueous outflow system of the cat, *Invest Ophthalmol Vis Sci* 22:319, 1982.

562. Riley MV: The sodium-potassium-stimulated adenosine triphosphatase of rabbit ciliary epithelium, *Exp Eye Res* 3:76, 1964.

563. Riley MV, Kishida K: ATPases of ciliary epithelium: cellular and subcellular distribution and probable role in secretion of aqueous humor, *Exp Eye Res* 42:559, 1986.

564. Ringvold A: Actin filaments in trabecular endothelial cells in eyes of the vervet monkey (*Cercopithecus aethiops*), *Acta Ophthalmologica* 56:217, 1978.

565. Rittig MG, Licht K, Funk RH: Innervation of the ciliary process vasculature and epithelium by nerve fibers containing catecholamines and neuropeptide Y, *Ophthalmic Res* 25:108, 1993.

566. Robinson JC, Kaufman PL: Effects and interactions of epinephrine, norepinephrine, timolol and betaxolol on outflow facility in the cynomolgus monkey, *Am J Ophthalmol* 109:189, 1990.

567. Robinson JC, Kaufman PL: Cytochalasin B potentiates epinephrine's outflow facility increasing effect, *Invest Ophthalmol Vis Sci* 32:1614, 1991.

568. Robinson JC, Kaufman PL: Dose-dependent suppression of aqueous humor formation by timolol in the cynomolgus monkey, *J Glaucoma* 2:251, 1993.

569. Robinson JC, Kaufman PL: Phalloidin inhibits epinephrine's and cytochalasin B's facilitation of aqueous outflow. *Arch Ophthalmol* 112:1610, 1994.

570. Rodriguez-Peralta L: The blood-aqueous barrier in five species, *Am J Ophthalmol* 80:713, 1975.

571. Rohen JW: The evolution of the primate eye in relation to the problem of glaucoma. In Lütjen-Drecoll E (ed): *Basic aspects of glaucoma research*. International symposium held at the Department of Anatomy, University Erlangen-Nürnberg, September 17 and 18, 1981, Stuttgart; New York, 1982, Schattauer.

572. Rohen JW: Why is intraocular pressure elevated in chronic simple glaucoma? Anatomical considerations, *Ophthalmology* 90:758, 1983.

573. Rohen JW, Futa R, Lütjen-Drecoll E: The fine structure of the cribriform meshwork in normal and glaucomatous eyes as seen in tangential sections, *Invest Ophthalmol Vis Sci* 21:574, 1981.

574. Rohen JW, Linner E, Witmer R: Electron microscopic studies on the trabecular meshwork in two cases of corticosteroid glaucoma, *Exp Eye Res* 17:19, 1973.

575. Rohen JW, Lütjen E, Bárány E: The relation between the ciliary muscle and the trabecular meshwork and its importance for the effect of miotics on aqueous outflow resistance. *Graefes Arch Clin Exp Ophthalmol* 172:23, 1967.

576. Rohen JW, Schachtschabel DO, Wehrmann R: Structural changes in human and monkey trabecular meshwork following in vitro cultivation, *Graefes Arch Clin Exp Ophthalmol* 218:225, 1982.

577. Rohen JW, Van der Zypen E: The phagocytic activity of the trabecular meshwork endothelium: an electron microscopic study of the vervet (*Cercopithecus ethiops*), *Graefes Arch Clin Exp Ophthalmol* 175:143, 1968.

578. Romano JH: Double-blind crossover comparison of aceclidine and pilocarpine in open-angle glaucoma, *Br J Ophthalmol* 54:510, 1970.

579. Rowlette LLS et al: High intraocular pressure induces expression of TIGR/MYOC and formation of extracellular matrix in the trabecular meshwork of human perfused anterior segments, *Invest Ophthalmol Vis Sci* 40:S666, 1999 (ARVO abstract 3517).

580. Ruskell GL: Facial parasympathetic innervation of the choroidal blood vessels in monkeys, *Exp Eye Res* 12:166, 1971.

581. Ruskell GL: The source of nerve fibres of the trabeculae and adjacent structures in monkey eyes, *Exp Eye Res* 23:449, 1976.

582. Ruskell GL: Innervation of the anterior segment of the eye. In Lütjen-Drecoll E (ed): *Basic aspects of glaucoma research*. International symposium held at the Department of Anatomy, University Erlangen-Nürnberg, September 17 and 18, 1981, Stuttgart; New York, 1982, Schattauer.

583. Sabany I et al: Effect of the protein kinase inhibitor H-7 on the structure and fluid conductance of the trabecular meshwork of live monkeys, *Arch Ophthalmol* 118:955, 2000.

584. Sagara T et al: Topical prostaglandin $F_{2\alpha}$ treatment reduces collagen types I, III, and IV in the monkey uveoscleral outflow pathway, *Arch Ophthalmol* 117:794, 1999.

585. Samuelsson-Almén M et al: Effects of atrial natriuretic factor (ANF) on intraocular pressure and aqueous humor flow in the cynomolgus monkey, *Exp Eye Res* 53:253, 1991.

586. Santafe J et al: A long-lasting hypotensive effect of topical diltiazem on the intraocular pressure in conscious rabbits, *Naunyn Schmiedebergs Arch Pharmacol* 355:645, 1997.

587. Sato A, Sato Y: Cholinergic neural regulation of regional cerebral blood flow, *Alzheimer Dis Assoc Disord* 9:28, 1995.

588. Schachtschabel DO, Bigalke B, Rohen JW: Production of glycosaminoglycans by cell cultures of the trabecular meshwork of the primate eye, *Exp Eye Res* 24:71, 1977.

589. Schachtschabel DO et al: Synthesis and composition of glycosaminoglycans by cultured human trabecular meshwork cells, *Graefes Arch Clin Exp Ophthalmol* 218:113, 1982.

590. Schenker JI et al: Fluorophotometric study of epinephrine and timolol in human subjects, *Arch Ophthalmol* 99:1212, 1981.

591. Schimek RA, Lieberman WJ: The influence of Cyclogyl and Neo-Synephrine on tonographic studies of miotic control in open angle glaucoma, *Am J Ophthalmol* 51:781, 1961.

592. Schmitt CJ et al: β-Adrenergic blockers: lack of relationship between antagonism of isoproterenol and lowering of intraocular pressure in rabbits. In Sears M (ed): *New directions in ophthalmic research*, New Haven, Conn, 1981, Yale University Press.

593. Schoenwald RD et al: Topical carbonic anhydrase inhibitors, *J Med Chem* 27:810, 1984.

594. Schutte M et al: Comparative adrenocholinergic control of intracellular Ca^{2+} in the layers of the ciliary body epithelium, *Invest Ophthalmol Vis Sci* 37:212, 1996.

595. Schwartz AL, Whitten ME, Bleiman B: Argon laser trabecular surgery in uncontrolled phakic open-angle glaucoma, *Ophthalmology* 88:203, 1981.

596. Schwartz B: The response of ocular pressure to corticosteroids. In Schwartz B (ed): *Corticosteroids and the eye*, Boston, 1966, Little, Brown and Co.

597. Schwartz B, Levene RZ: Plasma cortisol differences between normal and glaucomatous patients before and after dexamethasone suppression, *Arch Ophthalmol* 87:369, 1972.

598. Schwartz B, McCarty G, Rosner B: Increased plasma free cortisol in ocular hypertension and open-angle glaucoma, *Arch Ophthalmol* 105:1060, 1987.

599. Sears ML: The mechanism of action of adrenergic drugs in glaucoma, *Invest Ophthalmol* 5:115, 1966.

600. Sears ML: Autonomic nervous system: adrenergic agonists. In Sears ML (ed): *Pharmacology of the eye: handbook of experimental pharmacology,* Berlin, 1984, Springer-Verlag.

601. Sears ML, Neufeld AH: Adrenergic modulation of the outflow of aqueous humor, *Invest Ophthalmol* 14:83, 1975.

602. Seeman J et al: 3Alpha,5beta-tetrahydrocortisol effect on outflow facility, *J Ocular Pharmacol Ther* 18:35, 2002.

603. Seidël E: Weitre experimentelle untersuchungen über die quelle und den verlauf der introkulären saftströmung: IX. Uber der abfluss des kammerwassers aus der vorderen augenkammer, *Graefes Arch Clin Exp Ophthalmol* 104:357, 1921.

604. Seidël E: Weitre experimentelle untersuchungen über die quelle und den verlauf der introkularen saftsrömung: XII. Metteilung. Uber den manometrischen nachweis des physiologischen druckgefales zwishen vorderkammer und Schlemmshen kanal, *Graefes Arch Clin Exp Ophthalmol* 107:101, 1921.

605. Selbach JM et al: Efferent and afferent innervation of primate trabecular meshwork and scleral spur, *Invest Ophthalmol Vis Sci* 41:2184, 2000.

606. Sen DK, Saren GS, Saha K: Immunoglobulins in human aqueous humor, *Br J Ophthalmol* 61:216, 1977.

607. Serle JB et al: Corynanthine and aqueous humor dynamics in rabbits and monkeys, *Arch Ophthalmol* 102:1385, 1984.

608. Seufferlein T, Rozengurt E: Lysophosphatidic acid stimulates tyrosine phosphorylation of focal adhesion kinase, paxillin, and p130, *J Biol Chem* 269:9345, 1994.

609. Shabo AL, Maxwell DS, Kreiger AE: Structural alterations in the ciliary process and the blood-aqueous barrier of the monkey after systemic urea injections, *Am J Ophthalmol* 81:162, 1976.

610. Shade DL, Clark AF, Pang IH: Effects of muscarinic agents on cultured human trabecular meshwork cells, *Exp Eye Res* 62:201, 1996.

611. Shaffer RN: In Newell FW (ed): *Glaucoma: transactions of the fifth conference,* New York, 1960, Josiah Macy Jr. Foundation.

612. Shahidullah M, Wilson WS: Atriopeptin, sodium azide and cyclic GMP reduce secretion of aqueous humour and inhibit intracellular calcium release in bovine cultured ciliary epithelium, *Br J Pharmacol* 127:1438, 1999.

613. Shahidullah M, Wilson WS, Millar C: Effects of timolol, terbutaline and forskolin on IOP, aqueous humour formation and ciliary cyclic AMP levels in the bovine eye, *Curr Eye Res* 14:519, 1995.

614. Share NN et al: R-Enantiomer of timolol: a potential selective ocular antihypertensive agent, *Graefes Arch Clin Exp Ophthalmol* 221:234, 1984.

615. Shattil SJ et al: Tyrosine phosphorylation of pp125FAK in platelets requires coordinated signalling through integrin and agonist receptors, *J Biol Chem* 269:14738, 1994.

616. Shearer T, Clark E, Crosson CE: Adenosine A1 receptors regulate matrix metalloproteinase secretion from trabecular meshwork cells by a MAP kinase-dependent pathway. *Invest Ophthalmol Vis Sci* 41:S574, 2000 (ARVO abstract 3029).

617. Sheffield VC et al: Genetic linkage of familial open angle glaucoma to chromosome 1q21-q31, *Nat Genet* 4:47, 1993.

618. Shi XP et al: Adreno-cholinergic modulation of junctional communications between the pigmented and nonpigmented layers of the ciliary body epithelium, *Invest Ophthalmol Vis Sci* 37:1037, 1996.

619. Shibasaki H et al: Viscoelastic substance in the anterior chamber elevates intraocular pressure, *Ann Ophthalmol* 26:10, 1994.

620. Shibata T, Mishima H, Kurokawa T: Ocular pigmentation and intraocular pressure response to forskolin, *Curr Eye Res* 7:667, 1988.

621. Shiose Y: Electron microscopic studies on blood-retinal and blood-aqueous barriers, *Nippon Ganka Gakkai Zasshi* 73:1606, 1969.

622. Shiota N et al: Angiotensin II-generating system in dog and monkey ocular tissues, *Clin Exp Pharmacol Physiol* 24:243, 1997.

623. Shirato S et al: Kinetics of phagocytosis in trabecular meshwork cells: flow cytometry and morphometry, *Invest Ophthalmol Vis Sci* 30:2499, 1989.

624. Silver LH: Clinical efficacy and safety of brinzolamide (Azopt), a new topical carbonic anhydrase inhibitor for primary open-angle glaucoma and ocular hypertension: Brinzolamide Primary Therapy Study Group, *Am J Ophthalmol* 126:400, 1998.

625. Simon KA, Bonting SL: Possible usefulness of cardiac glycosides in treatment of glaucoma, *Arch Ophthalmol* 68:227, 1962.

626. Simon KA, Bonting SL, Hawkins NM: Studies on sodium-potassium-activated adenosine triphosphatase: II. Formation of aqueous humor, *Exp Eye Res* 1:253, 1962.

627. Sit AJ et al: Factors affecting the pores of the inner wall endothelium of Schlemm's canal, *Invest Ophthalmol Vis Sci* 38:1517, 1997.

628. Sit AJ et al: The role of soluble proteins in generating aqueous outflow resistance in the bovine and human eye, *Exp Eye Res* 64:813, 1997.

629. Smith BR et al: Forskolin, a potent adenylate cyclase activator, lowers rabbit intraocular pressure, *Arch Ophthalmol* 102:146, 1984.

630. Smith RS: Ultrastructural studies of the blood-aqueous barrier: 1. Transport of an electron dense tracer in the iris and ciliary body of the mouse, *Am J Ophthalmol* 71:1066, 1971.

631. Sommer A: Glaucoma: facts and fancies, *Eye* 10:295, 1996.

632. Sommer AE et al: Relationship between intraocular pressure and primary open angle glaucoma among white and black Americans: the Baltimore Eye Survey, *Arch Ophthalmol* 109:1090, 1991.

633. Southren AL, Hernandez AL, L'Hommedieu D: Potentiation of collagen synthesis in explants of the rabbit eye by 5 beta-dihydrocortisol, *Invest Ophthalmol Vis Sci* 27:1757, 1986.

634. Southren AL et al: Altered cortisol metabolism in cells cultured from trabecular meshwork specimen obtained from patients with primary open-angle glaucoma, *Invest Ophthalmol Vis Sci* 26:1413, 1983.

635. Southren AL et al: Intraocular hypotensive effect of a topically applied cortisol metabolite: 3α, 5β-tetrahydrocortisol, *Invest Ophthalmol Vis Sci* 28:901, 1987.

636. Southren AL et al: Treatment of glaucoma with $3\alpha,5\beta$-tetrahydrocortisol: a new therapeutic modality, *J Ocular Pharmacol* 10:385, 1994.

637. Sperber GO, Bill A: A method for near-continuous determination of aqueous humor flow: effects of anaesthetics, temperature and indomethacin, *Exp Eye Res* 39:435, 1984.

638. Sramek SJ et al: An ocular renin-angiotensin system: immunohistochemistry of angiotensinogen, *Invest Ophthalmol Vis Sci* 33:1627, 1992.

639. Steely HT, Browder S, Julian MB: The effects of dexamethasone on fibronectin expression in cultured trabecular meshwork cells, *Invest Ophthalmol Vis Sci* 33:2242, 1992.

640. Stelling JW, Jacob TJ: Functional coupling in bovine ciliary epithelial cells is modulated by carbachol, *Am J Physiol* 273:C1876, 1997.

641. Stewart RH, Kimbrough RL, Ward RL: Betaxolol vs. timolol: a six-month double-blind comparison, *Arch Ophthalmol* 104:46, 1986.

642. Stjernschantz J: Effect of parasympathetic stimulation on intraocular pressure, formation of aqueous humor and outflow facility in rabbits, *Exp Eye Res* 22:639, 1976.

643. Stjernschantz J, Uusitalo R, Palkama A: The aqueous proteins of the rat in the normal eye and after aqueous withdrawal, *Exp Eye Res* 16:215, 1973.

644. Stone EM et al; Identification of a gene that causes primary open angle glaucoma, *Science* 275:668, 1997.

645. Stone RA: Cholic acid accumulation by the ciliary body and by the iris of the primate eye, *Invest Ophthalmol Vis Sci* 18:819, 1979.

646. Stone RA: The transport of para-aminohippuric acid by the ciliary body and by the iris of the primate eye, *Invest Ophthalmol Vis Sci* 18:807, 1979.

647. Stumpff F, Wiederholt M: Regulation of trabecular meshwork contractility, *Ophthalmologica* 214:33, 2000.

648. Sugrue MF, Gautheron P, Grove J: MK-927: a topically active ocular hypotensive carbonic anhydrase inhibitor, *J Ocul Pharmacol* 6:9, 1990.

649. Sugrue MF, Mallorga P, Schwamm H: A comparison of L-671,152 and MK927, two topically effective ocular hypotensive carbonic anhydrase inhibitors, in experimental animals, *Curr Eye Res* 9:607, 1990.

650. Svedbergh B: Aspects of the aqueous humour drainage: functional ultrastructure of Schlemm's canal, the trabecular meshwork, and the corneal endothelium at different intraocular pressures, *Acta Univ Uppsl* 256:1, 1976.

651. Svedbergh B: Effects of intraocular pressure on the pores of the inner wall of Schlemm's canal: a scanning electron microscopic study. In Yamada E, Mishima S (eds), *The structure of the eye*, III, ed 3, Tokyo, 1976, Jpn J Ophthalmol.

652. Svedbergh B et al: Cytochalasin B-induced structural changes in the anterior ocular segment of the cynomolgus monkey, *Invest Ophthalmol Vis Sci* 17:718, 1978.

653. Swan K, Hart W: A comparative study of the effects of Mecholyl, Doryl, pilocarpine, atropine, and epinephrine on the blood-aqueous barrier, *Am J Ophthalmol* 23:1311, 1940.

654. Tamm E, Lütjen-Drecoll E: Ciliary body, *Microscop Res Tech* 33:390, 1996.

655. Tamm E, Rittig M, Lütjen-Drecoll E: Elektronenmikroskopische und immunhistochemische untersuchungen zur augendrucksenkenden wirkung von prostaglandin $F_{2\alpha}$. *Fortschr Ophthalmol* 87:623, 1990.

656. Tamm ER et al: Nerve endings with structural characteristics of mechanoreceptors in the human scleral spur, *Invest Ophthalmol Vis Sci* 35:1157, 1994.

657. Tamm ER et al: Modulation of myocilin/TIGR expression in human trabecular meshwork, *Invest Ophthalmol Vis Sci* 40:2577, 1999.

658. Tchernitchiv A et al: Glucocorticoid localization by radioautography in the rabbit eye following systemic administration of 3H-dexamethasone, *Invest Ophthalmol Vis Sci* 19:1231, 1980.

659. Teichmann I, Teichmann KD, Fechner PU: Glaucoma operation with the argon laser, *Eye Ear Nose Throat Mon* 55:58, 1976.

660. Ten Tusscher MP et al: Pre- and post-ganglionic nerve fibres of the pterygopalatine ganglion and their allocation to the eyeball of rats, *Brain Res* 517:315, 1990.

661. Thieme H et al: The effects of protein kinase C on trabecular meshwork and ciliary muscle contractility, *Invest Ophthalmol Vis Sci* 40:3254, 1999.

662. Thomas JV, Epstein DL: Timolol and epinephrine in primary open angle glaucoma: transient additive effect, *Arch Ophthalmol* 99:91, 1981.

663. Tian B, Gabelt BT, Kaufman PL: Effect of staurosporine on outflow facility in monkeys, *Invest Ophthalmol Vis Sci* 40:1009, 1999.

664. Tian B et al: Effects of adenosine agonists on intraocular pressure and aqueous humor dynamics in cynomolgus monkeys, *Exp Eye Res* 64:979, 1997.

665. Tian B et al: Effects of H-7 on the iris and ciliary muscle in monkeys, *Arch Ophthalmol* 116:1070, 1998.

666. Tian B et al: H-7 disrupts the actin cytoskeleton and increases outflow facility, *Arch Ophthalmol* 116:633, 1998.

667. Tian B et al: H-7 increases trabecular facility and facility after ciliary muscle disinsertion in monkeys, *Invest Ophthalmol Vis Sci* 40:239, 1998.

668. Tian B et al: Combined effects of H-7 and cytochalasin B on outflow facility in monkeys, *Exp Eye Res* 68:649, 1999.

669. Tian B et al: H-7 increases trabecular facility and facility after ciliary muscle disinsertion in monkeys, *Invest Ophthalmol Vis Sci* 40:239, 1999.

670. Tian B et al: Cytoskeletal involvement in the regulation of aqueous humor outflow, *Invest Ophthalmol Vis Sci* 41:619, 2000.

671. Ticho U, Zauberman H: Argon laser application to the angle structures in the glaucomas, *Arch Ophthalmol* 94:61, 1976.

672. Tokiwa T et al: Mechanism of cell dissociation with trypsin and EDTA, *Acta Med Okayama* 33:1, 1979.

673. Topper JE, Brubaker RF: Effects of timolol, epinephrine, and acetazolamide on aqueous flow during sleep, *Invest Ophthalmol Vis Sci* 26:1315, 1985.

674. Toris CB, Camras CB, Yablonski ME: Effects of PhXA41, a new prostaglandin F2 alpha, on aqueous humor dynamics in human eyes, *Ophthalmology* 100:1297, 1993.

675. Toris CB, Camras CB, Yablonski ME: Acute versus chronic effects of brimonidine on aqueous humor dynamics in ocular hypertensive patients, *Am J Ophthalmol* 128:8, 1999.

676. Toris CB, Pederson JE: Effect of intraocular pressure on uveoscleral outflow following cyclodialysis in the monkey eye, *Invest Ophthalmol Vis Sci* 26:1745, 1985.

677. Toris CB, Pederson JE: Aqueous humor dynamics in experimental iridocyclitis, *Invest Ophthalmol Vis Sci* 28:477, 1987.

678. Toris CB, Yablonski ME, Camras CB: Uveoscleral outflow and outflow facility are reduced in ocular hypertensive patients, *Invest Ophthalmol Vis Sci* 39:S489, 1998 (ARVO abstract).

679. Toris CB et al: Effects of apraclonidine on aqueous humor dynamics in human eyes, *Ophthalmology* 102:456, 1995.

680. Toris CB et al: Effects of brimonidine on aqueous humor dynamics in human eyes, *Arch Ophthalmol* 113:1514, 1995.

681. Toris CB et al: Effects of exogenous prostaglandins on aqueous humor dynamics and blood aqueous barrier function, *Surv Ophthalmol* 41(suppl 2):S69, 1997.

682. Toris CB et al: Aqueous humor dynamics in the aging human eye, *Am J Ophthalmol* 127:407, 1999.

683. Törnqvist G: Effect of cervical sympathetic stimulation on accommodation in monkeys: an example of a beta-adrenergic inhibitory effect, *Acta Physiol Scand* 67:363, 1966.

684. Townsend DJ, Brubaker RF: Immediate effect of epinephrine on aqueous formation in the normal human eye as measured by fluorophotometry, *Invest Ophthalmol Vis Sci* 19:256, 1980.

685. Tripathi BJ, Millard CB, Tripathi RC: Corticosteroids induce a sialated glycoprotein (Cort-GP) in trabecular cells in vitro, *Exp Eye Res* 51:735, 1990.

686. Tripathi BJ, Tripathi RC: Effect of epinephrine in vitro on the morphology, phagocytosis, and mitotic activity of human trabecular endothelium, *Exp Eye Res* 39:731, 1984.

687. Tripathi BJ, Tripathi RC, Swift HH: Hydrocortisone-induced DNA endoreplication in human trabecular cells in vitro, *Exp Eye Res* 49:259, 1989.

688. Tripathi RC: The functional morphology of the outflow systems of ocular and cerebrospinal fluids, *Exp Eye Res* 25(suppl):65, 1977.

689. Tripathi RC, Tripathi BJ: Contractile protein alteration in trabecular endothelium in primary open-angle glaucoma, *Exp Eye Res* 31:721, 1980.

690. Tripathi RC, Tripathi BJ: Human trabecular endothelium, corneal endothelium, keratocytes, and scleral fibroblasts in primary cell culture: a comparative study of growth characteristics, morphology, and phagocytic activity by light and scanning electron microscopy, *Exp Eye Res* 35:611, 1982.

691. Tsukahara S, Maezara N: Cytochemical localization of adenyl cyclase in the rabbit ciliary body, *Exp Eye Res* 26:99, 1978.

692. Uddman R et al: Vasoactive intestinal peptide nerves in ocular and orbital structures of the cat, *Invest Ophthalmol Vis Sci* 19:878, 1980.

693. Uehata M et al: Calcium sensitization of smooth muscle mediated by a rho-associated protein kinase in hypertension, *Nature* 389:900, 1997.

694. Underwood JL et al: Glucocorticoids regulate transendothelial fluid flow resistance and formation of intercellular junctions, *Am J Physiol* 277:C330, 1999.

695. Underwood-Hu JL et al: ZO-1 and TIGR expression in human trabecular meshwork cells, *Invest Ophthalmol Vis Sci* 40:S669, 1999 (ARVO abstract 3533).

696. Usukura J, Fain GL, Bok D: [3H]ouabain localization of Na-K ATPase in the epithelium of the rabbit ciliary body pars plicata, *Invest Ophthalmol Vis Sci* 29:606, 1988.

697. Uusitalo R: The action of physostigmine, morphine, cyclopentolate and homatropine on the secretion and outflow of aqueous humor in the rabbit eye, *Acta Physiol Scand* 86:239, 1972.

698. Uusitalo R: Effect of sympathetic and parasympathetic stimulation on the secretion and outflow of aqueous humor in the rabbit eye, *Acta Physiol Scand* 86:315, 1972.

699. Uusitalo R, Palkama A, Stjernschantz J: An electron microscopic study of the blood-aqueous barrier in the ciliary body and iris of the rabbit, *Exp Eye Res* 17:49, 1973.

700. Uusitalo R, Stjernschantz J, Palkama A: Studies on the ultrastructure of the blood-aqueous barrier in the rabbit, *Acta Ophthalmol* 123:61, 1974.

701. van Alphen GWHM, Kern R, Robinette SL: Adrenergic receptors of the intraocular muscles: comparison to cat, rabbit, and monkey, *Arch Ophthalmol* 74:253, 1965.

702. van Alphen GWHM, Robinette SL, Macri FJ: Drug effects on ciliary muscle and choroid preparations in vitro, *Arch Ophthalmol* 68:111, 1962.

703. van Alphen GWHM, Wilhelm PB, Elsenfeld PW: The effect of prostaglandins on the isolated internal muscles of the mammalian eye, including man, *Doc Ophthalmol* 42:397, 1977.

704. Van Buskirk EM: The ciliary vasculature and its perturbation with drugs and surgery, *Trans Am Ophthalmol Soc* 86:794, 1988.

705. Van Buskirk EM, Bacon DR, Fahrenbach WH: Ciliary vasoconstriction after topical adrenergic drugs, *Am J Ophthalmol* 109:511, 1990.

706. Van Buskirk EM, Grant WM: Lens depression and aqueous outflow in enucleated primate eyes, *Am J Ophthalmol* 76:632, 1973.

707. Vanlandingham BD, Maus TL, Brubaker RF: The effect of dorzolamide on aqueous humor dynamics in normal human subjects during sleep, *Ophthalmology* 105:1537, 1998.

708. Vareilles P et al: Comparison of the effects of timolol and other adrenergic agents on intraocular pressure in the rabbit, *Invest Ophthalmol* 16:987, 1977.

709. Vegge T: An epithelial blood-aqueous barrier to horseradish peroxidase in the ciliary processes of the vervet monkey (*Cercopithecus aethiops*), *Zeitschr Zellforsch Mikrosk Anat* 114:309, 1971.

710. Villumsen J, Alm A: Prostaglandin $F_{2\alpha}$ isopropylester eye drops: effects in normal human eyes, *Br J Ophthalmol* 73:419, 1989.

711. Villumsen J, Alm A: PhXA34: a prostaglandin $F_{2\alpha}$ analogue—effect on intraocular pressure in patients with ocular hypertension, *Br J Ophthalmol* 76:214, 1992.

712. Vogh BP, Godman DR: Effects of inhibition of angiotensin converting enzyme and carbonic anhydrase on fluid production by ciliary process, choroid plexus, and pancreas, *J Ocular Pharmacol* 5:303, 1989.

713. Volberg T et al: Effect of protein kinase inhibitor H-7 on the contractility, integrity and membrane anchorage of the microfilament system, *Cell Motil Cytoskeleton* 29:321, 1994.

714. Vuori ML et al: Concentrations and antagonist activity of topically applied betaxolol in aqueous humour, *Acta Ophthalmol* 71:677, 1993.

715. Wagner J et al: Demonstration of renin mRNA, angiotensinogen mRNA, and angiotensin converting enzyme mRNA expression in the human eye: evidence for an intraocular renin-angiotensin system, *Fr J Ophthalmol* 80:159, 1996.

716. Waitzman MB, Woods WB: Some characteristics of an adenyl cyclase preparation from rabbit ciliary process tissue, *Exp Eye Res* 12:99, 1971.

717. Wålinder P-E: Influence of pilocarpine on iodopyracet and iodide accumulation by rabbit ciliary body-iris preparations, *Invest Ophthalmol* 5:378, 1966.

718. Wålinder P-E, Bill A: Influence of intraocular pressure and some drugs on aqueous flow and entry of cycloleucine into the aqueous humor of vervet monkeys (*Cercopithecus ethiops*), *Invest Ophthalmol* 8:446, 1969.

719. Wallow IH et al: Ocular renin angiotensin: EM immunocytochemical localization of prorenin, *Curr Eye Res* 12:945, 1993.

720. Wan XL et al: Circadian aqueous flow medicated by beta-arrestin induced homologous desensitization, *Exp Eye Res* 64:1005, 1997.

721. Wang RF et al: The ocular hypotensive effect of the topical carbonic anhydrase inhibitor L-671,152 in glaucomatous monkeys, *Arch Ophthalmol* 108:511, 1990.

722. Watanabe K, Chiou GCY: Action mechanism of timolol to lower the intraocular pressure in rabbits, *Ophthalmic Res* 15:160, 1983.

723. Wax MB et al: Characterization of beta-adrenergic receptors in cultured human trabecular cells and in human trabecular meshwork, *Invest Ophthalmol Vis Sci* 30:51, 1989.

724. Wayman L et al: Comparison of dorzolamide and timolol as suppressors of aqueous humor flow in humans, *Arch Ophthalmol* 115:1368, 1997.

725. Weekers R, Prijot E, Gustin J: Recent advances and future prospects in the medical treatment of ocular hypertension, *Br J Ophthalmol* 38:742, 1954.

726. Weinreb RN, Bloom E, Baxter JD: Detection of glucocorticoid receptors in cultured human trabecular cells, *Invest Ophthalmol Vis Sci* 21:403, 1981.

727. Weinreb RN et al: Acute effects of dexamethasone on intraocular pressure in glaucoma, *Invest Ophthalmol Vis Sci* 26:170, 1985.

728. Weinstein BI et al: Defects in cortisol-metabolizing enzymes in primary open-angle glaucoma, *Invest Ophthalmol Vis Sci* 26:890, 1985.

729. Welling P, O'Neil R: Cell swelling activates basolateral membrane Cl and K conductances in rabbit proximal tubule, *Am J Physiol* 258:F951, 1990.

730. Wentworth WO, Brubaker RF: Aqueous humor dynamics in a series of patients with third neuron Horner's syndrome, *Am J Ophthalmol* 92:407, 1981.

731. Wentz-Hunter KK et al: Over- and under-expression of myocilin/TIGR in normal human trabecular meshwork cells, *Invest Ophthalmol Vis Sci* 41:S762, 2000 (ARVO abstract 4044).

732. Wheeler-Schilling TH et al: Angiotensin II receptor subtype gene expression and cellular localization in the retina and non-neuronal ocular tissues of the rat, *Eur J Neurosci* 11:3387, 1999.

733. White A, Handler P, Smith EL: Introduction to metabolism. In White A, Handler P, Smith EL (eds): *Principles of biochemistry*, ed 5, New York, 1973, McGraw-Hill.

734. Wickham MG, Worthen DM: Argon laser trabeculotomy: long-term follow-up, *Ophthalmology* 86:495, 1979.

735. Wiederholt M, Dörschner N, Groth J: Effect of diuretics, channel modulators, and signal interceptors on contractility of the trabecular meshwork, *Ophthalmologica* 211:153, 1997.

736. Wiederholt M et al: Regulation of outflow rate and resistance in the perfused anterior segment of the bovine eye, *Exp Eye Res* 61:223, 1995.

737. Wiederholt M et al: Contractile response of the isolated trabecular meshwork and ciliary muscle to cholinergic and adrenergic agents, *Ger J Ophthalmol* 5:146, 1996.

738. Wiggs JL et al: Genetic linkage of autosomal dominant juvenile glaucoma to 1q21-q31 in three affected pedigrees, *Genomics* 15:299, 1994.

739. Wilensky JT, Jampol LM: Laser therapy for open-angle glaucoma, *Ophthalmology* 88:213, 1981.

740. Wilke K: Early effects of epinephrine and pilocarpine on the intraocular pressure and the episcleral venous pressure in the normal human eye, *Acta Ophthalmol* 52:231, 1974.

741. Wilkerson M et al: Four-week safety and efficacy study of dorzolamide, a novel, active topical carbonic anhydrase inhibitor, *Arch Ophthalmol* 111:1343, 1993.

742. Wilson K et al: Dexamethasone induced ultrastructural changes in cultured human trabecular meshwork cells, *Exp Eye Res* 12:783, 1993.

743. Wilson WS, Shahidullah M, Millar C: The bovine arterially-perfused eye: an in vitro method for the study of drug mechanisms on IOP, aqueous humour formation and uveal vasculature, *Curr Eye Res* 12:609, 1993.

744. Wise JB: Long-term control of adult open-angle glaucoma by argon laser treatment, *Ophthalmology* 88:197, 1981.

745. Wise JB, Witter SL: Argon laser therapy for open-angle glaucoma: a pilot study, *Arch Ophthalmol* 97:319, 1979.

746. Wistrand PJ: Carbonic anhydrase in the anterior uvea of the rabbit, *Acta Physiol Scand* 24:144, 1951.

747. Woltersdorf OWJ, Schwam H, Bicking JB: Topically active carbonic anhydrase inhibitors: 1. O-acyl derivatives of 6-hydroxybenzothiazole-2-sulfonamide, *J Med Chem* 32:2486, 1989.

748. Worthen DM: Scanning electron microscopy after alpha chymotrypsin perfusion in man, *Am J Ophthalmol* 73:637, 1972.

749. Worthen DM, Wickham MG: Argon laser trabeculotomy, *Trans Am Acad Ophthalmol Otolaryngol* 78:OP371, 1974.

750. Worthen DM, Zimmerman TJ, Wind CA: An evaluation of the pilocarpine Ocusert, *Invest Ophthalmol* 13:296, 1974.

751. Yablonski ME, Cook DJ, Gray J: A fluorophotometric study of the effect of argon laser trabeculoplasty on aqueous humor dynamics, *Am J Ophthalmol* 99:579, 1985.

752. Yablonski ME, Novack GD, Burke PJ: The effect of levobunolol on aqueous humor dynamics, *Exp Eye Res* 44:49, 1987.

753. Yablonski ME, Zimmerman TJ, Waltman SR: A fluorophotometric study of the effect of topical timolol on aqueous humor dynamics, *Exp Eye Res* 27:135, 1978.

754. Yamada KM, Geiger B: Molecular interactions in cell adhesion complexes, *Curr Opin Cell Biol* 9:75, 1997.

755. Yamamoto R et al: The localization of nitric oxide synthase in the rat eye and related cranial ganglia, *Neuroscience* 54:189, 1993.

756. Yamamoto T et al: Clinical evaluation of UF-021 (rescula; isopropyl unoprostone), *Surv Ophthalmol* 41(suppl 2):S99, 1997.

757. Yanoff M: Glaucoma mechanisms in ocular malignant melanomas, *Am J Ophthalmol* 70:898, 1970.

758. Ye W et al: Interendothelial junctions in normal human Schlemm's canal respond to changes in pressure, *Invest Ophthalmol Vis Sci* 38:2460, 1997.

759. Yousufzai SY, Abdel-Latif AA: Effects of norepinephrine and other pharmacological agents on prostaglandin E2 release by rabbit and bovine irides, *Exp Eye Res* 37:279, 1983.

760. Yun AJ et al: Proteins secreted by human trabecular cells: glucocorticoid and other effects, *Invest Ophthalmol Vis Sci* 30:2012, 1989.

761. Zhan GL et al: Prostaglandin-induced iris color darkening: an experimental model, *Arch Ophthalmol* 116:1065, 1998.

762. Zhang X et al: Expression of muscarinic receptor subtype mRNA in the human ciliary muscle, *Invest Ophthalmol Vis Sci* 36:1645, 1995.

763. Zhang X et al: Expression of adenylate cyclase subtypes II and IV in the human outflow pathway, *Invest Ophthalmol Vis Sci* 41:998, 2000.

764. Zhang X et al: Expression of adenylate cyclase subtypes II and IV in the human outflow pathway, *Invest Ophthalmol Vis Sci* 41:998, 2000.

765. Ziai N et al: The effects on aqueous dynamics of PhXA41, a new prostaglandin F2α analogue, after topical application in normal and ocular hypertensive human eyes, *Arch Ophthalmol* 111:1351, 1993.

766. Zimmerman TJ: Topical ophthalmic beta blockers: a comparative review, *J Ocular Pharmacol* 9:373, 1993.

SECTION 7

VITREOUS

HENRIK LUND-ANDERSEN

CHAPTER 9

THE VITREOUS

HENRIK LUND-ANDERSEN AND BIRGIT SANDER

The vitreous body makes up approximately 80% of the volume of the eye and thus is the largest single structure of the eye (Figure 9-1). In the anterior segment of the eye, it is delineated by and adjoins the ciliary body, the zonules, and the lens. In the posterior segment of the eye, the vitreous body is delineated by and adjoins the retina.

The vitreous body has many normal physiological functions. This chapter focuses on the most important physiologic relationships, especially those that have a close clinical correlation. As background for the understanding of the physiology and the pathophysiology of the vitreous body, we focus on the main features of the anatomy, biochemistry, and biophysics.

The investigation of the vitreous body and its structure and function is hampered by two fundamental difficulties: First, any attempts to define vitreous morphology are in fact attempts to visualize a tissue, which by design is intended to be invisible. Second, the various techniques that have previously been used to define the structure of the vitreous body are combined with artifacts that make interpretations difficult in terms of the true in vivo physiologic situation.

ANATOMY
Embryology
Structural Considerations of Embryology. In the early stages the optic cup is mainly occupied by the lens vesicle. As the cup grows, the space formed is filled by a system of fibrillar material, presumably secreted by the cells of the embryonic retina. Later, with the penetration of the hyaloid artery, more fibrillar material, apparently originating from the cells of the wall of the artery and other vessels, con-

tributes to filling the space. The combined mass is known as *primary vitreous*.[21,22,35,102,117]

The secondary vitreous develops later, appearing at the end of the sixth week, and is associated with the increasing size of the vitreous cavity and the regression of the hyaloid vascular system. The main hyaloid artery remains for some time, but it eventually disappears and leaves in its place a tube of primary vitreous surrounded by the secondary vitreous, running from the retrolental space to the optic nerve (area of Martegiani). The tube is called *Cloquet's canal* (see Figure 9-1); this is not a liquid-filled canal, but simply a portion of differentiated gel devoid of collagen fibrils.

The term *tertiary vitreous* is related to the fibrillary material, which develops as the suspensor fibrils, the zonules, of the lens. During childhood the vitreous undergoes significant growth. The length of the vitreous body in the newborn eye is approximately 10.5 mm, and by the age of 13 years, the actual length of the vitreous increases to 16.1 mm in the male.[99] In the absence of refractive changes, the mean adult vitreous is 16.5 mm.[28,85]

Molecular and Cellular Considerations of Embryology. The two main components of the vitreous, collagen and hyaluronic acid, are produced in the primary and secondary vitreous. In the primary vitreous, however, there is initial production of substances other than hyaluronic acid, such as galactosaminoglycans; later hyaluronic acid becomes the predominate constituent.[25,103,117]

The primary vitreous contains cells that differentiate in the secondary vitreous as hyalocytes and fibroblasts. The hyalocytes are believed to be involved in the production of glycosaminoglycans, especially hyaluronic acid, a nonsulfated glycosaminoglycan.[103]

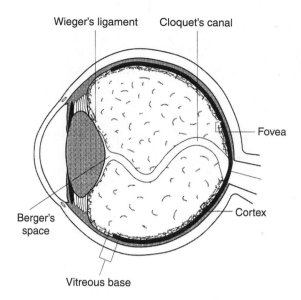

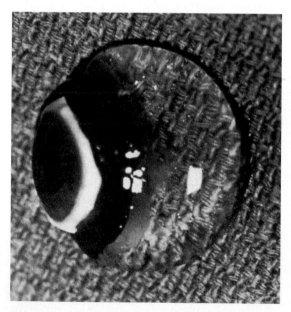

FIGURE 9-1   Sketch of the primate eye showing the vitreous body and its relations. Wieger's ligament is the attachment of the vitreous to the lens. Berger's space and Cloquet's canal are the former sites of the hyaloid artery. (From Heegaard S: *Acta Ophthalmol Scand Suppl 222,* 75:7, 1997.)

Although the function of the fibroblasts is not known exactly, they are probably involved in the formation of collagen. The retina may also be a source of collagen synthesis.[82,102] The hyalocytes are found in the vitreous cortex, approximately 30 μm from the internal limiting membrane (ILM), with the highest density near the vitreous base and the posterior pole.[8]

Anatomy of the Mature Vitreous Body

The mature vitreous body is a transparent gel that occupies the vitreous cavity. It has an almost spherical appearance, except for the anterior part, which is concave corresponding to the presence of the crystalline lens. The vitreous body is a transparent gel; however, it is not completely homogenous (Figure 9-2). The outermost part of the vitreous (or the hyaloid), called the *cortex,* is divided into an anterior cortex and a posterior cortex, the latter being approximately 100 μm thick (Figure 9-3). The cortex consists of densely packed collagen fibrils (Figure 9-4). The vitreous base (see Figure 9-1) is a three-dimensional zone. It extends approximately from 2 mm anterior to the ora serrata to 3 mm posterior to the ora serrata, and it is sev-

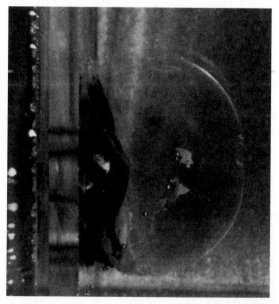

A   **B**

FIGURE 9-2   Human vitreous dissection. **A,** Vitreous of a 9-month-old child. The sclera, choroid, and retina were dissected off the vitreous, which remains attached to the anterior segment. A band of gray tissue can be seen posterior to the ora serrata. This is peripheral retina that was firmly adherent to the posterior vitreous base and could not be dissected. The vitreous is solid and, although on a surgical towel exposed to room air, maintains its shape because at this age the vitreous is almost entirely gel. **B,** Human vitreous dissected off the sclera, choroid, and retina and still attached to the anterior segment. The specimen is mounted on a lucite frame using sutures through the limbus and is then immersed in a lucite chamber containing an isotonic, physiologic solution that maintains the turgescence of the vitreous and prevents collapse and artifactual distortion of vitreous structure. (From Sebag J, Balazs EA: *Surv of Ophthalmol* 28[suppl]:493, 1984.)

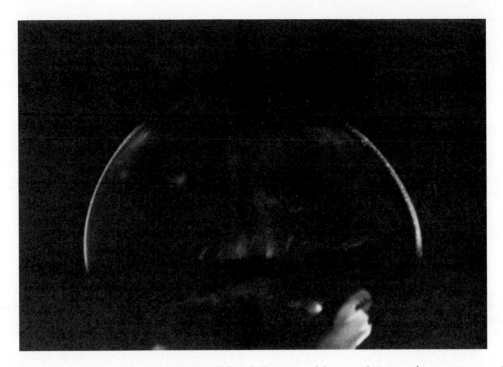

FIGURE 9-3 Human vitreous structure during childhood. This view of the central vitreous from an 11-year-old child demonstrates a dense vitreous cortex with hyalocytes. The posterior aspect of the lens is seen below, although dimly illuminated. No fibers are present in the vitreous.

eral millimeters thick. The collagen fibrils are especially densely packed in this region.

The Vitreoretinal Interface. The vitreoretinal interface can be defined from electron microscopy as the outer part of the vitreous cortex (posterior hyaloid), including anchoring fibrils of the vitreous body and the ILM of the retina[27,30,40-43,87] (Figure 9-5). This definition excludes the nonanchoring part of the vitreous cortex. The ILM is a retinal structure between 1 and 3 μm thick, consisting mainly of type IV collagen and proteoglycans. It contains several layers and can be considered the basal lamina of the Müller cells, the foot processes of which are in close contact with the membrane.

The vitreous cortex is firmly attached to the ILM in the vitreous base region, around the optic disc (Weiss ring), at the vessels, and in the area surrounding the foveola at a diameter of 500 μm.[44,83,98] Under normal conditions, the connection between the fibrils of vitreous cortex and the ILM is looser in the rest of the vitreoretinal interface. The adhesion is strong in young individuals, and dissection of the retina from the vitreous often leaves ILM tissue adherent to the vitreous cortex.[43,56,100-101] Under pathologic conditions, the tight connections between the vitreous cortex and the ILM play an im-

portant role, and imaging of the vitreoretinal interface has now been given a new dimension with the introduction of optical coherence tomography (OCT), as is discussed later in this chapter.

ULTRASTRUCTURAL, BIOCHEMICAL, AND BIOPHYSICAL ASPECTS
Ultrastructural and Biochemical Aspects
The vitreous contains more than 99% water; the rest is composed of solids. The vitreous acts as a gel (i.e., an interconnected meshwork) that surrounds and stabilizes a large amount of water compared with the amount of solids. The gel structure of the vitreous results from the arrangement of long, thick, nonbranching, collagen fibrils suspended in a network of hyaluronic acid, which stabilize the gel structure and the conformation of the collagen fibrils[7,9,99] (Figures 9-6 and 9-7).

In the human eye, the major part of the glycosaminoglycan is hyaluronic acid, with a molecular weight of 3 to 4.5×10^6.[103] The volume of nonhydrated hyaluronic acid is 0.66 cm^3/g, in contrast with the volume of the hydrated molecule, which is 2000 to 3000 cm^3/g.[7] The molecule forms into large, open coils, with the anionic sites spread apart. This arrangement of small-diameter fibers, which are

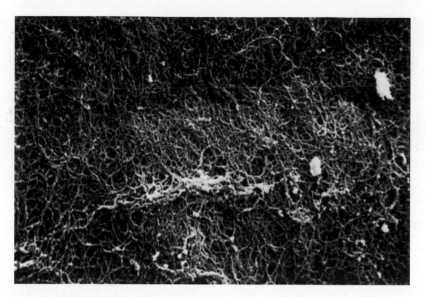

FIGURE 9-4 Ultrastructure of human vitreous cortex. Scanning electron microscopy demonstrates the dense packing of collagen fibrils in the vitreous cortex. To some extent this arrangement is exaggerated by the dehydration that occurs during specimen preparation for scanning electron microscopy. (Magnification × 3750.)

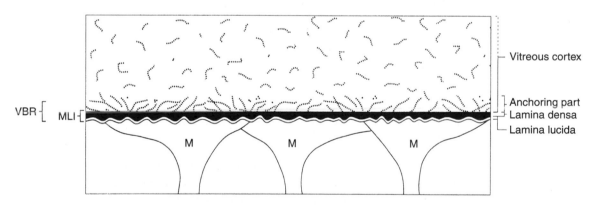

FIGURE 9-5 Sketch of the vitreoretinal interface/vitreoretinal border region (*VBR*). The VBR consists of two major components: the anchoring fibrils of the vitreous body and membrana limitans interna (*MLI*). The MLI is composed of three structures: the fusing point of the anchoring vitreous fibrils, lamina densa, and lamina lucida. *M*, Müller cell. (From Heegaard S: *Acta Ophthalmol Scand Suppl 222*, 75:9, 1997.)

separated by highly hydrated glycosaminoglycan chains, permits the transmission of light to the retina with minimal scattering. The collagen fibrils in the vitreous are thin, with diameters of approximately 10 to 20 nm. Collagen fibrils are mostly collagen type II. They are composed of three identical α-chains, which form a triple helix. The helix is stabilized by hydrogen bonds between opposing residues in different chains.[103] Collagen type IX is also present and may function as a bridge, linking type II collagen fibrils together.[9,29,110] Collagen V/XI is integrated with collagen II in the collagen fibers.[74] The collagen fibrils seem to interconnect with the hyaluronic acid, most likely via bridging glucoproteins.[103] The viscoelastic properties of the vitreous gel results from neither hyaluronic acid nor collagen alone but from the combination of the two molecules.[118]

Dissolved in the water of the vitreous gel are inorganic and organic substances, as shown in Table 9-1 (plasma values are also given for comparison).

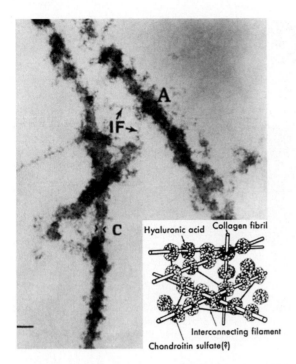

FIGURE 9-6 Ultrastructure of hyaluronic acid/collagen interaction in the vitreous. Specimen was fixed in glutaraldehyde/paraformaldehyde and stained with ruthenium red. Collagen fibrils (*C*) are coated with amorphous material (*A*) believed to be hyaluronic acid. The amorphous material may connect to the collagen fibril via another glycosaminoglycans, possibly chondroitin sulfate (*inset*). Interconnecting filaments (*IF*) appear to bridge between collagen fibrils, inserting or attaching at sites of hyaluronic acid adhesion to the collagen fibrils. (Bar = 0.1 μm.) (From Asakura A: *Acta Soc Ophthalmol J* 89:179, 1985.)

According to Table 9-1, it appears that gradients exist in both directions between vitreous and plasma. These gradients are a result of several mechanisms: presence of the blood-ocular barriers (i.e., active and passive passage across the barriers), metabolism in the retina and ciliary body, and diffusion processes in the vitreous body.

The values in Table 9-1 represent mean values for the whole vitreous. The methods used to quantitate vitreous concentrations are connected with methodologic difficulties and may differ between studies in absolute numbers. However, regional differences within the vitreous have been measured for some substances. Figures 9-8 to 9-10 show the regional difference for glucose (see Figure 9-8), lactate (see Figure 9-9), and oxygen (see Figure 9-10). The fall in vitreous oxygen tension toward the center, corresponding to the upper curve in Figure 9-10, was also found by Sakue[94] and seems to result from an oxygen flux from the retina toward the vitreous corresponding to arterioles; the flux goes in the opposite direction corresponding to the venules (lower curve). Several studies have found an increase in preretinal oxygen after photocoagulation, indicating that the oxygen supply to the inner retina improves after destruction of the outer retina and a concomitant decrease in tissue metabolism and oxygen needs.[36,79,88,112-114]

Biophysical Aspects

The gel structure acts as a barrier against movement of solutes. Basically, substances may move by two different processes: diffusion or bulk flow. The diffusion process can be illustrated in humans by using fluorescein as a tracer substance for the biophysical behavior of the gel. The fluorescein concentration in the vitreous body can be estimated by vitreous fluorophotometry. After intravenous (IV) injection of fluorescein, a certain amount (in healthy humans only a very small amount) passes through the ocular barriers into the anterior chamber and into the vitreous body. The ILM, the vitreoretinal interface, and the vitreous cortex cannot be regarded as a diffusion restriction to smaller molecules. In the vitreous the distribution versus time occurs according to the diffusion properties of a particular molecule in the vitreous gel.

An analysis of the fluorescein concentration gradient in the posterior part of the vitreous can be made with the aid of a simplified mathematical model of the relationship between the vitreous body and the blood-retinal barrier, as shown in Figures 9-11 to 9-14.[72]

In the model the vitreous body is considered as a globe with an outer delineation corresponding to the blood-retinal barrier (Figure 9-11). Fluorescein crosses the barrier passively with permeability *P*. Diffusion in the vitreous gel takes place with a diffusion coefficient *D*. The time-dependent plasma fluorescein concentration is given by *Co(t)*, and the concentration in the vitreous body dependent on time *t* and distance *r* from the center of the eye is given by *C(r,t)*.

The basic equations and the mathematical formalisms are as follows[72]:

EQUATION 1

$$c(r, t) = \int_0^t c_0(t - s) \cdot F(r, s; a, D, P) ds$$

where

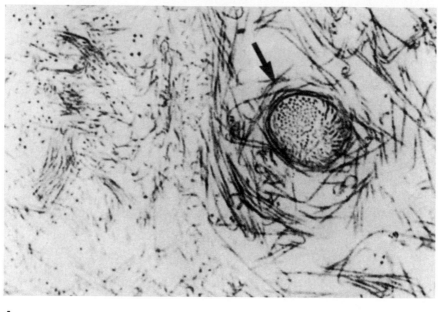

A

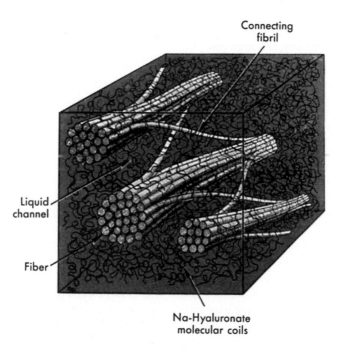

Connecting
fibril

Liquid
channel

Fiber

Na-Hyaluronate
molecular coils

B

Figure 9-7   Ultrastructure of human vitreous. **A,** Specimens were centrifuged to concentrate structural elements but contained no membranes or membranous structures. Only collagen fibrils were detected. There were also bundles of parallel collagen fibrils such as the one shown here in cross section (*arrow*). **B,** Schematic diagram of vitreous ultrastructure depicting the dissociation of HA molecules and collagen fibrils. The fibrils aggregate into bundles of packed parallel units. The HA molecules fill the spaces between the packed collagen fibrils and form "channels" of liquid vitreous. (From Sebag J, Balazs EA: *Invest Ophthalmol Vis Sci* 30:1867, 1989.)

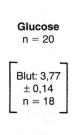

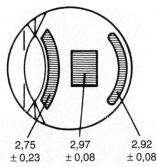

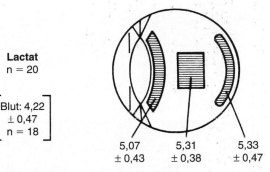

FIGURE 9-8 Glucose concentration in different parts of the vitreous body and in plasma. All values are in μmol/g tissue weight (mean ± standard deviation, *n* = 20). (*Blut* is the German word for *blood*.) (From Bourwieg H: *Graefes Arch Clin Exp Ophthalmol* 191:53, 1974.)

FIGURE 9-9 Lactate concentration in different parts of the vitreous body and in plasma. All values are in μmol/g tissue weight (mean ± standard deviation, *n* = 20). (From Bourwieg H: *Graefes Arch Clin Exp Ophthalmol* 191:53, 1974.)

TABLE 9-1

CONCENTRATION OF VARIOUS SUBSTANCES IN THE INTRAOCULAR FLUIDS OF THE RABBIT EYE (AVERAGES IN mmol/kg H$_2$O)

| | INORGANIC SUBSTANCES | | | | | | |
	SODIUM	POTASSIUM	CALCIUM	MAGNESIUM	CHLORIDE	PHOSPHATE	pH
Vitreous	134	9.5	5.4*	2.3*	105	2	7.29†
Plasma	143	5.6	9.9*	2.2*	97	0.4	7.41†

| | ORGANIC SUBSTANCES | | |
	ASCORBATE	GLUCOSE	LACTATE
Vitreous	0.46	3.0	12.0
Plasma	0.04	5.7	10.3

Modified from Reddy DVN: *Arch Ophthalmol* 63:715, 1960, by Kinsey VE: *Invest Ophthalmol Vis Sci* 6:395, 1967.
*From McNeil A, Gardner A, Stables S: *Clin Chem* 45:135, 1999.
†From Andersen MN: *Acta Ophthalmol* 69:193, 1991.

EQUATION 2

$$F(r, s; a, D, P) = \frac{aP}{r\sqrt{D}}$$

$$\times \left[G\left(\frac{a-r}{2\sqrt{D}}, s; k\right) - G\left(\frac{a+r}{2\sqrt{D}}, s; k\right) \right]$$

In Equation 2, *G* is given by

EQUATION 3

$$G(x, s; k) - e^{-x^2/4s}/\sqrt{\pi s}$$
$$- k \cdot e^{k(x+k \cdot s)} \, erfc(k\sqrt{s} + x/2\sqrt{s})$$

where *k* equals $(P/\sqrt{D}) - (\sqrt{D}/a)$ and *erfc* is the complementary error function. Radius *a* of the eye is determined experimentally. *P* and *D* are calculated from a set of experimental data by minimizing.

EQUATION 4

$$S = \sum_{i=1}^{N} w_i [c_m(r_i, t) - c(r_i, t)]^2$$

where $C_m(r_i, t)$ is the measured value at r = r$_i$, and *c* is the corresponding value given by Equation 1.

Equation 4 indicates that each point of the vitreous concentration profile is weighted equally during the fitting procedure. Larsen et al.[62] suggest another weighting procedure. However, this procedure adds too much weight to the low values toward the center of the eye, and accordingly, the present equal weighting procedure is preferred.

Figure 9-12 shows the fluorescein concentration in the bloodstream in relation to time after IV injection.[69] Figure 9-13 shows the fluorescein concentration in the vitreous body and the anterior chamber

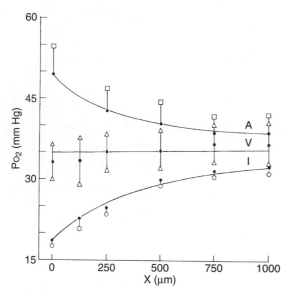

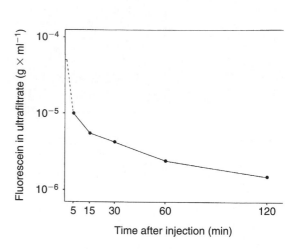

FIGURE 9-10 Heterogeneity of the P_{O_2} in the preretinal vitreous of a nonphotocoagulated eye. Graphic representation of the P_{O_2} (± SEM [standard error of the mean]) recorded when the O_2-sensitive microelectrode was withdrawn from the vitreal surface of the retina ($x = 0$) toward the vitreous. *Curve A,* Opposite an arteriole; *curve I,* opposite an intervascular zone; *curve V,* opposite a vein. These results are averages of measurements made on one or both eyes of 11 miniature pigs. (From Mohar I: *Invest Ophthalmol Vis Sci* 26:1410, 1985.)

FIGURE 9-12 Concentration of free (non–protein bound) fluorescein in ultrafiltrate of plasma over time after intravenous (IV) injection of the dye. The data were obtained in from a healthy subject. Fluorescein was injected at time 0. The first blood sample was obtained at 5 minutes, then 15, 30, 60, and 120 minutes after the injection. The concentration during the first minute after injection was not directly measured, but calculated (*dotted line*) (see method.) (From Lund-Andersen H, Krogsaa B, Jensen PK: *Acta Ophthalmol* 60:709, 1982.)

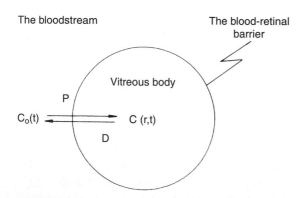

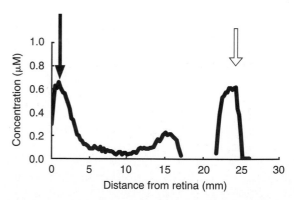

FIGURE 9-11 Simplified model of the eye used for the computerized calculation of a blood-retinal barrier permeability and vitreous body diffusion coefficient for the substance fluorescein. $C_o(t)$, Concentration of free (not protein-bound) fluorescein in plasma at time (t); $C(r,t)$, concentration of fluorescein in the vitreous body at time (t) and at the position (r) from the center of the eye; P, permeability of the blood-retinal barrier, symbolized by a single spherical shell; D, diffusion coefficient in the vitreous body. (From Lund-Andersen H: *Invest Ophthalmol Vis Sci* 26:698, 1985.)

FIGURE 9-13 Vitreous fluorophotometry scan along the optical axis of the eye obtained 60 minutes after injection of fluorescein. The black arrow indicates the retina; the open arrow represents the fluorescein concentration in the anterior chamber. The autofluorescence signal from the lens has been removed. Note a small peak behind the lens (approximately 15 mm from the retina) that results from fluorescein leaking from the anterior chamber into the vitreous body. (From Sander B, Larsen M, Moldow B: *Invest Ophthalmol Vis Sci* 42:433, 2001.)

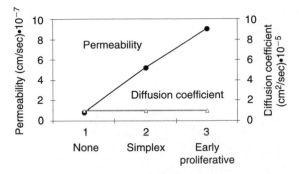

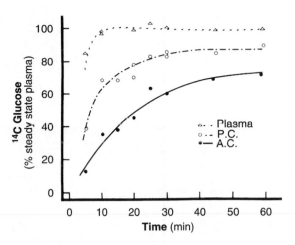

FIGURE 9-14 Diffusion coefficient for fluorescein in the vitreous body and fluorescein permeability of the blood-retinal barrier in diabetic patients with three different degrees of retinopathy. (Redrawn from Lund-Andersen H et al: Fluorophotometric evaluation of the vitreous body in the development of diabetic retinopathy. In Ryan S [ed]: *Retinal diseases*, Orlando, 1985, Grune & Stratton and Harcourt Brace Jovanovich.)

FIGURE 9-15 Entry of ^{14}C-glucose from the blood into the aqueous (*A.C.*) and vitreous (*P.C.*) humors. Blood and aqueous humor samples were fractionated on Sephadex columns before counting to separate glucose from its metabolic products. Curves are hand fitted to the data; 6 animals were used. Each point represents one tap; 12 animals were used. (From Riley MV: *Invest Ophthalmol Vis Sci* 11:600, 1972.)

60 minutes after the injection as determined by vitreous fluorophotometry. A combination of plasma and vitreous values by aid of the simplified mathematical model results by curve fitting in a diffusion coefficient of approximately 6×10^{-6} cm^2/sec. This is close to the diffusion coefficient that would be expected in an unstirred gel; experimentally, the diffusion coefficients for mannitol and inulin has been found to be 2.4 and 2.0×10^{-6} cm^2/sec, respectively.[68,70]

The diffusion coefficient for fluorescein in the vitreous in diabetic patients with different degrees of retinopathy is shown in Figure 9-14. Although the permeability of the blood-retina barrier increases in relation to the degree of retinopathy, the diffusion coefficient is unchanged, indicating that the spread of fluorescein in the vitreous gel occurs with the same kinetics and rate during the earlier phases of diabetic retinopathy.

The permeability for the blood-retinal barrier relates to low-molecular-weight substances and ions; is low in the healthy eye, as shown here for fluorescein; and is close to the permeability of the blood-brain barrier.[12,121] The blood-aqueous barrier (i.e., the barrier in the ciliary body and the iris) is looser, although it is still tighter than capillaries elsewhere, such as in the muscles.[17]

The presence of the ocular barriers and the "slow" diffusion process has the consequence that transient changes in the bloodstream are reflected slowly in the total vitreous body (see Figure 9-13). The slow change of the vitreous body concentra-

tion can be used in some aspects of legal medicine regarding postmortem diagnosis.[75] The time constants for many substances (Figures 9-15 and 9-16) are of the same magnitude as those describing glucose transport between the blood and brain; that is, half of the maximum is achieved in approximately 10 minutes.[67]

Bulk flow through the vitreous cavity as a result of a possible pressure gradient from the anterior part of the eye toward the posterior pole does not play any significant role for the distribution of low-molecular-weight substances in the intact vitreous; this aspect was not included in the mathematical model. However, high-molecular-weight substances or large particles are moving through the vitreous as a result of bulk flow (i.e., the flow of liquid that enters the vitreous body from the retrozonular space and leaves through the retina, as described by Fatt[26]). If such a compound is placed in the anterior part of the vitreous, it moves slowly toward the retina; the diffusion process is virtually zero for large molecules. In contrast, diffusion is more rapid for the movement of small molecules. Low-molecular-weight substances move faster, diffusing in all directions, and are virtually unaffected by bulk flow; if placed in the vitreous, a low-molecular-weight substance will also be found in the anterior chamber.

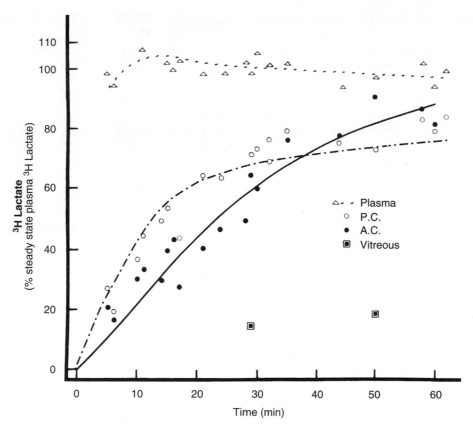

FIGURE 9-16   Entry of H-lactate from the blood into the aqueous (*A.C.*) and vitreous (*P.C.*) humors. The two lower curves in this figure are best-fit lines obtained by analog computer analysis in accordance with the theory of aqueous humor dynamics derived by Kinsey and Reddy. (From Riley MV: *Invest Ophthalmol Vis Sci* 11:600, 1972.)

AGING OF THE VITREOUS

The vitreous body goes through considerable physiologic changes during life, changes that have great significance for its function. A sliding transition exists between the physiologic aging changes and actual degenerative changes (e.g., retinitis pigmentosa, Wagner disease).

The normal postnatal vitreous body is a homogenous gel developed and biochemically constructed as described previously. The fundamental aging change is a disintegration of the gel structure, the so-called liquefaction or synchysis, especially notable in the center of the vitreous, where the collagen concentration is lowest.[117,118] Liquefaction starts early in life, and a linear increase in the volume of vitreous liquid is found with age.[7,109]

Molecular Mechanisms in Aging

The mechanisms behind liquefaction are not known exactly but might be linked to conformational changes of the collagen. The apparent molec-

ular weight of vitreous collagen increases with age because of the formation of new covalent cross-links between the peptide chains equivalent to the aging process in collagen elsewhere in the body.[1] Bundles of collagen fibrils are biomicroscopically visible as coarse fibrous opacities.[105] The common aging processes, such as the cumulative effect of light exposure and nonenzymatic glycosylation, seem to be important. Both hyaluronic acid and collagen may be affected by free radicals in the presence of a photosensitizer such as riboflavin (which is present in the eye) after irradiation with white light.[2] Enzymatic and nonenzymatic cross-linking have also been demonstrated.[107-108,124] Nonenzymatic glycosylation is well known from other tissues with a slow turnover of proteins, such as the lens.[54,115] Proteins are cross-linked because of the Maillard reaction, with the formation of a covalent bond between an amino group and a glucose leading to insoluble proteins (advanced glycation end products [AGEs]). The process is modulated by light accelerated in persons with diabetes mellitus.[95] The vitreous glucose concentration is doubled in persons with diabetes compared with that of healthy subjects.[73] Sebag et al.[108] have found that collagens in the vitreous are cross-linked because of nonenzymatic glycolysation.[103,108,123]

Other mechanisms are probably involved. The network density of collagen decreases in childhood with the growth of the eye, which could destabilize the gel. On the other hand, the hyaluronic acid concentration is increased, which leads to gel stabilization.[103] The concentration of electrolytes, soluble protein, and other substances such as metalloproteinase may change.[14,48] The soluble protein concentration increases with age because of an increase in the leakage through the blood-retina barrier, which may play a role both in the normal aging process and in pathologic conditions such as diabetic retinopathy.[117]

Structural Changes

Regardless of the exact nature of the molecular changes, the structure of the gel is dissolved and replaced with aqueous lacunae, which melt together over time. The hyaluronic acid is redistributed from the gel to the liquid vitreous with concomitant conformational changes.[5] The liquefaction is shown qualitatively in Figures 9-17 and 9-18 and quantitatively in Figure 9-19.[20]

Human vitreous structure can be observed using dark-field microscopy.[99,100,102,105] Using this technique reveals that in the young, the vitreous is optically empty, with the exception of the vitreous cortex. With time, fine parallel fibers appear, with anteroposterior fibers attached to the vitreous base and ora serrata. Peripheral fibers are circumferential with the vitreous. The fibers probably correspond to aggregated collagen fibers no longer separated by hyaluronic acid; with increasing age the fibers thicken and associate with pockets of liquid vitreous (lacunae).

In a series of investigations using an injection of India ink in the vitreous body, Worst[126] argued that the adult vitreous body is composed of a number of cisterns (Figure 9-20); the lining of the cisterns corresponds to the fibers found by Sebag.[50,51] A funnel-shaped cavity, the bursa premacularis, was found in front of the macula. Using fluorescein staining, Kishi[58] has described a similar structure termed *posterior precortical vitreous pocket* (PPVP). In that study the anterior part was found to be lined by the vitreous gel proper and the posterior part by the posterior hyaloid membrane. Sebag et al.[99-101,107]

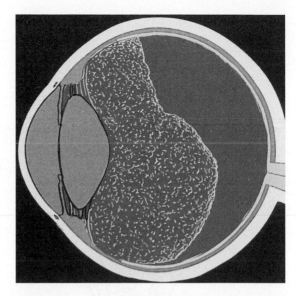

FIGURE 9-17 Schematic illustration of the vitreous body with lacunae. (From Kanski J: *Clinical ophthalmology,* ed 2, London, 1989. Butterworths.)

found a premacular hole in the cortex and observed herniation of the vitreous gel through the hole. The presence or absence of vitreous cortex in close apposition to the fovea is disputed and might be dependent on the age of the donor eye and the technique used.[37,56,58,104,117] Worst[126] proposed that anteroposterior traction of the collagen fibrils lining the cisternae is significant for the formation of macular holes.

Vitreoretinal Interface Imaging

Optical coherence tomography (OCT) is a clinical technique that is suitable both for measurement of retinal thickness and for imaging of the vitreoretinal interface[6,38-39,90] (Figure 9-21). Measurements of retinal thickness are comparable to those achieved with stereoscopic viewing and are reproducible, even in the presence of cataract.[45,116] The optimal resolution of the technique is close to 10 µm, and the distinction between high-reflectivity intravitreal membranes and nonreflective vitreous is favorable, although the exact nature of intravitreal strands cannot be deduced from the image.[15,125] Anteroposterior membranes will theoretically be more difficult to detect because of the minimal backscatter from the small cross section of such fibers.

The aging process of the vitreoretinal interface has been studied with OCT in 209 healthy subjects (ages 31 to 74 years).[122] Preretinal strands, presumably posterior cortex, were found in 60% of these

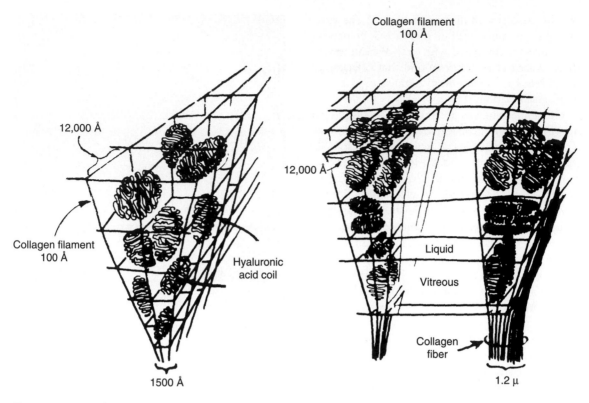

FIGURE 9-18   Schematic representation of the fine structure of the vitreous gel showing network reinforced with hyaluronic acid molecules. *Left,* Random distribution of the structural elements; *right,* formation of liquid pool and partial collapse of the network. (From Balazs EA, Denlinger JL: The vitreous. In Davson H [ed]: *The Eye,* vol 1A, New York, 1984, Academic Press.)

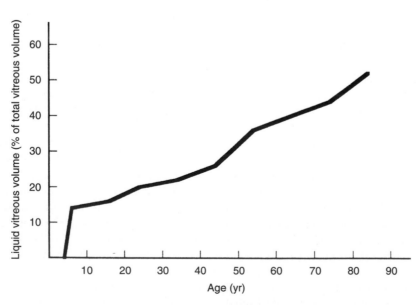

FIGURE 9-19   The formation of liquid vitreous (expressed as a percentage of the total vitreous space) during postnatal development and aging in the human eye. (From Seery M: Vitreous aging. In Albert DM, Jakobiec FA [eds]: *Principles and practice of ophthalmology,* Philadelphia, 1994, WB Saunders.)

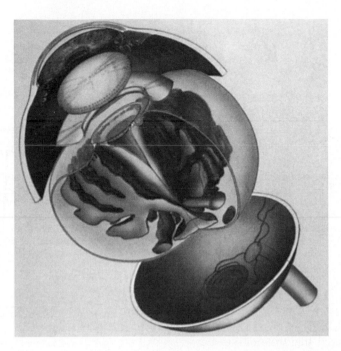

FIGURE 9-20   Schematic diagram of Worst's interpretation of vitreous structure. "Cisterns" are visualized using white India ink to fill areas of the vitreous that take up this opaque dye. There are retrociliary, equatorial, and perimacular cisternal rings and a bursa premacularis. (From Jongebloed WL, Worst JGF: *Doc Ophthalmol* 67:183, 1987.)

nonsymptomatic cases without biomicroscopic evidence of posterior vitreous detachment (PVD). Persistent attachment was found to the fovea, optic nerve head, and midperiphery. The study demonstrates that partial PVD found by OCT is common in healthy subjects.

Diffusion Kinetics as an Indicator of the Biophysical Status of the Vitreous

Using fluorophotometry examination of the fluorescein diffusion profile in the vitreous reveals three different profiles. These profiles provide information on how the vitreous body behaves during aging from a diffusion-kinetic point of view. The three different diffusion-kinetic relationships are shown in Figures 9-22 to 9-24. The upper curve (see Figure 9-22) shows a diffusion profile in the healthy vitreous body, in which the shape of the diffusion profile corresponds to the diffusion in an intact gel, and the diffusion coefficient corresponds to diffusion in a gel. Figure 9-23 shows that there is no diffusion profile, as is the case when degeneration and liquefaction of the vitreous body are present, as ob-

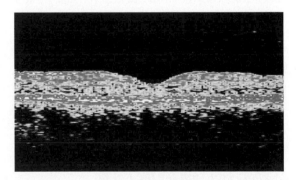

FIGURE 9-21   Optical coherence tomography scan from a healthy subject (6-mm scan through the fovea). The optically empty vitreous is in the top of the picture. The thin fovea is seen in the center of the retina. The retinal pigment epithelium/choriocapillaris is seen as the outermost part of the retina with a high reflectance (white and dark gray). The signal from the photoreceptors is less intensive (gray and black).

served in cases of retinitis pigmentosa. Figure 9-24 gives a diffusion profile interrupted by a convex hump, which can be related to a lacuna in the vitreous with high fluorescein concentration in the center.

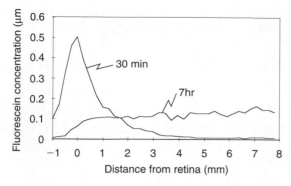

FIGURE 9-22 Preretinal vitreous concentration profiles for fluorescein in a subject with an intact vitreous gel. The profiles were measured after 30 minutes and 7 hours, which enable determination of passive permeability and outward, active transport. (From Moldow B et al: *Graefes Arch Clin Exp Ophthalmol* 236:881, 1998.)

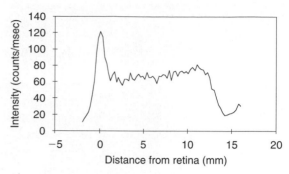

FIGURE 9-23 Fluorescein profile in the vitreous recorded at 30 minutes after fluorescein injection in a subject with vitreous liquefaction (retinitis pigmentosa). The peak to the left is the retinal peak. (From Moldow B et al: *Graefes Arch Clin Exp Ophthalmol* 236:881, 1998.)

In studies that compared the diffusion-kinetic relationships with a clinical evaluation of the vitreous body, a good correlation between the diffusion kinetic and the clinical evaluation was reported.[89,93]

PHYSIOLOGY OF THE VITREOUS BODY

In the following the most essential physiologic and pathophysiologic relationships of the vitreous body are illustrated. The normal physiology of the vitreous body can be divided into four main groups:

- Support function for the retina and filling-up function of the vitreous body cavity
- Diffusion barrier between the anterior and the posterior segment of the eye
- Metabolic buffer function
- Establishment of an unhindered path of light

Support Function for the Retina and Filling-Up Function of the Vitreous Body Cavity

Normal Conditions. The intact vitreous body protects the retina. An intact vitreous body, which fills up the entire vitreous cavity, may retard or prevent the development of a larger retinal detachment. Presumably, the vitreous body can also absorb external forces and reduce mechanical deformation of the eye globe. The intact vitreous body supports the lens during trauma to the eye. However, this mechanical support is only of limited significance. Thus eyes in which the vitreous has been removed during vitrectomy can still have a normal function, and the retina is not detached.

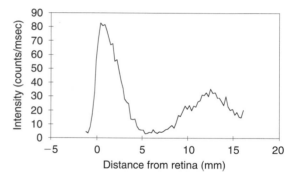

FIGURE 9-24 Vitreous fluorescein profile recorded from the right eye of a patient at 30 minutes after bolus injection. The figure illustrates a typical "camel hump," which has no visible influence on the preretinal gradient. (From Moldow B et al: *Graefes Arch Clin Exp Ophthalmol* 236:881, 1998.)

Pathologic/Pathophysiologic Correlations

Posterior Vitreous Detachment. As previously mentioned, degeneration of the vitreous body is a normal physiologic aging phenomenon. When the central degeneration is sufficiently large, this leads to a collapse of the rest of the vitreous body, which causes the cortex to sink into the center of the vitreous body. This leads to the condition PVD (Figures 9-25 and 9-26).

PVD is the most common pathophysiologic condition of the vitreous body and is considered a normal physiologic aging phenomenon that might be related to a decrease in anchoring fibrils at the vitreoretinal interface.[41,43,122,128] Vitreous detach-

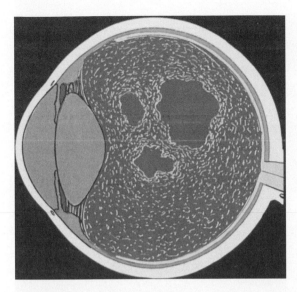

FIGURE 9-25 Schematic illustration of the vitreous body cavity with a posterior vitreous detachment. (From Kanski J: *Clinical ophthalmology,* ed 2, London, 1989, Butterworths.)

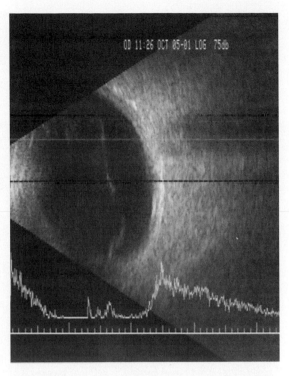

FIGURE 9-26 Ultrasound B-scan of a posterior vitreous detachment as shown schematically in Figure 9-25.

ment leads to opacities in the vitreous body, but otherwise it typically has no clinical consequences. However, if there is a strong attachment between the posterior cortex and the ILM, a PVD can result in a retinal tear. This is the first step in a rhegmatogenous retinal detachment.

PVD can also induce traction on the retina, especially in the foveal region, if there is a strong attachment between the vitreous cortex and the ILM. This is seen especially in eyes with diabetic retinopathy. A shrinking of the posterior cortex when it is attached to the ILM can induce various forms of surface retinopathy, such as macular holes or macular edema.

Perifoveal vitreous detachment has been argued as a primary pathogenic event in idiopathic macular hole formation. However, this phenomenon may be secondary to the formation of the macular hole.

Gass[31,32] has postulated a centrifugal retraction of retinal receptors as an early event that might be caused by an early vitreoretinal degeneration of foveal Müller cells and the overlying vitreous cortex with subsequent split of the Müller cells. According to this hypothesis, the photoreceptors are still present in the cuff around the hole and the large improvement in visual acuity often found after vitrectomy is to be expected.

Other studies, using OCT and B-scan ultrasonography, indicate that vitreous changes are the primary event.[33,49] Both techniques show a partial PVD, with attachment to the fovea, optic nerve, and midperiphery in early stages of macular holes. As the vitreous shrinks, a traction develops in the anteroposterior direction from the vitreous cortex to the fovea. An OCT image of a patient with a macular hole is shown in Figure 9-27, which clearly demonstrates the attachment sites of the posterior cortex. Although clearly seen in Figure 9-27, PVD is not found in all patients and the cause may not be the same in all patients.[34,39,46,57,59]

Intravitreal string formation also may be implicated in macular hole or retinal edema formation. The vitreous strand in Figure 9-28 seems to be intravitreal and not the result of partial PVD because the vitreous cortex was found to be attached to the retina during subsequent vitrectomy. This case illustrates the concept of a schisis in the vitreous cortex as a type of anomalous PVD described by Sebag.[16,102]

Tangential forces cannot be excluded in the pathogenesis of macular holes.[6,80] Traction is well known from proliferative diabetic retinopathy, and as illustrated in Figure 9-27, the posterior vitreous is still attached to the optic nerve and to the midperiphery, although the convex, slack shape of the

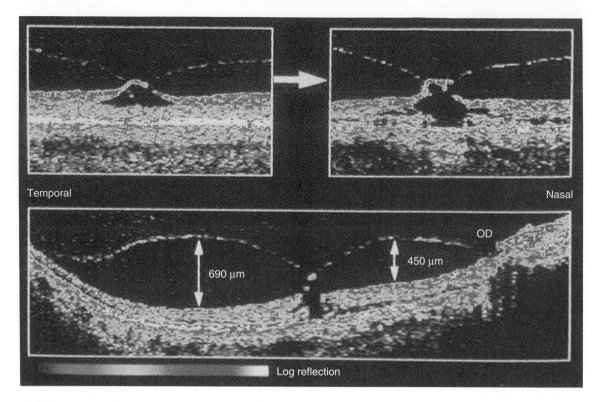

FIGURE 9-27   Evolution of an impending macular hole in a fellow eye to one with a stage 2 hole. *Top left*, Optical coherence tomogram showing a cyst formation in the inner part of the foveal center. The elevation of the foveal floor and the adherence of the partially detached posterior hyaloid suggest vitreoretinal traction. *Top right*, Two months later, the roof of the cyst has opened on the nasal side of the macula, constituting an incompletely detached operculum to which the posterior hyaloid adheres. *Bottom*, Composite optical coherence tomogram showing the convex elevation of the partially detached posterior hyaloid, suggesting anteroposterior vitreous traction. (From: Gaudric A et al: *Arch Ophthalmol* 117:744, 1999.)

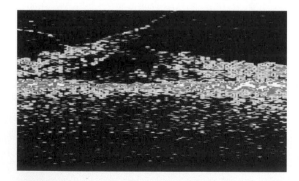

FIGURE 9-28   Optical coherence tomogram of a patient with macular hole. The scan shows an intravitreal string. During operation, the vitreous cortex was found to be adherent to the hole of the posterior pole, indicating that the intravitreal string could be to the result of a vitreoschisis.

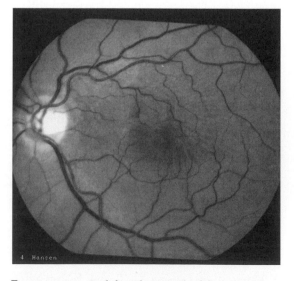

FIGURE 9-29   Red-free photograph of the patient from Figure 9-29 showing a macular hole and traction.

posterior cortex may present evidence for an argue in favor of an anteroposterior traction and against tangential traction.[33,52,80]

Development of Macular Edema. The basic principles behind the pathogenesis of macular edema are illustrated in Figure 9-31. The factors involved are the passive permeability and active transport across the blood-retina barrier, metabolic dysfunction with formation of osmotic equivalents and vitreoretinal traction. Under normal conditions, the blood-retinal barrier is tight (low passive permeability). An increase in the passive permeability or a decrease in the outward active transport may lead to edema formation (Table 9-2).

Although the major part of the pathophysiology seems to be related to a breakdown of the blood-retina barrier, vitreous traction is probably involved in some cases. In diabetic patients, OCT scans might have patterns similar to those seen in eyes with a macular hole, as shown in Figure 9-30. In several studies, eyes with otherwise untreatable edema have been shown to have partial PVD and vitrectomy seems to improve visual acuity in these eyes.[66,119-120,127] However, vitrectomy has also been helpful in cases without evidence of vitreomacular traction.[61]

As indicated earlier, the clinical significance of the tractional forces are complicated and difficult

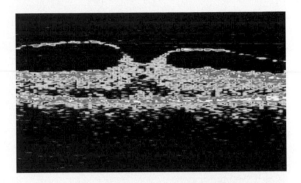

FIGURE 9-30 Optical coherence tomogram of a diabetic patient. The vitreous cortex is firmly attached to the fovea and the vascular arcades (not shown). After vitrectomy, normal anatomy and visual acuity were restored.

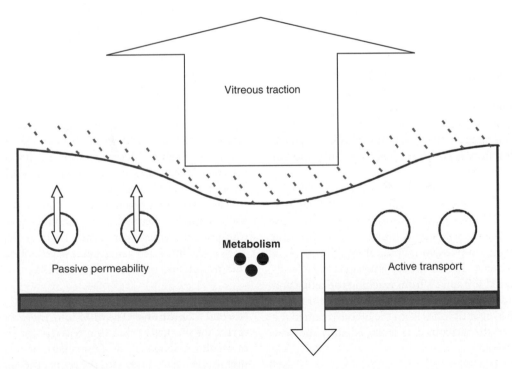

FIGURE 9-31 Schematic illustration of a retinal cross section through the fovea with the vitreous upward and the retinal pigment epithelium downward (*dark gray*); the retinal capillaries are shown as open circles. The factors related to the development of diabetic macular edema are vitreous traction, passive permeability (*bidirectional arrows*), active transport from the retina to the blood (*unidirectional arrow*), and metabolim (osmotic equivalents indicated with black dots).

TABLE 9-2

PASSIVE AND ACTIVE TRANSPORT
ACROSS THE BLOOD-RETINA BARRIER*

	PASSIVE PERMEABILITY (NM/SEC)	ACTIVE TRANSPORT (NM/SEC)
CSME		
Mean	11.32	62.20
95% confidence interval	8.7-14.7	48.2-80.2
Range	2-72	2-265
No CSME		
Mean	3.57	71.95
95% confidence interval	2.7-4.7	56.2-92.1
Range	1-13	23-195

From Sander B: *Br J Ophthalmol* 86:316, 2002.
*Passive and active transport of fluorescein through the blood-retina barrier in diabetic patients with and without clinically significant macular edema (CSME). Results are given nm/sec, equivalent to 10^{-7} cm/sec.

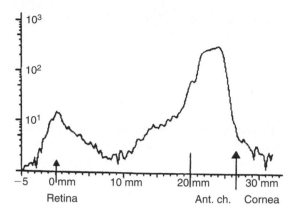

FIGURE 9-32   Fluorophotometric scan (30 minutes) in a patient after extracapsular cataract extraction with posterior chamber pseudophakos. Note the falling concentration of dye from the anterior and posterior toward the central vitreous. (From Ring K, Larsen M, Dalgaard P: *Acta Ophthalmol* 65:160, 1987.)

to quantitate, even if the effect of ILM peeling is ignored. Large randomized studies have not yet been finalized, and the involvement of the vitreous in the pathogenesis of these maculopathies is still a matter of debate.

Diffusion Barrier between the Anterior and the Posterior Segment of the Eye

Normal Conditions. The vitreous body is, as previously mentioned, a gel, and in that context it has a considerable barrier function for bulk movement of substances between the anterior and posterior part of the eye.

Substances that are liberated from the anterior segment of the eye have difficulties reaching high concentrations in the posterior part of the eye when the vitreous body is intact because diffusion is slow and movement by bulk flow is limited in a gel. An intact vitreous gel also prevents topically administered substances from reaching the retina and the optic nerve head in significant concentrations. Entrance of antibiotics from the bloodstream to the center of the vitreous also is impeded by the normal vitreous.

Pathologic/Pathophysiologic Correlations. If the vitreous body is partly removed, degenerated, or collapsed, the exchange between the anterior and posterior part of the eye is much faster and easier. This is the case when the lens is removed and anterior vitrectomy has been performed. Substances that are produced in the anterior segment of the eye or given topically enter the vitreous body through the looser barrier systems in the anterior part of the eye (blood-aqueous barrier) and can be expected to reach the retina in higher concentrations than in eyes with an intact vitreous and an intact iridolenticular barrier (Figures 9-32 and 9-33). The same is the case for topically administered, pharmacologically active substances. Whether this has any clinical significance is unknown, but the condition of the vitreous should always be taken into consideration in discussions on ocular pharmacokinetics, both for topically and systemically applied substances.

The preretinal oxygen tension is improved in diabetic patients after vitrectomy, indicating oxygen transport increases with faster fluid currents.[112] This is of clinical relevance because retinal neovascularization and macular edema regress.

Metabolic Buffer Function

Normal Conditions. The ILM and the posterior cortex do not act as diffusion barriers for smaller molecules. Because of the close anatomic relationship to the ciliary body and the retina, the vitreous body can act as a metabolic buffer and, to a certain degree, a reservoir for the metabolism of the ciliary body and especially the retina, as indicated in the

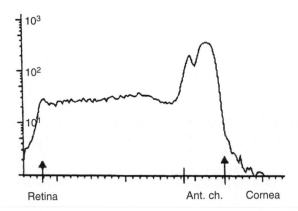

10^3

10^2

10^1

Retina   Ant. ch.   Cornea

FIGURE 9-33 Fluorophotometric scan (30 minutes) in a patient after intracapsular cataract extraction with anterior chamber pseudophakos. There is a high concentration of dye uniformly throughout the vitreous cavity caused by gross vitreous detachment. (From Ring K, Larsen M, Dalgaard P: *Acta Ophthalmol* 65:160, 1987.)

oxygen profiles in Figure 9-10. Because of the tight blood-retina barrier, water-soluble substances located in the retina have easier access to the vitreous cavity than to the bloodstream if the transport across the barrier is limited.

Substances present in or produced in the retina is thus diluted by diffusing into the vitreous body. Likewise glucose and glycogen in the vitreous body can supplement the metabolism of the retina, especially during anoxic conditions. The foot plates of the Müller cells also have close contact with the vitreous body. The vitreous body can thus act as a buffer in the physiologic function of the Müller cells, for example in the potassium homeostasis of the retina.[9,13,81]

Vitamin C is also present in the vitreous body in relative high concentrations, where it can act as a reservoir of antioxidants in stress situations, protecting the retina from metabolic- and light-induced free radicals[99] (see Table 9-1).

Pathologic/Pathophysiologic Correlation. Because normal function of the retina can be obtained after total vitrectomy, the metabolic buffer functions of the vitreous do not seem to play an important role. However, the condition of the vitreous may play a role for the effect of pathogenic factors produced in the retina.

The preretinal concentration of retinally produced vasoproliferation depends on the condition of the vitreous body. If the vitreous acts as a diffusion barrier to these substances, they are retained in high concentrations close to the retina.

Accordingly, one can speculate that vitrectomy can cure this condition, as can be seen in some aggressive cases of proliferative diabetic retinopathy. In other cases vitrectomy can lead to rapid movement of vasoproliferative factors from the posterior pole to the anterior pole, thus leading to neovascularization in the anterior segment of the eye (neovascular glaucoma).

Establishment of an Unhindered Path of Light

Normal Function. The normal physiologic function of the vitreous body allows an unhindered passage of light to the retina when visible light passes through the vitreous body. An important function for the vitreous body is to maintain this optimal transparency, which is primarily produced by the low concentration of structural macromolecules (less than 0.2% weight per volume) and soluble proteins.[118] The transparency may also be maintained by the specific collagen/hyaluronic acid configuration, in analogy with the cornea. The scattering properties of the vitreous are anisotropic, and the scatter decreases when the vitreous swells.[10]

Pathologic/Pathophysiologic Correlations. Degeneration of the vitreous body, as described earlier, with generation of opacities (so-called muches volantes) interferes with the path of light. This is also seen in connection with PVD, as has already been mentioned. Synchysis scintillations, asteroid degeneration, hemorrhages, inflammatory material, fibrous tissue in the vitreous body, and lack of regression of the hyaloid artery are examples of pathologic conditions that interfere with the normal path of light through the vitreous body.[111]

THE VITREOUS BODY AS SENSOR FOR THE PHYSIOLOGY OF SURROUNDING STRUCTURES

As previously described, neither the posterior cortex nor the ILM can be regarded as a diffusion barrier for smaller molecules. Because of the close anatomic relationship between the vitreous, the retina, and the ciliary body, changes in the concentrations of substances in the vitreous body mirror processes in these tissues. Typically, fluorescein is used as a tracer of salt (and water) movement. In vitro studies have shown both passive and active, outward transport through the blood-retina barrier.[18, 60,129-130] The passive movement (permeability) is bidirectional and probably results from fenestrations or leakage through tight junctions.[4,47] The outward transport from the retina to the blood, measured with fluorescein, is significantly reduced by metabolic and competitive inhibitors and is considered an active, carrier-mediated transport from the retina to the blood.[24,60,129] Thus active transport may be related to the metabolic activity of the pigment epithelium.

Determination of the Blood-Retinal–Barrier Transport for Fluorescein in Humans, Based on Concentration Changes in the Vitreous Body

Mathematical models that are able to determine the blood-retinal–barrier permeability in passive or active transport have been developed. The models are based on the assumption that the vitreous body is a globe surrounded by a homogenous blood-retinal barrier. The following assumptions are made: The diffusion of fluorescein in the vitreous body takes place in accordance with conventional diffusion kinetics with a diffusion coefficient (D), the passive permeability of fluorescein through the blood-retinal barrier ($P_{passive}$) follows the usual passive permeability rules, and the active transport ($T_{out,active}$) is carrier mediated and nonsaturable within the concentration range expected to be found in the vitreous body.

After IV injection of fluorescein, the concentration of fluorescein is determined in the bloodstream as the ultrafiltrated part in the plasma, and the concentration of fluorescein into the vitreous body is determined by vitreous fluorophotometry. The passive permeability and the diffusion coefficient is calculated as described earlier based on diffusion profiles obtained up to 60 minutes after fluorescein injection.[19,63-65,72] The outward, active transport is calculated from the preretinal fluorescein concentration curve 8 to 10 hours after fluorescein injection (see Figure 9-22). The basic equation is as follows:

$$J = P_{passive} \cdot C_p(t) - T_{out,active} \cdot C_r(t)$$

where

$$J = \text{Flux}$$
$$P_{passive} = \text{Permeability}$$
$$T_{out,active} = \text{Outward, active transport}$$
$$C = \text{Fluorescein concentration in the plasma and vitreous}$$

Many hours after fluorescein injection, the plasma concentration is low and the first term is small. Thus the outward (active) transport may be

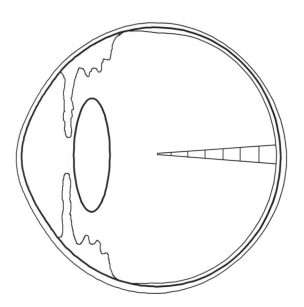

FIGURE 9-34 Simplified spherical model of the blood-retina barrier. The distance from the retina to the center of the eye is divided into a large number of conical cells. The fluorescein concentration in the cell next to the retina is estimated from the plasma fluorescein concentration curve and passive and active transport estimates. (From Sander B, Larsen M, Moldow B: *Invest Ophthalmol Vis Sci* 42:433, 2001.)

estimated from the preretinal gradient to equal $(D \cdot dC/dx) \cdot C_r^{-1}$, where dC/dx is the preretinal fluorescein gradient and C_r^{-1} is the fluorescein concentration at the retina.[23]

The calculation of outward transport is not possible earlier than approximately 5 to 7 hours after fluorescein injection, when the preretinal gradient is reversed (see Figure 9-22). The time of reversal varies according to the passive and active transport in the individual person, and the preceding equation does not take into account the nonsteady state of the whole diffusion process. With a mathematical model, the vitreous concentration curves can be simulated despite the nonsteady state of the system.[96] Fluorescein is metabolized to another fluorescent compound, fluorescein-glucuronide. In contrast to earlier studies, the system has thus to be modified to isolate the contribution of fluorescein from the metabolite in vivo.[84,86,129-132] The model in Figure 9-34 is based on a spherical geometry of the eye; however, the experimental and theoretical curves with this model did not fit in patients with high passive permeability. With a simpler, cylindrical model (Figure 9-35) the match to experimental curves improved. In the final model a correction for

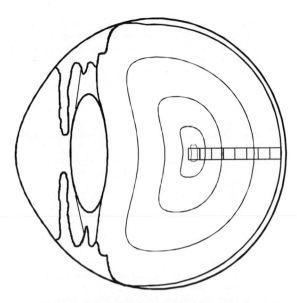

FIGURE 9-35 Simplified cylindrical model of the blood-retina barrier. Assuming diffusion from the anterior part of the eye into the vitreous and low leakage in the peripheral of the retina compared with the posterior pole, the concentration gradients will form ellipsoid curves in the vitreous (*thin lines*). The major direction of fluorescein flux is orthogonal to the concentration. (From Sander B, Larsen M, Moldow B: *Invest Ophthalmol Vis Sci* 42:433, 2001.)

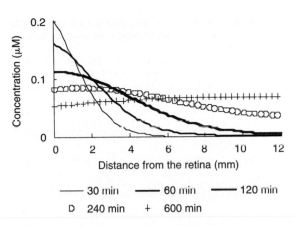

FIGURE 9-36 Vitreous curves calculated from 30 minutes to 8 hours after fluorescein injection (based on the model in Figure 9-35). Input data ($P_{passive}$ 2.5 nm/sec; T_{active} 25 nm/sec) corresponds to a healthy subject. (From Sander B, Larsen M, Moldow B: *Invest Ophthalmol Vis Sci* 42:433, 2001.

diffusion of fluorescein from the anterior chamber was also included because the concentration in the anterior chamber often exceeds the posterior concentration up to several hours after injection and diffuses into the vitreous. The concentration profiles over time with the final model is shown in Figure 9-36. With curve fitting it is possible to estimate the outward, active transport of fluorescein transport in the individual patient. The results are shown in Table 9-2.

It appears that the permeability for fluorescein in the healthy person is low and that the capacity of active transport process from vitreous to the blood is much larger than the passive permeability.[18,60,130] The passive permeability for fluorescein-glucuronide equals that of fluorescein despite a large difference in lipid solubility between these two substances, indicating that the transport is related to water-filled pores.

In healthy subjects the passive permeability of fluorescein is 1.9 nm/sec; the active, outward transport is 43 nm/sec.[78,96] The same parameters in diabetic patients with and without macular edema are shown in Table 9-2. The passive permeability increases significantly with macular edema, whereas the active transport is unaffected by edema, although it appears to increase in patients with early diabetes compared with persons with healthy eyes. The significance of this is unknown but may be related to an activation of the retinal pigment epithelium pump because of an increase of ions and nonionic compounds in the retina of diabetic patients.

CONCLUSION

Although the vitreous body can be removed and almost normal function of the eye will still be maintained, the vitreous body plays an important role in the physiology and pathophysiology of the eye. The "silent" vitreous body exerts many important physiologic functions with close parallel to pathophysiology. An important implication for the future will be intravitreal drug application and release; a further understanding of the physiology of the vitreous body will be important for a rational application of this new modality. The condition of the vitreous body is also important for movement of drugs within the eye and should be considered in discussions regarding the possibility that topically applied drugs will induce effects or side effects in the posterior segment of the eye.

REFERENCES

1. Akiba J, Ueno N, Chakrabarti B: Age-related changes in the molecular properties of vitreous collagen, *Curr Eye Res* 12:951, 1993.
2. Akiba J, Ueno N, Chakrabarti B: Mechanisms of photo-induced vitreous liquefaction, *Curr Eye Res* 13:505, 1994.

3. Andersen MN: Changes in the vitreous body pH of pigs after retinal xenon photocoagulation, *Acta Ophthalmol* 69:193, 1991.

4. Antoinetti DA et al: Vascular permeability in experimental diabetes is associated with reduced endothelial occludin content: vascular endothelial growth factor decreases occludin in endothelial cells, *Diabetes* 47:1953, 1998.

5. Armand G, Chakrabarti B: Conformational differences between hyaluronates of gel and liquid human vitreous: fractionation and circular dichroism studies, *Curr Eye Res* 6:445, 1987.

6. Asami T et al: Vitreoretinal traction maculopathy caused by retinal diseases, *Am J Ophthalmol* 131:134, 2001.

7. Balazs EA, Denlinger JL: The vitreous. In Davson H (ed): *The eye*, vol 1A, New York, 1972, Academic Press.

8. Balazs EA, Toth LZ, Eckl EA: Studies on the structure of the vitreous body. XII. Cytological and histochemical studies on the cortical tissue layer, *Exp Eye Res* 3:57, 1964.

9. Berman E: *Biochemistry of the eye,* New York, 1991, Plenum Press.

10. Bettelheim FA, Balazs EA: Light scattering patterns of the vitreous humor, *Biochem Biophysics Acta* 158:309, 1968.

11. Bourwieg H, Hoffmann K, Riese K: Über Gehalt and Verteilung nieder- und hochmolekularer substanzen im glaskörper, *Graefes Arch Clin Exp Ophthalmol* 191:53, 1974.

12. Bradbury MW, Lightman L: The blood-brain interface, *Eye* 4:249, 1990.

13. Brew H, Attwell D: Is the potassium channel distribution in glial cells optimal for spatial buffering of potassium, *Biophys J* 48:843, 1985.

14. Brown D et al: Cleavage of structural components of mammalian vitreous by endogenous matrix metalloproteinase-2, *Curr Eye Res* 13:639, 1994.

15. Chauhan DS et al: Papillofoveal traction in macular hole formation: the role of optical coherence tomography, *Arch Ophthalmol* 118:32, 2000.

16. Chu TG et al: Posterior vitreoschisis: an echographic finding in proliferative diabetic retinopathy, *Ophthalmology* 103:205, 1996.

17. Cunha-Vaz J: The blood-ocular barriers, *Surv Ophthalmol* 23:279, 1979.

18. Cunha-Vaz J, Maurice DM: The active transport of fluorescein by the retinal vessels and the retina, *J Physiol* 191:467, 1967.

19. Dalgaard P, Larsen M: Fitting numerical solutions of differential equations to experimental data: a case study and some general remarks, *Biometrics* 46:1097, 1990.

20. Davson: *Physiology of the eye,* ed 3, New York, 1972, Churchill Livingstone.

21. Duke-Elder WS: *Textbook of ophthalmology,* London, 1938, Henry Kimpton.

22. Eisner G: Zur anatomie des glaskörpes, *Graefes Arch Clin Exp Ophthalmol* 193:33, 1975.

23. Engler C et al: Fluorescein transport across the human blood-retina barrier in the direction vitreous to blood, *Acta Ophthalmol* 72:655, 1994.

24. Engler C et al: Probenecid inhibition of the outward transport of fluorescein across the human blood-retina barrier, *Acta Ophthalmol* 72:663, 1994.

25. Falbe-Hansen I, Ehlers N, Degn J: Development of the human foetal vitreous body. Biochemical changes, *Acta Ophthalmol* 47:39, 1969.

26. Fatt I: Flow and diffusion in the vitreous body of the eye, *Bull Math Biol* 37:85, 1975.

27. Fine BS, Tousimis AJ: The structure of the vitreous body and the suspensory ligaments of the lens, *Arch Ophthalmol* 65:95, 1961.

28. Fledelius HC: Ophthalmic changes from age 10 to 18 years: a longitudinal study of sequels to low birth weight. IV. Ultrasound oculometry of vitreous and axial length, *Acta Ophthalmol* 60:403, 1983.

29. Funderburgh J et al: Physical and biological properties of keratan sulphate proteoglycan, *Biochem Soc Trans* 19:871, 1991.

30. Gartner J: Vitreous electron microscopic studies on the fine structure of the normal and pathologically changed vitreoretinal limiting membrane, *Surv Ophthalmol* 9:291, 1964.

31. Gass JDM: Reappraisal of biomicroscopic classification of stages of development of macular hole, *Am J Ophthalmol* 119:752, 1995.

32. Gass JDM: Müller cell cone, an overlook of the anatomy if the fovea centralis, *Arch Ophthalmol* 117:821, 1999.

33. Gaudric A et al: Macular hole formation. New data provided by optical coherence tomography, *Arch Ophthalmol* 117:744, 1999.

34. Giovannini A, Amato G, Mariotti C: Optical coherence tomography in diabetic macular edema before and after vitrectomy, *Ophthal Surg Lasers* 31:187, 2000.

35. Gloor BP: The vitreous. In Moses RA (ed): *Adlers's physiology of the eye,* St Louis, 1981, Mosby.

36. Gottfredsdóttir M, Stefánsson E, Gíslason I: Retinal vasoconstriction after laser treatment for diabetic macular oedema, *Am J Ophthalmol* 115:64, 1993.

37. Grignoli A: Fibreous components of the vitreous body, *Arch Ophthalmol* 47:760, 1951.

38. Hee MR, Puliafito CA, Duker JS: Topography of diabetic macular edema with optical coherence tomography, *Ophthalmology* 105:360, 1998.

39. Hee MR, Puliafito CA, Wong C: Optical coherence tomography of macular holes, *Ophthalmology* 102:748, 1995.

40. Heegaard S: Structure of the human vitreoretinal border region, *Ophthalmologia* 208:82, 1994.

41. Heegaard S: Morphology of the vitreoretinal border region, *Acta Ophthalmol Scand Suppl 222,* 75:1, 1997.

42. Heegaard S, Jensen OA, Prause JA: Structure and composition of the inner limiting membrane of the retina, *Graefes Arch Clin Exp Ophthalmol* 224:355, 1986.

43. Hogan M: The vitreous, its structure, and relation to the ciliary body and retina, *Invest Ophthalmol Vis Sci* 2:418, 1963.

44. Hogan M: *Histology of the human eye,* Philadelphia, 1971, WB Saunders.

45. Hougaard J et al: Effects of pseudophakic lens capsule opacification on optical coherence tomography of the macula, *Curr Eye Res* 23:415, 2001.

46. Ib M et al: Anatomical outcomes of surgery for idiopathic macular hole as determined by optical coherence tomography, *Arch Ophthalmol* 120:29, 2002.

47. Ishibashi T, Inomata H: Ultrastructure of retinal vessels in diabetic patients, *Br J Ophthalmol* 77:574, 1993.

48. Jin M, Kachiwagi K, Iizuka Y: Matrix metalloproteases in human diabetic and non-diabetic vitreous, *Retina* 21:28, 2001.

49. Johnson MW, van Newkirk MR, Meyer KA: Perifoveal vitreous detachment is the primary pathogenic event in idiopathic macular hole formation, *Arch Ophthalmol* 19:215, 2001.

50. Jongebloed WL, Humalda D, Worst JFG: A SEM-correlation of the anatomy of the vitreous body: making visible the invisible, *Doc Ophthalmol* 64:117, 1986.

51. Jongebloed WL, Worst JFG: The cisternal anatomy of the vitreous body, *Doc Ophthalmol* 67:183, 1987.

52. Kaiser P et al: Macular traction detachment and diabetic macular edema associated with posterior hyaloidal traction, *Am J Ophthalmol* 131:44, 2001.

53. Kanski J: *Clinical ophthalmology,* ed 2, London, 1989, Butterworths.

54. Kasai K et al: Increased glycosylation of proteins from cataractous lenses in diabetes, *Diabetologia* 25:36, 1983.

55. Kinsey VE: Further study of the distribution of chloride between plasma and the intraocular fluids in the rabbit eye, *Invest Ophthalmol Vis Sci* 6:395, 1967.

56. Kishi S, Demaria C, Shimizu K: Vitreous cortex remnants at the fovea after spontaneous vitreous detachment, *Int Ophthalmol* 9:253, 1986.

57. Kishi S, Hagimura N, Shimizu K: The role of premacular liquified pocket and premacular vitreous cortex in idiopathic macular hole development, *Am J Ophthalmol* 122:622, 1996.

58. Kishi S, Shimizu K: Posterior precortical vitreous pocket, *Arc Ophthalmol* 108:979, 1990.

59. Kishi S, Takahashi B: Three-dimensional observations of developing macular holes, *Am J Ophthalmol* 130:65, 2000.

60. Koyano S, Arai M, Eguchi S: Movement of fluorescein and fluorescein glucuronide across retinal pigment epithelium choroid, *Invest Ophthalmol Vis Sci* 34:531, 1993.

61. La Heij EC et al: Vitrectomy results in diabetic macular oedema without evident vitreomacular traction, *Graefes Arch Clin Exp Ophthalmol* 239:264, 2001.

62. Larsen J, Lund-Andersen H, Krogsaa B: Transient transport across the blood-retina barrier, *Bull Math Biol* 45:749, 1983.

63. Larsen M, Dalgaard P, Lund-Andersen H: Determination of spatial coordinates in ocular fluorometry, *Graefes Arch Clin Exp Ophthalmol* 229:358, 1991.

64. Larsen M, Lund-Andersen H: Lens fluorometry: light attenuation effects and estimation of total lens transmittance, *Graefes Arch Clin Exp Ophthalmol* 229:363, 1991.

65. Larsen M et al: Fluorescein and fluorescein glucuronide in plasma after intravenous injection of fluorescein, *Acta Ophthalmol* 66:427, 1988.

66. Lewis H: The role of vitrectomy in the treatment of diabetic macular edema, *Am J Ophthalmol* 131:123, 2001.

67. Lund-Andersen H: Transport of glucose from blood to brain, *Physiol Rev* 59:305, 1979.

68. Lund-Andersen H, Kjeldsen S: Uptake of glucose analogues by rat brain cortex slices: a kinetic analysis based upon a model, *J Neurochem* 27:361, 1976.

69. Lund-Andersen H, Krogsaa B, Jensen PK: Fluorescein in human plasma in vivo, *Acta Ophthalmol* 60:709, 1982.

70. Lund-Andersen H, Moller M: Uptake of inulin by cells in rat brain cortex, *Exp Brain Res* 23:37, 1977.

71. Lund-Andersen H et al: Fluorophotometric evaluation of the vitreous body in the development of diabetic retinopathy. In Ryan S (ed): *Retinal diseases,* Orlando, 1985, Grune & Stratton and Harcourt Brace Jovanovich.

72. Lund-Andersen H et al: Quantitative vitreous fluorophotometry applying a mathematical model of the eye, *Invest Ophthalmol Vis Sci* 26:698, 1985.

73. Lundquist O, Österlin S: Glucose concentration in the vitreous of non-diabetic and diabetic human eyes, *Graefes Arch Clin Exp Ophthalmol* 232:71, 1994.

74. Mayne R et al: Isolation and characterization of type V/type XI collagen present in bovine vitreous, *J Biol Chem* 268:93, 1993.

75. McNeil A, Gardner A, Stables S: Simple method for improving the precision of electrolyte measurements in vitreous humor, *Clin Chem* 45:135, 1999.

76. Mohar I et al: Effect of laser photocoagulation on oxygenation of the retina in miniature pigs, *Invest Ophthalmol Vis Sci* 26:1410, 1985.

77. Moldow B et al: The effect of acetazolamide on passive and active transport of fluorescein across the blood-retinal barrier in retinitis pigmentosa complicated by macular edema, *Graefes Arch Clin Exp Ophthalmol* 236:881, 1998.

78. Moldow B et al: Effects of acetazolamide on passive and active transport of fluorescein across the normal BRB, *Invest Ophthalmol Vis Sci* 40:1770, 1999.

79. Molnar I et al: Effect of laser photocoagulation on oxygenation of the retina in miniature pigs, *Invest Ophthalmol Vis Sci* 26:1410, 1985.

80. Mori K, Bae T, Yoneya S: Dome-shaped detachment of premacular cortex in macular hole development, *Ophthalmic Surg Lasers* 31:203, 2000.

81. Newman EA: Regulation of potassium levels by Muller cells in the vertebrate retina, *Can J Physiol Pharmacol* 65:1028, 1987.

82. Newsome D, Linsenmayer T, Trelstad R: Vitreous body collagen, *J Cell Biol* 71:59, 1976.

83. Nork TM, Giola V, Hobson R: Subhyaloid hemorrhage illustrating a mechanism of macular hole formation, *Arch Ophthalmol* 109:884, 1991.

84. Ogura Y et al: Estimation of the permeability of the blood-retinal barrier in normal individuals, *Invest Ophthalmol Vis Sci* 26:969, 1985.

85. Oksala A: Ultrasonic findings in the vitreous at various ages, *Graefes Arch Clin Exp Ophthalmol* 207:275, 1978.

86. Palestine AG, Brubaker RF: Pharmacokinetics of fluorescein in the vitreous, *Invest Ophthalmol Vis Sci* 21:542, 1981.

87. Pedler C: The inner limiting membrane of the retina, *Br J Ophthalmol* 45:423, 1961.

88. Pournaras CJ et al: Experimental venous thrombosis: preretinal pO$_2$ before and after photocoagulation, *Klin Monatsbl Augenheilkd* 186:500, 1985.

89. Prager T et al: The influence of vitreous change on vitreous fluorometry, *Arch Ophthalmol* 100:594, 1982.

90. Puliafito C et al: Imaging of macular diseases with optical coherence tomography, *Ophthalmol* 102:217, 1995.

91. Reddy DVN, Kinsey VE: Composition of the vitreous humor in relation to that of plasma and aqueous humors, *Arch Ophthalmol* 63: 715, 1960.

92. Riley MV: Intraocular dynamics of lactic acid in the rabbit, *Invest Ophthalmol Vis Sci* 11:600, 1972.

93. Ring K, Larsen M, Dalgaard P: Fluorophotometric evaluation of ocular barriers and of the vitreous body in the aphakic eye, *Acta Ophthalmol* 65:160, 1987.

94. Sakaue H, Negi A, Honda Y: Comparative study of vitreous oxygen tension in human and rabbit eyes, *Invest Ophthalmol Vis Sci* 30:1933, 1989.

95. Sander B, Larsen M: Photochemical bleaching of fluorescent glycolysation products, *Int Ophthalmol* 18:195, 1994.

96. Sander B, Larsen M, Moldow B: Diabetic macular edema: passive and active transport of fluorescein through the blood-retinal barrier, *Invest Ophthalmol Vis Sci* 42:433, 2001.

97. Sander B et al: Diabetic macular oedema: a comparison between vitreous fluorometry, angiography and retinopathy, *Br J Ophthalmol* 86:316, 2002.

98. Schubert H: Cystoid macular edema: the apparent role of mechanical factors, *Prog Clin Biol Res* 312:299, 1989.

99. Sebag J: The vitreous. In Hart W (ed): *Adler's physiology of the eye,* ed 9, St Louis, 1985, Mosby.

100. Sebag J: Age-related differences in the vitreoretinal interface, *Arch Ophthalmol* 109:966, 1991.

101. Sebag J: Abnormalities of human vitreous structure, *Graefes Arch Clin Exp Ophthalmol* 231:257, 1993.

102. Sebag J: Surgical anatomy of the vitreous and the vitreo-retinal interface. In Tasman W (ed): *Duane's clinical ophthalmology,* Philadelphia, 1994, Lippincott.

103. Sebag J: Macromolecular structure of the corpus vitreum, *Prog Polym Sci* 23:415, 1998.

104. Sebag J: Letter to the editor, *Arch Ophthalmol* 100:1599, 1993.

105. Sebag J, Balazs EA: Morphology and ultrastructure of human vitreous fibers, *Invest Ophthalmol Vis Sci* 30:1867, 1989.

106. Sebag J, Balzac A: Pathogenesis of cystoid macular edema: an anatomical consideration of vitreoretinal adhesion, *Surv Ophthalmol* 28(suppl):493, 1984.

107. Sebag J et al: Biochemical changes in vitreous of humans with proliferative diabetic retinopathy, *Arch Ophthalmol* 110:1472, 1992.

108. Sebag J et al: Raman spectroscopy of human vitreous in proliferative retinopathy, *Invest Ophthalmol Vis Sci* 35:2976, 1994.

109. Seery M: Vitreous aging. In Albert DM, Jakobiec FA (eds): *Principles and practice of ophthalmology,* Philadelphia, 1994, WB Saunders.

110. Snowden J: The stabilization of in vivo assembled collagen fibrils by proteoglycans/glycosaminoglycans, *Biochem Biophys Acta* 703:21, 1982.

111. Spraul CW, Grossniklaus HE: Vitreous hemorrhage, *Surv Ophthalmol* 42:3, 1997.

112. Stefánsson E: The therapeutic effects of retinal laser treatment and vitrectomy: a theory based on oxygen and vascular physiology, *Acta Ophthalmol* 79:435, 2001.

113. Stefánsson E, Peterson J, Wang Y: Intraocular oxygen tension measured with a fiber-optic sensor in normal and diabetic dogs, *Am J Physiol* 256:H1127, 1989.

114. Stefánsson E et al: Retinal oxygenation and laser treatment in patients with diabetic retinopathy, *Am J Ophthalmol* 113: 36, 1992.

115. Stitt A: Advanced glycation: an important pathological event in diabetic and age related ocular disease, *Br J Ophthalmol* 85:746, 2001.

116. Strom C et al: Diabetic macular edema assessed with optical coherence tomography and stereo fundus photography, *Invest Ophthalmol Vis Sci* 43:241, 2002.

117. Swann D: Chemistry and biology of the vitreous body, *Int Rev Exp Pathol* 22:2, 1980.

118. Swann D, Constable I: Vitreous structure: I. Distribution of hyaluronate and protein, *Invest Ophthalmol Vis Sci* 11:159, 1972.

119. Tachi N: Surgical management of macular edema, *Semin Ophthalmol* 13:20, 1998.

120. Tachi N, Ogino N: Vitrectomy for diffuse macular edema in cases of diabetic retinopathy, *Am J Ophthalmol* 122:258, 1996.

121. Törnquist P, Alm A, Bill A: Permeability of ocular vessels and transport across the blood-retinal barrier, *Eye* 4:303, 1990.

122. Uchino E, Uemura A, Ohba N: Initial stages of posterior vitreous detachment in healthy eyes of older persons evaluated by optical coherence tomography, *Arch Ophthalmol* 119:1474, 2001.

123. Ueno N et al: Effects of visible-light irradiation on vitreous structure in the presence of a photosensitizer, *Exp Eye Res* 44:863, 1987.

124. Vaughan-Thomas A, Gilbert S, Duance C: Elevated levels of proteolytic enzymes in the aging human vitreous, *Invest Ophthalmol Vis Sci* 41:3299, 2000.

125. Wilkins JR, Puliafito CA, Hee MR: Characterization of epiretinal membranes using optical coherence tomography, *Ophthalmology* 103:2142, 1996.

126. Worst JGF: Cisternal systems of the fully developed vitreous in young adults, *Trans Ophthalmol Soc UK* 97:550, 1977.

127. Yamamoto T, Akabane N, Takeuchi S: Vitrectomy for diabetic macular edema: the role of posterior vitreous detachment and epimacular membrane, *Am J Ophthalmol* 132:369, 2001.

128. Yonomoto J et al: The age of onset of posterior vitreous detachment, *Graefes Arch Clin Ophthalmol* 232:67, 1994.

129. Yoshida A, Ishiko S, Kojima M: Outward permeability of the blood-retina barrier, *Graefes Arch Clin Exp Ophthalmol* 230: 84, 1992.

130. Yoshida A et al: Blood-ocular barrier permeability in monkeys, *Br J Ophthalmol* 76:84, 1992.

131. Zeimer R, Blair NP, Cunha-Vz JG: Pharmacokinetic interpretation of vitreous fluorophotometry, *Invest Ophthalmol Vis Sci* 24:1374, 1983.

132. Zeimer R, Blair NP, Cunha-Vz JG: Vitreous fluophotometry for clinical research, *Arch Ophthalmol* 101:1757, 1983.

SECTION 8

RETINA

ALBERT ALM AND BERNDT E.J. EHINGER

CHAPTER 10

DEVELOPMENT AND STRUCTURE
OF THE RETINA

RAJESH K. SHARMA AND BERNDT E.J. EHINGER

Perhaps as much as 80% of the sensory input in humans takes place through the retina, engaging about one third of the human brain for its processing, which makes the study of the retina interesting for clinicians and scientists alike. For clinicians the retina is an easily visible part of the central nervous system (CNS) and the only place in the body where blood vessels of the arteriolar level are visible, making the tissue a window for inspecting a part of the CNS and cardiovascular system. The retina reflects many of the changes in the CNS, such as increased intracranial tension, and in the cardiovascular system, such as vascular changes in hypertension and diabetes. For scientists the retina is the simplest and best-organized part of the CNS and has many remarkable features, making it an excellent tissue for research. It is not surprising that the retina has been so extensively investigated.

Eyes have passed through a long process of evolution. First, photosensitive intracellular organelles evolved to unicellular eyes and then to multicellular eyes. Even the most primitive vertebrate eyes are elaborate, although they have undergone mostly adaptive specialization rather than further evolution toward more complexities. The virtue of human vision lies not in the structure of the eye but in the ability of the mind to appreciate it. All vertebrate eyes have a three-layered retina, pigment epithelium, and identically derived dioptric and nutritional mechanisms. The evolution of color vision illustrates this point well. Vertebrates developed five major families of visual pigments (one rod and four spectrally distinct cone classes) early during development (350 to 400 million years ago) that enable tetrachromatic color vision. As mammals evolved, perhaps because of their nocturnal ancestral environment, color vision became less important and was reduced to dichromatic color vision, with only two spectral classes of cone cells. Much later (35 million years ago), as primates evolved, the need for distinguishing yellow-orange fruits from green foliage gave rise to a third pigment.[120] It was produced as a duplication and modification of one of the existing genes for longer-wavelength cone pigments. Spectral tuning of these pigments added one more dimension to their color perception, thus creating trichromatic vision.

EMBRYOGENESIS AND DEVELOPMENT OF THE RETINA

The neural plate, which is derived from the ectoderm, is the embryonic precursor of the entire nervous system, including the retina. The ectoderm has two regions; one will form the skin, and the other will form the neural plate. As the neural plate forms, different regions are predetermined to form individual parts of the CNS, including the neural elements of the eye. Soon after the neural plate is formed, it rolls up in the midline of the embryo to form the neural tube. This process is called *neurulation*. The neural tube formation involves movement of tissues and changes in the cellular shapes. The first signs of the developing eyes in humans appear by the third week of gestation (the 2.6-mm stage), when the brain is still in its three-vesicle stage. Two pits appear in the transverse neural folds; within a few days (the 3.2-mm stage), these pits develop into optic vesicles, which are connected to the brain by the optic stalks (Figure 10-1).

From the fourth to the sixth week (the 4- to 5-mm and 15- to 18-mm stages), the optic vesicles enlarge and start to invaginate their lateral parts. The concurrently developing lens is important for this and probably exerts its effect through extracel-

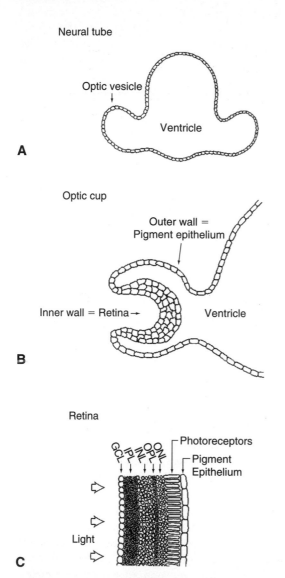

A

Neural tube

Optic vesicle

Ventricle

B

Optic cup

Outer wall =
Pigment epithelium

Inner wall = Retina →

Ventricle

C

Retina

Photoreceptors

Pigment
Epithelium

Light

FIGURE 10-1 Schematic diagrams showing the optic vesicles, which develop from the neural tube (**A**), the invagination of an optic vesicle to form an optic cup (**B**), and the layers of the retina, which develop from the cells of the inner wall of the optic cup (**C**). *GCL,* Ganglion cell layer; *INL,* inner nuclear layer; *IPL,* inner plexiform layer; *ONL,* outer nuclear layer; *OPL,* outer plexiform layer. (Redrawn from Dowling JE: *The retina: an approachable part of the brain,* Cambridge, 1987, The Belknap Press of the Harvard University Press.)

lular matrix components. The outer and the lower walls of the vesicle invaginate and come to rest on the upper and posterior walls, forming a two-layered cup that is open laterally and in its lower nasal quadrant, the fissure. If invagination fails, a congenital cystic eye forms. At later stages the fissure closes. If the fissure fails to close, a typical coloboma located in the inferior nasal quadrant of the eye results. Atypical colobomas comprise only one layer of atrophic retina and often are located in quadrants other than the inferior nasal. Different parts of the optic cup follow deviant paths of differentiation.

The invaginating portion (the inner wall lining the cup) gives rise to the neural retina along with most of its glial elements, and the outer wall produces the retinal pigment epithelium (RPE). The optic stalk gives rise to the glia of the optic nerve.

By the time the optic cup is formed (the 10-mm stage), the retinal differentiation is already in progress. Cell division in the outer wall of the optic cup occurs only in one plane, creating a single layer of cells. In these cells, pigment granules begin to appear by the 5- to 6-mm stage and are well formed by the 10-mm stage. By the end of the eighth week (the 30-mm stage), a single-layered pigmented epithelium can readily be identified. It continues to grow, but no further significant changes occur in it.

It seems that the developing neural retina influences the development of the RPE. In vertebrates (E 14 in rodents), with the help of certain growth factors such as fibroblast growth factors, the differentiating RPE cells can, for some time after the formation of the optic cup, be influenced into becoming neural retina.[152]

On the choroidal side, the RPE is firmly attached to Bruch's membrane. Both RPE and the choroid contribute to elements of this membrane, and Bruch's membrane thus has both ectodermal and mesodermal origins. It starts to develop by the 14- to 18-mm stage and is well demarcated by the sixth month.

By the 12-mm stage, two nuclear layers, called the *inner* and *outer neuroblastic layers,* are established at the posterior pole of the retina. A narrow acellular strip called the *Chievitz transient fiber layer* separates them. The development spreads radially through the optic cup, and by the 26-mm stage, two neuroblastic layers are developed out to its equator. Proliferation continues in the neuroretinal layer of the optic cup. The proliferating cells synthesize their DNA on the vitreal side of this neuroblastic cell mass. After synthesizing the DNA, they move toward the sclera and divide at the apical side of the neuroblastic cell mass. If the daughter cells do not leave the mitotic cycle, they move back to the vitreal side to synthesize more DNA.[129] Cells that leave the cell cycle migrate to locations determined at their birth and start to differentiate.

Only a few of the factors that control proliferation are understood, but some points have emerged. Proliferation appears to be both stimulatory and inhibitory. Transforming growth factor-α, acidic and basic fibroblast growth factors, and epidermal growth factors stimulate the proliferation of retinal progenitor cells in cultures. The growth factors regulate the cell proliferation through intracellular signaling cascades that ultimately influence the cell-cycle control system. Evidence also exists that conventional fast-acting neurotransmitter systems may inhibit or at least regulate proliferation. Some of these systems are more highly expressed during development and before any conventional nerve signaling occurs. Currently, the best examples are γ-aminobutyric acid (GABA) and acetylcholine.

The proliferation ceases in the central retina first and subsequently ceases in more peripheral parts.[129] The first cells to leave the cell cycle are the ganglion cells, cone cells, horizontal cells, and certain amacrine cells. More amacrine cells leave the cell cycle later. Rods then develop, and bipolar cells develop last. In humans the ganglion cells, horizontal cells, cone cells, and amacrine cells are present at birth, but some rods in the peripheral retina, together with some Müller and cone cells, may continue to be produced up to the third postnatal month. In species in which the retinal development takes place over a short time (such as in the frog, *Xenopus*), the birthdays of the cells overlap, whereas they are more sharply demarcated in species in which the retinal development is more extended, such as monkeys.

The birthday scheme of the retinal neurons is conserved during evolution, which perhaps reflects the evolutionary sequence of retinal neurons and the functional importance of this sequence. The neurons that evolved late may have found a function and organization secondary to already existing neurons (note the connections of rod pathways in later sections).

The development of the retinal nuclear and plexiform layers and the cellular differentiation of various cell types begins in the central retina and spreads peripherally. The ganglion cell layer appears first by the formation of the inner plexiform layer. Its development starts at 12 weeks, and it is well established by the fifth month. The outer plexiform layer forms at the fourth month, and cells located between the outer and the inner plexiform layers then consolidate to form the inner nuclear layer, erasing all of the Chievitz transient fiber layer except a remnant at the macula. This also disappears as the macula matures. The Chievitz layer leaves no identifiable mark in the adult retina.

The formation of the retinal layers depends on cells of different types developing in concert and forming appropriate connections with their partners. Different adhesion molecules are known to have important roles for this, and a number of such molecules have been identified. Some of these cell adhesion molecules (CAMs) control different generalized aspects of the development, whereas others have a more specific and restricted role. Neural CAMs and certain calcium-dependent CAMs (different cadherins) appear in the developing retina (including the pigment epithelium) and in the developing lens; these CAMs play a generalized role.[61,96,135] They may be responsible for the grouping of cells that is needed to form the tissue structure. Restricted CAMs are more numerous and are found only in the neural tissue in the eye. They are responsible for specialized types of cell adhesions. The CAMs associated with the axons of the retinal cells (such as G4, neurofascin, or F11) have distinct patterns of expression, implying they play a role in the growth of the axons.[132] Such molecules are also responsible for the affinity growth cones have for each other, and they eventually lead to the formation of axon fascicles. The specificity of the cell-to-cell adhesions seen during development probably results from different combinations of adhesion molecules creating a variety of surface properties of growth cone cells, a characteristic that allows the neurons to select complex pathways based on the combination of molecules on the surface of the cells along the way.

The cell distribution is not symmetric across the retina. This is partly the result of asymmetric growth after birth. In humans the retina grows by a factor of 1.8 after birth until 6 years of age. This is largely because of enlargement of the peripheral retina and results in decreased cell density peripherally. However, there are other asymmetries, such as the accumulation of cone cells in fovea and that of rods in the rod ring. The cone and ganglion cell density is also higher, even before birth, in the nasal retina than in the temporal retina. Furthermore, ganglion cells from different regions of the retina send their processes either to the ipsilateral or contralateral side of the brain to form topographic maps. This suggests the presence of important positional information already in the developing retina, but the details remain to be established.

Programmed cell death (apoptosis) is an important event during the development of most tissues, including retina tissue. During the early development of the eye, apoptosis is responsible for the sculpting of the optic primodium and the formation of the optic fissure. More important, it may be responsible for opening the extracellular channels and therefore creating passages where the optic fibers can grow.[131] Apoptosis is likely to fine-tune the number of cells of the different types at different locations. The process appears most prominent in ganglion cells. Approximately 70% of ganglion cells die in a developing human retina, but different subclasses of ganglion cells die at different rates.[20,103,111,112] Factors responsible for the control of apoptosis include the availability of trophic factors with different kinds of dendritic interactions and intrinsic or induced activity in the neurons.

The human central retina develops over a prolonged period. Histologic evidence for the development of the human fovea is already present between the eleventh and twelfth embryonic weeks on the temporal side of the disc.[88,121] In the early stages the macular region is actually elevated from the surface of the retina because the ganglion cells have accumulated there. By the sixth month of gestation, there are up to nine rows of ganglion cells in the macular region. This region then starts thinning, and ganglion cells and other cells of the inner retina become displaced centrifugally and develop elongated processes. The displacement results in a depression in the center of the macula. Migration of ganglion cells, cells of the inner nuclear layer, and Müller cells toward the periphery thus form the foveal pit. The cells maintain the synaptic contacts made at an earlier stage.[64] The foveal pit is fully formed by about 11 to 15 months postnatally. It is unclear how a rod-free fovea is produced. There is no evidence of selective rod apoptosis in it. It is possible that the progenitor cells produce only cone cells in the foveal region.

At the time of birth, the cone density of the human fovea is only 20% of the adult value, which it reaches only 4 to 5 years after birth. This is probably achieved by centripetal migration of cone cells toward the center of the fovea. The foveal area also decreases during development, contributing to increased cone density. As the fovea matures, the cone cells become thinner and therefore more compactly packed. Foveal cone cells continue to change their

shape and develop the outer segments well into adulthood.

ANATOMY OF THE RETINA

The neural retina consists of six neuron types: photoreceptor cells, horizontal cells, bipolar cells, amacrine cells, interplexiform cells, and ganglion cells (Figures 10-2 and 10-3). The neurons are in close contact with and supported by the radial glial cells, which are called the *Müller cells*. The photoreceptor outer segments are specialized to capture

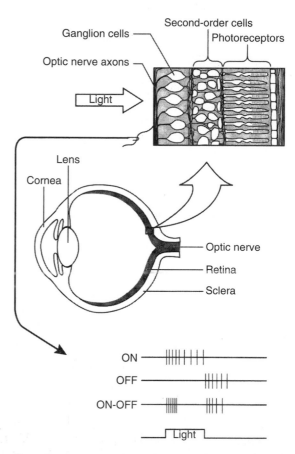

FIGURE 10-2   The retina, consisting of photoreceptors, second-order cells, and ganglion cells, lines the back (sclera) of the eye. The axons of the third-order ganglion cells run along the surface of the retina, forming the optic nerve to exit the eye. Light enters the eye through the transparent cornea and is focused on the retina by the lens. Recordings from single optic nerve axons (*bottom*) show three basic types of responses when the retina is diffusely illuminated. Some axons respond when the light is on, others when the light is turned off, and some at both times. (Redrawn from Dowling JE: *Creating mind: how the brain works,* New York, 1998, WW Norton.)

light and receive functional support from the RPE cells immediately outside of them.

The retina not only converts light into nerve signals but also processes some of the visual information, especially in birds and cold-blooded verte-brates. In mammals, much of the visual processing has been delegated to the cortex, resulting in decreased diversity in the amacrine and horizontal cell types, which were originally involved in visual processing at the retinal level.

Functional Organization of the Retina

Generally, the organization of the visual system is similar to that of other sensory systems in the body. They all have receptors that convey information to the brain through a series of neurons. In the eye the photoreceptor cells catch the external information (photons), convert it into a suitable cellular event (a membrane resistance change), and pass the information on to the brain through a series of neurons. In the simplest case the chain is first a bipolar cell (the second order neuron), which is followed by a ganglion cell (see Figures 10-2 and 10-3). Ganglion cells in turn carry the visual information up to the lateral geniculate body in the brain. Finally, the optic tracts carry the sensory impulse to the cerebral cortex. The signals are modified at each synaptic level. In the retina, predominantly static information is processed at the level of the first synapse (which is in the outer plexiform layer), whereas phasic information (movement) is dealt with at the second synapse, in the inner plexiform layer.

The signal does not always take the simplest path conceivable. In the rod pathway (for scotopic vision), the signal is not passed directly from the bipolar cells to the ganglion cells but through an intercalated neuron, the AII amacrine cell (Figure 10-4).

The retinal neurons form a network that permits extensive parallel processing of the visual stimuli, which is a hallmark of all sensory signal handling in the vertebrate nervous system. This makes it possible to derive many different kinds of information from the responses generated by photoreceptor cells, and this information is then sent in parallel channels to the higher visual centers.

The retina has separate channels for detecting the appearance and disappearance of light called the *ON* and *OFF channels*. They enhance the sensory input by providing excitatory signals to the CNS in response to any change in light intensities.

All photoreceptor cells in the vertebrate retina hyperpolarize to light. This is either passed on unchanged in the OFF bipolar cells by a sign-conserving synapse or passed on as a depolarization in the ON bipolar cells by a sign-inverting synapse. In cone pathways these channels often are already apparent at the level of the outer plexiform layer, where cone

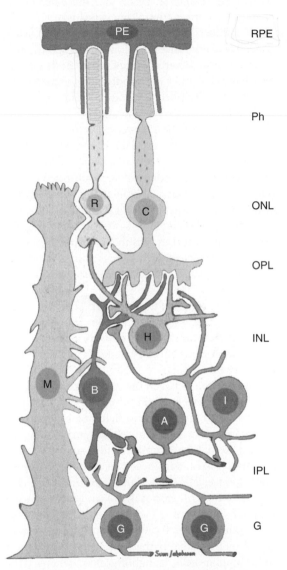

FIGURE 10-3 Schematic representation of different neurons in the retina and glial Müller cells. Cells: *A,* Amacrine cell; *B,* bipolar cell; *C,* cone photoreceptor cell; *G,* ganglion cell; *H,* horizontal cell; *I,* interplexiform cell; *M,* Müller cell; *PE,* pigment epithelium; *R,* rod photoreceptor cell. Layers: *G,* Ganglion cell layer; *INL,* inner nuclear layer; *IPL,* inner plexiform layer; *ONL,* outer nuclear layer (the cell bodies of the rods and cones); *OPL,* outer plexiform layer; *Ph,* photoreceptors (rods and cones); *RPE,* retinal pigment epithelium.

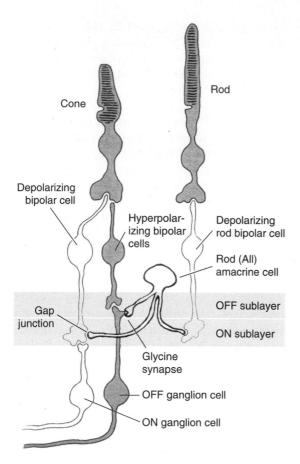

FIGURE 10-4   The pathway from rods to ganglion cells is complex, with the special AII glycinergic amacrine cell intercalated in the pathway. Cells that give depolarizing responses to light are shown as white; those that give OFF responses and hyperpolarize are shaded. Rods connect to specialized rod bipolar cells. When depolarized, these cells excite AII rod amacrine cells. This produces excitation through gap junctions of depolarizing cone bipolar cells (*left*), which influences the ON ganglion cell. At the same time the depolarization of the rod (AII) amacrine cells causes them to release inhibitory transmitter (glycine) onto the OFF-center ganglion cell. The glycinergic AII amacrine cell thus relays rod signals to both ON and OFF ganglion cells. (Redrawn from Daw NW, Jensen RJ, Brunken WJ: *Trends Neurosci* 13:110, 1990.)

cells connect to two types of bipolar cells that have either "flat" (OFF) or "invaginating" (ON) junctions and end up in sublamina *a* (OFF) or *b* (ON) of the inner plexiform layer, respectively. Rods are connected to only one type of bipolar cells, which are depolarizing. In the scotopic vision pathway, the ON/OFF division appears only when the signal is passed on to the ON and OFF cone channels by way of the AII amacrine cells. These cells receive input from the rod bipolar cells and pass it to OFF bipo-

lar cells through a chemical synapse and to the ON bipolar cells through an electrical synapse, a gap junction (see Figure 10-4).

Other vision tasks that are carried in separate channels within the cone pathways are the resolution of fine details in vision and the detection of changes in illumination. This is brought about by the P (midget) and M (parasol) cells; the P system codes for color, and the M system responds to a wide range of other stimulus types. Both systems also have ON and OFF subdivisions according to the scheme described previously. Color opponent mechanisms are likely generated by the ON and OFF channels of the P system. For red and green colors, both the ON and OFF channels have been identified, but these have not been identified for blue. Blue-sensitive cone cells are connected to only one type of bipolar cell, and this channel apparently does not have any OFF ganglion cell channel.

Other parallel signaling systems exist within the retina. One comprises cells that are direction selective, responding to slow velocities of image motion. The major planes for their direction selectivities correspond to the three principal planes of the semicircular canals of the inner ear. This system belongs to the accessory optic system and appears to detect self-motion so that appropriate corrective adjustments can be made for stabilizing the image on the central retina.

Interactions between the various parallel channels in the retina result in the center-surround organization of the receptive fields of bipolar cells and many of the ganglion cells (Figure 10-5). The central area of the receptive field is surrounded by an annular area, and these two areas have opposing responses.[38,83] Center and surround responses attenuate each other, but the central responses are generally dominating (see Figure 10-5). The center responses in the P cells of the primates are generated by the radial pathways (e.g., photoreceptor cells, bipolar cells, ganglion cells), whereas the antagonistic effect of surround illumination is generated in the outer plexiform layer by the inhibitory feedback of horizontal cells on photoreceptor cells.

Histologic Organization of the Retina

Retinal cells and their processes are stratified in 10 layers that can be identified histologically (Figure 10-6):

- The RPE
- The receptor layer comprising the outer and the inner segments of the photoreceptor cells

ON-center cell

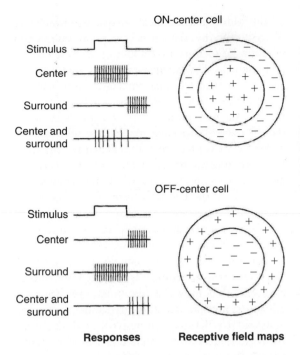

Responses   Receptive field maps

OFF-center cell

FIGURE 10-5 Idealized responses and receptive field maps for ON-center (*top*) and OFF-center (*bottom*) contrast-sensitive ganglion cells. The drawings on the left represent hypothetical responses to a spot of light presented in the center of the receptive field, in the surround of the receptive field, or in both the center and surround regions of the receptive field. A plus (+) symbol on the receptive field map indicates an increase in the firing rate of the cells (excitation); a minus (−) symbol indicates a decrease in the firing rate (inhibition). (From Dowling JE: *The retina: an approachable part of the brain*, Cambridge, 1987, The Belknap Press of the Harvard University Press.)

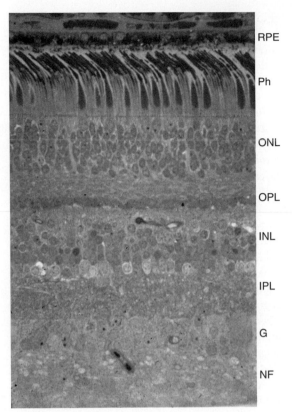

FIGURE 10-6 A radial section through the retina of a macaque monkey near the posterior pole. *G,* Ganglion cell layer; *INL,* inner nuclear layer; *IPL,* inner plexiform layer; *NF,* nerve fiber layer; *ONL,* outer nuclear layer (the cell bodies of the rods and cones); *OPL,* outer plexiform layer; *Ph,* photoreceptors (rods and cones); *RPE,* retinal pigment epithelium. (Courtesy J. Marshall.)

- The outer limiting membrane, which is not a true membrane but a narrow zone with numerous zonulae adherens between Müller cells and between Müller cells and the photoreceptor cells (The membranous appearance is an optical artifact in the light microscope.)
- The outer nuclear layer created by the photoreceptor cell bodies and their processes
- The outer plexiform layer formed by the synapses between photoreceptor cells, bipolar cells, and horizontal cells
- The inner nuclear layer containing the cell bodies of horizontal, bipolar, amacrine, and interplexiform cells and their fibers and the nuclei of the Müller cells
- The inner plexiform layer formed by synapses between bipolar, amacrine, and ganglion cells

- The ganglion cell layer, which also contains numerous "displaced" amacrine cells
- The nerve fiber layer containing axons from ganglion cells on their way to the optic nerve
- The inner limiting membrane formed by the Müller cell endfeet

Retinal Pigment Epithelium. RPE cells (see Figure 10-6) are regularly arranged as hexagonal tiles to form a single-layered cuboidal epithelium separating the photoreceptor outer segments from the choroid. This epithelium supports and maintains the functions of the photoreceptor outer segments. Each eye contains an estimated 4 to 6 million RPE cells. In the central retina the shape and size of the RPE cells are uniform, measuring about 14 μm in diameter. Toward the equator, the RPE cells become thinner and larger, and in the far periphery they lose their size constancy. Some cells may contain more than one nucleus, and at the ora serrata the retinal pigment epithelium cells may measure up to 60 μm in diameter.

The cell membrane of RPE cells is convoluted, with infoldings on their basal sides extending up to 1 μm into the cytoplasm. The basal membrane of these cells is narrowly separated from their basal lamina, which in reality forms the most proximal layer (layer 5) of Bruch's membrane. The basal infoldings increase the surface area of the cell membrane, suggesting that it is involved in transport functions. Facing the photoreceptor outer segments, the apical surfaces of the RPE cells are folded to form the 5- to 7-μm-long microvilli, which extend up to and surround one third of the photoreceptor outer segments. Because the outer segments of rods and cone cells are of different sizes, the villi surrounding the rod outer segments are smaller than those surrounding the cone outer segments. Two types of microvilli surround the rod and cone outer segments: large ones (5 to 7 μm), which extend in between the outer segments, and smaller ones (3 μm), which cover their tips. The microvilli seem to completely isolate the cone outer segments from those of rods.[54] The cytoplasm of RPE cells is laden with round or oval pigmented granules containing melanin, most of which is found on their apical side. Pigment granules can also be found in the villi. The granules measure up to 1 μm in diameter and are 2 to 3 μm long. Pigment granules are tyrosinase positive only in their immature stage, but as they mature, which happens long before birth, the granules become tyrosinase negative. The pigment granules absorb light, thus preventing scattered light or light coming through sclera from reaching the photoreceptor cells. Melanin pigments also scavenge free radicals. RPE cells in the equatorial and macular regions contain more melanin than do those in other regions.[51] There is no difference in the melanin contents in the RPE of Caucasians and those of African descent.[146] The melanin in the RPE cells comes from neuroepithelium, and this source of melanin does not show any racial differences. Choroidal melanin comes from the neural crest, which develops the peripheral nervous system. Melanocytes that derive their pigment from the neural crest and migrate to furnish pigments to skin, hair, and the uvea show a marked racial variance.

The cytoplasm also contains other organelles, especially smooth endoplasmic reticulum. The discs of the photoreceptor outer segments, which are phagocytized by the retinal pigment epithelium villi, can be seen in the cytoplasm of these cells as phagosomes. The phagosomes are gradually digested by the intracellular enzymes, and their end products are either deposited on Bruch's membrane or are retained within the cells as lipofuscin granules. These granules naturally increase with age.[148]

RPE cells contact each other laterally by junctional complexes, which create a diffusion barrier between the choroid and the retina. Toward the apical side of the lateral surface of these cells, the intracellular space of RPE cells is sealed off from the apical space by zonulae occludens and zonulae adherens. Desmosomes are found along the lateral membrane. The cells are also electrically coupled together by gap junctions. Retinal pigment epithelium cells thus have all three functional classes of cell junctions: the occluding type, the anchoring type, and the communicating type. Tight junctions are occluding junctions that play a role in maintaining the concentration difference of small hydrophilic molecules across the RPE sheet. They achieve this by joining the plasma membrane of adjacent cells, thus creating a continuous, impermeable or semipermeable barrier across the epithelium. They also act as a barrier in the lipid layer and restrict the diffusion of membrane transport proteins between the apical and the basolateral parts of RPE cell membranes. Cells are fastened to each other by anchoring junctions made up by zonulae adherens and desmosomes, which are connecting sites for intermediate filaments. There are no tight junctions in RPE on the basal side.

At the optic disc the RPE becomes thinner and terminates slightly before Bruch's membrane does. Peripherally, the RPE becomes continuous with the pigmented epithelium of the ciliary body.

The main functions of RPE include creating a barrier between the choroidal circulation and the retina; transporting ions, water, and metabolites between the retina and the choroid; and phagocytizing the shed-out photoreceptor outer segments. There is an increasing body of evidence that the RPE may also be involved in modulating the intraocular immunity. They also can differentiate into macrophages to remove debris from within the retina. Thus the RPE cells can function as epithelial cells, glial cells, and as macrophages.

Bruch's Membrane. Current work on the pathophysiology of age-related macular degeneration and possible surgical treatments suggests that Bruch's membrane deserves more attention than what it has hitherto received. It consists of five layers and reaches from the optic disc to the ora serrata. Its thickness varies in different parts of the eye; it is thickest in the vicinity of the optic disc (2 to 4 μm) and thinnest (1 to 2 μm) in the periphery.

The basement membrane of the RPE cells forms the innermost layer of Bruch's membrane. This is followed by an inner collagenous zone, an elastic layer, an outer collagenous zone, and finally the basement membrane of the choriocapillaris. Collagen and the elastin are the main structural proteins of Bruch's membrane. Certain kinds of collagens (types I, II, III, V, and XI) aggregate into long fibrils, which assemble into a variety of highly ordered bundles and sheets. Others (types IX and XII) are found on the surface of fibrils and influence their interactions with one another and with other matrix components. Type IV collagen forms sheetlike meshwork. Elastin fibers form an extensive network, imparting elasticity to the membrane. Fibronectin and laminin are large adhesive glycoproteins that, because of their multiple binding sites, help cells adhere to the membrane.

Outer Nuclear Layer. The cell bodies of the photoreceptor cells are located in the outer nuclear layer (see Figure 10-6). Cone perikarya tend to lie in its outermost part. The rod cell bodies outnumber the cone cell bodies in the periphery; the reverse is true for the central retina. In the latter part, the cone cells have oblique axons displacing their cell bodies from their synaptic pedicles in the outer plexiform layer. These oblique axons, with accompanying Müller cell processes, form a pale-staining fibrous-looking area known as the *Henle fiber layer*.

The outer nuclear layer is thickest in the foveal region, where it measures approximately 50 μm and contains approximately 10 rows of cone nuclei, and it becomes progressively thinner toward the periphery. At the nasal edge of the optic disc it is almost as thick as in the foveal region and contains eight to nine rows of nuclei. On the temporal side of the disc, the outer nuclear layer is about half the foveal-region size and contains only four rows of nuclei.

Photoreceptor Cells. Photoreceptor cells are highly specialized and convert light into nerve signals by a process called *phototransduction*. Their distal parts are adapted for capturing the light, and their proximal parts are adapted to transmit it. Two main types exist: rod cells and cone cells. The approximately 92 million rod cells are responsible for vision in dim light, whereas about 5 million cone cells are responsible for vision in bright illumina-

tion, in which color cues are important.[25] All rods contain the same rhodopsin, but human cone cells contain three different opsins sensitive to three different regions of the light spectrum. They have their peak absorptions at 420 (blue), 531 (green), and 588 nm (red).

Photoreceptor cells are organized in fairly exact hexagonal mosaics. Cone cells sensitive to green and red light predominate strongly in the primate foveola, but outside it, rods predominate and their density peaks in a ring at about 4.5 mm or approximately 20 degrees from the foveola (Figure 10-7). Blue-sensitive cone cells are absent from the very center of the foveola but reach their highest abundance on its slopes. The green- and red-sensitive cone cells remain rather evenly spaced throughout the retina but are surrounded by rings of rods.[24] The blue-sensitive cone cells are more unevenly spaced. The optic nerve (the blind spot) is devoid of photoreceptor cells.

The photoreceptor cells consist of a cell body, an outer and an inner segment, and an inner fiber (Figure 10-8). There may also be an outer fiber connecting the cell body to the outer and the inner segments. When no outer fiber is present, the inner segment connects directly with the cell body. The outer and the inner segments of the photoreceptor cells are located between the RPE and the outer limiting membrane. The inner segment is separated from the outer by a narrow connecting stalk, which actually has the structure of a cilium arising from a basal body in the inner segment. Nine cilium tubules arise from the basal body and reach varying distances into the outer segment, some reaching up to the tip. The outer segment is thus a highly modified cilium. From the other side of the cell body the equivalent of an axon, called the *inner fiber* (or *Henle's fiber*), projects to the outer plexiform layer and ends in a synaptic body. The lengths of the outer and the inner fibers vary depending on the position of the cell in the outer nuclear layer.

The cone nuclei are slightly larger than those of rods and contain less heterochromatin, which accounts for their fainter staining. The different kinds of cone cells are morphologically distinguishable in some vertebrates but usually are not in mammals. In humans red- and green-sensitive cone cells are indistinguishable by plain microscopy, but blue-sensitive cone cells can be identified to some extent. They have relatively long inner segments, and their synaptic endings are smaller.[3,113] Their distribution across the retina differs from the regular hexagonal mosaic typical of the other types. It is estimated

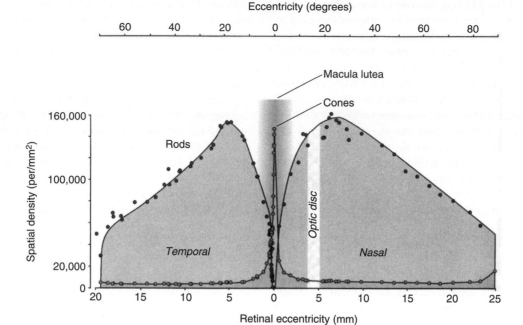

FIGURE 10-7   Rod and cone densities in the human retina. (Redrawn from Rodieck RW: *The first steps in seeing,* Sunderland, Mass, 1998, Sinauer Associates; modified from Sterberg G: *Acta Ophthalmol [Copenh]* 6:1, 1935.)

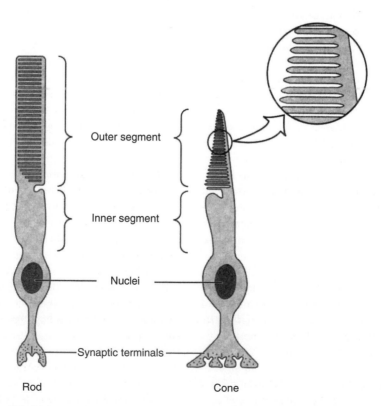

FIGURE 10-8   Simplified schematic representation of a cone and a rod. Light-sensitive visual pigment molecules are present in the membranous discs (rods) or infoldings (cones) of the outer segment regions of the cells. Information is passed on to second-order cells at the synaptic terminal regions of the cell. (From Dowling JE: *Creating mind: how the brain works,* New York, 1998, WW Norton.)

that 10% to 15% of all cone cells are blue sensitive. Agreement has not been reached on the proportions of the red and the green cone cells, but some histochemical studies suggest that approximately 50% to 54% of all cone cells are green sensitive and 33% to 35% are red sensitive.[91] Photoreceptor cells all use glutamate as their neurotransmitter.

The inner segments of cone cells are wider than those of rods, which are longer and cylindrical. The rod inner and outer segments have the same morphology across the retina, but cone outer segments become smaller toward the periphery. The inner segments of foveal cone cells are longer and more slender than those in extrafoveal cone cells.

The inner segments are separated from each other by Müller cell extensions called *fiber baskets*. The inner segments are subdivided into an outer part called the *ellipsoid*, which is joined to the outer segment by the cilium, and an inner part called the *myoid*, which connects with the cell body, directly or with the outer fiber. The ellipsoid is filled with mitochondria, particularly in cone cells, whereas the myoid is rich in glycogen particles and ribosomes. The inner segments synthesize the components for the renewal of the outer segments, and their mitochondria provide the energy required for the phototransduction.

The outer segments of rods are made up of approximately 600 to 1000 discs piled on each other. Each disc is actually a flattened sac made by a lipid membrane. Lobules are located at the rims of the discs and are aligned with each other by small filaments, which connect the discs to each other and to the plasma membrane covering them. Filaments also connect lobules in the same disc.[70]

The proximal third of the outer segments is covered by projections from the inner segments, called *calyces*, whereas the distal part of the outer segments are covered by microvilli from RPE cells. Only the central part of the outer segments has no cytoplasmic covering.

The rod outer segments are highly specialized for capturing photons, and they contain all the molecules needed for converting light into an electrical impulse.[8] The pigment molecule responsible for capturing light, rhodopsin, is embedded in high concentration in the flattened disc membranes. Rhodopsin is also found in the plasma membrane covering the discs, but at much lower concentrations.

Rhodopsin consists of a protein part, opsin, and a chromophore, 11-*cis*-retinal, which is a vitamin A derivative. The protein is made from 349 amino acids and folded so that it passes seven times through the membrane it sits in. Transducin and cyclic guanosine monophosphate (cGMP) phosphodiesterase (PDE), as well as other enzymes involved in the phototransduction cascade, are also thought to be associated with the disc membrane.

In cone cells the photopigment is not stored in membranous discs but rather in invaginations of the cytoplasmic membrane.[40] The outer segments are short in comparison with rods and are broader at the proximal end than at the apical end. They also have a looser contact with the RPE villi than rods have. Like in rods, the chromophore of the cone photopigment is 11-*cis*-retinal, but the opsin moieties differ so that the cone photopigments are maximally sensitive to blue, green, and red light.

The light absorbed by the photoreceptor outer segments also damages them to such an extent that they have to be replaced rapidly. Every morning, the rod outer segments shed their tips, which are then degraded by RPE phagocytosis. New discs are formed as cell membrane invaginations at the base of the outer segment (Figure 10-9). Replacement proteins and other cellular components for accomplishing this are synthesized in the rod inner segments. They are then transported to the outer segment through the cilium. Cone cells are also constantly renewed, in the evening rather than the morning, and less is known about the mechanism involved.

The outer segment regeneration is important for the survival of the photoreceptor cells, and disturbances in it are known to make the cells die. Many aspects of the regeneration remain to be clarified. Evidence exists that in amphibians, rhodopsin and another intrinsic membrane protein, the rim protein peripherin/rds, are carried to the membrane assembly site at the base of the outer segment by transport vesicles.[31] However, such vesicles have not been observed in mammals. Both passive diffusion and different active transport systems have been suggested, and at least one myosin type (VIIa) appears to be involved in the cilium.[89] Mutations in the gene for myosin VIIa result in photoreceptor degeneration of the Usher 1b type.

At the end of the disc generation, the disc rim is formed so that the disc becomes separated from the plasma membrane. This requires cytoskeletal proteins such as actin and actin-binding proteins.[21,22] In addition to rhodopsin, several other proteins are known and required in appropriate locations, including peripherin/rds at the disc rims, the cGMP channel protein in the outer plasma membrane, fodrin (a cytoskeletal protein), and calcium exchange proteins. The mechanisms needed for sorting these proteins to various locations are unknown.

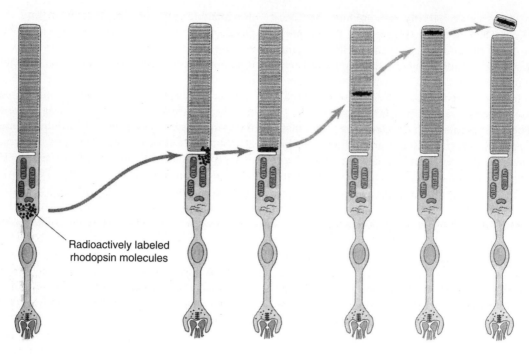

Radioactively labeled
rhodopsin molecules

FIGURE 10-9   Rod photoreceptor renewal. In a now classic experiment, newly formed photoreceptor proteins were radioactively labeled and the radioactivity was found to form a band that appeared first at the base of the outer segments and then moved outward until shed and digested by the retinal pigment epithelium (RPE). (Modified from Rodieck RW: *The first steps in seeing,* Sunderland, Mass, 1998, Sinauer Associates; and Young RW: *Sci Am* 223:81, 1970.)

Mutations in the rhodopsin gene are a common cause of hereditary retinal degenerations, and more than 100 different mutations have now been identified.[28] Some of these may interfere with the transport of the protein, causing membrane instability and photoreceptor death.

Outer Plexiform Layer. Photoreceptor cells form synapses with the bipolar and horizontal cells in the outer plexiform layer. The long Henle fibers make the outer plexiform layer thick (about 50 μm) in the macular region, but in other areas it is only a few microns thick and thins out more toward the periphery (see Figure 10-6). Its most distal part is occupied predominantly by the inner fibers (axons) of the photoreceptor cells. Their synaptic bodies (rod spherules and cone pedicles) occupy the middle of the layer, and dendrites of bipolar and horizontal cells, together with Müller cell processes, occupy the innermost part.

Rod Spherules. Processes from bipolar and horizontal cells invaginate the rod spherules, and the three components form a structure called a *triad,* usually one per spherule (Figure 10-10). The rod spherule contains mitochondria, microtubules, and numerous presynaptic 300- to 500-Å vesicles. A narrow (about 150 Å) synaptic cleft separates the cell's presynaptic and postsynaptic membranes. Inside the spherule there is a sickle-shaped penta-laminar synaptic ribbon, which abuts the synapse and lies perpendicular to the cell surface facing the enclosed postsynaptic nerve processes.[19] Between the ribbon and the cell membrane, there is a dense curved structure called the *arcuate density.* The ribbons and the arcuate densities are surrounded by synaptic vesicles and are involved in the release of neurotransmitters from the synaptic vesicles. The lateral, more deeply inserted processes in the invaginations belong to horizontal cells, and the centrally placed processes belong to rod bipolar cells.[37]

Conventional vesicular neurotransmitter release carries information from the photoreceptor to the postsynaptic bipolar and horizontal cell processes. The latter also pass information to both photoreceptor cells and bipolar cell processes, but the mechanism for this information transfer is not well known.

Cone Pedicles. Cone pedicles have an organization that is similar to that of rod spherules, but they are larger and contain several triads, up to about 25 (see Figure 10-10). The synaptic ribbons are smaller

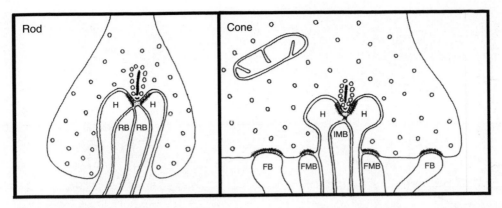

FIGURE 10-10   Schematic drawings showing the arrangements and kinds of junctions made by bipolar cell dendrites and horizontal cell processes with rod (*left*) and cone (*right*) receptor terminals in the primate retina. Horizontal cell processes (*H*) always end laterally and deeper in the invaginations of both the rod and cone terminals. The invaginating midget bipolar dendrites (*IMB*) end as the central element in the cone terminal invaginations, whereas the rod bipolar dendrites (*RB*) end as the central elements in the rod terminal invagination. The flat midget bipolar dendrites (*FMB*) terminate at basal junctions that are close to an invagination, whereas the dendrites of the other flat bipolar cells (*FB*) usually contact the basal surface of the cone terminal somewhat distant from the invaginations. (Redrawn from Dowling JE: *The retina: an approachable part of the brain,* Cambridge, 1987, The Belknap Press of the Harvard University Press.)

and more numerous. This is consistent with the large number of synaptic contacts the cone pedicles make. These are of three types: invaginating contacts (triads), flat surface contacts, and interreceptor contacts.[74] The triads have the organization seen also in rods. The flat surface contacts are shallow indentations by bipolar cell processes in the basal surface of cone pedicles (see Figure 10-10). They have also been called *basal junctions*.[85] Up to 500 such contacts may be seen on each pedicle. No synaptic vesicles or ribbons lie in their vicinity. The membranes of the cone pedicle and the bipolar cell processes are slightly thickened at the site of contacts. The biochemical mechanisms involved in passing the signal at these flat contacts are unknown.

From each pedicle protrudes up to a dozen small lateral extensions (telodendria), which extend to similar expansions of neighboring pedicles or rod spherules. Small gap junctions are present on these telodendria, forming contacts between cone pedicles and between cone pedicles and rod spherules.[116] Tight junctions have also been seen between neighboring telodendria, but no conventional synapses exist between them. Up to about five gap junctions can occur on a single rod spherule from neighboring cone telodendria, and a single cone pedicle can have as many as 10 contacts with the neighboring rods. Blue-sensitive cone cells tend to have fewer such electrical contacts than the other cone types. The anatomic observations have been verified with

electrophysiologic recordings, which prove there are direct electrical contacts between photoreceptor cells; however, the significance of these contacts remains debated.

Inner Nuclear Layer. The inner nuclear layer contains four types of cells: horizontal cells, bipolar cells, amacrine cells, and Müller cells. Horizontal cells are located in the distal part of the inner nuclear layer, whereas amacrine cells are in the most proximal part of this layer. Bipolar cells' and Müller cells' nuclei occupy the outer intermediate and the inner intermediate parts of the layer, respectively. The location of the cells in the different parts of the inner nuclear layer is not strict.

Horizontal Cells. Horizontal cells have long processes that arborize exclusively in the outer plexiform layer. Their dendritic fields increase with eccentricity, but the shapes of the fields remain the same. The narrow single axon of horizontal cells does not transmit any electrical signals, and the telodentric part of the cell is thus electrically insulated from the dendritic part. The mammalian retina has two types of horizontal cells (Figure 10-11). The HII subtype (which is axonless in some mammalian species) contacts cone cells alone. In the other subtype (HI), the dendrites contact the cone cells and the axons of the rods.[12,27,53]

The axon-bearing HI subtype is found in all mammalian retinas and has identical connectivity

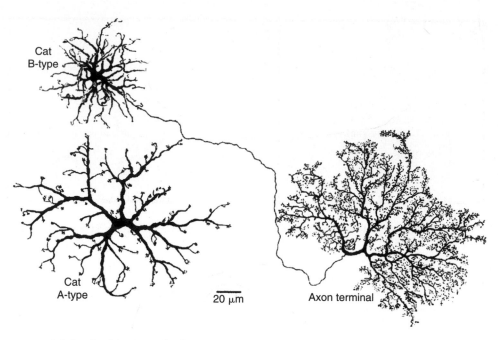

Cat
B-type

Cat
A-type

20 μm

Axon terminal

FIGURE 10-11   Golgi-stained horizontal cells in whole mounted cat retina, one with an axon and one axonless. The axon-bearing (B-type) cell has a dendritic end that is cone connected and an axon-terminal portion contacting rods. The axonless A-type horizontal cells are believed to be cone driven. (From Fisher SK, Boycott BB: *Proc R Soc Lond B Biol Sci* 186:317, 1974.)

and function, regardless of whether the animal has dichromatic or trichromatic vision. The axon in these cells arises from a dendrite and is thin at the origin (0.5 μm in diameter) but increases in thickness as the axon branches out. The axon branches end with clusters of telodendrons, which enter rod triad synapses.[12] The dendrites of the HI horizontal cells radiate in all directions, branch little, and at their terminations give out clusters of small processes with tiny end swellings, which form the lateral processes of cone pedicle triads.

Gap junctions also connect horizontal cells to each other, and proteins called *connexons* are involved in the formation of such contacts. Certain connexons have been identified in nonprimate mammalian retinas, but none have been identified in the human retina. Gap junctions not only form electrical circuits but also allow low-molecular-weight substances to pass from one cell to another. They can be slowly modulated by a number of factors, including dopamine and pH, and the gap junction coupling of horizontal cells is among the first and best examples of this.

Horizontal cells may use GABA as their neurotransmitter. The release mechanism is not the conventional one with synaptic vesicles, but rather

some other form of facilitated transport. Horizontal cells provide inhibitory feedback to photoreceptor cells or inhibitory feed-forward to bipolar cells.

Bipolar Cells.   Bipolar cells carry the signal from photoreceptor cells to ganglion cells or amacrine cells. They are best classified according to anatomic features, and the most important one is whether they contact rods or cone cells (hence the distinction of rod bipolar cells and cone bipolar cells). The dendrites of the rod bipolar cells enter rod triad synapses. In the parafoveal region, rod bipolar cells may contact as many as 18 to 70 rods and have a dendritic field measuring 15 to 30 μm. The cone bipolar cell dendrites make flat contacts (basal junctions) or enter into cone triads as their central element.[12,23,72]

Both rod and cone bipolar cells of the invaginating type mostly send their axons into sublamina *b* of the inner plexiform layer, where the dendrites of ON ganglion cells terminate. Rod bipolar cell axons descend without much branching and extend small numbers of synaptic terminal, called *dyads,* which are postsynaptic at ribbon synapses and contact a pair of amacrine cell processes.[37,119] The axons of bipolar cells that make basal junctions with photoreceptors descend to sublamina *a,* where dendrites of OFF ganglion cells terminate.

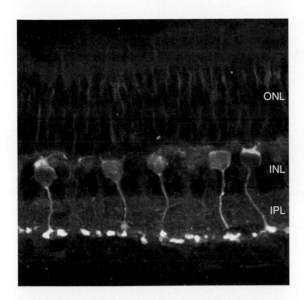

FIGURE 10-12 Fluorescence micrograph of rod bipolar cells labeled with an antibody against PKC, an enzyme which specifically occurs in these cells. Rabbit retina. *INL,* Inner nuclear layer; *IPL,* inner plexiform layer; *ONL,* outer nuclear layer.

Only one variety of rod bipolar cells has been described in mammals, including humans (Figure 10-12), and it is easily identified by its high content of the enzyme protein kinase C (PKC).[58,80] Primate cone bipolar cells can be divided into 8 to 10 different types according to their dendritic branching pattern, the number of cone cells contacted, and the shape and stratification of their processes in the inner plexiform layer.[47]

Only limited information is available concerning the role of the different types of cone bipolar cells of mammalian retinas. About five of them collect information from many cone cells and have been called *diffuse bipolar cells.* Certain bipolar cells contact only a few cone cells each, and in the fovea, bipolar cells contact only a single cone each. These cells are comparatively small and are called *midget bipolar cells.*[11] Each cone contacts an invaginating and a basal junction–type midget bipolar cell. The axons of midget bipolar cells mostly form synapses on a single midget ganglion cell.

Bipolar cells contacting blue-sensitive cone cells are immunoreactive to cholecystokinin. They form triad synapses with one to three such cone cells and reach sublamina *b* of the inner plexiform layer.[81,92]

Diffuse cone bipolar cells make basal junction or triad contacts with a number of cone cells, and their axons terminate in sublamina *a* or *b,* respectively.[72,76]

Giant bipolar cells make flat contacts with large numbers of cone cells, and their axons terminate in both sublaminas of the inner plexiform layer.[92]

Both rod and cone bipolar cells use glutamate for their neurotransmission. Glycine and, to some extent, GABA have also been advocated as bipolar cell neurotransmitters, but the evidence is controversial.

Amacrine Cells. Most amacrine cell neurons are located in the proximal part of the inner nuclear layer, but some can also be found in the ganglion cell layer (in which case they are called *displaced amacrine cells*) or rarely in the inner plexiform layer (in which case they are called *interstitial amacrine cells*). They all modulate signals in the inner plexiform layer and are diverse in both their morphology and neurochemistry.[76] As many as 40 or 50 different types may exist, but only few have been well characterized. The diversity is more pronounced in cold-blooded vertebrates and birds than in mammals.

Broadly, amacrine cells can be classified according to their dendritic field diameters as narrow-field (30 to 150µm), small-field (150 to 300µm), medium-field (300 to 500µm), or wide-field (300 to 500µm) cells. According to the distribution of the dendrites in the inner plexiform layer, they can also broadly be classified as stratified or diffuse. Amacrine cells typically do not have axons, and this is reflected in their name; however, certain large-field amacrine cells of the vertebrate retina can have long axonlike output processes that project exclusively within the retina.[122]

Neuroactive substances detected in amacrine cells include glycine, GABA, acetylcholine, 5-hydroxytryptamine (serotonin), dopamine, nitric oxide (NO), neurotensin, enkephalins, somatostatin, substance P, vasoactive intestinal peptide (VIP), and glucagon. Colocalization of these substances and their morphologic and functional correlation is a useful method for characterizing amacrine cells. The neurochemicals mediate both classical fast neurotransmission and more remanent signal modulation.

Most amacrine cells contain glycine or GABA, two structurally related inhibitory neurotransmitters, and are referred to as *glycinergic* or *GABAergic* amacrine cells. Approximately 40% to 50% of all amacrine cells are likely to be glycinergic (Figure 10-13) and comprise several different morphologic classes.[15,43,76]

One of the best-characterized glycinergic amacrine cells is a narrow-field type called *AII.*[109] As discussed, these cells form an important part of the rod pathway, relaying signals from the rods to ON

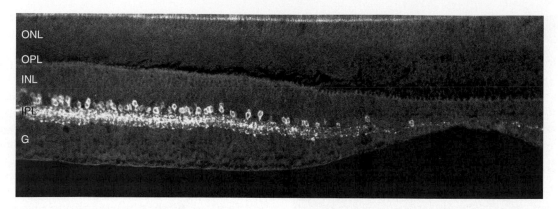

FIGURE 10-13　Fluorescence micrograph of glycinergic neurons in the foveolar region of the squirrel monkey retina, visualized by immunolabeling the glycine transporter GLYT1. Note the high number of neurons and the spread of their processes throughout the inner plexiform layer, which they are restricted to. *G,* Ganglion cell layer; *INL,* inner nuclear layer; *IPL,* inner plexiform layer; *ONL,* outer nuclear layer; *OPL,* outer plexiform layer. (Courtesy K. Warfvinge.)

cone bipolar cells through gap junctions in sublamina *b* and relaying signals to OFF cone bipolar cells through a chemical synapse in sublamina *a*.[76] A large number of AII amacrine cells occur in the retina (10% of all amacrine cells and 25% of the glycinergic amacrine cells in cats), and their fields do not overlap much. AII amacrine cells typically contain the calcium-binding protein calretinin.[142] Each AII amacrine cell in the central retina may receive input from as many as 30 rod bipolar cells.[56,133]

A second type of glycinergic amacrine cells, called DAPI-3 cells, comprise less than 2% of the amacrine cells in rabbits (Figures 10-14 and 10-15). They were the third type of cells identified with the special nuclear dye DAPI (hence the name).[149] They are bistratified and medium-field cells and are similar to the type A8 cell described by Kolb.[77] They appear to have synaptic associations with the cholinergic starburst amacrine cells thought to be involved in the important motion detection system of the retina.

An estimated 40% of the amacrine cells are GABAergic.[2] Small populations of GABA-ergic amacrine cells (approximately 12% of all amacrine cells) are presumed also to use a second neurotransmitter or neuromodulator such as 5-hydroxytryptamine (serotonin), dopamine, acetylcholine, substance P, or NO. All or almost all the substance P–containing cells also contain GABA, but the functional significance of this precise coexistence is unknown.[110] Generally, the GABA-ergic amacrine cells in mammals have medium to wide, overlapping, and stratified fields, contrasting the more narrow fields of most glycinergic amacrine cells. One well-studied and com-

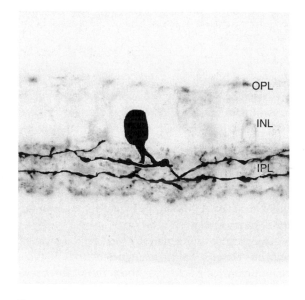

FIGURE 10-14　Schematic drawing of the cell body and distribution of the processes of a glycinergic DAPI-3 cell in the rabbit retina. *INL,* Inner nuclear layer; *IPL,* inner plexiform layer; *OPL,* outer plexiform layer. (Redrawn from Zucker CL, Ehinger B: *J Comp Neurol* 393:309, 1998.)

mon amacrine cell type that contains GABA and also is capable of taking up indoleamines is called *A17*.[44,97,105,127,138] These wide-field cells form reciprocal synapses with the rod bipolar cells in the inner plexiform layer, modifying signal transmission from rod bipolar to AII amacrine cells. They account for most of the reciprocal connections at the rod bipolar dyads.[45,55]

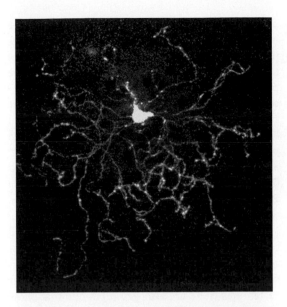

FIGURE 10-15 A DAPI-3 cell in a whole-mounted rabbit retina, injected with Lucifer yellow, showing the characteristic distribution of its undulating and entangled processes. (From Zucker CL, Ehinger B: *J Comp Neurol* 393:309, 1998.)

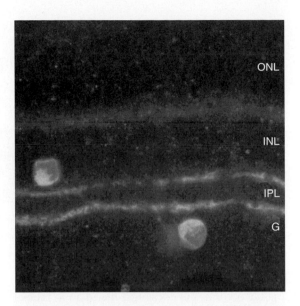

FIGURE 10-16 Confocal micrograph, visualized with choline acetyl transferase (ChAT) immunolabeling, of two cholinergic amacrine cell bodies: one in the position of classic amacrine cells in the inner nuclear layer (*INL*) and the other, a so-called displaced amacrine cell, in the ganglion cell layer (*G*). The inner plexiform layer (*IPL*) contains two narrow bands of cholinergic processes. *ONL,* Outer nuclear layer. (From Zucker CL, Ehinger B: *J Comp Neurol* 393:309, 1998.)

Starburst amacrine cells (Figure 10-16) are the only cholinergic neurons in the retina. They have a characteristic wide-field morphology with radiating dendrites resembling a starburst firecracker (Figure 10-17), and they are found in mirror-image locations in the inner nuclear layer and the ganglion cell layer. Those in the ganglion cell layer are often referred to as *displaced amacrine cells,* which is somewhat inappropriate and misleading because they are not really misplaced. In humans and in cats there are more of these cells in the ganglion cell layer than in the inner nuclear layer.[67] The processes of the starburst cholinergic neurons form two distinct sublayers in the inner plexiform layer.[95,136] In addition to acetylcholine, cholinergic amacrine cells also appear to contain GABA, suggesting that they are both excitatory and inhibitory in function. Starburst amacrine cells are involved in the important motion detection system of the retina, but their exact role in it remains to be established.[5,62]

Dopamine-containing cells are very few (approximately 8000; Figure 10-21), and to cover the entire retinal surface they have long processes.[93] At least two distinct types of dopaminergic neurons can be identified.[7,42,102] Type 1 cells synapse on the numerous AII amacrine cells (in layer 1 of the inner plexiform layer), which form the connecting link

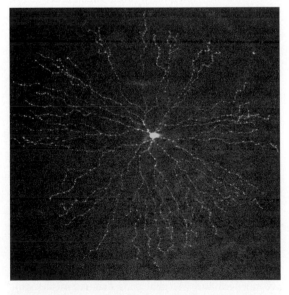

FIGURE 10-17 Confocal micrograph of a cholinergic starburst amacrine cell with its characteristic radiating and dichotomously dividing processes, injected with Lucifer Yellow. (Confocal micrograph, Zucker and Ehinger, unpublished.)

between rod bipolar cells and ganglion cells. Type 1 cells thus seem to modulate the flow of information about scotopic vision, perhaps by regulating the gap junctions of the AII amacrine cells. Type 2 cells arborize in the inner layers of the inner plexiform layer, and some of them may also contain VIP.

NADPH-diaphorase activity is found in amacrine cells that contain nitric oxide synthase (NOS) immunoreactivity.[130] They are therefore presumed to use NO as a neurotransmitter or neuromodulator. Two types of such cells have been identified, but the precise functions of NO in retinal neurotransmission remain to be established.

Somatostatin immunoreactivity is present in certain rare amacrine cells whose processes run for long distances (up to 20 mm in humans). A rabbit retina contains about 1000 such cells.[125,126,147] They mainly occur in the horizontal meridian in rabbits and cats and in the ventral retina in humans. Certain other amacrine cells also have long-range processes like that of somatostatin-containing cells.[26,73,139] The exact role of these cells is not established, but light stimulation of the retina does cause effects far away from the area of stimulation, and the cells with long processes may participate in such activities.[52,82]

Interplexiform Cells. The cell bodies of the interplexiform cells are located in the inner nuclear layer, and they send their processes to both the outer and inner plexiform layers (See Figure 10-3). In the inner plexiform layer, these processes are both presynaptic and postsynaptic to amacrine cells and presynaptic to both rod and the cone bipolar cells. In the outer plexiform layer the cells are presynaptic to rod or cone bipolar cells.[39,79,87,102] They use GABA or dopamine as their neurotransmitter. The interplexiform cells carry feedback signals between the inner plexiform layer and the outer plexiform layer, but further details about their physiology remain to be established.

Glial Cells. Four kinds of glial cells exist in the retina: (1) the Müller cells, which are by far the most numerous; (2) the astrocytes that mainly appear in the innermost parts of the retina; (3) the microglial cells, which are phagocytic, vary considerably in number, and appear whenever and wherever they are needed; and (4) glial cells that surround ganglion cell axons when they are myelinated. In primates the ganglion cell axons normally are myelinated only in the optic nerve.

Müller Cells. Müller cells are the main glial cells of the retina. They extend through the whole thickness of the neural retina, with their perikarya in the inner nuclear layer (see Figure 10-3), and they issue many fine processes, which cover most surfaces of the neuron cell bodies in the nuclear layers. In the plexiform layers, Müller cell processes similarly cover the dendritic processes of the neurons to the synaptic clefts, insulating them both electrically and chemically. In the nerve fiber layer, the Müller cell processes cover most ganglion cell axons.[104] Similarly, blood vessels within the retina are covered by Müller cells. The vessels on the vitreal side of the ganglion cell layer are also covered by astrocytes, which form a second class of glial cells in the retina.

Distally, Müller cells form a series of junctional complexes with themselves and with the photoreceptor cells. In primates these junctional complexes consist mainly of zonulae adherens, but in lower vertebrates there are also gap junctions that allow electrical coupling between the Müller cells.[98,115,118] In the light microscope, these junctional complexes appear like a membrane and therefore somewhat inappropriately but irrevocably are called the *outer limiting membrane*.[16] Müller cells extend beyond the outer limiting membrane into the subretinal space, forming microvilli. Their surface is thereby increased so that they can more easily handle metabolites and ions in the subretinal space. The proximal end of the Müller cells terminate in an expansion called the *endfoot,* which rests on its basal lamina, called the *inner limiting membrane.* Vitreous collagen fibrils merge with this membrane and contribute to its thickness, which is 1 to 2 µm. It covers the whole retina, even the fovea, from the ora serrata to the optic disc.

In addition to the structural support Müller cells offer neurons, these cells regulate the extracellular environment of the retina by buffering the light-evoked variations of particularly the K^+ concentrations in the extracellular space. They also remove glutamate from the extracellular space by active uptake. Specific ion channels and transport systems are located in the specific parts of the Müller cells. The presence of cellular retinol and retinal-binding proteins in them suggests that they may participate in the visual cycle of retinoid metabolism.[9,30,46] Müller cells are thought to perform many of the functions provided in the brain by oligodendroglia and astrocytes, which are absent or at least sparse in mammalian retinas. For instance, they synthesize and store glycogen, and they can provide glucose to the retinal neurons.

Investigations have shown that Müller cells respond to various growth factors and cytokines.

Under normal conditions, RPE cells, retinal neurons, and Müller cells themselves are the source of these molecules. In pathologic conditions molecules from inflammatory cells, platelets, and plasma may activate the receptors in Müller cells, which are likely to play an active role in various pathophysiologic conditions. In response to these stimuli, Müller cells may proliferate, express glial fibrillary acidic protein, induce major histocompatability molecules, and synthesize intracellular adhesion molecules. However, the precise significance of these changes for the pathobiology of the retina is not understood.

Other Glial Cells. Star-shaped astrocytes sparsely occur in the ganglion cell layer and the inner plexiform layers. Their processes contact ganglion cells and capillary surfaces. Most of the astrocytes in the nerve fiber layer send out two types of processes, one around nerve fibers and other to blood vessel walls. These cells also have star-shaped bodies located close to blood vessels. Most of their processes wind around the retinal blood vessels, but some also reach out for the neighboring nerve fibers.[114]

Reticuloendothelial microglial cells normally are found only in small numbers in the nerve fiber layer. However, under pathologic conditions these mobile phagocytic cells can be found anywhere in the retina.

Inner Plexiform Layer. The inner plexiform layer is where bipolar, amacrine, and ganglion cells form connections (see Figures 10-3 and 10-6). Its thickness varies between about 18 and 36 μm, and it is absent in the center of the foveola. Occasional cells found in this layer are either displaced amacrine or displaced ganglion cells, which are then called *interstitial cells.* Rarely, astroglial cells can also be found in it.

Bipolar cell terminals and dendrites of amacrine and ganglion cells branch in different levels of the inner plexiform layer. This results in the division its into five sublamina (S1 to S5), with S1 being the most distal (closest to the scleral) and S5 the most proximal (closest to the vitreous).[122] Rod bipolar cell terminals occupy sublamina S5, whereas those of cone bipolar cells reach sublayers S1 to S4. The inner plexiform layer can also be divided into sublamina *a* (S1 and S2) and *b* (S3-S5), a division first made for cats. The OFF and ON ganglion cell processes occupy the sublamina *a* and *b*, respectively, and the ON/OFF ganglion cells appear in both. The distribution of ON and OFF ganglion cells in different sublamina of the inner plexiform layer demonstrates the anatomic basis of these channels in the retina, but the physiologic implications of this sublayering are not fully understood.

Ultrastructurally, three types of processes and synapses occur in the inner plexiform layer. Bipolar cell processes are rounded and contain an abundance of neurotubules and neurofilaments and only a few mitochondria. Their synapses are characterized by a synaptic ribbon and sometimes also an arcuate density similar to the one seen in photoreceptor triad synapses. The synaptic ribbons are smaller and are surrounded by denser synaptic vesicles than those in photoreceptor triad synapses.[117] No other synapses are known to contain ribbon synapses in the inner plexiform layer. Amacrine cell processes possess electron-microscopic properties of both axons and dendrites; nevertheless they usually can be distinguished from bipolar cell axons. Synaptic vesicles aggregate at the site of synaptic contacts, forming so-called conventional synapses. Ganglion cell dendrites lack specific features and are therefore difficult to identify.

The bipolar ribbon synapses usually have two postsynaptic members: either two amacrine cell processes or one ganglion cell and one amacrine cell process (Figure 10-18). These synapses are called *dyads.*[37] Both the presynaptic and especially the postsynaptic membranes are thickened in dyad synapses. Occasionally, the amacrine cell processes form reciprocal contacts back to the bipolar cell terminals within 0.5 to 1.0 μm of its postsynaptic position. Bipolar cells occasionally form synapses with a single postsynaptic process, which by analogy is called a *monad.* Bipolar cell processes also sometimes make synapses on amacrine cell somata.

Apart from their participation in dyad synapses, amacrine cell processes also often make synapses of the conventional type with bipolar cell processes and their terminals as well as ganglion cell processes or somata. These synapses are similar to the ones found in most other parts of the CNS. They show thickening of the presynaptic and postsynaptic membranes, a widened synaptic cleft, and aggregation of vesicles along the presynaptic membrane (Figure 10-19).

Gap junctions were first noted only occasionally with electron microscopy, but more recent dye injection studies have shown they are a regular and common structure in the inner plexiform layer, joining amacrine cells of like kind.[7] As already described, they also join the AII amacrine cells with bipolar cells.

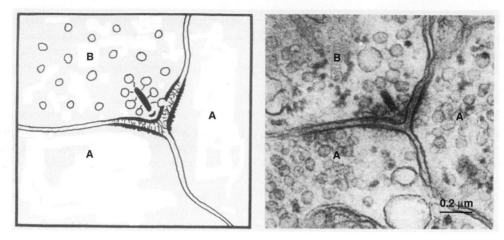

FIGURE 10-18 Drawing and electron micrograph of the characteristic synaptic ribbon in a bipolar cell dyad (*B*) in the inner plexiform layer of a frog retina. Both postsynaptic processes belong to amacrine cells (*A*), and one is making a reciprocal synapse back to the bipolar cell process. (Redrawn from Dowling JE: *The retina: an approachable part of the brain,* Cambridge and London, 1987, The Belknap Press of the Harvard University Press.)

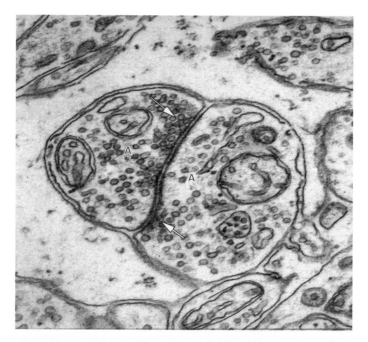

FIGURE 10-19 Two amacrine cell processes (*A*) in the inner plexiform layer of a cynomolgus monkey retina making synaptic contacts with each other (reciprocal synapses; *arrows*). The synapses are of the conventional type, with an accumulation of synaptic vesicles and membrane thickenings at the synaptic sites.

Ganglion Cell Layer. This layer contains ganglion cells and so-called displaced amacrine cells. It is thickest in the macular region, where it measures between 60 and 80 μm and contains 8 to 10 rows of nuclei. In the foveal region this layer is completely lacking. Elsewhere, the ganglion cell layer typically contains a single row of cells and is about 10 to 20 μm thick. On the temporal side of the disc, the ganglion cell layer may contain two rows. Consistent with the distribution of photoreceptor cells, ganglion cells are more densely packed in the central retina than in the peripheral retina.

Ganglion Cells. Ganglion cells are neurons that collect all visual information processed in the retina and send it to the brain. Their perikarya are located mainly in the ganglion cell layer, and their dendrites form synapses with bipolar and amacrine cells in the inner plexiform layer (see Figure 10-3). Rarely, ganglion cells can also be found in the inner nuclear layer or the inner plexiform layer. The axons of ganglion cells form the optic nerve, and they terminate predominantly in the lateral geniculate body or its equivalents. Approximately 10% are estimated to project to subthalamic structures, serving for nonvisual processes such as the pupillary reflexes or the circadian rhythm.[128] Like many long axon cells in the CNS, the ganglion cells use glutamate for their neurotransmission, but some of these cells also contain substance P.[13,18,41] The classification of ganglion cells is both incomplete and confusing, mostly because they have been named differently in different species and because the functional characteristics of various morphologic types of cells are poorly understood.

One type of ganglion cell, which has increasingly become more important and prominent with the evolution of primates, is the midget ganglion cell type. These are small cells that send a single dendritic process to the inner plexiform layer, where they branch in either sublamina *a* or *b*, and in the central retina they make single synapses with midget cone bipolar cells. They are thus each responsible for carrying visual information from a single cone.[75] These cells are also called *P cells* because they project to the parvicellular part of the lateral geniculate body. It is estimated that approximately 80% of the ganglion cells in the monkey retina are of this type.[108] These cells probably carry information regarding form and color perception.

Another type of ganglion cell called *parasol ganglion cells* have a larger cell body. One or more dendrite arising from these cells form a large horizontally spread arbor either in the proximal or the distal part of the inner plexiform layer.[124,143] These cells are conserved across the species. Physiologically, they comprise more than one type of cell. Some of them probably correspond to the blue ON-center ganglion cells. Other parasol ganglion cells seem to receive input from all chromatic types of cone cells and terminate at the magnocellular part of the lateral geniculate body; these are therefore said to be of the M type. They can be identified by neurofibrillar stain, and it is estimated that

they comprise approximately 10% of the ganglion cells. Their wide dendritic fields allow them to cover the entire retina. M ganglion cells respond to moving or changing stimuli and are thus presumably responsible for carrying such information to the brain.

The Nerve Fiber Layer and the Optic Nerve. The axons of ganglion cells form the nerve fiber layer as they converge from all parts of the retina toward the optic disc. As the nerve fibers from different regions of the retina continue joining, the nerve fiber layer becomes thick near the optic disc, where it measures 20 to 30 μm. Peripherally, it becomes thinner, until at the extreme periphery it is indistinguishable. The ganglion cell axons vary in size from 0.6 to 2.0 μm, depending on the size and type of ganglion cell from which they originate.

The ganglion cell axons form small bundles in the nerve fiber layer; these bundles are often surrounded by glial cell processes belonging to Müller cells or astrocytes. Generally, the nerve fibers approach the optic disc radially, but fibers may come from the temporal side arch above or below the fovea. Fibers from the macula and the retina between the macula and the optic disc reach the optic disc in a straight structure called the *maculopapillar bundle*. Because the temporal part of the disc receives nerve fibers only from a small part of the retina, the thickness of the nerve fiber layer is here reduced (10 μm). Nerve fibers in the retina normally are not myelinated, but myelinated fibers can sometimes be seen near the optic disc, an anomaly that is benign.

Rod Photoreceptor Pathways

The rod photoreceptor pathways in the retina are concerned with vision in dim light: scotopic vision. Rods outnumber photoreceptors in most vertebrates by a factor of about 10 to 20, so even though there is a high degree of convergence in the rod pathways, the rod pathway neurons outnumber those of the cone system everywhere but in the central fovea. The convergence is a way of increasing the sensitivity of the system at the expense of resolution. It has been estimated that about 75,000 rod photoreceptors drive 5000 rod bipolar cells and then 250 AII amacrine cells before converging to a single large ganglion cell.*

Some completely nocturnal animals have lost some of their cone types and their associated

---

*References 55, 56, 78, 101, 133, 134.

neurons and rely much more on the rod system than mammals do. Even though humans can do well without scotopic vision, night blindness is a symptom that is prominent enough to make it one of the earliest symptoms that become apparent in children with retinitis pigmentosa.

Morphologically, only a single type of bipolar cell makes connections with rod photoreceptors. Their responses are always of the ON-center depolarizing type, which is mediated predominantly by the metabotropic glutamate receptor, mGluR6.[140] They have a characteristic morphology, which is most easily demonstrated with immunohistochemistry for PKC, which these neurons for unknown reasons selectively contain (see Figure 10-12). Depending on species and retinal location, rod bipolar cells each contact between 15 and 80 rod spherules in the outer plexiform layer, entering the triad as its central element. They send their processes to the inner plexiform layer, where they terminate in the sublayers closest to the ganglion cell bodies. Here they make ribbon synapses in dyads, and the postsynaptic elements are invariably two amacrine cells. There are several such dyads on a single rod bipolar cell terminal, making the system divergent at this level, but it is also convergent in the sense that several rod bipolar cells can contact a given amacrine cell. Most commonly, one of the two postsynaptic elements in a rod bipolar cell dyad is an AII glycinergic amacrine cell and the other is a type A17 indoleamine accumulating reciprocal amacrine cell.[97]

The AII Amacrine Cell Type. The AII amacrine cell is a small-field type that extensively makes gap junctions with cone bipolar cells or other AII amacrine cells in sublamina b[76] (see Figures 10-4 and 10-20). It receives approximately 30% of its input from rod bipolar terminals in lower sublamina b of the inner plexiform layer. Most of its conventional chemical synapses are to center-hyperpolarizing (OFF-center) ganglion cells whose dendrites appear only in sublamina a of the inner plexiform layer.

Rod bipolar cells respond to light with center-depolarizing (ON-center) responses, as do the important subsequent neurons, the AII amacrine cells (see Figure 10-4). This is expected for events in sublamina b of the inner plexiform layer, where ganglion cells also have depolarizing or ON-center responses. The cone bipolar cells contacted by AII amacrine gap junctions are of a variety that synapses with ON-center ganglion cell processes in sublamina b.

The AII cell thus directly drives OFF-center ganglion cells through their conventional synapses in sublamina a and ON-center ganglion cells through their gap junctions with cone bipolar cells that contact the ON-center ganglion cells. The system makes it possible for rod signals to reach both ON- and OFF-center types of ganglion cells. Because the rod photoreceptor system presumably evolved after

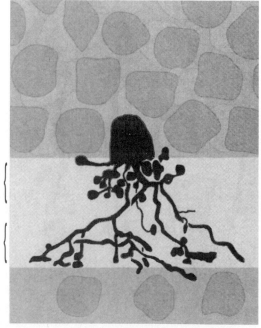

FIGURE 10-20   An AII amacrine cell at 3 mm eccentricity. The cell type is glycinergic and relays rod bipolar cell signals into the cone pathways. It spreads its two kinds of processes to two different parts of the inner plexiform layer. (Modified from Rodieck RW: *The first steps in seeing,* Sunderland, Mass, 1998, Sinauer Associates; after Grünert U, Martin PR: *J Neurosci* 11:2742, 1991.)

Lobular appendages

Dendrites

the cone system, it has been suggested that as the rod pathways evolved, they took advantage of the already-present signal processing systems in the inner plexiform layer by linking to them. As a result, a given ganglion cell can relay the same kind of visual information to the brain regardless of whether it originates in rod or cone cells or both. This appears simpler and better than maintaining separate systems for scotopic and photoptic vision at the inner plexiform and ganglion cell levels.[10]

The Indoleamine Accumulating Amacrine Cell Type (A17). A17 is a wide-field amacrine cell that usually makes reciprocal synapses with the rod bipolar cell terminal in sublamina *b*.[97,100] It is most likely GABA-ergic, but it is also able to accumulate indoleamines selectively; hence it is called an *indoleamine-accumulating cell*. It contacts a large number of bipolar cell terminals, perhaps 1000, but apparently no other cell types. The A17 indoleamine-accumulating neuron thus integrates information of a rather large part of the retina, perhaps setting sensitivity levels over the area it controls. They are very sensitive at low light intensities and respond to light flashes with a center depolarizing response.

Dopaminergic Retinal Neurons. The dopaminergic neurons in humans and Old World monkeys are located almost exclusively in the outermost fifth of the inner plexiform layer, stratum 1 (Figure 10-21). They are sparse but have wide dendritic fields with thin varicose processes than can extend for hundreds of microns.[76,77] Dopaminergic neurons are of type A18. Originally found in the 1960s with formaldehyde-induced dopamine fluorescence, they are now usually demonstrated by immunolabeling for the dopamine-synthesizing enzyme tyrosine hydroxylase, although this procedure may be less specific. Their fine terminals surround cell bodies and dendrites of several different kinds of amacrine cells, most notably the AII and A17 types, which are closely linked to the rod pathways (see previous discussion). Like the indoleamine-accumulating A17 type, the dopaminergic neurons are likely to integrate information over wide regions of the retina. However, they are not as exclusively linked to the rod pathway as the indoleamine-accumulating neurons are.

The dopaminergic neurons most likely close the gap junctions that the AII cells have with each other and with cone bipolar cells in sublamina *b*, perhaps increasing receptive field sizes of ganglion cells under scotopic conditions and increasing the signal gain in the rod pathways.[60,69] Dopaminergic amacrine cells may also modulate the retinal circadian cycle in at least some species.[86,90]

Cone Photoreceptor Pathways
Cone photoreceptor cells contact bipolar cells, which contact ganglion cells, forming a three-neuron chain

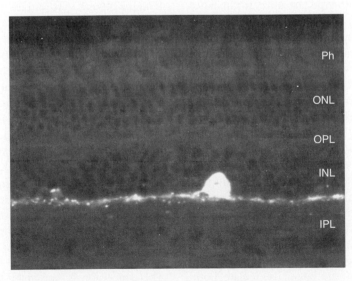

FIGURE 10-21 Dopaminergic amacrine cell and processes in the macaque retina, demonstrated by tyrosine hydroxylase immunohistochemistry. *INL,* Inner nuclear layer; *IPL,* inner plexiform layer; *ONL,* outer nuclear layer; *OPL,* outer plexiform layer; *Ph,* photoreceptors. (From Marshak DW: *Prog Brain Res* 131:83, 2001.)

through the retina (see Figure 10-3). In this respect, the cone pathways are simpler than the rod pathways, which form a four-neuron chain (see Figure 10-4). However, there are three different types of cone cells, which are predominantly sensitive to blue, green, and red light, and cone cells can induce two types of responses in bipolar cells: hyperpolarization or depolarization. In this respect, the cone pathways are more complicated than the rod pathways, in which there is only one kind of bipolar cell. Furthermore, the pathways for blue-sensitive cone cells are different from those for the other two types.

Cone cells elicit two fundamentally different responses in bipolar cells: They either hyperpolarize or depolarize. Cone bipolar cells thus come in two varieties according to how they respond: the OFF-center hyperpolarizing and the ON-center depolarizing ones. Different kinds of glutamate receptors (ionotropic and metabotropic) are responsible for the two response types. The OFF receptors are ionotropic and typically sensitive to AMPA (α-amino-3-hydroxy-5-methyl-4-isoxazole proprionic acid) or kainate and occur in bipolar cells that make basal junctions with cone cells.[32] These bipolar cells have electrical responses similar to those in their photoreceptors (i.e., they are of OFF-center [center-hyperpolarizing] types). The synapse is said to be sign conserving. In the inner plexiform layer, OFF-center bipolar cells have their terminals in sublamina *a*, where OFF–ganglion cell processes occur.

The ON receptors are metabotropic, predominantly of the mGluR6 type (sensitive, for instance, to APB), and occur in bipolar cells that contact photoreceptors in triad synapses in rod and cone cells. This synapse is sign inverting, and the bipolar cells are of ON-center (center-depolarizing) types. In the inner plexiform layer, ON-center bipolar cells have their terminals in sublamina *b*, where ON–ganglion cell processes occur.

The Midget Cell System. Obtaining the highest possible resolution requires that foveal cone cells connect to a system of small bipolar and ganglion cells, forming the midget cell system. The convergence of this system is small and is absent in the absolute center of the fovea. The low degree of convergence is also maintained by the midget ganglion cells, each of which project to an individual parvocellular layer cell of the lateral geniculate body. Midget ganglion cells thus belong to the P-cell class. The foveal cone cells need to elicit responses in both OFF and ON bipolar cells, so each connects to

one of each type, which contact one OFF and one ON midget ganglion cell. With this organization, each foveal midget path carries information exclusively for either the green or the red color vision channel.

In monkey retinas, midget ganglion cells respond to light with an opponent chromatic center-surround organization. If the center shows red-sensitive cone ON responses, there is an inhibitory surround provided by green-sensitive cone cells and vice versa. There may be a similar color-opponency system for blue and yellow, although less evidence exists to support this idea. The midget ganglion cells are small, and their receptive fields are also always small. It is apparent that the midget pathways are important for both high-resolution vision and color vision.

Gross Anatomy and Histologic Correlations

In the vertebrate retina the photoreceptor cells are located near the RPE and the nerve fiber layer is located near the vitreous; the vertebrate retina is therefore said to be an inverted retina. Some invertebrate retinas (e.g., in the squid) are not inverted. Even though the squid eye resembles a mammalian eye, the two have evolved differently and independently. Therefore light entering the mammalian eye has to pass through the whole thickness of the retina to reach the photosensitive part of the photoreceptor cells. This is not necessarily a disadvantage. For instance, the retinal ganglion cells and, to some extent, the bipolar cells contain pigments (mainly two carotenoids: lutein and zeaxanthine) that protect retinal neurons against oxidative stress, which is especially intense in the center of the tissue. The pigments are found throughout the retina, but they are most concentrated in its central region, which is therefore called the *macula lutea.* Macroscopically, this is a spot about 5 to 6 mm in diameter, subtending a visual field of about 18 degrees.

The central part of the retina is most important for visual functions and therefore has certain structural modifications. The *fovea centralis* is a small depression measuring approximately 1.5 mm in diameter at the edge and approximately 400 μm at the floor; it sustains an angle of 5 degrees at the nodal point of the eye. The posterior focal point of the optical system of the eye lies within this area. The depression is caused by centrifugal displacement of the cells of the inner retina. This highly specialized area of the retina is designed for the highest visual acuity. It is rod free and extends approximately 500 to 700 μm. Blue-sensitive cone cells are absent from the centralmost part of the fovea, probably as an adaptation to minimize the effects of chromatic aberrations. The term *foveal vision* refers to the vision brought about by the rod-free area of the fovea.

Cone cells in the fovea centralis have elongated outer segments, so they resemble rods. No blood vessels reach the fovea, and the foveal cone cells are thus exclusively nourished by the choriocapillaris.

The resolving power of the fovea depends (among other things) on the density of the photoreceptor cells or the mosaic formed by the inner segments.[99] In humans the inner segments of foveal cone cells make a triangular lattice and have a diameter of 1.6 to 2.2 μm with a minimal center-to-center spacing of about 2.5 μm.[65] Even 1.25 to 2.5 degrees outside the foveal center, as the rods start appearing, the mosaic becomes more irregular, but not random.[66] Away from the center, their number rapidly increases.

The parafoveal and perifoveal regions surround the fovea. The parafoveal region extends up to about 1.25 mm and the perifoveal region to about 2.75 mm from the center of the fovea. The density of cone cells decreases with increasing eccentricity, whereas that of rods increases sharply. The density of rods reaches 100,000 rods/mm² at a distance of 1.2 to 1.7 mm away from the foveal center. The parafoveal region has a large accumulation of cells in the inner nuclear and the ganglion cell layers. The ganglion cell layer becomes single layered at the end of perifovea, which also marks the end of the central retina.

Aging Changes

In the neural retina the most important age changes take place in the Müller cells and the axons of the ganglion cells forming the optic nerve. A number of ultrastructural and functional changes have been described in Müller cells, which also become hypertrophic with increasing age.[14,106] In the optic nerve the number of nerve fibers decreases and are replaced by connective tissue.[33] Hyaline bodies (corpora amylacea) appear in the peripapillary nerve fiber layer, optic nerve head, and optic nerve.[6] Ganglion cells and bipolar cells accumulate lipids.

An estimated one third to one half of the neurons in the CNS may be lost during the human life span.[63,145] It therefore appears reasonable to assume that the number of retinal neurons also decreases with age, but for obvious technical reasons counting them in the same primate eye at different times is almost impossible, which affects the reliability of the counts. Some studies suggest that the foveal cone cells decrease in number with age.[24,48,151]

An age-dependent displacement of the photoreceptor nuclei from their normal location to the inner segments has been described.[57,84] The inner segment of cone cells will accumulate lipofuscins, which are lipid oxidation end products.[68,137] They are stored in lysosomal residual bodies. The photoreceptor outer segments tend to become convoluted with age, possibly because aging RPE cells are progressively unable to phagocytize the photoreceptor outer segments properly.[94]

The RPE cells exhibit obvious signs of aging. This happens because these cells not only have to deal with the wastes of their own already high metabolism but also have to take the burden of removing the outer segments of photoreceptor cells. When unable to cope properly, the aging RPE cells accumulate abnormal molecules that result from incomplete digestion, such as lipofuscin. This further interferes with the metabolism of the cells, which develops into a vicious circle and causes the loss of photoreceptor cells.[34,141] Waste products from the RPE are partially deposited on the basal lamina and Bruch's membrane in the form of drusen.[1,4,59,150]

The number of RPE cells in the central retina decrease and become pleomorphic with age.[34,144] Other changes in the RPE are also common. These changes include atrophy and depigmentation, as well as hyperplasia, hypertrophy, and cell migration. The melanin concentration in the RPE cells decreases with age, particularly in Caucasians but also in persons of African descent. The melanin granules are slowly (over decades) digested by lysosomes.[17,49,51,146]

Debris deposits from RPE cells as the result of aging are prominent in Bruch's membrane and start to appear already in childhood.[17] At this age only occasional deposits are seen in the inner collagenous zone of the membrane. With age, deposits become more frequent and can be found in the outer layers of Bruch's membrane.[50] This results in a thickening of Bruch's membrane, hyalinization, and basophilia.[71] The lipid contents of Bruch's membrane increase throughout life.[107]

REFERENCES

1. Abdelsalam A, Del Priore L, Zarbin MA: Drusen in age-related macular degeneration: pathogenesis, natural course, and laser photocoagulation-induced regression, *Surv Ophthalmol* 44:1, 1999.

2. Agardh E et al: GABA immunoreactivity in the retina, *Invest Ophthalmol Vis Sci* 27:674, 1986.

3. Ahnelt PK, Kolb H, Pflug R: Identification of a subtype of cone photoreceptor, likely to be blue sensitive, in the human retina, *J Comp Neurol* 255:18, 1987.

4. Anderson DH et al: Local cellular sources of apolipoprotein E in the human retina and retinal pigmented epithelium: implications for the process of drusen formation, *Am J Ophthalmol* 131:767, 2001.

5. Ariel M, Daw NW: Pharmacological analysis of directionally sensitive rabbit retinal ganglion cells, *J Physiol (Lond)* 324:161, 1982.

6. Avendano J et al: Corpora amylacea of the optic nerve and retina: a form of neuronal degeneration, *Invest Ophthalmol Vis Sci* 19:550, 1980.

7. Baldridge WH, Vaney DI, Weiler R: The modulation of intercellular coupling in the retina, *Semin Cell Dev Biol* 9:311, 1998.

8. Baylor DA: Photoreceptor signals and vision: proctor lecture, *Invest Ophthalmol Vis Sci* 28:34, 1987.

9. Bok D, Ong DE, Chytil F: Immunocytochemical localization of cellular retinol binding protein in the rat retina, *Invest Ophthalmol Vis Sci* 25:877, 1984.

10. Boycott B, Wässle H: Parallel processing in the mammalian retina: the proctor lecture, *Invest Ophthalmol Vis Sci* 40:1313, 1999.

11. Boycott BB, Dowling JE: Organization of the primate retina: light microscopy, *Philos Trans R Soc Lond Biol* 255:109, 1969.

12. Boycott BB, Kolb H: The horizontal cells of the rhesus monkey retina, *J Comp Neurol* 148:115, 1973.

13. Brecha NC et al: Identification and localization of biologically active peptides in the vertebrate retina, *Progr Retinal Res* 3:185, 1984.

14. Bringmann A et al: Age- and disease-related changes of calcium channel-mediated currents in human Muller glial cells, *Invest Ophthalmol Vis Sci* 41:2791, 2000.

15. Bruun A, Ehinger B: Uptake of certain possible neurotransmitters into retinal neurons of some mammals, *Exp Eye Res* 19:435, 1974.

16. Bunt-Milam AH et al: Zonulae adherentes pore size in the external limiting membrane of the rabbit retina, *Invest Ophthalmol Vis Sci* 26:1377, 1985.

17. Burns RP, Feeney-Burns L: Clinico-morphologic correlations of drusen of Bruch's membrane, *Trans Am Ophthalmol Soc* 78:206, 1980.

18. Canzek V et al: In vivo release of glutamate and aspartate following optic nerve stimulation, *Nature* 293:572, 1981.

19. Carter-Dawson L et al: Structural and biochemical changes in vitamin A-deficient rat retinas, *Invest Ophthalmol Vis Sci* 18:437, 1979.

20. Catsicas S, Catsicas M, Clarke PG: Long-distance intraretinal connections in birds, *Nature* 326:186, 1987.

21. Chaitin MH: Immunogold localization of actin and opsin in rds mouse photoreceptors, *Prog Clin Biol Res* 314:265, 1989.

22. Chaitin MH, Burnside B: Actin filament polarity at the site of rod outer segment disk morphogenesis, *Invest Ophthalmol Vis Sci* 30:2461, 1989.

23. Cohen E, Sterling P: Convergence and divergence of cones onto bipolar cells in the central area of cat retina, *Philos Trans R Soc Lond B Biol Sci* 330:323, 1990.

24. Curcio CA et al: Distribution of cones in human and monkey retina: individual variability and radial asymmetry, *Science* 236:579, 1987.

25. Curcio CA et al: Human photoreceptor topography, *J Comp Neurol* 292:497, 1990.

26. Dacey DM: Monoamine-accumulating ganglion cell type of the cat's retina, *J Comp Neurol* 288:59, 1989.

27. Dacheux RF, Raviola E: Horizontal cells in the retina of the rabbit, *J Neurosci* 2:1486, 1982.

28. Daiger SP, Sullivan LS, Rossiter BJ: Laboratory for the Molecular Diagnosis of Inherited Eye Diseases: Retnet— cloned and/or mapped genes causing retinal diseases. Available at: http://www.sph.uth.tmc.edu/Retnet/. Accessed April 2002.

29. Daw NW, Jensen RJ, Brunken WJ: Rod pathways in mammalian retinae, *Trends Neurosci* 13:110, 1990.

30. de Leeuw AM et al: Immunolocalization of cellular retinol-, retinaldehyde- and retinoic acid-binding proteins in rat retina during pre- and postnatal development, *J Neurocytol* 19:253, 1990.

31. Deretic D, Papermaster DS: Polarized sorting of rhodopsin on post-Golgi membranes in frog retinal photoreceptor cells, *J Cell Biol* 113:1281, 1991.

32. Devries SH, Schwartz EA: Kainate receptors mediate synaptic transmission between cones and 'Off' bipolar cells in a mammalian retina, *Nature* 397:157, 1999.

33. Dolman CL, McCormick AQ, Drance SM: Aging of the optic nerve, *Arch Ophthalmol* 98:2053, 1980.

34. Dorey CK et al: Cell loss in the aging retina: relationship to lipofuscin accumulation and macular degeneration, *Invest Ophthalmol Vis Sci* 30:1691, 1989.

35. Dowling JE: *The retina: an approachable part of the brain,* Cambridge, 1987, The Belknap Press of the Harvard University Press.

36. Dowling JE: *Creating mind: how the brain works,* New York, 1998, WW Norton.

37. Dowling JE, Boycott BB: Organization of the primate retina: electron microscopy, *Proc Roy Soc (Lond) Ser B* 166:80, 1966.

38. Dowling JE, Boycott BB: Retinal ganglion cells: a correlation of anatomical and physiological approaches, *UCLA Forum Med Sci* 8:145, 1969.

39. Dowling JE, Ehinger B: Synaptic organization of the amine-containing interplexiform cells of the goldfish and cebus monkey retinas, *Science* 188:270, 1975.

40. Eckmiller MS: Distal invaginations and the renewal of cone outer segments in anuran and monkey retinas, *Cell Tissue Res* 260:19, 1990.

41. Ehinger B: Glutamate as a retinal neurotransmitter. In Osborne NN, Weiler R (eds): *Neurobiology of the inner retina,* Berlin-Heidelberg, 1989, Springer-Verlag.

42. Ehinger B, Falck B: Morphological and pharmacohistochemical characteristics of adrenergic retinal neurons of some mammals, *Albrecht Von Graefes Arch Klin Exp Ophthalmol* 178:295, 1969.

43. Ehinger B, Falck B: Autoradiography of some suspected neurotransmitter substances: GABA glycine, glutamic acid, histamine, dopamine, and L-dopa, *Brain Res* 33:157, 1971.

44. Ehinger B, Florén I: Indoleamine-accumulating neurons in the retina of rabbit, cat and goldfish, *Cell Tissue Res* 75:37, 1976.

45. Ehinger B, Holmgren I: Electron microscopy of the indoleamine-accumulating neurons in the retina of the rabbit. *Cell Tissue Res* 197:175, 1979.

46. Eisenfeld AJ, Bunt-Milam AH, Saari JC: Immunocytochemical localization of retinoid-binding proteins in developing normal and RCS rats, *Prog Clin Biol Res* 190:231, 1985.

47. Euler T, Wässle H: Immunocytochemical identification of cone bipolar cells in the rat retina, *J Comp Neurol* 361:461, 1995.

48. Farber DB et al: Distribution patterns of photoreceptors, protein, and cyclic nucleotides in the human retina, *Invest Ophthalmol Vis Sci* 26:1558, 1985.

49. Feeney L: Lipofuscin and melanin of human retinal pigment epithelium: fluorescence, enzyme cytochemical, and ultrastructural studies, *Invest Ophthalmol Vis Sci* 17:583, 1978.

50. Feeney-Burns L, Ellersieck MR: Age-related changes in the ultrastructure of Bruch's membrane, *Am J Ophthalmol* 100:686, 1985.

51. Feeney-Burns L, Hilderbrand ES, Eldridge S: Aging human RPE: morphometric analysis of macular, equatorial, and peripheral cells, *Invest Ophthalmol Vis Sci* 25:195, 1984.

52. Fischer B, Kruger J: Continuous movement of remote patterns and shift-effect of cat retinal ganglion cells, *Exp Brain Res* 40:229, 1980.

53. Fisher SK, Boycott BB: Synaptic connections made by horizontal cells within the outer plexiform layer of the retina of the cat and the rabbit, *Proc R Soc Lond B Biol Sci* 186:317, 1974.

54. Fisher SK, Steinberg RH: Origin and organization of pigment epithelial apical projections to cones in cat retina, *J Comp Neurol* 206:131, 1982.

55. Freed MA, Smith RG, Sterling P: Rod bipolar array in the cat retina: pattern of input from rods and GABA-accumulating amacrine cells: *J Comp Neurol* 266:445, 1987.

56. Freed MA, Sterling P: The ON-alpha ganglion cell of the cat retina and its presynaptic cell types, *J Neurosci* 8:2303, 1988.

57. Gartner S, Henkind P: Aging and degeneration of the human macula. 1. Outer nuclear layer and photoreceptors, *Br J Ophthalmol* 65:23, 1981.

58. Greferath U, Grunert U, Wässle H: Rod bipolar cells in the mammalian retina show protein kinase C-like immunoreactivity, *J Comp Neurol* 301:433, 1990.

59. Hageman GS, Mullins RF: Molecular composition of drusen as related to substructural phenotype, *Mol Vis* 5:28, 1999.

60. Hampson EC, Vaney DI, Weiler R: Dopaminergic modulation of gap junction permeability between amacrine cells in mammalian retina, *J Neurosci* 12:4911, 1992.

61. Hatta K, Takeichi M: Expression of N-cadherin adhesion molecules associated with early morphogenetic events in chick development, *Nature* 320:447, 1986.

62. He S, Jin ZF, Masland RH: The nondiscriminating zone of directionally selective retinal ganglion cells: comparison with dendritic structure and implications for mechanism, *J Neurosci* 19:8049, 1999.

63. Henderson G, Tomlinson BE, Gibson PH: Cell counts in human cerebral cortex in normal adults throughout life using an image analysing computer, *J Neurol Sci* 46:113, 1980.

64. Hendrickson AE, Yuodelis C: The morphological development of the human fovea, *Ophthalmology* 91:603, 1984.

65. Hirsch J, Hylton R: Quality of the primate photoreceptor lattice and limits of spatial vision, *Vision Res* 24:347, 1984.

66. Hirsch J, Miller WH: Does cone positional disorder limit resolution? *J Opt Soc Am A* 4:1481, 1987.

67. Hutchins JB: Acetylcholine as a neurotransmitter in the vertebrate retina, *Exp Eye Res* 45:1, 1987.

68. Iwasaki M, Inomata H: Lipofuscin granules in human photoreceptor cells, *Invest Ophthalmol Vis Sci* 29:671, 1988.

69. Jensen RJ, Daw NW: Effects of dopamine and its agonists and antagonists on the receptive field properties of ganglion cells in the rabbit retina, *Neuroscience* 17:837, 1986.

70. Kajimura N, Harada Y, Usukura J: High-resolution freeze-etching replica images of the disk and the plasma membrane surfaces in purified bovine rod outer segments, *J Electron Microsc (Tokyo)* 49:691, 2000.

71. Killingsworth MC: Age-related components of Bruch's membrane in the human eye, *Graefes Arch Clin Exp Ophthalmol* 225:406, 1987.

72. Kolb H: Organization of the outer plexiform layer of the primate retina: electron microscopy of Golgi-impregnated cells, *Phil Trans Roy Soc (Lond) Ser B* 258:261, 1970.

73. Kolb H: The morphology of the bipolar cells, amacrine cells and ganglion cells in the retina of the turtle Pseudemys scripta elegans, *Philos Trans R Soc Lond B Biol Sci* 298:355, 1982.

74. Kolb H: The architecture of functional neural circuits in the vertebrate retina: the proctor lecture, *Invest Ophthalmol Vis Sci* 35:2385, 1994 (published erratum appears in *Invest Ophthalmol* 35:3576, 1994).

75. Kolb H, Dekorver L: Midget ganglion cells of the parafovea of the human retina: a study by electron microscopy and serial section reconstructions, *J Comp Neurol* 303:617, 1991.

76. Kolb H, Fernandez E, Nelson R: The organization of the vertebrate retina. Available at: http://webvision.med.utah.edu/. Accessed April 2002.

77. Kolb H, Linberg KA, Fisher SK: Neurons of the human retina: a Golgi study, *J Comp Neurol* 318:147, 1992.

78. Kolb H, Nelson R: OFF-alpha and OFF-beta ganglion cells in cat retina: II. Neural circuitry as revealed by electron microscopy of HRP stains, *J Comp Neurol* 329:85, 1993.

79. Kolb H, West RW: Synaptic connections of the interplexiform cell in the retina of the cat, *J Neurocytol* 6:155, 1977.

80. Kolb H, Zhang L, Dekorver L: Differential staining of neurons in the human retina with antibodies to protein kinase C isozymes, *Vis Neurosci* 10:341, 1993.

81. Kouyama N, Marshak DW: Bipolar cells specific for blue cones in the macaque retina, *J Neurosci* 12:1233, 1992.

82. Kruger J, Fischer B, Barth R: The shift-effect in retinal ganglion cells of the rhesus monkey, *Exp Brain Res* 23:443, 1975.

83. Kuffler SW, Nicholls JG: *From neuron to brain: a cellular approach to the function of the nervous system,* Sunderland, Mass, 1976, Sinauer Associates.

84. Lai YL et al: Subretinal displacement of photoreceptor nuclei in human retina, *Exp Eye Res* 34:219, 1982.

85. Lasansky A: Basal junctions at synaptic endings of turtle visual cells, *J Cell Biol* 40:577, 1969.

86. Li L, Dowling JE: Effects of dopamine depletion on visual sensitivity of zebrafish, *J Neurosci* 20:1893, 2000.

87. Linberg KA, Fisher SK: An ultrastructural study of interplexiform cell synapses in the human retina, *J Comp Neurol* 243:561, 1986.

88. Linberg KA, Fisher SK: A burst of differentiation in the outer posterior retina of the eleven-week human fetus: an ultrastructural study, *Vis Neurosci* 5:43, 1990.

89. Liu X et al: Myosin VIIa, the product of the Usher 1B syndrome gene, is concentrated in the connecting cilia of photoreceptor cells, *Cell Motil Cytoskeleton* 37:240, 1997.

90. Mangel SC, Wang Y: Dopamine acts as a circadian clock effector by activating D4 receptors in fish retina, *Soc Neurosci Abstr* 21:903, 1995.

91. Marc RE, Sperling HG: Chromatic organization of primate cones, *Science* 196:454, 1977.

92. Mariani AP: Bipolar cells in monkey retina selective for the cones likely to be blue-sensitive, *Nature* 308:184, 1984.

93. Mariani AP, Kolb H, Nelson R: Dopamine-containing amacrine cells of rhesus monkey retina parallel rods in spatial distribution, *Brain Res* 322:1, 1984.

94. Marshall J et al: Convolution in human rods: an ageing process, *Br J Ophthalmol* 63:181, 1979.

95. Masland RH, Mills JW, Hayden SA: Acetylcholine-synthesizing amacrine cells: identification and selective staining by using radioautography and fluorescent markers, *Proc R Soc Lond B Biol Sci* 223:79, 1984.

96. Matsunaga M et al: Guidance of optic nerve fibres by N-cadherin adhesion molecules, *Nature* 334:62, 1988.

97. Menger N, Wässle H: Morphological and physiological properties of the A17 amacrine cell of the rat retina, *Visual Neurosci* 17:769, 2000.

98. Miller RF, Dowling JE: Intracellular responses of the Müller (glial) cells of mudpuppy retina: their relation to b-wave of the electroretinogram, *J Neurophysiol* 33:323, 1970.

99. Miller WH, Bernard GD: Averaging over the foveal receptor aperture curtails aliasing, *Vision Res* 23:1365, 1983.

100. Nelson R, Kolb H: A17: a broad-field amacrine cell in the rod system of the cat retina, *J Neurophysiol* 54:592, 1985.

101. Nelson R, Kolb H, Freed MA: OFF-alpha and OFF-beta ganglion cells in cat retina. I: Intracellular electrophysiology and HRP stains, *J Comp Neurol* 329:68, 1993.

102. Nguyen-Legros J, Versaux-Botteri C, Savy C: Dopaminergic and GABAergic retinal cell populations in mammals, *Microsc Res Tech* 36:26, 1997.

103. O'Leary DD, Fawcett JW, Cowan WM: Topographic targeting errors in the retinocollicular projection and their elimination by selective ganglion cell death, *J Neurosci* 6:3692, 1986.

104. Ogden TE: Nerve fiber layer of the primate retina: thickness and glial content, *Vision Res* 23:581, 1983.

105. Osborne NN, Beaton DW: Direct histochemical localisation of 5,7-dihydroxytryptamine and the uptake of serotonin by a subpopulation of GABA neurones in the rabbit retina, *Brain Res* 382:158, 1986.

106. Paasche G et al: Mitochondria of retinal Müller (glial) cells: the effects of aging and of application of free radical scavengers, *Ophthalmic Res* 32:229, 2000.

107. Pauleikhoff D et al: Aging changes in Bruch's membrane: a histochemical and morphologic study, *Ophthalmology* 97:171, 1990.

108. Perry VH, Oehler R, Cowey A: Retinal ganglion cells that project to the dorsal lateral geniculate nucleus in the macaque monkey, *Neurosci* 12:1101, 1984.

109. Pourcho RG, Goebel DJ: A combined Golgi and autoradiographic study of (3H)glycine-accumulating amacrine cells in the cat retina, *J Comp Neurol* 233:473, 1985.

110. Pourcho RG, Goebel DJ: Colocalization of substance P and gamma-aminobutyric acid in amacrine cells of the cat retina, *Brain Res* 447:164, 1988.

111. Provis JM, van Driel D: Retinal development in humans: the roles of differential growth rates, cell migration and naturally occurring cell death, *Aust NZ J Ophthalmol* 13:125, 1985.

112. Provis JM et al: Development of the human retina: patterns of cell distribution and redistribution in the ganglion cell layer, *J Comp Neurol* 233:429, 1985.

113. Pum D, Ahnelt PK, Grasl M: Iso-orientation areas in the foveal cone mosaic, *Vis Neurosci* 5:511, 1990.

114. Ramirez JM et al: Structural specializations of human retinal glial cells, *Vision Res* 36:2029, 1996.

115. Rasmussen KE: The Müller cell: a comparative study of rod and cone retinas with and without retinal vessels, *Exp Eye Res* 19:243, 1974.

116. Raviola E, Gilula NB: Gap junctions between photoreceptor cells in the vertebrate retina, *Proc Natl Acad Sci USA* 70:1677, 1973.

117. Raviola E, Raviola G: Structure of the synaptic membranes in the inner plexiform layer of the retina: a freeze-fracture study in monkeys and rabbits, *J Comp Neurol* 209:233, 1982.

118. Raviola G: The structural basis of the blood-ocular barriers, *Exp Eye Res* 25(suppl):27, 1977.

119. Raviola G, Raviola E: Light and electron microscopic observations on the inner plexiform layer of the rabbit retina, *Am J Anat* 120:403, 1967.

120. Regan BC et al: Fruits, foliage and the evolution of primate colour vision, *Philos Trans R Soc Lond B Biol Sci* 356:229, 2001.

121. Rhodes RH: A light microscopic study of the developing human neural retina, *Am J Anat* 154:195, 1979.

122. Rodieck RW: *The vertebrate retina,* San Francisco, 1973, WH Freeman.

123. Rodieck RW: *The first steps in seeing,* Sunderland, Mass, 1998, Sinauer Associates.

124. Rodieck RW, Binmoeller KF, Dineen J: Parasol and midget ganglion cells of the human retina, *J Comp Neurol* 233:115, 1985.

125. Sagar SM: Somatostatin-like immunoreactive material in the rabbit retina: immunohistochemical staining using monoclonal antibodies, *J Comp Neurol* 266:291, 1987.

126. Sagar SM, Marshall PE: Somatostatin-like immunoreactive material in associational ganglion cells of human retina, *Neuroscience* 27:507, 1988.

127. Sandell JH, Masland RH: A system of indoleamine-accumulating neurons in the rabbit retina, *J Neurosci* 6:3331, 1986.

128. Schiller PH, Malpeli JG: Properties and tectal projections of monkey retinal ganglion cells, *J Neurophysiol* 40:428, 1977.

129. Sharma RK, Ehinger B: Mitosis in developing rabbit retina: an immunohistochemical study, *Exp Eye Res* 64:97, 1997.

130. Sharma RK, Perez MT, Ehinger B: Immunocytochemical localisation of neuronal nitric oxide synthase in developing and transplanted rabbit retinas, *Histochem Cell Biol* 107:449, 1997.

131. Silver J, Hughes AF: The role of cell death during morphogenesis of the mammalian eye, *J Morphol* 140:159, 1973.

132. Silver J, Rutishauser U: Guidance of optic axons in vivo by a preformed adhesive pathway on neuroepithelial endfeet, *Dev Biol* 106:485, 1984.

133. Sterling P, Freed MA, Smith RG: Architecture of rod and cone circuits to the *on*-beta ganglion cell, *J Neurosci* 8:623, 1988.

134. Sterling P et al: Microcircuitry of the on-beta ganglion cell in daylight, twilight, and starlight, *Neurosci Res Suppl* 6:S269, 1987.

135. Takeichi M: The cadherins: cell-cell adhesion molecules controlling animal morphogenesis, *Development* 102:639, 1988.

136. Tauchi M, Masland RH: The shape and arrangement of the cholinergic neurons in the rabbit retina, *Proc R Soc Lond* 223:101, 1984.

137. Tucker GS: Refractile bodies in the inner segments of cones in the aging human retina, *Invest Ophthalmol Vis Sci* 27:708, 1986.

138. Vaney DI: Morphological identification of serotonin-accumulating neurons in the living retina, *Science* 233:444, 1986.

139. Vaney DI, Peichl L, Boycott BB: Neurofibrillar long-range amacrine cells in mammalian retinae, *Proc R Soc Lond Ser B Biol Sci* 235:203, 1988.
140. Vardi N et al: Localization of mGluR6 to dendrites of ON bipolar cells in primate retina, *J Comp Neurol* 423:402, 2000.
141. Wassell J et al: The photoreactivity of the retinal age pigment lipofuscin, *J Biol Chem* 274:23828, 1999.
142. Wässle H et al: The rod pathway of the macaque monkey retina: identification of AII-amacrine cells with antibodies against calretinin, *J Comp Neurol* 361:537, 1995.
143. Watanabe M, Rodieck RW: Parasol and midget ganglion cells of the primate retina, *J Comp Neurol* 289:434, 1989.
144. Watzke RC, Soldevilla JD, Trune DR: Morphometric analysis of human retinal pigment epithelium: correlation with age and location, *Curr Eye Res* 12:133, 1993.
145. Weale RA: Senile changes in visual acuity, *Trans Ophthalmol Soc U K* 95:36, 1975.
146. Weiter JJ et al: Retinal pigment epithelial lipofuscin and melanin and choroidal melanin in human eyes, *Invest Ophthalmol Vis Sci* 27:145, 1986.
147. White CA et al: Somatostatin-immunoreactive cells in the adult cat retina, *J Comp Neurol* 293:134, 1990.
148. Wing GL, Blanchard GC, Weiter JJ: The topography and age relationship of lipofuscin concentration in the retinal pigment epithelium, *Invest Ophthalmol Vis Sci* 17:601, 1978.
149. Wright LL et al: The DAPI-3 amacrine cells of the rabbit retina, *Vis Neurosci* 14:473, 1997.
150. Young RW: Pathophysiology of age-related macular degeneration, *Surv Ophthalmol* 31:291, 1987.
151. Yuodelis C, Hendrickson A: A qualitative and quantitative analysis of the human fovea during development, *Vision Res* 26:847, 1986.
152. Zhao S, Thornquist SC, Barnstable CJ: In vitro transdifferentiation of embryonic rat retinal pigment epithelium to neural retina, *Brain Res* 677:300, 1995.
153. Zucker CL, Ehinger B: Gamma-aminobutyric acid A receptors on a bistratified amacrine cell type in the rabbit retina, *J Comp Neurol* 393:309, 1998.

CHAPTER 11

THE RETINAL PIGMENT EPITHELIUM

MORTEN LA COUR

The retinal pigment epithelium (RPE) is a monolayer of cuboidal epithelial cells that separates the photoreceptors from their choroidal blood supply. The human RPE incorporates approximately 3.5 million epithelial cells arranged in a regular hexagonal pattern. The RPE cell density is approximately 5000 cells/mm^2 in the fovea. In the periphery the RPE cell density is lower, approximately 2000 cells/mm^2. The individual peripheral RPE cells are larger and more pleomorphic than central cells.[34] In the primate retina, each RPE cell faces 30 to 40 photoreceptors, a number that is rather constant throughout the retina.[70,86] In fully developed primate retinas, no mitoses are seen in the RPE and the epithelium is believed to consist of a stable, nondividing pool of cells.[78]

The retinal membrane of the RPE forms numerous long microvilli that interdigitate with the rod outer segments (Figure 11-1). In mammals, the cone outer segments are ensheathed by multilamellar specializations of RPE retinal membrane, the so-called cone sheaths.[77] The epithelial cells are bound together by junctional complexes with prominent tight junctions. These junctions divide the cells in an apical half that faces the retina and a basal half that faces the choroid.[36] The nucleus and numerous mitochondria are located in the basal half of the cell. Numerous pigment granules, located predominantly in the apical cytoplasm, give the epithelium its macroscopic black appearance, from which it derives its name.[12]

The choroidal side of the RPE resides on Bruch's membrane, which is a pentilaminar elastic membrane that is approximately 2 μm thick. The innermost part of Bruch's membrane is the basement membrane of the RPE. The outer part of Bruch's membrane is the basement membrane of the choriocapillaries. Between are two collagenous layers and a central elastic layer.[32]

The retinal side of the epithelium faces the subretinal space, which is the extracellular space that surrounds the outer and inner segments of the photoreceptors (see Figure 11-1). The outer border of the subretinal space is formed by the tight junctions of the RPE. These effectively hinder diffusion of water-soluble substances between the subretinal space and extracellular space of the choroid.[67,80] The external limiting membrane constitutes the internal border of the subretinal space. This membrane is freely permeable to molecules with diameters of less than 30 Å, but it restricts diffusion of larger molecules such as albumin, γ-globulin, and interphotoreceptor matrix retinoid-binding protein (IRBP) (see later discussion).[14] The subretinal space is no actual cleft but is a domain at the level of the photoreceptor outer segments with more loosely organized extracellular space than the narrow clefts that separate the densely packed cells in the inner retina. The subretinal space is filled with the interphotoreceptor matrix, which consists of a combination of proteins and proteoglycans.[33] Apart from the interphotoreceptor matrix, no anatomic contacts exist between the photoreceptors and the RPE. Under the pathologic condition of retinal detachment, fluid accumulates within the subretinal space and the photoreceptors become separated from the RPE. This causes a loss of photoreceptor function, which is potentially reversible, if the nor-

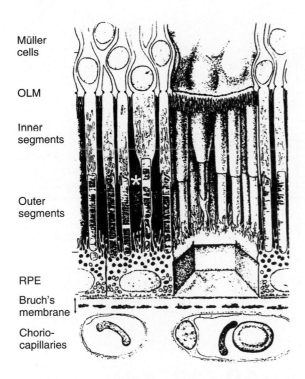

Müller cells

OLM

Inner segments

Outer segments

RPE

Bruch's membrane

Chorio-capillaries

FIGURE 11-1   Diagram of the subretinal space showing the relationship between the retinal pigment epithelium (*RPE*), the outer and inner segments of the photoreceptors, the outer limiting membrane (*OLM*), Bruch's membrane, and the choriocapillaries. The *asterisk* denotes the subretinal space. (From Steinberg RH, Linsenmeier RA, Griff ER: *Vision Res* 23:1315, 1983.)

mal anatomic contacts between the neurosensory retina and the RPE can be restored.

RPE FUNCTION

Both photoreceptors and choriocapillaries depend on the RPE for their survival. If the RPE is destroyed by chemical or mechanical means, the photoreceptors and the choriocapillaries atrophy.[21,42] The RPE produces a host of cytokines, including basic fibroblast growth factor (bFGF), which has been shown to promote survival of photoreceptors in an animal model of retinal dystrophy (RCS rats).[26] Despite considerable progress in the study of RPE cytokines, it is still not clear which of the many compounds secreted by the RPE are important for the survival of photoreceptors and choriocapillaries in vivo.[15]

The retinal pigment epithelial cells mainly function as supportive cells for the photoreceptors. The best studied of these supportive functions are the participation of the RPE in photoreceptor outer segment renewal, the storage and metabolism of vi-

tamin A, and the transport and barrier functions of the epithelium. These three aspects of RPE physiology are discussed in later sections.

Other, less-well-characterized functions of the RPE are the absorption of stray light by the melanin pigment in the epithelium, the scavenging of free radicals by the melanin pigment, and the drug detoxification by the smooth endoplasmic reticulum cytochrome P-450 system found in RPE cells.[12,73]

Photoreceptor Outer Segment Turnover

It has been known for more than 20 years that the outer segments of both rod and cone photoreceptors undergo continuous renewal. New membrane material is added at the base of the outer segments, and old membrane material is removed from the tip of the outer segments by RPE phagocytosis.[6,88] RPE phagocytosis is important for photoreceptor survival. In RCS rats, RPE phagocytosis of outer segment material is defective. In these rats, rod outer segments become elongated with debris piling up in the subretinal space. After postnatal day 15, progressive photoreceptor death and retinal dystrophy are apparent.[18,64]

In rods the rate of membrane renewal can be followed by pulse labeling with radioactive amino acids and subsequent autoradiography.[85] The radioactive label is incorporated in the discs as a reaction band that can be followed as it travels outward through the rod outer segments (Figure 11-2). From this type of experiment, it can be assessed that the renewal time for rod outer segments in rhesus monkeys is 13 days in the parafoveal region and 9 days in the peripheral retina.[87] A similar outer segment renewal process takes place in cones. However, contrary to the situation in rods, the rate of cone outer segment membrane renewal cannot be assessed by pulse labeling and autoradiography. Evidence from phagosome counts suggest that the rate of outer segment renewal is slower in cones than in rods.[4] Outer segment disc shedding is characterized by a circadian rhythm. In rods a burst of disc shedding and phagocytosis occurs in the morning, immediately after light onset.[48] In cones there seems to be some species variability in the pattern of disc shedding.[6] In rhesus monkeys, a burst of disc shedding is associated with light onset, although discs are also shed during the dark period in this species.[4]

The amount of membrane material ingested and degraded by the RPE cells is impressive. According to a quantitative study in the rhesus monkey, it can be calculated that, every day, each extrafoveal RPE cell must ingest and degrade a vol-

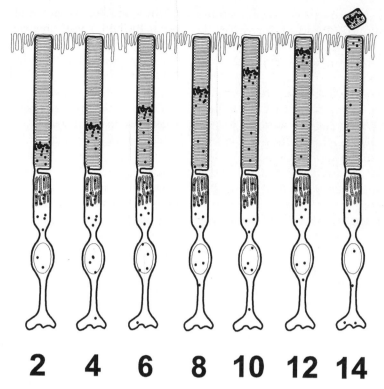

FIGURE 11-2   Diagram of parafoveal primate rod outer segment renewal. At day 0, radioactive-labeled leucine was injected intravenously. Numbers below each rod indicate days after injection of label. Based on the autoradiographic studies of Young.The actual experiments included measurements after 2 and 4 days. (Modified from Young RW: *Invest Ophthalmol Vis Sci* 15:700, 1976.)

ume of rod outer segment material that corresponds to 7% of the volume of the RPE cell itself.[86] Because the RPE cells normally do not divide, the burden of membrane material that these cells must ingest and degrade in their lifetime far exceeds that of any other phagocytic cell.[78] Probably as a consequence of this massive phagocytic load on the RPE cells, lipofuscin granules accumulate with age in these cells.[24] Exocytosis through the RPE choroidal cell membrane of lipofuscin and other waste products of phagocytosis may lead to the accumulation of hydrophobic material in Bruch's membrane and reduced water permeability of this membrane.[60] Early accumulation of lipofuscin in the RPE is seen in Stargardt's disease, which is a macular dystrophy caused by a defective *ABCR* gene.[3] The *ABCR* gene product seems to be involved in the transfer of all-*trans-retinal* from the disc lumen and into the cytosol of outer segments in rods. Accumulation of indigestible retinoid metabolites in the rods has been hypothesized as the cause of the excess RPE lipofuscin accumulation in this disease.[10]

Retinoid Metabolism and the Visual Cycle

The RPE plays an important role in uptake, storage, and metabolism of vitamin A and related compounds—the so-called retinoids. It has been known for more than 100 years that photoreception involves bleaching of the visual pigments and that the RPE is required for the regeneration of these pigments.[59] The underlying mechanisms are now known in considerable detail.[17,68,71] The retinoid 11-*cis*-retinaldehyde is the chromophore of the visual pigments in mammals. When light is absorbed in a photoreceptor, the visual pigments are degraded and the chromophore is converted to all-*trans*-retinol, which finds its way to the RPE.[22] Within the RPE, all-*trans*-retinol is reisomerized to 11-*cis*-retinol and oxidized to 11-*cis*-retinaldehyde, which is then transported back to the photoreceptor outer segments. The light-induced movement of retinoids between the photoreceptors and the RPE and the involved transformations between the different retinoids is denoted as the *visual cycle*.[68]

Retinol enters the retina through the choroidal membrane of the RPE. It circulates in the blood bound to a small (21-kD) carrier protein, serum *retinol-binding protein* (RBP), which is complexed to another and larger protein, *transthyretin*.[74] Autoradiographic studies have demonstrated specific membrane binding sites for RBP on the RPR choroidal membrane.[11] However, the receptor has not been identified with certainty, and the retinol uptake mechanism in the RPE choroidal membrane remains to be elucidated.[17] Retinol also enters the RPE cell through the retinal membrane of the epithelium. The all-*trans*-retinol that is liberated from the outer segments is shuttled to the RPE through the subretinal space. The extracellular protein that carries retinoids through the subretinal space is probably the IRBP, which is a large extracellular protein of approximately 135 kD. IRBP is the most abundant protein in the subretinal space and is capable of binding retinol and retinal in both their all-*trans* and their 11-*cis* configurations.* The role of IRBP as the obligate carrier of retinoids in the subretinal space has been challenged by a recent report, in which the kinetics of retinoid transfer between the RPE and the neurosensory retina was studied in mice with a targeted disruption of the *IRBP* gene (*IRBP*−/− gene knockout mice). It was found that the kinetics of 11-cis-retinal and visual pigment (rhodopsin) recovery after a flash of light was only marginally slower in IRBP−/− mice than in normal wild-type mice.[66]

The fate of retinol inside the RPE cell has recently been reviewed and is illustrated in Figure 11-3.[9,17] Once inside the RPE cell, the retinol is bound to a small (16-kD) carrier protein, cellular retinol-binding protein (CRBP), which is a relative ubiquitous protein, not specific for the RPE. To be isomerized to the 11-*cis* isomer, all-*trans*-retinol must first be esterified because the retinol ester rather than the retinol itself is the substrate for the isomerization reaction.[5] The esterification is catalyzed by a lecithin/retinol acyltransferase (LRAT). The acyl group is derived from lecithin, a membrane phospholipid. The retinyl ester is a stable, nontoxic form of the retinoid that can be stored in the RPE cell or that can act as a substrate for the isomerohydrolase enzyme that catalyzes the combined hydrolysis of the ester bond and isomerization of the all-*trans*-retinol to 11-*cis*-retinol. The energy-rich ester bond in the retinyl ester provides the energy required for the isomerization.[23,68] The isomerohydrolase enzyme has not been purified or cloned. Once 11-*cis*-retinol is formed,

it is bound by the cellular retinaldehyde-binding protein (CRALBP), a 36-kD protein localized mainly in RPE cells and Müller cells. It binds retinol and retinal, but only in their 11-*cis* configurations. 11-*cis*-retinol can be reesterified by LRAT and stored in the RPE cell as 11-*cis*-retinyl ester, or it can be oxidized to 11-*cis*-retinal by 11-*cis*-retinol dehydrogenase. While bound to CRALBP, 11-*cis*-retinaldehyde travels to the retinal membrane of the RPE cell from where it is released. The mechanism for this is unclear.

Another protein thought to be involved in retinoid metabolism is RPE65, a microsomal protein exclusively found in the RPE. Reports concerning the necessity of this protein for the reisomerization of all-*trans*-retinoid to 11-*cis*-retinoid are conflicting.[19,69]

Proteins involved in retinoid metabolism seem to be important for photoreceptor survival. Lack of IRBP causes early-onset photoreceptor death in *IRBP*−/− mice.[53,66] IRBP abnormality may be the cause of some forms of human autosomal recessive retinitis pigmentosa.[81] Defects in *RPE65* cause an early-onset autosomal recessive retinitis pigmentosa in humans and retinal dystrophy in the Briard-Beagle dog.[31,55,82] In humans, mutations in the *RLBP1* gene that encodes CRALBP seems to be a rare cause of autosomal recessive retinal degeneration of the retinitis punctata albescens phenotype.[63]

Transport

The vertebrate outer retina is avascular, and the choriocapillary layer is the main source of oxygen and nutrients for the photoreceptors. The RPE is interposed between the choriocapillary layer and the photoreceptors, and it controls the exchange of water-soluble nutrients and metabolites between the choroid and the subretinal space. The epithelial cells exert this control because tight junctions bind the cells together and effectively hinder transfer of water-soluble compounds between the cells (i.e., via the paracellular route).

In vitro experiments have shown that the RPE has a retina-positive transepithelial potential between 2 and 15 mV. This potential is responsible for the cornea-positive standing potential of the eye, which can be recorded by direct current (DC) electroretinography.[29] The transepithelial electrical resistance across isolated RPE preparations has been measured to be between 79 and 350 Ω cm.[2,39] The isolated epithelium in vitro absorbs Na^+, Cl^-, HCO_3^-, and K^+. The transepithelial transport of these ions has been studied extensively in isolated

---

*References 1, 13, 16, 17, 47, 52.

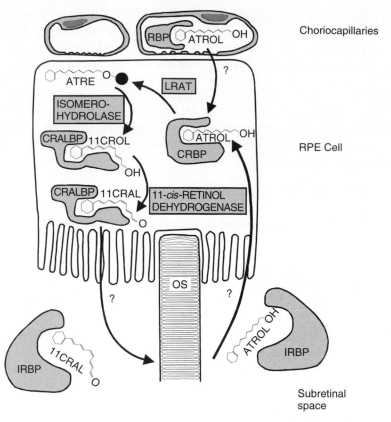

Choriocapillaries

RPE Cell

Subretinal space

FIGURE 11-3 Diagram of retinoid trafficking in and around the retinal pigment epithelium (*RPE*) cell. *ATRE,* All-*trans*-retinylester; *ATROL,* all-*trans*-retinol; *11CRAL,* 11-*cis*-retinal; *CRALBP,* cellular retinaldehyde-binding protein; *CRBP,* cellular retinol-binding protein; *11CROL,* 11-*cis*-retinol; *IRBP,* interphotoreceptor matrix retinoid-binding protein; *LRAT,* lechitin/retinol acyl transferase; *OS,* photoreceptor outer segment; *RBP,* retinol-binding protein. (Modified from Bok D: *J Cell Sci* 17[suppl]:189, 1993.)

preparations of frog and bovine RPE. In both preparations, several transport mechanisms have been identified in the RPE membranes, and models that explain quantitatively the transepithelial transport of the major ions in these species have been proposed[39,45] (Figure 11-4). The retinal membrane of the RPE incorporates an electrogenic Na^+/K^+ pump that pumps Na^+ out the cell and K^+ into the cell at the expenditure of metabolic energy.[62] The Na^+/K^+ pump lowers the intracellular activity of Na^+ below the electrochemical equilibrium for this ion. Secondary active transport systems use the energy invested in the inwardly directed Na^+ gradient to drive transport of other ions. The retinal membrane incorporates three such secondary active transport systems: (1) an $Na^+/K^+/2Cl^-$ cotransport system, (2) an Na^+/H^+ exchange mechanism, and (3) an $Na^+/2HCO_3^-$ cotransport system.* These

transport systems accumulate Cl^- and HCO_3^- intracellularly above their electrochemical equilibrium. The choroidal membrane incorporates a Cl^- conductance that serves as an exit mechanism for this ion.[30,41,44] Bicarbonate exit is mediated by Cl^-/HCO_3^- exchangers in the RPE choroidal membrane.[51] Most of the potassium that is pumped into RPE cells is recycled across the retinal membrane, probably through an adenosine triphosphate (ATP)–dependent, inward-rectifying K^+ conductance.[37,38,46,72] Some potassium exits the RPE cells through a smaller K^+ conductance in the choroidal membrane.[61]

Other transport mechanisms, including transport systems for lactic acid, glucose, γ-aminobutyric acid (GABA), ascorbic acid, fluorescein, and amino acids, have also been described in the RPE.[39] The absorption of fluorescein by the RPE can be assessed noninvasively in humans with vitreous fluorophotometry. This method may yield clinically

*References 2, 8, 40, 41, 43, 44, 50.

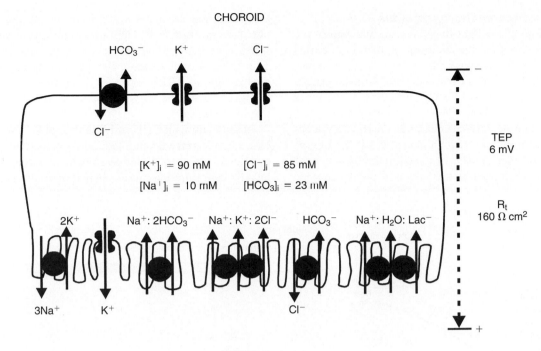

CHOROID

RETINA

Figure 11-4 Model of mammalian retinal pigment epithelium (RPE) ion transport mechanisms. The retinal membrane incorporates an active Na^+/K^+ pump, a K^+ channel, $Na^+/2HCO_3^-$ cotransport system, an $Na^+/K^+/2Cl^-$ cotransport system, a Cl^-/HCO_3^- exchange mechanism, and an $Na^+/water/lactate$ cotransport mechanism. The choroidal membrane incorporates a K^+ channel, a Cl^- channel, and a Cl^-/HCO_3^- exchange mechanism. There are yet uncharacterized efflux mechanisms for Na^+, HCO_3^-, lactate, and water across the choroidal membrane. This model shows the intracellular concentrations of the major ions in mammalian RPE cells. Also shown are the transepithelial potential *(TEP)* and the transepithelial electrical resistance across the epithelium R_t. (Modified from Hughes BA, Gallemore RP, Miller SS: Transport mechanisms in the retinal pigment epithelium. In Marmor MF, Wolfensberger TJ [eds]: *The retinal pigment epithelium: function and disease,* New York, 1998, Oxford University Press.)

valuable information about the health of the RPE in patients with retinal disease.[25]

The RPE from several species has been shown to absorb water.[39] This is consistent with the clinical experience that fluid under a rhegmatogenous retinal detachment is absorbed once the holes in the neurosensory retina are surgically closed. The rate of subretinal fluid resorption across the entire RPE in this setting has been estimated to be 2 ml per 24 hours. This corresponds to more than 50% of the aqueous secretion in that period.[56] This rate of water transport is probably not present under physiologic conditions.[79] Nevertheless, the RPE has a large reserve capacity for removal of excess fluid from the subretinal space.[56] The RPE water transport may have a role in the maintenance of normal retinal adhesion by exerting suction on the neurosensory retina. However, other mechanisms also seem to contribute to retinal adhesion.[57,58] In vivo experiments show that the carbonic anhydrase inhibitor acetazolamide stimulates

fluid absorption across the RPE, but the mechanism behind this is not understood.[39,58]

The mechanisms underlying RPE water transport have only begun to be elucidated. It is a clinical experience, confirmed in laboratory experiments, that subretinal fluid can be absorbed despite a high protein content.[56] Proteinaceous retinal exudates can eventually be dehydrated to the extent that lipoprotein crystals precipitate in the retina as the so-called hard exudates.[20] Proposed mechanisms for RPE fluid transport must therefore be able to account for the apparent ability of the RPE to transport fluid against an osmotic gradient. An $H^+/lactate$ cotransport system in the retinal membrane of frog RPE has been shown to be linked to water transport at the molecular level. This $H^+/lactate/water$ cotransport system has been shown in vitro to be able to transport water into the RPE cells against an osmotic gradient.[89] However, the physiologic significance of this finding is uncertain at present.

Light-Induced Responses of the RPE

Because of the light-dependent metabolism of the photoreceptors, the composition of the subretinal space is affected by light. In dark-adapted retinas the dark current of the photoreceptors demands a high rate of active Na^+/K^+ pumping in the inner segments of these cells. Light onset causes a decrease in the dark current and, consequently, a decrease in the rate of photoreceptor Na^+/K^+ pumping and metabolism. In the subretinal space, light onset is followed by a decrease in the K^+ concentration, an increase in pH, and a decrease in the lactate concentration.[65,83,84] Light onset also causes an increase in the volume of the subretinal space.[49] The RPE responds to these changes, and some of the light-induced RPE responses generate electrical changes that can be measured with electroretinographic techniques.[29]

In the mammalian retina the subretinal K^+ concentration decreases from 5 to 2 mM within 10 seconds after light onset.[76] This decrease in the extracellular K^+ concentration causes a hyperpolarization of

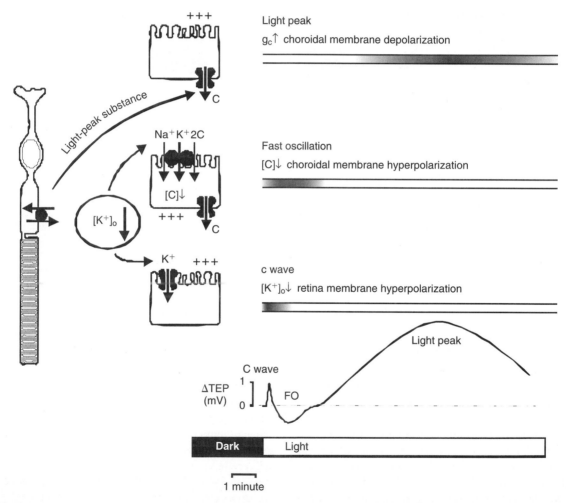

FIGURE 11-5 Diagram of three light-induced responses of the retinal pigment epithelium (RPE). The changes in the transepithelial potential (*ΔTEP*) across the RPE is shown as it develops after light onset. Initially, the cornea-positive c wave is generated by a hyperpolarization of the membrane potential across the RPE retinal membrane. The c wave is terminated by the cornea-negative fast oscillation (FO) that is generated by a delayed hyperpolarization of the membrane potential across the RPE choroidal membrane. The light peak is apparent after several minutes and is generated by delayed depolarization of the membrane potential across the RPE choroidal membrane. The c wave and the FO are consequences of the light-induced decrease in the K^+ concentration in the subretinal space, and it can be reproduced in isolated RPE preparations in vitro after a reduction in the retinal extracellular K^+ concentration. The light peak is caused by a "light-peak substance" secreted by the neuroretina after light onset. The light-peak substance has remained elusive, and the light peak has not been reproduced in vitro in the absence of the neuroretina.

membrane potential across the predominantly K^+ permeable retinal membrane of the RPE. This increases the cornea-positive transepithelial potential across the RPE and is reflected as the c wave in the electroretinogram[65,75] (Figure 11-5). The light-induced decrease in the subretinal K^+ concentration also results in a reduced rate of $Na^+/K^+/2Cl^-$ cotransport across the RPE retinal membrane.[7,44] This in turn causes a decrease in the intracellular Cl^- activity in the RPE cells that develops within 1 to 2 minutes after light onset. The decrease in intracellular Cl^- activity causes a hyperpolarization of the membrane potential across the predominantly Cl^- permeable choroidal membrane in the RPE. This results in a reduction of the cornea-positive transepithelial potential across the RPE and is reflected electroretinographically as the fast oscillation that terminates the c wave in the electroretinogram.[7] The fast oscillation is too slow to be apparent in standard clinical electroretinography, but it can be measured in DC-coupled electroretinography. Several minutes after light onset, the Cl^- permeability of the choroidal membrane increases. This causes delayed depolarization of the membrane potential across this membrane and results in the development of the cornea-positive light peak, which can be measured clinically with electrooculography or DC electroretinography. The increased Cl^- permeability of the choroidal membrane is mediated by an elusive "light-peak substance" that is secreted by the neuroretina after light onset[28,29] (see Figure 11-5).

THE RPE IN PROLIFERATIVE VITREORETINAL DISEASE

RPE cells normally do not divide; however, after retinal trauma or rhegmatogenous retinal detachment, they can proliferate vigorously and be liberated from the epithelium as free RPE cells.[27] In the setting of a rhegmatogenous retinal detachment, these free RPE cells can be observed clinically as "tobacco dust" in the vitreous by slit-lamp examination. The free RPE cells settle on all inner surfaces of the posterior segment of the eye, where they transdifferentiate into a fibroblast-like phenotype and participate in the formation of fibrocellular contracting membranes. This condition is called *proliferative vitreoretinopathy* (PVR) and is feared by vitreoretinal surgeons because retinal detachments complicated with PVR are difficult to repair.[54] RPE proliferation is also important in the formation of some cases of epiretinal membranes, particularly if a retinal hole is present.[35]

REFERENCES

1. Adler AJ, Martin KJ: Retinol-binding proteins in bovine interphotoreceptor matrix, *Biochem Biophys Res Commun* 108:1601, 1982.
2. Adorante JS, Miller SS: Potassium-dependent volume regulation in retinal pigment epithelium is mediated by Na, K, Cl cotransport, *J Gen Physiol* 96:1153, 1990.
3. Allikmets R: A photoreceptor cell-specific ATP-binding transporter gene (ABCR) is mutated in recessive Stargardt macular dystrophy, *Nat Genet* 17:122, 1997.
4. Anderson DH et al: Rod and cone disc shedding in the rhesus monkey retina: a quantitative study, *Exp Eye Res* 30:559, 1980.
5. Bernstein P, Law W, Rando R: Isomerization of all-trans-retinoids to 11-cis-retinoids in vitro, *Proc Natl Acad Sci USA* 84:1849, 1987.
6. Besharse JC, Defoe DM: Role of the retinal pigment epithelium in the photoreceptor membrane turnover. In Marmor MF, Wolfensberger TJ (eds): *The retinal pigment epithelium,* Oxford, 1998, Oxford University Press.
7. Bialek S, Joseph DP, Miller SS: The delayed basolateral membrane hyperpolarization of the bovine retinal pigment epithelium: mechanism of generation, *J Physiol (Lond)* 484(pt 1):53, 1995.
8. Bialek S, Miller SS: K^+ and Cl^- transport mechanisms in bovine pigment epithelium that could modulate subretinal space volume and composition, *J Physiol* 475:401, 1994.
9. Bok D: The retinal pigment epithelium: a versatile partner in vision, *J Cell Sci* 17(suppl):189, 1993.
10. Bok D: Photoreceptor "retinoid pumps" in health and disease, *Neuron* 23:412, 1999.
11. Bok D, Heller J: Transport of retinal from the blood to the retina: an autoradiographic study of the pigment epithelial cell surface receptor for plasma retinol-binding protein, *Exp Eye Res* 22:395, 1976.
12. Boulton M: Melanin and the retinal pigment epithelium. In Marmor MF, Wolfensberger TJ (eds): *The retinal pigment epithelium,* Oxford, 1998, Oxford University Press.
13. Bunt-Milam AH, Saari C: Immunocytochemical localization of two retinoid-binding proteins in vertebrate retina, *J Cell Biol* 97.703, 1983.
14. Bunt-Milam AH et al: Zonulae adherentes pore size in the external limiting membrane of the rabbit retina, *Invest Ophthalmol Vis Sci* 26:1377, 1985.
15. Campochiaro PA: Growth factors in the retinal pigment epithelium and retina. In Marmor MF, Wolfensberger TJ (eds): *The retinal pigment epithelium,* Oxford, 1998, Oxford University Press.
16. Carlson A, Bok D: Polarity of 11-cis retinal release from cultured retinal pigment epithelium, *Invest Ophthalmol Vis Sci* 40:533, 1999.
17. Chader GJ, Pepperberg DR, Crouch R: Retinoids and the retinal pigment epithelium. In Marmor MF, Wolfensberger TJ (eds): *The retinal pigment epithelium,* Oxford, 1998, Oxford University Press.
18. Chaitin MH, Hall MO: Defective ingestion of rod outer segments by cultured dystrophic rat pigment epithelial cells, *Invest Ophthalmol Vis Sci* 24:812, 1983.
19. Choo DW, Cheung E, Rando RR: Lack of effect of RPE65 removal on the enzymatic processing of all-trans-retinol into 11-cis-retinol in vitro, *FEBS Lett* 440:195, 1998.
20. Christoffersen N, Sander B, Larsen M: Precipitation of hard exudate after resorption of intraretinal edema after treatment of retinal branch vein occlusion, *Am J Ophthalmol* 126:454, 1998.

21. del Priore LV et al: Retinal pigment epithelial debridement as a model for the pathogenesis and treatment of macular degeneration, *Am J Ophthalmol* 122:629, 1996.

22. Dowling JE: Chemistry of visual adaptation in the rat, *Nature* 188:114, 1960.

23. Dreigner P et al: Membranes as the energy source of in the endogenic transformation of vitamin A to 11-cis-retinol, *Science* 244:968, 1989.

24. Eldred GE: Lipofuscin and other lysosomal storage deposits in the retinal pigment epithelium. In Wolfensberger TJ, Marmor MF (eds): *The retinal pigment epithelium,* Oxford, 1998, Oxford University Press.

25. Engler CB et al: Fluorescein transport across the human blood-retina barrier in the direction vitreous to blood: quantitative assessment in vivo, *Acta Ophthalmol Scand* 72: 655, 1994.

26. Faktorovich EG et al: Photoreceptor degeneration in inherited retinal dystrophy delayed by basic fibroblast growth factor, *Nature* 347:83, 1990.

27. Fisher SK, Anderson DH: Cellular responses of the retinal pigment epithelium to retinal detachment and reattachment. In Wolfensberger TJ, Marmor MF (eds): *The retinal pigment epithelium,* Oxford, 1998, Oxford University Press.

28. Gallemore RP, Griff ER, Steinberg RH: Evidence in support of a photoreceptoral origin for the "light-peak substance," *Invest Ophthalmol Vis Sci* 29:566, 1988.

29. Gallemore RP, Hughes BA, Miller SS: Light-induced responses of the retinal pigment epithelium. In Wolfensberger TJ, Marmor MF (eds): *The retinal pigment epithelium,* Oxford, 1998, Oxford University Press.

30. Gallemore RP et al: Basolateral membrane Cl⁻ and K⁺ conductances of the dark-adapted chick retinal pigment epithelium, *J Neurophysiol* 70:1656, 1993.

31. Gu SM et al: Mutations in RPE65 cause autosomal recessive childhood-onset severe retinal dystrophy, *Nat Genet* 17:194, 1997.

32. Guymer R, Luthert PJ, Bird AC: Changes in Bruch's membrane and related structures with age, *Prog Retin Eye Res* 18:59, 1999.

33. Hageman GS, Kuehn MK: Biology of the interphotoreceptor matrix-retinal pigment epithelium-retina interface. In Wolfensberger TJ, Marmor MF (eds): *The retinal pigment epithelium,* Oxford, 1998, Oxford University Press.

34. Harman AM et al: Development and aging of cell topography in the human retinal pigment epithelium, *Invest Ophthalmol Vis Sci* 38:2016, 1997.

35. Hiscott P et al: Matrix and the retinal pigment epithelium in proliferative retinal disease, *Prog Retin Eye Res* 18:167, 1999.

36. Hudspeth AJ, Yee AG: The intercellular junctional complexes of retinal pigment epithelia, *Invest Ophthalmol Vis Sci* 12:354, 1973.

37. Hughes BA, Takahira M: Inwardly rectifying K⁺ currents in isolated human retinal pigment epithelial cells, *Invest Ophthalmol Vis Sci* 37:1125, 1996.

38. Hughes BA, Takahira M: ATP-dependent regulation of inwardly rectifying K+ current in bovine retinal pigment epithelial cells, *Am J Physiol* 275:C1372, 1998.

39. Hughes BA et al: Transport mechanisms in the retinal pigment epithelium. In Marmor MF, Wolfensberger TJ (eds): *The retinal pigment epithelium,* Oxford, 1998, Oxford University Press.

40. Hughes BA et al: Apical electrogenic NaHCO3 cotransport: a mechanism for HCO₃ absorption across the retinal pigment epithelium, *J Gen Physiol* 94:125, 1989.

41. Joseph DP, Miller SS: Apical and basal membrane ion transport mechanisms in bovine retinal pigment epithelium, *J Physiol* 435:439, 1991.

42. Korte GE, Perlman JI, Pollack A: Regeneration of mammalian retinal pigment epithelium, *Int Rev Cytol* 152:223, 1994.

43. la Cour M: Rheogenic sodium-bicarbonate cotransport across the retinal membrane of the frog retinal pigment epithelium, *J Physiol* 419:539, 1989.

44. la Cour M: Cl⁻ transport in frog retinal pigment epithelium, *Exp Eye Res* 54:921, 1992.

45. la Cour M: Ion transport in the retinal pigment epithelium: a study with double barrelled ion-selective microelectrodes, *Acta Ophthalmol* 71(suppl):1, 1993.

46. la Cour M, Lund-Andersen H, Zeuthen T: Potassium transport of the frog retinal pigment epithelium: autoregulation of potassium activity in the subretinal space, *J Physiol* 375:461, 1986.

47. Lai YL et al: Interphotoreceptor retinol-binding proteins: possible transport vehicles between compartments of the retina, *Nature* 298:848, 1982.

48. LaVail MM: Rod outer segment disc shedding in rat retina: relationship to cyclic lightning, *Science* 194:1071, 1976.

49. Li JD, Govardovskii VI, Steinberg RH: Light-dependent hydration of the space surrounding photoreceptors in the cat retina, *Vis Neurosci* 11:743, 1994.

50. Lin H, Miller SS: pHᵢ regulation in frog retinal pigment epithelium: two apical membrane mechanisms, *Am J Physiol* 261:C132, 1991.

51. Lin H, Miller SS: Phᵢ-dependent Cl-HCO₃ exchange at the basolateral membrane of frog retinal pigment epithelium, *Am J Physiol* 266:C935, 1994.

52. Liou GI et al: Vitamin A transport between retina and pigment epithelium: an interstitial protein carrying endogenous retinol (interstitial retinol-binding protein), *Vision Res* 22:1457, 1982.

53. Liou GI et al: Early onset photoreceptor abnormalities induced by targeted disruption of the interphotoreceptor retinoid-binding protein gene, *J Neurosci* 18:4511, 1998.

54. Machemer R: Proliferative vitreoretinopathy (PVR): a personal account of its pathogenesis and treatment, *Invest Ophthalmol Vis Sci* 29:1771, 1988.

55. Marlhens F et al: Autosomal recessive retinal dystrophy associated with two novel mutations in the RPE65 gene, *Eur J Hum Genet* 6:527, 1998.

56. Marmor MF: Control of subretinal fluid and mechanisms of serous detachment. In Wolfensberger TJ, Marmor MF (eds): *The retinal pigment epithelium,* Oxford, 1998, Oxford University Press.

57. Marmor MF: Mechanisms of retinal adhesion. In Wolfensberger TJ, Marmor MF (eds): *The retinal pigment epithelium,* Oxford, 1998, Oxford University Press.

58. Marmor MF, Maack T. Enhancement of retinal adhesion and subretinal fluid resorption by acetazomamide, *Invest Ophthalmol Vis Sci* 23:121, 1982.

59. Marmor MF, Martin LJ: 100 years of the visual cycle, *Surv Ophthalmol* 22:279, 1978.

60. Marshall J et al: Aging and Bruch's membrane. In Wolfensberger TJ, Marmor MF (eds): *The retinal pigment epithelium,* Oxford, 1998, Oxford University Press.

61. Miller SS, Steinberg RH: Passive ionic properties of frog retinal pigment epithelium, *J Membrane Biol* 36:337, 1977.

62. Miller SS, Steinberg RH, Oakley B II: The electrogenic sodium pump of the frog retinal pigment epithelium, *J Membrane Biol* 44:259, 1978.

63. Morimura H, Berson EL, Dryja TP: Recessive mutations in the RLBP1 gene encoding cellular retinaldehyde-binding protein in a form of retinitis punctata albescens, *Invest Ophthalmol Vis Sci* 40:1000, 1999.

64. Mullen RJ, LaVail MM: Inherited retinal dystrophy: primary defect in pigment epithelium determined with experimental rat chimeras, *Science* 192:799, 1976.

65. Oakley BII, Green DG: Correlation of light-induced changes in retinal extracellular potassium concentration with c-wave of the electroretinogram, *J Neurophysiol* 39:1117, 1976.

66. Palczewski K et al: Kinetics of visual pigment regeneration in excised mouse eyes and in mice with a targeted disruption of the gene encoding interphotoreceptor retinoid-binding protein or arrestin, *Biochemistry* 38:12012, 1999.

67. Peyman GA, Bok D: Peroxidase diffusion in the normal and laser-coagulated primate retina, *Invest Ophthalmol* 11:35, 1972.

68. Rando RR, Bernstein PS, Barry RJ: New insights into the visual cycle. In Osborne N, Chader G (eds): *Progress in retinal research*, vol 10, New York, 1991, Pergamon Press.

69. Redmond TM et al: Rpe65 is necessary for production of 11-cis-vitamin A in the retinal visual cycle, *Nat Genet* 20:344, 1998.

70. Robinson SR, Hendrickson A: Shifting relationships between photoreceptors and pigment epithelial cells in monkey retina: implications for the development of retinal topography, *Vis Neurosci* 12:767, 1995.

71. Saari JC: Retinoids in photosensitive systems. In Sporn MB, Roberts AB, Goodman DS (eds): *The retinoids: biology, chemistry, and medicine*, New York, 1994, Raven Press.

72. Segawa Y, Hughes BA: Properties of the inwardly rectifying K^+ conductance in the toad retinal pigment epithelium, *J Physiol (Lond)* 476:41, 1994.

73. Shichi H, Nebert DW: Drug metabolism in ocular tissues. In Gram TE (ed): *Extrahepatic metabolism of drugs and other foreign compounds*, Lancaster, 1980, MTP Press Limited.

74. Soprano DR, Blaner WS: Plasma retinol-binding protein. In Sporn MB, Roberts AB, Goodman DS (eds): *The retinoids: biology, chemistry, and medicine*, New York, 1994, Raven Press.

75. Steinberg RH, Linsenmeier RA, Griff ER: Retinal pigment epithelial cell contribution to the electroretinogram and electrooculogram. In Osborne NN, Chader GJ (eds): *Progress in retinal research*, vol 4, New York, 1985, Pergamon.

76. Steinberg RH, Oakley BII, Niemeyer G: Light-evoked changes in $[K^+]_o$ in retina of intact cat eye, *J Neurophysiol* 44:897, 1980.

77. Steinberg RH, Wood I, Hogan MJ: Pigment epithelial ensheathment and phagocytosis of extrafoveal cones in human retina, *Philos Trans R Soc Lond B Biol Sci* 277:459, 1977.

78. Tso MOM, Friedman E: The retinal pigment epithelium. I. Comparative histology, *Arch Ophthalmol* 78:641, 1967.

79. Tsuboi S: Measurement of the volume flow and hydraulic conductivity across the isolated dog retinal pigment epithelium, *Invest Ophthalmol Vis Sci* 28:1776, 1987.

80. Törnquist P: Capillary permeability in cat choroid, studied with the single injection technique (II), *A Physiol Scand* 106:425, 1979.

81. Valverde D et al: Analysis of the IRBP gene as a cause of RP in 45 spanish families. Autosomal recessive retinitis pigmentosa. Interstitial retinol binding protein: Spanish multicentric and multidiciplinary group for research into retinitis pigmentosa, *Ophthalmic Genet* 19:197, 1998.

82. Veske A et al: Retinal dystrophy of Swedish briard/briard-beagle dogs is due to a 4-bp deletion in RPE65, *Genomics* 57:57, 1999.

83. Wang L, Tornquist P, Bill A: Glucose metabolism in pig outer retina in light and darkness, *Acta Physiol Scand* 160:75, 1997.

84. Yamamoto F, Steinberg RH: Effects of systemic hypoxia on pH outside rod photoreceptors in the cat retina, *Exp Eye Res* 54:699, 1992.

85. Young RW: The renewal of photoreceptor cell outer segements, *J Cell Biol* 33:61, 1967.

86. Young RW: The renewal of rod and cone outer segments in the rhesus monkey, *J Cell Biol* 49:303, 1971.

87. Young RW: Shedding of discs from rod outer segements in the rhesus monkey, *J Ultrastructure Res* 34:190, 1971.

88. Young RW, Bok D: Participation of the retinal pigment epithelium in the rod outer segment renewal process, *J Cell Biol* 42:392, 1969.

89. Zeuthen T, Hamann S, la Cour M: Cotransport of H^+, lactate and H_2O by membrane proteins in retinal pigment epithelium of bullfrog, *J Physiol (Lond)* 497:3, 1996.

CHAPTER 12

GENETICS AND BIOLOGY OF THE INHERITED RETINAL DYSTROPHIES

DAVID A.R. BESSANT, SHALESH KAUSHAL, AND SHOMI S. BHATTACHARYA

The powerful techniques of modern molecular genetics have revolutionized the understanding of the molecular biologic basis of the inherited retinal dystrophies. Collectively, this large group of phenotypically and genetically heterogeneous retinal disorders represents the most common inherited form of human visual handicap, with an estimated prevalence of 1 in 3000.

The eye and its disorders have often been involved in important breakthroughs in mammalian genetics, probably by virtue of the relative ease with which ocular phenotypes can be determined. The earliest and best documented autosomal dominant pedigree in human genetics involves the descendants of Jean Nougaret (1637-1719), a southern French butcher who had congenital stationary night blindness (CSNB). In 1911, Wilson localized the locus for color blindness, the first gene ever mapped, to the human X chromosome. The first mammalian genetic linkage, between the mouse pink-eye dilute (p) and albino (c) loci, was demonstrated by Haldane in 1915.

In 1984, using newly developed molecular genetic techniques, Bhattacharya[19] described the linkage of X-linked retinitis pigmentosa (xlRP) to a specific location (locus) on the short arm of the X chromosome. In 1989, Humphries' group[99] reported the linkage of autosomal dominant retinitis pigmentosa (adRP) to a locus on chromosome 3. This permitted Dryja,[39] in 1990, to discover the first adRP-causing mutations in the *rhodopsin* gene. In the 10 years since

that breakthrough, a variety of inherited retinal disorders have been linked to more than 120 loci, and more than 60 of the disease-causing genes have been identified. A comprehensive list of these genes and loci can be obtained from two excellent electronic databases: "RetNet" (www.sph.uth.tmc.edu/Retnet/disease.htm) and "Online Mendelian Inheritance in Man" (www.ncbi.nlm.nih.gov/Omim/).

CLINICIAN'S PERSPECTIVE ON INHERITED EYE DISEASE

An ophthalmologist caring for a patient or family affected by an inherited eye disease must offer both prognostic advice and genetic counseling. To do this, the ophthalmologist must make an accurate clinical diagnosis and determine the pattern of inheritance of the disease trait within the family.

Clinical Classification

The inherited retinal dystrophies demonstrate extensive variations in phenotype. These may represent (1) mutations in different genes, (2) different mutations in the same gene (allelic heterogeneity), (3) variability in the genetic background on which a gene is expressed, or (4) modulation by environmental factors. Accurate diagnosis may also be hindered by changes to the disease phenotype that occur as a result of disease progression. In their early stages, both Best macular dystrophy and X-linked retinoschisis (XLRS) result in distinctive macular lesions. With time, however, both may progress to leave a nonspecific macular scar (Figure 12-1). The situation may be further confused in X-linked disorders in which female carriers may manifest a milder form of the disease, presumably resulting from an imbalance of X chromosome inactivation (e.g., X-linked retinitis pigmentosa) or have abnormal ocular findings in the absence of symptoms, such as carriers of mutations in the choroideremia gene *CHM*.[34]

Collectively, these factors may, at times, make it difficult for even the skilled clinician to make the correct diagnosis. A flexible approach, using clinical examination, additional investigations, and examination of other family members may often yield a definitive diagnosis in these situations.

Peripheral Dystrophies. Retinal dystrophies can be classified clinically according to whether they are stationary (e.g., CSNB, rod monochromatism) or progressive and according to which photoreceptor system—rods or cones—is primarily affected. Cones operate under conditions of bright light (photopic) and provide trichromatic color vision, whereas rods can function in near darkness (scotopic). The cone-rich macular region, located in the center of the retina, is structured to maximize detailed vision, and the rod-dominated periphery provides adequate field of vision and motion detection.

Disorders primarily affecting the rod system (e.g., retinitis pigmentosa [RP], choroideremia) initially present with night blindness (nyctalopia) and may progress to involve substantial loss of the peripheral visual field; however, central vision is preserved, at least until late in the course of the disease. These disorders can be classified as peripheral dystrophies.

Central Dystrophies. In contrast, primary diseases of the cone system (cone dystrophies) manifest initially with loss of central visual acuity (discrimination) and color vision and should not significantly affect peripheral vision unless the rod system is also involved (cone-rod dystrophies).[101] Some disorders affect both photoreceptor populations within the specialized central part of the retina while leaving the peripheral rods and cones intact; these disorders are called *macular dystrophies.*

Further classification, especially of the central dystrophies, is based on typical or, rarely, pathognomonic clinical features such as the fundal appearance (Best disease, XLRS) or on a combination of ocular findings and further clinical analysis.

Syndromic Dystrophies. Although most patients with a retinal dystrophy have an isolated retinal degeneration, there are a number of syndromic forms

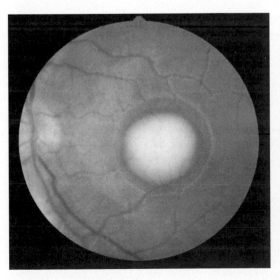
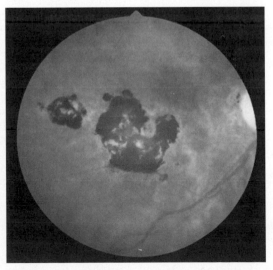

A   **B**

FIGURE 12-1   Fundus photographs of a boy (12 years of age) and his mother (30 years of age) with Best macular dystrophy, demonstrating the classic egg-yolk or vitelliform lesion at the macula in the son (**A**) and an area of nonspecific macular atrophy in his mother (**B**).

of retinal dystrophy in which a systemic disease is associated with progressive retinal degeneration[68] (Table 12-1). In some instances these systemic diseases are caused by known metabolic disorders, and as such, many provide insights into the basic pathogenetic mechanisms of the retinal disease. A clinician must be aware of these associations when examining a patient with retinal dystrophy so that the presence or absence of systemic features, often of a neurologic nature, can be ascertained by careful history taking, examination, and clinical (e.g., audiologic) or laboratory (e.g., phytanic acid levels in Refsum disease) testing. Usher syndrome, the association of hearing loss and RP, is the most prevalent of the syndromic dystrophies.

When used appropriately, these clinical classifications not only supply prognostic guidelines for clinicians but also served to provide scientists with relatively "pure" samples of disease for molecular genetic and biochemical analysis.

Clinical Examination and Investigations

Investigation of a patient with a suspected inherited retinal disorder begins with a thorough clinical and genetic (family) history and is followed by detailed examination of the fundus. This may then be supplemented by a number of relevant investigations, of which electrophysiology is often the most important.

Electrophysiology. Electroretinography enables objective functional evaluation of different retinal cell types and layers.[122] The full-field electroretinogram (ERG) measures the mass response of the whole retina, reflects photoreceptor and inner nuclear layer retinal function, and allows separate functional assessment of the photopic (cone) and scotopic (rod) systems. The a wave of the scotopic ERG arises in the rod photoreceptors, and the b wave is generated by the bipolar and Müller cells. Most laboratories perform ERG studies according to guidelines established by the International Society for Clinical Electrophysiology of Vision. Standard responses include (1) a bright white flash (the mixed rod-cone maximal response); (2) the scotopic rod response recorded under full dark adaptation; and (3) light-adapted photopic transient and 30-Hz flicker ERGs, which assess cone function.

The pattern ERG (PERG) provides a sensitive measure of macular function.[6] Significant reduction of the PERG can be observed during the progression of any dystrophy that involves the macula and may be a predictor of subsequent visual acuity loss. Macular, cone, and cone-rod dystrophies all commonly present with loss of central vision and reduction in PERG. In a macular dystrophy, however, the full-field ERG is unaffected, whereas in cone dystrophy the 30-Hz flicker is abnormal and

TABLE 12-1

SYNDROMIC RETINAL DYSTROPHIES

SYNDROME	SYSTEMIC FEATURES	INHERITANCE	REFERENCE
Neurologic Disorders			
Usher	Neurosensory deafness, vestibular dysfunction in Usher type 1	AR	Smith et al., 1994 (*Am J Med Genet* 50:32)
Laurence-Moon/Bardet-Biedl	Polydactyly, short stature, mental retardation, hypogonadism, obesity, and spastic paraplegia	AR	Green et al., 1989 (*N Engl J Med* 321:1002)
Friedreich ataxia	Cerebellar dysfunction, ataxia, sensory loss	AR	
Kearns-Sayre	Chronic progressive external ophthalmoplegia, cardiomyopathy, heart block, deafness	M	Kearns, 1965 (*Trans Am Ophthalmol Soc* 63:559)
Metabolic Disorders			
Abetalipoproteinemia	Acanthocytosis, ataxia, sensory neuropathy, fat intolerance	AR	Bassen and Kornzweig, 1950 (*Blood* 5:381)
Refsum (phytanic acid α-hydroxylase deficiency)	Cerebellar ataxia, quadriplegia, cardiomyopathy, dry skin	AR	Refsum, 1981 (*Arch Neurol* 38:605)
Batten (ceroid-lipofuscinosis)	Mental retardation, hypotonia, ataxia	AR	Zeman, 1976 (In Bergsma D, Bron AJ, Collier E [eds]: *The eye and inborn errors of metabolism*, New York, Alan R Liss)

in a cone-rod phenotype the scotopic response is also reduced.

The electrooculogram (EOG) records the light-induced rise in standing potential across the retinal pigment epithelium (RPE) following a period of dark adaptation.[11] In Best macular dystrophy a reduction in the EOG light rise, accompanied by a normal ERG, provides excellent confirmation of the diagnosis and can even be used to identify asymptomatic carriers of mutations in the *VMD2* gene (see p. 376).

Psychophysics. An individual's field of vision can be assessed separately under both photopic and scotopic conditions to determine his or her subjective ability to see in different lighting conditions.[75] Dark adaptometry can quantitatively determine the kinetics of cone and rod recovery following a bright flash of light sufficient to bleach of the retina.[126] Patients with a sectorial form of RP, for example, may demonstrate profoundly delayed rod adaptation.[102] Fine matrix mapping determines threshold responses within the macular region and is used to assess localized retinal dysfunction.

Fundus Imaging. Fluorescein angiography can be useful to detect the "dark choroid" that characterizes Stargardt disease or fundus flavimaculatus and to ascertain the presence of cystoid macular edema (CME), and choroidal neovascularization (CNV), which may occur in certain other dystrophies.[93]

The confocal scanning laser ophthalmoscope (cSLO) can be used to image fundus autofluorescence, which originates largely from the RPE, and hence to evaluate the interaction of photoreceptors with the RPE.[138] Regions of increased autofluorescence may be observed during retinal degeneration, possibly resulting from overloading of the RPE by products of photoreceptor metabolism. Subsequently, loss of photoreceptors and/or RPE results in areas of hypofluorescence.[139]

Optical coherence tomography (OCT) is a recently introduced method for determining retinal thickness and for evaluating structural retinal pathologic changes by laser interferometry, which may be of increasing value as its resolution improves.[63]

Inheritance Pattern

Retinal dystrophies may be inherited as autosomal dominant, autosomal recessive, sex-linked (X-linked) recessive, digenic, and mitochondrial traits. The prevalence of these dystrophies varies with the country and race being studied, and the proportion ac-

counted for by each of the different patterns of inheritance reflects population variables such as the level of consanguinity. The overall incidence of RP in the United States has been calculated to be approximately 1 in 3700, with the inheritance averaging 10% autosomal dominant, 84% autosomal recessive (including simplex cases), and 6% X-linked recessive.[24] In the United Kingdom, adRP accounts for approximately 20%, autosomal recessive retinitis pigmentosa (arRP) for 70%, and xlRP for up to 10% of all RP cases.[77] The highest known frequency of RP is among the Native American Navaho, with 1 in 1800 affected.[69] Simplex cases, with no previous family history of RP, constitute up to 50% of all patients. Most of these are presumed to be cases of arRP, with a smaller proportion resulting from digenic RP, incompletely penetrant adRP, and rare new dominant mutations. From the preponderance of males among simplex cases, it has been calculated that approximately 1 in 10 males with simplex RP have inherited an X-linked form of the disease (xlRP).[76]

In some instances there is an extensive history of the retinal disorder within the family, and this may define a particular mode of inheritance, usually autosomal dominant or X-linked recessive. Alternatively, the clinical diagnosis may be one of a disorder that is inherited in only a single pattern, such as choroideremia (X-linked recessive), gyrate atrophy (autosomal recessive), or Kearns-Sayre syndrome (mitochondrial). Consanguinity in the parents of affected individuals suggests an autosomal recessive pattern of inheritance.

In some families, determination of the inheritance pattern may prove more difficult. A single male affected by RP, for example, is most likely to have inherited an autosomal recessive form of the disease, which would be associated with a minimal risk to future generations. However, he may have inherited the disorder as an X-linked trait, passed down to him through a series of asymptomatic female gene carriers. In this case both the prognostic and the genetic ramifications would be different because xlRP is often more severe and rapidly progressive than arRP, and all the man's daughters would be obligate carriers of xlRP. The genetic possibilities in this scenario also include adRP with incomplete penetrance, such as that associated with mutations at the chromosome 19q locus,[4] and digenic RP, caused by synergistic mutations in *peripherin-RDS* and *ROM-1* (see p. 371). In both situations there would be a direct risk to the affected man's children, male or female. Last, in a few cases the added complications of adoption and nonpaternity may make genetic counseling impossible without the benefit of molecular genetic analysis.

In some circumstances the clinician is unable to offer the patient satisfactory prognostic and/or genetic advice. For example, clinical examination and electrophysiology often fail to determine whether the daughter of a female xlRP carrier is herself a carrier of the disease gene. Mutation screening of the known xlRP genes, *RPGR*[100] and *RP2*,[123] and/or haplotype analysis of the xlRP critical disease intervals within the woman's family may determine the answer to this important question.

MOLECULAR GENETIC TECHNIQUES

Molecular genetics seeks either to locate disease genes on genetic and physical maps of the human genome (linkage mapping) and subsequently identify the gene responsible or to analyze potential "candidate" genes directly. The international Human Genome Project, initiated in the late 1980s, has now determined virtually the entire nucleotide sequence of the human genome, greatly facilitating the isolation of the remaining genes responsible for human retinal dystrophies.[33]

Genetic Linkage Mapping

In human molecular genetics, linkage mapping is used to determine linkage between a specific disease trait and markers of known chromosomal location by demonstrating that they are inherited together (cosegregate) in all affected members of a pedigree or pedigrees[106] (Figure 12-2).

Each copy of the same human chromosome contains many small variations (deoxyribonucleic acid [DNA] polymorphisms) that together constitute an individual's unique genetic identity; these polymorphisms can be used individually as polymorphic markers to determine the parental origin of a particular genetic locus. During meiotic cell division, each pair of homologous chromosomes undergoes at least one recombination (crossover) between nonsister chromatids. If two loci are physically located close together on the same chromosome, there is a greater chance that they will not be separated by random recombination events during meiosis and will appear "linked." To demonstrate linkage, one selects representative markers for each locus. Ideally, these markers should be highly polymorphic within a given human population to maximize the probability that they will be different in any two copies of that chromosome.

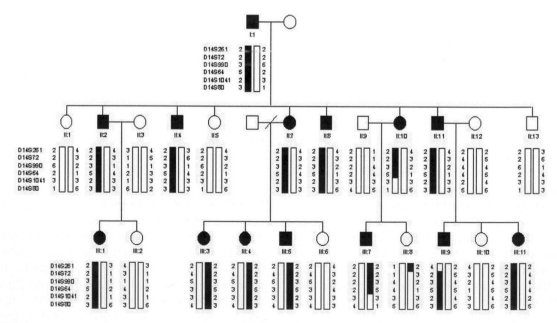

FIGURE 12-2   Linkage analysis. The pedigree of a family in which 14 individuals are affected by autosomal dominant retinitis pigmentosa, showing haplotypes for polymorphic markers in the centromeric region of chromosome 14q. Centromeric recombination events in individuals III-8 and III-9, and a telomeric recombination in affected individual II-10 define D14S261 and D14S1041 as the flanking markers for this adRP locus. The affected haplotype is indicated by black shading of the bars situated between the marker alleles.

Successful linkage analysis requires a high-density genetic map, with large numbers of polymorphic markers mapped at regular intervals.[36]

The extent of genetic linkage between two loci is measured by the recombination fraction *(θ), which is the proportion of recombinations that occur between these loci in a given number of meioses (opportunities for recombination).* As the physical distance between two loci decreases, there is less chance of recombination and the observed recombination fraction falls. A *θ* value of 0 implies tight linkage, and a *θ* value of 0.5 indicates two loci that segregate independently. This is the maximum value that can be achieved because each sister chromatid has only a 50% chance of being involved in any one crossover. The recombination fraction can be used as a measure of the "genetic distance" between loci.

The probability of linkage over a range of recombination fractions can be measured quantitatively and expressed on a logarithmic scale to produce a lod ($\log_{10}$ of odds) score. This is the ratio of the probability that the data would have arisen if the loci were linked (*θ* has a given value less than 0.5) to the probability that the data would have arisen if the loci were unlinked (*θ* = 0.5). The *θ* value that gives the maximum lod score (Z_{max}) best estimates of the degree of linkage between the two loci. A lod score of 3 (odds of 1000:1) is accepted as proof of linkage. In practice, Z_{max} is calculated by dedicated computer programs.

A relatively large family, consisting of at least 11 informative meioses, is required to obtain a lod score of 3. Accurate diagnosis of affectation status is essential, and the number of meioses that can be included in the analysis may have to be reduced if the disease onset occurs in late age and cannot be detected presymptomatically. Therefore linkage analysis is best suited to the study of extended, multigenerational pedigrees segregating fully penetrant autosomal dominant traits.

Once linkage to a single marker has been obtained, the critical genetic interval, within which the disease gene must lie, can be defined; this is done by genotyping the pedigrees with further genetic markers in the vicinity of the first to identify key recombinant individuals.

Candidate Gene Analysis

As information regarding the function of newly identified genes is discovered, the genes may become candidates for involvement in a particular retinal disease, either because they demonstrate a functional relationship with the underlying metabolic defect (functional candidates) or because they are exclusively expressed in the involved tissue (tissue-specific candidates). Occasionally, these candidate genes may be human homologs of genes responsible for a similar disease phenotype in other organisms (comparative candidates). Alternatively, they may be identified as members of a gene family of which other members have been implicated in a related disorder.

The candidate gene approach is particularly well suited to the study of recessive disease traits because in the absence of extensive consanguinity, autosomal recessive pedigrees that are sufficiently large to be suitable for linkage analysis are rare. This is illustrated by the fact that many of the loci for arRP were identified by this approach, whereas all the loci for adRP were demonstrated by linkage analysis.

Mutation analysis of candidate genes is usually carried out as a two-stage process, beginning with relatively simple, rapid, and inexpensive screening tests and proceeding to direct sequencing when an anomaly is detected[83] (see Color Plate 3). Screening methods aim to detect a difference between the sequence of wild-type and mutant DNA amplified by the polymerase chain reaction (PCR).[119] The screening stage is particularly important in the initial analysis of large genes, such as *ABCR* (see p. 373). However, because all screening tests fail to detect a proportion of sequence changes, it is essential to directly sequence every exon, or coding region, of a gene before excluding it as a cause of disease. Once a sequence change in a particular exon has been detected, direct sequencing can be used to identify the exact mutation. This can then be confirmed by restriction enzyme digest analysis.

RETINITIS PIGMENTOSA

RP is recognized as the most common of the inherited retinal dystrophies. In reality it is a generic name for a group of diffuse, usually bilaterally symmetric, retinal dystrophies primarily affecting the rod photoreceptors.[21] These conditions exhibit great phenotypic and genetic heterogeneity (Table 12-2), with a substantial variation in both the age of onset and the severity of the disease.

Clinical Features of Retinitis Pigmentosa

The ophthalmoscopic features of classical RP include depigmentation or atrophy of the RPE, pigment

TABLE 12-2
GENES AND LOCI FOR RETINITIS PIGMENTOSA

PROTEIN	GENE	LOCUS	INHERITANCE	REFERENCES*
RPE65	*RPE65*	1p31	AR	Morimura, 1998
RP18		1q13-q23	AD	Xu, 1996
Crumbs homolog	*CRB1*	1q31-q32.1	AR	den Hollander, 1999
RP28		2p11-p16	AR	Gu, 1999
c-mer receptor tyrosine kinase	*MERTK*	2q14.1	AR	Gal, 2000
RP26		2q31-q33	AR	Bayés, 1998
Rhodopsin	*RHO*	3q21-q24	AD	Dryja, 1990
Prominin (mouse)–like-1	*PROML1*	4p	AR	Maw, 2000
cGMP phosphodiesterase-β	*PDEβ*	4p16.3	AR	Huang, 1995
cGMP gated channel protein	*CNGCα*	4p14-q13	AR	Dryja, 1995
cGMP phosphodiesterase-α	*PDEα*	5q31.2-qter	AR	Huang, 1995
RP29		4q32-q34	AR	Payne, 2000
Peripherin-RDS	*RDS*	6p21.1	AD Digenic	Kajiwara, 1991, 1994
Tubby-like protein	*TULP1*	6p21.3	AR	Hagstrom, 1998
RP25		6cen-q15	AR	Khaliq, 1999
RP9		7p15-p13	AD	Inglehearn, 1993
RP10		7q31.3	AD	Jordan, 1993
RP1 protein	*RP1*	8p11-q21	AD	Pierce/Sullivan, 1999
Rod outer membrane protein-1	*ROM1*	11q13	Digenic	Kajiwara, 1994
Neural retina leucine zipper	*NRL*	14q11.1-12.1	AD	Bessant, 1999
Retinaldehyde-binding protein	*RLBP1*	15q26	AR	Maw, 1997
RP22		16p12.1-p12.3	AR	Finckh, 1998
RP13		17p13.3	AD	Greenberg, 1994
RP17		17q22	AD	Bardien, 1995
RP11		19q13.4	AD	Al-Maghtheh, 1994
RP23		Xp22	XL	Hardcastle, 2000
RP6		Xp21.3-p21.2	XL	Breuer, 2000
RP GTPase regulator	*RGPR (RP3)*	Xp21	XL	Meindl, 1996
RP2 protein	*RP2*	Xp11.3-p11.2	XL	Schwahn, 1998
RP24		Xq26-q27	XL	Gieser, 1998

AD, Autosomal dominant; *AR,* autosomal recessive; *cGMP,* cyclic guanine monophosphate; *XL,* X-linked.
*In the case of genes not referred to in detail in the text of the article, the full reference can be obtained from "RetNet" (www.sph.uth.tmc.edu/Retnet/disease. htm).

deposition in the retina, narrowing of the retinal arterioles, and pallor of the optic nerve head (Figure 12-3). These changes are evident first in the midperiphery of the retina and may extend both centrally and peripherally as the disease progresses. The pigmentary disturbance may take the form of clumps and strands of black pigment (sometimes described as a bone corpuscular pattern), but small irregular clumps and spots of pigment are also common.

Pigmentation may also be more prominent in a perivascular distribution because of pigment deposition within vessel walls. The macular area is relatively spared and in some cases may appear entirely normal. Histologic studies of RP retinas indicate that the observed pigment arises from the RPE.

Although pigment deposition has given RP its name, it appears to be a result of the underlying degenerative process and is not thought to contribute

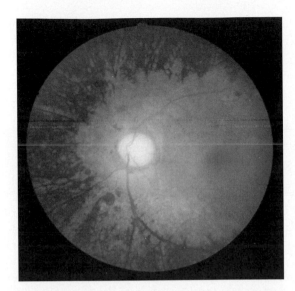

FIGURE 12-3 Retinitis pigmentosa. Fundus photograph showing extensive "bone-spicule" intraretinal pigmentation throughout the periphery of the retina, narrowing of retinal vessels, and optic atrophy.

to the visual loss. In addition, a number of noninherited disorders may present with a pigmentary retinopathy that mimics RP, presumably because of the limited number of ways in which the RPE can react to disease processes. The causes of pseudo-retinitis pigmentosa include infections (e.g., syphilis, rubella), acute zonal occult outer retinopathy (AZOOR), ocular injury, spontaneous retinal reattachment, uveal effusion syndrome, drug toxicity (e.g., thioridazine, desferrioxamine), and vascular occlusions. Some of these conditions present unilaterally, strongly suggesting a noninherited cause, but others may have to be distinguished from RP by electrophysiologic testing.

In typical RP, the onset of night blindness dates back to early childhood, and this may remain the only symptom for many years. This subjective complaint can be substantiated with dark adaptometry. The next stage of the disease is usually progressive loss of peripheral visual field. The patient usually notices this in the form of clumsiness or bumping into things rather than an actual awareness of a diminishing field of vision. Initially, there may be a midperipheral ring scotoma (corresponding to the midperipheral retinal degeneration), but with time, this area of visual field loss extends both peripherally and centrally until only a small area of central vision remains (tunnel vision), sometimes in association with a temporal island of peripheral vision.

In most individuals with RP the visual acuity is not significantly affected until later stages of the disease. In some cases a decrease in central vision is not the result of progression of the retinal disease, but rather the result of one of the recognized complications of RP, such as the formation of posterior subcapsular cataracts or the development of CME.

The diagnosis of RP can be confirmed by psychophysical (visual field) and electrodiagnostic testing. Visual field changes are best determined by studies of the perimetric light thresholds under dark-adapted conditions. This method can demonstrate a generalized elevation of the rod thresholds, even in early cases, and in areas of the visual field that appear normal on routine testing, which is performed under light-adapted conditions. The attenuation of the ERG, which is a recording of the electrical signals generated by the retina in response to light stimuli, is the most sensitive indicator of the presence of RP or a related inherited retinal degeneration. It may be diagnostic in childhood, even before the onset of symptoms associated with visual field loss or the development of fundal changes.

Autosomal Dominant Retinitis Pigmentosa. adRP is itself both clinically and genetically heterogeneous and may be characterized by diffuse loss of rod function, with relative preservation of cone function in the early stages of the disease, or it may display regional loss of rod function accompanied by concomitant loss of cone function in the affected areas.[96]

Autosomal Recessive Retinitis Pigmentosa. If most simplex cases are presumed to be recessive, arRP is numerically the most important form of RP, and like adRP, it exhibits extensive genetic heterogeneity. No specific clinical features of arRP exist that can be used to reliably distinguish it from adRP or xlRP.

X-Linked Retinitis Pigmentosa. The phenotype observed in males affected by any of X-linked forms of RP is usually more severe, both in terms of earlier age of onset and more rapid progression, than that associated with adRP or arRP. Onset is typically in the first decade, and the disease progresses to partial or complete blindness by the third or fourth decade of life.[20] This and the need to offer accurate genetic advice to female carriers and potential carriers means that members of xlRP families may be involved in a disproportionate number of attendances at ophthalmology clinics.

The inheritance pattern may be obvious from pedigree analysis, but it can be confused with incomplete penetrance of adRP or mitochondrial inheritance. In addition, some male patients with simplex RP have inherited an X-linked form of the disease. Pedigree analysis is further complicated by the fact that carrier females may also manifest symptoms and signs of RP to varying degrees, presumably resulting from *lyonization* (random inactivation of the X chromosome during early development). Confirmation of the inheritance pattern is achieved by comparison of affected males and females within a pedigree, which always reveals an earlier age of onset and more rapidly progressive disease in males.

Digenic Retinitis Pigmentosa. Digenic RP is caused by the simultaneous segregation of heterozygous mutations in two different genes, *RDS-peripherin* and *ROM-1,* and is discussed in a later section (see p. 371).

Mechanisms of Cell Death in Retinitis Pigmentosa

Photoreceptor loss in the retinal dystrophies occurs primarily through programmed cell death (apoptosis).[113] In both human RP and mouse models of RP caused by rod-specific gene defects, loss of rod photoreceptors is accompanied by eventual loss of cones from the affected part of the retina. This suggests that degenerating photoreceptor cells induce apoptosis in adjacent genetically normal cells.[71] In developed countries, where many people live in well-illuminated cities with good transport facilities, the loss of cone-mediated reading vision has a far greater impact on quality of life than does the night blindness and visual field loss caused by loss of rod function.

MOLECULAR GENETICS OF THE INHERITED RETINAL DYSTROPHIES

For the clinician it may be useful to tabulate the genes responsible for retinal dystrophies according to the clinical phenotype and inheritance pattern observed. Table 12-2, for example, catalogs all of the currently known genes and loci responsible for the various forms of RP. Table 12-3 lists the genes associated with central retinal dystrophies, and Table 12-4 lists the genes responsible for CSNB.

A better understanding of how the protein products of these genes relate to one another and to the pathogenesis of retinal degeneration can be obtained from a functional classification. The prod-

ucts of most of these genes can be placed into one of four categories: (1) phototransduction proteins, (2) photoreceptor structural proteins, (3) proteins involved in photoreceptor and retinal pigment epithelial (particularly vitamin A) metabolism, and (4) proteins regulating gene expression (transcription factors).

Proteins of the Phototransduction Cascade

The phototransduction cascade is discussed in detail in Chapter 13 and summarized in Color Plate 4. Rhodopsin, the rod photopigment, and all other phototransduction proteins are located in the rod outer segment (ROS), a specialized photoreceptor structure that contains large numbers of flat membranes (discs), which provide an extensive surface area for the capture of incoming photons. Rhodopsin consists of an opsin molecule (a seven-transmembrane helix G protein–coupled receptor) covalently bound to the chromophore 11-*cis*-retinal. Incident light induces isomerization of the retinal and dissociation into opsin and all-*trans*-retinal. In addition, light-induced conformational changes in the opsin molecule expose binding sites for the photoreceptor G protein transducin.

Within the cytoplasm the activated α-subunit of transducin activates the heterotetrameric enzyme cyclic guanine monophosphate (cGMP) phosphodiesterase (PDE), which then hydrolyses cGMP. The resulting fall in cGMP levels results in closure of cGMP-gated cation channels on the plasma membrane of the ROS. This reduces the influx of sodium and calcium ions, and the subsequent hyperpolarization of the entire rod cell plasma membrane curtails the release of the rod's neurotransmitter, glutamate, at its synaptic terminal.

Termination of the photoresponse is largely mediated by the decline in ROS calcium concentration. This leads to inactivation of photoactivated rhodopsin, transducin, and PDE and to stimulation of retina-specific guanylate cyclases (RetGC-1 and RetGC-2) to increase intracellular cGMP levels.

Mutations causing human retinal disease have been identified in many of the proteins that participate in the photoactivation and the recovery processes.

Rhodopsin. Mutations in the rhodopsin gene, situated on chromosome 3q, are reported to be responsible for approximately 25% of all cases of adRP in the United Kingdom,[74] Europe,[27] and the United States, making this numerically the most important of all the known RP genes. More than

TABLE 12-3
CONE, CONE-ROD, AND MACULAR DYSTROPHY GENES

PROTEIN	PHENOTYPE	GENE	LOCUS	INHERITANCE	REFERENCES*
RPE65	Leber amaurosis	*RPE65*	1p31	AR	Gu/Mahlens, 1997
Rim protein (ABCR)	Stargardt disease Cone-rod dystrophy	*ABCR*	1p21-p13	AR	Allikmets, 1997; Cremers, 1998
EGF-containing fibrillin-like extracellular matrix protein 1	Malattia Leventinese/ Doyne retinal dystrophy	*EFEMP1*	2p16-p21	AD	Stone, 1999
Peripherin-RDS	Macular, pattern, and cone-rod dystrophy	*RDS*	6p21.1	AD	Keen, 1996
GCAP-1	Cone dystrophy	*GUCA1A*	6p21.1	AD	Payne, 1998
Bestrophin	Best disease	*VMD2*	11q13	AD	Petrukhin, 1998
Retinal guanylate cyclase (RetGC-1)	Cone-rod dystrophy Leber amaurosis	*GUC2D*	17p13.1	AD AR	Kelsell, 1998; Perrault, 1996
Aryl hydrocarbon-interacting receptor protein-like 1	Leber amaurosis	*AIPL1*	17p13.1	AR	Sohocki, 2000
Cone-rod homeobox (CRX)	Cone-rod dystrophy Leber amaurosis	*CRX*	19q13.3	AD AR	Freund, 1997, 1998
Tissue inhibitor of metallo-proteinases-3	Sorsby fundus dystrophy	*TIMP3*	22q13-qter	AD	Weber, 1994
Retinoschisin	Retinoschisis	*XLRS1*	Xp22	XL	Sauer, 1997

AD, Autosomal dominant; *AR,* autosomal recessive; *EGF,* epidermal growth factor; *XL,* X-linked.
*In the case of genes not referred to in detail in the text of the article, the full reference can be obtained from "RetNet" (www.sph.uth.tmc.edu/Retnet/disease.htm).

TABLE 12-4
CONGENITAL STATIONARY NIGHT BLINDNESS (CSNB) GENES

PROTEIN	PHENOTYPE	GENE	LOCUS	INHERITANCE	REFERENCES*
Arrestin (S-antigen)	Oguchi disease	*SAG*	2q37.1	AR	Fuchs, 1995
Rhodopsin	CSNB	*RHO*	3q21-q24	AD	Dryja, 1993
Transducin α-subunit	CSNB	*GNAT1*	3p22	AD	Dryja, 1996
Phospho-diesterase-β	CSNB	*PDE6B*	4p16.3	AR	Gal, 1994
Rhodopsin kinase	Oguchi disease	*RHOK*	13q34	AR	Yamamoto, 1995
Nyctalopin	CSNB1 (complete)	*NYX*	Xp11.4	XL	Pusch, 2000
L-type voltage-gated calcium channel, α_1-subunit	CSNB2 (incomplete)	*CACNA1F*	Xp11.23	XL	Bech-Hansen, 1998

AD, Autosomal dominant; *AR,* autosomal recessive; *XL,* X-linked.
*In the case of genes not referred to in detail in the text of the article, the full reference can be obtained from "RetNet" (www.sph.uth.tmc.edu/Retnet/disease.htm).

100 different mutations of the rhodopsin gene (*RHO*) have been identified, most of which produce single amino acid substitutions[54] (see Color Plate 5). The vast majority are associated with adRP, but mutations causing arRP and autosomal dominant congenital stationary night blindness (adCSNB) have also been reported.

Because the rhodopsin molecule accounts for nearly 50% of the protein content of the outer segments and 80% of the proteins in the discs, it must also be considered as an important structural protein of the ROS.[65] Mice lacking one copy of the rhodopsin gene have short, disorganized outer segments and suffer a very slow retinal degeneration, similar to that observed in mice lacking one copy of the *peripherin/RDS* gene[73] (see p. 371). This is in contrast to the rapid degeneration observed in mice expressing various adRP rhodopsin transgenes, suggesting that adRP is caused by a rhodopsin protein with a deleterious gain-of-function rather than a lack of functioning protein (haploinsufficiency). Although human rhodopsin and *peripherin/RDS* mutations almost exclusively cause dominantly inherited retinal dystrophies, all of the RP mutations

observed in genes encoding other proteins of the phototransduction pathway give rise to arRP. Therefore, in both mice and humans, most rhodopsin mutations behave as though they disrupt the structure of the ROS rather than the function of the phototransduction pathway.

Considerable phenotypic heterogeneity has been observed with different rhodopsin mutations. One particularly interesting subgroup of mutations (e.g., Thr58Arg, Gly106Asp) produce a form of adRP that has been defined as sectorial, characterized by retinal degeneration affecting only the lower half of the fundus in association with loss of the corresponding superior visual field[16] (Figure 12-4).

Structural and Functional Characteristics of Rhodopsin. Biochemical and mutagenesis studies of rhodopsin have elucidated many key structural and functional aspects of this molecule. These include the following: (1) 11-*cis*-retinal is attached by a Schiff base linkage to lysine 296 within the seventh transmembrane helix[26]; (2) parts of the transmembrane domain form the retinal binding pocket and, as such, alter the spectral properties of rhodopsin[103]; (3) the cytoplasmic loops, especially

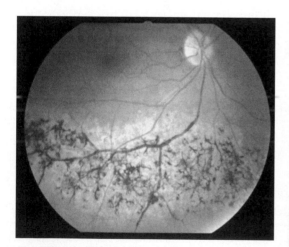

A

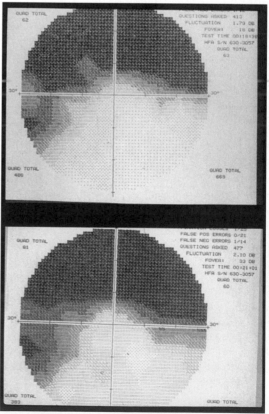

B

FIGURE 12-4　Sectorial retinitis pigmentosa. Fundus photograph (**A**) and visual field plot (**B**) of a patient with a rhodopsin Thr58Arg mutation. Intraretinal pigmentation is seen only in the inferior retina, with loss of the corresponding superior visual field.

those above the third and fourth and fifth and sixth helices, are critical for transducin binding[46]; (4) glutamine residue 113 appears to be the counterion of the Schiff base and critically regulates the spectral properties of rhodopsin[120]; (5) the intradiscal domain is the site of a disulfide bond between cysteines 110 and 187[80]; and (6) the C-terminal region has multiple serine and threonine residues that are phosphorylated during the deactivation of visual transduction.[144]

The human adRP mutation Lys296Glu renders rhodopsin incapable of binding 11-*cis*-retinal and produces a particularly severe adRP phenotype. In vitro this mutant opsin was shown to be active even in the absence of 11-*cis*-retinal, possibly reflecting the loss of the salt bridge between residues 113 and 296, which is essential for maintaining the opsin in an inert state.[116] However, the same mutation introduced into transgenic mice did not give rise to constitutive activation of rhodopsin.[88]

Human adRP mutations have also been reported involving the cysteine residues 110 and 187, which form the disulfide bond essential for maintaining the tertiary structure of rhodopsin (e.g., Cys110Tyr, Cys187Tyr). A cluster of missense mutations in the region of these cysteines may also have a similar effect by preventing the apposition of residues 110 and 187.

Functional Analysis of Mutations. Heterologous expression studies, in which constructs of wild-type and mutated rhodopsin genes were transfected in cultured cells, have defined two or three classes of mutant based on the effect of the mutation on rhodopsin biosynthesis, regeneration with 11-*cis*-retinal, and glycosylation pattern.[81,131] Although class I mutants tend to cluster in the first transmembrane domain and at the extreme carboxy-terminus, the mutants found in each class are not generally located in one region of the protein.

Class I Mutants. In vitro class I mutants (20%) are similar to wild-type rhodopsin in terms of yield, localization to the plasma membrane, regeneration, transducin activation, and phosphorylation by rhodopsin kinase. In transgenic mice, however, the class I mutant Gln344Ter opsin is inefficiently localized to the ROS, and the Pro347Ser mutant gives rise to a massive accumulation of vesicles at the base of the ROS.[89,132] The amino acids valine345 and proline347 may form part of a protein sorting signal that is not essential for movement of protein from endoplasmic reticulum (ER) to plasma membrane in cultured cells but that is required for transport of rhodopsin to the ROS. The dynein light-chain protein Tctex-1 may mediate this transport. Although the wild-type carboxy-terminus of rhodopsin binds to Tctex-1, several carboxy-terminal mutations responsible for adRP cause failure of the mutant opsin to bind.[134]

Class II Mutants. Class II mutants (20%) are expressed at low levels, do not form chromophore, are retained in the ER, bind 11-*cis*-retinal variably, and are abnormally glycosylated. These mutants (e.g., Tyr178Cys, Ser186Pro) either grossly alter the structure of the retinal-binding pocket and prevent the binding of 11-*cis*-retinal or configure this pocket in such a way that the Schiff base linkage is not stable.

Class III Mutants. Many of the mutants (60%) are expressed at intermediate levels, form some chromophore, are also retained in the ER, and are abnormally glycosylated. These class III mutants have abnormal bleaching kinetics and also trigger transducin inefficiently.

In studies of the common Pro23His mutation, a large fraction of the purified protein did not regenerate. Furthermore, the mutant was abnormally glycosylated and retained in the ER, suggesting that it did not fold efficiently or that certain nonnative structures were favored. Proteins that fold slowly or are misfolded are retained in the ER and are eventually degraded. The abnormality in glycosylation most likely then reflects the protein's inability to leave the ER rather than a true defect in the inability of the mutant to acquire the mature glycosylation. Pro23His is an N-terminal mutation, but there are many mutations within the transmembrane region, typically clustered in helices A and B (e.g., Pro53Arg) and the intradiscal loops (e.g., Gly106Arg) that also have a similar phenotype.

Rhodopsin and Congenital Stationary Night Blindness. The rhodopsin mutations Gly90Asp and Ala292Glu have both been associated with CSNB[111] (see p. 370). In both instances it has been demonstrated that the purified mutant protein is active in the absence of the chromophore 11-*cis*-retinal, and this behavior would be expected to limit the light sensitivity of the rods. It is believed both substitutions lead to the disruption of the important salt bridge between glutamine 113 and lysine 296.

Rhodopsin and Autosomal Recessive Retinitis Pigmentosa. There is a single reported rhodopsin mutation (Glu249Ter) that, in the homozygous state, causes arRP. Retinal degeneration presumably results from a loss of function, comparable to that seen in mice homozygous for rhodopsin gene knockouts, who sustain rapid degeneration of the retina.[73]

Rod cGMP Phosphodiesterase. PDE is a heterotetrameric enzyme consisting of two large subunits (α and β) that become active when the two inhibitory γ-subunits are removed by activated transducin. After the discovery that a homozygous loss-of-function mutation in *pdeb* (the gene encoding the β-subunit of rod cGMP PDE) is responsible for the classic murine retinal degeneration *rd,* mutations were found in *PDE6B* (the human homologue of *pdeb*) in patients with arRP.[98] Additional *PDE6B* mutations have since been identified, and these are currently one of the most commonly identified causes of arRP, accounting for 4% to 5% of cases. Subsequently, mutations in *PDE6A,* the gene encoding the α-subunit of rod cGMP PDE, have also been found in patients with arRP.[72]

Most *PDE6B* mutations are located in the C-terminal half of the protein, which contains the catalytic domain, and are predicted to decrease PDE activity. This leads to an increase in intracellular cGMP levels, which may be toxic to the rods. No mutations in *PDE6G* (the gene encoding the PDE γ-subunit) have been found, despite the fact that mutations introduced by gene targeting into the murine homolog *pdeg* produced a retinal degeneration phenotype resembling RP.[136]

cGMP-Gated Cation Channel Proteins. As with many other components of the phototransduction cascade, two variants of the cGMP-gated cation channel protein exist: one specific for rod and one for cone photoreceptors. These channel proteins are heterotetramers of two homologous α- and β-subunits. Mutations responsible for arRP were first identified in *CNCG1*, the gene encoding the α-subunit of the rod-specific cGMP-gated cation channel protein, and subsequently in the gene encoding the β-subunit of this protein (*CNGB1*).[7,41] Mutations causing achromatopsia, or rod monochromacy, have been demonstrated in both the α- and β-subunits of the cone cGMP-gated channel protein.[85,130]

Retinal Guanylate Cyclases and Guanylate Cyclase Activating Proteins. The enzymatic activity of the retinal guanylate cyclases RetGC-1 and RetGC-2 is modulated by calcium, increasing as the calcium concentration falls during light exposure and decreasing when calcium levels rise in the dark. This is mediated by two calcium-binding guanylate cyclase activating proteins: GCAP-1 and GCAP-2. Both of these proteins contain four calcium-binding domains (EF-hands). When photoactivation causes closure of the cGMP-gated cation channels, entry of calcium into the photoreceptor is prevented. At these low calcium concentrations, calcium dissociates from the GCAPs, permitting them to stimulate RetGC-1 and RetGC-2 to increase cGMP production.

Mutations in the gene encoding RetGC-1 (*GUCD2*) are one cause of the severe recessive cone-rod dystrophy (CRD) Leber congenital amaurosis (LCA).[108] An animal model for this form of LCA is provided by a naturally occurring null mutation in the chicken ortholog of RetGC-1, which also gives rise to a recessive photoreceptor degeneration.[125]

Several missense mutations at codon 838, which lies within a putative intracellular dimerization domain of RetGC-1, are responsible for a later-onset dominant CRD phenotype.[43] Functional characterization of these mutations indicates that they have a higher affinity for GCAP-1 than wild-type RetGC-1 and marked residual activity at high calcium concentrations.[145] It is proposed that the resulting elevation of cGMP levels in the dark leads to persistently high intracellular calcium levels, which may disrupt the membrane potential of the mitochondrial outer membrane and initiate an apoptotic pathway.

A single missense mutation (Y99C) in the third calcium-binding domain of GCAP-1 has been shown to cause dominant cone dystrophy.[107] In high calcium concentrations (2 μM), at which wild-type GCAP-1 shows no RetGC stimulatory activity, the GCAP-1 (Y99C) mutant continues to exhibit 30% to 50% of the stimulatory activity seen in low (50 nM) calcium. This mutation may have a similar, although milder, deleterious effect as the RetGC1 mutations and may lead to preferential cone death because of higher levels of RetGC-1 expression in cones.

Congenital Stationary Night Blindness. CSNB, like RP, is a clinically and genetically heterogenous disorder primarily affecting the rod photoreceptors; patients with CSNB become aware of night blindness (nyctalopia) in early childhood.[28] In contrast to RP, however, the disease is nonprogressive, there is no apparent rod degeneration, and affected individuals retain photopic vision throughout life.

CSNB may be inherited as an autosomal dominant, autosomal recessive, or X-linked trait. Analysis of the molecular genetics of CSNB may result in the identification of genes for RP because many CSNB loci have proven to be allelic with RP loci.

adCSNB has been found in association with several mutations in genes encoding components of the phototransduction cascade: rhodopsin (Ala292Glu); *PDE6B* (His258Asp); and the α-subunit of transducin, *GNAT1* (Gly38Asp).[40,42,53] The *GNAT1* mutation is interesting because it is responsible for the CSNB that affects the famous Nougaret family. In each case the proposed effect of the mutation is a constitutive activation of the phototransduction cascade leading to desensitization of rod photoreceptors.

Oguchi disease is a rare autosomal recessive form of CSNB characterized by a normal fundus appearance following full dark adaptation that gives way to a golden or gray-white coloration of the retina on light exposure (the Mizuo phenomenon). Homozygous *null* mutations of the genes encoding Arrestin and rhodopsin kinase, both of which play a role in deactivating rhodopsin, have been identified in patients with Oguchi disease.[50,147] Once again, prolonged activation of rod photoreceptors may lead to desensitization, but in contrast to the dominant forms of CSNB, in Oguchi disease, rod sensitivity eventually returns to normal after extended dark adaptation.

Three X-linked CSNB loci have been identified. *CSNB1* is associated with severe myopia and undetectable rod function ("complete" CSNB). Up to 50% of complete X-linked CSNB cases are caused by mutations in the *NYX* gene, which encodes the protein nyctalopin.[10,110] Nyctalopin is an extracellular glycosylphosphatidyl (GPI)–anchored member of the small leucine-rich proteoglycan (SLRP) protein family and is expressed in retina and brain. Families linked to the *CSNB2* locus are described as having "incomplete" CSNB to indicate that they have subnormal but measurable rod function. Several different mutations in the gene *CACNA1F*, which encodes a retina-specific voltage-gated calcium channel α1-subunit, have been found in patients with *CSNB2*.[9,128] These mutations are predicted to cause a decrease in neurotransmitter release from photoreceptors. *CSNB3* is allelic with *RP3*, and a novel mutation in *RPGR* has been identified in a patient with CSNB.[70]

Photoreceptor Structural Proteins
Peripherin/RDS and ROM-1. Mutations in the *peripherin/RDS* gene, which is located at 6p21 and encodes the protein peripherin/RDS, are estimated to account for 5% of all adRP cases.[79] Peripherin/RDS is an abundant transmembrane protein that is localized to the outer segment disc rims in both rods and cones and that may play an important role in maintaining rim curvature and possibly in anchoring rod discs to the adjacent plasma membrane.[135] In rods, peripherin/RDS forms a heterotetrameric complex with another structural protein, ROS protein 1 (ROM-1), with which it has 55% nucleotide sequence homology.[8] Because no cone-specific equivalent of ROM-1 has been identified thus far, it has been suggested that four peripherin/RDS molecules bind together to form a homotetramer in cones.

A large insertion mutation in the murine *peripherin/rds* gene was found to be responsible for the naturally occurring mouse retinal dystrophy *rds* (retinal degeneration slow). This acts as a null mutation, resulting in a complete lack of *peripherin/rds* in homozygous *rds⁻/rds⁻* mice, which fail to develop outer segments.[32] In heterozygous mice, which have a 50% reduction in *peripherin/rds* (haploinsufficiency), outer segments are produced but are shortened and structurally disorganized.

More than 40 different mutations of the human homolog *peripherin/RDS* have been identified, and these are associated with a wide phenotypic variety of dominantly inherited photoreceptor dystrophies that differ in the extent of rod or cone involvement, including adRP, CRD, and several macular dystrophies.[84] In contrast to the murine *rds* mutation, the human mutations are assumed to cause retinal dystrophy by a dominant negative effect of the mutant peripherin/RDS protein on photoreceptor function and stability. This has been demonstrated by the introduction of a mutated (Pro216Leu) *peripherin/RDS* transgene into *rds⁻/rds⁻* mice. Transgenic Pro216Leu mice sustained increased outer segment dysplasia and accelerated photoreceptor cell death, when compared with heterozygous *rds⁺/rds⁻* mice with one wild-type copy of *peripherin/rds*.[82]

Further studies have shown that some *peripherin/RDS* mutations, which are associated with human adRP, prevent peripherin/RDS and ROM-1 from forming a tetramer; although the Arg172Trp mutation, responsible for autosomal dominant macular dystrophy, behaves normally with respect to subunit assembly.[58] It is possible that mutations causing macular dystrophy either affect *RDS-RDS* binding or the binding of *peripherin/RDS* to an unidentified cone counterpart of ROM-1. Individual *RDS* mutations can also be associated with marked intrafamilial phenotypic variation. One family segregating a deletion in codons 153-154 has been reported to have affected members with adRP, pattern macular dystrophy, and fundus flavimaculatus, suggesting that the eventual phenotype may depend on the interaction of *peripherin/RDS* with one or more as yet unidentified proteins.[141]

The important structural relationship between peripherin/RDS and ROM-1 is underlined by a small number of families with RP in whom affected individuals are compound heterozygotes for both a specific *RDS* mutation (Leu185Pro) and one of a number of *ROM1* mutations.[78] In contrast, family members who possess the *RDS* or the *ROM1* mutation alone are not affected, providing the first definite example of a digenic disorder in human genetics.

Because *peripherin/RDS* is located on chromosome 6 and *ROM1* on chromosome 11, the two mutations in digenic RP will segregate independently and may both be inherited by the offspring of an affected individual (25% chance), resulting in a pseudodominant pattern of inheritance. This is in contrast to the situation in arRP, in which meiosis prevents two mutated copies of the same gene from both being transmitted to an offspring. The digenic pattern of inheritance must therefore be taken into account when carrying out genetic counseling of small, apparently dominant pedigrees and in all cases of sporadic RP.

Heterologous expression of peripherin/RDS and ROM-1 in cultured cells has revealed that Leu185Pro peripherin/rds does not form *RDS-RDS* homotetramers but can form heterotetramers with ROM-1.[59] RP appears to result when this mutation is combined with a 50% reduction in ROM-1 concentration.

Usher Syndrome. The Usher syndromes are the most common of the syndromic retinal dystrophies, with a prevalence of approximately 1 in 25,000.[25] This clinically and genetically heterogeneous group of recessively inherited disorders is characterized by the combination of congenital sensorineural deafness and RP.[45] The Usher syndromes are subdivided on the basis of the severity of auditory and vestibular dysfunction: Individuals with Usher syndrome type I (USH1) are profoundly deaf and lack vestibular function, but subjects with Usher syndrome type II (USH2) have mild nonprogressive hearing loss and normal vestibular function. Usher syndrome type III is rare and includes progressive hearing loss associated with variable vestibular function.

Usher Syndrome Type 1: MYO7A and CDH23. At least six genetic loci (*USH1A-F*) have been identified for USH1, of which *USH1B* (located at 11q13.5) accounts for approximately 75% of all cases of USH1. The gene for *USH1B* (*MYO7A*) was identified when the recessive mouse mutant *shaker-1*, which manifests a progressive cochlear and vestibular degeneration (but not retinal dystrophy), was found to be caused by mutations in the murine homolog *myo7a*.[57]

A large number of nonsense mutations, deletions, and missense mutations in *MYO7A* have since been demonstrated, both in *USH1B* families and in individuals with isolated (nonsyndromic) deafness.[140] *MYO7A* encodes the protein myosin VIIA, which belongs to a family of unconventional myosins involved in phagocytosis, endocytosis, vesicular transport, chemotactic movement, and other motilities associated with actin. Myosin VIIA has been immunolocalized to the base of rod and cone outer segments and to the apical microvilli of the RPE.[92] One study reported myosin VIIA immunoreactivity in primate, but not rodent, photoreceptors and suggested that this might explain the phenotypic difference between *shaker-1* mice and humans.

Mutations in the *CDH23* gene have been identified in consanguineous Pakistani, Indian, and Turkish families as a cause of USH1 at the *USH1D* locus and of recessive nonsyndromic deafness.[23] *CDH23* encodes a cadherin-like protein of unknown function that, like myosin VIIA, is expressed in both retina and cochlea. Cadherins function as intercellular adhesion molecules, suggesting a role for *CDH23* in the maintenance of interactions between retinal cells.

Usher Syndrome Type 2: USH2A. Usher syndrome type 2 is also genetically heterogeneous with three loci identified (*USH2A-C*), of which *USH2A* accounts for at least 90% of affected individuals. The *USH2A* gene encodes a putative extracellular matrix protein, usherin, that is expressed in the retina and inner ear and that contains laminin epidermal growth factor (EGF) and fibronectin type III domains that may be involved in cell adhesion.[44] A 2299delG mutation is particularly common in *USH2A* patients, whereas other mutations in *USH2A* give rise to recessive RP without hearing loss.[115]

X-Linked Retinoschisis. XLRS, a juvenile-onset macular dystrophy, is characterized by cystic lesions within the nerve fiber layer (macular schisis cavities); these lesions are thought to arise from a defect in Müller cells. XLRS is one of the few dystrophies that give rise to an electronegative ERG, suggestive of a postreceptoral defect. Macular schisis is associated with peripheral retinoschisis in approximately 50% of cases. The *XLRS1* gene encodes the protein retinoschisin, which shares homology with discoidin and other proteins implicated in cell-to-cell interactions.[121] In murine retina this protein is expressed exclusively in photoreceptor cells, but it is also secreted into the inner retina and may have a role in photoreceptor-to-Müller cell interaction.[60] More than 80 different mutations of *XLRS* have been observed.[114]

Retinol (Vitamin A) Metabolism

Regeneration of 11-*cis*-retinal (the "visual cycle") is a complex process involving several enzymes and retinoid-binding proteins in both the rod photoreceptor and the RPE (see Color Plate 6). This process is facilitated by the interdigitation of ROSs and the apical microvilli of the RPE, which increases the surface area across which metabolites can be transported.

During photoactivation, opsin-bound 11-*cis*-retinal is isomerized to all-*trans*-retinal, released from its binding pocket, and then transported out of the ROS disc by the adenosine triphosphate (ATP)–binding cassette transporter of rods (*ABCR*). In the ROS cytoplasm, a rod-specific dehydrogenase (*t*-RDH) converts retinal to all-*trans*-retinol, which then crosses the interphotoreceptor space bound to interphotoreceptor retinoid-binding protein (IRBP) and enters the RPE. In the RPE, all-*trans*-retinol binds to cellular retinoid-binding protein (CRBP) and is esterified by lecithin retinol acyl transferase (LRAT) to produce an all-*trans*-retinyl ester. This ester is transformed into 11-*cis*-retinol by an isomerohydrolase enzyme, which may be the protein RPE65. Retinol is then bound by cellular retinaldehyde-binding protein (CRALBP), which also promotes the oxidation of retinol to 11-*cis*-retinal by 11-*cis*-retinol dehydrogenase (*c*-RDH) and inhibits the esterification of 11-*cis*-retinol.[118] Regenerated 11-*cis*-retinal is then returned, via the interphotoreceptor space, to the rods. Mutations involving visual cycle proteins have now been identified in several retinal dystrophies, all of which are recessively inherited.

ABCR, Rim Protein, and Stargardt Disease/Fundus Flavimaculatus.

Stargardt disease/fundus flavimaculatus (STGD1) is an autosomal recessive retinal dystrophy characterized by the presence of yellow-white flecks at the level of the RPE, which may be concentrated at the fovea (Stargardt disease) or be scattered throughout the peripheral retina with minimal macular involvement (fundus flavimaculatus)[104] (Figure 12-5). The severity of visual loss depends on the degree of macular involvement. Stargardt disease typically presents in late childhood, often with a relatively rapid loss of visual acuity occurring over a few weeks or months. Foveal flecks give way to macular atrophy as the disease progresses, resulting in severely reduced central vision (20/200). Fundus flavimaculatus tends to present in later life and is often associated with preservation of central vision. Fluorescein angiography in both conditions is characterized by a dark choroid resulting from blocking of normal choroidal fluorescence by the RPE deposits. Both angiography and electrophysiology indicate that there may be widespread retinal dysfunction even when fundal changes are limited to the macular area.

Histopathology in early Stargardt disease indicates that the characteristic flecks and dark choroid result from deposition of lipofuscin pigment granules in RPE cells.[22] With disease progression, degeneration of the RPE occurs and photoreceptor loss occurs at a late stage.

Autosomal recessive Stargardt disease/fundus flavimaculatus (STGD1) is genetically homogeneous, with all affected families linking to a locus at 1p21-p13. Causative mutations have been demonstrated in the gene *ABCR*, which encodes Rim protein (RmP), a photoreceptor-specific ATP-binding transporter protein.[3] Although Stargardt disease

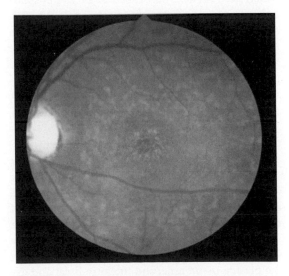

FIGURE 12-5 Stargardt disease/fundus flavimaculatus. Fundus photograph demonstrating yellow flecks at the level of the retinal pigment epithelium, both at the fovea and scattered in the surrounding retina.

primarily affects the cone-rich macula, RmP is expressed exclusively in rod photoreceptor outer segments, where it colocalizes with peripherin/RDS at the disc rim.[5]

A valuable insight into the function of RmP in the pathogenesis of STGD1 has recently been gained from a study using *abcr* knockout mice as a model of the human disorder.[142] Levels of critical outer segment proteins (rhodopsin, rds/peripherin, and ROM-1) were similar in *abcr*[-/-] and wild-type mice. Abnormalities demonstrated in mice with the *abcr*[-/-] null mutation included (1) delayed rod dark adaptation; (2) delayed clearance of all-*trans*-retinaldehyde following a photobleach; (3) a 1.6-fold increase in phosphatidylethanolamine (PE) levels in ROSs; (4) presence of protonated *N*-retinylidene-PE (the condensation product of retinaldehyde and PE) in preference to the nonprotonated form; (5) a tenfold to twentyfold increase in the RPE levels of *N*-retinylidene-*N*-retinylethanolamine (A2-E, the condensation product of two retinaldehydes with ethanolamine), which is the major fluorescent constituent of lipofuscin; and (6) accumulation of dense bodies in RPE cells associated with thickening of Bruch's membrane.

On the basis of these findings, the authors propose that *abcr/ABCR* acts as an outwardly directed flippase for protonated *N*-retinylidene-PE, located at the rim of ROS discs. This would be consistent with the biology of other members of the ABC (ATP-binding cassette) transporter family, some of which have been demonstrated to act as phospholipid flippases.[37] Several retinoids, including all-*trans*-retinaldehyde, have been shown to increase the adenosine triphosphatase (ATPase) activity of RmP, but only when RmP was reconstituted in the presence of PE.[129] This implies that all-*trans*-retinaldehyde may be reacting with PE to form *N*-retinylidene-PE, the proposed substrate for RmP.

RmP may speed up the recovery of retinal sensitivity (dark adaptation) following a photobleach by accelerating transfer of all-*trans*-retinaldehyde from the disc interior to the cytoplasm. Because the disc rim is adjacent to the plasma membrane, the location of RmP may increase the efficiency of retinoid recycling by minimizing the diffusion path via the extracellular space to the RPE. In cone outer segments the disc membranes are continuous with the plasma membrane, and the intradiscal and extracellular spaces are contiguous. Therefore there may be no requirement for RmP in these cells.

Because RPE cells are responsible for the phagocytosis of ROSs, elimination of *N*-retinylidene-PE from the interior of discs may also protect the RPE from lipofuscin accumulation. A2-E has been shown to induce apoptosis in mammalian RPE.[133] In *abcr*[-/-] mice high concentrations A2-E may act as a positively charged lysomotrophic detergent, dissolving cellular membranes and potentially leading to the death of RPE cells, with secondary degeneration of photoreceptors. Because the perifoveal retina in humans contains a ringlike area of high rod density, the predilection of STGD1 for the macula may be attributable to rod-mediated damage to the macular RPE. This hypothesis correlates well with the histopathologic and clinical findings in Stargardt disease.

RPE65 (All-*trans*-Retinyl Ester Isomerohydrolase). The *RPE65* gene encodes a 65-kD microsomal protein (RPE65), which is expressed exclusively in the RPE, where it accounts for approximately 10% of total membrane protein.[64] Mutations in *RPE65* have been demonstrated in LCA and autosomal recessive childhood-onset severe retinal dystrophy.[61,94] The latter phenotype is poorly defined and may include early-onset forms of both arRP and recessive CRD. *Rpe65*[-/-] mice lack rhodopsin, despite the presence of the opsin apoprotein in ROS.[112] Rod function, as measured by electroretinography, is abolished, although cone function persists. In these mice, excess all-*trans* retinyl esters accumulate in the RPE, whereas 11-*cis* retinyl esters are absent. These data suggest that RPE65 acts as, or in conjunction with, an all-*trans*-retinyl ester isomerohydrolase and that cone pigment regeneration may be dependent on a separate pathway.

Administration of oral 9-*cis*–retinal to *Rpe65*[-/-] mice has been shown to result in rhodopsin formation and an improvement in the ERG, implying that pharmacologic intervention might be successful in individuals with retinal dystrophies caused by defects in RPE65.[137]

Cellular Retinaldehyde-Binding Protein. Mutations in CRALBP cause retinitis punctata albescens, a form of arRP in which white dots are found scattered across the retina.[97] One recombinant CRALBP mutant (R150Q) was demonstrated to be unable to bind 11-*cis*-retinal, which presumably impairs oxidation of 11-*cis*-retinol to 11-*cis*-retinal in vivo, limiting the quantity of retinal available to the photoreceptors. A similar phenotype, with small white deposits at the level of the RPE, night blindness, and visual field loss, also characterizes chronic retinol (vitamin A) deficiency. Photoreceptor degeneration is also observed in animal models of chronic retinol deficiency.[67]

11-*cis*-Retinol Dehydrogenase. Conversion of 11-*cis*-retinol to 11-*cis*-retinal within the RPE is catalyzed by 11-*cis*-retinol dehydrogenase, encoded by the gene *RDH5*. Two recessive missense mutations of *RDH5* have been identified in patients with fundus albipunctatus, a form of CSNB also characterized by the presence of white deposits in the retina and delayed dark adaptation.[146] In vitro, mutant *RDH5* had a tenfold decreased yield and a greatly reduced specific activity compared with the wild-type enzyme.

Interestingly, the retina develops normally, without white deposits, in mice homozygous for a targeted disruption of the *RDH5* gene.[38] These mice displayed normal rod and cone ERG responses and normal dark adaptation kinetics at bleaching levels under which patients with fundus albipunctatus could be detected unequivocally. Only at high bleaching levels was delayed dark adaptation observed, suggesting that the murine RPE contains an alternative mechanism for the biosynthesis of 11-*cis*-retinal.

Serum Retinal-Binding Protein. The *RBP4* gene encodes SRBP, which is the specific carrier for retinol in the blood. Two siblings, who were compound heterozygous for missense mutations in *RBP4*, were observed to have nyctalopia since early childhood, atrophy of the RPE, elevated dark adaptation thresholds, and abnormal scotopic and photopic ERGs.[124] The absence of detectable SRBP in these individuals was associated with serum retinol levels less than 20% of normal, which would severely limit the availability of retinol to the RPE for formation of chromophore.

Transcription Factors

Many transcription factors (proteins that regulate gene expression) are required for normal ocular development, and some remain essential for maintenance of the mature retina.[47]

Cone Rod Homeobox (CRX). The photoreceptor-specific transcription factor CRX, derived from the homeobox gene *CRX* (19q13.3), is expressed both during retinal development and in adult retina. Mice homozygous for a targeted disruption of the murine *Crx* gene do not elaborate photoreceptor outer segments and lack electroretinographic evidence of rod and cone activity.[52] Rat photoreceptors expressing a dominant-negative *Crx* mutation also fail to develop normal outer segments,[51] suggesting that *Crx* is essential for photoreceptor morphogenesis. In mature retinas, CRX acts synergistically with the transcription factor neural retina leucine zipper (NRL) to control expression of photoreceptor-specific genes such as rhodopsin and the cone opsins.[31]

Dominant mutations in the human *CRX* gene (e.g., Glu80Ala and Glu168 1bp deletion) have been found in adCRD.[48] These may be pathogenic by a dominant-negative (gain of function) mechanism or result in haploinsufficiency of CRX. Recessive mutations in *CRX* are one cause of LCA, a severe CRD in which retinal degeneration may be present at birth.[49] Affected individuals have severe visual loss associated with nystagmus in the first few months of life and a significantly reduced or undetectable ERG. The early onset and relative severity of these dystrophies may reflect the essential role of CRX in retinal development.

Neural Retina Leucine Zipper. In vitro the transcription factor NRL also binds to sequences present in or near the promoters of many photoreceptor-specific genes and regulates their expression, both alone and in synergy with *CRX*. A Ser50Thr missense mutation in the *NRL* gene (chromosome 14q11.2) has been identified in several ancestrally related families with adRP.[18] Serine50 is located in one of two highly conserved regions of the transactivation (TA) domain of NRL and is conserved in other members of the Maf family of proteins that contain a TA domain. When coexpressed with *CRX* in transient transfection experiments, NRL^{S50T} demonstrated significantly enhanced synergistic transactivation of the rhodopsin promoter, resulting in increased transcriptional activity.[17] Rhodopsin is the major structural protein of ROS, and in animal models, overexpression of rhodopsin has been shown to cause photoreceptor cell death.[105] A similar mechanism may be responsible for the retinal degeneration resulting from the NRL^{S50T} mutation.

Photoreceptor-Specific Nuclear Receptor (*NR2E3*). Patients with recessive enhanced S-cone syndrome (ESCS) exhibit increased sensitivity to blue light, mediated by what is normally the least populous cone photoreceptor subtype, the S (short wavelength, blue) cones. Ninety-four percent of a cohort of ESCS probands was found to have mutations in the gene *NR2E3*, which encodes photoreceptor cell-specific nuclear receptor (PNR), one of a large family of nuclear receptor transcription factors involved in signaling pathways.[62] These nuclear receptors have been shown to be involved in embryonic development and in the maintenance of cellular function in adult life. Abnormal determination of cone cell fate during retinal development may therefore lead to an altered ratio of short-wavelength to long- and medium-wavelength cone photoreceptors in ESCS.

A homozygous missense mutation in *PNR* (Arg311Gln) has also been identified as the cause of late-onset RP in the highly consanguineous population of Portuguese Crypto-Jews.[56] These individuals did not undergo electrophysiologic assessment of S-cone function. A deletion in the murine homolog of *NR2E3* gives rise to the late-onset autosomal recessive retinal degeneration of the *rd7* mouse, which provides a naturally occurring animal model for the human diseases.[1]

Proteins of Undetermined Function

Although many of the earliest retinal dystrophy genes (e.g., rhodopsin, *PDE6B*) were identified by mutation analysis of functional candidates, recent advances in molecular genetic techniques have resulted in the isolation of genes encoding proteins of unknown function, which may be members of as yet unrecognized protein families. Many of these are not uniquely expressed in photoreceptors and may instead be RPE proteins, such as bestrophin, or indeed are ubiquitously expressed like *EFEMP1* and the RP GTPase regulator (RPGR), responsible for xlRP at the *RP3* locus.[117]

Bestrophin in Best Vitelliform Macular Dystrophy. Best macular dystrophy is a dominantly inherited disorder with variable expressivity.[14] The characteristic vitelliform lesion is a round or oval yellow subretinal deposit in the macular region. Histopathologic examination demonstrates the aberrant accumulation of lipofuscin-like material in RPE cells. As the disease progresses, the yellow material is reabsorbed, leaving a large area of RPE atrophy at the macula and an associated reduction of central vision. Although some carriers of mutations in the *VMD2* gene may not have symptoms and may have normal fundus examination results, they can be identified clinically by the combination of an abnormal EOG results and a normal ERG results.

Characterization and mutation screening of potential candidate genes within the Best disease critical interval (located at 11q12-q13) lead to the identification of mutations in a novel RPE-specific gene, designated *VMD2*, in patients with Best disease.[109] The product of the *VMD2* gene, bestrophin, has been localized by immunocytochemistry to the basolateral plasma membrane of RPE cells.[95] On the basis of histologic evidence and structural analysis, it has been suggested that the bestrophin

may have a role in the transport or metabolism of polyunsaturated fatty acids within the retina. Mutations in *VMD2* have also been reported in the phenotypically similar, but later-onset, adult vitelliform macular dystrophy.[143]

EFEMP1 *in Malattia Leventinese and Doyne Honeycomb Retinal Dystrophy.* Malattia Leventinese and Doyne honeycomb retinal dystrophy are phenotypically similar, dominantly inherited dystrophies characterized by yellow-white deposits (drusen) beneath the RPE in the macular region and around the optic disc. Central vision may be preserved, but there is a significant risk of serious visual loss resulting from choroidal neovascularization.

In a spectacular example of a "founder effect,"[39] apparently unrelated pedigrees from several different countries with dominant drusen of the Doyne/Malattia Leventinese type were all found to have an Arg345Trp mutation in the gene *EFEMP1*.[127] *EFEMP1* (EGF-containing fibrillin-like extracellular matrix protein 1) is a widely expressed protein with homology to the fibulin family of extracellular matrix glycoproteins.

THERAPY OF THE INHERITED RETINAL DYSTROPHIES

Current Management

Individuals affected by a retinal dystrophy should be provided with good prognostic and genetic counseling to enable them to plan their future with the maximum amount of relevant information available. Suitable employment often depends on adequate central vision, and if this becomes significantly impaired, assistance with reading and writing is essential. This may include standard low visual aids (reading glasses, handheld and stand magnifiers), closed-circuit television cameras, and suitable personal computing technology (large monitors, e-mail, voice recognition software, and scanners with optical character recognition [OCR] software).

Loss of visual field and/or central vision in people with retinal dystrophies often results in failure to conform to local legal requirements for driving. This may be particularly disabling if the individual lives in remote area or relies on a car for work. Night blindness and color blindness are less likely to affect a person's employment prospects and leisure activities but usually prevent the person from obtaining satisfactory posts in the armed forces.

Social support for people with visual disability varies from country to country and may involve both statutory authorities (social and welfare services, formal blind or partial-sight registration) and charitable organizations (e.g., Retinitis Pigmentosa Society). These bodies may provide social, educational, employment, and in some cases, financial support to persons with retinal dystrophy.

Some individuals with RP have cataracts and CME as complications of their condition. When appropriate, these patients can be managed by cataract extraction and the use of carbonic anhydrase inhibitors (e.g., acetazolamide), respectively.

Future Prospects

Virtually no disease-specific treatment is currently available for patients with retinal dystrophy. Dietary management, which should be initiated as soon as possible to minimize irreversible retinal damage, exists for just three rare recessive dystrophies: Refsum disease, abetalipoproteinemia, and gyrate atrophy.[15] Current research projects seek to develop treatments based on (1) the manipulation of photoreceptor apoptosis, (2) the introduction of functional genes into photoreceptor or RPE cells, and (3) transplantation of photoreceptors and/or RPE cells.

Manipulation of Photoreceptor Apoptosis.

Several growth factors (basic fibroblast growth factor [bFGF], brain-derived neurotrophic factor [BDNF], and ciliary neurotrophic factor [CNTF]) have been used therapeutically to modify the apoptotic pathway and delay photoreceptor degeneration in animal models of retinal dystrophy.[86] This form of therapy can be applied to retinal disorders of unknown genetic origin, but the beneficial effects of treatment are relatively short lived.

Gene Therapy Strategies.

The basic methodology of introducing functional genes, with a variety of viral vectors, has been used in four different techniques to successfully rescue photoreceptors in rodent models of RP.

Gene Augmentation in Recessive and X-Linked Diseases. The classic approach of delivering a normal gene to compensate for loss-of-function mutations has been used to rescue both the *rd* mouse and the *rds* mouse.[2,12] In the *rds-/-* mouse the introduction of an *rds* transgene resulted in the production of outer segments containing both peripherin/rds and rhodopsin and significantly improved ERG responses.

Ribozyme Treatment in Dominant Disorders. Treatment of disorders caused by dominantly inherited gain-of-function mutations is more complex because it requires the elimination of the mutant gene product. Ribozymes (ribonucleic acid [RNA] enzymes) are RNA-cleaving RNA molecules, the recognition sequences of which can be designed to identify and cleave mutant RNA while leaving wild-type RNA intact.[66] The introduction of mutation-specific ribozymes achieved long-term rescue of photoreceptors in the rhodopsin P23H transgenic rat, which models the most common form of adRP found in North America.[87]

Regulation of Apoptosis. Delivery into photoreceptors of additional copies of the *bcl-2* gene, which is involved in the regulation of apoptosis, has been used to delay photoreceptor loss in the *rd* mouse.[13]

Growth Factor Therapy. Gene transfer of a secretable form of CNTF has been used as an alternative to direct intravitreal injection to increase the longevity of treatment and delay photoreceptor loss in both *rd* and *rds* mice.[29,30]

Transplantation of Photoreceptors and Retinal Pigment Epithelium.

Successful transplantation of functional photoreceptors has yet to be achieved.[90] However, subretinal transplantation of RPE cells has been used to delay loss of photoreceptors in the RCS rat, in which a mutation of the receptor tyrosine kinase gene *Mertk* results in failure of RPE to phagocytose shed outer segments, with subsequent photoreceptor cell death.[35,91] Mutations in the human *MERTK* gene are responsible for some cases of arRP.[55] This form of treatment may be applicable to the increasing number of human dystrophies that are recognized to be caused by mutations in RPE-specific genes.

REFERENCES

1. Akhmedov NB et al: A deletion in a photoreceptor-specific nuclear receptor mRNA causes retinal degeneration in the *rd7* mouse, *Proc Natl Acad Sci USA* 97:5551, 2000.
2. Ali R et al: Restoration of photoreceptor ultrastructure and function in retinal degeneration slow mice by gene therapy, *Nat Genet* 25:306, 2000.
3. Allikmets R et al: A photoreceptor cell-specific ATP-binding transporter gene (*ABCR*) is mutated in recessive Stargardt's macular dystrophy, *Nat Genet* 15:236, 1997.
4. Al-Maghtheh M et al: Evidence for a major retinitis pigmentosa locus on 19q13.4 (RP11), and association with a unique bimodal expressivity phenotype, *Am J Hum Genet* 59:864, 1996.
5. Azarian SM, Travis GH: The photoreceptor rim protein is an ABC transporter encoded by the gene for recessive Stargardt's disease (ABCR), *FEBS Lett* 409:247, 1997.

6. Bach M et al: Standard for pattern electroretinography. International Society for Clinical Electrophysiology of Vision, *Doc Ophthalmol* 101:11, 2000.

7. Bareil C et al: Segregation of a mutation in *CNGB1* encoding the beta-subunit of the rod cGMP-gated channel in a family with autosomal recessive retinitis pigmentosa, *Hum Genet* 108:328, 2001.

8. Bascom RA et al: Molecular cloning of the cDNA for a novel photoreceptor-specific membrane protein (rom-1) identifies a disk rim protein family implicated in human degenerative retinopathies, *Neuron* 8:1171, 1992.

9. Bech-Hansen NT et al: Loss-of-function mutations in a calcium-channel alpha1-subunit gene in Xp11.23 cause incomplete X-linked congenital stationary night blindness, *Nat Genet* 19:264, 1998.

10. Bech-Hansen NT et al: Mutations in *NYX*, encoding the leucine-rich proteoglycan nyctalopin, cause X-linked complete congenital stationary night blindness, *Nat Genet* 26:319, 2000.

11. Behrens F, Weiss LR: An automated and modified technique for testing the retinal function (Arden test) by use of the electro-oculogram (EOG) for clinical and research use, *Doc Ophthalmol* 96:283, 1998.

12. Bennett J et al: Photoreceptor cell rescue in retinal degeneration (rd) mice by in vivo gene therapy, *Nat Med* 2:649, 1996.

13. Bennett J et al: Adenovirus-mediated delivery of rhodopsin-promoted bcl-2 results in a delay in photoreceptor cell death in the rd/rd mouse, *Gene Ther* 5:1156, 1998.

14. Benson WE et al: Best's vitelliform macular dystrophy, *Am J Ophthalmol* 79:59, 1975.

15. Berson EL: Nutrition and retinal degenerations, *Int Ophthalmol Clin* 40:93, 2000.

16. Berson EL, Howard J: Temporal aspects of the electroretinogram in sector retinitis pigmentosa, *Arch Ophthalmol* 86:653, 1971.

17. Bessant DA et al: NRL S50T mutation and the importance of "founder effects" in inherited retinal dystrophies, *Eur J Hum Genet* 8:783, 2000.

18. Bessant DAR et al: A mutation in NRL is associated with autosomal dominant retinitis pigmentosa, *Nat Genet* 21:355, 1999.

19. Bhattacharya SS et al: Close genetic linkage between X-linked retinitis pigmentosa and a restriction fragment length polymorphism identified by recombinant DNA probe L1.28, *Nature* 309:253, 1984.

20. Bird AC: X-linked retinitis pigmentosa, *Br J Ophthalmol* 59:177, 1975.

21. Bird AC: Retinal photoreceptor dystrophies, *Am J Ophthalmol* 119:543, 1995.

22. Birnbach CD et al: Histopathology and immunocytochemistry of the neurosensory retina in fundus flavimaculatus, *Ophthalmology* 101:1211, 1994.

23. Bork JM et al: Usher syndrome 1D and nonsyndromic autosomal recessive deafness DFNB12 are caused by allelic mutations of the novel cadherin-like gene CDH23, *Am J Hum Genet* 68:26, 2001.

24. Boughman JA, Conneally PM, Nance WE: Population genetic studies of retinitis pigmentosa, *Am J Hum Genet* 32:223, 1980.

25. Boughman JA, Vernon M, Shaver KA.: Usher syndrome: definition and estimate of prevalence from two high-risk populations, *J Chronic Dis* 36:595, 1983.

26. Bownds D: Site of attachment of retinal in rhodopsin, *Nature* 216:1178, 1967.

27. Bunge S et al: Molecular analysis and genetic mapping of the rhodopsin gene in families with autosomal dominant retinitis pigmentosa, *Genomics* 17:230, 1993.

28. Carr RE: Congenital stationary night blindness, *Trans Am Ophthalmol Soc* 74:448, 1974.

29. Cayouette M, Gravel C: Adenovirus-mediated gene transfer of ciliary neurotrophic factor can prevent photoreceptor degeneration in the retinal degeneration (rd) mouse, *Hum Gene Ther* 8:423, 1997.

30. Cayouette M et al: Intraocular gene transfer of ciliary neurotrophic factor prevents death and increases responsiveness of rod photoreceptors in the retinal degeneration slow mouse, *J Neurosci* 18:9282, 1998.

31. Chen S et al: Crx, a novel Otx-like paired homeodomain protein, binds to and transactivates photoreceptor cell-specific genes, *Neuron* 19:1017, 1997.

32. Cohen AI: Some cytological and initial biochemical observations on photoreceptors in retinas of rds mice, *Invest Ophthalmol Vis Sci* 24:832, 1983.

33. Collins FS, Mansoura MK: The Human Genome Project, *Cancer* 91:221, 2000.

34. Cremers FPM et al: Cloning of a gene that is rearranged in patients with choroideraemia, *Nature* 347:674, 1990.

35. D'Cruz PM et al: Mutation of the receptor tyrosine kinase gene Mertk in the retinal dystrophic RCS rat, *Hum Mol Genet* 9:645, 2000.

36. Dib C et al: A comprehensive genetic map of the human genome based on 5,264 microsatellites, *Nature* 380:152, 1996.

37. Dogra S et al: Asymmetric distribution of phosphatidylethanolamine in *C. albicans:* possible mediation by CDR1, a multidrug transporter belonging to ATP binding cassette (ABC) superfamily, *Yeast* 15:111, 1999.

38. Driessen CA et al: Disruption of the 11-*cis*-retinol dehydrogenase gene leads to accumulation of *cis*-retinols and *cis*-retinyl esters, *Mol Cell Biol* 20:4275, 2000.

39. Dryja TP et al: A point mutation of the rhodopsin gene in one form of retinitis pigmentosa, *Nature* 343:364, 1990.

40. Dryja TP et al: Heterozygous missense mutation in the rhodopsin gene as a cause of congenital stationary night blindness, *Nat Genet* 4:280, 1993.

41. Dryja TP et al: Mutations in the gene encoding the alpha subunit of the rod cGMP-gated channel in autosomal recessive retinitis pigmentosa, *Proc Natl Acad Sci USA* 92:10177, 1995.

42. Dryja TP et al: Missense mutation in the gene encoding the alpha subunit of rod transducin in the Nougaret form of congenital stationary night blindness, *Nat Genet* 13:358, 1996.

43. Duda T et al: Impairment of the rod outer segment membrane guanylate cyclase dimerization in a cone-rod dystrophy results in defective calcium signalling, *Biochemistry* 39:12522, 2000.

44. Eudy JD et al: Mutation of a gene encoding a protein with extracellular matrix motifs in Usher syndrome type IIa, *Science* 280:1753, 1998.

45. Fishman GA et al: Usher's syndrome, *Arch Ophthalmol* 101:1367, 1983.

46. Franke RR et al: Rhodopsin mutants that bind but fail to activate transducin, *Science* 250:123, 1990.

47. Freund C, Horsford DJ, McInnes RR: Transcription factor genes and the developing eye: a genetic perspective, *Hum Mol Genet* 5:1471, 1996.

48. Freund CL et al: Cone-rod dystrophy due to mutations in a novel photoreceptor-specific homeobox gene (CRX) essential for maintenance of the photoreceptor, *Cell* 91:543, 1997.

49. Freund CL et al: De novo mutations in the CRX homeobox gene associated with Leber congenital amaurosis, *Nat Genet* 18:311, 1998.

50. Fuchs S et al: A homozygous 1-base pair deletion in the Arrestin gene is a frequent cause of Oguchi disease in Japanese, *Nat Genet* 10:360, 1995.

51. Furukawa T, Morrow EM, Cepko CL: Crx, a novel Otx-like homeobox gene, shows photoreceptor-specific expression and regulates photoreceptor differentiation, *Cell* 91:531, 1997.

52. Furukawa T et al: Retinopathy and attenuated circadian entrainment in Crx-deficient mice, *Nat Genet* 23:466, 1999.

53. Gal A et al: Heterozygous missense mutation in the rod cGMP phosphodiesterase beta-subunit gene in autosomal dominant stationary night blindness, *Nat Genet* 13:358, 1994.

54. Gal A et al: Rhodopsin mutations in inherited retinal dystrophies and dysfunctions, *Prog Retinal Eye Res* 16:51, 1997.

55. Gal A et al: Mutations in MERTK, the human orthologue of the RCS rat retinal dystrophy gene, cause retinitis pigmentosa, *Nat Genet* 26:270, 2000.

56. Gerber S et al: The photoreceptor cell-specific nuclear receptor gene (PNR) accounts for retinitis pigmentosa in the Crypto-Jews from Portugal (Marranos), survivors from the Spanish Inquisition, *Hum Genet* 107:276, 2000.

57. Gibson F et al: A type VII myosin encoded by the mouse deafness gene shaker-1, *Nature* 374:62, 1995.

58. Goldberg AF, Molday RS: Expression and characterization of peripherin/rds-rom-1 complexes and mutants implicated in retinal degenerative diseases, *Methods Enzymol* 316:671, 2000.

59. Goldberg AFX, Molday RS: Defective subunit assembly underlies a digenic form of retinitis pigmentosa linked to mutations in peripherin/rds and rom-1, *Proc Natl Acad Sci USA* 93:13726, 1996.

60. Grayson C et al: Retinoschisin, the X-linked retinoschisis protein, is a secreted photoreceptor protein, and is expressed and released by Weri-Rb1 cells, *Hum Mol Genet* 9:1873, 2000.

61. Gu S-M et al: Mutations in RPE65 cause autosomal recessive childhood severe onset retinal dystrophy, *Nat Genet* 17:194, 1997.

62. Haider NB et al: Mutation of a nuclear receptor gene, NR2E3, causes enhanced S cone syndrome, a disorder of retinal cell fate, *Nat Genet* 24:127, 2000.

63. Hamada S, Yoshida K, Chihara E: Optical coherence tomography images of retinitis pigmentosa, *Ophthalmic Surg Lasers* 31:253, 2000.

64. Hamel CP et al: Molecular cloning and expression of RPE65, a novel retinal pigment epithelium-specific microsomal protein that is post-transcriptionally regulated in vitro, *J Biol Chem* 268:15751, 1993.

65. Hargrave PA, McDowell JH: Rhodopsin and phototransduction: a model system for G protein-linked receptors, *FASEB J* 6:2323, 1992.

66. Hauswirth WW, Lewin AS: Ribozyme uses in retinal gene therapy, *Prog Retinal Eye Res* 19:689, 2000.

67. Hayes KC: Retinal degeneration in monkeys induced by deficiencies of vitamin E or A, *Invest Ophthalmol Vis Sci* 13:499, 1974.

68. Heckenlively JR: *Retinitis pigmentosa,* Philadelphia, 1988, Lippincott.

69. Heckenlively JR et al: Retinitis pigmentosa in the Navajo, *Metab Pediatr Ophthalmol* 4:155, 1980.

70. Hermann K et al: RPGR mutation analysis in patients with retinitis pigmentosa and congenital stationary night blindness, *Am J Hum Genet* 59:A263, 1996.

71. Huang PC et al: Cellular interactions implicated in the mechanism of photoreceptor degeneration in transgenic mice expressing a mutant rhodopsin, *Proc Natl Acad Sci USA* 90:8484, 1993.

72. Huang SH et al: Autosomal recessive retinitis pigmentosa caused by mutations in the alpha subunit of rod cGMP phosphodiesterase, *Nat Genet* 11:468, 1995.

73. Humphries M et al: Retinopathy induced in mice by targeted disruption of the rhodopsin gene, *Nat Genet* 15:216, 1997.

74. Inglehearn CF et al: A completed screen for mutations of the rhodopsin gene in a panel of patients with autosomal dominant retinitis pigmentosa, *Hum Mol Genet* 1:41, 1992.

75. Jacobsen SG, Boight WJ, Parel JM: Automated light and dark adapted perimetry for evaluating retinitis pigmentosa, *Ophthalmology* 93:1604, 1986.

76. Jay BS, Bird AC: X-linked retinitis pigmentosa, *Trans Am Acad Ophthalmol Otolaryngol* 77:641, 1973.

77. Jay M: On the heredity of retinitis pigmentosa, *Br J Ophthalmol* 66:405, 1982.

78. Kajiwara K, Berson EL, Dryja TR: Digenic retinitis pigmentosa due to mutations at the unlinked peripherin/RDS and ROM1 loci, *Science* 264:1604, 1994.

79. Kajiwara K et al: Mutations in the human retinal degeneration slow gene in autosomal dominant retinitis pigmentosa, *Nature* 354:480, 1991.

80. Karnik SS et al: Cysteine residues 110 and 187 are essential for the formation of correct structure in bovine rhodopsin, *Proc Natl Acad Sci USA* 85:8459, 1988.

81. Kaushal S, Khorana HG: Structure and function in rhodopsin: point mutations associated with autosomal dominant retinitis pigmentosa, *Biochemistry* 33:6121, 1994.

82. Kedzierski W et al: Generation and analysis of transgenic mice expressing P216L-substituted Rds/peripherin in rod photoreceptors, *Invest Ophthalmol Vis Sci* 38:498, 1997.

83. Keen J et al: Rapid determination of single base pair mismatches as heteroduplexes on Hydrolink gels, *Trends Genet* 7:5, 1991.

84. Keen TJ, Inglehearn CF: Mutations and polymorphisms in the human peripherin-RDS gene and their involvement in inherited retinal degeneration, *Hum Mutat* 8:297, 1996.

85. Kohl S et al: Total colour blindness is caused by mutations in the gene encoding the alpha-subunit of the cone photoreceptor cGMP-gated cation channel, *Nat Genet* 19:257, 1998.

86. LaVail MM et al: Protection of mouse photoreceptors by survival factors in retinal degenerations, *Invest Ophthalmol Vis Sci* 39:592, 1998.

87. LaVail MM et al: Ribozyme rescue of photoreceptor cells in P23H transgenic rats: long-term survival and late-stage therapy, *Proc Natl Acad Sci USA* 97:11488, 2000.

88. Li T et al: Constitutive activation of phototransduction by K296E opsin is not a cause of photoreceptor degeneration, *Proc Natl Acad Sci USA* 92:3551, 1995.

89. Li T et al: Transgenic mice carrying the dominant rhodopsin mutation P347S: evidence for defective vectorial transport of rhodopsin to the outer segments, *Proc Natl Acad Sci USA* 93:14176, 1996.

90. Litchfield TM, Whiteley SJ, Lund RD: Transplantation of retinal pigment epithelial, photoreceptor and other cells as treatment for retinal degeneration, *Exp Eye Res* 64:655, 1997.

91. Little CW et al: Transplantation of human fetal retinal pigment epithelium rescues photoreceptor cells from degeneration in the Royal College of Surgeons rat retina, *Invest Ophthalmol Vis Sci* 37:204, 1996.

92. Liu X et al: Myosin VIIa, the product of the Usher 1B syndrome gene, is concentrated in the connecting cilia of photoreceptor cells, *Cell Motil Cytoskel* 37:240, 1997.

93. Marano F et al: Hereditary retinal dystrophies and choroidal neovascularization, *Graefes Arch Clin Exp Ophthalmol* 238:760, 2000.

94. Marlhens F et al: Mutations in RPE65 cause Leber's congenital amaurosis, *Nat Genet* 17:139, 1997.

95. Marmorstein AD et al: Bestrophin, the product of the best vitelliform macular dystrophy gene (VMD2), localizes to the basolateral plasma membrane of the retinal pigment epithelium, *Proc Natl Acad Sci USA* 97:12758, 2000.

96. Massof RW, Finkelstein D: Two forms of autosomal dominant primary retinitis pigmentosa, *Doc Ophthalmol* 51:289, 1987.

97. Maw MA et al: Mutations in the gene encoding cellular retinaldehyde-binding protein in autosomal recessive retinitis pigmentosa, *Nat Genet* 17:198, 1997.

98. McLaughlin ME et al: Recessive mutations in the gene encoding the beta-subunit of rod phosphodiesterase in patients with retinitis pigmentosa, *Nat Genet* 4:130, 1993.

99. McWilliams P et al: Autosomal dominant retinitis pigmentosa (ADRP): localization of an ADRP gene to the long arm of chromosome 3, *Genomics* 5:619, 1989.

100. Meindl A et al: A gene (RPGR) with homology to the RCC1 guanine nucleotide exchange factor is mutated in X-linked retinitis pigmentosa (RP3), *Nat Genet* 13:35, 1996.

101. Moore AT: Cone and cone-rod dystrophies, *J Med Genet* 29:289, 1992.

102. Moore AT et al: Abnormal dark adaptation kinetics in autosomal dominant sector retinitis pigmentosa due to rod opsin mutation, *Br J Ophthalmol* 76:465, 1992.

103. Nakayama TA, Khorana HG: Mapping of the amino acids in membrane-embedded helices that interact with the retinal chromophore in bovine rhodopsin, *J Biol Chem* 266:4269, 1991.

104. Noble KG, Carr RE: Stargardt's disease and fundus flavimaculatus, *Arch Ophthalmol* 7:1281, 1979.

105. Olsson JE et al: Transgenic mice with a rhodopsin mutation (Pro23His): a mouse model of retinitis pigmentosa, *Neuron* 9:815, 1992.

106. Ott J: *Analysis of human genetic linkage,* Baltimore, 1991, Johns Hopkins University Press.

107. Payne A et al: GCAP1 mutation in an autosomal dominant cone dystrophy pedigree mapping to a new locus on chromosome 6p21.1, *Hum Mol Genet* 7:273, 1998.

108. Perrault I et al: Spectrum of retGC1 mutations in Leber's congenital amaurosis, *Eur J Hum Genet* 8:578, 2000.

109. Petrukhin K et al: Identification of the gene responsible for Best macular dystrophy, *Nat Genet* 19:241, 1998.

110. Pusch CM et al: The complete form of X-linked congenital stationary night blindness is caused by mutations in a gene encoding a leucine-rich repeat protein, *Nat Genet* 26:324, 2000.

111. Rao VR, Cohen G, Oprian D: Rhodopsin mutation G90D and a molecular mechanism for congenital stationary night blindness, *Nature* 367:639, 1994.

112. Redmond TM et al: Rpe65 is necessary for production of 11-*cis*-vitamin A in the retinal visual cycle, *Nat Genet* 20:344, 1998.

113. Reme C et al: Apoptotic cell death in retinal degenerations, *Prog Retinal Eye Res* 17:443, 1998.

114. The Retinoschisis Consortium: Functional implications of the spectrum of mutations found in 234 cases with X-linked juvenile retinoschisis, *Hum Mol Genet* 7:1185, 1998.

115. Rivolta C et al: Missense mutation in the USH2A gene associated with recessive retinitis pigmentosa without hearing loss, *Am J Hum Genet* 66:1975, 2000.

116. Robinson PR et al: Opsins with mutations at the site of chromophore attachment constitutively activate transducin but are not phosphorylated by rhodopsin kinase, *Proc Natl Acad Sci USA* 91:5411, 1994.

117. Roepman R et al: The retinitis pigmentosa GTPase regulator (RPGR) interacts with novel transport-like proteins in the outer segments of rod photoreceptors, *Hum Mol Genet* 9:2095, 2000.

118. Saari JC, Bredberg DL, Noy N: Control of substrate flow at a branch in the visual cycle, *Biochemistry* 33:3106, 1994.

119. Saiki RK, Gelfand DH, Stoffel S: Primer-directed enzymatic amplification of DNA with a thermostable DNA polymerase, *Science* 239:487, 1988.

120. Sakmar TP, Franke RR, Khorana HG: Glutamic acid-113 serves as the retinylidene Schiff base counterion in bovine rhodopsin, *Proc Natl Acad Sci USA* 86:8309, 1989.

121. Sauer CG et al: Positional cloning of the gene associated with X-linked juvenile retinoschisis, *Nat Genet* 17:164, 1997.

122. Scholl HP, Zrenner E: Electrophysiology in the investigation of acquired retinal disorders, *Surv Ophthalmol* 45:29, 2000.

123. Schwahn U et al: Positional cloning of the gene for X-linked retinitis pigmentosa 2, *Nat Genet* 19:327, 1998.

124. Seeliger MW et al: Phenotype in retinol deficiency due to a hereditary defect in retinol binding protein synthesis, *Invest Ophthalmol Vis Sci* 40:3, 1999.

125. Semple-Rowl SL et al: A null mutation in the photoreceptor guanylate cyclase gene causes the retinal degeneration chicken phenotype, *Proc Natl Acad Sci USA* 95:1271, 1998.

126. Steinmetz RL et al: Symptomatic abnormalities of dark adaptation in patients with age-related Bruch's membrane change, *Br J Ophthalmol* 77:549, 1993.

127. Stone EM et al: A single EFEMP1 mutation associated with both Malattia Leventinese and Doyne honeycomb retinal dystrophy, *Nat Genet* 22:199, 1999.

128. Strom TM et al: An L-type calcium-channel gene mutated in incomplete X-linked congenital stationary night blindness, *Nat Genet* 19:260, 1998.

129. Sun H, Molday RS, Nathans J: Retinal stimulates ATP hydrolysis by purified and reconstituted ABCR, the photoreceptor-specific ATP-binding cassette transporter responsible for Stargardt disease, *J Biol Chem* 274:8269, 1999.

130. Sundin OH et al: Genetic basis of total colour blindness among the Pingelapese islanders, *Nat Genet* 25:289, 2000.

131. Sung C-H, Davenport C, Nathans J: Rhodopsin mutations responsible for autosomal dominant retinitis pigmentosa, *J Biol Chem* 268:26645, 1993.

132. Sung C-H et al: A rhodopsin gene mutation responsible for autosomal dominant retinitis pigmentosa results in a protein that is defective in localization to the photoreceptor outer segment, *J Neurosci* 14:5818, 1994.

133. Suter M et al: Age-related macular degeneration: the lipofuscin component N-retinyl-N-retinylidene ethanolamine detaches proapoptotic proteins from mitochondria and induces apoptosis in mammalian retinal pigment epithelial cells, *J Biol Chem* 275:39625, 2000.

134. Tai AW et al: Rhodopsin's carboxy-terminal cytoplasmic tail acts as a membrane receptor for cytoplasmic dynein by binding to the dynein light chain Tctex-1, *Cell* 97:877, 1999.

135. Travis GH, Sutcliffe G, Bok D: The retinal degeneration slow (rds) gene product is a photoreceptor disc membrane associated glycoprotein, *Neuron* 6:61, 1991.

136. Tsang SH et al: Development of an animal model of retinitis pigmentosa generated by a targeted disruption of the murine cGMP phosphodiesterase gamma-subunit gene, *Am J Hum Genet* 57:A253, 1995.

137. Van Hooser JP et al: Rapid restoration of visual pigment and function with oral retinoid in a mouse model of childhood blindness, *Proc Natl Acad Sci USA* 97:8623, 2000.

138. von Ruckmann A, Fitzke FW, Bird AC: Distribution of fundus autofluorescence with a scanning laser ophthalmoscope, *Br J Ophthalmol* 79:407, 1995.

139. von Ruckmann A et al: In vivo fundus autofluorescence in macular dystrophies, *Arch Ophthalmol* 115:609, 1997.

140. Weil D et al: The autosomal recessive isolated deafness, DFNB2, and the Usher 1B syndrome are allelic defects of the myosin-VIIA gene, *Nat Genet* 16:191, 1997.

141. Weleber RG et al: Phenotypic variation including retinitis pigmentosa, pattern dystrophy and fundus flavimaculatus in a single family with a deletion of codon 153 or 154 of the peripherin/rds gene, *Arch Ophthalmol* 111:1531, 1993.

142. Weng J et al: Insights into the function of Rim protein in photoreceptors and etiology of Stargardt's disease from the phenotype in *abcr* knockout mice, *Cell* 98:13, 1999.

143. White K, Marquardt A, Weber BHF: VMD2 mutations in vitelliform macular dystrophy (Best disease) and other maculopathies, *Hum Mutat* 15:301, 2000.

144. Wilden U, Kuhn H: Light-dependent phosphorylation of rhodopsin: number of phosphorylation sites, *Biochemistry* 21:3014, 1982.

145. Wilkie SE et al: Functional characterization of missense mutations at codon 838 in retinal guanylate cyclase correlates with disease severity in patients with autosomal dominant cone-rod dystrophy, *Hum Mol Genet* 9:3065, 2000.

146. Yamamoto H et al: Mutations in the gene encoding 11-*cis* retinol dehydrogenase cause delayed dark adaptation and fundus albipunctatus, *Nat Genet* 22:188, 1999.

147. Yamamoto S et al: Defects in the rhodopsin kinase gene in the Oguchi form of stationary night blindness, *Nat Genet* 15:175, 1997.

CHAPTER 13

RETINAL BIOCHEMISTRY

SERGE PICAUD

As part of the central nervous system (CNS), the vertebrate retina shares many common metabolic and biochemical features with other CNS structures. However, it has also acquired a strong specificity to allow the circuit to safely fulfill its visual task. Vision starts with photon absorption by the visual pigments in cone and rod photoreceptor outer segments (OS). Excited pigments then trigger the phototransduction cascade that results in a change of membrane potential graded with respect to the light intensity. This spatiotemporal information provided by the photoreceptor matrix is then processed in parallel by the neural network. This neural processing compiles the information at the ganglion cell level under rates of action potentials. The retinal circuit thus integrates the graded analog-like information of photoreceptors in a digital-like signal at the ganglion cell level.

This chapter focuses on the biochemical specificity of the retina that lies not only in phototransduction but also on the subsequent neuronal information processing. Graded synaptic transmission is peculiar because neurons are physiologically depolarized for prolonged periods. Photoreceptors are depolarized in the dark and therefore continuously release the excitotoxic transmitter glutamate onto postsynaptic cells. Therefore specific molecular mechanisms are required to maintain the ionic homeostasis of the cell and to control the external glutamate concentration. Recent advances are integrated with more classic works to explain (1) how photoreceptors transform the photic stimulus into a graded electric signal; (2) how the retinal network has coped with the burden of graded neuronal processing; and finally, (3) how energy is supplied, stored, and consumed to support retinal parallel processing. Because it is not possible to provide a complete review of all pertinent and important studies generated in this field, readers are referred to recent reviews at each section heading to obtain more thorough coverage of the field and to find specific references.

PHOTOTRANSDUCTION*

The visual cycle starts with photon absorption by visual pigments at the level of the photoreceptor OS. In the human retina, each photoreceptor cell, rods and the three types of cones, expresses a specific visual pigment with a different spectral sensitivity[35] (Figure 13-1). All of these visual pigments are formed by a cell-specific apoprotein, opsin, and a common attached chromophore, the 11-*cis*-retinaldehyde derived from vitamin A (Figure 13-2). The rod visual pigment rhodopsin exhibits an absorption spectrum that matches almost perfectly the wavelength sensitivity curve of dark-adapted human retina, with an absorption peak at 500 nm, provided the appropriate corrections are made for the partial absorption of the shorter wavelengths by the slightly yellow human lens. The three cone pigment absorption spectra must be combined to fit the photopic luminosity curves of trichromats that have normal color vision.

Rhodopsin Activation

Rhodopsin, the most abundant visual pigment of the retina, has been studied in more details than cone pigments. Early biochemical studies demonstrated that the protein is integrated in the disc membranes contained in rod outer segments (ROS). The complete amino acid sequence of the

---

*References 37, 55, 70, 106, 115, 136, 155, 161, 212.

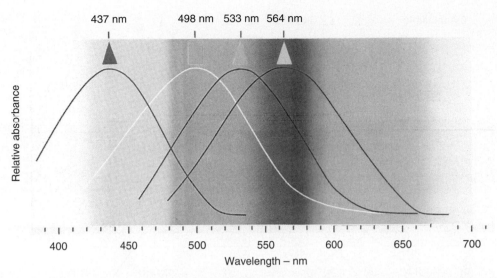

FIGURE 13-1 Absorption spectra of human rhodopsin (*black curve*) and of the three human and monkey cone opsins (*white curve*). These spectra were obtained by subtracting light absorption before and after bleaching on small retinal areas (see Brown and Wald[21]). (From Dowling JE: *The retina: an approachable part of the brain,* Cambridge, Mass, 1987, Harvard University Press.)

protein has been determined, allowing scientists to define its molecular structure in the membrane (Figure 13-3) and to study its structure function. The protein is thought to contain seven transmembrane domains producing three cytoplasmic and intradiscal loops; a fourth cytoplasmic loop is produced by the binding of cysteines 322 and 323 to palmitoyl residues inserted in the membrane lipid bilayer. The chromophore 11-*cis*-retinaldehyde is covalently linked to the protein by lysine 296 residue (Lys296) in the seventh transmembrane domain by a protonated Schiff base. At the other end, the β-ionone ring of the molecule is oriented toward the tryptophan 265 (Trp265) residue in helix VI. Its C9 methyl group was also found to interact with the glycine residue Gly121.[53] The chromophore thus lies near the center of the lipid bilayer with its delocalized π-electron system oriented in a plane parallel to the disc membrane. Formation of the Schiff base shifts the absorption peak of the chromophore from the ultraviolet (UV) to the visible. This shift is exacerbated to 500 nm by the glutamic acid 113 residue (Glu113) in the third transmembrane helix, which acts as a counterion for the protonated Schiff base. These ionic interactions increase the degree of delocalization for retinal π-electron system. Site-directed mutation of this Glu113 residue to glutamine induces a shift in the absorbance maximum from 500 to 380 nm.[52]

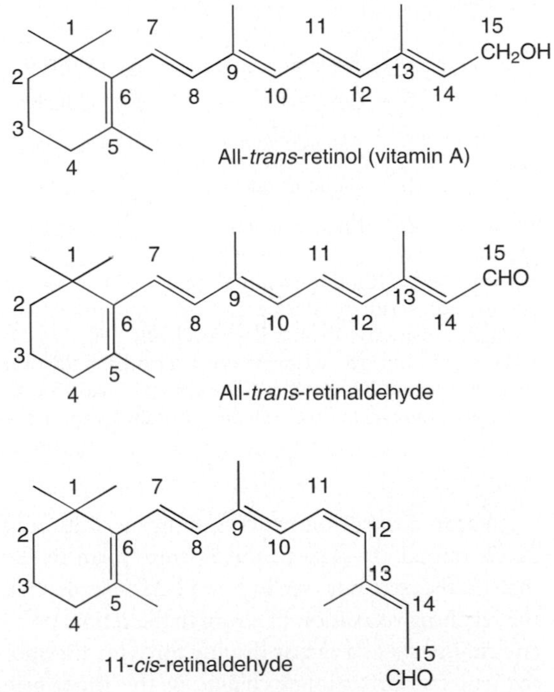

FIGURE 13-2 Retinoid structures. During light absorption the opsin chromophore 11-*cis*-retinal, which is synthesized from all-*trans*-retinol (vitamin A) in the retinal pigment epithelium, is converted to all-*trans*-retinal.

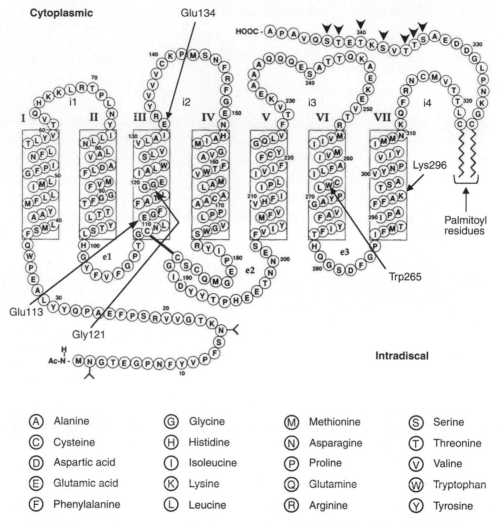

FIGURE 13-3 Rhodopsin amino acid sequence. Sites phosphorylated by the rhodopsin kinases (RK) are indicated by arrowheads, serine residues are in *black,* and threonine residues are in gray. The lysine residue 296 (Lys296) is crucial for light sensitivity because it is covalently linked to 11-*cis*-retinal by a protonated Schiff base with the glutamic acid residue 113 (Glu113) acting as a counterion. On the other end, the β-ionone ring of retinal is oriented toward the tryptophane residue 265 (trp265). The glutamic acid 134 (Glu134) and arginine 135 residues were proposed to provide the signal for transducin GDP release. (Modified from Hargrave PA: *Invest Ophthal Vis Sci* 42:3, 2001.)

Photon absorption triggers an isomerization of 11-*cis*-retinal (11-Ral) to the all-*trans* form in less than 20 picoseconds (see Figure 13-2). It seems that the resulting relaxation of strain in the retinal polyene chain acts as a major driving force for the subsequent conformational change in the rhodopsin molecule (R). This conformational change involves a relative movement of helix IV with respect to helix III. More specifically, it may result from steric interactions between the chromophore and glycine 121 residue (Gly121) in helix III and from rotations with modifications of hydrogen bonds for several residues, including Lys296 at one end of the chromophore and Trp265 at the other end. Among the

formed intermediates, metarhodopsin II is the catalytically active form (R*) for the following transducin activation (Figure 13-4). Formation of this active molecule is obtained by deprotonation of the Schiff base and concurrent protonation of the Glu113 residue, which suppresses its stabilizing ionic interaction. This whole conformational change requires 10 milliseconds following photon absorption; the active molecule stores 27 kcal mol^{-1} of the energy carried by the absorbed photon (57 kcal mol^{-1} for a photon at 500 nm).

Each catalytically active rhodopsin can freely move within the lipid bilayer and activate several hundreds of transducin molecules at a rate of about

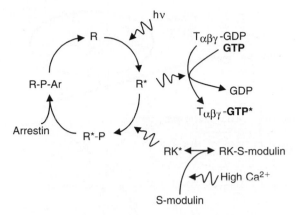

Figure 13-4 The rhodopsin cycle. Rhodopsin (*R*) is first activated by light (*hv*). The activated rhodopsin (*R**) can thus activate transducin molecules (*$T_{\alpha\beta\gamma}$*) by inducing a GTP-GDP exchange. The deactivation of the rhodopsin molecule then requires its phosphorylation by the rhodopsin kinase (*RK**). High Ca^{2+} prevents this phosphorylation step by promoting S-modulin interaction with rhodopsin kinase. The phosphorylation step increases arrestin affinity to rhodopsin, thereby preventing further transducin activation and speeding up rhodopsin recovery.

---

one per millisecond. This activation includes a guanine diphosphate (GDP)–to–guanine triphosphate (GTP) exchange, with the consecutive release of transducin α-subunit (Tα) from both rhodopsin and transducin βγ-subunit dimer (Tβγ) (see Figure 13-4). Following photon absorption, the relative motion of rhodopsin helices III and IV modifies the third cytoplasmic loop, allowing the third and second cytoplasmic loops of the protein to interact with transducin. The conserved residues' glutamic acid 134 (Glu134), which was found to rotate during rhodopsin photoactivation, was proposed to provide (with residue arginine 135) the signal for transducin GDP release.[1] The conserved disulfide bond between cysteine 110 (Cys110, helix III) and cysteine 187 (Cys187, second intradiscal loop) was also reported to participate in stabilizing the rhodopsin-transducin complex.[27] A cross-link may even be formed between rhodopsin at position 240 and transducin.[152]

Rhodopsin Inactivation

To prevent further transducin activation, the active rhodopsin molecules are inactivated in a time scale of a few hundred milliseconds, whereas rhodopsin activation occurs within a few milliseconds. During this inactivation process, rhodopsin is phosphorylated by rhodopsin kinase in a sequential manner near its C terminus to allow arrestin binding (see

Figure 13-4). It is still unclear whether protein kinase C (PKC) participates in this phosphorylation step. Rhodopsin is first triphosphorylated predominantly at serine residues Ser334, Ser338, and Ser343 and subsequently at threonine residues including Thr335, Thr336, Thr340, and Thr342 (see Figure 13-3). This phosphorylation step in the rhodopsin cycle is regulated by a 26-kD calcium-binding protein, called *S-modulin,* that suppresses rhodopsin kinase activity on Ca^{2+} binding[24] (see Figure 13-4). Recoverin is suspected to be this protein, although its distribution does not restrict to ROS. Its N terminus is acylated by a fatty acid that targets the protein to the membrane on Ca^{2+} binding. In fact, under conditions of high free Ca^{2+}, the soluble rhodopsin kinase associates to the membrane-bound recoverin and loses its activity.[164] Recoverin would thus prolong the lifetime of activated rhodopsin by preventing its phosphorylation. Rhodopsin phosphorylation greatly increases the affinity for arrestin, which thus competes with transducin (see Figure 13-4). If rhodopsin phosphorylation is mandatory for a full recovery, this arrestin binding simply speeds up the recovery phase, as indicated by the use of an arrestin-binding inhibitor or by the knockout of the arrestin gene.[130,209] Dephosphorylation of rhodopsin is probably achieved by a type 2A phosphatase or more precisely by a Ca^{2+}-dependent opsin phosphatase (CAOP) with a similar pharmacologic profile.[86] Ca^{2+} stimulates the latter protein with an affinity of 400 to 500 nM, which is in the physiologic range encountered in rods.

The Chromophore Cycle

After a pulse of intense light, activation and regeneration of the visual pigment occurs with a time constant of approximately 400 seconds for rhodopsin and approximately 100 seconds for cone pigments. After rhodopsin inactivation, the Schiff base is hydrolyzed to release free all-*trans*-retinal (t-Ral) (Figure 13-5). This retinoid molecule appears to be shuttled through the disc membrane from the lumenal side to the cytoplasmic side by a member of the adenosine triphosphate (ATP)–binding cassette family (ABCR).[3,67] This transporter, also called the *Rim protein* (RmP), was previously found at the incisures and edges of ROS discs.[112,132] Although passive diffusion could be sufficient, ABCR may facilitate transport of t-Ral as a Schiff base with phosphatidyl ethanolamine (PE), a complex found in lipofuscin deposits that accumulate in *ABCR* gene knockout mice.[178,205] t-Ral is then reduced to all-*trans*-retinol (t-Rol) by the nicotinamide ade-

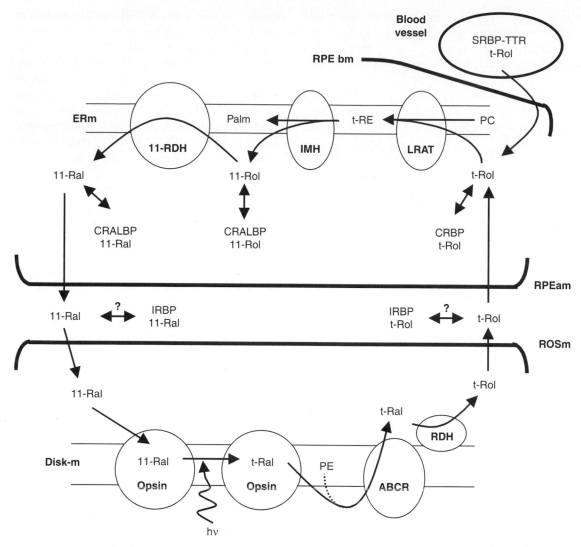

FIGURE 13-5   The retinoid cycle. The rhodopsin chromophore 11-*cis*-retinal (*11-Ral*) is isomerized by light (*hν*) to all-*trans*-retinal (*t-Ral*). After its dissociation from rhodopsin, t-Ral is transported across the disc membrane (*disk-m*); the ABCR transporter may facilitate this transport of t-Ral as a Schiff base with phosphatidyl ethanolamine (*PE*). On the cytoplasmic side, t-Ral is then reduced to all-*trans*-retinol (*t-Rol*) by the NADPH-dependent all-*trans*-retinol dehydrogenase (*RDH*). T-Rol leaves the cell to enter the interphotoreceptor space, where it may interact with the interphotoreceptor retinoid-binding protein (*IRBP*) to finally enter the pigment epithelial cells at their apical membrane (*RPEam*). T-Rol is also provided to RPE cells at their basal membrane (*RPEbm*) from choroid blood vessels, where it circulates as a complex with the serum retinol-binding protein (RBP) and transthyretin (*TTR*). In RPE cells, t-Rol binds to the cellular retinol-binding protein type I (*CRBP*) or is esterified as an all-*trans*-retinyl ester (*t-RE*) by the lecithin retinol acyltransferase (*LRAT*). Phosphatidylcholine (*PC*) usually provides palmitate (*palm*) for the esterification. An isomerohydrolase (*IMH*) finally hydrolyses t-RE to 11-*cis*-retinol (*11-Rol*) and a free fatty acid. The 11-Rol is oxidized to 11-Ral by 11-*cis*-retinol dehydrogenase (11-RDH). Both 11-Ral and 11-Rol can interact with cellular retinaldehyde-binding protein (*CRALBP*). 11-Ral can diffuse across the RPEam and the rod outer segment membrane (*ROSm*) to re-associate with the opsin molecule.

nine dinucleotide phosphate—reduced form (NADPH)–dependent all-*trans*-retinol dehydrogenase (RDH) (see Figure 13-5). Because RDH can hydrolyze retinal Schiff base, the retinal-PE complex transported by ABCR could provide a physiologically relevant substrate for the photoreceptor-specific RDH.[149] The retinal-to-retinol reduction reaction appears to be the limiting step in the visual pigment cycle because t-Ral is the only intermediate to accumulate following 40% rhodopsin bleaching in mice.[162] However, the sequential appearance and disappearance of the subsequent retinoid intermediates were detected in rats by Dowling[34] and Zimmerman, Yost, and Daemen[224] following 100% bleaching of the visual pigment. t-Rol can subsequently diffuse to the subretinal space, where it may bind to the retinoid-binding sites of the interphotoreceptor retinoid-binding protein (IRBP), a protein secreted in the interphotoreceptor matrix (IPM) by photoreceptors themselves (see Figure 13-5). IRBP, which has a great affinity (30 to 80 nM) for t-Rol and 11-Ral, can stabilize and facilitate the movement of these two ligands that must cross the IPM back and forth, respectively. However, pigment regeneration appears normal in the IRBP−/− knockout mice despite the observed photoreceptor degeneration.[154]

t-Rol then enters retinal pigment epithelial (RPE) cells at their apical membrane (RPEam). It can also be supplied from the blood flow at the opposite side through RPE cells' basal membrane (RPEbm) (see Figure 13-5). t-Rol, also called *vitamin A,* circulates in the blood flow as a complex formed with serum retinol-binding protein (RBP) and transthyretin (TTR; prealbumin). Retinoid-binding proteins are important to transport retinoids extracellularly and intracellularly because retinoids are hydrophobic and chemically unstable; the RBP-TTR complex may further prevent glomerular filtration. For t-Rol uptake into RPE cells, specific RBP binding sites have been located at the RPEbm. The glycoprotein P63, which is mainly expressed on basolateral RPE membranes, was found to have a high affinity for RBP (30 to 70 nM) and thus proposed to be its receptor on RPE cells.[14]

When entering RPE cells, t-Rol binds to the cytosolic retinoid-binding protein type I (CRBP-I), which is also expressed in Müller cells and has a specific affinity for t-Rol. t-Rol is thus delivered to the lecithin retinol acyltransferase (LRAT) for its esterification into an all-*trans*-retinyl ester (t-RE) (see Figure 13-5). This ester is formed by a preliminary LRAT acetylation mainly from phosphatidylcholine (PC), leading to the subsequent esterification of t-Rol with palmitate (palm). t-REs are then immediately converted by an isomerohydrolase into 11-*cis*-retinol (11-Rol) and a free fatty acid; the hydrolysis provides the energy for the isomerization of the retinoid from the all-*trans* to the *cis-trans* configuration ($\Delta G = 4.7$ kcal/mol). The enigmatic protein RPE65 located in the RPE cells and possibly in cones could be a component of the isomerohydrolase because t-REs accumulate and 11-*cis* retinoids are undetectable in RPE65 knockout

mice.[150] After the isomerization, 11-Rol can bind to the cellular retinaldehyde-binding protein (CRALBP) expressed in the RPE and Müller cells. CRALBP binds 11-Ral and 9-*cis*-retinal in 1:1 stoichiometry, but also to a lesser extent, 11-Rol and 9-*cis*-retinol. The binding to CRALBP facilitates the final oxidation of 11-Rol into 11-Ral by the 11-*cis*-retinol dehydrogenase (11-RDH) (see Figure 13-5). Retinoids can be stored in the RPE cells after esterification by LRAT of either t-Ral or 11-Ral. Hydrolysis of the stored 11-*cis* retinyl-ester in 11-Rol and the subsequent dehydrogenation in 11-Ral could occur at the apical plasma membrane, whereas all other reactions of t-Rol appear to occur in the endoplasmic reticulum.[104] On its way back to photoreceptors, where it recombines with opsin, 11-Ral binding to extracellular IRBP was found to stimulate 11-Ral release from RPE cells and increase its delivery to photoreceptors.

An alternative production pathway for 11-Ral could be its direct photoisomerization from t-Ral by the retinal G protein–coupled receptor (RGR).[69] RGR is a membrane-bound opsin more closely related to invertebrate opsin than to rhodopsin that is expressed within the smooth endoplasmic reticulum in RPE cells and in Müller cell endfeet and their radiating processes. It specifically binds t-Ral and can convert it into 11-Ral on irradiation at 470 nm or in the near-UV light. If the function of RGR resides in this photoisomerization, it remains unclear how t-Ral is obtained in RPE and Müller cells.

Cone Visual Pigments

The different human cone opsins have approximately 56% to 58% homology with rhodopsin at the nucleotide level and 43% to 47% at the amino acid level. In contrast, red and green cone opsins exhibit a high homology of their amino acid sequence (95.9%), whereas their proportions of identical amino acids fall to 44% and 42.8%, respectively, with the blue opsin. This high homology between red and green opsins, which is also evident from their close absorption spectra (see Figure 13-1), indicates that their genes originated from a recent duplication (30 millions years), in contrast to duplications at the origin of their ancestors, blue cone opsin and rhodopsin. Most vertebrates apart from primates have only blue and green cones. Although the amino acid sequences of these proteins are somewhat different from that of rhodopsin, they nonetheless exhibit similar protein structures with seven-transmembrane helices. They all have a glutamic acid residue in the third transmembrane domain, which corresponds to Glu113 in rhodopsin and can serve as a counterion to the protonated Schiff base.

The biochemical events of the visual pigment cycle appear identical in cones to that described previously in rods. However, it has been suggested that cones may obtain their regenerated chromophore from Müller cells because cones appear to resensitize in the absence of RPE cells. Furthermore, chick glial cells can take up exogenous t-Rol and convert it to all-*trans*-retinyl palmitate and subsequently to 11-*cis*-retinyl palmitate to finally generate 11-Rol. The latter molecule is certainly produced for visual function because 11-*cis*-retinoids, unlike all-*trans*-retinoids and 9-*cis*-retinoids, do not participate in other physiologic processes such as binding to retinoid nuclear receptors. Furthermore, CRALBP and CRBP were both strictly localized to Müller cells in the neuroretina (retina without RPE cells), and CRALBP was isolated from the neuroretina as a complex with either 11-Rol or 11-Ral. Finally, cones may also resensitize with 11-Rol, in contrast to rods that strictly require 11-Ral.

Transducin and Phosphodiesterase Activation

Photoinduced metarhodopsin II (R*) activates G protein and transducin ($T_{\alpha\beta\gamma}$) by promoting a GDP-to-GTP exchange (Figure 13-6). After this nucleotide exchange, the active α-subunit of transducin (T_α) dissociates from rhodopsin and from transducin βγ-subunit dimer ($T_{\beta\gamma}$). The activated transducin can bind to the cyclic guanine monophosphate (cGMP) phosphodiesterase (PDE), which is composed of one α-, one β-, and two γ-subunits. Addition of the δ PDE subunits appears to render the protein soluble. The activated transducin α binds to one $PDE_{\alpha\beta\gamma\gamma}$ protein and removes one γ inhibitory subunit, thereby activating the catalytic site of either the α- or the β-subunit. Two activated transducins α are therefore required to remove the two PDEγ inhibitory subunits and fully activate the α and β catalytic sites of the enzyme. In contrast to the transducin activation that represents an amplification step, this complex formation between the activated transducin α and the PDEγ subunit correspond to a 1:1 interaction. The active $PDE_{\alpha\beta}$** subunits can then hydrolyze cGMP to GMP with a 1500-fold increase in activity when both γ-subunits are dissociated.

Shutting off the transducin activity is achieved by the intrinsic GTPase activity of the transducin, which cleaves its bound GTP to GDP (see Figure 13-6). This GTPase activity of transducin was re-

ported to be increased by a GTPase-activating protein (GAP), consisting of the regulator of G protein signaling (RGS9) and Gβ, which may act independently or in concert with PDEγ itself. Transducin and PDE regeneration may be further delayed in low Ca^{2+} by phosducin sequestration of transducin βγ. The protein phosducin binds to the transducin βγ only when dephosphorylated, and its ROS content is similar to that of transducin. Phosducin phosphorylation, which increases by a factor of 3 in high Ca^{2+} (dark adaptation), thus may facilitate transducin regeneration. This phosphorylation process is attributed to a cyclic adenosine monophosphate (cAMP)–dependent protein kinase A. Ca^{2+} would indirectly regulate the enzyme by modulating the level of cAMP through a Ca^{2+}-calmodulin–sensitive adenylate cyclase. The final step in regenerating transducin requires the interaction of transducin βγ with the complex (PDEγ/inactivated transducin α) to release PDEγ. PDE recovery is also modulated by a PKC phosphorylation of PDEγ that increases its affinity for PDEαβ.

Regulation of cGMP-Dependent Channels

After its activation by transducin, PDE hydrolyzes cGMP to 5′-GMP at a rate of approximately 4000 molecules per second, providing a second step of amplification after the transducin activation (Figure 13-7). The consecutive decrease in intracellular cGMP induces the closure of cGMP-dependent cationic channels in ROS. In the dark these cGMP-dependent cationic channels are constantly open, thereby inducing a dark current that produces a continuous photoreceptor depolarization. After light activation of the phototransduction cascade, the cGMP hydrolysis by PDE triggers the channel closure, resulting in a reduction of the dark current (Figure 13-8, *A*) and a consequent photoreceptor hyperpolarization[15,16,167] (Figure 13-8, *B*). The current amplitude decrease is graded with respect to the light intensity of the stimulus (see Figure 13-8, *A*), and it therefore generates a graded hyperpolarization in photoreceptors (Figure 13-8, *B* and *C*). The cGMP-dependent channels are unselective to monovalent and divalent cations, although the channel conductance greatly decreases in the presence of divalent cations. Under physiologic conditions these channels mostly carry Na^+, Mg^{2+}, and Ca^{2+}, with Ca^{2+} producing up to 15% of the dark current. If α-subunits can form functional channels when expressed alone, β-subunit coexpression is required to recover the l-*cis*-diltiazem

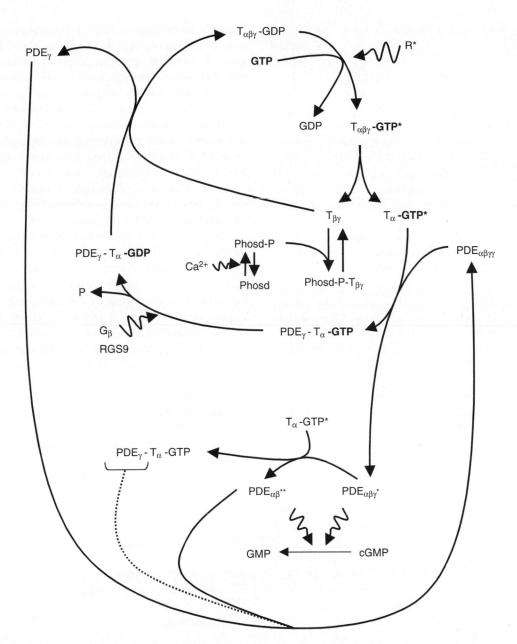

FIGURE 13-6 The transducin and phosphodiesterase (*PDE*) cycles. The activated rhodopsin (*R**) facilitates the GTP-GDP exchange in the transducin molecule ($T_{\alpha\beta\gamma}$). This activation of the transducin molecule induces the dissociation of the α-subunit (T_α-*GTP**). This active T_α-GTP* associates with one inhibitory γ-subunit of the phosphodiesterase ($PDE_{\alpha\beta\gamma\gamma}$). To activate the other catalytic site of the PDE, another active transducin is required to remove the second PDE γ-subunit. These active forms of PDE ($PDE_{\alpha\beta\gamma}$* and $PDE_{\alpha\beta}$**) hydrolyze cyclic guanine monophosphate (*cGMP*) into GMP. The subsequent inactivation of transducin results from its intrinsic GTPase activity, which can be stimulated by proteins G_β and RGS9. The release of PDEγ is obtained after interaction with βγ transducin subunits ($T_{\beta\gamma}$). This reassociation for the recovery of transducin and PDE is modulated by phosducin (*Phosd*), which can bind to $T_{\beta\gamma}$ and thus prevents its reassociation to T_α when phosducin is phosphorylated (*Phosd-P*) in high Ca^{2+}.

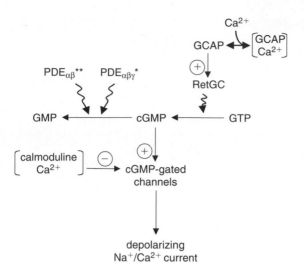

FIGURE 13-7 Regulation of cyclic guanine monophosphate–gated channels. The concentration of cyclic guanine monophosphate (*cGMP*) is a continuous balance between synthesis by the guanylate cyclases (*RetGC*) and hydrolysis by the two active forms of the phosphodiesterase (*PDE$_{\alpha\beta\gamma}$* * and *PDE$_{\alpha\beta}$* **). RetGC are upregulated by guanylate cyclase activating proteins (*GCAP*) that lose their properties on Ca^{2+} binding. The cGMP concentration controls the activation of cGMP-gated channels, which are also under the negative control of Ca^{2+}-calmoduline. These channel generate an Na$^+$- and Ca^{2+}-depolarizing current that reaches its maximum on dark adaptation (dark current).

blockade of the native channel. Sequence analysis of the subunits suggests that they may both participate to form the pore for the native channels. Although both subunits contain a cGMP-binding domain, four subunits are thought to comprise the native channels to explain the Hill coefficient for cGMP, which varies between 1.7 and 3.5. Binding of one to four cGMP molecules produces increasing levels of channel activation, reaching the higher level with four cGMP-bound molecules.[92,159] In the presence of Ca^{2+} and calmodulin, the cGMP affinity of the channel decreases from 19 to 33 M, whereas Ca^{2+} alone has no effect.

The recovery of the photoresponse requires an increase in cGMP concentration. This concentration is a continuous balance between hydrolysis by PDE, the activity of which greatly increases during light stimuli, and synthesis by two retinal guanylate cyclases (human: RetGC1 and RetGC2; rat: GC-E and GC-F) (see Figure 13-7). RetGC subunits consist of an extracellular receptor-like domain, a transmembrane domain, a kinaselike domain, a dimerization motif, and a catalytic domain. To synthesize cGMP, RetGCs are activated at least tenfold by guanylate cyclase activating proteins (GCAPs). These GCAPs are 23-kD acidic proteins belonging to the calmodulin family and exhibiting three

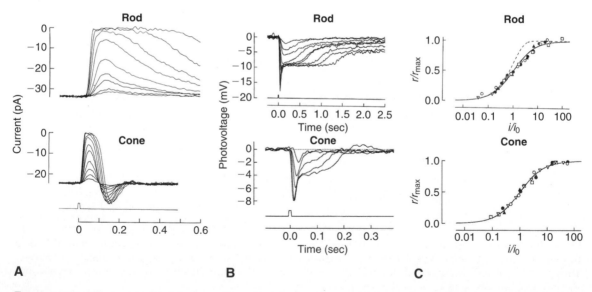

FIGURE 13-8 Photocurrents and photovoltages from rods and cones of the monkey *Macaca fascicularis*. **A,** Current responses to light flashes of increasing intensities. Flash strengths were increased by a factor of 2 and were expected to cause between 2.9 and 860 photoisomerizations for the rod and between 190 and 36,000 photoisomerizations for the illustrated red cone. **B,** Photovoltage responses to light flash of increasing intensities. Note that the time scale for the red cone is different than that for the rod. **C,** Normalized peak hyperpolarization as a function of flash strength. These diagrams illustrate that the voltage response is graded with respect to light intensities in both photoreceptor types. Each symbol denotes a different cell (three green cones and two red cones). (**A** from Baylor DA: *Invest Ophthalmol Vis Sci* 28:34, 1987; **B** and **C** from Schneeweis DM, Schnapf JL: *Science* 268:1053, 1995.)

EF-hand Ca^{2+}-chelating motifs. GCAP1 is characterized by its hydrophobicity, certainly related to the myristylation of its N terminus. It appears to interact continuously and specifically with RetGC1, which is either activated at low intracellular Ca^{2+} or conversely inactivated at high Ca^{2+}. RetGC1 is therefore inactivated in the dark when high cGMP levels open cGMP-dependent channels, thereby allowing a continuous Ca^{2+} flux in OS. Its activation results from light stimulation that produces a reduced Ca^{2+} influx through cGMP-dependent channels because of cGMP hydrolysis by PDE. The GCAP1 distribution parallels that of RetGC1 and is restricted to the photoreceptor OS but is higher in cones than in rods. GCAP2 and GCAP3 are unselective for the two RetGCs.

Calcium Homeostasis

In the photoreceptor OS, free intracellular Ca^{2+} can fall from 500 nM in dark-adapted rods to 50 nM on illumination. This Ca^{2+} drop is essential for light adaptation and for the recovery from a light stimulation. In the dark, Ca^{2+} enters continuously into the ROS through cGMP-dependent cationic channels. When these channels close, the ROS intracellular Ca^{2+} concentration decreases because Ca^{2+} extrusion in the photoreceptor OS exclusively relies on the Na^+/Ca^{2+}-K^+ exchanger. This exchanger has a stoichiometry of 1 Ca^{2+} and 1 K^+ extruded for 4 Na^+ imported, resulting in one inward positive charge per cycle. Surprisingly, when expressed in a cell line, the cloned exchanger does not carry K^+ similar to all other Ca^{2+}/Na^+, suggesting that the K^+ sensitivity is conferred by an additional subunit.[116] The power of this mechanism is attested by the exchanger's ability to control the intracellular Ca^{2+} concentration even when isolated ROS are recorded with the patch-clamp technique and thus dialyzed with the recording pipette solution. However, under physiologic conditions this exchanger does not reach its thermodynamic equilibrium, estimated at a cytoplasmic Ca^{2+} concentration to be as low as 1 nM. Another Ca^{2+}-ATPase was found on ROS disc membrane, but it appears not to load Ca^{2+} into discs where the luminal Ca^{2+} concentration is in the millimolar levels. Its affinity on the cytoplasmic side is low (10 μM) and above the cytoplasmic Ca^{2+} concentration (50 to 500 nM).

The physiologic relevance of the Ca^{2+} homeostasis is attested by the change in light-response amplitudes and kinetics when loading the ROS intracellular cytoplasm with Ca^{2+} chelators. As mentioned previously, many biochemical steps in the phototransduction cascade are affected by the Ca^{2+} concentration. High Ca^{2+} prevents rhodopsin phosphorylation by rhodopsin kinase by means of S-modulin (or recoverin), thus protecting rhodopsin from deactivation (see Figure 13-4). It can further increase the light response by speeding up transducin recovery by releasing transducin $\beta\gamma$ from phosducin sequestration, which facilitates its reassociation to inactivated transducin α (see Figure 13-6). On the other hand, high Ca^{2+} limits Ca^{2+} entry through cGMP-gated channels by decreasing its cGMP affinity and by suppressing GCAP activation of RetGC, thereby preventing cGMP synthesis (see Figure 13-7). These events are all essential for light adaptation and for the light-response recovery.

INFORMATION PROCESSING AND RETINAL NEUROCHEMISTRY[74,147]

Following phototransduction by photoreceptors, the retinal network extracts useful information such as motion or contrast edge that are coded at the ganglion cell level in rates of action potentials. On a given stimulation, different ganglion cell populations were thus found to generate different spatiotemporal patterns of action potential depending on the level of their dendritic arborization in the inner plexiform layer (IPL).[156] This information processing is generated by vertical connections from photoreceptors to bipolar cells then to ganglion cells and by lateral interactions by means of horizontal cells in the outer plexiform layer (OPL) and amacrine cells in the IPL. The focus of the following is not to describe the physiology of this information processing but to examine the retinal neurochemistry of this transformation from a graded light response of photoreceptors (see Figure 13-8, *B* and *C*) to a phasic ganglion cell activity. Photoreceptor and bipolar cells are classically considered to release the excitatory transmitter glutamate, whereas horizontal cells and most amacrine cells were described to release inhibitory transmitters, mainly γ-aminobutyric acid (GABA) and also glycine. However, some amacrine cells were found to release other neurotransmitters such as acetylcholine or dopamine or peptides like somatostatin (see Chapter 15). Finally, unconventional transmitters such as nitric oxide (NO) were also found to be released in the retina.

Glutamatergic Transmission[105,113,183,191]

Although photoreceptors and bipolar cells were recently found to express Na^+ channels that allow them to generate spikes, they mainly produce graded potential responses and, as a consequence, tonically release glutamate at their terminals.[75,131,218,220] This release of transmitter is mediated by exocytosis or vesicular release, as supported by the capacitance measurement in presynaptic cells, fluorescent observations, or the miniature currents observed in presynaptic and postsynaptic cells.* However, transporter-mediated release has also been considered in photoreceptors (see following discussion). The vesicular release of glutamate occurs at specialized synapses called *the ribbon synapses* (Figure 13-9), which are also present at other graded potential synapses in saccular and vestibular hair cells from the inner ear. These ribbon synapses were so named because they exhibit an electron-dense bar (approximately 0.5 μm) extending into the cytoplasm perpendicular to the plasma membrane. In fact, this synaptic ribbon is horseshoe-shaped above the active zones (approximately 2 μm). These ribbon synapses differ not only structurally but also functionally from conventional synapses.

Synaptic Release at Ribbon Synapses. At ribbon synapse, the rate of transmitter release can be higher than 100 vesicles per second per synapse in salaman-

---

*References 23, 61, 101, 139, 158, 192.

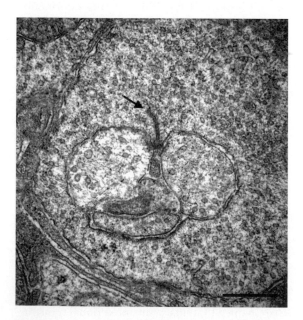

Figure 13-9   Rod photoreceptor ribbon synapse. The ribbon in the photoreceptor terminal is indicated by an arrow. The two large lateral postsynaptic elements are horizontal cell processes, whereas the central elements are from a ON rod bipolar cell. (Bar = 0.5 μm.) (Courtesy Noëlle Hanoteau.)

der rods or goldfish bipolar cells, whereas this rate averaged only 20 vesicles per second per synapse at a conventional synapse.[61,153,174,192] Accordingly, more than 100 synaptic vesicles can be tethered to the ribbon and thus participate in the readily releasable pool of vesicles, whereas the pool of docked vesicles per active zone is only 8 to 10 vesicles at hippocampal button-type conventional synapses.[195] At ribbon synapses, glutamate release is characterized by an ultrafast component (τ approximately 1.5 millisecond or less), followed by a delayed and larger releasable pool (τ approximately 300 milliseconds).[108] This delayed exocytosis represents more than 80% of the total glutamate release, in contrast to conventional synapses, where it accounts for less than 20%. These two components of the readily releasable pool of vesicles can rapidly and completely fuse with the plasma membrane within 200 milliseconds on large depolarization provided sufficient ATP is available at the terminal, or it can be released tonically during weaker depolarizations. However, endocytosis occurs with similar time constants at both synapses to regenerate synaptic vesicles from the plasma membrane. Therefore ribbon synapses have a high rate of synaptic release compared with conventional synapses.

Glutamate is loaded into synaptic vesicles by the vesicular glutamate transporter (VGLUT1/BNPI) that is expressed in both plexiform layers.[175] This uptake relies on an electrochemical gradient generated by a V-type H^+-ATPase that needs a Cl^- conductance in parallel for efficient acidification of the lumen. This Cl^- conductance seems to be mediated by the ClC-3 channel (the mutation of this gene in mice results in photoreceptor degeneration and hippocampus loss).[175] Docking the synaptic vesicle to the membrane normally involves the GTPase rab3. Interestingly, Rim, a putative rab3-effector protein, was specifically localized to the ribbon, suggesting its role in the vesicle recruitment.

The localization of KIF3A, a kinesin motor protein, to synaptic ribbons and to their attached synaptic vesicles suggests an ATP-dependent translocation of synaptic vesicles along the ribbon. The ribbon-specific antigen B16 was also recently identified, but it was found to have homology with the family of adapter protein (AP1 to AP4); these proteins, such as AP2, are involved in clathrin binding to vesicles in clathrin-mediated endocytosis. This homology thus may appear difficult to reconcile with the potential docking function of the ribbon synapse. After its docking to the plasma membrane, the synaptic vesicle is classically primed for exocytosis by assembly of an exocitosome comprised of synaptobrevin (VAMP) on the synaptic vesicle and SNAP25 and syntaxin 1 on the plasma membrane.[176] Surprisingly, syntaxin 1, which also binds to Ca^{2+} channels, is not expressed in photoreceptor and bipolar cell terminals, but it is replaced by syntaxin 3, which was not found elsewhere in the brain. This finding may underline molecular interactions specifically tailored for tonic glutamate release at ribbon synapses. The complex then binds α-SNAP and an *N*-ethylmaleimide–sensitive ATPase (NSF). Finally, the vesicle priming ends by ATP hydrolysis, disruption of the complex, and a possible hemifusion of the membrane.

Endocytosis also consumes energy by the GTPase dynamin 1. Because docking, priming, recycling synaptic vesicles, and especially loading them with glutamate are all ATP- or GTP-consuming steps in synaptic transmission, the high rate of vesicle exocytosis at ribbon synapses should be a great energy concern for the cells.

Calcium Homeostasis at Synaptic Terminals. At ribbon and conventional synapses, both exocytosis and endocytosis are regulated by the Ca^{2+} concentration. Exocytosis was first found to require an increase of Ca^{2+} concentration above 50 μM close to the active zone.[61,192] Subsequently, the required concentration was measured in both photoreceptors and bipolar cells and reported to be in a lower range between 0.8 and 20 μM.[153,158] The recycling of the plasma membrane by endocytosis is triggered by lower Ca^{2+} concentrations below 1 μM and showed a high Ca^{2+} cooperativity, with a Hill coefficient of 4.[193]

This difference in Ca^{2+} sensitivity between exocytosis and endocytosis could rely on the different distributions of Ca^{2+} channels and the mechanisms of Ca^{2+} extrusion. Photoreceptors and bipolar cells express L-type Ca^{2+} channels that do not inactivate or that inactivate only very slowly on prolonged depolarization, in contrast to other Ca^{2+} channels found in the nervous system.[194] Their molecular compositions appear cell specific for rods, the different cones, and bipolar cells. A retina-specific α1F-subunit, the mutation of which is responsible for X-linked congenital stationary night blindness, was already identified and localized to rods and, possibly, some bipolar cells. These noninactivating Ca^{2+} channels are obviously essential to sustain tonic transmitter release, but the continuous Ca^{2+} flux could easily become toxic and thus requires efficient Ca^{2+} extrusion mechanisms.

The two known mechanisms for Ca^{2+} exclusion mechanisms in the plasma membrane are Ca^{2+}-ATPases and Na^+-Ca^{2+} exchangers. In contrast to the OS, Na^+-Ca^{2+} exchangers do not contribute significantly to Ca^{2+} homeostasis at ribbon synapses, but instead, a plasma membrane Ca^{2+}-ATPase was found to extrude Ca^{2+} at photoreceptor and bipolar cell terminals, as well as in the photoreceptor IS.[79,83,114,219] These plasma membrane ATPases were located as a belt around the cone photoreceptor terminal, whereas L-type Ca^{2+} channels occupy the base of the terminals. In yellow or green cones, these channels even exhibit a patchy distribution that suggests a specific localization at active zones close to the ribbon.[113,114] Intracellular stores can also have a great influence on synaptic transmission by regulating the Ca^{2+} homeostasis in the terminal. For instance, inositol phosphate-3 receptors (IP3) that can trigger Ca^{2+} release from intracellular stores were located in photoreceptor and bipolar cell terminals.[135] Caffeine-sensitive intracellular Ca^{2+} stores were found to modulate the intracellular Ca^{2+} concentration and consequently to regulate glutamate synaptic transmission in salamander rod photoreceptors and goldfish bipolar cells.[78,84] Although mitochondria can participate in Ca^{2+} uptake from the cytoplasm, their main contribution to Ca^{2+} homeostasis at the ribbon terminal seems to be ATP production for the plasma membrane Ca^{2+}-ATPase.[219] In contrast to conventional synapses, the continuous Ca^{2+} flux into retinal terminals and the subsequent ATP-dependent Ca^{2+} extrusion may impose another specific energy burden on ribbon synapses.

Glutamate Transporters. Photoreceptors and OFF bipolar cells continuously release glutamate in the dark; light stimuli are therefore mediated by a decrease in glutamate concentration in the synaptic cleft. This concentration is under the control of release, diffusion, and uptake by glutamate transporters, which have a stoichiometry of 1glut$^-$/3 Na^+/1 H^+ transported for 1 K^+ antiported, generating a two-charge movement. Excitatory amino acid transporters EAAT1 (GLAST) were localized in Müller glial cells and RPE cells; EAAT2 (GLT-1) in cone photoreceptors and bipolar cells; EAAT3 (EAAC1) in horizontal, amacrine, and ganglion cells; and finally, the retina-specific transporter EAAT5 in rod photoreceptors and occasionally in some bipolar cell bodies.

Glutamate transporters clearly affect synaptic transmission at the photoreceptor terminal, as evidenced by the blockade of the light response in postsynaptic neurons when applying glutamate transport blockers.[42] In the absence of glutamate vesicular release, neuronal glutamate transporters were even reported to efficiently control the synaptic glutamate concentration.[42] However, although glutamate transporters were estimated to be as many as 10,000 to 20,000 in salamander cone terminals, it is still difficult to reconcile how they could lower the glutamate concentration within 100 milliseconds based on a turnover of 14 molecules per second.[88,196] Only a faster glutamate translocation, as recently reported in the cerebellum, could allow glutamate transporters to rapidly clear glutamate from the synaptic cleft at light onset.[9]

Neuronal glutamate transporters could play other functional roles apart from glutamate uptake. First, transporters were thought to release glutamate, a property that could be uncovered under conditions unfavorable for Ca^{2+}-mediated release.[168] However, this hypothesis was criticized because of the difficulty to completely suppress Ca^{2+} flux during cell depolarization.[143] Second, retinal glutamate transporters could act as presynaptic and postsynaptic receptors thanks to their coupled Cl^- conductance.[50,140,180] The molecular cloning of glutamate transporters confirmed that these proteins can generate large leak Cl^- conductance.[39] The Cl^- conductance was proposed to play an important role as a feedback mechanism.[165] It was shown that a cone photoreceptor can respond to its own glutamate release; the glutamate transporter generates miniature currents carried by Cl^-.[139] By regulating the cell membrane potential, this negative-feedback mechanism could thus control voltage-dependent Ca^{2+} channel activation and hence glutamate release.[139] The glutamate transporter would act as a presynaptic ionotropic receptor. Such a feedback mechanism may be particularly important in photoreceptors to control and adjust the tonic release of glutamate and thus prevent its excitotoxicity on postsynaptic neurons. The existence of such a feedback in mammalian rod photoreceptor is supported by the biophysical properties of EAAT5.[8] It is interesting to note that a glutamate transporter with a large Cl^- conductance acts as a postsynaptic receptor in a white perch ON bipolar cell.[50] In the mammalian retina, a metabotropic glutamate receptor, mGluR8, was also reported to act as a presynaptic feedback mechanism regulating Ca^{2+} flux at the photoreceptor terminal.[81] Similarly, a group III mGluR was found to regulate glutamate release from salamander bipolar terminals.[10]

Müller glial cells efficiently take up glutamate leaking out from the synaptic cleft. This glutamate uptake is such that high glutamate concentrations must be applied exogenously to affect synaptic transmission. The EAAT1 (GLAST) knockout mice and antisense knockdown further demonstrate the influence of this glial glutamate uptake on synaptic transmission.[13,54] In these models, the electroretinogram (ERG) b wave, which provides a global measure of ON bipolar cell light response, exhibited a drastic decrease. In addition, retinal neurons were more susceptible to ischemic insults. In contrast, the EAAT2 (GLT-1) knockout did not induce any major retinal dysfunction.

Glutamate Homeostasis. Glutamate taken up in Müller glial cells is partly converted to glutamine (Figure 13-10) by glutamine synthetase and partly transformed by glutamate dehydrogenase (GD) into α-ketoglutarate (Figure 13-11), which is an intermediate in the tricarboxylic acid (TCA) cycle (Krebs cycle). Conversely, glutamate (30%) is synthesized de novo by glial cells from pyruvate and CO_2 by means of the TCA cycle to release glutamine. First, pyruvate is transformed to oxaloacetate by the anaplerotic enzyme pyruvate carboxylase, specifically found in glial cells. Glutamate is then synthesized from α-ketoglutarate by GD and finally converted to glutamine by glutamine synthetase (GS).

Glutamate and glutamine could also be exogenously supplied to the glial cells because they can cross the blood-brain barrier. Consistent with such an exogenous supply, RPE cells were reported to express EAAT1 (GLAST) and to have a high glutamate content. As a consequence of this glutamate-glutamine conversion, glutamine appears as a specific amino acid signature of Müller cells in cat and monkey.[73,103] Glutamine produced in glial cells is then released into the extracellular space to be taken up by neurons and reconverted to glutamate. The conversion from glutamine to glutamate is achieved by the phosphate-activated glutaminase (PAG) (see Figure 13-11), which was demonstrated histochemically and immunocytochemically in photoreceptor inner segment and terminals, as well as in other retinal neurons.[43,49,182] Glutamine hydrolysis to glutamate produces a nitrogen group that may be shuttled back to glial cells via branched-chain aminotransferase.[90]

Glutamine transport across the membranes certainly occurs through known neutral amino acid transporters not specified so far for retinal Müller glial cells. This glutamine-glutamate cycle between

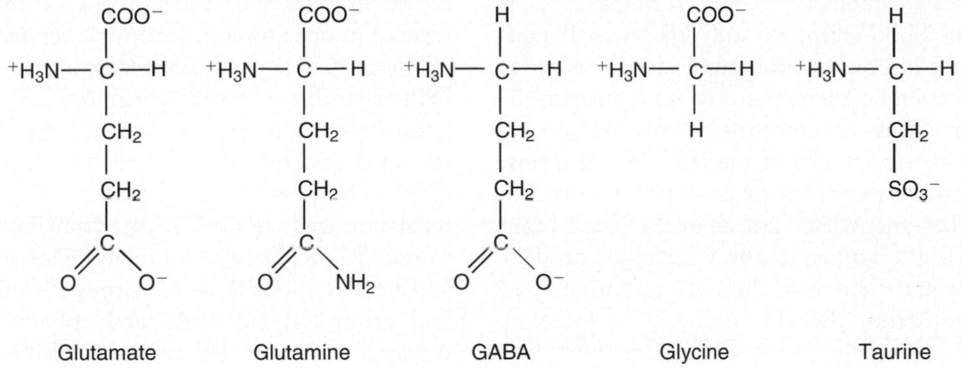

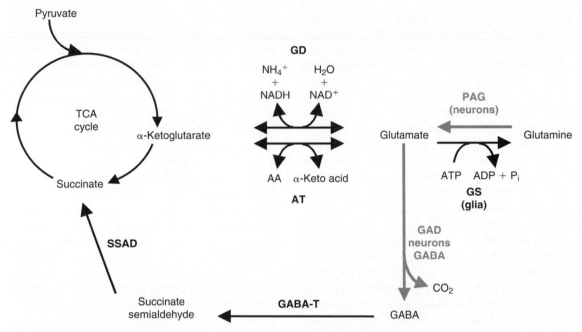

FIGURE 13-10 Structure of the major retinal neurotransmitters and their metabolites.

FIGURE 13-11 Glutamate/GABA metabolism. Glutamate is synthesized or catabolized by glutamate dehydrogenase (*GD*) or aminotransferases (*AT*) into α-ketoglutarate, an intermediate in the Krebs cycle (tricarboxylic acid cycle [*TCA cycle*]). These reactions are thought to occur mainly in glial cells, where glutamate can be converted to glutamine by glutamine synthetase (*GS*). Glial cells are also in responsible for the degradation of GABA to succinate by GABA-transaminase and succinate semialdehyde dehydrogenase (*SSAD*). In neurons, glutamate is obtained by transporter uptake and by synthesis through phosphate-activated glutaminase (*PAG*) from glutamine released by glial cells. In GABA-ergic neurons, glutamate is converted to GABA by glutamate acid decarboxylase (*GAD*). Specific neuronal functions are written in gray for better distinction from glial activity.

neurons and glial cells (see Figure 13-11) appears crucial for glutamatergic transmission as demonstrated by GS inhibition using methionine sulfoximine. After the drug was applied, retinal neurons lost their glutamate content and synaptic transmission was suppressed, as indicated by the drastic decrease in recorded b wave of the ERG. However, neurons may synthesize glutamate from α-ketoglutarate, an intermediate of the TCA cycle, either with GD as in photoreceptors or by transamination reactions that occur in all retinal neurons. For instance, aspartate aminotransferase (AAT), which possesses the highest activity of all glutamate-manufacturing enzyme, is found in photoreceptors and other retinal neurons. In addition, alanine aminotransferase may have a metabolic interest because it produces pyruvate. Ornithine aminotransferase dysfunction results in gyrate atrophy of the choroid and retina, which can be prevented by an arginine-restricted diet.[200] Leucine, which can cross the blood-brain barrier, is also known to affect glutamate production through the branched-chain amino acid aminotransferase (BCAT).

Glutamate Receptors. Glutamate activates different ionotropic and metabotropic receptors on postsynaptic bipolar, horizontal, amacrine, and ganglion cells. This part is extensively reviewed in Chapter 15 and elsewhere.[129,183] Therefore this paragraph is intended to briefly summarize data on ionotropic receptors and to focus on recent data reported on the transduction pathway of the glutamate metabotropic receptor mediating the light response in ON bipolar cells. Glutamate ionotropic receptors are all gating cation channels, and they were classified in three groups named after their respective preferred agonist: AMPA receptors (subunits GluR1-4), kainate receptors (subunits GluR5-7 and KA1-2), and NMDA receptors (subunits NMDAR1 and NMDAR2A-D also called *NR1* and *NR2A-D*). All subunits of AMPA and kainate receptors were detected in OFF bipolar, amacrine, and ganglion cells, although different subpopulations can be discriminated physiologically on the basis of their specific receptor subtypes.[29] For instance, in the monkey retina, horizontal cells were found to express GluR2-4 and the H1 horizontal cell subpopulation also expressed GluR6-7.[58,59] Most OFF bipolar cells expressed kainate receptors instead, either GluR5 or GluR6/7. KA2 receptors were also found in these cell types in the rat retina.[19] GluR2 is considered to generate the Ca^{2+} permeability of AMPA receptors described in bipolar cells.[46] NMDA receptors, which exhibit a higher Ca^{2+} permeability and use glycine as a coagonist, are expressed in many amacrine and ganglion cells and occasionally in horizontal and glial cells.

By gating cation channels, these ionotropic receptors are acting at sign-preserving synapses. In contrast, ON bipolar cells receive their visual information at a glutamatergic sign-inversing synapse and hyperpolarize in the dark when photoreceptors tonically release glutamate. This sign-inversing synapse relies on a metabotropic glutamate receptor, whose activation causes the closing of a cation channel instead of its opening as in ionotropic receptors.

Metabotropic glutamate receptors are classified in three groups on the basis of amino acid sequence homology.[129] In expression systems, group I (mGluR1 and mGluR5) stimulates phospholipase C (PLC) by means of $G_{q/11}$, and the subsequent IP3 formation leads to Ca^{2+} release from intracellular stores. mGluR1 can also stimulate cAMP formation and arachidonic acid release. Group II (mGluR2-3) and group III (mGluR4 and mGluR6-8) are thought to be coupled to the inhibition of the adenylate cyclase. Because this coupling is strongly sensitive to pertussis toxin, it is likely to involve G proteins from the G_i family. In ON bipolar cells the metabotropic receptor mediating the light response was identified as mGluR6, which seems retina specific. In contrast to other group III metabotropic receptors, mGluR6 was first thought to use a pathway similar to the phototransduction cascade in which a G protein would activate a cGMP-specific PDE, which would then close cGMP-dependent channels and trigger membrane hyperpolarization. GTP and cGMP were found to increase conductance that was suppressed by l-2-amino-4-phosphonobutyrate (APB or L-AP4), a selective agonist of group III mGluR. Furthermore, inhibitors of both G proteins and PDE appeared to decrease the APB response.[119,120,171] However, all the main components of the phototransduction cascade (transducin, PDE, and cGMP-gated channels) were absent from ON bipolar cell dendrites. Then, mGluR6 was reported to couple to pertussis-sensitive G protein and more efficiently to the G protein G_0 than to transducin.[76,172,204] The subunit $G_0\alpha$ was also colocalized with mGluR6 in bipolar dendrites.[187,189] This subunit suppressed the APB-sensitive current when introduced in recorded ON bipolar cells through the recording pipette solution, whereas dialysis with $G_i\alpha$ or transducin $G\beta\gamma$ had no significant effect.[117]

The demonstration that $G_0\alpha$ is required by mGluR6 to mediate the light response was obtained in $G_0\alpha$ knockout mice. These mice showed no b-wave ERG as was seen in mGluR6 knockout mice.[30] The target for G_0 is still unknown, but a potential activation of a cGMP-specific PDE was recently excluded by using nonhydrolyzable analogs of cGMP and PDE inhibitors.[117] The cGMP activation of the current may instead indicate a modulatory effect of the cation channel. It is still unclear whether $G_0\beta\gamma$, as in other systems, or $G_0\alpha$ itself regulates this unidentified channel.[33]

This molecular pathway is regulated by two mechanisms. First, NO stimulates guanylyl cyclase and thus increases cGMP levels, which positively regulate the currents. Second, Ca^{2+} entering the cell through the channel itself could decrease the amplitude of the APB-sensitive current, thereby providing a mechanism of adaptation to dim light background.[118,175] The mGluR6 pathway could be further modulated in rod bipolar cells by group I mGluR (mGluR1a and mGluR5a) that were immunodetected in their dendritic tips and that could stimulate PLC and the subsequent release of IP3-sensitive intracellular Ca^{2+} stores. These group I mGluR may also be responsible for the reduction of $GABA_C$ receptor current (see later discussion) that resulted from an enhanced activity of PKC caused by PLC stimulation. ON and OFF cone bipolar cells express mGluR7 in their synaptic terminals, where mGluR7 could act as an autoreceptor. This hypothesis is further supported by recent physiologic observations on salamander bipolar cell terminals.[10]

As mentioned previously, mGluR8 was histologically and physiologically detected in rod photoreceptor terminals, where it decreases intracellular Ca^{2+}. However, although the underlying molecular mechanism has not been elucidated, it does not involve protein phosphorylation or modulation of the cAMP concentration.[81] In fish horizontal cells, expression of mGluR was controversial and their agonists induced three specific actions: (1) suppression of inwardly rectifying K^+ currents (I_{Kir}), (2) an inhibition of ionotropic glutamate receptors, and (3) an enhancement and a shift in voltage dependence of L-type I_{Ca}. Although the molecular mechanism was demonstrated only for K^+ current, all effects could be explained by a cGMP increase and activation of a cGMP-dependent protein kinase (PKG). All mGluR were reported in ganglion and amacrine cells, except for mGluR6 and mGluR3. For instance, mGluR2 was reported in starburst amacrine cells, where it seemed to play a role in directional selectivity. In amphibian ganglion cells, mGluR, possibly from group I, was found to suppress L-type Ca^{2+} channel currents by a mechanism involving IP3 production and release of Ca^{2+} from intracellular stores. In rat ganglion cells, mGluR were also regulating positively or negatively Ca^{2+} current that was generated by N-type Ca^{2+} channels through a different intracellular mechanism. Although there is no histologic evidence of mGluR in rat Müller cells, application of mGluR agonists on salamander cells suggests that these receptors could control intracellular Ca^{2+} release and K^+ currents. K^+ current regulation partly resulted from activation of a pertussis toxin-sensitive G protein with stimulation of adenylate cyclase.

Inhibitory Transmission[142,211]

Horizontal cells and most amacrine cells are classically considered to release an inhibitory transmitter, mainly GABA and glycine for some amacrine cells (see Figure 13-10). Although GABA was described as an amino acid signature for horizontal cells in fish, cat, and central monkey retina, its role as a transmitter in horizontal cells is still a matter of controversy.[73,102,103] GABA and glycine not only have their inhibitory action in common but also share the same vesicular inhibitory amino acid transporter (VIAAT or VGAT).[107,163] It has even been demonstrated that both transmitters could be released at a single synapse.[72]

GABA Synaptic Release. In the fish retina, GABA release from amacrine cells was found to be Ca^{2+} dependent, whereas it was Ca^{2+} independent in horizontal cells. In fact, several lines of evidence suggest that GABA is released from horizontal cells by a GABA transporter. Such a transporter-mediated release could be particularly adapted for horizontal cells, which are graded potential neurons like photoreceptors and bipolar cells. However, GABA-transporter–mediated release has also been reported to occur in amacrine cells, although amacrine cells can propagate spikes along their dendrites.[7,25,36]

In contrast to the fish retina, different observations do not support GABA-transporter release in mammalian horizontal cells, but instead support a classic vesicular release. First, neither GABA uptake nor cloned GABA transporters were detected in horizontal cells (see later discussion). Furthermore, VIAAT was localized to horizontal cell terminals, which suggests GABA loading in synaptic vesicles.[57] The synaptic vesicle protein synaptoporin was also located in horizontal cells in the rabbit retina.[20] Cloned GABA transporters were not expressed in horizontal cells; GAT1 and rat GAT3 (mouse GAT4) are expressed in specific amacrine cells and in Müller cells, whereas rat GAT2 (mouse GAT3) is found selectively in RPE cells.[71] However, this distribution can differ depending on the animal species. In the salamander retina, for example, Müller cells were not immunolabeled for GAT1 or for GAT3, and surprisingly, some bipolar cells appeared immunopositive.[210] To support vesicular release, Ca^{2+} influx are mediated by L-type Ca^{2+} channels in both horizontal and amacrine cells, although in some fish horizontal cells, Ca^{2+} currents were sensitive to omega-agatoxin and not to dihydropyridine antagonists like P-type Ca^{2+} channels.[47,109,138,141] In these cell populations, Ca^{2+} homeostasis is mainly controlled by an Na^+-Ca^{2+} exchanger in the plasma membrane and caffeine-sensitive intracellular Ca^{2+} stores.[47,48,109]

As mentioned previously, two cloned Na^+-Cl^-–dependent transporters can take up GABA in glial cells after its synaptic release. Glial cells then convert GABA to succinate by the mitochondrial enzymes, GABA transaminase (GABA-T), and succinate semialdehyde dehydrogenase (SSAD)[45] (see Figure 13-11). This glial cell pathway for GABA metabolism is supported by the great increase in GABA content when GABA transaminase is inhibited with vigabatrin.[122] In neurons, GABA can directly reenter synaptic vesicles after its uptake from the extracellular space, or it can be synthesized from glutamate by the enzyme glutamate acid decarboxylase (GAD) (see Figure 13-11). Glutamate is provided directly from uptake through the glutamate transporter (EAAT3) specifically expressed in these cells postsynaptic to glutamatergic neurons (see previous discussion), or it could be produced from glutamine. The two isoforms GAD-65 and GAD-67 were reported to be localized in different amacrine cells, as well as in horizontal cells, with some changes (depending on the animal species).[18,188] In primate amacrine cells, GABA-transporter release (see previous discussion) was correlated to GAD-67 expression.[7]

Glycine Homeostasis. After its vesicular release, glycine is also taken up by an Na^+-Cl^-–dependent transporter, Glyt-1, which is expressed in glycinergic amacrine and interplexiform cells.[216] Uptake of radioactive glycine also labels bipolar cells, but this labeling is attributed to the diffusion of glycine through gap junctions between glycinergic amacrine cells (AII) and bipolar cells. The expression of Glyt-1 in amacrine cells was somehow unexpected because, in other structures of the CNS, this transporter is located in glia, whereas Glyt-2 is found in neurons. This differential distribution was correlated with a different stoichiometry that imposes uptake in neurons and allows release and uptake from glial cells to possibly regulate NMDA receptor activity.[157] Glycine can be synthesized from serine by the enzyme serine hydroxymethyl transferase (SHMT). However, the activity of this enzyme appears very low in retina previously depleted of their glycine content. This glycine depletion was obtained in vitro by applying methylglycine (sarco-

sine), a competitive substrate for Glyt-1. Because glycine can easily enter the retina from blood vessels and from the vitreous humor, these observations suggest that retinal glycine is mainly provided exogenously to amacrine neurons.[146]

Postsynaptic Receptors. Inhibitory transmitters activate different ionotropic and metabotropic receptors on retinal neurons, except on rods. GABA and glycine receptor physiology is extensively reviewed in Chapter 15 and elsewhere.[98] The ionotropic receptors $GABA_A$, $GABA_C$, and glycine all gate Cl^- channels such that physiologic responses are dependent on the Cl^- equilibrium potential set by Cl^- transporters. The K^+-Cl^- cotransporter (KCC2) that normally extrudes chloride was localized in ganglion cells, bipolar axons, and OFF bipolar dendrites, whereas the Na^+-K^+-Cl^- cotransporter (NKCC) that normally accumulates chloride was expressed in horizontal cells and ON bipolar dendrites.[190] These distributions suggest that inhibitory transmitters could depolarize horizontal cells and ON bipolar dendrites, whereas they would more classically hyperpolarize other cells and ON bipolar axons.

In contrast to $GABA_A$ and glycine receptors, $GABA_C$ receptors slowly desensitize during long transmitter application, which is particularly well adapted to the tonic release of transmitter occurring in the retina. This property could explain the restricted expression of these receptors to the retina and few other CNS structures, as compared with the ubiquitous distribution of $GABA_A$ and glycine receptors. $GABA_C$ receptors are also one order of magnitude more sensitive to GABA than $GABA_A$ receptors, and their pharmacology is also distinct: It is not potentiated by benzodiazepines and barbiturates; it is not blocked by bicuculline; and it is not, or often only partially, suppressed by picrotoxin. Depending on the species, these $GABA_C$ receptors were found in bipolar cells from rat and salamander, in fish horizontal cells, in salamander ganglion cells, and in mammalian cone photoreceptors.[41,97,134,148,222] In rat bipolar cells these $GABA_C$ receptors were modulated by PLC through activation of a G protein. Because the $GABA_C$ responses were also sensitive to L-AP4 and other mGluR agonists, they may be regulated by mGluR or serotonin receptors (5-HT$_2$).[40] $GABA_A$ receptors are not only expressed in horizontal, bipolar, amacrine, and ganglion cells as glycine receptors but are also expressed in cone photoreceptors (turtle and mice) and occasionally on Müller glial cells (fish and monkey).[99,134,151,179]

Metabotropic GABA$_B$ receptors that can modulate Ca^{2+} and K$^+$ channel activity through G protein coupling were located presynaptically or postsynaptically in horizontal, amacrine, and ganglion cells.[80] Their presence on frog Müller glial cells was also reported.[223] In salamander ganglion cells, two receptors modulate either the L- or N-type Ca^{2+} channels through G protein activation. Modulation of N-type Ca^{2+} channels appears direct and indirect by protein kinase A pathway.[170,221] These GABA$_B$ receptors can be either downregulated by a Ca^{2+}-calmodulin pathway that alters the GABA apparent affinity or upregulated by NO and cGMP levels.[169] Finally, the recent finding of GABA$_B$ receptor interaction with the transcription factor ATF-4 and its coclustering in amacrine cells suggest that the receptor could control gene expression in these cells.[123]

Taurine[94]

The physiologic function of taurine, an amino acid closely related to GABA and glycine (see Figure 13-10), is still unclear in the retina and brain. However, its critical role in the retina is demonstrated by the photoreceptor degeneration that occurs in the central cat retina (mainly cones) fed a taurine-free diet or in rat retina after injections of taurine-transporter blockers.[60,133] Carnivores, like cats, are fully dependent on their diet for taurine, whereas herbivores have to synthesize it and omnivores are in an intermediate position. Taurine is generally considered to play a role in osmoregulation and also regulates protein phosphorylation, especially during osmotic stress.[166] In addition, it activates glycine receptors, but with a low affinity. In the retina it was further shown to regulate Ca^{2+} uptake in ROS, retinal synaptosomes, and mitochondrial fractions.[93,111]

Taurine was consistently found in photoreceptors, but depending on the animal species, it was also localized in some bipolar and amacrine cells, as well as in astrocytes surrounding blood vessels, RPE cells, and Müller glial cells.[73,87,103,145] This distribution is consistent with the localization of taurine transporters to RPE cells; photoreceptors, especially cones; bipolar cells; astrocytes; and Müller cells.[137,147] High-affinity transporters (approximately ~ 7 µM) that were demonstrated biochemically in ROS preparation might be responsible for taurine accumulation in photoreceptors.[110] In contrast, low-affinity transporters (approximately ~ 330 µM) located in RPE cells and presumably in astrocytes and Müller cells may allow taurine transport from the bloodstream into the retina.[137,147]

When taurine is not uniquely provided from the diet, it can be produced from cysteine. Cysteine is first transformed by cysteine dioxygenase in cysteinesulfinate, which is then decarboxylated in hypotaurine by cysteine sulfinic acid decarboxylase (CSAD). Hypotaurine is finally oxidized in taurine by hypotaurine dehydrogenase. These enzymes were localized in the retina and cornea.[62] CSAD, which appears as a key enzyme in taurine synthesis, was found to have its activity decreased by light stimulation.[66]

Taurine release can be stimulated by light and K$^+$ elevation, but in the latter case, it is observed on removing the elevated K$^+$ solution. Taurine seems to be released from ROS in a Ca^{2+}-independent mechanism, possibly through transporters.[95] This Ca^{2+}-independent release requires Cl$^-$ and is correlated to an increase in cell volume, which supports taurine function in cellular osmoregulation. However, further studies are required to fully understand the critical physiologic role of taurine for photoreceptor survival.

Arginine and Nitric Oxide Synthesis[26]

The amino acid arginine has metabolic functions common to all cells, but it also participates to an important signaling pathway in the brain and the retina as a precursor for NO synthesis. NO is generated by nitric oxide synthases (NOS), which are either constitutive (endothelial and neuronal) or inducible. Neuronal NOS was consistently observed in two types of amacrine cells and in displaced amacrine cells.[68,124] Depending on the species investigated, it was also detected in some horizontal, bipolar, interplexiform, and ganglion cells. Finally, photoreceptors were occasionally reported to express neuronal NOS. Because NOS use reduced NADPH as a cofactor to oxidize arginine and generate NO, the NADPH-diaphorase histochemical staining has been used to selectively label NO-synthesizing neurons. This histochemical staining generally confirmed the neuronal NOS distribution in the retina.[68]

Continuous or flickering lights stimulate NO production.[121] NO is not released like a classical transmitter, but rather freely diffuses through membrane, even retrogradely. In cells, NO activates a soluble guanylate cyclase to produce cGMP. The cGMP molecules can then act on cGMP-gated channels found in photoreceptor OS, in amphibian photoreceptor terminals, and in ganglion cells. In ON bipolar cells, cGMP was also found to greatly increase the glutamate-sensitive current. The cGMP-dependent protein kinase G (PKG) pathway can be stimulated, controlling the gap-junction conductance between horizontal cells. NO was reported to generate other effects such as a Ca^{2+} channel modulation in photoreceptors and an increased ADP ribosylation of G proteins like transducins and other rod photoreceptor proteins. Increase in NO levels during flickering light stimulation was also correlated to an increase in retinal blood flow.[22]

RETINAL ENERGY METABOLISM[136,185,186,207]

Energy Supply

Glucose Metabolism. The energy demand for phototransduction and visual information processing is high. As in other structures of the CNS, this energy is provided from glucose metabolism rather than from fat or protein degradation. Glucose metabolism starts with glycolysis in which glucose is metabolized to 2 pyruvate molecules with formation of 2 ATP and the reduction of 2 NAD^+ into NADH. The regeneration of NAD^+ can then occur either by conversion of pyruvate into lactate or by the mitochondrial respiratory chain. Under aerobic conditions, pyruvate enters the TCA cycle (see Figure 13-11), which requires the mitochondrial respiratory chain and oxygen consumption to generate 36 additional ATP per glucose. The retina can switch from glycolysis to oxidative metabolism, or vice versa, to generate its ATP energy needs, depending on the glucose and oxygen supply. The isolated retina can produce 75% of its normal ATP production by glycolysis in the absence of oxygen, whereas in hypoglycemic conditions (1 mM glucose), it generates 85% of its normal ATP needs by oxidative metabolism.[207] Activities of these metabolic pathways were estimated following blood measurements of flow rate and lactate and oxygen levels. In the outer retina, most of the glucose (approximately 80%) is consumed by lactate formation to produce only 26% of the ATP need.[197,198] Light dramatically decreases glucose consumption, mainly by reducing lactate formation; the ratio of ATP production for this metabolic pathway remains at 20%. In the inner retina the figures are different; 69% of the glucose is oxidized, and the metabolic pathways are not affected by light.[199]

Metabolic transformation of glucose can also follow the pentose pathway (or hexose monophosphate pathway), which was found to be particularly active in ROS for rhodopsin regeneration and ROS protection from oxidative damage. Glucose is degraded to CO_2 without oxygen consumption but with reduction of $NADP^+$ in NADPH. The redox potential of NADPH can then be used by different enzymes, including glutathione reductase, which, in concert with the glutathione peroxidase, can decompose hydrogen peroxide into water. This pentose pathway can also provide ribose as an intermediate for nucleotide synthesis.

Glucose Supply. Glucose enters the retina from the choroid through the RPE and from retinal blood vessels. A facilitated diffusion of glucose was demonstrated at the level of the retinal pigment epithelium that is lying on the fenestrated blood vessels of the choroid.[184] This facilitated diffusion was attributed to the presence of the glucose transporter GLUT1 on both the apical and basal side of the retinal pigment epithelium.[177,181] This transporter was also located at the luminal and contraluminal plasma membranes of endothelial cells of retinal blood vessels, whereas it was absent from the fenestrated endothelial cells of the choriocapillaries.[181] It was also detected in rod and cone photoreceptor OS, where its activity was measured.[64,89,96] In the human retina, the transporter was located in the same subcellular compartments and in Müller glial cells, the nerve fiber layer, and photoreceptor cell bodies.[85,100] In contrast, GLUT3, the neuron-specific glucose transporter, was expressed only in the IPL.[100] In the rat retina, its distribution is extended to the OPL and some cell bodies of both the inner nuclear and ganglion cell layer.[202] A subpopulation of GLUT3-positive cells (30% to 50%) was identified as cholinergic amacrine cells by choline acetyltransferase immunolabeling.[203] Finally, the other glucose transporter, GLUT2, was found in the rat retina only at the apical ends of the Müller glial cells, where these cells face the interphotoreceptor space.[201] The transporters GLUT4 and GLUT5 were not detected in the human retina.[100]

After entering retinal cells, glucose can be stored as glycogen in Müller glial cells and also in some retinal neurons, including rod bipolar cells, some amacrine cells, and cone photoreceptors.[127,160] Glycogen content in cones was consistent with the selective localization of the brain glycogen phosphorylase in these photoreceptors but not in rods.[126] Diffuse staining for this enzyme was also located in the two plexiform layers, whereas the muscle glycogen phosphorylase was detected only in the IPL.

Lactate Metabolism. From the distribution of glucose transporters, it is unclear whether all retinal neurons express at least one glucose transporter and take up glucose in their cytoplasm. A study by Poitry-Yamate, Poitry, and Tsacopoulos[144] suggests that retinal neurons may instead use lactate released by Müller glial cells as an alternative source of energy. Cultured human Müller cells consume 99% of their glucose by glycolysis and lactate production.[208] Although Muller cells can shift to oxidative metabolism under hypoglycemic conditions, they may spare oxygen for retinal neurons under normal conditions. The need for oxygen is supported by its high consumption in photoreceptors, three to four times that of other retinal or brain neurons. Retinal neurons, especially photoreceptors, prefer lactate to glucose for their oxidative metabolism and consequently take up lactate released by glial cells.[144] This view is in agreement with the prevalence of H-lactate dehydrogenase, which transforms lactate into pyruvate, in the photoreceptor layer. The ability of lactate to prevent retinal damage and ATP and amino acid depletion during aglycemia further supports the role of lactate as an adequate energy supply to retinal neurons.[217]

The retinal distribution of the monocarboxylate transporters MCT1 and MCT2 that transport monocarboxylates such as lactate, pyruvate, and ketone bodies is in agreement with the use of lactate as an energy source in retinal neurons and photoreceptors.[17,44] MCT1 is observed in ROS, the Müller cell microvilli, the outer nuclear layer, and the plexiform layers, whereas MCT2 is distributed in the plexiform layers and the Müller glial cell endfeet at the inner limiting membrane. MCT1 and MCT2 are also associated with cells of the retinal blood barrier. MCT1 was localized at the apical side of the retinal pigment epithelium and in endothelial cells from retinal blood capillaries in the OPL at both the luminal and abluminal side, whereas MCT2 was associated only with glial cell processes surrounding microvessels.

Energy Consumption in Rod Outer Segment

A high energy demand is required to sustain the phototransduction cascade reactions in ROS. ATP and GTP are needed not only for rhodopsin phosphorylation, transducin GTPase, cGMP synthesis, and ABCR retinal transport but also for Na^+ extrusion by the Na^+-K^+ pump. Na^+ enters through the cGMP-dependent channels together with Ca^{2+}, as well as through the Na^+/Ca^{2+}-K^+ exchanger. Mitochondria that usually provide most of the cellular energy by aerobic glucose metabolism are absent from ROS but are densely packed in the photoreceptor inner segments. As seen from the oxygen consumption (see later discussion), ATP is obviously produced in the inner segment to support ROS, but the ATP diffusion to ROS is certainly hampered at the connecting cilium. Furthermore, nucleotide diffusion in ROS (time course in seconds) appears difficult to reconcile with the need of phototransduction reactions occurring in time scales of milliseconds.[82,128] A phosphocreatine shuttle may in fact facilitate this energy transfer from the inner segment to the ROS. A creatine kinase that transfers high-energy phosphate groups from creatine phosphate to ATP was located in the ROS. Furthermore, the photoreceptor content of phosphocreatine was found to be regulated by light.

Although photoreceptors obtain most of their energy by oxidative metabolism, they can shift to glycolysis under anaerobic conditions.[4,206] The ratio between these two sources of ATP seems to depend on the species and on the external conditions. Severe hypoxemia does not alter the photocurrent in vivo, as indicated by the measure of the a-wave ERG.[28] Similarly, suppressing aerobic metabolism with potassium cyanide decreased the photoreceptor current by only 50%.[206] Glucose is directly taken up by the glucose transporter, GluT1 into ROS, where all of the enzymes of the glycolytic pathway were located.[64] Glyceraldehyde-3-phosphate dehydrogenase was found to be a major protein associated with ROS, whereas other proteins were detected in ROS preparations by enzymatic assays.[63] This glycolytic pathway provides approximately 100 µM per second of ATP based on ROS lactate production; it therefore covers the basal cGMP synthesis and Na^+ extrusion, but it does not provide enough energy to recover from illumination. In the dark the basal cGMP turnover was estimated at 14 µM per second in the rabbit retina. Because 2 ATP molecules are needed to regenerate 1 molecule of cGMP from 5'-GMP, 28 µM of ATP are consumed for the basal turnover of cGMP. After illumination, the synthesis of cGMP increases by a factor of 4.5, reaching approximately 126 µM ATP per second. Na^+ extrusion was calculated to consume 55 µM ATP per second. This excess in energy demand is supplied by the oxidative metabolism, but it has also been proposed that the Ca^{2+} stores in ROS could provide an energy reserve. Ca^{2+} is at millimolar concentrations in the disc lumen and a Ca^{2+}-ATPase was found on the disc membrane with a low Ca^{2+} affinity above the cytoplasmic concentration. This ATPase could function in the inverse mode by synthesizing ATP while releasing Ca^{2+} from the disc lumen.

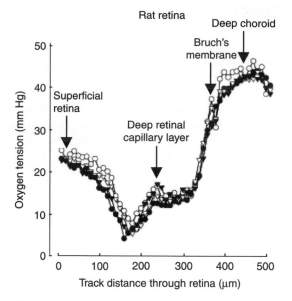

A

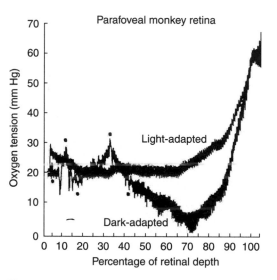

B

FIGURE 13-12　Oxygen tension in the rat (**A**) and parafoveal monkey retina (**B**). These profiles of oxygen tension as a function of retinal depth reflect the oxygen sources and consuming layers in the retina and choroids. It further illustrates the higher oxygen consumption in dark-adapted retina. These measures were obtained during both penetration and withdrawal of oxygen-sensitive electrodes in (**A**) and withdrawal in (**B**). (**A** from Yu DY et al: *Am J Physiol* 36:H2498, 1994; **B** from Ahmed J et al: *Invest Ophthal Vis Sci* 34:516, 1993.)

Rhodopsin regeneration requires the reduction of the aldehyde t-Ral to the alcohol t-Rol. This reaction is achieved by retinol dehydrogenase found in ROS using the redox potential provided by NADPH. Because the transhydrogenase that transfer the redox potential from NADH produced by glycolysis to NADPH was not found in ROS, it is more likely that NADPH is restored from $NADP^+$ in the pentose phosphate pathway. This cycle was found to generate enough NADPH for the reduction of t-Ral into t-Rol.[65] This metabolic pathway in the ROS was also sufficient to stimulate glutathione reduction by the antioxidative enzymes glutathione peroxidase and glutathione reductase, which also require NADPH.[65]

Oxygen Supply and Consumption[213]

Oxygen consumption by the retina for the oxidative metabolism was described as higher than that of the brain on a per-gram basis, thereby suggesting that the retina is one of highest consuming tissue of the body.[4-6] Early experiments with dystrophic retina in which photoreceptors degenerate suggest that photoreceptors are the main energy-consuming cells in the retina.[51] Retinal oxygen distribution was then measured with oxygen-sensitive electrodes to estimate oxygen consumption in the retina.

For the oxygen supply, unvascularized retina (rabbit) rely only on the rich vascular bed lying in the choroid, whereas vascularized retina (e.g., primate, mouse, pig) can also receive oxygen from capillaries, mostly in the OPL and in the ganglion cell and nerve fiber layer. In vascularized retina the highest oxygen tension remains at the Bruch's membrane close to the choroid vasculature, but a small rebound is associated with the deep retinal capillary layer in the OPL before reaching a minimum level. The oxygen tension slowly increases in the superficial retina toward the inner limiting membrane[214] (Figure 13-12, *A*). In avascularized retina the oxygen level gradually decreases from the outer retina at the Bruch's membrane to a minimum at the vitreal side as in the monkey parafoveal retina[2] (Figure 13-12, *B*). However, this pattern changes under dark adaptation, with a greater consumption in the outer retina (see Figure 13-12, *B*). All these data indicate that oxygen is mainly consumed in photoreceptor inner segments, the OPL, and the outer part of the IPL, where OFF bipolar cells have their terminal endings. These locations in the plexiform layers (OPL and IPL) correspond to the localization of synaptic terminals from neurons depolarized in the dark. The specific energy demand results from the maintained Ca^{2+} influx in the depolarized terminals and its continuous glutamate release that triggers a sustained activation of postsynaptic glutamate receptors (see previous discussion).

Activation of the Ca^{2+} exchanger, the glutamate transporter, and the glutamate receptors generates Na^+ influx, which must be balanced by Na^+-K^+ pump activity. As in other parts of the CNS, maintenance of ionic gradients across the plasma membrane is greatly increased in depolarized or active neurons.[38] In avascularized retina the inner retina may function in anoxic conditions with glycolysis, the anaerobic metabolism providing all of the required energy.[4,215] The high flow rate and low oxygen extraction associated with the choroidal vascularization appears ideally adapted to sustain the steep oxygen gradient in the outer retina and thus provide all the required oxygen to the inner segments.[91]

pH Regulation
Energy metabolism is a proton-producing process with 1 CO_2 molecule (HCO_3^- + H^+) produced for 6 ATP generated in the TCA cycle or 1 lactic acid per ATP during glycolysis. In contrast, neuronal glutamatergic and GABA-ergic activity are generally associated with an alkalinization of the extracellular space. For instance, glutamate uptake is associated with the cotransport of a proton H^+. In the retina this modulation of the extracellular pH may significantly affect signal processing. For example, Ca^{2+} channels are blocked by protons.[11] Thus synaptic transmission between photoreceptors and second-order neurons is substantially reduced by extracellular acidification.[12,56,77] In the fish and rabbit retina, a circadian clock was shown to regulate the pH with a decrease at night.[31,32]

In the retina, pH gradually decreases from the vitreal side to the outer limiting membrane and then increases slightly before the RPE cells.[32] The minimum at the outer limiting membrane close to photoreceptor IS, where photoreceptor mitochondria are concentrated, is consistent with a location of high metabolic activity. Glial Müller cells were found to play a major role in the regulation of retinal extracellular pH.[125] These cells express high amounts of extracellular and intracellular carbonic anhydrase, which catalyses the transformation of CO_2 molecules into HCO_3^- and H^+. Furthermore, these cells express an Na^+-HCO_3^- cotransport system that acidifies the extracellular space in response to an increase in extracellular K^+. The localization of this cotransport system, mainly at the Müller cell endfeet, supports the hypothesis of a glial regulation of blood flow because blood vessels dilate on acidification of the extracellular space and retinal astrocyte and Müller cell endfeet usually contact retinal blood vessels.

CONCLUSIONS
This chapter has focused on some major and specific biochemical events that occur during the phototransduction cascade and the subsequent information processing of the graded signals. It may provide some explanations to the origin of retinal dystrophies. The specific molecular and cellular mechanisms developed for vision are at the origin of a great diversity in retinal hereditary dystrophies. The retinal specificity of the proteins directs the dysfunction to the retina, as in retinitis pigmentosa, or to the retina and related organs, as in Usher syndrome. On the other hand, the high energy demand required for retinal information processing may explain other visual deficits occurring with aging or under ischemic conditions, as in diabetic retinopathy, glaucoma, or possibly age-related macular degeneration.

ACKNOWLEDGMENTS
I thank Professor Alm, Dr. David Cia, Dr. Jie Gong, and Dr. Michel Roux for helpful comments on the manuscript.

REFERENCES
1. Acharya S, Karnik SS: Modulation of GDP release from transducin by the conserved Glu134-Arg135 sequence in rhodopsin, *J Biol Chem* 271:25406, 1996.
2. Ahmed J et al: Oxygen distribution in the macaque retina, *Invest Ophthal Vis Sci* 34:516, 1993.
3. Allikmets R: A photoreceptor cell-specific ATP-binding transporter gene (ABCR) is mutated in recessive Stargardt macular dystrophy, *Nat Genet* 17:122, 1997.
4. Ames A III, Li YY: Energy requirements of glutamatergic pathways in rabbit retina, *J Neurosci* 12:4234, 1992.
5. Anderson B Jr: Ocular effects of changes in oxygen and carbon dioxide tension, *Trans Am Ophthalmol Soc* 66:423, 1968.
6. Anderson B Jr, Saltzman HA: Hyperbaria, hybaroxia, and the retinal and cerebral vessels, *Headache* 5:73, 1965.
7. Andrade da Costa BL, de Mello FG, Hokoc JN: Transporter-mediated GABA release induced by excitatory amino acid agonist is associated with GAD-67 but not GAD-65 immunoreactive cells of the primate retina, *Brain Res* 863:132, 2000.
8. Arriza JL et al: Excitatory amino acid transporter 5, a retinal glutamate transporter coupled to a chloride conductance, *Proc Natl Acad Sci USA* 94:4155, 1997.
9. Auger C, Attwell D: Fast removal of synaptic glutamate by postsynaptic transporters, *Neuron* 28:547, 2000.
10. Awatramani GB, Slaughter MM: Intensity-dependent, rapid activation of presynaptic metabotropic glutamate receptors at a central synapse, *J Neurosci* 21:741, 2001.
11. Barnes S, Bui Q: Modulation of calcium-activated chloride current via pH-induced changes of calcium channel properties in cone photoreceptors, *J Neurosci* 11:4015, 1991.
12. Barnes S, Merchant V: Modulation of transmission gain by protons at the photoreceptor output synapse, *PNAS* 90:10081, 1993.
13. Barnett NL, Pow DV: Antisense knockdown of GLAST, a glial glutamate transporter, compromises retinal function, *Invest Ophthalmol Vis Sci* 41:585, 2000.

14. Bavik CO, Busch C, Erikson U: Characterization of a plasma retinol-binding protein membrane receptor expressed in the retinal pigment epithelium, *J Biol Chem* 267:23035, 1992.

15. Baylor DA: Photoreceptor signals and vision, *Invest Ophthalmol Vis Sci* 28:34, 1987.

16. Baylor DA, Nunn BJ: Electrical properties of the light-sensitive conductance of rods of the salamander *Ambystoma tigrinum, J Physiol* 371:115, 1986.

17. Bergersen L et al: Cellular and subcellular expression of monocarboxylate transporters in the pigment epithelium and retina of the rat, *Neuroscience* 90:319, 1999.

18. Brandon C, Criswell MH: Displaced starburst amacrine cells of the rabbit retina contain the 67-kDa isoform, but not the 65-kDa isoform, of glutamate decarboxylase, *Vis Neurosci* 12:1053, 1995.

19. Brandstätter JH, Koulen P, Wässle H: Selective synaptic distribution of kainate receptor subunits in the two plexiform layers of the rat retina, *J Neurosci* 17:9298, 1997.

20. Brandstätter JH et al: Distributions of two homologous synaptic vesicle proteins, synaptoporin and synaptophysin, in the mammalian retina, *J Comp Neurol* 370:1, 1996.

21. Brown PK, Wald G: Visual pigments in human and monkey retinas, *Nature* 200:37, 1963.

22. Buerk DG, Riva CE, Cranstoun SD: Nitric oxide has a vasodilatory role in cat optic nerve during flicker stimuli, *Microvasc Res* 55:13, 1996.

23. Burrone J, Lagnado L: Synaptic depression and the kinetics of exocytosis in retinal bipolar cells, *J Neurosci* 20:568, 2000.

24. Chen CK et al: Ca-dependent interaction of recoverin with rhodopsin kinase, *J Biol Chem* 270:18060, 1995.

25. Cook PB, Werblin FS: Spike initiation and propagation in wide field transient amacrine cells of the salamander retina, *J Neurosci* 14:3852, 1994.

26. Cudeiro J, Rivadulla C: Sight and insight: on the physiological role of nitric oxide in the visual system, *TINS* 22:3, 1999.

27. Davidson FF, Loewen PC, Khorana HG: Structure and function of rhodopsin: replacement by alanine of cysteine residue 110 and 187 affects the light-activated metarhodopsin II state, *Proc Natl Acad Sci USA* 91:4029, 1994.

28. Derwent JJ, Linsenmeier RA: Intraretinal analysis of the a-wave of the electroretinogram (ERG) in dark-adapted intact cat retina, *Vis Neurosci* 18:353, 2001.

29. DeVries SH: Bipolar cells use kainate and AMPA receptors to filter visual information into separate channels, *Neuron* 28:847, 2000.

30. Dhingra A et al: The light response of ON bipolar neurons requires Gαo, *J Neurosci* 20:9053, 2000.

31. Dmitriev AV, Mangel SC: Circadian clock regulates of Ph of the fish retina, *J Physiol* 522:77, 2000.

32. Dmitriev AV, Mangel SC: Circadian clock regulation of Ph in the rabbit retina, *J Neurosci* 21:2897, 2001.

33. Dolphin AC: Mechanisms of modulation of voltage-dependent calcium channels by G proteins, *J Physiol Lond* 506:3, 1998.

34. Dowling JE: The chemistry of visual adaptation in the rat, *Nature* 188:114, 1960.

35. Dowling JE: *The retina: an approachable part of the brain,* Cambridge, Mass, 1987, Harvard University Press.

36. Duarte CB, Santos PF, Carvalho AP: Corelease of two functionally opposite neurotransmitters by retinal amacrine cells: experimental evidence and functional significance, *J Neurosci Res* 58:475, 1999.

37. Ebrey T, Koutalos Y: Vertebrate photoreceptors, *Prog Retin Eye Res* 20:49, 2001.

38. Erecinska M, Silver IA: Ions and energy in mammalian brain, *Prog Neurobiol* 43:37, 1994.

39. Fairman WA et al: An excitatory amino-acid transporter with properties of a ligand-gated chloride channel, *Nature* 375:599, 1995.

40. Feigenspan A, Bormann J: Modulation of GABA$_C$ receptors in rat retinal bipolar cells by protein kinase C, *J Physiol* 481:325, 1994.

41. Feigenspan A, Wässle H, Bormann J: Pharmacology of GABA receptor Cl$^-$ channels in rat retinal bipolar cells, *Nature* 361:159, 1993.

42. Gaal L et al: Postsynaptic response kinetics are controlled by a glutamate transporter at cone photoreceptors, *J Neurophysiol* 79:190, 1998.

43. Gebhard R: Histochemical demonstration of glutamate dehydrogenase and phosphate-activated glutaminase activities in semithin sections of the rat retina, *Histochemistry* 97:101, 1992.

44. Gerhart DZ, Leino RL, Drewes LR: Distribution of monocarboxylate transporters MCT1 and MCT2 in rat retina, *Neuroscience* 92:367, 1999.

45. Germer A et al: Distribution of mitochondria within Müller cells: I. Correlation with retinal vascularization in different mammalian species, *J Neurocytol* 27:329, 1998.

46. Gilbertson TA, Scobey R, Wilson M: Permeation of calcium ions through non-NMDA glutamate channels in retinal bipolar cells, *Science* 251:1613, 1991.

47. Gleason E, Borges S, Wilson M: Control of transmitter release from retinal amacrine cells by Ca^{2+} influx and efflux, *Neuron* 13:1109, 1994.

48. Gleason E, Borges S, Wilson M: Electrogenic Na-Ca exchange clears Ca^{2+} loads from retinal amacrine cells in culture, *J Neurosci* 15:3612, 1995.

49. Godfrey DA et al: Aspartate aminotransferase and glutaminase activities in rat olfactory bulb and cochlear nucleus; comparisons with retina and with concentrations of substrate and product amino acids, *Neurochem Res* 19:693, 1994.

50. Grant GB, Dowling JE: A glutamate-activated chloride current in cone-driven ON bipolar cells of the white perch retina, *J Neurosci* 15:3852, 1995.

51. Graymore CN: Metabolic survival of the isolated retina, *Br Med Bull* 26:130, 1970.

52. Han M, Smith SO: High-resolution structural studies of the retinal–Glu113 interaction in rhodopsin, *Biophys Chem* 56:23, 1995.

53. Han M et al: The C9 methyl group of retinal interacts with glycine-121 in rhodopsin, *Proc Natl Acad Sci USA* 94:13442, 1997.

54. Harada T et al: Functions of the two glutamate transporters GLAST and GLT-1 in the retina, *Proc Natl Acad Sci USA* 95:4663, 1998.

55. Hargrave PA: Rhodopsin structure, function, and topography, *Invest Ophthal Vis Sci* 42:3, 2001.

56. Harsanyi K, Mangel SC: Modulation of cone to horizontal cell transmission by calcium and pH in the fish retina, *Vis Neurosci* 10:81, 1993.

57. Haverkamp S, Grunert U, Wässle H: The cone pedicle, a complex synapse in the retina, *Neuron* 27:85, 2000.

58. Haverkamp S, Grunert U, Wässle H: Localization of kainate receptors at the cone pedicles of the primate retina, *J Comp Neurol* 436:471, 2001.

59. Haverkamp S, Grunert U, Wässle H: The synaptic architecture of AMPA receptors at the cone pedicle of the primate retina, *J Neurosci* 21:2488, 2001.

60. Hayes KC, Carey RE, Schmidt SY: Retinal degeneration associated with taurine deficiency in the cat, *Science* 188:949, 1975.

61. Heidelberger R et al: Calcium dependence of the rate of exocytosis in a synaptic terminal, *Nature* 371:513, 1994.

62. Heinamaki AA: Endogenous synthesis of taurine and GABA in rat ocular tissues, *Acta Chem Scand B* 42:39, 1988.

63. Hsu SC, Molday RS: Glyceraldehyde-3-phosphate dehydrogenase is a major protein associated with the plasma membrane of retinal photoreceptor outer segments, *J Biol Chem* 265:13308, 1990.

64. Hsu SC, Molday RS: Glycolytic enzymes and a GLUT-1 glucose transporter in the outer segments of rod and cone photoreceptor cells, *J Biol Chem* 266:21745, 1991.

65. Hsu SC, Molday RS: Glucose metabolism in photoreceptor outer segments. Its role in phototransduction and in NADPH-requiring reactions, *J Biol Chem* 269:17954, 1994.

66. Ida S et al: Alteration of metabolism of retinal taurine following prolonged light and dark adaptation: a quantitative comparison with gamma-aminobutyric acid (GABA), *J Neurosci Res* 6:497, 1981.

67. Illing M, Molday LL, Molday RS: The 220-kDa rim protein of retinal rod outer segments is a member of the ABC transporter superfamily, *J Biol Chem* 272:10303, 1997.

68. In-Beom K, Su-Ja O, Myung-Hoon C: Neuronal nitric oxide synthase immunoreactive neurons in the mammalian retina, *Microsc Res Tech* 50:112, 2000.

69. Jiang M, Pandey S, Fong HK: An opsin homologue in the retina and pigment epithelium, *Invest Ophthalmol Vision Sci* 34:3669, 1993.

70. Jindrova H: Vertebrate phototransduction: activation, recovery, and adaptation, *Physiol Res* 47:155, 1998.

71. Johnson J et al: Multiple gamma-aminobutyric acid plasma membrane transporters (GAT-1, GAT-2, GAT-3) in the rat retina, *J Comp Neurol* 375:212, 1996.

72. Jonas P, Bischofberger J, Sandkuhler J: Corelease of two fast neurotransmitters at a central synapse, *Science* 281:419, 1998.

73. Kalloniatis M, Marc RE, Murry RF: Amino acid signatures in the primate retina, *J Neurosci* 16:6807, 1996.

74. Kalloniatis M, Tomisich G: Amino acid neurochemistry of the vertebrate retina, *Prog Retin Eye Res* 18:811, 1999.

75. Kawai F et al: Na+ action potentials in human photoreceptors, *Neuron* 30:451, 2001.

76. Kikkawa S et al: GTP-binding protein couples with metabotropic glutamate receptor in bovine retinal on-bipolar cell, *Biochem Biophys Res Commun* 195:374, 1993.

77. Kleinschmidt J: Signal transmission at the photoreceptor synapse: role of calciumions and protons, *Ann NY Acad Sci* 635:468, 1994.

78. Kobayashi K, Sakaba T, Tachibana M: Potentiation of Ca^{2+} transients in the presynaptic terminals of goldfish retinal bipolar cells, *J Physiol* 482:7, 1995.

79. Kobayashi K, Tachibana M: Ca^{2+} regulation in the presynaptic terminals of goldfish retinal bipolar cells, *J Physiol* 483:79, 1995.

80. Koulen P et al: Presynaptic and postsynaptic localization of GABAB receptors in neurons of the rat retina, *Eur J Neurosci* 10:1446, 1998.

81. Koulen P et al: Modulation of the intracellular calcium concentration in photoreceptor terminals by a presynaptic metabotropic glutamate receptor, *Proc Natl Acad Sci USA* 96:9909, 1999.

82. Koutalos Y et al: Diffusion coefficient of the cyclic GMP analog 8-(fluoresceinyl)thioguanosine 3′,5′ cyclic monophosphate in the salamander rod outer segment, *Biophys J* 69:2163, 1995.

83. Krizaj D, Copenhagen DR: Compartmentalization of calcium extrusion mechanisms in the outer and inner segments of photoreceptors, *Neuron* 21:249, 1998.

84. Krizaj D et al: Caffeine-sensitive calcium stores regulate synaptic transmission from retinal rod photoreceptors, *J Neurosci* 19:7249, 1999.

85. Kumagai AK, Glasgow BJ, Pardridge WM: GLUT1 glucose transporter expression in the diabetic and nondiabetic human eye, *Invest Ophthalmol Vis Sci* 35:2887, 1994.

86. Kutuzov MA, Bennett N: Calcium-activated opsin phosphatase activity in retinal rod outer segments, *Eur J Biochem* 238:613, 1996.

87. Lake N, Verdone-Smith C: Immunocytochemical localization of taurine in the mammalian retina, *Curr Eye Res* 8:163, 1989.

88. Larsson HP et al: Noise analysis of the glutamate-activated current in photoreceptors, *Biophys J* 70:733, 1996.

89. Li XB, Szerencsei RT, Schnetkamp PP: The glucose transporter in the plasma membrane of the outer segments of bovine retinal rods, *Exp Eye Res* 59:351, 1994.

90. Lieth E et al: Nitrogen shuttling between neurons and glial cells during glutamate synthesis, *J Neurochem* 76:1712, 2001.

91. Linsenmeier RA, Padnick-Silver L: Metabolic dependence of photoreceptors on the choroid in the normal and detached retina, *Invest Ophthalmol Vis Sci* 41:3117, 2000.

92. Liu D T et al: Constraining ligand-binding site stoichiometry suggests that a cyclic nucleotide-gated channel is composed of two functional dimers, *Neuron* 21:235, 1998.

93. Lombardini JB: Effects of taurine and mitochondrial metabolic inhibitors on ATP-dependent Ca^{2+} uptake in synaptosomal and mitochondrial subcellular fractions of rat retina, *J Neurochem* 51:200, 1988.

94. Lombardini JB: Taurine: retinal function, *Brain Res Brain Res Rev* 16:151, 1991.

95. Lombardini JB: Spontaneous and evoked release of [3H]taurine from a P2 subcellular fraction of the rat retina, *Neurochem Res* 18:193, 1993.

96. Lopez-Escalera R et al: Glycolysis and glucose uptake in intact outer segments isolated from bovine retinal rods, *Biochemistry* 30:8970, 1991.

97. Lukasiewicz PD, Maple BR, Werblin FS: A novel GABA receptor on bipolar cell terminals in the tiger salamander retina, *J Neurosci* 14:1202, 1994.

98. Lukasiewicz PD, Shields CR: A diversity of GABA receptors in the retina, *Semin Cell Dev Biol* 9:293, 1998.

99. Malchow RP, Qian HH, Ripps H: Gamma-aminobutyric acid (GABA)-induced currents of skate Müller (glial) cells are mediated by neuronal-like GABA_A receptors, *Proc Natl Acad Sci USA* 86:4226, 1989.

100. Mantych GJ, Hageman GS, Devaskar SU: Characterization of glucose transporter isoforms in the adult and developing human eye, *Endocrinology* 133:600, 1993.

101. Maple BR, Werblin FS, Wu SM: Miniature excitatory postsynaptic currents in bipolar cells of the tiger salamander retina, *Vis Res* 34:2357, 1994.

102. Marc RE, Murry RF, Basinger SF: Pattern recognition of amino acid signatures in retinal neurons, *J Neurosci* 15:5106, 1995.

103. Marc RE et al: Amino acid signatures in the normal cat retina, *Invest Ophthalmol Vis Sci* 39:1685, 1998.

104. Mata N, Villazana ET, Tsin AT: Colocalization of 11-*cis* retinyl esters and retinyl ester hydrolase activity in retinal pigment epithelium plasma membrane? *Invest Ophthalmol Vis Sci* 39:1312, 1998.

105. Matthews G: Synaptic mechanisms of bipolar terminals, *Vis Res* 39:2469, 1999.

106. McBee JK et al: Confronting complexity: the interlink of phototransduction and retinoid metabolism in the vertebrate retina, *Prog Retin Eye Res* 20:469, 2001.

107. McIntire SL et al: Identification and characterization of the vesicular GABA transporter, *Nature* 389:870, 1997.

108. Mennerick S, Matthews G: Ultrafast exocytosis elicited by calcium current in synaptic terminals of retinal bipolar neurons, *Neuron* 17:1241, 1996.

109. Micci MA, Christensen BN: Na$^+$/Ca^{2+} exchange in catfish retina horizontal cells: regulation of intracellular Ca^{2+} store function, *Am J Physiol* 274:C1625, 1998.

110. Militante JD, Lombardini JB: Taurine uptake activity in the rat retina: protein kinase C-independent inhibition by chelerythrine, *Brain Res* 818:368, 1999.

111. Militante JD, Lombardini JB: Stabilization of calcium uptake in rat rod outer segments by taurine and ATP, *Amino Acids* 19:561, 2000.

112. Molday RS, Molday LL: Identification and characterization of multiple forms of rhodopsin and minor proteins in frog and bovine outer segment disc membranes. Electrophoresis, lactin labeling, and proteolysis studies, *J Biol Chem* 254:4653, 1979.

113. Morgans CW: Neurotransmitter release at ribbon synapses in the retina, *Immunol Cell Biol* 78:442, 2000.

114. Morgans CW et al: Calcium extrusion from mammalian photoreceptor terminals, *J Neurosci* 18:2467, 1998.

115. Nathans J: The evolution and physiology of human color vision: insights from molecular genetic studies of visual pigments, *Neuron* 24:299, 1999.

116. Navanglone A et al: Electrophysiological characterization of ionic transport by the retinal exchanger expressed in human embryonic kidney cells, *Biophys J* 73:45, 1997.

117. Nawy S: The metabotropic receptor mGluR6 may signal through G$_o$, but not phosphodiesterase, in retinal bipolar cells, *J Neurosci* 19:2938, 1999.

118. Nawy S: Regulation of the on bipolar cell mGluR6 pathway by Ca^{2+}, *J Neurosci* 20:4471, 2000.

119. Nawy S, Jahr CE: Suppression by glutamate of cGMP-activated conductance in retinal bipolar cells, *Nature* 346:269, 1990.

120. Nawy S, Jahr CE: cGMP-gated conductance in retinal bipolar cells is suppressed by the photoreceptor transmitter, *Neuron* 7:677, 1991.

121. Neal M, Cunningham J, Matthews K: Selective release of nitric oxide from retinal amacrine and bipolar cells, *Invest Ophthalmol Vis Sci* 39:850, 1998.

122. Neal MJ et al: Immunocytochemical evidence that vigabatrin in rats causes GABA accumulation in glial cells of the retina, *Neurosci Lett* 98:29, 1989.

123. Nehring RB et al: The metabotropic GABA$_B$ receptor directly interacts with the activating transcription factor 4, *J Biol Chem* 275:35185, 2000.

124. Neufeld AH, Shareef S, Pean J: Cellular localization of neuronal nitric oxide synthase (NOS-1) in the human and rat retina, *J Comp Neurol* 416:269, 2000.

125. Newman EA: Acid efflux from retinal glial cells generated by sodium bicarbonate cotransport, *J Neursci* 16:159, 1996.

126. Nihira M et al: Primate rod and cone photoreceptors may differ in glucose accessibility, *Invest Ophthalmol Vis Sci* 36:1259, 1995.

127. Okubo A et al: Ultracytochemical demonstration of glycogen in cone, but not in rod, photoreceptor cells in the rat retina, *Anat Anz* 180:307, 1998.

128. Olson A, Pugh EN: Diffusion coefficient of cyclic GMP in salamander rod outer segments estimated with two fluorescent probes, *Jr Biophys* 65:1335, 1993.

129. Ozawa S, Kamiya H, Tsuzuki K: Glutamate receptors in the mammalian central nervous system, *Prog Neurobiol* 54:581, 1998.

130. Palczewski K, Rispoli G, Detwiler PB: The influence of arrestin (48K protein) and rhodopsin kinase on visual transduction, *Neuron* 8:117, 1992.

131. Pan ZH, Hu HJ: Voltage-dependent Na(+) currents in mammalian retinal cone bipolar cells, *J Neurophysiol* 84:2564, 2000.

132. Papermaster DS et al: Immunocytochemical localization of a large intrinsic membrane protein to the incisures and margins of frog rod outer segment disks, *J Cell Biol* 78:415, 1978.

133. Pasantes-Morales H et al: Effects of the taurine transport antagonist, guanidinoethane sulfonate, and β-alanine on the morphology of rat retina, *J Neurosci Res* 9:135, 1983.

134. Pattnaik B et al: GABAC receptors are localized with microtubule-associated protein 1B in mammalian cone photoreceptors, *J Neurosci* 20:6789, 2000.

135. Peng YW et al: Localization of the inositol 1,4,5-trisphosphate receptor in synaptic terminals in the vertebrate retina, *Neuron* 6:525, 1991.

136. Pepe IM: Rhodopsin and phototransduction, *J Photochem Photobiol B* 48:1, 1999.

137. Peterson WM, Miller SS: Identification and functional characterization of a dual GABA/taurine transporter in the bullfrog retinal pigment epithelium, *J Gen Physiol* 106:1089, 1995.

138. Pfeiffer-Linn CL, Lasater EM: Whole cell and single-channel properties of a unique voltage-activated sustained calcium current identified in teleost retinal horizontal cells, *J Neurophysiol* 75:609, 1996.

139. Picaud SA et al: Cone photoreceptors respond to their own glutamate release in the tiger salamander, *Proc Natl Acad Sci USA* 92:9417, 1995.

140. Picaud SA et al: Glutamate-gated chloride channel with glutamate-transporter-like properties in cone photoreceptors of the tiger salamander, *J Neurophysiol* 74:1760, 1995.

141. Picaud SA et al: Adult human retinal neurons in culture: Physiology of horizontal cells, *Invest Ophthalmol Vis Sci* 13:2637, 1998.

142. Piccolino M: The feedback synapse from horizontal cells to cone photoreceptors in the vertebrate retina, *Prog Retin Eye Res* 14:141, 1995.

143. Piccolino M, Pignatelli A, Rakotobe LA: Calcium-independent release of neurotransmitter in the retina: a "copernican" viewpoint change, *Prog Retin Eye Res* 18:1, 1999.

144. Poitry-Yamate CL, Poitry S, Tsacopoulos M: Lactate released by Müller glial cells is metabolized by photoreceptors from mammalian retina, *J Neurosci* 15:5179, 1995.

145. Pow DV: Taurine, amino acid transmitters, and related molecules in the retina of the Australian lungfish *Neoceratodus forsteri*: a light-microscopic immunocytochemical and electron-microscopic study, *Cell Tissue Res* 278:311, 1994.

146. Pow DV: Transport is the primary determinant of glycine content in retinal neurons, *J Neurochem* 70:2628, 1998.

147. Pow DV: Amino acids and their transporters in the retina, *Neurochem Int* 38:463, 2001.

148. Qian H, Dowling JE: Novel GABA responses from rod-driven retinal horizontal cells, Nature 361:162, 1993.

149. Rattner A, Smallwood PM, Nathans J: Identification and characterization of all-*trans*-retinol dehydrogenase from photoreceptor outer segments, the visual cycle enzyme that reduces all-*trans*-retinal to all-*trans*-retinol, *J Biol Chem* 275:11034, 2000.

150. Redmond TM et al: RPE is necessary for production of 11-*cis*-vitamin A in the retinal visual cycle, *Nat Genet* 20:344, 1998.

151. Reichelt W et al: GABA$_A$ receptor currents recorded from Mueller glial cells of the baboon (*Papio cynocephalus*) retina, *Neurosci Lett* 203:159, 1996.

152. Resek JF, Farrens D, Khorana HG: Structure and function in rhodopsin: covalent cross-linking of the metarhodopsin II-transducin complex, *Proc Natl Acad Sci USA* 91:7643, 1994.

153. Rieke F, Schwartz EA: Asynchronous transmitter release: control of exocytosis and endocytosis at the salamander rod synapse, *J Physiol* 493:1, 1996.

154. Ripps H et al: The rhodopsin cycle id preserved in IRBP "knockout" mice despite abnormalities in retinal structure and function, *Vis Neurosci* 17:97, 2000.

155. Rispoli G: Calcium regulation of phototransduction in vertebrate rod outer segments, *J Photochem Photobiol B* 44:1, 1998.

156. Roska B, Werblin F: Vertical interactions across ten parallel, stacked representations in the mammalian retina, *Nature* 410:583, 2001.

157. Roux MJ, Supplisson S: Neuronal and glial glycine transporters have different stoichiometries, *Neuron* 25:373, 2000.

158. Rouze NC, Schwartz EA: Continuous and transient vesicle cycling at a ribbon synapse, *J Neurosci* 18:8614, 1998.

159. Ruiz ML, Karpen JW: Single cyclic nucleotide-gated channels locked in different ligand-bound states, *Nature* 389:389, 1997.

160. Rungger-Brandle E, Kolb H, Niemeyer G: Histochemical demonstration of glycogen in neurons of the cat retina, *Invest Ophthalmol Vis Sci* 37:702, 1996.

161. Saari JC: Biochemistry of visual pigment regeneration, *Invest Ophthalmol Vis Sci* 41:337, 2000.

162. Saari JC et al: Reduction of all-*trans*-retinal limits regeneration of visual pigments in mice, *Vis Res* 38:1325, 1998.

163. Sagne C et al: Cloning of a functional vesicular GABA and glycine transporter by screening of genome databases, *FEBS Lett* 10 417:177, 1997.

164. Sanada K et al: Calcium-bound recoverin targets rhodopsin kinase to membranes to inhibit rhodopsin phosphorylation, *FEBS Lett* 384:227, 1996.

165. Sarantis M, Everett K, Attwell D: A presynaptic action of glutamate at the cone output synapse, *Nature* 332:451, 1988.

166. Schaffer S, Takahashi K, Azuma J: Role of osmoregulation in the actions of taurine, *Amino Acids* 19:527, 2000.

167. Schneeweis DM, Schnapf JL: Photovoltage of rods and cones in the macaque retina, *Science* 268:1053, 1995.

168. Schwartz EA: Calcium-independent release of GABA from isolated horizontal cells of the toad retina, *J Physiol* 323:211, 1982.

169. Shen W, Slaughter MM: Internal calcium modulates apparent affinity of metabotropic GABA receptors, *J Neurophysiol* 82:3298, 1999.

170. Shen W, Slaughter MM: Metabotropic GABA receptors facilitate L-type and inhibit N-type calcium channels in single salamander retinal neurons, *J Physiol* 516:711, 1999.

171. Shiells RA, Falk G: Glutamate receptors of rod bipolar cells are linked to a cyclic GMP cascade via a G-protein, *Proc R Soc Lond B Biol Sci* 242:91, 1990.

172. Shiells RA, Falk G: The glutamate-receptor linked cGMP cascade of retinal on-bipolar cells is pertussis and cholera toxin-sensitive, *Proc R Soc Lond B Biol Sci* 247:17, 1992.

173. Shiells RA, Falk G: A rise in intracellular Ca^{2+} underlies light adaptation in dogfish retinal "on" bipolar cells, *J Physiol* 15:343, 1999.

174. Stevens CF, Tsujimoto T: Estimates for the pool size of releasable quanta at a single central synapse and for the time required to refill the pool, *Proc Natl Acad Sci USA* 92:846, 1995.

175. Stobrawa SM et al: Disruption of ClC-3, a chloride channel expressed on synaptic vesicles, leads to a loss of the hippocampus, *Neuron* 29:185, 2001.

176. Sudhöf TC: The synaptic vesicle cycle: a cascade of protein protein interactions, *Nature* 375:645, 1995.

177. Sugasawa K et al: Immunocytochemical analyses of distributions of Na, K-ATPase and GLUT1, insulin and transferrin receptors in the developing retinal pigment epithelial cells, *Cell Struct Funct* 19:21, 1994.

178. Sun H, Molday RS, Nathans J: Retinal stimulates ATP hydrolysis by purified and reconstituted ABCR, the photoreceptor specific ATP-binding cassette transporter responsible for Stargardt disease, *J Biol Chem* 274:8269, 1999.

179. Tachibana M, Kaneko A: Gamma-aminobutyric acid acts at axon terminals of turtle photoreceptors: difference in sensitivity among cell types, *Proc Natl Acad Sci USA* 81:7961, 1984.

180. Tachibana M, Kaneko A: L-glutamate-induced depolarization in solitary photoreceptors: a process that may contribute to the interaction between photoreceptors in situ, *Proc Natl Acad Sci USA* 85:5315, 1988.

181. Takata K et al: Ultracytochemical localization of the erythrocyte/HepG2-type glucose transporter (GLUT1) in cells of the blood-retinal barrier in the rat, *Invest Ophthalmol Vis Sci* 33:377, 1992.

182. Takatsuna Y et al: Distribution of phosphate-activated glutaminase-like immunoreactivity in the retina of rodents, *Curr Eye Res* 13:629, 1994.

183. Thoreson WB, Witkovsky P: Glutamate receptors and circuits in the vertebrate retina, *Prog Retin Eye Res* 18:765, 1999.

184. To CH, Hodson SA: The glucose transport in retinal pigment epithelium is via passive facilitated diffusion, *Comp Biochem Physiol A Mol Integr Physiol* 121:441, 1998.

185. Tsacopoulos M, Magistretti PJ: Metabolic coupling between glia and neurons, *J Neurosci* 16:877, 1996.

186. Tsacopoulos M et al: Trafficking of molecules and metabolic signals in the retina, *Prog Retin Eye Res* 17:429, 1998.

187. Vardi N: Alpha subunit of Go localizes in the dendritic tips of ON bipolar cells, *J Comp Neurol* 395:43, 1998.

188. Vardi N, Kaufman DL, Sterling P: Horizontal cells in cat and monkey retina express different isoforms of glutamic acid decarboxylase, *Vis Neurosci* 11:135, 1994.

189. Vardi N et al: Identification of a G-protein in depolarizing rod bipolar cells, *Vis Neurosci* 10:473, 1993.

190. Vardi N et al: Evidence that different cation chloride cotransporters in retinal neurons allow opposite responses to GABA, *J Neurosci* 20:7657, 2000.

191. Von Gersdorff H: Synaptic ribbons: versatile signal transducers, *Neuron* 29:7, 2001.

192. Von Gersdorff H, Matthews G: Dynamics of synaptic vesicle fusion and membrane retrieval in synaptic terminals, *Nature* 367:735, 1994.

193. Von Gersdorff H, Matthews G: Inhibition of endocytosis by elevated internal calcium in a synaptic terminal, *Nature* 370:652, 1994.

194. Von Gersdorff H, Matthews G: Calcium-dependent inactivation of calcium current in synaptic terminals of retinal bipolar neurons, *J Neurosci* 16:115, 1996.

195. Von Gersdorff H et al: Evidence that vesicles on the synaptic ribbon of retinal bipolar neurons can be rapidly released, *Neuron* 16:1221, 1996.

196. Wadiche JI et al: Kinetics of a human glutamate transporter, *Neuron* 14:1019, 1995.

197. Wang L, Kondo M, Bill A: Glucose metabolism in cat outer retina: effects of light and hyperoxia, *Invest Ophthalmol Vis Sci* 38:48, 1997.

198. Wang L, Tornquist P, Bill A: Glucose metabolism in pig outer retina in light and darkness, *Acta Physiol Scand* 160:75, 1997.

199. Wang L, Tornquist P, Bill A: Glucose metabolism of the inner retina in pigs in darkness and light, *Acta Physiol Scand* 160:71, 1997.

200. Wang T et al: Correction of ornithine accumulation prevents retinal degeneration in a mouse model of gyrate atrophy of the choroid and retina, *Proc Natl Acad Sci USA* 97:1224, 2000.

201. Watanabe T et al: GLUT2 expression in the rat retina: localization at the apical ends of Müller cells, *Brain Res* 655:128, 1994.

202. Watanabe T et al: Localization and ontogeny of GLUT3 expression in the rat retina, *Brain Res Dev Brain Res* 94:60, 1996.

203. Watanabe T et al: Colocalization of GLUT3 and choline acetyltransferase immunoreactivity in the rat retina, *Biochem Biophys Res Commun* 256:505, 1999.

204. Weng K et al: Functional coupling of a human retinal metabotropic glutamate receptor (hmGluR6) to bovine rod transducin and rat Go in an in vitro reconstitution system, *J Biol Chem* 272:33100, 1997.

205. Weng J et al: Insights into the function of Rim protein in photoreceptors and etiology of Stargardt's disease from the phenotype in ABCR knockout mice, *Cell* 98:13, 1999.

206. Winkler BS: Glycolytic and oxidative metabolism in relation to retinal function, J Gen Physiol 77:667, 1981.

207. Winkler BS: *A quantitative assessment of glucose metabolism in the isolated retina. Les séminaires ophtalmologiques IPSEN,* vol 6, New York, 1995, Elsevier.

208. Winkler BS et al: Energy metabolism in human retinal Müller cells, *Invest Ophthalmol Vis Sci* 41:3183, 2000.

209. Xu J et al: Prolonged photoresponses in transgenic mouse rods lacking arrestin, *Nature* 389:423, 1997.

210. Yang CY, Brecha NC, Tsao E: Immunocytochemical localization of gamma-aminobutyric acid plasma membrane transporters in the tiger salamander retina, *J Comp Neurol* 389:117, 1997.

211. Yazulla S: Neurotransmitter release from horizontal cells. In Djamgoz MBA et al (eds): *Neurobiology and clinical aspects of the outer retina,* London, 1995, Chapman and Hall.

212. Yokoyama S: Molecular evolution of vertebrate visual pigments, *Prog Retin Eye Res* 19:385, 2000.

213. Yu DY, Cringle SJ: Oxygen distribution and consumption within the retina in vascularised and avascular retinas and in animal models of retinal disease, *Prog Retin Eye Res* 20:175, 2001.

214. Yu DY et al: Intraretinal oxygen distribution in rats as a function of systemic blood pressure, *Am J Physiol* 36:H2498, 1994.

215. Yu DY et al: Intraretinal oxygen levels before and after photoreceptor loss in the RCS rat, *Invest Ophthalmol Vis Sci* 41:3999, 2000.

216. Zafra F et al: Glycine transporters are differentially expressed among CNS cells, *J Neurosci* 15:3952, 1995.

217. Zeevalk GD, Nicklas WJ: Lactate prevents the alterations in tissue amino acids, decline in ATP, and cell damage due to aglycemia in retina, *J Neurochem* 75:1027, 2000.

218. Zenisek D, Matthews G: Calcium action potentials in retinal bipolar neurons, *Vis Neurosci* 15:69, 1998.

219. Zenisek D, Matthews G: The role of mitochondria in presynaptic calcium handling at a ribbon synapse, *Neuron* 25:229, 2000.

220. Zenisek D et al: Voltage-dependent sodium channels are expressed in nonspiking retinal bipolar neurons, *J Neurosci* 21:4543, 2001.

221. Zhang J, Shen W, Slaughter MM: Two metabotropic gamma-aminobutyric acid receptors differentially modulate calcium currents in retinal ganglion cells, *J Gen Physiol* 110:45, 1997.

222. Zhang J, Slaughter MM: Preferential suppression of the ON pathway by GABA$_C$ receptors in the amphibian retina, *J Neurophysiol* 74:1583, 1995.

223. Zhang J, Yang XL: GABA$_B$ receptors in Müller cells of the bullfrog retina, *Neuroreport* 10:1833, 1999.

224. Zimmerman WF, Yost MT, Daemen FJ: Dynamics and function of vitamin A compounds in rat retina after a small bleach of rhodopsin, *Nature* 250:66, 1974.

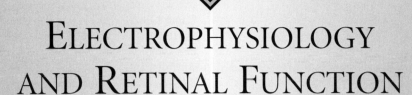

ELECTROPHYSIOLOGY AND RETINAL FUNCTION

VESNA PONJAVIC AND STEN ANDRÉASSON

BACKGROUND AND HISTORY

The electroretinogram (ERG) is a recording of action potentials produced within the retina on stimulation with light. A Swedish ophthalmologist, Frithiof Holmgren, reported the first ERG in 1865. He noticed a change in the resting potential of the eye in response to light[24] (Figure 14-1). The first retinal potential from human eyes was recorded by Dewar.[15] Nevertheless, mainly animal models were studied for many years. In 1908, Einthoven and Jolly[20] discovered that the recorded retinal potential consisted of three different components. Granit[23] continued the studies of different component in the ERG, and later Rodieck[37] also analyzed its components, recording with microelectrodes in the retina.

Riggs[35] initiated further studies of the human ERG after the introduction of a practical corneal electrode for human use in 1941. During the twentieth century, many researchers have contributed to the development of the clinical ERG methods, which today are essential for the diagnosis of retinal degenerations. In 1945, Karpe[25] reported the results of a study on 64 normal and 87 abnormal eyes, providing the initial groundwork for clinical investigations. Another important step for improving the understanding of the retinal function was when Brown[13] described the early receptor potential (ERP), which is an early response that reflects changes in rhodopsin at the photoreceptor level. Gouras[22] emphasized the importance of isolating separate rod and cone responses in the ERG as a basis for analyses of the retinal potentials. This analysis became possible by using different color filters when testing with full-field stimulation, both for the testing light and for the background light. From a historical point of view, it is interesting that Holmgren[24] had already tested the effect of different colors in his first report in 1865 on electric activity in the eye. Berson[10] stressed the importance of the temporal aspect of the ERG. He observed that in patients with progressive retinal degeneration, the full-field ERG often demonstrated a delayed cone b-wave implicit time.

The clinical value of measuring small remaining b-wave amplitudes in patients with severe retinal degenerations was a matter of opinion for a long time. When Karpe[25] published his clinical study, the ERGs in patients with retinitis pigmentosa showed a flat response. At that time, amplitudes below 10 μV, were not measurable. Goodman and Gunkel[21] reported that it was possible to measure residual b-wave responses in some patients with early forms of retinitis pigmentosa. The use of full-field stimulation and computer averaging made it possible to detect residual b-wave amplitudes as small as 1 μV.[7] Later, Berson[11] used computer averaging in combination with an analog narrow-band electronic filter in his full-field ERG recordings, and thereby extended the lower limit for detectable responses to 0.1 μV (Figure 14-2). Another method for measuring submicrovolt flicker amplitude responses and statistical estimates of measurement uncertainty was recently described by Sieving et al.[40]

Because different laboratories have chosen different examination procedures and because it is important to compare recordings from different patients with each other, a basic standard clinical protocol was created in 1989 (the International

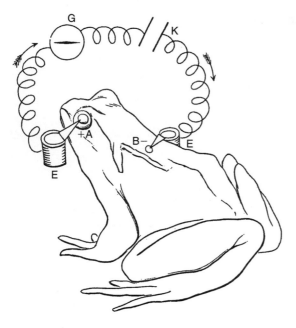

FIGURE 14-1 Diagram showing the arrangement of the experiment on eye of a frog. *A,* Eye showing the electrode (*E*), in contact with it. *B,* Skin removed and subcutaneous tissue in contact with other electrode (*E*). *G,* Galvanometer; *K,* key. *Arrows* indicate direction of current. Cornea positive. Back negative. (From Dewar J: *Nature* 15:433, 1877.)

Society for Clinical Electrophysiology of Vision [ISCEV] standard) so that responses could be recorded comparably throughout the world.[29] This document, which contains description and information of basic technology, different cornea electrodes, light sources, light adjustment, and a clinical protocol, was later updated and has been of great value.[29] According to the ISCEV standard, additional testing procedures may be added for better and more specific interpretation of the ERG (Figure 14-3).

ORIGIN OF THE RETINAL RESPONSES

The ERG is a sum of different complicated action potentials occurring simultaneously in different structures of the retina. Granit[23] was first to analyze these different components. He based his studies on the changes in the ERG on administration of ether. This anesthetic first led to a disappearance of a slow cornea-positive response (PI) and then to a loss of the earlier cornea-positive response (PII), leaving only a negative potential (PIII). After continued administration of ether, this component fi-

nally also disappeared. Asphyxia, on the other hand, led first to a loss of the fast, transient cornea-positive response (PII). Granit[23] thought this positive waveform (PII) was responsible for the b wave (Figure 14-4).

Rodieck[37] continued this work, emphasizing that the ERG is the summation of several considerably disparate potentials. The separation of the ERG-response into different waveforms is important for understanding the origin of these responses. For many years it has been disputed which specific cell layer dominantly contributes to a certain waveform. The first part of the response is the negative a wave. It has been agreed that the a wave represents photoreceptor activity, even though the ERP before the a wave is a more precise photoreceptor response.[14]

The Müller cells have previously been considered important for the generation of the b wave in the ERG, but more recent studies show that the bipolar cells may produce the b wave directly either selectively or in association with the Müller cells.

The slow response, also called the *c wave,* which can be measured with special methods, originates from the pigment epithelium cells.

Activity in the inner plexiform layer probably produces the small oscillatory potentials, which are subcomponents of the ERG and are superimposed on the b wave. Previous studies have shown that the oscillatory potentials are affected in vascular retinal diseases and may be important for predicting proliferative diabetic retinopathy.[47]

The scotopic threshold response (STR) is a prominent component of the dark-adapted ERG. It is a second negative potential generated by the Müller cells in response to light.[41]

Because of the possibility of modifying testing procedures in an almost unlimited way during ERG recordings, there may be wide variations in the waveform of ERGs. In clinical practice the most important components are the a and the b waves. The amplitudes of the responses are measured in microvolts (μV) for the a and b waves and the implicit times in microseconds (ms). The b-wave implicit time is, by definition, the time from stimulus onset to the b-wave response maximum. The amplitudes in the ERG show marked variations in both normal and diseased populations, whereas the b-wave implicit time varies less.

It is important to remember that the ERG represents the activity of the outer retinal layers (photoreceptor cells and bipolar cells) and that the gan-

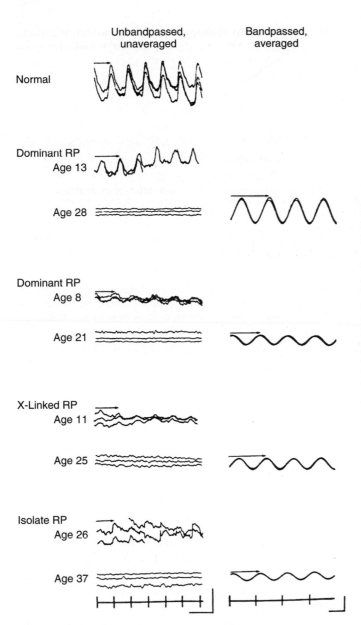

Figure 14-2 Full-field 30-Hz electroretinograms from a normal subject and four patients with retinitis pigmentosa tested at an 11- to 15-year interval. Stimulus onset, vertical markers; calibration symbol (*left column, lower right*) designated 100 μV vertically for the normal subject and top three patients and 40 μV vertically for the bottom patient and 50 msec horizontally for all traces; calibration (*right column, lower right*) designated 2 μV vertically for the dominant, X-linked, and isolated patients and 20 msec horizontally for all traces. B-wave implicit times are designated with *arrows*. *RP,* Retinitis pigmentosa. (From Andréasson S, Sandberg M, Berson E: *Am J Ophthalmol* 105:500, 1988.)

glion cell layer does not give any contribution to the ERG. Diseases of the inner cell layers and of the optic nerve, such as glaucoma, are associated with a completely normal ERG.

METHODS OF MEASUREMENT

The full-field ERG is the retinal response to a brief flash of light from the Ganzfeld sphere, and it reflects the total retinal function. It can be detected with skin electrodes placed around the eye, but the most accurate recording is achieved by using a corneal contact lens electrode centered on the cornea. Several different types of corneal electrodes are available, but the Burian-Allen bipolar contact lens and the Doran Gold lens seem to be the most favorable and the most commonly used in clinical practice. Before an ERG is recorded, the pupil should be maximally dilated and the retina dark adapted for 30 to 45 minutes. The entire retina is then illuminated through the lens using different wavelengths, intensities, and rates of light stimuli. The electric responses are obtained through the bipolar lens and then analyzed by different electronic and

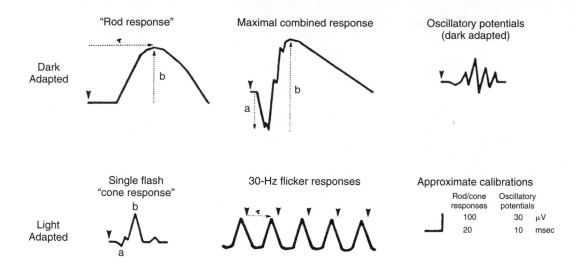

FIGURE 14-3 Diagram of the five basic electroretinogram responses defined by standard. These waveforms are exemplary only and are not intended to indicate minimum, maximum, or even average values. *Large arrowheads* indicate the stimulus flash. *Dotted arrows* exemplify how to measure time-to-peak (*t,* implicit time), a-wave amplitude, and b-wave amplitude. (From Marmor MF, Zrenner E: *Doc Ophthalmol* 97:143, 1998/1999.)

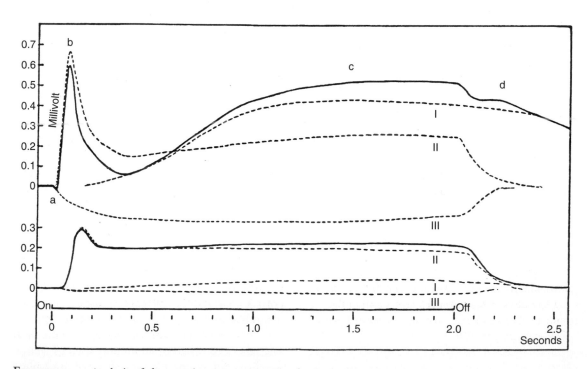

FIGURE 14-4 Analysis of electroretinogram at two stimulus intensities. *Upper tracing,* 14 L. *Lower tracing,* 0.14 mL. The a wave has been broadened slightly out of proportion to demonstrate its derivation more clearly. Duration of stimulus was 2 seconds. A slow cornea-positive response (*I*), an earlier cornea-positive response (*II*), and a negative potential (*III*). (From Granit R: *J Physiol [Lond]* 77:207,1993.)

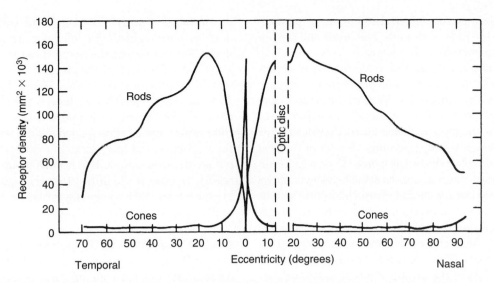

FIGURE 14-5   Topography of the layer of rods and cones in the human retina. (From Osterberg G: *Acta Ophthal* [suppl 6]:1,1935.)

computer analysis systems. ERG responses are obtained under both light-adapted and dark-adapted conditions.

During interpretation of the retinal responses, it is important to understand the structure of the retina. Figure 14-5 demonstrates the distribution of rods and cones in the retinal layers. The normal retina consists of several layers, including the photoreceptor layer, where the photosensitive rods and cones are localized. In a single healthy retina, there are approximately 120 million rods and 9 million cones. Even though there is a maximum concentration of the cones in the macula region 90% of the cones are outside the macula. There are no rods in the foveola (the central 1 degree), and the highest concentration of rods is about 15 degrees from the foveola, with fewer rods toward the periphery.

The proportion of rods and cones is about 13:1, and it is important to remember that, when evaluating the ERG, approximately 75% of the total response is emanating from circuits driven by rods.

The clinical protocol for evaluating an ERG can be divided into several parts. The single-flash dark-adapted rod response consists mainly of a b wave, which reflects the function of the rods. The b-wave amplitude is reduced early in the natural course of rod and rod-cone dystrophies and may be absent in patients with different forms of nyctalopia.

The combined dark-adapted rod and cone responses reveal information about the total retinal function. The contribution of the rods and the

cones to the b-wave amplitudes is approximately 75% and 25%, respectively. This response is especially interesting for monitoring the total retinal function in different retinal disorders over time.

Single-flash light-adapted cone responses demonstrate cone function and are valuable in clinical practice, especially in patients in whom 30-Hz flicker-stimulus ERG cannot be obtained (e.g., in children who do not cooperate because of photophobia). Stimulation with repeated 30-Hz flickering light results in an isolated cone response in which the amplitude reveals the amount of remaining healthy cones. The cone response in the ERG is selectively affected early in the course of cone degenerations.

The implicit time of the full-field cone b wave is believed to be normal in patients with stationary forms of retinal disorders and prolonged in patients with progressive tapetoretinal degenerations.[9]

Electroretinogram during General Anesthesia

Full-field ERGs are important for detecting retinal diseases in children and infants. In this age group, the fundus may appear normal or have only minor pathologic changes, even when the retinal function is extremely reduced. However, it is not always possible to obtain full-field ERGs in children younger than 4 years of age when using only topical anesthesia. These children can be given a general anesthetic and examined with full-field ERG. However, sedation is known to affect the ERG and general anesthesia can therefore alter important parameters in the ERG, such as the amplitude and the implicit time of the cone b wave.

Whitacre and Ellis[46] surveyed the use of several anesthetic drugs for sedation before an ocular examination. They concluded that there is no ideal sedative and that different compounds can influence the ERG examination in different ways. Previous studies have demonstrated only minor changes in the ERG response when using propofol (Diprivan).[5] This anesthetic drug seems to be suitable for obtaining a good baseline for clinical electrophysiologic investigations of retinal function (Figure 14-6).

Clinical electroretinography in infants also demands consideration of changes resulting from maturation. Previous reports have demonstrated an increase of the b-wave amplitudes at least during the first 6 months of life. Birch and Anderson[12] described that at birth the rod response is barely detectable, but during the first 4 months, there is a rapid development of the rod response, with a tenfold increase of its amplitude. From the age of 4 months up to adulthood, there is a further increase in the rod response and a decrease in the rod b-wave implicit time. Selective cone responses show a similar but less prominent change in amplitude between birth and 4 months of age. These reports emphasize the difficulties when interpreting the electric activity during the first 4 months of life.

Isolated Rod and Cone Responses

One of the major goals with full-field ERG is to demonstrate isolated cone and rod responses. In

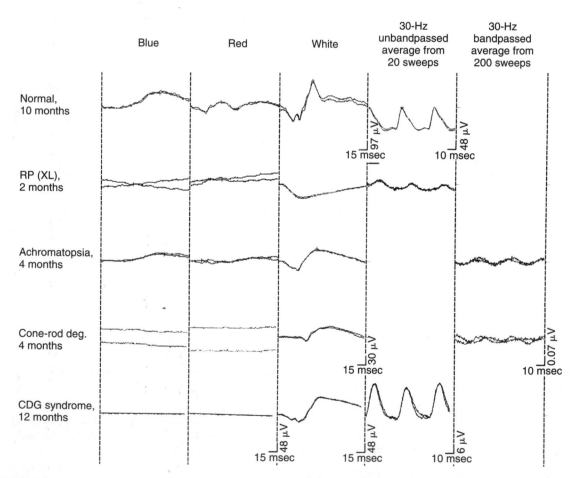

FIGURE 14-6   Full-field electroretinograms (ERGs) from four infants with different types of retinal degeneration and one normal infant. The three panels to the left show two superimposed single-flash recordings from blue, red, and white light. The two right panels show the responses to 30-Hz flickering light. (Normal ERG value [2 standard deviation] for children during general anesthesia with white flash, 191 ± 70 μV; 30-Hz flickering white light cone b-wave amplitude, 54.3 ± 30 μV; and cone b-wave implicit time, 30.4 ± 2.8 msec). *CDG,* Congenital disorder of glycosylation; *RP,* retinitis pigmentosa. (From Andréasson S, Ponjavic V: *Acta Ophthalmol Scand* 74[suppl]:219, 1996.)

previous studies, authors have used the terms *photopic* and *scotopic* responses, depending on the state of retinal adaptation, but this is not equivalent to isolated rod or cone responses. One way to separate the responses from rods and cones is to use different filters with different wavelengths in the Ganzfeldt sphere. The ISCEV standard notes that the isolated rod response can also be obtained by stimulation with a dim white light.

The full-field ERG may also be used to quantify the amount of remaining function for each of the three cone mechanisms. The middle-wavelength, or green-sensitive, cone system and the long-wavelength, or red-sensitive, cone system may be evaluated by comparing cone ERGs elicited by a short-wavelength flash or a photopically matched long-wavelength flash superimposed on a photopic background. Full-field 30-Hz cone ERG responses can also be examined with orange light (λ greater than 550 nm, Cinemoid No. 5), and blue-green light (λ less than 550 nm, Cinemoid No. 16). The amplitude of the responses of the two light stimuli is known to be different in deuteranopia and protanopia.

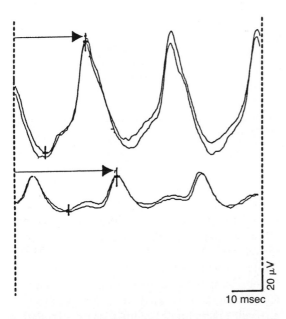

Figure 14-7 Thirty-Hz flicker electroretinogram of a typical nonrubeotic eye (*top*) and a rubeotic eye (*bottom*) 8 days after onset of central vein occlusion. Each panel contains two averaged curves generated from 20 sweeps. The *arrow* shows the cone b-wave implicit time in the 30-Hz flicker electroretinogram. The crosses are at the lowest point of the curve and at its peak; the vertical distance between them represents the amplitude. (From Larsson J, Andréasson S, Bauer B: *Am J Ophthalmol* 125:247, 1998.)

Temporal Aspects of the Electroretinogram

The implicit time for the isolated cone b-wave responses mediated by 30-Hz flicker stimulation is valuable for assessing retinal functions. Berson[9] demonstrated that the cone b-wave implicit time is often prolonged in the full-field ERG from patients with retinal degenerations. This parameter is important for the early detection of retinal disorders, and it is a valuable prognostic factor. It has also recently been shown that the cone b-wave implicit time may be a diagnostic tool even in the evaluation of patients with central vein occlusion.[28] A prolonged implicit time indicates an increased risk for developing neovascular glaucoma (Figure 14-7).

Electrooculography

An electrical potential exists between the front and the back of the eye, originating from the pigment epithelium, and the eye could actually be described as a dipole. The electrooculogram (EOG) is an objective method for measuring this standing potential in the eye, using skin electrodes on both sides of it. When an eye (a dipole) moves, an electrical potential change is picked up by the skin electrodes. The standing potential of a human eye varies from 1 to 6 mV, depending on the illumination and its state of adaptation. Emil DuBois Reymond first described the potential, but it was Riggs[36] who first demonstrated in 1954 that the potential is decreased in certain retinal degenerations.

The purpose of the EOG is to assess changes seen in the standing potential during a dark-light adaptation cycle, which reflects the function of the retinal pigment epithelium. This is done by asking the patient to fixate two alternating left and right fixation lights, most conveniently mounted in a so-called Ganzfeld illumination sphere. This induces a standardized and steadily alternating horizontal gaze shift. The testing is first performed in darkness while the patient is adapting to the dark and is then performed with a standard light turned on. During dark adaptation, a steady decline of the recorded amplitude can be measured for several minutes and the minimum reached is called the *dark trough*. When the eye is then exposed to light, the recorded amplitude shows a significant increase and its maximum is called the *light peak* (Figure 14-8).

Arden[6] calculated the ratio of the amplitude of the light peak over the dark trough (Lp/Dt), and today this calculation is called the *Arden index*. With reservation for different EOG equipment in different laboratories, it is believed that the Arden index should exceed 1.5 in eyes with a healthy retinal pigment epithelium.

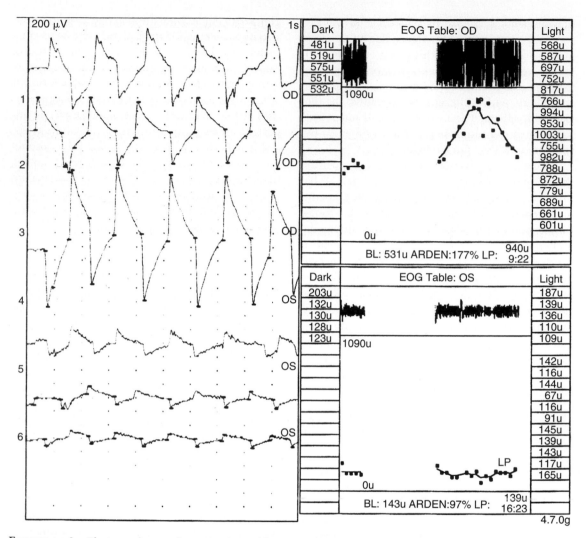

Dark	EOG Table: OD	Light
481u		568u
519u		587u
575u		697u
551u		752u
532u	1090u	817u
		766u
		994u
		953u
		1003u
		755u
		982u
		788u
		872u
		779u
		689u
		661u
		601u
	0u	
	BL: 531u ARDEN:177% LP: 940u 9:22	

Dark	EOG Table: OS	Light
203u		187u
132u		139u
130u		136u
128u		110u
123u	1090u	109u
		142u
		116u
		144u
		67u
		116u
		91u
		145u
		139u
		143u
		LP 117u
		165u
	0u	
	BL: 143u ARDEN:97% LP: 139u 16:23	

4.7.0g

FIGURE 14-8   Electrooculogram from a patient with one normal eye with an Arden index of 1.8 and the other eye with abnormal function of the pigment epithelium and an Arden index of 1.0.

Different disorders affecting the pigment epithelium can be analyzed with this test. In patients with Best disease (vitelliform macular dystrophy), the EOG demonstrates a pathologic change with an Arden index less than 1.5.[44] Although the full-field ERG reflects the activity from the inner retinal layers, the EOG is a valuable supplement for measuring the function of the pigment epithelium.

Multifocal and Focal Electroretinogram Examination

The full-field ERG is a reliable method for measuring the responses from the rods and cones throughout the entire retina, but it is less useful for examination of focal changes in the macula.

Different kinds of equipment have been used for obtaining responses from localized areas of the retina and especially the macular region. One of the most widespread early methods was the Doran focal ERG, which can be characterized as a method for obtaining the cone ERG from the macular region. The method is based on a technique that uses a rebuilt ophthalmoscope for focused stimulation of the macula, as well as the area between the macula and the optic disc. The responses are assessed using a Burian Allen bipolar electrode on the cornea. The ERG amplitude from the macular region is then compared with the responses from the paramacular area, which are known to be lower than those from the fovea. Recently, a new technique for recording the cone response in the central part of the retina has been developed—the multifocal ERG.[8,43] With this method, it is possible to record more than 100 focal cone ERGs from each eye within 8 minutes. The screen presents a stimulus pattern of usually 61 to 241 hexagons covering up to 25 degrees of the visual field; an underlying mathematical system calculates the true signal from each location. The responses are measured by using a bipolar contact lens electrode attached to the eye. The components that mainly generate a multifocal ERG response are believed to be the cones. There is also a small contribution from ganglion cell and from the optic nerve head. Use of a multifocal ERG makes it possible to assess the local cone function in different areas of the central retina (Figure 14-9).

Separate rod and cone responses can be achieved with conventional full-field ERG, but the cone response then reflects the function of all existing cones throughout the retina. Therefore the multifocal ERG adds further knowledge about the cone function, especially in the macular region.

ELECTROPHYSIOLOGIC RESPONSES IN PATIENTS WITH DIFFERENT DEFECTS IN RETINAL PROTEINS

In recent years the progress in the field of molecular genetics has significantly extended our knowledge concerning different proteins in the retina. Several new proteins of importance for normal retinal function have been identified. These findings help in the understanding of the electric phenomena that happen in the retina. Today it is possible to study the electric phenomena, in both humans and animals, when these proteins are defective, when they malfunction, or when they are absent. Some of these proteins seem to be of particular importance for normal retinal function.

Bestrophin

The function of the retinal pigment epithelium is assessed by EOG. A defect in the recently identified protein called *bestrophin* leads to changes in the EOG responses.[32,34] Bestrophin probably plays a major role in the transport mechanisms of the pigment epithelium cell membrane. It has at least four putative transmembrane domains; therefore a defective protein may be responsible for the changes in the electrical potential during the light-adaptation phase of the EOG test. The light-induced rise in the EOG originates from both cone and rod activity and is associated with the extracellular K^+ ion concentration. Changes in bestrophin function affect the electric resistance between the photoreceptors and the choroid and must therefore be involved in this activity. The full-field ERG is not affected in eyes with a defect bestrophin protein, which is as expected because the full-field ERG predominantly reflects the function of the retina proximal to the retinal pigment epithelium, where bestrophin is not present. The protein is present in all retinal pigment epithelium cells, which explains why it affects a mass response like the EOG, but it is not understood why the mutated protein in most other respects affects only the macula (see Color Plate 7).

The ABCR Protein

Recently, another protein responsible for macular function has been identified.[2] The ABCR protein is present in the disc membrane of rod outer segments and is expressed exclusively in photoreceptor cells.[42] It is believed that the *ABCR* gene product mediates the transport of an essential molecule across the photoreceptor cell membrane. Different mutations in the *ABCR* gene are responsible for the Stargardt disease.[1] Both focal ERG and the multifocal ERG analyses show a dysfunction of the cones in the macular region, even though the mutated protein is present throughout the retina and exclusively in rods.[27,38] The reason for this seeming discrepancy is not fully known.

The RS protein

Another recently identified protein is the RS protein, which is involved in congenital retinoschisis.[39] The full-field ERGs in patients with juvenile retinoschisis characteristically demonstrate a reduced b-wave amplitude, and in severe cases, a reduction in the a-wave amplitude is also noted.[31] The b/a ratio is often less than 1.0. The Müller cells are involved in generating the STR of the ERG. The reductions of STR amplitudes in juvenile retinoschisis implicate Müller cells in the pathophysiology in at least some cases of juvenile retinoschisis.

The RS protein contains a discoid domain, shared with a number of other proteins, which is involved in cell-to-cell adhesion and phospholipid binding. This function is in agreement with the observed splitting of the retina in retinoschisis patients, indicating that the *RS* gene is important during retinal development. The electric response from patients with a defect or no RS protein demonstrates a specific influence on the ERG recordings (see Color Plates 8 and 9).

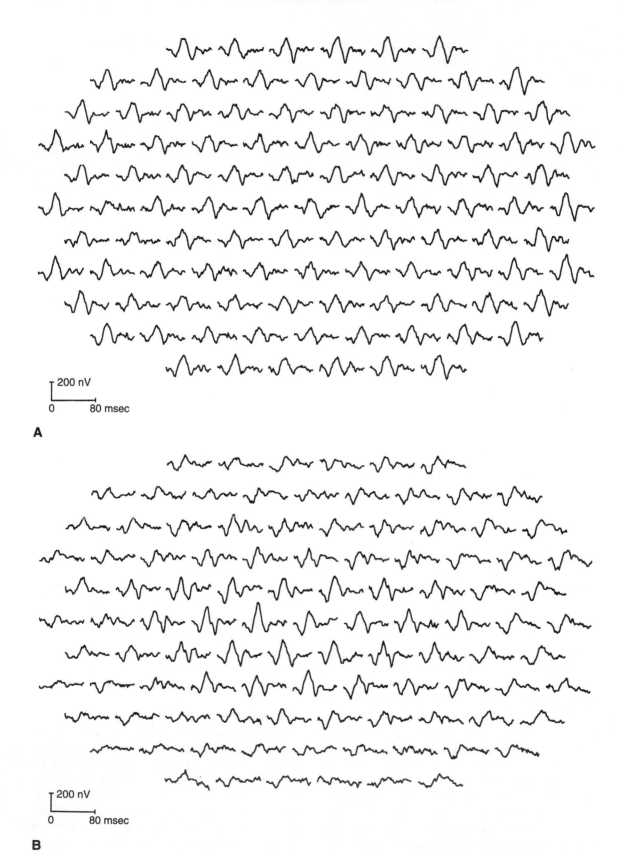

200 nV

0   80 msec

A

200 nV

0   80 msec

B

FIGURE 14-9   Multifocal electroretinograms from a normal patient (**A**) and a patient with Vigabatrin treatment (**B**). The reduced responses in the 25-degree periphery are clearly seen.

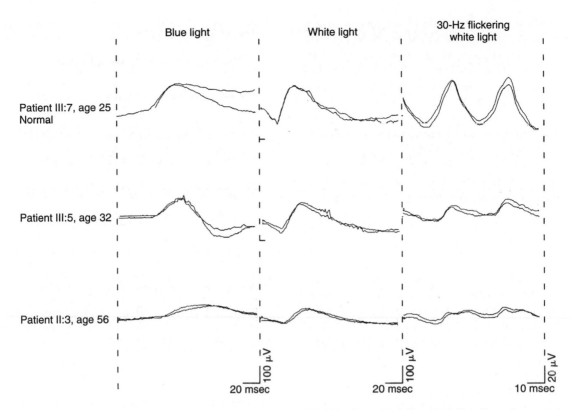

FIGURE 14-10 Full-field electroretinograms from a family with a slowly progressive retinal disorder and a mutation in the peripherin/RDS gene (Arg-172-Trp). Shown are rod response to dim blue light (*left column*), mixed cone-rod responses to white flashes (*middle column*), and isolated cone responses to a 30-Hz flickering light (*right column*). (From Ekström U et al: *Ophthalmic Genetics* 19:149, 1998.)

Rhodopsin and Peripherin/RDS

Peripherin/RDS and rhodopsin are the two most important and the most frequently examined of all proteins involved in retinal degeneration.[17]

Both proteins seem to have a major role in the pathogenesis of autosomal dominant forms of retinitis pigmentosa.[16] Rhodopsin is a seven-helix membrane protein of rod photoreceptor outer segments and plays a major role in the visual cascade on perception of light. The RDS protein is a membrane-associated glycoprotein restricted to photoreceptor outer segment discs.

Several mutations in the rhodopsin and the peripherin/RDS gene have been described, as have the electric responses from a retina with a defect or absent rhodopsin and peripherin/RDS protein. The clinical phenotype associated with these different mutations demonstrates an extreme variability, but a frequent and prominent feature is the early prolongation of the cone b-wave implicit time in the full-field 30-Hz flicker ERG.

Defects in the peripherin/RDS protein seem to be of special importance because alterations in this protein may cause either an isolated macular pathologic condition or a predominantly peripheral retinal dysfunction. However, some described clinical phenotypes include both macular and peripheral pathology. This has resulted in a confusingly diverse group of reported diagnoses associated with peripherin/RDS gene mutations[45] (Figure 14-10).

Other Proteins

The full-field ERG in patients with achromatopsia demonstrates an absence of cone responses. One protein reported to be responsible for this disease is the cyclic guanine monophosphate (cGMP)–gated cation channel in cone photoreceptors (CNGA3).[26] This protein is important for the visual transduction cascade in the cone photoreceptors. A defect or absent protein leads to reduced or diminished changes the electric responses from the cones, as assessed by full-field ERG.[9]

Defects in the rhodopsin kinase gene cause a diminished rod response in the full-field ERG.[18] In rod photoreceptors, rhodopsin kinase (RHOK) phosphorylates rhodopsin in bright light, which initiates the regeneration of the light-activated photoreceptor. Absent or defective rhodopsin kinase alters this phosphorylation of the visual pigment rhodopsin, which seems to cause an absence of rod responses in full-field ERG.

Rhodopsin kinase also interacts with arrestin in shutting off rhodopsin after it has been activated by a photon of light. Therefore it is possible that defective or absent arrestin may be responsible for rod dysfunction. No electric activity can be derived from the rods in a retina in which rhodopsin kinase or arrestin is defective or absent.

Choroideremia is a degenerative disease mainly involving the choroid. However, the electric responses from the retina, measured by the full-field ERG, demonstrate an early reduction of the amplitudes and a delayed cone 30-Hz flicker response, indicating a widespread retinal degeneration.[33] The disease is caused by mutations in the Rab escort protein REP-1, which facilitates the transfer of geranylgeranyl moieties in tissues, but the precise biochemical mechanisms leading to retinal degeneration are still under investigation (see Color Plate 10).

REFERENCES

1. Allikmets R et al: Mutation of the Stargardt disease gene (ABCR) in age-related macular degeneration, *Science* 277:1805, 1997.
2. Allikmets R et al: A photoreceptor cell-specific ATP-binding transporter gene (ABCR) is mutated in recessive Stargardt macular dystrophy, *Nat Genetics* 15:236, 1997.
3. Andréasson S, Ponjavic V: Full-field electroretinograms in infants with hereditary tapetoretinal degeneration, *Acta Ophthalmol Scand* 74(suppl):219, 1996.
4. Andréasson S, Sandberg M, Berson E: Narrow-band filtering for monitoring low-amplitude cone electroretinograms in retinitis pigmentosa, *Am J Ophthalmol* 105:500, 1988.
5. Andréasson S, Tornqvist K, Ehinger B: Full-field electroretinograms during general anesthesia in normal children compared to examination with topical anesthesia, *Acta Ophthalmol* 71:491, 1993.
6. Arden GB, Barrada A, Kelsey JH: New clinical test of retinal function based on the standing potential of the eye, *Br J Ophthalmol* 46:449, 1962.
7. Armington JC et al: Detection of the electroretinogram in retinitis pigmentosa, *Exp Eye Res* 1:74, 1961.
8. Bearse MA, Sutter EE: Imaging localized retinal dysfunction with the multifocal electroretinogram, *J Opt Soc Am A* 13:634, 1996.
9. Berson EL: Retinitis pigmentosa: the Friedenwald lecture, *Invest Ophthalmol Vis Sci* 34:1659, 1993.
10. Berson EL, Gouras P, Hoff M: Temporal aspects of the electroretinogram, *Arch Ophthalmol* 81:207, 1969.
11. Berson EL, Sandberg MA, Maguire A: Electroretinograms in carriers of blue cone monochromatism, *Am J Ophthalmol* 102:254, 1986.
12. Birch DG, Anderson JL: Standardized full-field electroretinography: normal values and their variation with age, *Arch Ophthalmol* 110:1571, 1992.
13. Brown KT, Murakami M: A new receptor potential of the monkey retina with no detectable latency, *Nature* 201:626, 1964.
14. Carr RE, Siegel IM: Action spectrum of the human early receptor potential, *Nature* 225:88, 1970.
15. Dewar J: The physiological action of light, *Nature* 15:433, 1877.
16. Dryja TP et al: Mutation spectrum of the rhodopsin gene among patients with autosomal dominant retinitis pigmentosa, *Proc Natl Acad Sci USA* 88:9370, 1991.
17. Dryja TP, Li T: Molecular genetics of retinitis pigmentosa, *Hum Mol Genet* 4(spec no):1739, 1995.
18. Eksandh L et al: Phenotypic expression of juvenile X-linked retinoschisis in Swedish families with different mutations in the XLRS1 gene, *Arch Ophthalmol* 118:1098, 2000.
19. Ekström U et al: A Swedish family with a mutation in the peripherin/RDS gene (Arg-172-Trp) associated with a progressive retinal degeneration, *Ophthalmic Genetics* 19:149, 1998.
20. Einthoven W, Jolly WA: The form and magnitude of the electrical response of the eye to stimulation by light at various intensities, *Q J Exp Physiol* 1:373, 1908.
21. Goodman G, Gunkel RD: Familial electroretinographic and adaptometric studies in retinitis pigmentosa, *Am J Ophthalmol* 46:142, 1958.
22. Gouras P: Electroretinography: some basic principles, *Invest Ophthalmol* 9:557, 1970.
23. Granit R: The components of the retinal action potential in mammals and their relation to the discharge in the optic nerve, *J Physiol (Lond)* 77:207, 1933.
24. Holmgren F: Metod att objectivera effecten af ljusintryck på retina, *Upsala Läkaref Förh* 1:184, 1865.
25. Karpe G: The basis of clinical electroretinography, *Acta Ophthalmol* 23(suppl):84, 1945.
26. Kohl S et al: Mutations in the CNGB3 gene encoding the beta-subunit of the cone photoreceptor cGMP-gated channel are responsible for achromatopsia (ACHM3) linked to chromosome 8q21, *Hum Mol Genet* 9:2107, 2000.
27. Kretschmann U et al: Multifocal electroretinography in patients with Stargardt's macular dystrophy, *Br J Ophthalmol* 82:267, 1998.
28. Larsson J, Andréasson S, Bauer B: Cone b-wave implicit time in the 30 Hz flicker ERG as an early predictor for rubeosis in central retinal vein occlusion, *Am J Ophthalmol* 125:247, 1998.
29. Marmor MF, Zrenner E: Standard for clinical electroretinography (1999 update), *Doc Ophthalmol* 97:143, 1998/1999.
30. Österberg G. Topography of the layer of rods and cones in the human retina, *Acta Ophthal* (suppl 6):1, 1935.
31. Peachey NS et al: Psychophysical and electroretinographic findings in X-linked juvenile retinoschisis, *Arch Ophthalmol* 105:513, 1987.
32. Petrukhin K et al: Identification of the gene responsible for Best's macular dystrophy, *Nat Genetics* 19:241, 1998.
33. Ponjavic V et al: Phenotype variations within a choroideremia family lacking the entire CMH gene, *Ophthalmic Genetics* 16:143, 1995.
34. Ponjavic V et al: Clinical expression of Best's vitelliform macular dystrophy in Swedish families with mutations in the *bestrophin* gene, *Ophthalmic Genetics* 20:251, 1999.

35. Riggs LA: Continuos and reproducible records of the electrical activity of the human retina, *Proc Doc Exper Biol Med* 48:204, 204.
36. Riggs LA: Electroretinography in cases of night blindness, *Am J Ophthalmol* 38:70, 1954.
37. Rodieck RW: Components of the electroretinogram: a reappraisal, *Vis Res* 12:773, 1972.
38. Sandberg MA, Jacobson SG, Berson EI: Foveal cone electroretinograms in retinitis pigmentosa and juvenile macular degeneration, *Am J Ophthalmol* 88:702, 1979.
39. Sauer GS et al: Positional cloning of the gene associated with X-linked juvenile retinoschisis, *Nat Genetics* 17:164, 1997.
40. Sieving PA et al: Submicrovolt flicker electroretinogram: cycle-by-cycle recording of multiple harmonics with statistical estimation of measurement uncertainty, *Invest Ophthalmol Vis Sci* 39:1462, 1998.
41. Sieving PA, Frishman LR, Steinberg RH: Scotopic threshold response of proximal retina in cat, *J Neurophysiol* 56:1049, 1986.
42. Sun H, Nathans J: Stargardt's ABCR is localized to the disc membrane of retinal rod outer segments, *Nat Genetics* 17:15, 1997.
43. Sutter EE, Tran D: The field topography of ERG components in man, I: the photopic luminance response, *Vision Res* 32:433, 1992.
44. Thorburn W, Nordström S: EOG in a large family with hereditary macular degeneration. (Best's vitelliform macular dystrophy) identification of gene carriers, *Acta Ophthalmol (Copenh)* 56:455, 1978.
45. Weleber RG et al: Phenotypic variation including retinitis pigmentosa, pattern dystrophy, and fundus flavimaculatus in a single family with a deletion of codon 153 or 154 of the peripherin/RDS gene, *Arch Ophthalmol* 111:1531, 1993.
46. Whitacre MM, Ellis PP: Outpatient sedation for ocular examination, *Surv Ophthalmol* 28:643, 1984.
47. Yonemura D, Aoki T, Tsuzuki K: Electroretinogram in diabetic retinopathy, *Arch Ophthalmol* 68:19, 1962.

CHAPTER 15

INTRACELLULAR LIGHT RESPONSES AND SYNAPTIC ORGANIZATION OF THE VERTEBRATE RETINA

SAMUEL M. WU

ORGANIZATION AND LIGHT RESPONSES OF RETINAL NEURONS

All vertebrate retinas are constructed according to the same basic plan. The outermost layer contains the photoreceptors, with outer segments embedded in the pigment epithelium and cell bodies that form the outer nuclear layer (ONL). Next is the inner nuclear layer (INL), which contains the cell bodies of horizontal cells (HCs), bipolar cells, and amacrine cells. The innermost layer is the ganglion cell layer (GCL), which contains cell bodies of the ganglion cells. Interspersed between the ONL and INL is the outer plexiform layer (OPL), which contains photoreceptor synaptic terminals, processes of HCs, and the dendrites of bipolar cells. Between the INL and GCL is the inner plexiform layer (IPL), which contains axons of bipolar cells and dendrites of amacrine cells and ganglion cells.[17,26]

In addition to structural similarities, electrical responses of retinal neurons in all vertebrates are very much alike.[26] For this reason, although retinal responses and synaptic organization described in this chapter are largely derived from the lower vertebrates (because they have relatively large retinal neurons, suitable for detailed electrophysiologic analysis), the patterns of neuronal light responses and functional organizations presented here can be generalized to all vertebrates,[7,58,86] including humans.[93]

Rod and cone photoreceptors absorb light and transduce its energy into electrical signals in the form of membrane hyperpolarization.[110] Signals in rods and cones are transmitted to higher retinal neurons through a complex but highly organized network of electrical and chemical synapses in the OPL and IPL. Photoreceptors make electrical synapses with other nearby photoreceptors, sign-preserving chemical synapses on dendrites of HCs and hyperpolarizing bipolar cells (HBCs), and sign-inverting chemical synapses on the depolarizing bipolar cells (DBCs). HCs make feedback synapses on cones and feed-forward synapses on bipolar cell dendrites, and they are electrically coupled with one another. Bipolar cells relay signals from the outer retina to the inner retina, and they make sign-preserving chemical synapses on amacrine cell and ganglion cell dendrites. Amacrine cells make inhibitory chemical synapses on bipolar cell axon terminals and dendrites of ganglion cells and other amacrine cells. Ganglion cells send retinal signals to the brain.[26,130]

Figure 15-1 is a composite diagram showing light responses of the major types of neurons in the tiger salamander retina to 500-nm light steps of dim, moderate, and high intensities. Rods are about 2 to 3 log units more sensitive to the 500-nm light than the cones are. The bipolar cells are separated

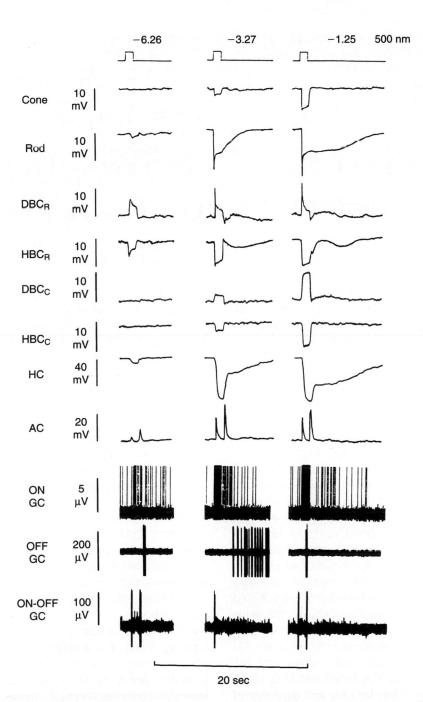

FIGURE 15-1 Voltage responses of major types of neurons in the tiger salamander retina to 500-nm light steps of dim, moderate, and high intensities.[44] Rods are about two to three log units more sensitive to the 500-nm light than the cones are. The bipolar cells are separated into four classes: the rod-dominated depolarizing bipolar cell (DBC_R) and the hyperpolarizing bipolar cell (HBC_R) and the cone-dominated depolarizing bipolar cell (DBC_C) and the hyperpolarizing bipolar cell (HBC_C). Ganglion cells are divided into three main types: the ON-center, OFF-center, and ON-OFF ganglion cells (*ON GC, OFF GC,* and *ON-OFF GC*). *AC*, ON-OFF amacrine cell; *HC*, horizontal cell.

into four classes: the rod-dominated DBC and HBC (DBC$_R$ and HBC$_R$) and the cone-dominated DBC and HBC (DBC$_C$ and HBC$_C$). Ganglion cells are divided into three main types: the ON-center, OFF-center, and ON-OFF ganglion cells (ON GC, OFF GC, and ON-OFF GC, respectively). Detailed descriptions of light responses of individual retinal neurons and the synaptic organization of the retina are given in the following sections.

PHOTORECEPTOR RESPONSES AND SYNAPSES

Phototransduction

The primary function of photoreceptors is to convert light energy into electrical signals, a process called *phototransduction*. There are two types of photoreceptors: rods and cones. Although they differ in structure, function, and synaptic outputs, the basic phototransduction strategies used by these two photoreceptors are similar. In rods the light sensitive molecule is rhodopsin, which consists of a protein named *opsin* and a chromophore, the 11-*cis*-retinal. Opsin consists of 348 amino acids, with seven transmembrane helices, and 11-*cis*-retinal is attached to the center of opsin by *Schiff-base linkage*.[104,116] The 11-*cis*-retinal has a high absorption coefficient and broad absorption band in the visible region. When light enters the retina, an absorbed photon isomerizes the 11-*cis*-retinal to all-*trans*-retinal and moves the Schiff-base linkage of the retinal by about 5 Å, resulting in conformation changes of rhodopsin through several photolytic intermediates. One conformation of the protein, metarhodopsin II, or photoexcited rhodopsin (R*), is crucial for the phototransduction process. R* acts on the G protein transducin and activates its α-subunit, which separates from the β- and γ-subunits and in turn activates a membrane-bound phosphodiesterase (PDE), the enzyme that hydrolyzes cyclic guanine monophosphate (cGMP). When the intracellular level of cGMP falls, fewer cGMP-gated channels in the rod outer segment plasma membrane are open and the rods hyperpolarize. Termination of the light-response cascade is mediated by inactivation of R* by phosphorylation catalyzed by rhodopsin kinase, inactivation of PDE by hydrolysis, synthesis of cGMP by guanylyl cyclase, and regeneration of rhodopsin.[8,89,146]

The cGMP-gated channels in the rod outer segment plasma membrane are tetramers made up of at least two different subunit proteins, α and β, with molecular sizes of 63 and 249 kD.[104] Noise analysis of the rods' dark current indicates that the single-channel current is about 3 fA under physiologic conditions,[13,34,38] and it is about 1 pA in the absence of divalent ions.[42,148] Two conductances, whose mean values are 24 pS and 8 pS, were found in single-channel currents.[148] In the rod outer segment, light-sensitive cGMP-gated channels comprise the predominant, perhaps exclusive, ion conductance in the plasma membrane. The current-voltage relation of the rod outer segment membrane in darkness is strongly outward, rectifying with a reversal potential near 8.5 mV; in bright light the current-voltage (I-V) relation is almost flat, with a conductance of only 0.78 pS.[12]

In cones the phototransduction process is similar to that in rods, with three main differences: (1) Although the chromophore in all cones is the 11-*cis*-retinal, the opsins have different structures. This leads to different absorption spectra and light sensitivity.[81,82] (2) The I-V relation of the cGMP-gated channels is different from that of the rod, and it exhibits strong inward rectification at negative potentials.[43] (3) The cone light sensitivity is about 100 to 1000 times lower than that of the rods, but the response kinetics are several times faster.[146]

Figure 15-2 shows photocurrents elicited by light flashes of increasing intensity and recorded with suction electrodes from a rod and a cone from the monkey retina.[8] It is evident that the rod is much more sensitive to light than the cone, and the response waveform and kinetics of the two photoreceptors are different. Electrical coupling, voltage responses, and spectral sensitivity of the two photoreceptors are described in the following sections.

Photoreceptor Coupling

Electrical synapses between photoreceptors were first discovered in the turtle retina.[10] Electron microscopic studies revealed that gap junctions exist between photoreceptors in many vertebrate species.[23,37,90,103] In the primate retina, anatomic data have shown large gap junctions between cones and smaller junctions between rods and cones, suggesting that cone-cone coupling is stronger than rod-cone coupling.[90,91,112] In the turtle retina, couplings are found between cones of the same spectral sensitivity and between rods,[10,22,24,95] whereas in amphibians, rods are strongly coupled to each other but cones are not.[4,5,37] Coupling between rods and cones has been observed in turtles and tiger sala-

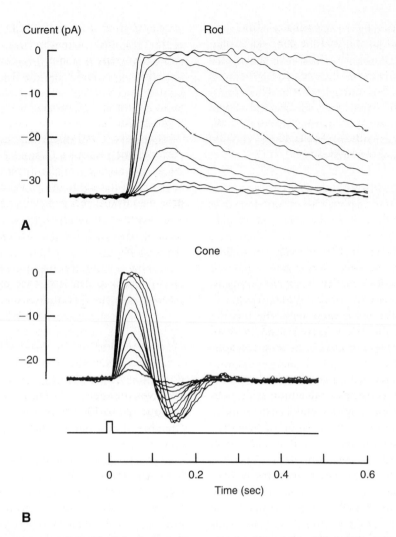

FIGURE 15-2 Photocurrents elicited by light flashes of increasing intensity and recorded with suction electrodes from a rod (**A**) and a cone (**B**) from the monkey retina.[8] The number of photoisomerizations per flash varied between 2.9 and 860 for the rod and between 190 and 36,000 for the cone.

manders, but the coupling resistance is higher than that between cones (in turtles) and between rods (in tiger salamander).[5,94] Although most rods are weakly coupled with cones in the tiger salamander retina, a small fraction of rods (10% to 15%) are strongly coupled with adjacent cones.[126,134] Voltage responses of these rods (named rod_Cs) to current injection into a next-neighbor cone are about three to four times larger than those of the other rods.[134] Rod_Cs behave like hybrids of rods and cones, and their function is not completely understood.

Photoreceptor coupling decreases resolution (visual acuity) of the visual system by spatially averaging photoreceptor signals over some lateral dis-

tance in the retina.[60] However, the advantage of this arrangement is that it improves the signal/noise ratio of the photoreceptor output when the retina is uniformly illuminated.[31,98] This is especially important for the rods to detect dim images under dark-adapted conditions when the voltage noise is high.[11,98] Rod and cone photoreceptors operate in different ranges of illumination and exhibit different spectral sensitivities.[8,111] Electrical coupling between rods and cones broadens the operating ranges and spectral sensitivity spans of both types of photoreceptor by mixing their light-evoked signals. In addition, when the signal in one type of photoreceptor is suppressed (e.g., rod response in the presence of background light), its output synapse can be used to transmit signal from the other type of photoreceptor (e.g., cones).[128] It has been shown that rod-cone coupling in the tiger salamander retina is enhanced by background light.[141] This allows transmission of cone signals through the rod output synapses. Such "synapse sharing" minimizes the amount of neural hardware and facilitates cone inputs in second-order retinal cells.[128]

Rod and Cone Voltage Responses

In darkness the resting potentials of rods and cones are near −40 mV, far from the potassium equilibrium potential (near −80 mV). This is because a continuous dark current, carried mainly by sodium ions, flows into the outer segments through the cGMP-gated channels. Light closes the cGMP-gated channels, suppresses the inward dark current, and hyperpolarizes the photoreceptors.[12] The top two traces of Figure 15-1 are salamander rod and cone voltage responses elicited by light steps of increasing intensity. A major difference between the waveform of these voltage responses and the current responses (see Figure 15-2) of photoreceptors is that the voltage responses exhibit large sags (especially in rods), whereas the current responses are sustained. The voltage sag is mediated by a delayed inward current activated by membrane hyperpolarization (I_H).[3,4]

Although both cones and rods are hyperpolarized by light, their responses are easily distinguishable. In the salamander retina, for example, the rod spectral sensitivity peaks at about 520 nm and cone sensitivity peaks at about 622 nm; the rods are about 1000 times more sensitive to 500-nm light than the cones.[144,145] When the peak voltage responses are plotted against light intensity, data points can be fitted by the following equation:

$$V/V_M = I^N/(I^N + \sigma^N) \qquad (1)$$

When the responses are plotted against the logarithm of the light intensity, equation 1 becomes

$$V/V_M = 0.5 \ [1 + 1.15N \tanh (\log I - \log \sigma)] \quad (2)$$

where

V = Response amplitude
V_M = Maximum response amplitude
σ = Light intensity that elicits a half-maximal response
N = Constant
$\tanh$ = Hyperbolic tangent function
$\log$ = Logarithmic function of base 10

The V-Log I plot is used not only for photoreceptor responses but also for light-evoked responses of other retinal neurons.[79,107,108,145] It can be shown by equation 2 that the dynamic range (the light-intensity range span for eliciting responses between 0.05% and 0.95% of V_M) of a cell equals to 2.56/N.[108]

Figure 15-3, *A*, shows the response-intensity (V-Log I) relations of a rod and a cone in the tiger salamander retina to 500- and 750-nm lights.[145] It is evident that the rod is more sensitive to the 500-nm light than the cone, but the two photoreceptors exhibit nearly equal sensitivity to the 750-nm light. The spectral sensitivities of the two photoreceptors are plotted in Figure 15-3, *B*. In the human retina, there is one type of rod and three types of cones with peak sensitivities near 520, 480, 550, and 680 nm.[8] The spectral sensitivity curves are shown in Figure 15-3, *C*.

Horizontal Cell and Bipolar Cell Responses and Synapses
Glutamatergic Synapses between Photoreceptors and Second-Order Retinal Neurons

Glutamate is the neurotransmitter used by all vertebrate photoreceptors, with a possible exception of blue cones, whose neurotransmitter identity is still unknown.[21,72,75,133] Light responses of the HBCs and HCs are mediated primarily by kainate (KA) and/or α-amino-3-hydroxy-5-methylisoxazole-4-propionic acid (AMPA) receptors,[25,67,99,100,142] and the responses of the DBCs are mediated mainly by L-α-amino-4-phosphonobutyrate (L-AP4) receptors.[83,84,96,97,99] In darkness, glutamate released from photoreceptors binds to the KA/AMPA receptors in HBCs and HCs and opens postsynaptic cation channels.[6,25,67] It also binds to the L-AP4 receptors in DBCs, which results in an increase of cGMP hydrolysis by a G protein–mediated process, thus leading to a fall of intracellular cGMP and closure of cation channels.[84,96] Light reduces glutamate release from photoreceptors, closes the KA/AMPA receptor–gated channels, and hyperpolarizes HBCs and HCs. The light-induced decrease of glutamate release also leads to opening of cGMP-gated channels and depolarizing responses in DBCs.

Glutamate is released from photoreceptors through a calcium-dependent vesicular process. Calcium entry into photoreceptor synaptic terminals triggers exocytosis of glutamatergic vesicles,[92] releasing packages of glutamate, each of which activate a number of glutamate receptors that initiate transient

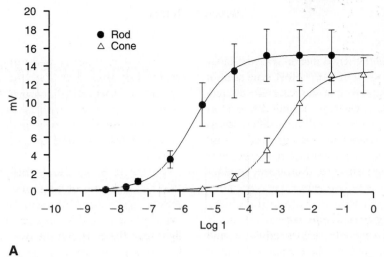

A

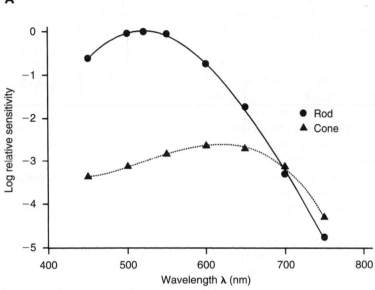

B

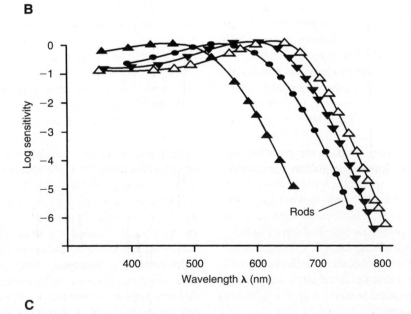

C

FIGURE 15-3 **A,** Response-intensity (V-Log I) relations of a rod and a cone in the tiger salamander retina to 500- and 750-nm lights.[146] **B,** Spectral sensitivity curves of the two photoreceptors in A. The peak sensitivity near 520 nm for the rod and near 620 nm for the cone.[145] **C,** The spectral sensitivity curves of the rods, blue, green, and red cones of the human retina, with peak sensitivity near 520, 480, 550, and 680 nm, respectively.[8]

postsynaptic currents termed *spontaneous excitatory postsynaptic currents* (sEPSCs).[68] sEPSCs are seen in most HBCs, but analogous (sign inverted) discrete postsynaptic currents generally are not observed in DBCs.[67,132,133] This probably reflects a difference in the kinetics of the glutamate receptors in DBCs and HBCs. DBCs utilize L-AP4 metabotropic glutamate receptors, which generate relatively slow conductance changes via a second messenger system.[84,85] Therefore the postsynaptic response to transmitter release from a single vesicle or cluster of vesicles is likely to be heavily filtered in DBCs. HBCs, on the other hand, utilize rapidly activating ionotropic AMPA receptors and are capable of generating sEPSCs with a rise time of about 1 millisecond.[2,101]

Horizontal Cell Responses

Intracellular recordings from the HCs were first made by Svaetichin[105] in the bream retina, and thus the light responses of these cells were termed *S-potentials.* Two major types of HCs that receive cone inputs may be distinguished: the L-type (luminosity), which hyperpolarizes to light stimuli of all wavelengths, and the C-type (chromaticity or color), which hyperpolarizes to light stimuli within certain ranges of wavelength but depolarizes to light in other wavelength ranges.[78,80,106,110] The C-type HCs may be divided into the biphasic and the triphasic cells. Two kinds of biphasic C cells have been reported: the green/blue cells, which depolarize to red and green flashes and hyperpolarize to blue light, and the red/green cells, which depolarize to red light and hyperpolarize to green and blue lights.[78,106] The triphasic C cells, on the other hand, hyperpolarize to both blue and red lights and depolarize to green light.[110,122] Figure 15-4 shows the voltage responses of an L-type HC, a biphasic C-type HC, and a triphasic C-type HC recorded from the carp retina to light steps of different wavelengths. HCs that receive input from only rods are found in many species.[26,53] The light responses of these cells differ from those of the cone HCs in two ways: Rod S-potentials in the carp are found to have peak spectral sensitivity around 520 nm, whereas the L-type cone S-potentials peak around 600 nm. The sensitivity to light is much higher in rod S-potentials than in L-type S-potentials.[53] The receptive fields of HCs are much larger than those of the photoreceptors. Naka and Rushton[80] showed that the amplitude of the L-type HC response continued to increase up to a light spot diameter of 1.2 mm. Similar results have been obtained in the mudpuppy and cat HCs.[102,108]

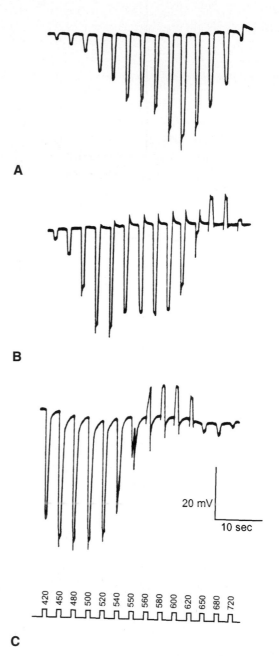

A

B

20 mV

10 sec

420 450 480 500 520 540 550 560 580 600 620 650 680 720

C

FIGURE 15-4   Voltage responses of a L-type horizontal cell (HC) (**A**), a biphasic C-type HC (**B**), and a triphasic C-type HC (**C**) recorded from the carp retina in response to light steps of different wavelengths.

Horizontal Cell Synapses

HCs mediate bipolar cell surround responses through a feedback synaptic pathway (horizontal cell → cone → bipolar cell)[9,16,127] and through feedforward synapses (horizontal cell → bipolar cell).[40,41,129,143] Two major synaptic mechanisms have been proposed for the feedback actions of HCs on cones. A long-standing hypothesis is that HCs release an inhibitory neurotransmitter (γ-aminobutyric acid [GABA], in several species) in darkness and that this neurotransmitter binds to receptors on cone synaptic terminals and opens chloride channels in the cone plasma membrane. In this scheme, when illumination of the receptive field surround hyperpolarizes the HCs and suppresses feedback transmitter release, the cones are depolarized, causing depolarization in HBCs and hyperpolarization in DBCs.[40,51,129] A second proposed mechanism is that HCs directly modulate calcium currents in cones, resulting in an increase of the calcium-dependent glutamate release that depolarizes the HBCs and hyperpolarizes the DBCs.[54] One study suggests that hemichannels on the HC dendrites are involved in modulating calcium-dependent glutamate release from the cones.[55] It is possible that the HC-to-cone feedback synapses in different species or under different conditions favor one or the other mechanisms. The two mechanisms may also coexist in some feedback synapses in which both GABA$_A$-gated chloride channels and calcium current modulation are involved.

Properties of the feed-forward synapses are less well understood. Studies of the salamander retina have suggested that feed-forward synapses contribute significantly to the surround antagonism of DBC light responses.[40,41,129,143] However, application of GABA to the dendrites of salamander bipolar cells elicits no response (in Co^{2+} Ringer's), so if HCs make feed-forward synapses on bipolar cells in the salamander retina, GABA is probably not the neurotransmitter used at these synapses.[69] Histochemical evidence suggests that only about 50% to 60% of the HCs in the salamander retina are GABA-ergic,[128,131] the identity of neurotransmitter (or neurotransmitters) used by the rest of the HCs is unknown but unlikely to be glycine.[133,135] A feed-forward synapse from HCs to DBCs would require an excitatory synaptic conductance mechanism, but no such mechanism has been found on the dendrites of DBCs.

HCs in the vertebrate retina are electrically coupled to one another. In fish retina the electrical (gap) junctions between HCs are extensive. Gap junctions are observed between HC perikarya or between HC processes, but the couplings are made only between HCs of homologous types. For example, the H1 cone HCs in the fish couple only with other H1 cells, H2 couple only with other H2 cells, and HC axon terminals couple only with other HC axon terminals.[123]

Bipolar Cell Responses

Two major types of bipolar cells are found in all vertebrates, based on their receptive field properties.[49,121] The DBCs depolarize to central illumination and hyperpolarize to concentric surround illumination; the HBCs hyperpolarize to central illumination and depolarize to concentric surround illumination. In the mudpuppy retina, annular illumination does not polarize the bipolar cells unless the centers of their receptive fields are simultaneously illuminated.[121] The dynamic range of the light-evoked responses in these cells is reported to be about 2.2 log units in the mudpuppy retina and the value of N is close to 1.2.[108] In many species, bipolar cells do not register color information. In the goldfish retina, however, Kaneko[50] reported a type of color-opponent bipolar cell with red ON-center and red and green OFF-surround (or vice versa) responses.

Rod and Cone Synaptic Pathways

Rods are responsible for vision under conditions of dim illumination, when the cones are not responsive. Cones operate under conditions of bright illumination, and they mediate color vision and provide high spatial resolution, features that rods do not handle.[26] Synaptic organization of the rod and cone pathways in the outer retina varies from species to species. In mammals, rod and cone signals are transmitted separately to rod and cone bipolar cells, which send the segregated signals to the higher-order visual cells.[15] HCs in the fish retina also receive rod and cone signals separately. There is one type of rod-driven HC and three types of cone-driven HCs, and each type of the cone HCs exhibits a distinct pattern of color responses.[53,78] Bipolar cells in the fish retina, on the other hand, receive mixed inputs from rods and cones.[50,103] The second-order neurons in the amphibian retinas are thought to receive mixed inputs from rods and cones.[28,39,61] However, evidence suggests that bipolar cells in the tiger salamander, either ON-center or OFF-center, fall into two groups: one rod dominated and the other cone dominated.[44,145] These two types of bipolar cells relay rod- or cone-dominated (although not exclusively rod- or cone-driven) signals to higher-order visual neurons.[44] It seems that the tiger salamander retina adopts a compromised strategy between mixing and segregating the rod and cone signals at the bipolar cell level. Figure 15-1 shows typical light responses of DBC_R, HBC_R, DBC_C, and HBC_C. Similar to the sensitivity difference between rods and cones, DBC_Rs and HBC_Rs are more sensitive to 500-nm light than are DBC_Cs and HBC_Cs. It has been shown that wide variations in light sensitivity and axonal morphology are present within each of the four classes of bipolar cells.[132] Figure 15-5, *A*, shows variations of the V-Log I relations of a sample of 41 bipolar cells recorded from dark-adapted salamander retina. Comparing Figure 15-5, *A*, with Figure 15-3, *A*, reveals that the left group of V-Log I relations in Figure 15-5, *A,* lies within the sensitivity range of the rod; thus they are rod-dominated cells. The right group lies within the sensitivity range of the cone; thus they are the cone-dominated cells.[145] In addition, the spectral sensitivity of the rod- and cone-dominated bipolar cells corresponds well with the spectral sensitivity of the rod and cone (Figure 15-5, *B*). Although postsynaptic responses of both HBC_Rs and HBC_Cs are mediated by AMPA receptors, their kinetics and desensitization properties are different.[67] Moreover, sEPSCs in dark-adapted HBC_Rs are larger than those in HBC_Cs.[132]

Center-Surround Antagonistic Receptive Field Organization

Center-surround antagonistic receptive fields (CSARFs) form the basic alphabet for encoding spatial information in the visual system. CSARF was first discovered by Kuffler[58] in 1953, who demonstrated that light falling on the central region of the receptive field of cat retinal ganglion cells elicited a response of opposite sign as that elicited by light falling on the surround region of the receptive field. Later studies showed that such CSARFs also exist upstream in retinal bipolar cells and downstream in cells in the lateral geniculate nucleus and the primary visual cortex.[47-49,121] Furthermore, complex receptive fields of neurons in higher visual centers are probably mediated by arrays of upstream neurons that exhibit CSARF organization.[47]

The first neurons along the visual pathway that exhibit CSARF organization are the retinal bipolar cells. The center input of a bipolar cell is mediated by direct photoreceptor output synapses made on its dendrites (and the dendrites of adjacent bipolar cells electrically coupled).[14,28,40] The surround input is mediated by the HCs in the OPL and by amacrine cells in the IPL.[28,121] HCs make sign-inverting feedback synapse on cones and feed-

forward synapses on bipolar cells.[9,127,129,143] Color Plate 11 is a summary diagram of major synapses that mediate CSARF of the four types of bipolar cells. It also summarizes the synaptic circuitry mediating the CSARF of ganglion cells and the major neurotransmitter systems in the retina that are described later in this chapter.

CSARF organization is ubiquitous in all vertebrate species. According to the computational theory of Marr, it is essential for detecting edges in visual images.[73] Marr and colleagues point out that the CSARF of retinal bipolar cells, for example, acts like a filter for visual images and that the filter constitutes an approximation of taking the second spatial derivative of the light intensity ($\nabla^2 I$). At the edge of an image, $\nabla^2 I$ gives a large positive value on one side of the edge, a large negative value on the other side, and a zero-crossing in the middle. This type of filter (e.g., CSARF) can register intensity changes efficiently and therefore is an excellent edge detector. In addition, Marr's theory also suggests that CSARFs play a crucial role in the detection of moving edges in visual images.[74] CSARFs are also major vehicles for carrying color information in the visual system. In some species the receptive field of certain bipolar cells and ganglion cells exhibit "double-opponent" organization. For instance, the receptive field center of a bipolar cell is depolarized by red and hyperpolarized by green, whereas the surround is depolarized by green and hyperpolarized by red.[52] In other species, bipolar cells have other color-coding organizations that include opponent receptive field centers with nonopponent surround or vice versa.[50,147] These types of color-coded CSARF organizations help the visual system detect stationary and moving color edges.

Bipolar Cell Output Synapses

Electrical coupling between bipolar cells has been reported in several vertebrate retinas. Electron microscopic studies have revealed that gap junctions are made between bipolar cell axon terminals in the IPL.[71,124] Current injection into fish bipolar cells elicits sign-preserving responses in adjacent bipolar cells.[59] In the tiger salamander retina, the diameter of the bipolar cell receptive field center is about 10 to 20 times larger than the diameter of the dendritic arbors of these cells.[14] These results suggest that bipolar cells of the same type are extensively coupled to one another at least in certain species or certain areas of the retina. The primary function of bipolar cell coupling is to increase the receptive field center of these cells. In addition, bipolar cell

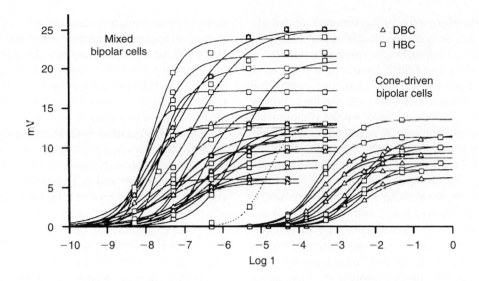

A

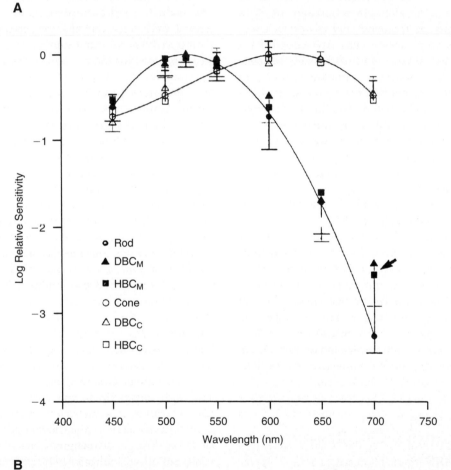

B

FIGURE 15-5 **A,** V-Log I relations of 41 bipolar cells recorded from dark-adapted salamander retina. The left group of V-Log I relations lies within the sensitivity range of the rod (see Figure 15-3, *A*), and thus they are rod-dominated cells; the right group lies within the sensitivity range of the cone (see Figure 15-3, *A*), and thus they are the cone-dominated cells.[146] **B,** Spectral sensitivity of the rod- and cone-dominated of bipolar cells (*circles* and *triangles*), and the spectral sensitivity of the rods and cones (*solid lines*).

coupling also improves the signal/noise ratio of the bipolar cell output signals. The disadvantage of bipolar cell coupling, however, is that it reduces the spatial resolution of bipolar cell outputs.

Bipolar cells make chemical synapses on amacrine cells and ganglion cells in an orderly fashion. Within the IPL, axon terminals of DBCs make synaptic contacts with the dendrites of amacrine cells and ganglion cells predominantly in the lower half (sublamina B) of the IPL, whereas HBCs make synapses mainly in the upper half (sublamina A) of the IPL.[32,33,86] One study shows that there are at least 12 different types of bipolar cells in the salamander retina, each with synaptic processes that terminate at a unique depth (or combination of depths) within the IPL.[132] The stratification of bipolar cell axon terminals leads to an orderly mapping of visual signals within the IPL. In addition to a segregation of visual information into OFF-center and ON-center layers (sublaminas A and B, respectively), there is an overlying mapping of spectral information along the depth of the IPL, with cone signals being transmitted predominantly to the central IPL and rod signals predominantly to the margins of the IPL. Superimposed on these two mappings is a more complex set of inhibitory interactions involving other interneurons in the inner retina. This orderly segregation of visual signals along the depth of the IPL provides the substrate for computation of visual information in the retina, and it begins a chain of parallel information processing in the visual system.[46-48]

Glutamate is the neurotransmitter used by all vertebrate bipolar cells, except for a subpopulation of salamander bipolar cells that may release GABA.[72,75,136,139] Postsynaptic responses of amacrine cells and ganglion cells are mediated primarily by the KA, AMPA, and *N*-methyl-D-aspartate (NMDA) receptors.[45,77] The KA/AMPA receptors mediate the early component, whereas the NMDA receptors mediate the late component of the light responses.[77]

AMACRINE CELL AND INTERPLEXIFORM CELL RESPONSES AND SYNAPSES

Amacrine Cell Light Responses

Most amacrine cells respond to light with depolarizing transients at the onset and cessation of the stimulus.[113,140] A few action potentials at the peak of these transient depolarizations are sometimes observed.[140] In the goldfish and catfish retina, a sustained type of amacrine cell response has been reported: Cells

showing these responses depolarize to green light and hyperpolarize to red light.[50] The light responses of the ON amacrine cells and the ON responses of the transient ON-OFF amacrine cells are driven by the DBCs, and the responses of the OFF cells and the OFF responses of the ON-OFF cells are driven by the HBCs.[76] The V-Log I relation of the ON response of the transient ON-OFF amacrine cells under dark-adapted conditions is mediated by rod-dominated inputs of very-high-voltage gain, and that of the OFF response is N-shaped: It exhibits a peak at low light intensity, a dip at intermediate intensity, and a second peak at high intensity.[140]

Amacrine Cell Synapses

Amacrine cells make chemical synapses on bipolar cell axon terminals (feedback synapses), ganglion cell dendrites (feed-forward synapses), and other amacrine cells.[28,125] Most amacrine cells use GABA or glycine as their neurotransmitter.[135,137,138] Whereas the GABA receptors on amacrine cells and ganglion cells are largely GABA$_A$ receptors, those on bipolar cell axon terminals are largely GABA$_C$ receptors (although GABA$_A$- and GABA$_B$-mediated responses have also been observed in bipolar cells).[57,63-65]

Discrete inhibitory postsynaptic currents (sIPSCs) mediated by glycinergic amacrine cells and interplexiform cells have been observed in bipolar cells.[35,36,70,109] It has been shown in the tiger salamander retina that the sIPSCs in approximately 69% of bipolar cells were mediated by glycinergic amacrine cell inputs that make synapses on bipolar cell axon terminals. These axonal sIPSCs can be reversibly abolished by 500-nM strychnine, but they persist in 10-μM tetrodotoxin (TTX).[70]

Interplexiform Cell Responses and Synapses

Interplexiform cells have been found to make chemical synapses on amacrine cells in the IPL and HCs and bipolar cells in the OPL.[27] With use of whole-cell voltage clamp and Lucifer yellow fluorescent techniques, it has been found that the many interplexiform cells in the salamander retina exhibit transient depolarizing responses at the light onset and offset, similar to the transient ON-OFF amacrine cells (Gao F, Wu SM, unpublished results). In the fish and New World monkeys, dopamine is a major interplexiform cell neurotransmitter.[27] Dopamine is found to modulate HC coupling and glutamate receptors in the outer retina.[56,62] It also plays important roles in mediating circadian rhythm and visual adaptation in the

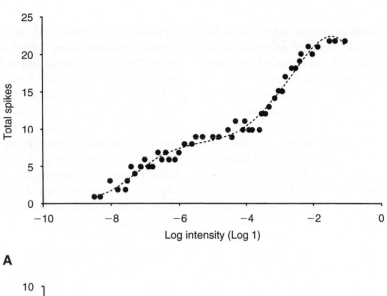

A

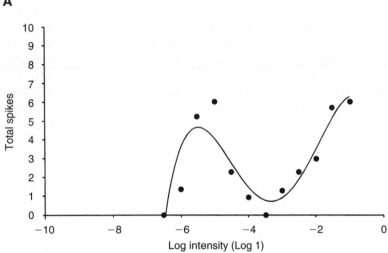

B

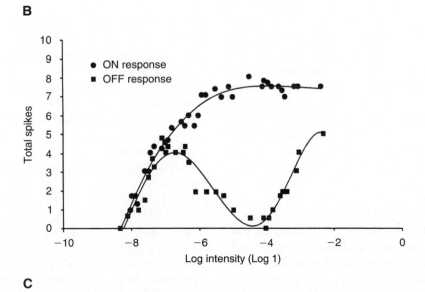

C

FIGURE 15-6 The response-intensity relations (V-Log I) of sustained ON ganglion cells (**A**), sustained OFF ganglion cells.[44] (**B**), and transient ON-OFF ganglion cells (**C**) recorded from the dark-adapted salamander retina in response to 500-nm light steps.[44]

retina.[66] In the amphibian and fish, glycine is the neurotransmitter used by some interplexiform cells.[128] Through study of the sIPSCs in bipolar cells, it has been found that a subpopulation of bipolar cells in the salamander retina receive active synaptic inputs from glycinergic interplexiform cells that make synapses on bipolar cell dendrites in the OPL.[70]

GANGLION CELL RESPONSES

Intracellular recordings of ganglion cell activity were first made from the retinas of mudpuppy.[121] To a steady step of light spot at the receptive field center, ganglion cells give rise to three types of responses: one with an increase of spike activity at the onset of the light step (ON cells), the second with a spike increase at the light offset (OFF cells), and the third with spike activity at both light onset and offset (ON-OFF cells). The light responses of the ON ganglion cells and the ON responses of the ON-OFF ganglion cells are driven by the ON-center DBCs, and those of the OFF cells and the OFF responses of the ON-OFF cells are driven by the OFF-center HBCs.[76,88,121] To a steady step of light annulus, the ON cells exhibit an OFF response and the OFF cells exhibit an ON response, reflecting the center-surround antagonism of these cells.[119] These surround responses are mediated partially by the surround responses of bipolar cells generated by the lateral synapses made by HCs in the outer retina and by amacrine cells on bipolar cell axon terminals in the inner retina.[107,108] Surround responses of ganglion cells are also mediated by the inhibitory synapses between amacrine cells and ganglion cells.[119] In the salamander retina, it has been shown that the surround responses of ON-center ganglion cells with small receptive fields are mediated mainly by sustained GABA-ergic amacrine cells and that the transient lateral inhibition (TLI), or the suppression of ganglion cell center response by *changes* of surround illumination, is mediated by the wide-field transient glycinergic amacrine cells.[19,20]

The response-intensity relations (V-Log I) of sustained ON ganglion cells, sustained OFF ganglion cells, and transient ON-OFF ganglion cells recorded from the dark-adapted salamander retina to 500-nm light steps are given in Figure 15-6.[44] The V-Log I curve of the sustained ON cells is composed of two limbs, with the lower limb resulting from rod-dominated inputs and the upper limb resulting from cone-dominated inputs. The V-Log I relation of sustained OFF ganglion cells is N-shaped. It shows an initial peak at low light intensity, a dip at intermediate intensity, and a second peak at high intensity. The V-Log I relation of the ON response of ON-OFF ganglion cells is monophasic, with dynamic range near that of the rods. Similar to the sustained OFF ganglion cells, the V-Log I curve of the OFF response of the transient ON-OFF ganglion cells is N-shaped. The suppression of the OFF responses in OFF and ON-OFF ganglion cells at intermediate light intensity has been reported in the frog and cat ganglion cells, and thus this may be a general trait of dark-adapted vertebrate retinas.[18,87]

In response to flickering lights or moving stimuli, ON-OFF ganglion cells exhibit sustained spike activity.[7,118] A spinning light annulus with black and white bands (windmill) elicits sustained inhibition in these cells.[120] In some animals, such as rabbits, subpopulations of ganglion cells exhibit directional selectivity: They respond to a moving light stimulus in a given direction with high spike activity, but they respond to the same stimulus moving in the opposite direction with poor spike activity.[7,117] Synaptic mechanisms mediating directional selectivity are not completely understood, although synaptic inputs from cholinergic amacrine cells to ganglion cells are probably involved.[1,114]

Retinal ganglion cells can also be classified in accordance with their cell and dendritic field size, as well as loci of axon projection. Such a scheme is most commonly used for mammalian retinas, and cells are divided into the x, y, and w types. The x cells have medium-size cell bodies and small dendritic fields, whereas y cells have large cell bodies and large dendritic fields. Both x and y cells project to the lateral geniculate nucleus. The w cells have small cell bodies and large dendritic fields, and they project to the superior colliculus.[29,30,115]

ACKNOWLEDGMENTS

This work was supported by grants from NIH (EY 04446), NIH Vision Core (EY 02520), the Retina Research Foundation (Houston), and the Research to Prevent Blindness, Inc.

REFERENCES

1. Amthor FR, Grzywacz NM: Inhibition in ON-OFF directionally selective ganglion cells of the rabbit retina, *J Neurophysiol* 69:2174, 1993.
2. Ashmore JF, Copenhagen DR: An analysis of transmission from cones to hyperpolarizing bipolar cells in the retina of the turtle, *J Physiol* 340:569, 1983.

3. Attwell D, Werblin FS, Wilson M: The properties of single cones isolated from the tiger salamander retina, *J Physiol* 328:259, 1982.

4. Attwell D, Wilson M: Behaviour of the rod network in the tiger salamander retina mediated by membrane properties of individual rods, *J Physiol* 309:287, 1980.

5. Attwell D, Wilson M, Wu SM: A quantitative analysis of interactions between photoreceptors in the salamander (*Ambystoma*) retina, *J Physiol* 352:703, 1984.

6. Attwell D et al: Neurotransmitter-induced currents in retinal bipolar cells of the axolotl, *Ambystoma mexicanum*, *J Physiol* 387:125, 1987.

7. Barlow HB, Levick WR: The mechanisms of directionally selective units in rabbit's retina, *J Physiol* 178:477, 1965.

8. Baylor DA: Photoreceptor signals and vision. Proctor lecture, *Invest Ophthalmol Vis Sci* 28:34, 1987.

9. Baylor DA: Lateral interaction between vertebrate photoreceptors, *Fed Proc* 33:1074, 1974.

10. Baylor DA, Fuortes MG, O'Bryan PM: Receptive fields of cones in the retina of the turtle, *J Physiol* 214:265, 1971.

11. Baylor DA, Lamb TD, Yau KW: The membrane current of single rod outer segments, *J Physiol* 288:589, 1979.

12. Baylor DA, Nunn BJ: Electrical properties of the light-sensitive conductance of rods of the salamander *Ambystoma tigrinum*, *J Physiol* 371:115, 1986.

13. Bodia RD, Detwiler PD: Patch-clamp recordings of the light-sensitive dark noise in retinal rods from the lizard and frog, *J Physiol* 367:183, 1985.

14. Borges S, Wilson M: Structure of the receptive fields of bipolar cells in the salamander retina, *J Neurophysiol* 58:1275, 1987.

15. Boycott BB, Wassle H: Parallel processing in the mammalian retina, *Invest Ophthalmol Vis Sci* 40:1313, 1999.

16. Burkhardt DA: Responses and receptive-field organization of cones in perch retinas, *J Neurophysiol* 40:53, 1977.

17. Cajal SY: La retine des vertebres, *La Cellule* 9:119, 1893.

18. Chino YM, Sturr JF: Rod and cone contributions to the delayed response of the on-off ganglion cell in the frog, *Vis Res* 15:193, 1975.

19. Cook PB, Lukasiewicz P, McReynolds J: Action potentials are required for the lateral transmission of glycinergic transient inhibition in the amphibian retina, *J Neurosci* 18:2301, 1998.

20. Cook PB, McReynolds J: Lateral inhibition in the inner retina is important for spatial tuning of ganglion cells, *Nat Neurosci* 1:714, 1998.

21. Copenhagen DR, Jahr CE: Release of endogenous excitatory amino acids from turtle photoreceptors, *Nature* 341:536, 1988.

22. Copenhagen DR, Owen WG: Functional characteristics of lateral interactions between rods in the retina of the snapping turtle, *J Physiol* 259:251, 1976.

23. Custer NV: Structurally specialized contacts between the photoreceptors of the retina of the axolotl, *J Comp Neurol* 151:35, 1973.

24. Detwiler PB, Hodgkin AL: Electrical coupling between cones in turtle retina, *J Physiol* 291:75, 1979.

25. DeVries SH: Bipolar cells use kainate and AMPA receptors to filter visual information into separate channels, *Neuron* 28:847, 2000.

26. Dowling JE: *The retina, an approachable part of the brain*, Cambridge, Mass, 1987, Harvard University Press.

27. Dowling JE, Ehinger B: Synaptic organization of the amine-containing interplexiform cells of the goldfish and Cebus monkey retinas, *Science* 188:270, 1975.

28. Dowling JE, Werblin FS: Organization of retina of the mudpuppy, *Necturus maculosus*. I. Synaptic structure, *J Neurophysiol* 32:315, 1969.

29. Enroth-Cugell C, Robson JG: The contrast sensitivity of retinal ganglion cells of the cat, *J Physiol* 187:517, 1966.

30. Enroth-Cugell C, Shapley RM: Cat retinal ganglion cells: correlation between size of receptive field centre and level of field adaptation, *J Physiol* 225:58P, 1972.

31. Falk G, Fatt P: Physical changes induced by light in the rod outer segments of vertebrates. In Dartnall HJA (ed): *Handbook of sensory physiology*, vol VII/I, *Photochemistry of vision*, Berlin, 1972, Springer-Verlag.

32. Famiglietti EV Jr, Kaneko A, Tachibana M: Neuronal architecture of on and off pathways to ganglion cells in carp retina, *Science* 198:1267, 1977.

33. Famiglietti EV Jr, Kolb H: Structural basis for ON-and OFF-center responses in retinal ganglion cells, *Science* 194:193, 1976.

34. Fesenko EE, Kolesnikov SS, Lyubarsky AL: Induction by cyclic GMP of cationic conductance in plasma membrane of retinal rod outer segment, *Nature* 313:310, 1985.

35. Gao F, Wu SM: Characterization of spontaneous inhibitory synaptic currents in salamander retinal ganglion cells, *J Neurophysiol* 80:1752, 1998.

36. Gao F, Wu SM: Multiple types of spontaneous excitatory synaptic currents in salamander retinal ganglion cells, *Brain Res* 21:487, 1999.

37. Gold GH, Dowling JE: Photoreceptor coupling in retina of the toad, *Bufo marinus*. I. Anatomy, *J Neurophysiol* 42:292, 1979.

38. Gray P, Attwell D: Kinetics of light-sensitive channels in vertebrate photoreceptors, *Proc R Soc B*, 223:379, 1985.

39. Hanani M, Vallerga S: Rod and cone signals in the horizontal cells of the tiger salamander retina, *J Physiol* 298:397, 1980.

40. Hare WA, Owen WG: Spatial organization of the bipolar cell's receptive field in the retina of the tiger salamander, *J Physiol* 421:223, 1990.

41. Hare WA, Owen WG: Effects of 2-amino-4-phosphonobutyric acid in the distal layers of the tiger salamander's retina, *J Neurophysiol* 445:741, 1992.

42. Haynes LW, Kay AR, Yau KW: Single cyclic GMP-activated channel activity in excised patches of rod outer segment membrane, *Nature* 321:66, 1986.

43. Haynes L, Yau KW: Cyclic GMP-sensitive conductance in outer segment membrane of catfish cones, *Nature* 317:61, 1985.

44. Hensley SH, Yang XL, Wu SM: Relative contribution of rod and cone inputs to bipolar cells and ganglion cells in the tiger salamander retina, *J Neurophysiol* 69:2086, 1993.

45. Hensley SH, Yang XL, Wu SM: Identification of glutamate receptor subtypes mediating inputs to bipolar cells and ganglion cells in the tiger salamander retina, *J Neurophysiol* 69:2099, 1993.

46. Hubel DH, Livingstone MS: Segregation of form, color, and stereopsis in primate area 18, *J Neurosci* 7:3378, 1987.

47. Hubel DH, Wiesel TN: Receptive fields, binocular interaction and functional architecture in the cat's visual cortex, *J Physiol* 160:106, 1962.

48. Hubel DH, Wiesel TN: Brain mechanisms of vision, *Sci Am* 241:150, 1979.

49. Kaneko A: Physiological and morphological identification of horizontal, bipolar and amacrine cells in goldfish retina, *J Physiol* 207:623, 1970.

50. Kaneko A: Receptive field organization of bipolar and amacrine cells in the goldfish retina, *J Physiol* 235:133, 1973.

51. Kaneko A, Pinto LH, Tachibana, M: Transient calcium current of retinal bipolar cells of the mouse, *J Physiol* 410:613, 1989.

52. Kaneko A, Tachibana M: Retinal bipolar cells with double colour-opponent receptive fields, *Nature* 293:220, 1981.

53. Kaneko A, Yamada M: S-potentials in the dark-adapted retina of the carp, *J Physiol* 227:261, 1972.

54. Karmermans M, Spekreijse H: The feedback pathway from horizontal cells to cones, a mini review with a look ahead, *Vis Res* 39:2449, 1999.

55. Karmermans M et al: Hemichannel-mediated inhibition in the outer retina, *Science* 292:1178, 2001.

56. Knapp AG, Dowling JE: Dopamine enhances excitatory amino acid-gated conductances in cultured retinal horizontal cells, *Nature* 325:437, 1987.

57. Koulen P et al: Immunocytochemical localization of the GABAc receptor rho subunits in the cat, goldfish and chicken retina, *J Comp Neurol* 380:520, 1997.

58. Kuffler SW: Discharge patterns and functional organization of the mammalian retina, *J Neurophysiol* 16:37, 1953.

59. Kujiraoka T, Saito T: Electrical coupling between bipolar cells in carp retina, *Proc Natl Acad Sci USA* 83:4063, 1986.

60. Lamb TD, Simon EJ: The relation between intercellular coupling and electrical noise in turtle photoreceptors, *J Physiol* 263:257, 1976.

61. Lasansky A: Organization of the outer synaptic layer in the retina of the larval tiger salamander, *Philos Trans R Soc Lond B Biol Sci* 265:471, 1973.

62. Lasater EM, Dowling JE: Dopamine decreases conductance of the electrical junctions between cultured retinal horizontal cells, *Proc Natl Acad Sci USA* 82:3025, 1985.

63. Lukasiewicz P, Shields CR: Different combinations of GABAa and GABAc receptors confer distinct temporal properties to retinal synaptic responses, *J Neurophysiol* 79:3157, 1998.

64. Lukasiewicz PD: GABA$_C$ receptors in the vertebrate retina, *Mol Neurobiol* 12:181, 1996.

65. Maguire G et al: Gamma-aminobutyric type B receptor modulation of L-type calcium channel current at bipolar cell terminals in the retina of the tiger salamander, *Proc Natl Acad Sci USA* 86:10144, 1989.

66. Mangel SC, Dowling JE: Responsiveness and receptive field size of carp horizontal cells are reduced by prolonged darkness and dopamine, *Science* 229:1107, 1985.

67. Maple BR, Gao F, Wu SM: Glutamate receptors differ in rod- and cone-dominated off-center bipolar cells, *Neuroreport* 10:1, 1999.

68. Maple BR, Werblin FS, Wu SM: Miniature excitatory postsynaptic currents in bipolar cells of the tiger salamander retina, *Vis Res* 34:2357, 1994.

69. Maple BR, Wu SM: Synaptic inputs mediating bipolar cell responses in the tiger salamander retina, *Vis Res* 36:4015, 1996.

70. Maple BR, Wu SM: Glycinergic synaptic inputs to bipolar cells in the tiger salamander retina, *J Physiol* 506:731, 1998.

71. Marc RE, Liu WL, Muller JF: Gap junctions in the inner plexiform layer of the goldfish retina, *Vis Res* 28:9, 1988.

72. Marc RE et al: Patterns of glutamate immunoreactivity in the goldfish retina, *J Neurosci* 10:4006, 1990.

73. Marr D, Hildreth E: Theory of edge detection, *Proc R Soc B* 207:187, 1980.

74. Marr D, Ullman S: Directional selectivity and its use in early visual processing, *Proc R Soc B* 211:151, 1981.

75. Massey SC, Maguire G: The role of glutamate in retinal circuitry. In Wheal M, Thomson T (eds): *Excitatory amino acid and synaptic transmission,* London, 1995, Academic Press.

76. Miller RF: The neuronal basis of ganglion cell receptive field organization and the physiology of amacrine cells. In Schmidt FO, Worden FG (eds): *The neuroscience fourth study program,* Cambridge, Mass, 1979, MIT Press.

77. Mittman S, Taylor WR, Copenhagen DR: Concomitant activation of two types of glutamate receptor mediates excitation of salamander retinal ganglion cells, *J Physiol* 428:175, 1990.

78. Naka KI, Rushton WA: S-potentials from colour units in the retina of fish (*Cyprinidae*), *J Physiol* 185:536, 1966.

79. Naka KI, Rushton WA: S-potentials from luminosity units in the retina of fish (*Cyprinidae*), *J Physiol* 185:587, 1966.

80. Naka KI, Rushton WA: The generation and spread of S-potentials in fish (*Cyprinidae*), *J Physiol* 192:437, 1967.

81. Nathans J: The genes for color vision, *Sci Am* 260:42, 1989.

82. Nathans J, Thomas D, Hogness DS: Molecular genetics of human color vision: the genes encoding blue, green, and red pigments, *Science* 232:193, 1986.

83. Nawy S: The metabotropic receptor mGluR6 may signal through G$_o$, but not phosphodiesterase, in retinal bipolar cells, *J Neurosci* 19:2938, 1999.

84. Nawy S, Jahr CE: Suppression by glutamate of cGMP-activated conductance in retinal bipolar cells, *Nature* 346:269, 1990.

85. Nawy S, Jahr CE: cGMP-gated conductance in retinal bipolar cells is suppressed by the photoreceptor transmitter, *Neuron* 7:677, 1991.

86. Nelson R, Famiglietti EV Jr, Kolb H: Intracellular staining reveals different levels of stratification for on- and off-center ganglion cells in cat retina, *J Neurophysiol* 41:472, 1978.

87. Olsen BT, Schneider T, Zrenner E: Characteristics of rod driven off-responses in cat ganglion cells, *Vis Res* 26:835, 1986.

88. Pang JJ, Gao F, Wu SM: Relative contributions of bipolar cell and amacrine cell inputs to light responses on ON, OFF and ON-OFF retinal ganglion cells, *Vis Res* 2002 (in press).

89. Pugh EN, Lamb TD: Phototransduction in vertebrate rods and cones: molecular mechanisms of amplification, recovery and light adaptation. In Stavenga DG, Degrip WJ, Pugh EN Jr (eds): *Handbook of biological physics,* New York, 2000, Elsevier Science.

90. Raviola E, Gilula NB: Gap junctions between photoreceptor cells in the vertebrate retina, *Proc Natl Acad Sci USA* 70:1677, 1973.

91. Raviola E, Gilula NB: Intramembrane organization of specialized contacts in the outer plexiform layer of the retina: a freeze-fracture study in monkeys and rabbits, *J Cell Biol* 65:192, 1975.

92. Rieke F, Schwartz EA: A cGMP-gated current can control exocytosis at cone synapses, *Neuron* 13:863, 1994.

93. Schnapf JL, Kraft TW, Baylor DA: Spectral sensitivity of human cones, *Nature* 296:439, 1987.

94. Schwartz EA: Cones excite rods in the retina of the turtle, *J Physiol* 246:639, 1975.

95. Schwartz EA: Rod-cone interaction in the retina of the turtle, *J Physiol* 246:617, 1975.

96. Shiells RA, Falk G: The glutamate-receptor linked cGMP cascade of retinal on-bipolar cells is pertussis and cholera toxin-sensitive, *Proc R Soc Lond B Biol Sci* 247:17, 1992.

97. Shiells RA, Falk G: Responses of rod bipolar cells isolated from dogfish retinal slices to concentration-jumps of glutamate, *Vis Neurosci* 11:1175, 1994.

98. Simon EJ, Lamb TD, Hodgkin AL: Spontaneous voltage fluctuations in retinal cones and bipolar cells, *Nature* 256:661, 1975.

99. Slaughter MM, Miller RF: 2-amino-4-phosphonobutyric acid: a new pharmacological tool for retina research, *Science* 211:182, 1981.

100. Slaughter MM, Miller RF: An excitatory amino acid antagonist blocks cone input to sign-conserving second-order retinal neurons, *Science* 219:1230, 1983.

101. Smith BN, Dudek FE: Amino acid-mediated regulation of spontaneous synaptic activity patterns in the rat basolateral amygdala, *J Neurophysiol* 76:1958, 1996.

102. Steinberg RH: Rod and cone contributions to S-potentials from the cat retina, *Vis Res* 9:1319, 1969.

103. Stell WK: The structure and relationships of horizontal cells and photoreceptor-bipolar synaptic complexes in goldfish retina, *Am J Anat* 121:401, 1967.

104. Stryer L: *Biochemistry,* New York, 1995, WH Freeman.

105. Svaetichin G: The cone action potential, *Acta Physiol Scand* 29:565, 1953.

106. Svaetichin G, MacNichol EF Jr: Retinal mechanisms for chromatic and achromatic vision, *Ann NY Acad Sci* 74:385, 1958.

107. Thibos LN, Werblin FS: The properties of surround antagonism elicited by spinning windmill patterns in the mudpuppy retina, *J Physiol* 278:101, 1978.

108. Thibos LN, Werblin FS: The response properties of the steady antagonistic surround in the mudpuppy retina, *J Physiol* 278:79, 1978.

109. Tian N, Hwang TN, Copenhagen DR: Analysis of excitatory and inhibitory spontaneous synaptic activity in mouse retinal ganglion cells, *J Neurophysiol* 80:1327, 1998.

110. Tomita T: Electrophysiological study of the mechanisms subserving color coding in the fish retina, *Cold Spring Harb Symp Quant Biol* 30:559, 1965.

111. Tomita T et al: Spectral response curves of single cones in the carp, *Vis Res* 7:519, 1967.

112. Uga S et al: Some new findings on the fine structure of human photoreceptor cells, *J Electron Microsc* 19:71, 1970.

113. Vallerga S: Physiological and morphological identification of amacrine cells in the retina of the larval tiger salamander, *Vis Res* 21:1307, 1981.

114. Vaney DI: Territorial organization of direction-selective ganglion cells in rabbit retina, *J Neurosci* 14:6301, 1994.

115. Victor JD, Shapley RM: Receptive field mechanisms of cat X and Y retinal ganglion cells, *J Gen Physiol* 74:275, 1979.

116. Wald G: Molecular basis of visual excitation, *Science* 162:230, 1968.

117. Werblin F et al: Neural interactions mediating the detection of motion in the retina of the tiger salamander, *Vis Neurosci* 1:317, 1988.

118. Werblin FS: Response of retinal cells to moving spots: intracellular recording in Necturus maculosus, *J Neurophysiol* 33:342, 1970.

119. Werblin FS: Lateral interactions at inner plexiform layer of vertebrate retina: antagonistic responses to change, *Science* 175:1008, 1972.

120. Werblin FS: Regenerative amacrine cell depolarization and formation of on-off ganglion cell response, *J Physiol* 264:767, 1977.

121. Werblin FS, Dowling JE: Organization of the retina of the mudpuppy, *Necturus maculosus*. II. Intracellular recording, *J Neurophysiol* 32:339, 1969.

122. Witkovsky P: A comparison of ganglion cell and S-potential response properties in carp retina, *J Neurophysiol* 30:546, 1967.

123. Witkovsky P, Owen WG, Woodworth M: Gap junctions among the perikarya, dendrites, and axon terminals of the luminosity-type horizontal cell of the turtle retina, *J Comp Neurol* 216:359, 1983.

124. Witkovsky P, Stell WK: Retinal structure in the smooth dogfish *Mustelus canis:* electron microscopy of serially sectioned bipolar cell synaptic terminals, *J Comp Neurol* 150:147, 1973.

125. Wong-Riley MTT: Synaptic organization of the inner plexiform layer in the retina of the tiger salamander, *J Neurocytol* 3:1, 1974.

126. Wu SM: The off-overshoot responses of photoreceptors and horizontal cells in the light-adapted retinas of the tiger salamander, *Exp Eye Res* 47:261, 1988.

127. Wu SM: Input-output relations of the feedback synapse between horizontal cells and cones in the tiger salamander retina, *J Neurophysiol* 65:1197, 1991.

128. Wu SM: Signal transmission and adaptation-induced modulation of photoreceptor synapses in the retina, *Prog Retinal Res* 10:27, 1991.

129. Wu SM: Feedback connections and operation of the outer plexiform layer of the retina, *Curr Opin Neurobiol* 2:462, 1992.

130. Wu SM: Synaptic transmission in the outer retina, *Ann Rev Physiol* 56:141, 1994.

131. Wu SM, Dowling JE: Effects of GABA and glycine on the distal cells of the cyprinid retina, *Brain Res* 199:401, 1980.

132. Wu SM, Gao F, Maple BR: Functional architecture of synapses in the inner retina: segregation of visual signals by stratification of bipolar cell axon terminals, *J Neurosci* 20:4462, 2000.

133. Wu SM, Maple BR: Amino acid neurotransmitters in the retina: a functional overview, *Vis Res* 38:1371, 1998.

134. Wu SM, Yang XL: Electrical coupling between rods and cones in the tiger salamander retina, *Proc Natl Acad Sci USA* 85:275, 1988.

135. Yang CN, Yazulla S: Light-microscopic localization of putative glycinergic neurons in the larval tiger salamander retina by immunocytochemical and autoradiographic methods, *J Comp Neurol* 272:343, 1988.

136. Yang CY: Gamma-aminobutyric acid transporter-mediated current from bipolar cells in tiger salamander retinal slices, *Vis Res* 38:2521, 1998.

137. Yang CY, Yazulla S: Light microscopic localization of putative glycinergic neurons in the larval tiger salamander retina by immunocytochemical and autoradiographical methods, *J Comp Neurol* 272:343, 1988.

138. Yang CY, Yazulla S: Localization of putative GABAergic neurons in the larval tiger salamander retina by immunocytochemical and autoradiographic methods, *J Comp Neurol* 277:96, 1988.

139. Yang CY, Yazulla S: Glutamate-, GABA-, and GAD-immunoreactivities co-localize in bipolar cells of tiger salamander retina, *Vis Neurosci* 11:1193, 1994.

140. Yang XL, Gao F, Wu SM: Non-linear, high-gain and sustained-to-transient signal transmission from rods to amacrine cells in dark-adapted retina, *J Physiol* 2002 (in press).

141. Yang XL, Wu SM: Modulation of rod-cone coupling by light, *Science* 244:352, 1989.

142. Yang XL, Wu SM: Coexistence and function of glutamate receptor subtypes in the horizontal cells of the tiger salamander retina, *Vis Neurosci* 7:377, 1991.

143. Yang XL, Wu SM: Feedforward lateral inhibition in retinal bipolar cells: input-output relation of the horizontal cell-depolarizing bipolar cell synapse, *Proc Natl Acad Sci USA* 88:3310, 1991.

144. Yang XL, Wu SM: Response sensitivity and voltage gain of the rod- and cone-horizontal cell synapses in dark- and light-adapted tiger salamander retina, *J Neurophysiol* 76:3863, 1996.

145. Yang XL, Wu SM: Response sensitivity and voltage gain of rod- and cone-bipolar cell synapses in dark-adapted tiger salamander retina, *J Neurophysiol* 78:2662, 1997.

146. Yau KW, Baylor DA: Cyclic GMP-activated conductance of retinal photoreceptor cells, *Ann Rev Neurosci* 12:289, 1989.

147. Yazulla S: Cone input to bipolar cells in the turtle retina, *Vis Res* 16:737, 1976.

148. Zimmerman AL, Baylor DA: Cyclic GMP-sensitive conductance of retinal rods consists of aqueous pores, *Nature* 321:70, 1986.

SECTION 9

VISUAL PERCEPTION

PAMELA A. SAMPLE AND CHRIS A. JOHNSON

ENTOPTIC PHENOMENA*

GERALD WESTHEIMER

Entoptic (literally, "within the eye") imagery refers to visual perceptions that have their origin in the structure of an observer's own eye. The structures responsible for these images may be normal anatomic components of the eye, or they may be pathologic imperfections, such as opacities in the media of the eye. The images are not ordinarily visible on casual observations but rather require special circumstances of illumination, as well as the direct visual attention of the observer. Using the concept somewhat loosely, one may also include those visual experiences that result from stimulation of the retina by inadequate (nonlight) stimuli, including the unformed images produced by mechanical stimulation of the retina, so-called phosphenes.

An appreciation of entoptic phenomena and their origins is useful to clinicians and students as a means of improving their understanding of the physiology of vision. Occasionally, the phenomena are of clinical utility by allowing a subjective confirmation of some capacity for visual function in which objective findings may not be available. Because of their subjective nature, however, entoptic phenomena require observer skills of perception and articulate description of their appearance before they can be clinically useful.

This chapter is arranged so that entoptic images are discussed in an order roughly corresponding to the anatomic distribution of the structures related to the images. The first phenomena to be considered are those arising from opacities in the media, including the cornea, lens, and vitreous. The latter part of the chapter deals with images determined by the structure of the retina.

IMPERFECTIONS IN THE OCULAR MEDIA

When the ocular fundus is illuminated by a focal source of light held close to the examiner's eye and within 1 m or so distant from the eye being observed, the pupil of the eye appears to be filled with a diffuse reddish glow. This phenomenon is commonly termed the *fundus reflex,* not to be confused with the neurally mediated reactions of the pupil to light stimulation of the retina. The reddish glow of the fundus reflex is the result of diffuse reflection of light by the retina and choroid. The reflected light exits from the eye through the pupil and serves to reveal in the ocular media any imperfections that prevent light from returning through the pupil toward the examiner's eye. Such imperfections are seen as dark areas within the otherwise diffusely illuminated pupil (Figure 16-1). The imperfections need not be true opacities in the sense of blocking the passage of light completely, but they may be only local variations in the refractive index of the media. For example, a streak of mucus across the corneal surface is seen as a dark line because it refracts the light of the fundus reflex away from the examiner's view. Localized variations in the refractive index of the media are also commonly produced by surface irregularities in the corneal epithelium, by defects in Descemet's membrane, or by changes in the state of hydration of the lens.

Small, discrete opacities of the cornea and lens reduce the optical clarity of the media by scattering light. They appear as fine dark specks when retroilluminated by the fundus reflex. Larger opacities produce dark areas in the red fundus reflection seen by the examiner. For example, clumps of pigmented cells on the anterior lens capsule may be torn loose from adhesions of the posterior iris sur-

---

*Based on the chapter "Entoptic Imagery" by William H. Hart, Jr., M.D., Ph.D., in the previous edition.

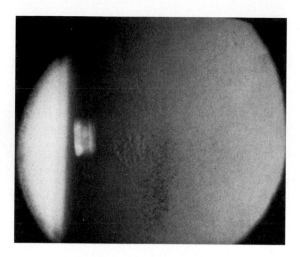

FIGURE 16-1   Slit-lamp view of the fundus reflex through dilated pupil. Illuminating beam enters pupil at left. In the center of the pupil a small central disc of a posterior subcapsular cataract is visible. To its right there is a vertical spindle-shaped pattern of dark particles in which pigment granules have been deposited on the corneal epithelium (so-called Krukenberg's spindle).

face to the lens (posterior synechia). These appear to the examiner as black spots within the pupillary aperture. This sort of opacity in the ocular media may significantly reduce the amount of light reaching the retina, but it will scatter only a small fraction of the light.

The various types of optical defects produce entirely different effects on the patient's vision. Translucent defects, which are local discontinuities in the index of refraction of the optical media, do not completely block the passage of light. They spread or scatter the light and are often damaging to vision by reducing the contrast of images at the retina. Numerous small opacities produce the same effect. In an apparent paradox, although a larger opacity reduces the total amount of light reaching the retina, it may not appreciably reduce the contrast of the image by light scatter. Before the development of corneal transplantation for the treatment of corneal scarring, an effective form of therapy was to convert an area of corneal translucency into a true opacity by means of tattooing. If an adequate aperture of clear tissue remained, considerable improvement in visual acuity often resulted.

With reversal of the passage of light and use of the observer's visual system, the same phenomena can be seen and reported on by a patient. The ideal method here is to place a point source of light at the anterior focal point of the eye, about 17 mm in front of the cornea. After refraction by the cornea

and lens, the light becomes a parallel bundle, which is limited in size by the pupil. Any defect in the media produces a shadow or unevenness of illumination detectable by the patient in much the same way as would be seen by the examiner as just described. A good approximation of this method of illumination is a small pinhole a fraction of a millimeter in diameter that is placed in the anterior focal point of the eye, admitting light from the sky or diffusely illuminated wall (Figure 16-2). The observer then sees a patch of light, the border of which is the shadow of the pupillary margin of the iris. The patch varies in size with changes in pupillary diameter. Optical discontinuities in the ocular media are then seen as shadows or bright areas within the circular patch. The shape, position, and movement of these light and dark areas correspond to their density and position within the eye.

The more sophisticated method of relative entoptic parallax permits the localization of a media defect that casts a shadow on the retina[7] (see Figure 16-2). As the pinhole is moved with respect to the eye, shadows change their position with respect to the outlined papillary margins. Those resulting from defects located posterior to the pupil lag and those in front lead.

Use of the pinhole method allows entoptic visualization of a number of both normal and pathologic phenomena arising from the anterior corneal surface and its tear film. Occasionally, horizontal bands of light, apparently caused by folds in the corneal epithelium, may be seen. They course in unbroken lines across the entire width of the pupillary image and change their position as the margins of the eyelids are slowly approximated or separated. They can be distinguished easily from the entoptic image of the tear film. The tear film that adheres to the lid margins produces a longitudinal stripe that can be seen as the pupillary fissure is narrowed. This image appears first along the inferior portions of the pupillary image (because of the inversion of the perceived direction of retinal images).

Droplets and threads of mucus on the surface of the tear film of the cornea likewise can be seen as bright spots surrounded by a dark ring. These move up and down in a slow swimming fashion as the palpebral fissure is widened or narrowed. A variety of folds and channels may also be seen. These consist of vertical lines that are gently curved in some locations, and in other regions they may bend more angularly. The curved lines and the channels that separate them can be observed on repetitive examinations at different times, suggesting that they represent definite anatomic structures. Their

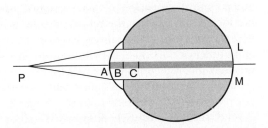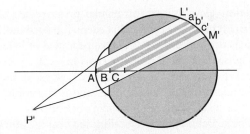

FIGURE 16-2   A small light source, *P*, in the anterior focal plane of the eye gives rise to a parallel beam of light in the eye. The size and shape of the illuminated retinal patch LM are determined by the pupil. Opacities cast shadows that can be seen entoptically. *Right,* The position of the shadows within the illuminated patch varies with the angle of incidence of the beam. This permits the observer to judge the location of opacities in the eye with respect to the plane of the pupil by the method of relative entoptic parallax. As the light source is moved up and down, the shadow *a′* of target *A*, which is in front of the pupil, moves faster than the bundle of light admitted by the pupil; the shadow *c′* of target *C* moves more slowly.

origin is not certain, but they may represent vitreous membranes or folds in the surface of the corneal epithelium underlying the tear film. Staining of the tear film with fluorescein dye sometimes shows a mosaic pattern outlined by straight and curved lines in the corneal epithelium (Figure 16-3). This anterior corneal mosaic pattern is easily produced by a brief period of gentle digital pressure on the cornea through the closed upper lid. It is thought to be caused by the formation of shallow, linear channels in the corneal epithelium; these are produced by elevated ridges in Bowman's membrane that are created during the period of corneal flattening. Corneal flattening by hard contact lenses often produces this phenomenon.[5]

PHYSIOLOGIC AND PATHOLOGIC HALOS

A small bright light source situated at some distance from the eye, such as a street light at night, can give rise to halos. Their origin is the diffraction of light at small structures within the eye. When there are many small apertures of approximately the same size within a larger one of the pupil, the diffraction pattern from each of the smaller ones will sum. Circular structures, such as round cells or intercellular spaces in the cornea, will produce circular Fraunhofer diffraction patterns of a size proportional to the wavelength of light and inversely to their diameter. The first ring of the diffraction pattern can easily become visible against a dark background. Because its diameter varies with wavelength, there is a spectral distribution in the halos (violet to red) when the light source is white. With a monochromatic source, such as a sodium light street lamp, the halo diameter can be estimated in

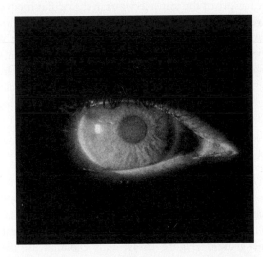

FIGURE 16-3 Anterior corneal mosaic pattern stained with fluorescein dye. Pattern is most visible in pupillary area.

angular measure and allow the calculation of the size of the structure inducing it. The radius θ of the first diffraction ring of an aperture of diameter a for light of wavelength λ is given by the formula $tan\ \theta = 1.22\lambda/a$. This yields, for example, a value of 3.5 degrees for the sodium wavelength of 589 nm and a 10-μm structure. Physiologic halos have diameter of this magnitude and are thought to arise from the typical normal structure of the corneal epithelium.

Halos also are reported by patients who have the severe photophobia of ultraviolet radiation keratopathy, which results in damage to corneal epithelial cells. Similarly, persons with endothelial corneal dystrophies that result in corneal edema often notice halos as a first symptom of their disorder. In patients with otherwise normal endothelial function, elevations of intraocular pressure can be sufficient to produce epithelial edema. In such individuals the appearance and disappearance of halos can be seen to parallel fluctuations in ocular pressure. When the intraocular pressure is elevated, microscopic spaces of fluid appear among the epithelial cells just anterior to Bowman's membrane.

The structure of the crystalline lens, on the other hand, is more like that of a circular grating, giving rise to diffraction images that are radial spokes; they are apparent to most observers even in the optimally focused image of a point source.

The pinhole method previously described for viewing opacities in the cornea and tear film also readily shows defects in the optical qualities of the lens.

Under ordinary circumstances, observers are not aware of the imperfections in the ocular media. Even large opacities of the cornea or lens may not produce noticeable defects in the retinal image if they only block, rather than scatter, the light entering the eye. However, the closer an opacity is to the retina, the more prominent will the shadow be that it casts and the more likely that a patient will notice and report it.[18]

ENTOPTIC IMAGES PRODUCED WITHIN THE VITREOUS

Posteriorly located opacities that cast sharp umbral shadows on the retina appear as positive scotomas when seen against an evenly illuminated white background (Figure 16-4). This explains the ex-

treme annoyance caused by even very small opacities located adjacent to the retinal surface. It likewise explains the occasional very large opacity lying in the anterior portion of the vitreous, which is surprisingly inconspicuous to the patient.

Small vitreous opacities are present even in the normal eye. They are seen against a bright background, such as a diffusely illuminated wall or the blue sky, as small specks or dots and move as the eye is moved. Because of the gel-like consistency of the vitreous, they usually lag behind a fast saccade. The dots may be seen as single round globules or sometimes chains of little bright spots of light resembling a string of pearls. Fine dark lines in amorphous masses that appear like pieces of dust or small branching twigs are also occasionally seen and may become annoying when they cross the center of the field of view. Although they usually do not interfere with vision, they may sometimes be a source of discomfort and alarm to the patient. They are called *muscae volitantes* because they seem to dart about like flies as the eye moves.

Most of the vitreous opacities that are seen entoptically are entirely harmless. However, when a sudden increase in opacities with accompanying flashes of light is noted, these symptoms may be caused by vitreoretinal traction or the creation of retinal breaks that may eventually lead to retinal detachment.

Occasionally, a large vitreous opacity may be seen with an ophthalmoscope as a disc-shaped structure floating in the posterior vitreous. This is

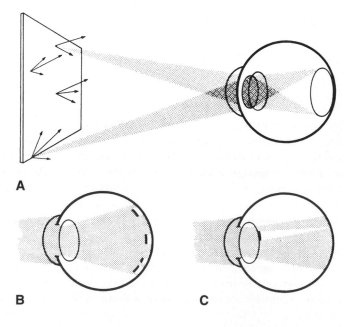

FIGURE 16-4   **A,** Light from any point in a uniform extended source entering the pupil generates a large brightly illuminated image. Each image point is at the apex of a light cone based in the pupil. **B,** Opacities near the retina cast a sharp shadow that is conspicuous to the patient. **C,** A small opacity directly behind lens, on the other hand, obscures only part of the beam destined for each retinal point; its shadow is not sharp. This explains how even very small opacities lying near retina can be annoying while a much larger one in the anterior segment can remain unnoticed. (From Rubin ML, Walls CL: *Studies in physiological optics,* Springfield, Ill, 1965, Charles C Thomas.)

probably caused by detachment of the posterior vitreous from the margin of the optic disc (separation of the so-called posterior vitreous base), or it may represent a transverse tear across the posterior portion of the hyaloid canal.[19] By itself, this finding is of little consequence. However, it should be emphasized that, despite the generally benign nature of vitreous floaters, a distinction should be made between those that develop slowly and those that appear abruptly. The latter are more likely to be related to retinal breaks or hemorrhage into the vitreous body. Patients should not be reassured about the generally benign nature of floaters until complications have been ruled out by appropriate examination for posterior vitreous separation, retinal breaks, and possible retinal detachment.

Perhaps the most striking demonstration of the relative insignificance of optical effects of vitreous opacities is provided by patients who have asteroid hyalosis. Asteroid bodies in the vitreous are caused by local accumulations of calcium soaps. Patients with this disorder are rarely aware of the opacities, which serve only to reduce the total amount of light reaching the retina, without degrading the image. Only rarely do such patients experience a reduction in their visual acuity. When seen with an ophthalmoscope, however, these structures reflect considerable light back toward the observer, creating the image of a swarm of brightly illuminated dots within the vitreous body. Indeed, the observer's view of the fundus may be obscured entirely and yet the patient may experience only a minor disturbance of vision.

VITREORETINAL SOURCES OF ENTOPTIC IMAGES: MOORE'S LIGHTNING STREAKS

Moore[11] originally described an entoptic phenomenon consisting of flashes of light that were likened to the appearance of flashes of lightning. These lightning streaks, which are now recognized as common, are seen most often in the temporal visual field and are largely vertical in orientation. They are sometimes accompanied by the simultaneous development of a shower of small vitreous opacities and occur most often in middle-aged patients, more often among women than among men. Moore originally believed that this phenomenon did not imply the presence of a serious underlying disorder. However, it has since been stressed that this common syndrome is of more serious import than Moore originally believed.[22] The phenomenon is

thought to result from degenerative changes in the vitreous body that lead to detachment of the posterior vitreous from the surface of the retina. As a separation occurs between the posterior vitreous face and the internal limiting membrane of the retina, traction on the retina at some points produces phosphenes (flashes of light). The preference of these phosphenes for the temporal visual field may be a result of the asymmetry of retinal sensitivity. Traction on the temporal retina near the ora serrata (subserving nasal visual field) may not be noticed subjectively. Similar traction on the seeing portions of the peripheral nasal retina produces phosphenes that are seen in the temporal visual field.

Patients seeking attention for the sudden appearance of lightning flashes should be examined carefully, particularly if the symptom is recent or has been associated with the appearance of a large number of bothersome floaters. A dilated examination of the fundus by indirect ophthalmoscopy is required to rule out the presence of retinal breaks that might subsequently lead to the development of retinal detachment. Although most patients reporting such phosphenes do not develop serious retinal disease, a small but significant proportion do.

PHOSPHENES OF QUICK EYE MOVEMENT

Nebel[13] has described an entoptic phenomenon that appears to be related to, although distinct from, Moore's lightning streaks. He named the phenomenon *flick phosphene* (Figure 16-5). It is best seen in a completely dark-adapted eye, such as when awaking from sleep in a still darkened room. If the eyes are then rapidly moved from one side to the other, one can observe in the visual field of each eye bright patterns in the region of the blind spot. Each eye produces its own individual phosphene, which lasts only a fraction of a second.

The retina seems to "fatigue," so repeated observations produce a gradual fading of the phosphenes. The images may have the shape of a sheaf, the truncated apex of which points toward either the physiologic blind spot or the center of fixation. When first seen, the pattern is bright yellow or orange with sharp borders. Repeated attempts to elicit the images cause them to become indistinct, blurred, and less brightly colored. Nebel[13] attributed these phosphenes to physical deformation of the retina by the posterior surface of the vitreous body. Abrupt saccadic motion of the eye causes the inertial drag of the vitreous body to be transmitted directly to the

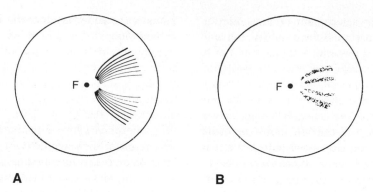

Figure 16-5   Phosphene of right eye in right-to-left flick. **A,** Phosphene pattern in rested eye. **B,** Pattern after fatigue. *F,* Fovea, as identified by afterimage of fixated inducing light. (From Nebel B: *Arch Ophthalmol* 58:236, 1957.)

Figure 16-6   Phosphenes of right-to-left flick and interpretation relating to topography of their origin. **A** and **C,** Phosphenes as seen by the observer. **B** and **D,** Projection of phosphenes back to retina. *Dashed arrows* represent shearing force by inertial retardation of vitreous. Projected phosphene is tilted and displaced slightly to make it visible. *F,* Fovea; *N,* optic nerve. (From Nebel B: *Arch Ophthalmol* 58:237, 1957.)

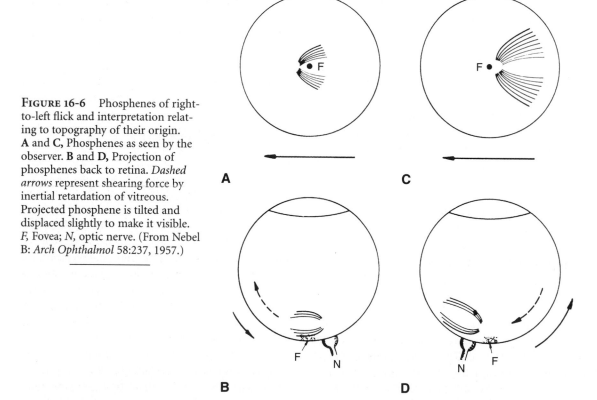

retina (Figure 16-6). The resulting deformation of the cellular structures within the retina results in a mechanical phosphene. Support for this interpretation lies in the observation that the images are more easily elicited in the eyes of individuals undergoing the early senescent changes of vitreous liquefaction (syneresis).

RETINAL VASCULATURE: PURKINJE FIGURES

The retinal arteries and veins lie in the inner layers and hence in the light path to the receptors. Because they are close to the receptors, they cast shadows on them. However, because they always remain in fixed locations, they are ordinarily invisible. Powerful adapting mechanisms in the retina change sensitivity locally to factor them out, equalizing and reestablishing uniform activity across a patch of retina that would, in the absence of shadows of the blood vessels, have been evenly illuminated. When the direction of the incident light is changed quickly, the shadows fall on neighboring areas that have not been adapted, exposing them to added stimulation. The shadows now suddenly become visible and produce a vivid percept of the retinal vascular tree. However, as local adaptation proceeds, this quickly fades again unless it is revived by further movement. The phenomenon is named for its discoverer, Johannes Purkinje, in whose 1823 classical treatise[16] this and many other subjective visual phenomena are described in much detail.

A slit-lamp beam that directs bright light to the retina at an unusual angle is a prominent way of inducing the Purkinje figure. It can also be generated by suitable transscleral illumination, which does not involve the eye's optics and can therefore be used in patients with severe media opacities. It has been suggested that it might have promise as a means of evaluating the integrity of retinal function before cataract surgery. Unfortunately, just where it matters most—in and around the macula—there is no visible vasculature, and hence the procedure has little value for this purpose.

The large vessels around the optic disc can be as wide as 1 degree of arc of visual angle, and in their shadow, there is no detectable visual function. Careful plotting of the visual fields around the blind spot with small targets can be used to map out the scotomas resulting from vessels in the vicinity of the optic disc—a procedure called *angioscotometry.*

Another phenomenon associated with retinal circulation has been widely reported. When viewing a large uniform field of light, one can occasionally see small tumbling discs following fixed curve paths in the perifovea. The consensus is that they are individual blood corpuscles darting through retinal capillaries one at a time. Calculations of corpuscle diameter (about 10 µm) and location of capillaries within the retina, as well as the their added prominence in light wavelengths absorbed by hemoglobin, make this the most likely interpretation.

If pressure is applied to the eye, induced pulsations in the retinal vessels can sometimes be seen entoptically, especially after physical exercise.[8] Rapid expansions of the arteriolar vessels, synchronous with cardiac systole, can be observed. These are followed by a second, diastolic phase in which slower contractile movements are seen along the paths of the same vessels. If the subject has not exercised before this examination, the pulsations are usually too small to be entoptically apparent.

ENTOPTIC IMAGES INFLUENCED BY THE DISTRIBUTION OF RETINAL NERVE FIBERS: BLUE ARCS OF THE RETINA

During the nineteenth century Purkinje described numerous important visual phenomena. In addition to his observations on the shift of the spectral sensitivity of the eye during dark adaptation and his description of visualization of the retinal vascular tree, he was also the first to describe the phenomenon known as *blue arcs.*

When a small rectangular stimulus, preferably red, is placed in the nasal visual field on the horizontal meridian near the fovea in darkness and with dark-adapted vision, one can see a fleeting light pattern arching over and under the fovea toward the blind spot (Figure 16-7.) The pattern follows the arcuate trajectory of the optic nerve fibers in the retina between the horizontal raphe and the optic disc (Figure 16-8). Because of their bluish appearance, they are called *blue arcs* but the actual color depends on the state of the eye's adaptation.

In a rigorous analysis, Alpern and Dudley[1] have shown that the blue arcs originate from stimulation of the cones by the rectangular inducing light pattern, but the action spectrum of the blue arcs themselves is that of the rods. The optimal stimulus conditions have been described by Moreland.[12] Because the entoptic pattern follows the trajectory of the retinal nerve fibers from the inducing region to the optic disc and circumnavigates the fovea, the best interpretation of the phenomenon is that conduction of activity in the nonmyelinated fibers from the site of light stimulation to the optic nerve head generates some activity in the retina along its curved pathway. The fact that the blue arcs are caused by the rod pathway might lead one to conclude that action potentials passing along nerve fibers cause the emission of light, albeit with energy so low as to be seen only by dark-adapted rods. However, this seems not to be the case. Rather the cause is some activity induced in the underlying neural layers of the retina by the conduction of impulses in the optic nerve fiber layer. These fibers do not become myelinated until passing into the optic nerve, and this lack of insulation probably allows electrical signals, or more likely changes in ion concentration in the extracellular space, to leak into the

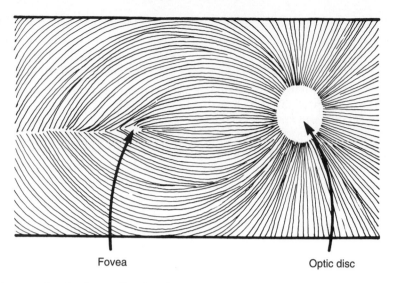

Fovea   Optic disc

Figure 16-7 Diagram of path of nerve fiber bundles of retina in and around the macula and optic disc. Note horizontal raphe temporal to fovea and arcuate paths taken by fibers.

Figure 16-8 Typical patterns created by the blue arcs phenomenon for a right eye. *Rectangles* represent shape and orientation of the red-inducing stimuli that are most effective in eliciting the arcs. Compare arcs to the distribution of retinal nerve bundles in Figure 16-7. (Modified from Moreland JD: *Vision Res* 8:99, 1968.)

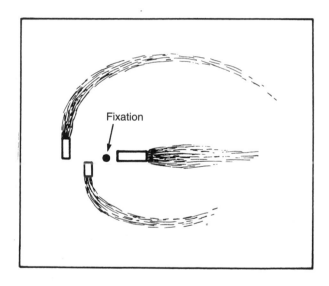

Fixation

more distal neural network of the retina. The color appearance of the blue arc has been used in hypotheses delineating the contribution of rods to color vision.[9]

Maxwell's Spot

When an evenly illuminated surface is viewed through alternating yellow and blue filters, a circular dark pattern is seen around the fovea for the first few seconds of looking through the blue filter. Most often it has a doughnut shape with an outer diameter of 2 to 3 degrees. As the eye becomes adapted to the blue light, the spot fades but it can be re-stored by readapting to new alternations between yellow and blue.[4] Its description goes back to James Clerk Maxwell,[10] who developed the electromagnetic theory, contributed to color vision, and originated the method of retinal illumination now known as *Maxwellian view*. The conjecture that the spot is associated with a paucity of blue receptors in the fovea is no longer accepted. It is now understood that Maxwell's spot results from impregnation of the macular region with a carotenoid pigment related to xanthophylls, whose distribution matches the entoptic appearance of Maxwell's spot.[20] It is absent or at least attenuated in the center of the macula. It has been speculated that the

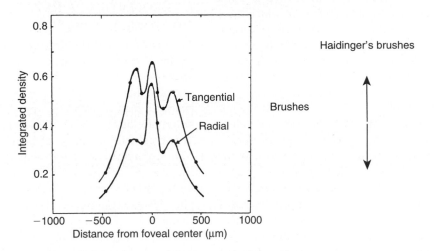

FIGURE 16-9 Appearance of Haidinger's brushes is determined by differential absorption of plane-polarized light by xanthophyll pigment molecules oriented about the center of the foveal macula. *Left,* Microdensitometry scans of tissue sections for tangentially and radially oriented plane-polarized light. Absorption is lower for radially oriented plane of polarization. *Right,* Dark portion of brush pattern results from greater absorption of tangentially oriented light (vertically oriented plane of polarization). (From Snodderly DM, Auran JD, Delori FC: *Invest Opthalmol Vis Sci* 25:674, 1984.)

pigment has protective properties with respect to foveal receptors, but this raises the question why it is not most concentrated in the fovea.

ENTOPTIC IMAGES ARISING FROM THE OUTER PLEXIFORM LAYER: HAIDINGER'S BRUSHES

If one views a diffusely illuminated source of plane-polarized light, brushes or sheaves radiating from the point of fixation in the form of an hourglass can be seen. The brushes have contrasting yellow and blue hues and rotate with the plane of polarization. This entoptic phenomenon is known as *Haidinger's brushes.* DeVries et al.[6] and Stanworth and Naylor[21] have demonstrated that this phenomenon is caused by variations in absorption of plane-polarized light by oriented molecules of xanthophyll pigment in the foveal retina. Stanworth measured threshold for the appearance of the brush effect as a function of the extent of polarization of the light and found that the strength of the effect varied with the wavelength of light in a manner directly paralleling the optical density of carotenoid pigments such as xanthophyll. The yellow pigment preferentially blocks the blue light, producing a dark central spot in the inner layers of the fovea. Scanning densitometry with plane-polarized light shows that the optical density of Henle's fiber layer in the macular

retina of a monkey varies with the rotational orientation of the plane of polarization (Figure 16-9). Assuming central symmetry in the orientation of the pigment molecules, this effect would explain the entoptic appearance of Haidinger's brushes.

Because the brush effect is determined by the orientation of the pigment molecules in front of the photoreceptor layer, any process that disturbs this orientation may lead to a loss of the brush image, even though the photoreceptor layer itself is normal. For this reason, loss of the Haidinger brush image may indicate the presence of macular disease, such as edema, at a time when visual acuity is normal and the macula appears normal by direct ophthalmoscopy.

PHOSPHENES

A luminous sensation arising from direct stimulation of the retina is called *phosphene,* and it may be induced by mechanical or electrical forces.

Mechanical deformation, for example by pressure on the eyeball with a small blunt probe, produces a localized bright sensation called a *pressure* or *deformation phosphene.* Its location in the opposite visual field is a telling demonstration of the concept of local sign of the retina and the inversion of the retinal image. The threshold force for producing a deformation image is about four times higher in darkness than in bright light. Negative deformation phosphenes, in which there is an area of darkening, can occur under certain circumstances when the retina is well illuminated. They are caused by local disturbances of the light-gathering properties of photoreceptors because they cannot be induced when the retina is illuminated transsclerally.[4]

Current passing through the eye can induce electrical phosphenes. The effectiveness of electric currents to stimulate the retina depends on the component of the current density perpendicular to the retinal surface; the components along the retinal surface are ineffective. This implicates radial retinal structures, such as the receptors and bipolar cells. More detailed analysis revealed that the optimal direction of current near the macula does not favor the cone outer segments, which remain radial in this location, but does favor the inner segments and bipolar cells, which here lean outward with respect to the visual axis. Interesting experiments can be performed using the interaction of electrical and photic stimuli.

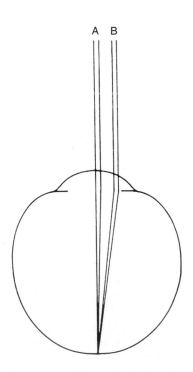

A B

FIGURE 16-10 Normal retinal directional sensitivity effect. Light in bundle entering through center of the pupil (**A**) is more effective in stimulating retinal cones than in bundle coming into eye near edge of dilated pupil and hence reaching retinal cones obliquely (**B**). (From Westheimer G: *Arch Ophthalmol* 79:584, 1968.)

ENTOPTIC PHENOMENA CAUSED BY PROPERTIES OF RETINAL PHOTORECEPTORS

Intrinsic Gray of the Retina

In complete darkness one does not have the visual sensation of blackness, but rather of a definite grayness that is actually subjectively lighter in appearance than the sensation produced by looking at a matte black surface of near-zero reflectance. This persistent sensation of light probably arises from spontaneous neural activity evidenced in ganglion cell discharges in the normal retina even in the absence of light. It has been used to underpin Hering's opponent theory of light, which claims the sensation of black results not from the absence of light but from the inhibition of the light/dark opponency mechanism. It has also been proposed that bleached rhodopsin, which remains after exposure to bright light and is gradually reduced in the recovery process of dark adaptation, generates signals in the retina that are in some respects similar to real light and have been called *dark light*.[3]

Stiles-Crawford Effect

The Stiles-Crawford effect is a phenomenon related to the directional sensitivity of retinal photoreceptors. Parallel rays of light entering the pupil through its center are more effective in stimulating retinal cones than are those that enter the eye near the edge of a dilated pupil, reaching the retinal cones somewhat more obliquely (Figure 16-10). If the strength of an adapting light beam is measured at various points of entry through the pupillary aperture according to its ability to bring a constantly bright flickering test light to the threshold of perception (Figure 16-11), its effectiveness is found to vary in a systematic fashion. Its peak effectiveness is near the center of the pupillary aperture for the normal eye and falls steadily toward the periphery of the pupillary aperture in a symmetric fashion. Eyes that are not normal, such as those having irregular posterior staphylomas or myopia, may have an asymmetric arrangement of foveal cone receptors in relation to the pupillary aperture. In such eyes (Figure 16-12) there may be marked asymmetry of the Stiles-Crawford effect. Westheimer[23] has demonstrated for his own eye that by deliberately throwing the image of a point source of light out of focus (Figures 16-13 and 16-14), the brightness of the foveal blur patch can itself be seen to be asymmetric. The asymmetry can be predicted from the known foveal cone tilt.

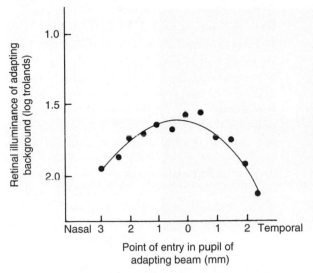

FIGURE 16-11   Normal retinal directional sensitivity pattern. Abscissae: point of entry along horizontal meridian of pupil of bundle of light providing background; ordinates: relative sensitivity of retina, measured by inverse of amount of light necessary in background field to bring constant increment stimulus to threshold. Background (7.5 degrees) was exposed continuously, and ordinates give its retinal illuminance in trolands of green light. Incremental stimulus was circular, 12 minutes of arc in diameter, 0.05 second in duration, and 30 trolands of red light and was placed at threshold by adjustment of wedge in background beam. (From Westheimer G: *Arch Ophthalmol* 79:584, 1968.)

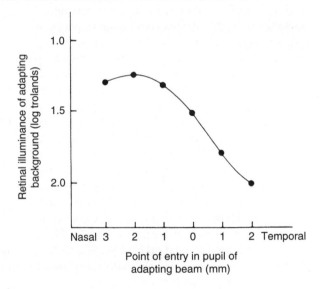

FIGURE 16-12   Asymmetric retinal directional sensitivity pattern in author's right eye, foveal vision. Abscissae: point of entry of bundle of light providing background; ordinates: relative sensitivity of retina, measured by inverse of amount of light necessary in background field to bring constant increment stimulus to threshold. (From Westheimer G: *Arch Ophthalmol* 79:584, 1968.)

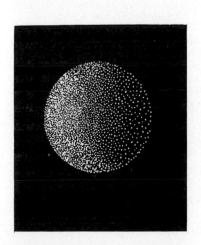

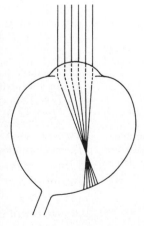

FIGURE 16-13   *Left,* Appearance of foveal blur patch of bright star against dark sky seen with uncorrected myopic right eye with large pupil. Stiles-Crawford pattern of this eye, illustrated in Figure 16-12, is asymmetric. *Right,* Schematic diagram illustrating path of rays making up blur patch. That the seen pattern is brightest near its left border implies that receptors in region of fovea point in direction of nasal edge of dilated pupil. (From Westheimer G: *Arch Ophthalmol* 79:584, 1968.)

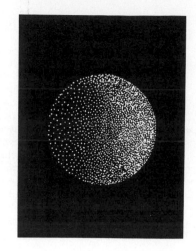 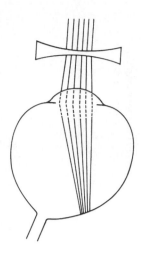

FIGURE 16-14   Appearance of foveal blur patch of bright star against dark sky seen under artificially hyperopic condition with large pupil in right eye with asymmetric Stiles-Crawford effect (see Figures 16-11 and 16-12). *Right,* Schematic diagram illustrating path of rays making up blur patch. Right edge of seen pattern corresponds to nasal edge of retinal blur patch. That it is brightest implies that receptors in foveal region are pointing to nasal edge of dilated pupil. (From Westheimer G: *Arch Ophthalmol* 79:584, 1968.)

Entoptic Perimetry

A television monitor or computer monitor filled with a dynamic random light pattern, when viewed by someone with a normal visual system, appears as "visual noise." Circumscribed defects caused by peripheral retinal lesions are readily seen in the white-noise field if the patient is capable of stable fixation. Those areas corresponding to the damaged retina appeared to have no random motion and are gray or motionless in appearance.[2] That the defect is not ordinarily apparent to the patient in normal vision has been ascribed to a "filling in" process, which is also used to explain the absence of a noticeable blind spot.[17] Subjects can be made to outline scotomas, and it has been found that for retinal, but not central defects, those areas in which subjects reported no white noise corresponded to retinal lesions.[14,15] There seems to be a close correlation between this method of entoptic perimetry and the more conventional ways of mapping visual field defect.

REFERENCES

1. Alpern M, Dudley D: The blue arcs of the retina, *J Gen Physiol* 49:405, 1966.
2. Aulhorn E, Köst G: Rauschfeldkampimetrie. Eine neuartige perimetrische Untersuchungsweise, *Klin Monatsbl Augenheilkd* 192:284, 1988.
3. Barlow HB: Dark adaptation: a new hypothesis, *Vis Res* 4:47, 1964.
4. Brindley GS: *Physiology of the retina and visual pathway,* ed 2, London, 1970, Edward Arnold.
5. Dangle ME, Kracher OD, Stark WJ: Anterior corneal mosaic in eyes with keratoconus wearing hard contact lenses, *Arch Ophthalmol* 102:888, 1984.
6. De Vries H, Spoor A, Jielif R: Properties of the eye with respect to polarized light, *Physica* 19:419, 1953.
7. Emsley HH: *Visual optics,* ed 2, London, 1939, Hatton Press.
8. Friedman B: Observations on entoptic phenomena, *Arch Ophthalmol* 28:285, 1942.
9. Ingling CR Jr, Drum BA: Why the blue arcs of the retina are blue, *Vis Res* 17:498, 1977.
10. Maxwell JC: On the unequal sensibility of the foramen centrale to light of different colours. In *The scientific papers of James Clerk Maxwell,* New York, 1965, Dover (originally published in 1856).
11. Moore RF: Subjective lightning streaks, *Br J Ophthalmol* 19:545, 1935.
12. Moreland JD: On demonstrating the blue arcs phenomenon, *Vis Res* 8:99, 1968.
13. Nebel B: The phosphene of quick eye motion, *Arch Ophthalmol* 58:235, 1957.
14. Plummer DJ, Azen SP, Freeman WR: Scanning laser entoptic perimetry for the screening of macular and peripheral retinal disease, *Arch Ophthalmol* 118:1205, 2000.
15. Plummer DJ et al: Correlation between static automated and scanning laser entoptic perimetry in normal subjects and glaucoma patients, *Ophthalmology* 107:1693, 2000.
16. Purkinje JE: *Beobachtungen und Versuche zur Physiologie der Sinne,* vol 1, Prague, 1823, J Calve, vol 2, Berlin, 1825, G Riemer.
17. Ramachandran VS, Gregory RL, Aiken W: Perceptual fading of visual texture borders, *Vis Res* 33:717, 1993.
18. Rubin ML, Walls CL: *Studies in physiological optics,* Springfield, Ill, 1965, Charles C Thomas.
19. Schepens CL, Trempe CL, Takahashi M: *Atlas of vitreous biomicroscopy,* Boston, 1999, Butterworth.
20. Snodderly DM, Auran JD, Delori FC: The macular pigment, II, spatial distribution in primate retinas, *Invest Ophthalmol Vis Sci* 25:674, 1984.
21. Stanworth A, Naylor E: The measurement and clinical significance of the Haidinger effect, *Trans Ophthalmol Soc UK* 75:67, 1955.
22. Verhoeff F: Are Moore's lightning streaks of serious portent? *Am J Ophthalmol* 41:837, 1956.
23. Westheimer G: Entoptic visualization of Stiles-Crawford effect, *Arch Ophthalmol* 79:584, 1968.

CHAPTER 17

VISUAL ACUITY

GERALD WESTHEIMER

Visual acuity refers to the spatial limit of visual discrimination. It is surely the single most significant measure of functional integrity of the biologic apparatus to which the eye professions are dedicated. If restricted to expressing a patient's visual status in only one number, most practitioners would opt for one of the form 20/20.

Technically speaking, a visual acuity measurement involves the determination of a threshold; therefore our discussion has to deal with the problems typically associated with sensory thresholds: specification of the physical stimulus, transduction in the sense organ, anatomic and physiologic substrates, criteria and scales of measurements, techniques of obtaining threshold values, and influence of interacting variables.

Fechner,[14] who claimed to have invented his psychophysical law on October 22, 1850 (in the morning, in bed), made the distinction between outer and inner psychophysics. By *outer psychophysics,* he meant the relationship between the physical stimulus outside the body and the associated mental state; he applied the term *inner psychophysics* to the relationship between the physiologic state at the level of the sense cells and the mental state. Leaving aside the emphasis Fechner placed on the mental, or psychologic, aspect, the distinction between outer and inner psychophysics focuses attention on the role of transduction of the physical stimulus in the sense organ. Nowhere does this distinction assume greater significance than in spatial vision. Later generations of students of sensation have used the terms *distal* and *proximal* stimulus, the former denoting, in our case, the light distribution in object space as a physicist might describe it, and the latter the pattern of photon absorption in retinal receptors. The intervening processes of optical

image formation, including refraction, diffraction, absorption, and scattering, are at least as important in understanding visual acuity and what can interfere with it as any of the succeeding stages: photochemical transduction in the retinal receptors, sorting and transmission of neural signals in the retina and visual pathways, and higher cortical processing. There is no need at present to define the end stage of visual acuity. Depending on the situation, we may seek a patient's verbal response, a "voluntary" motor response such as a gesture or a button press, or an "involuntary" response such as pupil contraction or optokinetic nystagmus, or we may be satisfied with a set of electric signals from some part of the central nervous system.

SPECIFICATION OF THE STIMULUS (PHYSICAL BASIS)

The retinal receptor cells are not exposed directly to the light from the objects, but rather to the energy distribution in the image formed by the eye's optical system. The first step in dealing with visual acuity then is the specification of the relationship between objects and their retinal images. The schema for this relationship has two aspects: the relative spacing of the images of sequential object points and the light spread in the image of each point. Choosing the chief ray as the reference facilitates the discussion. Of the light emanating from any object, only the bundle that is admitted by the pupil matters as far as the retinal image is concerned. To save the effort of tracing all the rays through the cornea and checking which the iris intercepts, we use the artifice of finding the image of the iris formed by the cornea: the entrance pupil. Any ray from any object that passes through the entrance pupil also ends up in the retinal image. The ray from the object to the center of the entrance pupil is called the *chief ray* because it identifies the center of the light bundle from that particular object. To examine the situation in any region of the retina in which reasonable homogeneity of imagery applies, it suffices to study the locations of the intercept of the chief rays with the retina because the light spread associated with the image of each point is centered around the chief ray.

The entrance pupil is situated about 3 mm behind the corneal vertex. When one looks at an eye and measures the pupil size, one is in reality measuring the size of the entrance pupil, which is about 10% larger. Each chief ray uniquely defines a retinal position. Therefore it is a satisfactory procedure to transfer specification of retinal distances (in linear measure along the retina) into the measure of angular separation of object-sided chief rays. In a typical emmetropic eye, a retinal distance of 1 mm corresponds to angular separation of chief rays of about 3.5 degrees. The convention of expressing retinal distance in angular measure of chief rays in object space is almost universal.

A significant feature of the chief ray method of specifying retinal image position is that, because the bundle of rays converging onto the image plane is centered on the chief ray, the method retains its validity even with focus changes caused by lenses or accommodation (so long as the pupil center stays put). The image patch may change size with focus changes, but the location of its center (the chief ray intercept) does not move. If the eye were an ideal

optical instrument without diffraction or aberrations, no more need be said about imagery than what angle the chief rays of the objects make with each other and where the objects are situated with respect to the plane conjugate to the retina. In actual practice, additional considerations center on the extent of departure of the image quality from the ideal of a point image for a point object.

In optical instrument design it is customary to partition the deviations from point imagery into a variety of classes. However, the significant datum is the total effect of all of them, that is, the actual light spread in the image of a point object or the point-spread function. Once this basic information is available, it is possible to describe the light distribution in any object merely by superposing the spread functions centered on all the elements making up the object.

It is difficult to ascertain the value for the light spread in the retinal image of a given eye, but indirect measurements have shown it to have the general shape shown in Figure 17-1. The following factors contribute to the spread:

1. *Diffraction:* According to the wave theory of light, limitation of the aperture causes a spread of light even in a fully focused system. The Fraunhofer diffraction image of a point object by a circular aperture has the familiar bell shape with oscillating fringes shown in textbooks of physics (Figure 17-2). It comes to its first zero at a radial distance of 1.22 λ/a radians (angle in object space), where λ is the wavelength of the light and a is the diameter of the

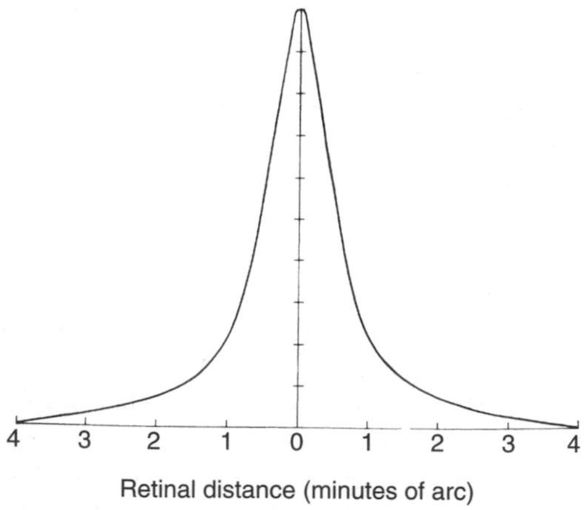

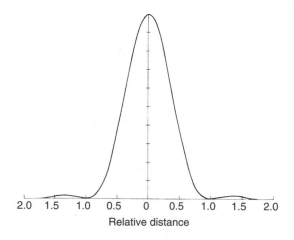

FIGURE 17-1 Line-spread function (i.e., light distribution in the image of a thin line object) for a human eye in best focus and moderate pupil diameter.

FIGURE 17-2 Fraunhofer's diffraction pattern for a point object. Abscissae are in normalized coordinates, where 1.00 is equal to an angle of 1.22 λ/a radians in object space. Pupil diameter = a, wavelength of light = λ.

entrance pupil. The central patch of the pattern is called the *Airy disc* and contains most of the light energy; the height of the first ring is only 1.75% of the central peak. Whenever the eye's pupil is less than 2 mm in diameter, the actual image spread is equal to the diffraction image, and the other factors (see following discussion) can usually be ignored.

2. *Aberrations:* Because of a variety of factors that may vary from one eye to the next, rays entering through the periphery of the pupil may not converge on the geometric image point, therefore contributing to the spread of light in the image beyond that caused by diffraction. These effects become more prominent as the pupil widens, more or less offsetting the resulting reduction of the diffraction effects. As a consequence, the image quality usually does not improve much beyond that of a diffraction-limited instrument with a 2.5-mm pupil diameter. For pupil diameters larger than 5 mm, the spread is usually increased because the peripheral regions of the cornea and lens are often afflicted with optical aberrations while contributing heavily to the total light entering the eye. For example, enlarging the pupil from 6 to 7 mm contributes 6.5 times more additional light than enlarging it from 2 to 3 mm. For cone vision, the Stiles-Crawford effect would reduce this to a factor of about 2.

   Recent technologic advances have made it possible to create aberration-free images for large pupils in experimental observers. Resolution and contrast sensitivity for fine gratings is enhanced somewhat by this method of image optimization.[30]

3. *Scatter:* Because the ocular media have some microscopic and ultramicroscopic structure, light is scattered in its passage from the cornea to the retina. An examiner uses backward scatter when examining an eye with the slit lamp, but forward scatter can be more serious. Its effect can be extensive, spreading light from even a narrow incident beam over a considerable portion of the retina. Complaints of glare can have their origin in scattered light, which increases in prominence with age (see Aging later in this chapter). Shielding the eyes from the direct rays of intense light sources (wearing the green eyeshades of older days) is good advice, although not easily put into effect for automobile headlights at night.

4. *Absorption:* The media are not uniformly transparent to incoming light. In general, the shorter the wavelength of the entering light, the smaller the proportion that reaches the retinal receptors.

5. *Focus factors:* The effect of defocus on visual acuity is dealt with separately and has been characterized adequately. However, it must be remembered that when a person has active accommodation, it cannot be taken for granted that the accommodative stance is always appropriate to the stimulus distance. This is a problem, especially when no sharply delineated targets are available to anchor accommodation. Night and instrument myopia are well-known instances of the phenomenon, but it also can occur when "fogging" during a refractive examination.

Altogether, it is only conjecture to assume that a given eye under a given set of circumstances would display the optimal point-spread function. The procedures needed to deduce the light spread in images other than points have been outlined elsewhere.[48] They have to be followed for each particular target when the relative effect of the various factors on visual acuity is being determined. Light spread, the first in a sequence of transformations, needs special attention, lest phenomena be assigned to complex neural interaction when, for example, they may have a simple explanation in light scatter or accommodation instability.

RETINAL ANATOMY

One unavoidable bottleneck in the processing of spatial information in the retina is the finite size of the retinal receptors. In the fovea the cones are packed approximately two to the linear minute of arc, and each cone's local sign is indivisible.[8,9] Electrical coupling of photoreceptors has been reported, but this is probably not an issue in the primate fovea. Therefore, in principle, it is impossible to resolve patterns whose spacing demands separate sampling of intensity at intervals smaller than half a minute of arc (Figure 17-3).

Other limits are set by the neural connectivity of retinal cells at their various layers.[7] This applies particularly in the retinal periphery, where many rod connections converge on a ganglion cell. Although the rods themselves are small, the fact that summation of their signals takes place over areas up to several degrees in diameter sets upper bounds to the partitioning of spatial information.

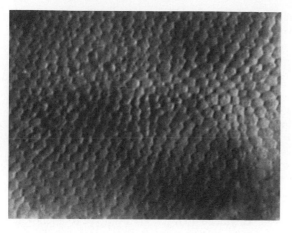

FIGURE 17-3 Optical section through the cone inner segments of the human fovea. Width of section is about 55 μ (i.e., it covers a substantial fraction of the rod-free area). (From Curcio CA et al: *Science* 236:579, 1987.)

Although there is no question of the role played by the elements of the retinal mosaic in limiting resolution, certain spatial distinctions can be made that appear to have a finer grain—the hyperacuities. Because the diameter of the retinal receptors constitutes an unavoidable limitation to partitioning spatial information except at defined intervals, as does the extended dimension of the image of a point object, sophisticated neural processing must interrelate signals from adjoining cells to provide the information regarding location.

PHYSIOLOGIC FACTORS

Because visual acuity is conceptually and operationally well anchored in psychophysics, the detailed dissection of its physiologic substrates is not an issue central to its discussion. In fact, current electrophysiology has not yet demonstrated neural processing mechanisms that approach the best human thresholds.

Nevertheless, spatial differentiation is inevitably coupled to light difference detection. If for any reason this is deficient, spatial resolution suffers. Thus one finds that visual acuity follows pari passu intensity discrimination sensitivity for the small stimulus areas involved.[39] For example, the detection of a double star as composed of two separate stimuli requires that the trough between the two light peaks be deep enough that an intensity discrimination ($\Delta I/I$) for such a small stimulus area can be carried out. Because $\Delta I/I$ has to be larger when the luminance gets lower, resolution deteriorates; that is, the peaks have to be separated farther

to create a trough that delivers a $\Delta I/I$ value sufficiently large to be detected for that area at the prevailing luminance.

Many other variables that influence visual acuity (e.g., adaptation and exposure duration) exert their effect predominantly on the light discrimination sense and only through it on resolution. In many cases the effects can be traced for some distances through the optical, anatomic, and physiologic stages and the threshold identified by a prevailing limitation along the way. Before returning to a brief survey of some of these interacting variables, we need to outline the procedures involved in actual measurements of visual acuity.

ACUITY CRITERIA

Within the general definition of visual acuity, that is, thresholds in which spatial dimension is the variable, some obvious subdivisions can be recognized; these subdivisions are outlined best by the different criteria set for the response of the observer (Table 17-1):

1. The criterion of the presence of a single feature ("minimum visible")
2. The criterion of the presence, or internal arrangement, of identifying features in a visible target ("minimum resolvable" or ordinary visual acuity)
3. The criterion of the relative location of visible features (the "spatial minimum discriminable," or hyperacuity)

Minimum Visible

What is involved in minimum visibility is the detection of the presence of a visual stimulus, but the stimulus variation is carried out by manipulating the contrast of the target through the medium of varying its size. The most typical example of this remains the experiments in which one measures the minimum width of a telegraph wire that can be seen against a uniform sky. The threshold value is of the order of 1 second of arc, that is, a small fraction of the diameter of a retinal receptor. However, the situation is not as startling as it sounds because it has a simple basis in the variation of the physical stimulus. The retinal light spread for a single, thin dark line seen against a uniform bright background is a dimple with the cross-sectional outline of the line-spread function. In the human eye this has a width at half height of at least 1 minute of arc. For all targets that have a width of about this value or less, the shape of the light distribution remains about the same; variations of target width manifest

TABLE 17-1

CLASSIFICATION OF VISUAL ACUITY ACCORDING TO CRITERIA

CRITERION	MINIMUM VISIBLE	MINIMUM RESOLVABLE (ORDINARY VISUAL ACUITY)	MINIMUM DISCRIMINABLE (HYPERACUITY)
Task	Determine presence or absence of a target	Determine presence of, or distinguish between more than one, identifying feature in a visible target	Determine relative location of two or more visible features with respect to each other
Typical forced choice psychophysical question	Is there a line in this field? If there was a line in the field, was it horizontal or vertical?	Is this a *C* or an *O*? Is the gap in the *C* up, down, right, or left?	Is the upper line to the right or the left of the lower line?
Physiologic basis	Local brightness difference threshold (ΔI)	Detection of brightness differences between several adjoining small areas	Assignment of relative local signs to two or more suprathreshold visual features
Method of measurement	Vary object size	Vary object size or spacing between object components	Vary relative location of features
Magnitude of best threshold	~1 second of arc	~30 seconds of arc	~3 seconds of arc
Effect of image degradation	Moderate	Serious	Slight (except in stereoacuity)

themselves purely as variations of dimple depth. Threshold measurements for the minimum visible (e.g., where a dark line is widened progressively until its presence is detected) in reality are merely ΔI thresholds for a more or less fixed retinal light distribution whose contrast is varied by varying the target width (Figure 17-4). The situation is analogous to one in the time domain, when one can let a light pulse reach threshold by increasing either the intensity of a stimulus or its duration, so long as the pulse length remains within the limits of the critical duration of the Bunsen-Roscoe-Bloch law (see Chapter 20).

A definitive study by Hecht and Mintz[19] showed that variations in contrast sensitivity as a function of luminance, for example, can fully account for variations in the minimum visible spatial threshold. Although the stimulus change is effected in the dimension of space, the minimum visible threshold really does not approach the essence of visual acuity because the subject's judgment does not demand the making of any spatial differentiations, except in the trivial sense of whether a field is uniform. However, the other two subdivisions of visual acuity demand just that differentiation.

Minimum Resolvable or Ordinary Visual Acuity

Most commonly associated with visual acuity is the concept of Snellen's letters or Landolt's C's. A high-contrast, clearly visible target is shown, and the

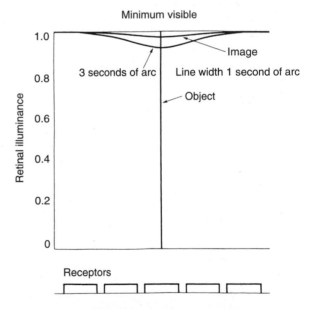

FIGURE 17-4 Schematic diagram to illustrate that the *minimum visible* is a brightness rather than a spatial visual threshold. A single dark line seen against a uniform background is widened until it can be detected. As the line is widened, the retinal image pattern, which has the outline of the complement of the eye's line-spread function, increases in contrast but remains invariant in shape. Detection occurs when the ΔI threshold is reached for the prevailing adaptation level. Although the object is changed in a spatial dimension, detection is purely that of a brightness change. For threshold line width (approximately 1 second of arc), the retinal image contrast is just a few percentage point. (From Westheimer G: *Invest Ophthalmol* 18:893, 1979.)

subject has to make a spatial judgment best exemplified by the distinction between a *P* or an *F*, a *B* or an *R*, and a *C* or an *O*. That is, either the presence of a gap or the relative arrangement of components of a letter has to be detected. Because we are dealing with a resolution task, more pointed tests of this capacity than Snellen's letters are available, such as a double star that is being separated until seen double or a grating whose spatial frequency is being reduced until its structure becomes apparent. However, Snellen's letters have the virtue of not requiring a binary decision that is subject to guessing; they belong to a moderately sized ensemble of well-known patterns and optimize information transfer between patient and examiner.

Conceptually, the simplest situation is one in which members of a point or line pair are moved apart until the observer can judge them to be separate. Each of the two bright points or lines would be imaged on the retina with the light distribution of the point- or line-spread function. Initially, the two spread functions overlap thoroughly, but as the target pair is separated, overlap is only partial. A pattern emerges, characterized by two humps with an inter-

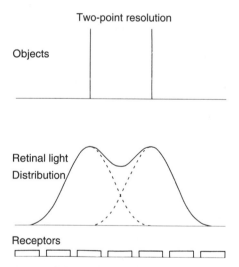

Figure 17-5 Example of ordinary visual acuity is the detection of doubleness for a stimulus consisting of two points, each of which is imaged on the retina as a point-spread function. The amount of overlap depends on the point separation. The essential elements for detecting doubleness (i.e., for resolution) are (1) an underlying retinal image pattern with two peaks separated by a trough, (2) a retinal illuminance difference between the peaks and the trough and the trough that is within the ΔI capability of the visual system in the prevailing state of adaptation, and (3) separate localization of the differentially stimulated regions.

vening trough (Figure 17-5). Resolution (i.e., correct judgment of doubleness) can be achieved when the peak/trough ratio of retinal illuminance is accommodated by the $\Delta I/I$ ratio of the visual system for the stimulus area involved at the prevailing level of adaptation. In addition, the effective grain of the visual system has to be small enough for the peaks and trough to fall in separate detecting units, regardless of whether they are defined by the limitations of retinal anatomic structure or synaptic organization.

In a normal observer in best focus, the resolution limit or, as it is usually called, the *minimum angle of resolution (MAR)*, is between 30 seconds of arc and 1 minute of arc. There is remarkable concordance between the observed minimum angle of resolution, the expected resolving capacity of the eye's optics, and the predicted performance of a system that has a manifest visual acuity of 20/20 or better. The requirements are good optical imagery, foveal fixation, intact receptor structure and function, photopic luminance levels, and of course, full integrity of the involved neural pathways.

For the actual determination of the resolution limit in a clinical or physiologic setting, the most widely used procedure involves gratings. The period of a high-contrast grating is reduced (i.e., the spatial frequency increased) until the observer can no longer resolve it. It is acceptable to use a square-wave grating because, at the resolution limit, it does not differ in practice from a sinusoidal grating. The third-harmonic component, which is present in a square-wave grating, is, by definition, already beyond the resolution limit.

In most clinical situations, conceptually pure tests such as two-line or grating resolution are not practicable and one prefers to have a patient read letters or numerals. It must be realized, however, that factors other than resolution enter into discrimination between letters of the alphabet. These are generally classified as belonging to form perception, about which little is known as yet at the physiologic and psychophysical levels.[52] As shown later in this chapter, in some abnormalities of visual acuity, the decrement in letter acuity is higher than in grating resolution, implying that, in the end, a distinction must be made between these two kinds of tasks.

Minimum Discriminable or Hyperacuity

Certain spatial distinctions can be made by a normal observer when the threshold is much lower than ordinary acuity, and therefore these must have a fundamentally different basis. The best known of these is alignment or vernier acuity.[63] The tasks share with ordinary acuity the presence of a clearly delineated target and therefore should never be confused with the threshold for the minimum visible, in which merely the presence or absence of a target is being judged. However, in a hyperacuity test the subject is asked to make a judgment about the location of an element, usually relative to another element of the same target. Typical examples of hyperacuity configurations are shown in Figure 17-6. They all share the property of allowing spatial judgments whose thresholds in normal observers are 2 to 10 seconds of arc.

The mechanism subserving hyperacuity is still being explored, but so much is clear: No contradiction is involved with the optical and receptor mosaic factors that limit ordinary visual acuity.[50] Localization of a feature can be achieved with arbitrary precision as long as enough light quanta are available. However, the neural processing required for these judgments must be sophisticated.

Stereoscopic acuity also has a threshold of a few seconds of arc and therefore may be included under this heading. However, its processing probably differs somewhat from that in ordinary hyperacuity.

Measurement of Ordinary Visual Acuity (Minimum Angle of Resolution)

Various patterns have been used to ascertain a patient's minimum angle of resolution. The major feature of all of them is that a given pattern is enlarged bodily or reduced to find the threshold size at which the judgment can be made correctly.

The most familiar of these tests is the Snellen chart. In a normal observer in best focus, the reso-

lution limit is between 30 seconds of arc and 1 minute of arc. The standard testing procedure is to enlarge the pattern until resolution can be achieved. Commonly, the overall size of the letter is five times the width of each limb (Figure 17-7). The Landolt C affords the easiest description. The reference letter is a ring with an outer diameter subtending 5 minutes of arc at the observer's eye and an inner diameter subtending 3 minutes of arc. A gap 1 minute of arc wide is made in the ring, and the ring is presented with its opening in one of, say, four possible positions: up, down, right, or left. The subject has to indicate in which direction the C is pointing. At an observation distance of 6 m (20 feet), the overall size of the letter is 8.73 mm and the gap is 1.75 mm. If this is the subject's threshold, that is, if his or her minimum angle of resolution is 1 minute of arc, the visual acuity is identified as 6/6 or 20/20. However, suppose that the subject has a minimum angle of resolution of 0.75 minute of arc, that is, at 6 m he or she can resolve a letter with a

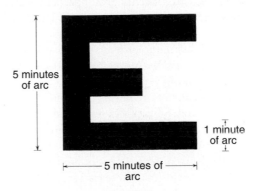

Figure 17-7 20/20 Snellen letter.

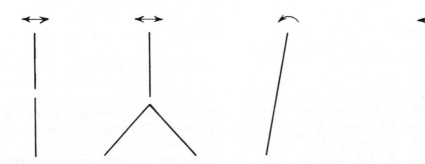

Figure 17-6 Typical target configurations, which demonstrate the hyperacuity capability of the visual system (i.e., the detection of small differences in relative localization of features). *Arrows* indicate the direction of displacement, which in each case can be judged to a few seconds of arc under optimal conditions. From left to right, vernier offset detection of two vertical lines; offset detection of the tip of a chevron from a line; detection of orientation change of a line; detection of lateral displacement of a target.

feature that subtends 1.3 mm and whose overall size is 6.5 mm; such a letter has a gap that subtends 1 minute of arc at 4.5 m (15 feet) and would be resolvable by an observer with 1 minute of arc resolution at such a distance. The subject is then said to have visual acuity of 6/4.5 or 20/15.

Illiterate E and Landolt's C tests are based on the same principle as Snellen's charts. One may distinguish these from certain repetitive patterns such as gratings or checkerboards. In these the corresponding feature size must always be clearly understood; in a grating it is half the length of a period; in a checkerboard it is the side length of a square.

On the whole, single features such as individual-style letter charts are to be preferred because, under certain conditions of defocus, repetitive patterns may at times be spuriously resolved at a size for which a patient cannot consistently make correct judgments on letters.

All letters in the alphabet are not equally legible.[42] In addition, most charts do not use the whole alphabet. Test charts have been created with letters in other scripts. Instruments have occasionally been designed to permit zooming of letters until they can be resolved, but the multiple-choice psychophysical technique of letter charts with several letters to the row has never been bettered in the practical situation.

The procedure of requiring a patient to read a letter chart rests on facilities for verbal communication that may not always be satisfied. A patient may not be able to understand the request or to indicate to the examiner what his or her performance actually is. For this reason, several so-called objective techniques of measuring visual acuity have been devised. They use a nonverbal response mode, but it cannot always be guaranteed that the results would be equivalent because they may be channeled through different neural circuits. This has been made clear particularly by the case of one patient who was manifestly blind by all observable criteria, but whose grating "resolution" measured by evoked potentials was normal.[4]

The two most prominent objective measuring techniques for the minimum angle of resolution involve neural electrical potentials and oculomotor responses. The evoked potential technique is based on the presentation of a differentiated spatial pattern to the subject and measuring the changes in the electroencephalogram (EEG) that accompany the presentation.[35] In the most sophisticated modern versions of this test, the stimulus consists of a change merely in the internal light distribution in the pattern, without any overall changes in total light reaching the eye. Examples are the instantaneous exchange of light and dark squares in a checkerboard or the replacement of a uniform field with a grating of the same average luminance. Whenever the pattern dimension is too small to be resolved, no changes are expected in the evoked potential on stimulus presentation. Use of temporal repetition and a signal averager can allow good measurements of resolution.

Pursuit and optokinetic eye movements are released by target movements, usually with little or no "voluntary" components. Here again, targets with spatial differentiations too small to be resolved would not be expected to lead to associated smooth eye movements, and we clearly have a good principle for acuity measurement.[16] A variant of the eye movement method, observation of the relative frequency of voluntary fixations, has recently been the primary vehicle for accumulating information about the developments of visual acuity in infants.[13] In one of two equivalent but separated patches of the infant's visual field, a grating is shown and an observer notes the relative frequency of voluntary fixations on the two; the expectation is that a field with a differentiated pattern is favored for fixation. However, one needs to remember that this technique presupposes access to and integrity of the oculomotor pathways. When concordance of results with the various measuring techniques is lacking, the origin obviously has to be sought in difference in the pathways used in them.[10] Evoked potential recordings with electrode placements favoring the visual cortex would probe the most elementary pathways, but letter recognition and verbalization involve many other cortical areas. Whatever technique is applied, attention has to be given to the method of identifying a threshold. Even when there is no resolution, an EEG blip occasionally may occur synchronously with a stimulus, a randomly occurring saccade (although a smooth movement is unlikely) may land on the target, or a subject may guess correctly the letter presented or the target's direction if it is an illiterate E or a grating. Special procedures have been devised to ensure that objective techniques separate "signal" from "noise." Threshold determination is, of course, one of the time-honored problems of psychophysics. The method of constant stimuli with forced choice has been applied effectively, as has the method of staircases. In either case the usual value of thresholds is the target size at which the subject responds correctly on 75% of occasions. In clinical practice it works well to indicate the number of letters a patient misses in a line of Snellen's letters or can read beyond it (e.g., 20/15 − 1 or 20/20 + 2).

Thresholds obtained with a rigorous psychophysical method give not only a mean value of, say, the minimum angle of resolution but also a standard error of this mean. Such a number has the virtue of permitting conclusions about whether the threshold is significantly different statistically in one situation compared with another. It has been found that the standard error of the minimum angle of resolution, in common with that of other sensory limits, remains an approximately constant proportion of the mean (Weber's law).[49]

This finding suggests that a logarithmic scale be applied to the minimum angle of resolution; for example, the size of the letters in a visual acuity chart increase in geometric proportion as follows: 20/16, 20/20, 20/31, 20/39, 20/48, 20/61, 20/76, 20/95, 20/120, 20/149, 20/186, and 20/232. In practice, variations of such a scheme have been followed for nearly 100 years.[40] The identification of the percentage loss of visual acuity as a consequence of disease or injury is medicolegally significant. An earlier attempt by Snell and Sterling[43] led to a system of measurement in which any increase by 1 minute of arc in the minimum angle of resolution was regarded as reducing the visual efficiency to 86% of its previous value. Table 17-2 indicates several ways for specifying visual acuity levels: minimum angle of resolution, Snellen's acuity, Snell-Sterling's efficiency rating, Snellen's fraction (i.e.,

the reciprocal of the minimum angle of resolution), and the logarithm of Snellen's fraction. Identical numbers can give considerably different impressions, depending on the mode of presentation. As mentioned before, because the ratio Δ MAR/mean MAR is approximately constant, the logarithmic scale is the most appropriate. In it, all reductions of acuity by a given factor constitute equivalent decrements. For example, the step from 20/10 to 20/20 is equivalent to the steps from 20/20 to 20/40, or from 20/200 to 20/400.

FACTORS INFLUENCING VISUAL ACUITY

Because all optical, anatomic, and physiologic elements are at or near their peak performance when a subject exhibits what we call *normal* visual acuity, a diminution of function in any of these constituent elements manifests itself in a reduction in visual acuity. The list of factors influencing visual acuity is legion, and no attempt is made to give an exhaustive account of them here.[47] However, the effects of some stimulus variables are of more universal interest and have been well documented.

Refractive Error

As soon as the optics of the eye are defocused, the point-spread function widens and two stars, to be identified as separate, need to be farther apart than in the fully focused state. The width of the defocused point-spread function depends directly on

TABLE 17-2
VISUAL ACUITY EQUIVALENTS IN DIFFERENT NOTATIONS

MAR (MINUTES OF ARC)	SNELLEN'S VISUAL ACUITY		SNELL-STERLING'S VISUAL EFFICIENCY (%)	SNELLEN'S FRACTION	LOG VISUAL ACUITY RELATIVE TO 20/20
	FEET	METERS			
0.5	20/10	6/3	109	2.0	0.3
0.75	20/15	6/4.5	104	1.33	0.1
1.00	20/20	6/6	100	1.0	0
1.25	20/25	6/7.5	96	0.8	−0.1
1.5	20/30	6/9	91	0.67	−0.18
2.0	20/40	6/12	84	0.5	−0.3
2.5	20/50	6/15	76	0.4	−0.4
3.0	20/60	6/18	70	0.33	−0.5
4.0	20/80	6/24	58	0.25	−0.6
5.0	20/100	6/30	49	0.2	−0.7
6.0	20/120	6/36	41	0.17	−0.78
7.5	20/150	6/45	31	0.133	−0.88
10.0	20/200	6/60	20	0.10	−1.0
20.0	20/400	6/120	3	0.05	−1.3

the amount of defocus and inversely on the pupil size. For normal observation of a Snellen chart, the data in Figure 17-8 are typical. However, there are some complications. Because of optical peculiarities, some repetitive patterns (e.g., gratings, checkerboards) can occasionally be resolved with a defocused optical system when letters of a similar size cannot. Another important variable is pupil size. Depth of focus increases with reduction in pupil size; thus the curve in Figure 17-8 is less steep in a patient with a 2-mm pupil than shown. That a young hyperope can compensate for the refractive error by accommodation and hence may have no deficit in unaided acuity needs no special mention. However, it also must be remembered that retention of the state of zero accommodation is an active process. Thus blurring a young emmetropic eye with a +2-diopters lens may not make it exactly 2 diopters myopic—with good anchor points missing, accommodation may be active and the defocus could be more than 2 diopters and, more important, unstable. In astigmatic imagery the point-spread function has different dimensions in the various directions. Meridional variation in acuity leads to a choppy performance on letter charts.

Retinal Eccentricity

Only in the center of the fovea are the conditions appropriate for maximum acuity. Even 1 degree away from it there is a reduction to about 60% of maximum.[60] The function of visual acuity with eccentricity is shown in Figure 17-9. Data on the fall-off of cone and ganglion cell density with eccentricity in the human retina have recently become available.[7,9] It is true that cones are farther apart as distance from the fovea increases, but rods remain closely packed and, in theory, could have been connected to carry good spatial information. The reduction in image quality in the retinal periphery is certainly nowhere near as severe as the reduction in acuity.[24] The immediate cause is an increase in retinal summation areas, that is, the area from which excitatory signals converge on a ganglion cell. Because the visual cortex appears to be organized in processing modules, each presumably with a constant number of input lines, one seeks concordance with the cortical magnification ratio (i.e., the number of degrees of visual field represented in a millimeter of visual cortex).[22,36]

Visual acuity and hyperacuity seem to fall off at different rates with eccentricity, but both exhibit better values for a given angle of eccentricity in the temporal than in the nasal visual field.[12,51]

Luminance

Data from Shlaer's definitive study[39] of the effect of luminance on visual acuity are shown in Figure 17-10. The evidence points to a separate rod and cone branch of the curve. Rods asymptote at a value of about 8 minutes of arc, and this acuity

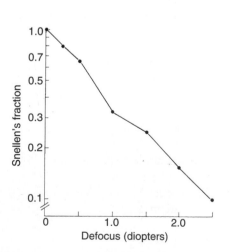

Figure 17-8 Visual acuity (Snellen's fraction) as a function of defocus for a typical eye. The ordinates are plotted on logarithmic coordinates. (Data from Laurance L: *Visual optics and sight testing,* ed 3, London, 1926, School of Optics.)

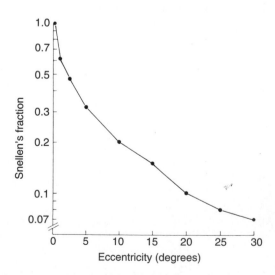

Figure 17-9 Visual acuity (Snellen's fraction) as a function of retinal eccentricity. (Data from Wertheim T: *Z Psychol* 7:172, 1894.)

usually is found in the absence or complete dysfunction of cones.[41] Visual acuity remains constant over a wide range of photopic luminances, extending from the level of full moonlight to that of a bright sky on a sunny day. High luminances cause an unexplained reduction in acuity, even in adjoining zones of moderate luminance.[62]

Contrast

When contrast is reduced, resolution is reduced. This occurs over a large range of retinal illuminance levels, particularly in the range below 90 trolands.[44] Although stereoscopic acuity also suffers seriously when contrast is reduced, vernier alignment acuity is less severely affected.[57]

Weston,[58] studying accuracy and speed in detecting Landolt C orientation near the resolution threshold, found performance over a wide range of luminance and contrast levels to be better with what he called *reverse* contrast (i.e., white letter against a dark background). The difference was 11%.

Reduced-contrast letter charts have been designed to quantify performance deficits in patients whose contrast sensitivity has been compromised by either increased intraocular scatter of impairment of retinal function or a combination of both factors. To distinguish between the two would require objective evaluation of stray light in the eye and more sophisticated tests of contrast sensitivity (see Chapter 18).[18,34,54]

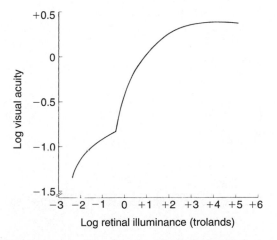

FIGURE 17-10 Visual acuity (Snellen's fraction) as a function of luminance. (Data from Shlaer S: *J Gen Physiol* 21:165, 1937.)

Pupil Size

With pupil size less than about 2.5 mm, the eye's point-spread function in good focus becomes progressively wider and a reciprocal relationship is expected between minimum angle of resolution and pupil size. Depending on the quality of the optics of the peripheral zones of the pupil, visual acuity remains approximately constant, in the range of 2.5 to 6 mm, beyond which the aberrations begin to widen the point-spread function again.[27]

Exposure Duration

Although reduction of visual acuity is progressive with decreasing exposure duration in the millisecond range, this can be offset by increasing illumination to ensure constancy of the number of absorbed quanta.[17] However, visual acuity in most observers is not as good for target exposures in the range of 100 to 500 msec as for longer durations, even though retinal summation is no longer a factor.[2] Vernier acuity seems relatively immune to reduction in exposure duration, but this is not the case for stereoscopic acuity.[57]

Target and Eye Movements

There is a decrement in certain visual functions during saccades and also in the general case in which there is significant movement of the retinal image. A target moving at moderate velocities, a few tens of degrees per second for at least half a second, can induce good enough pursuit eye movement to ensure acuity not far from normal. However, small movements of the image do not detract from acuity—strict stability of the retinal image is not a requirement for optimum resolution.[25,56]

Meridional Variations in Acuity

Differences in acuity in the various retinal meridians have been reported widely. They require grating or similar targets that permit the selective evaluation of the function one meridian at a time. The usual finding is that horizontal and vertical meridians are favored, although this is not universally so. The differences rarely exceed 15%, and there are claims for an etiologic influence connected with uncorrected astigmatism.[11]

Interaction Effects

Visual acuity suffers when targets are too close together, a phenomenon often referred to as *crowding*. Thresholds rise and occasionally may even double when a competing target is presented within a few minutes of arc. That this is not purely optical in origin is demonstrated by the non-monotonic relationship between threshold and intertarget distance; the diminution of performance is maximal at a distance of 2 to 5 minutes of arc and disappears for larger and smaller distances. The effect can be observed with ordinary visual acuity and also vernier and stereoscopic acuity.[5,15,53]

Developmental Aspects

For a long time, the difficulties of assessing the resolving capacity of the infant had left the time course of visual acuity development unclear. By the time ordinary methods—illiterate E's, for example—can be used, visual acuity is normal. It takes several months after birth for the full development of pursuit eye movement; therefore it is not easy to differentiate between inability to resolve a pattern and inability to execute the movement that would betray resolution. Preferential-looking methods, using the frequency of intersaccadic fixation in regions containing a pattern as compared with those not containing a pattern, have yielded fairly consistent results in the hands of dedicated experimentalists. Reasonable indication of the state of development of visual acuity with infant age is given in Figure 17-11. The subject has been reviewed thoroughly by Dobson and Teller.[10] When evoked potential is used as the measure, the data routinely come up with thresholds that are lower. This may be because evoked potentials tap off at an earlier state of elaboration of the visual acuity signal than do eye movements or verbal responses; however, it must not be forgotten that evoked responses are based on an averaging procedure often effectively summing many hundreds of stimuli. Active research is in progress on the possible interference with normal development (e.g., by patching one eye or failing to correct the optical defects engendered by aphakia or aniridia). The interest was sparked by Wiesel and Hubel's observation[61] in 1963 that cats whose eyes were kept artificially closed in their first few weeks of life had visual behavior and single-cell responses in the visual cortex that differed from the norm. There appears to be a clear need for the visual system to be exposed to appropriate optical stimuli during a critical period of development, but it is as yet too early to identify the exact period and the nature of the needed stimuli in the human infant. See the following discussion of amblyopia.

Hyperacuity development in infants proceeds at a rate different than that of visual acuity.[38] In early infancy, vernier acuity can in fact be poorer than visual acuity; however, this reverses as development proceeds.

Aging

Because good visual acuity depends on the integrity of various structures in the eye and visual path-

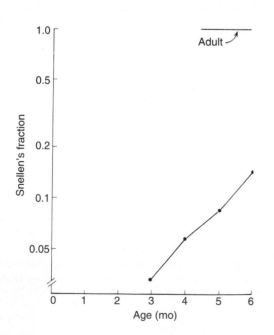

FIGURE 17-11 Visual acuity (Snellen's fraction) as a function of age in the infant. (Data from Dobson V, Teller D: *Vision Res* 18:1469, 1978.)

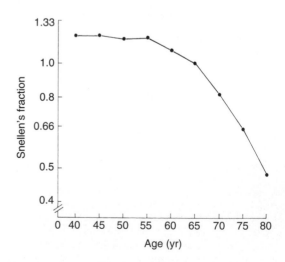

FIGURE 17-12 Fiftieth percentile of distribution of measured visual acuity in the population, graphed as a function of age. (Data from Weymouth FW: The effect of age on visual acuity. In Hirsch MJ, Wick RE [eds]: *Vision of the aging patient*, Radnor, 1960, Chilton.)

ways, it is natural to expect its maintenance into old age to be an exception rather than the rule. Figure 17-12, showing the 50th percentile of the measured visual acuity of a population as a function of age greater than 40 years, may be used as a guide.

Increased intraocular scatter of light is almost universally associated with the aging eye.[23,55] It interferes with visual acuity because it reduces contrast in retinal images of small targets (Figure 17-13). This becomes a problem when trying to detect a small dim feature or when resolving dark letters against a bright background (Figure 17-14).

Sinusoidal Grating Targets

As discussed earlier, the optical spread in the eye constitutes one possible limit to resolution. It would be advantageous to have a test that probes the retinal and neural stages of the visual acuity processing alone, bypassing, so to speak, the eye's optics. As it happens, one mode of illuminating the retina creates a pattern largely independent of the optical quality of the eye: Young's interference fringes (Figure 17-15). When two monochromatic coherent point sources are imaged in the pupil, light diverging from them into the vitreous forms a system of interference fringes whose angular spacing in object space is given by the formula λ/a, in which λ is the wavelength and a is the separation of the sources in the plane of the pupil. When laser

light of wavelength 623 nm is used, fringe spacing of 1 minute of arc occurs, with a source separation of 2.14 mm in the pupil; fringe spacing of 2 minutes of arc occurs (minimum angle of resolution = 1 minute of arc), with a source separation of 1.07 mm; and so on. The retinal image is a sinusoidal grating, that is, a grating whose intensity profile is sinusoidal. Its major virtue is that it retains high

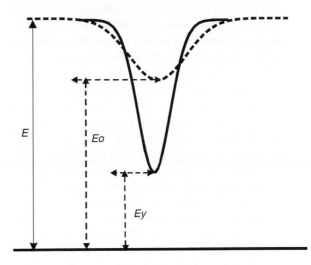

Figure 17-14 Because of the larger extent of the point-spread function in an older eye, the retinal illuminance *Eo* in the center of the image of a small dark disc is much higher than the equivalent value *Ey* in a young eye. In the example shown, the Michelson contrast in the older eye is 0.29 and is 0.61 in the young one. To reach the same contrast in the older eye, the target would have to be several times larger. (From Westheimer G, Liang J: *J Opt Soc Am A* 12:1417, 1995.)

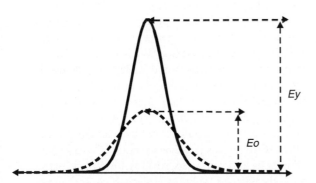

Figure 17-13 Light distribution in the center of the retinal image of a bright point object in young eyes (*Ey*) and in an older eye (*Eo*), normalized to the total quantity of light. Because intraocular scatter in the older eye spreads the image over a larger area and the outlying annular zones receive more light than in the young eye, the light intensity in the center is much reduced. The performance of older eyes is further compromised by higher absorption in the media. (From Westheimer G, Liang J: *J Opt Soc Am A* 12:1417, 1995.)

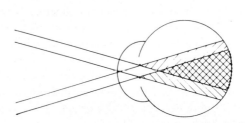

Figure 17-15 Basis for the interference fringe method of measuring resolution of retinal and central stages of the visual system, bypassing the refractive stage. A pair of coherent point sources is imaged in the plane of the pupil. Wherever the two bundles overlap in the image space, a system of interference fringes is formed. Spacing of the fringes in angular measure in the eye's object space is given by λ/a radians, where λ represent the wavelength of light and a represents the separation of the two point sources. When $\lambda = 623$ nm and $a = 1.0$ mm, fringe peaks are 2.14 minutes of arc apart.

contrast and constant fringe spacing regardless of the state of refraction or aberrations. The procedure has been used to find the resolution limit of the visual system when the optical factors have been eliminated, disclosing that retinal resolution matches that of good optics with a 2- to 2.5-mm pupil.[6,46] Gratings with finer fringes, created by separating the source images beyond 2.5 mm, are not resolved. However, the clinical utility of the test is still an open matter. Careful ophthalmoscopic and retinoscopic examination gives an excellent indication of the optics of an eye, making it unnecessary to bypass the eye's optics just to ascertain whether they caused an acuity deficit.

A much more important question concerns the capacity for resolution of the retinal and central stages when they cannot be reached by means of the standard optical imaging route because of opacities in the media. If it were possible to smuggle a system of interference fringes into the vitreous, in principle, one could reach a conclusion regarding the integrity of the neural stages before instituting surgical relief for the opacities of the media. The difficulty in the way of this approach is apparent from Figure 17-15. Fringes of a given spacing arise from the interference of coherent beams from two points in the pupil a fixed distance apart. For maximum contrast the intensity of the two beams must be equal. When the effective intensity of one beam is reduced to k times the other ($1 > k > 0$), the interference fringe contrast is reduced to $2\sqrt{k}/(1 + k)$. The essential precondition for the application of a sinusoidal grating interference fringe test that bypasses the optics of the eye is that pairs of locations can be found in the media that allow the admission of twin coherent beams whose image-sided intensities are not excessively different. The psychophysical safeguards when using a grating ("Do you now see a set of stripes?") are somewhat more cumbersome than when using letters ("Please read the letters on this line of the chart") but do not constitute a crippling disadvantage for such a test.

Sinusoidal grating targets used by way of the ordinary optics of the eye have generated a great deal of interest. In 1956, Schade[37] found that sinusoidal gratings with fringe spacing of 5 to 8 minutes of arc can be seen when they have a remarkably low contrast, often much less than 1%, while fringes with finer spacing (i.e., higher spatial frequency) and also with coarser spacing (i.e., lower spatial frequency) have to have higher contrast to be visible. The basic element of the test is a grating target of

given spatial frequency, expressed in cycles per degree of visual angle. Its contrast is changed by keeping the mean luminance constant and varying the difference between the luminance at the peaks (L_{max}) and troughs (L_{min}) of the sinusoidal luminance profile of the grating target until the observer's threshold is reached. The modulation M is given by the following expression:

$$M = \frac{L_{max} - L_{min}}{L_{max} + L_{min}}$$

This formula originally was proposed by Michelson[31] for the visibility of interference fringes and gives what should be called the *Michelson contrast*, which is applicable to repetitive patterns. For a single target with peak luminance L_{max} seen against a uniform background of luminance L, the Weber fraction $(L_{max} - L)/L = \Delta L/L$ has become the standard.

Modulation sensitivity measurements are made in the spatial frequency range of 0.5 cycles/degree (where each sinusoidal fringe covers 2 degrees of visual angle) and 20 or 30 cycles/degree (where it covers 3 or 2 minutes of arc). Thresholds usually are plotted as the reciprocal of the Michelson contrast on logarithmic coordinates. Thus the situation where $L_{max} = 101$, $L_{min} = 99$, and $M = 2/200 = 0.01$ would be represented by a modulation sensitivity of 100. Similarly, when $L_{max} = 110$ and $L_{min} = 90$, $M = 20/200 = 0.1$ would mean a modulation sensitivity of 10. Modulation sensitivity curves, which combine the effect of optical, neural, and behavioral stages of vision, can be obtained under a variety of conditions; a typical one for central fixation and photopic luminance is shown in Figure 17-16. The curve exemplifies the band-pass characteristics of the human visual system, which also is apparent in the temporal domain (see Chapter 20). Its origin is largely in the center-surround organization of neural elements in the retina and visual projection. An excitatory center flanked by inhibitory surrounds is a characteristic of retinal ganglion cells and also of cortical neurons, and these are well matched by light patterns such as gratings that can deliver the appropriate stimulus to the various components of the receptive field at the same time. Unless only a few cycles are shown at a time, gratings are not localized sufficiently to probe, for example, the fovea that has a diameter of 30 minutes of arc.

In one application of the modulation sensitivity approach, the target modulation is set at 1 (i.e., $L_{min} = 0$) and a threshold is obtained by varying the spatial frequency until the field is no longer seen as striped.

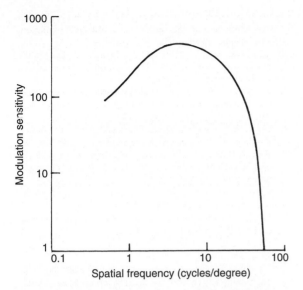

FIGURE 17-16 Modulation sensitivity curve for normal human observer at high photopic luminance and foveal vision. Axis of abscissae refers to spatial frequency of grating targets with sinusoidal luminance profile (i.e., number of complete grating cycles in each degree of visual angle). Modulation sensitivity is reciprocal measure of grating contrast needed for threshold. The curve shows the spatial bandpass characteristics of the visual system: Contrast sensitivity is higher in intermediate range and falls off for both higher and lower spatial frequencies.

The test then is a determination of visual acuity for a grating target. On the other hand, when the spatial frequency is set at values below this cut-off spatial frequency and the modulation is varied until the field begins to appear uniform and no longer striped, thresholds map the contrast detection for coarser-than-resolution targets, in this case, sinusoidal gratings. A great deal of work is in progress to determine whether such stimulus manipulation in the domain of contrast can aid in the diagnosis of ophthalmic disorders, but the results are not yet definite.[1]

AMBLYOPIA

Amblyopia is a condition in which reduced visual acuity in the eye does not exhibit any explicit abnormality on detailed examination. It is usually unilateral, and specific etiologic factors have been identified, including the presence, at an early formative stage of visual development, of an uncorrected difference in refractive state between the two eyes (anisometropic amblyopia) or a sustained lack of binocular fixation (strabismic amblyopia). Other factors such as congenital cataract or oculomotor instability (e.g., nystagmus) may also be involved.

Animal models of amblyopia exist. They have their basis in the pioneering work of Wiesel and Hubel,[61] who raised kittens with one eye sutured and observed changes in the organization of the visual cortex. This had led to many studies concerning the so-called critical period (i.e., the time span during which visual functional integrity is needed for subsequent development of normal adult vision) (see Mitchell and Timney[33] for review). More recently, a thorough study was conducted on monkeys, who were raised from infancy with one eye optically blurred, induced by atropinization.[20] Resolution and contrast sensitivity, measured behaviorally, were reduced, but the retina and all other eye tissues were histologically normal. In the lateral geniculate nuclei, however, cells belonging to the parvocellular stream from the affected eye were smaller, and in the visual cortex, anatomic and physiologic changes were found in structures associated with the processing of fine spatial detail originating in the blurred eye.

As discussed earlier, one can differentiate between simple resolving capacity, localizing ability, and letter or feature recognition. Grating resolution, vernier acuity, and Snellen acuity, respectively, are individual tests for these capabilities. Ordinarily, the diagnosis of amblyopia would be based on simple Snellen acuity alone. It is therefore of interest to inquire about the extent to which reductions in this measure are mirrored also by reductions in the others. It turns out that a fundamental difference exists between anisometropic and strabismic amblyopia.

Insofar as it has been measured, contrast discrimination for small fields or high spatial frequency gratings is reduced in all kind of amblyopia.[21,32] Vernier alignment and bisection of spatial intervals, which fall into the category of hyperacuity, are also poorer in all kinds of amblyopia than in the normal. In persons with anisometropic amblyopia the ratio between hyperacuity and ordinary visual acuity is the same as that in a normal eye.[29] In strabismic amblyopia, hyperacuity and grating resolution also are down in proportion, but in addition, letter acuity is more severely reduced. This extra loss in strabismic amblyopia emphasizes the point made earlier about the need to invoke a further mechanism, specifically, form vision, to distinguish between pure resolution and Snellen letter performance.

In reviewing the cause of the amblyopias, Levi[28] comes to the conclusion that the origin of the difference between anisometropic and strabismic amblyopia lies in the ontology of visual acuity and hyperacuity. Visual acuity develops more slowly than hyperacuity in infancy.[38] Strabismic amblyopia becomes manifest at an earlier age than anisometropic amblyopia, at a time when the ratio between hyperacuity and visual acuity is still rather low. Persons with anisometropic amblyopia, on the other hand, have a little longer span of normal development before their pathology emerges. Therefore they have a chance to achieve a stage in which the ratio between the two acuities has already reached a normal level, although their development is arrested before either of these two functions has gained the full adult capability, which may be at age 6 or even later.

REFERENCES

1. Arden GB: Recent developments in clinical contrast sensitivity testing. In Breinin GM, Siegel IM (eds): *Advances in diagnostic visual optics,* Berlin, 1983, Springer-Verlag.
2. Artal P et al: Effects of aging on retinal image quality, *J Opt Soc Am A* 10:1656, 1993.
3. Baron WS, Westheimer G: Visual acuity as a function of exposure duration, *J Opt Soc Am* 63:212, 1973.
4. Bodis-Wollner I et al: Visual association cortex and vision in man: pattern evoked occipital potentials in a blind boy, *Science* 198:629, 1977.
5. Butler T, Westheimer G: Interference with stereoscopic acuity: spatial, temporal and disparity tuning, *Vision Res* 18:1387, 1978.
6. Campbell FW, Green DG: Optical and retinal factors affecting visual resolution, *J Physiol (Lond)* 181:576, 1965.
7. Curcio CA, Allen KA: Topography of ganglion cells in the human retina, *J Comp Neurol* 300:5, 1990.
8. Curcio CA et al: Distribution of cones in human and monkey retina: individual variability and radial symmetry, *Science* 236:579, 1987.
9. Curcio CA et al: Human photoreceptor topography, *J Comp Neurol* 292:497, 1990.
10. Dobson V, Teller D: Visual acuity in human infants: a review and comparison of behavioral and electrophysiological studies, *Vision Res* 18:1469, 1978.
11. Emsley HH: Irregular astigmatism of the eye, effect of correcting lenses, *Trans Opt Soc Lond* 27:28, 1925.
12. Fahle M: Zum Einfluss von Gesichtsfeldort und Reizorientierung auf verschiedene Wahrnehmungsleistungen. In Herzau W (ed): *Pathophysiologie des Sehens,* Stuttgart, 1984, Ferdinand Enke.
13. Fantz RL: Pattern vision in young infants, *Psychol Record* 8:43, 1958.
14. Fechner GT: *Elemente der Psychophysik,* Leipzig, 1860, Breitkopf & Härtel.
15. Flom MC, Weymouth FW, Kahneman D: Visual resolution and contour interaction, *J Opt Soc Am* 53:1026, 1963.
16. Goldmann H: Objektive Sehschärfenbestimmung, *Ophthalmologica* 105:240, 1942.
17. Graham CH, Cook C: Visual acuity as a function of intensity and exposure time, *Am J Psychol* 49:654, 1937.
18. Haegerstrom-Portnoy G et al: The SKILL card: an acuity test of reduced luminance and contrast, *Invest Ophthalmol Vis Sci* 38:207, 1997.
19. Hecht S, Mintz EU: The visibility of single lines at various illuminations and the retinal basis of visual resolution, *J Gen Physiol* 22:593, 1939.
20. Hendrickson AE et al: Effects of early unilateral blur on the macaque's visual system. II. Anatomical observations, *J Neuro Science* 7:1327, 1987.
21. Hess RF, Howell ER: The threshold contrast sensitivity function in strabismic amblyopia: evidence for a two-type classification, *Vision Res* 17:1049, 1977.
22. Hubel H, Wiesel TN: Functional architecture of macaque monkey visual cortex, *Proc R Soc Lond B* 198:1, 1977.
23. IJspeert JK et al: The intraocular straylight function in 129 healthy volunteers: dependence on angle, age and pigmentation, *Vision Res* 30:699, 1990.
24. Jennings JAM, Charman WN: Off-axis image quality in the human eye, *Vision Res* 21:445, 1981.
25. Keesey UT: Effects of involuntary eye movements on visual acuity, *J Opt Soc Am* 50:769, 1960.
26. Laurance L: *Visual optics and sight testing,* ed 3, London, 1926, School of Optics.
27. Leibowitz H: The effect of pupil size on visual acuity for photometrically equated test fields at various levels of luminance, *J Opt Soc Am* 42:416, 1952.
28. Levi DM: Visual acuity in strabismic and anisometropic amblyopia, *Pediatr Ophthalmol* 3:289, 1990.
29. Levi DM, Klein SA: Hyperacuity and amblyopia, *Nature* 298:268, 1982.
30. Liang J, Williams DR, Miller DT: Supernormal vision and high resolution retinal imaging through adaptive optics, *J Opt Soc Am A* 14:2884, 1997.
31. Michelson AA: On the application of interference methods to spectroscopic measurements, *Phil Mag Series V* 27:484, 1891.
32. Miller EF II: The nature and cause of impaired vision in the amblyopic eye of a squinter, *Am J Optom Arch Am Acad Optom* 32:10, 1955.
33. Mitchell DE, Timney B: Postnatal development of function in the mammalian visual system. In Darian-Smith I (ed): *American physiological society handbook of physiology,* vol III, part I, *The nervous system,* Oxford, 1984, American Physiological Society and Oxford University Press.
34. Pelli DG, Robson JG, Wilkins AJ: The design of a new letter chart for measuring contrast sensitivity, *Clin Vision Sci* 2:187, 1988.
35. Regan D: *Evoked potentials in psychology, sensory physiology, and clinical medicine,* London, 1972, Chapman & Hall.
36. Rolls ET, Cowey A: Topography of the retina and striate cortex and its relationship to visual acuity in rhesus and squirrel monkeys, *Exp Brain Res* 10:298, 1970.
37. Schade OH Sr: Optical and photoelectric analog of the eye, *J Opt Soc Am* 46:721, 1956.
38. Shimoyo S, Held R: Vernier acuity is less than grating acuity in 2- and 3-month-olds, *Vision Res* 17:77, 1977.
39. Shlaer S: The relation between visual acuity and illumination, *J Gen Physiol* 21:165, 1937.
40. Sloan LL: Measurement of visual acuity, *Arch Ophthalmol* 45:704, 1951.
41. Sloan LL: Congenital achromatopsia: a report of 19 cases, *J Opt Soc Am* 44:117, 1954.
42. Sloan LL, Rowland WM, Altman A: Comparison of three types of test target for the measurement of visual acuity, *Q Rev Ophthalmol* 8:4, 1952.
43. Snell AC, Sterling S: Percentage evaluation of macular vision, *Arch Ophthalmol* 54:443, 1925.
44. Van Nes FL, Bouman MA: Spatial modulation transfer in the human eye, *J Opt Soc Am* 57:401, 1967.
45. Wertheim T: Uber die indirekte Sehschärfe, *Z Psychol* 7:172, 1894.

46. Westheimer G: Modulation thresholds for sinusoidal light distributions on the retina, *J Physiol* 152:67, 1960.

47. Westheimer G: Visual acuity, *Ann Rev Psychol* 16:359, 1965.

48. Westheimer G: Optical properties of vertebrate eyes. In Fuortes M (ed): *Handbook of sensory physiology,* vol 7/2, *Physiology of photoreceptor organs,* Berlin, 1972, Springer-Verlag.

49. Westheimer G: The scaling of visual acuity measurements, *Arch Ophthalmol* 97:327, 1979.

50. Westheimer G: The spatial sense of the eye, Proctor Lecture, *Invest Ophthalmol Vis Sci* 18:893, 1979.

51. Westheimer G: The spatial grain of the perifoveal retina, *Vision Res* 22:157, 1982.

52. Westheimer G: The Prentice Lecture, visual acuity and hyperacuity: resolution, localization, form, *Am J Optom Physiol Optics* 64:567, 1987.

53. Westheimer G, Hauske G: Temporal and spatial interference with vernier acuity, *Vision Res* 15:1137, 1975.

54. Westheimer G, Liang J: Evaluating diffusion of light in the eye by objective means, *Invest Ophthalmol Vis Sci* 35:2652, 1994.

55. Westheimer G, Liang J: Influence of light scatter on the eye's optical performance, *J Opt Soc Am A* 12:1417, 1995.

56. Westheimer G, McKee SP: Visual acuity in the presence of retinal-image motion, *J Opt Soc Am* 65:847, 1975.

57. Westheimer G, Pettet MW: Contrast and duration of exposure differentially affect vernier and stereoscopic acuity, *Proc R Soc London B* 241:42, 1990.

58. Weston HC: The relationship between illumination and visual efficiency—the effect of brightness contrast, MRC Industrial Health Research Board, Report No 87, London, 1945, HMSO.

59. Weymouth FW: The effect of age on visual acuity. In Hirsch MJ, Wick RE (eds): *Vision of the aging patient,* Radnor, Pa, 1960, Chilton.

60. Weymouth FW et al: Visual acuity within the area centralis and its relation to eye movements and fixation, *Am J Ophthalmol* 11:947, 1928.

61. Wiesel TN, Hubel DH: Single-cell responses in striate cortex of kittens deprived of vision in one eye, *J Neurophysiol* 26:1003, 1963.

62. Wilcox WW: The basis of the dependence of visual acuity on illumination, *Proc Natl Acad Sci USA* 18:47, 1932.

63. Wülfing EA: Über den kleinsten Gesichtswinkel, *Z Biol* 29:199, 1892.

EARLY VISUAL PROCESSING OF SPATIAL FORM

DAVID REGAN

FIVE WAYS OF BREAKING CAMOUFLAGE

The human visual system can segregate an object from its surroundings (i.e., break an object's camouflage) in five ways. Normally sighted individuals can see an object and process its spatial characteristics if it differs sufficiently from its surroundings in any one of the following five respects: luminance, color, texture, motion, and binocular disparity. In this sense the human visual system contains five distinct subsystems for processing the spatial characteristics of objects.

The luminance-contrast subsystem does not have a special advantage, except in the case of very fine detail; apart from this special situation, when spatial sampling (i.e., the number of texture elements per degree of subtense) is matched, all the spatial discrimination thresholds that have been reported are little, if at all, different for texture-defined, motion-defined, disparity-defined, and luminance-defined forms.[49] However, because most basic and clinical research on the processing of spatial form has been restricted to spatial form that is rendered visible by being brighter or dimmer than its surroundings, this review focuses mainly on luminance contrast.

EARLY VISUAL PROCESSING OF LUMINANCE-DEFINED OBJECTS

Low-, Medium-, and High-Contrast Letter Acuity

High-contrast letter charts are called *Snellen charts*. There are many kinds of Snellen charts, one of which is shown as Figure 18-1, *A*. The smaller the letters that can be read, the better the (high-contrast) visual acuity. It is conventional to regard 20/20 (i.e., 6/6 or

1.0) acuity as the norm. However, mean acuity in control subjects is somewhat better than 20/20, although to assess acuities better than 20/20 it is necessary to have very sharp letters, and some projector displays fail in this respect.[18,75] High-contrast letter acuity is reduced not only by refractive errors (myopia, hyperopia, astigmatism) but also by several pathway disorders, including amblyopia, optic neuritis, and macular degeneration.

It was once assumed that an ability to read small high-contrast letters meant that foveal vision was satisfactory. During the last 25 years, however, studies using low-contrast test stimuli such as gratings (see later discussion) and letters have shown this assumption to be invalid.[25,40,44] A comparison of low-contrast letter acuity chart results with the results of a sine wave grating test in a group of patients with neuroophthalmologic disorders showed good agreement. Both tests picked up visual loss in patients with normal Snellen acuities.[58] Figure 18-1, *B*, shows a Regan low-contrast letter acuity chart that differs from the high-contrast chart in Figure 18-1, *A*, in that letter contrast is less than 100%. Figure 18-2, *A* and *C*, shows the way in which visual acuity varies with letter contrast in a young and an older group of control subjects. Note the considerable individual variation within each group.

An indication that a patient has a visual pathway dysfunction (as distinct from a refractive disorder) is that the ratio between acuity scores on high- and low-contrast letter charts is more than 2.5 standard deviations from the mean ratio for a group of age-matched control subjects. This indication has been reported in patients with a variety of ophthalmologic and neuroophthalmologic disorders, includ-

Z R D O V C N S

H R V C O S K Z 2

N D C O H R V S   3

K V R Z C O H S   4

Z N V K D S O R   5

D C R V H N Z K   6

O S K C V R Z N   7

S N H K C D V O   8

N R D C O K S Z   9

V H C O R Z D N   10

H R O S C V K N   11

A

FIGURE 18-1   Regan high- and low-contrast visual acuity charts. Letter size increases by a constant fraction (1.26:1) in successive ascending rows so that letter size doubles every third line. Thus a fall in acuity of, say, one line means the same thing, whatever the observer's initial visual acuity. The third line from the bottom has letters that subtend 5 minutes of arc when viewed from 20 feet (approximately 6 m). An observer who can read this line from 20 feet (or 6 m) is said to have 20/20 (or 6/6 in metric measure, or 1.0 decimal) visual acuity. If the smallest letters that can be read from a distance of 20 feet (or 6 m) by a particular observer are twice the size of those on the 20/20 line and could be read from 40 feet by a second observer with 20/20 acuity, the first observer is said to have 20/40 acuity. The five letter charts have contrast of 100%, 50%, 25%, 11%, and 4%. **A,** High-contrast chart. (From Regan D: *Clin Vis Sci* 2:235, 1988.)

B

FIGURE 18-1, CONT'D   Regan high- and low-contrast visual acuity charts. Letter size increases by a constant fraction (1.26:1) in successive ascending rows so that letter size doubles every third line. Thus a fall in acuity of, say, one line means the same thing, whatever the observer's initial visual acuity. The third line from the bottom has letters that subtend 5 minutes of arc when viewed from 20 feet (approximately 6 m). An observer who can read this line from 20 feet (or 6 m) is said to have 20/20 (or 6/6 in metric measure, or 1.0 decimal) visual acuity. If the smallest letters that can be read from a distance of 20 feet (or 6 m) by a particular observer are twice the size of those on the 20/20 line and could be read from 40 feet by a second observer with 20/20 acuity, the first observer is said to have 20/40 acuity. The five letter charts have contrast of 100%, 50%, 25%, 11%, and 4%. **B,** Low-contrast chart. (From Regan D: *Clin Vis Sci* 2:235, 1988.)

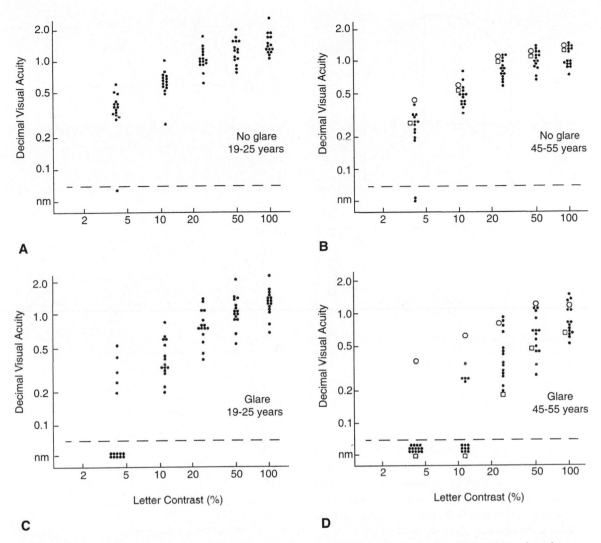

FIGURE 18-2 Effect of glare on low- and high-contrast letter acuity. Decimal visual acuity (ordinate) is plotted versus letter contrast (abscissa) without glare and with glare for 15 control subjects aged 19 to 25 years (**A** and **B**) and for 15 control subjects aged 45 to 55 years (**C** and **D**). Viewing was monocular, and one eye per subject was tested. Each symbol represents one eye. In the 45 to 55 age group, the *open circle* marks the eye least affected by glare and the *open square* marks the eye most affected by glare. (From Regan D: *Optom Vis Sci* 68:489, 1991.)

ing diabetes, amblyopia, multiple sclerosis, and Parkinson's disease.[58,59]

Glare Susceptibility

For many individuals the ability to see objects of low and moderate contrast fails in high-glare situations, such as when driving into low sun or at night on crowded roads, walking on a summer beach, or even being in a white-walled bathroom.[1,14,38,80] Especially on the road, this is a potent cause of accidents. The problem is caused by light scattering within the eye and thereby reducing the contrast of the retinal image. A notorious consequence of early

cataract is an increase in glare susceptibility, but susceptibility varies considerably even among normally sighted individuals, and as shown in Figure 18-2, *B* and *D*, some 19 to 25-year-old individuals show high susceptibility.[47,81]

Susceptibility can be quantified in terms of the glare susceptibility ratio (GSR), defined as visual acuity with no glare source divided by visual acuity in the presence of a standard glare source.[47] This index provides a direct impression of the effect of glare. For example, suppose the GSR were 5 for a letter chart of 10% contrast. This would imply that, for the amount of glare used in the test, a car of 10% contrast, when

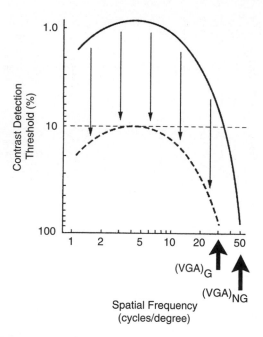

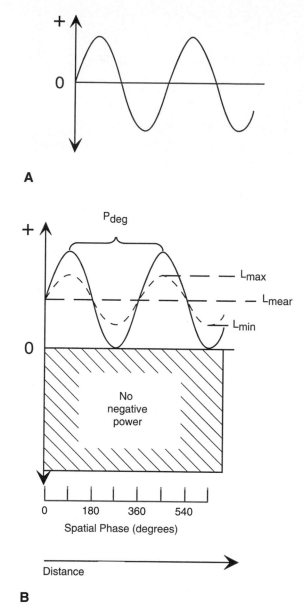

FIGURE 18-3   The shape of the contrast sensitivity function explains why moderate glare causes objects of moderate contrast to be invisible while having little effect on visual acuity. *G*, With glare; *NG*, no glare; *VGA*, visual grating acuity. (From Regan D, et al: *Ophthalmol Physiol Optom* 13:115, 1993.)

---

seen against a road that could be seen at 1000 m in low-glare conditions, would not be seen until it was 200 m away in high-glare conditions. A similar method was developed independently by Bailey and Bullimore.[5] Elliot and Bullimore[15] compare different methods for assessing glare susceptibility.

Figure 18-3 shows that the reason glare can render low-contrast objects invisible while having comparatively little effect on visual acuity is no more than a straightforward consequence of the shape of the contrast sensitivity function.

The causes of glare susceptibility include lens opacities, light entering through the iris (especially for those with blue eyes), and corneal scarring.[14,38,80] Note that the slit-lamp technique for examining lens opacities is based on light scattered back from lens opacities, whereas the disabling effect of glare is caused by the light that is scattered forward onto the retina. Consequently, slit-lamp examination does not necessarily indicate the degree of glare disability experienced by individual patients.[16,17,61]

The (Luminance) Contrast Sensitivity Function

Figure 18-4 shows how luminance varies across the bars of a sinusoidal grating for which *spatial (luminance) contrast* is defined as $100(L_{max} - L_{min})/(L_{max} +$

FIGURE 18-4   A sine wave grating. **A,** A sine wave is as often negative as positive. **B,** The variation of luminance across the bars of a sinewave grating follows a sine wave superimposed on a steady level. The *continuous line* is for a grating of 100% contrast. The *broken line* is for a grating of about 50% contrast.

L_{min}) and can range from 0% to 100%. Figure 18-4 also depicts the *period* (P deg) of the grating. Provided the grating contains a sufficient number of complete cycles (five is a rule of thumb), the *spatial frequency* of the grating is approximately equal to P^{-1} cycles/degree. For caveats, see Regan.[49]

The dashed line in Figure 18-5, *A,* shows a typical plot of the contrast required to render the bars

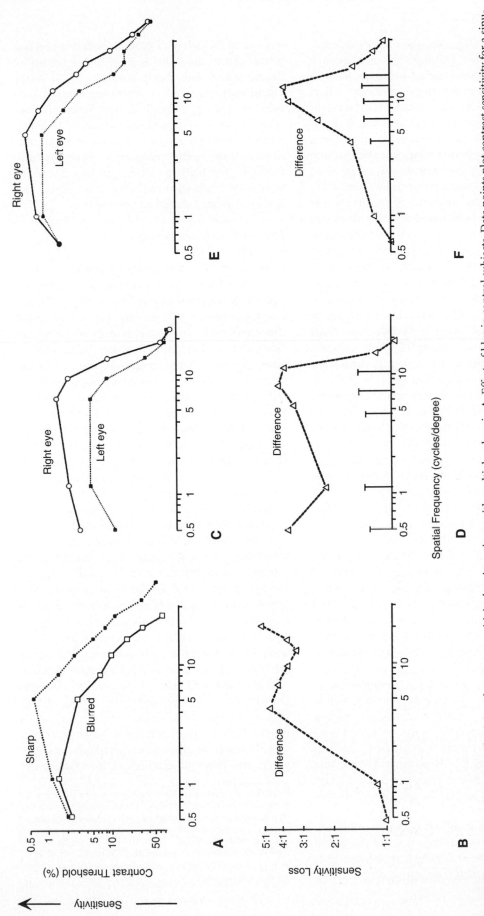

Figure 18-5 Spatial-frequency selectivity of contrast-sensitivity loss in patients with multiple sclerosis. **A,** Effect of blur in control subjects. Data points plot contrast sensitivity for a sinusoidal grating (ordinate) versus the grating's spatial frequency with the grating sharply accommodated (*solid symbols*) and with the retinal image blurred by viewing through a +1 diopter lens (*open symbols*). Data are means for 19 eyes. **B,** Difference between the *continuous* and *dotted lines* in panel **A. C,** Data points plot contrast sensitivity for the left (*solid symbols*) and right (*open symbols*) eyes of a patient with multiple sclerosis. **D,** The difference curve reveals selective loss at low and intermediate spatial frequencies, the mirror image of the pattern of loss in panel **B. E,** Data points plot contrast sensitivity for the left (*solid symbols*) and right (*open symbols*) eyes of a patient with multiple sclerosis. **F,** The difference curve reveals bandpass selective loss at intermediate spatial frequencies. The heavy T-shaped bars in panels **D** and **F** show data obtained from 29 control subjects. They indicate the standard deviations of the difference between contrast sensitivities in the left and right eye. (From Regan D, Silver R, Murray TJ: *Brain* 100:563, 1977.)

of a grating just visible (i.e., the *contrast detection threshold*) versus the grating's spatial frequency. This plot is called the *contrast sensitivity function* (CSF). It is considerably more informative than Snellen acuity because Snellen acuity expresses sensitivity to fine detail only, whereas the CSF expresses sensitivity to coarse and intermediate detail as well as sensitivity to fine detail. The Pelli-Robson letter chart offers a convenient way of assessing contrast sensitivity over a range of low spatial frequencies.[40] The spatial frequency of a grating whose patterning can just be detected at 100% contrast is called *grating acuity*. It is 35 to 50 cycles/degree at everyday photopic levels of illumination.[11,70,82] High grating acuity is requisite for high Snellen acuity.

Figure 18-5, *A* and *B*, depicts a loss of contrast sensitivity that is selective for high spatial frequencies. This pattern of loss can be caused by refractive error that blurs the retinal image or by retinal and visual pathway disorders and is associated with a reduction of Snellen acuity. Figure 18-5, *C* and *D*, illustrates a mirror-image pattern of loss that spares Snellen acuity. This unusual pattern has been reported in patients with multiple sclerosis.[62] Figure 18-5, *E*, depicts contrast sensitivity loss that extends over a broad range of spatial frequencies and spares Snellen acuity. The contrast sensitivity loss may be selective for grating orientation.[63] The visual world of a patient with such a loss is distorted as distinct from its being blurred. This pattern of loss can result in a curiosity: A patient's ability to read letters of a certain size can be improved by moving *farther away* from the test chart.[64]

Although examples of the extreme patterns depicted in Figure 18-5, *C* and *E*, have been reported in patients with neurologic disorders, it is unclear whether, taken together with commonly observed reduction of visual acuity (i.e., reduction of contrast sensitivity at high spatial frequencies), they represent three different types of loss or merely extremes of a continuum.[7,8]

A kind of sharply notched loss of contrast sensitivity is observed in some control subjects, as well as in some patients. It is caused by monocular diplopia rather than by a visual pathway dysfunction. It is selective for grating orientation, as can be the loss depicted in Figure 18-5, *E*.[2,57] However, it differs in that the kind of loss shown in Figure 18-5, *E*, can vary over the visual field and can be selective for temporal frequency.[9,57]

The just-noticeable difference between the spatial frequencies of two gratings is called the *spatial frequency discrimination threshold*. At high contrasts it remains approximately constant (at about 5%) up to a spatial frequency of 20 to 30 cycles/degree, and it has risen to only 13% at 50 cycles/degree before discrimination fails precipitously.[12,27,66,74] It is approximately independent of grating contrast provided the grating is clearly visible.[65] A selective loss of sensitivity to low spatial frequencies (e.g., associated with multiple sclerosis) produces a substantial elevation of spatial frequency discrimination threshold for high spatial frequencies for which there is no sensitivity loss.[65] The vision of such patients is distorted as distinct from blurred.

Spatial Fourier Analysis and Spatial Filters

A perusal of the vision research literature can leave one confused about the significance of spatial Fourier analysis for understanding the functioning of the human visual system. It is certainly true that the spatial characteristics of any spatial pattern of luminance can be described in terms of a power spectrum and a phase spectrum, that the spatial-domain and spatial-frequency-domain descriptions are complementary, and that this fact is central to a branch of optical physics.*,[49] For our present purpose, the crucial fact is that the phase spectrum is essential when describing a complex image such as a face (Figure 1-20 in Regan[49] illustrates this point). In addition, psychophysical evidence indicates that the human visual system does not encode the phase spectrum; rather, it encodes the spatial pattern of local contrast.[3,4,10]

Rather than thinking in terms of the Fourier transform of the retinal image when attempting to understand the functioning of the human visual system, it is useful to regard the earliest stage of processing the spatial attributes of an object as a parallel array of spatial filters, each of which passes a limited range of spatial frequencies and orientations and has a strictly local receptive field. From this point of view, the contrast sensitivity function (see Figure 18-5, *A*) can be regarded as the envelope of many narrow subunits.[6,13] Filters of narrow spatial width determine sensitivity to gratings of high spatial frequencies and support visual acuity; wider filters support visual sensitivity to intermediate spatial frequencies; the widest spatial filters support visual sensitivity to gratings of low spatial fre-

---

*Note that any given spatial frequency component is determined by the entire image being analyzed. Thus it incorrect to state that high spatial frequency information is located at sharp edges. In addition, because the luminance profile of a sine wave grating is not a sine wave (Figure 18-4 illustrates that the profile is a sine wave superimposed on a constant level), it is not correct to say that any given spatial pattern can be synthesized by superimposing sine wave gratings.

quency. The output of each filter carries three labels: its location, its preferred orientation, and its preferred spatial frequency.[71,76]

In effect, these spatial filters perform parallel analyses of the retinal image at a fine scale (fine detail), intermediate scale (medium detail), and coarse scale (coarse detail). It has been proposed that the visual losses illustrated in Figure 18-5, *C* and *E,* can be understood in terms of selective functional damage to large- and medium-width filters, respectively. It is widely supposed that the physiologic basis for these psychophysical filters is the spatial filtering properties of cortical neurons.

Evidence that the sensitivity profile of first-stage spatial filters follows a "Mexican-hat" shape has been obtained by using an aperiodic test stimulus such as a single thin line superimposed on either subthreshold flanking lines or a subthreshold grating.[26,33,86] The solid circles in Figure 18-6 show results from an experiment in which thresholds for a central line were measured as a function of the position of a pair of flanking lines (see inset).[86] When the flanking lines were within about 0.05 degree of the central test line, sensitivity was greatly increased; however, when the flanking lines were between 0.05 to 0.20 degree of the test line, a sensitivity reduction (indicative of inhibition) occurred. According to Wilson,[87] each small retinal area is served by a parallel array of at least 72 orientation-tuned spatial filters with Mexican-hat sensitivity profiles; there are at least 6 widths of filter for each of about 12 different preferred orientations.

The Mexican-hat sensitivity profile has the property of being insensitive to a uniform luminance. The outputs of a parallel array of such filters approximate the second spatial derivative of luminance, that is, the spatial variation of local contrast across an image. (A minimally mathematical explanation of this point is offered on pp. 145 to 149 in Regan.[49])

Hyperacuities

The shortest distance between the centers of foveal cones is approximately 25 arcsec (i.e., 0.007 degree of visual angle). This determines the limit of visual resolution. It has long been known that several visual discriminations can transcend this limit. For example, the best values of vernier step acuity can be as low as 2 to 5 arcsec, up to 10 times less than the distance between foveal cones. Westheimer[83,84] termed these discriminations *hyperacuities.* They include line separation discrimination, bisection acuity, and for short lines, orientation discrimina-

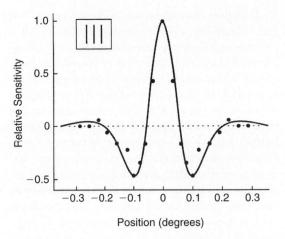

FIGURE 18-6   Data from an experiment measuring subthreshold summation between a center line and two flanking lines. The data show a central excitatory zone with inhibitory zones on either side. (From Wilson HR: *Vision Res* 18:971, 1978.)

tion. They are based on the pattern of activity among excited neurons.

It is well known that the just-noticeable difference in wavelength is far less than the range of wavelengths to which any of the three cone types responds. In this sense, wavelength (hue) discrimination is also a kind of hyperacuity. In this same sense, orientation discrimination and spatial frequency discrimination are also kinds of hyperacuity because their discrimination threshold (0.2 to 0.6 degree and roughly 5%) are far less than the orientation and spatial frequency tuning band width of first-stage spatial filters. A proposed explanation for this discrepancy is that the discriminations are based on the relative activity among populations of neurons that prefer different orientation and different spatial frequencies, respectively, and that this relative activity is extracted at opponent-orientation and opponent-size stages of processing.[12,85] Experimental evidence consistent with this idea has been reported.[41,50,52]

Early Visual Processing of Two-Dimensional Images

All of the research reviewed so far was restricted to visual processing along one dimension (e.g., perpendicular to the bars of a grating). In an early study on the processing of two-dimensional form, Kelly and Magnuski[32] compared contrast detection thresholds for circular targets with thresholds for gratings. They concluded that the visual processing of a two-dimensional pattern is not a linear, isotropic, homogeneous process.

A further indication that a knowledge of the early processing of one-dimensional stimuli such as gratings and Gabor patterns is insufficient to understand the early processing of two-dimensional stimuli is that individuals can discriminate trial-to-trial variations in the aspect ratio of a rectangle or ellipse when the area of the target is subjected to large trial-to-trial variations so as to remove either height or width as a reliable cue to the task.[54] The conclusion was that the human visual system contains a neural mechanism that is sensitive to the aspect ratio of a figure somewhat independently of its area. This finding could not have been predicted from a knowledge of visual responses to one-dimensional variations of luminance. Experimental psychophysical research on the early processing of two-dimensional form is still in its infancy.

MOTION-DEFINED FORM

Figure 18-7, *A,* illustrates a camouflaged stationary spatial letter. The letter can be rendered visible by moving the texture elements within it at a different velocity to the texture elements outside it. Figure 18-7, *C* and *D,* illustrates that if the two sets of texture elements move at different speeds or in different directions, the letter is rendered visible in a photograph by orientation-texture contrast. Presumably,

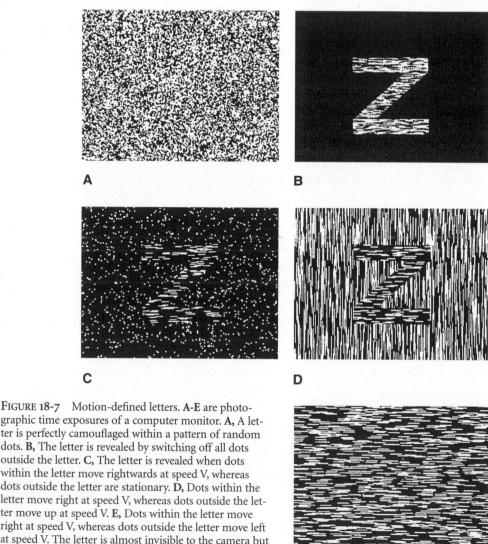

FIGURE 18-7   Motion-defined letters. **A-E** are photographic time exposures of a computer monitor. **A,** A letter is perfectly camouflaged within a pattern of random dots. **B,** The letter is revealed by switching off all dots outside the letter. **C,** The letter is revealed when dots within the letter move rightwards at speed V, whereas dots outside the letter are stationary. **D,** Dots within the letter move right at speed V, whereas dots outside the letter move up at speed V. **E,** Dots within the letter move right at speed V, whereas dots outside the letter move left at speed V. The letter is almost invisible to the camera but is clearly evident when viewed by normally sighted individuals. (From Regan D, et al: *J Neurosci* 12:2198, 1992.)

the finite integration times of cortical neurons tuned to line length and orientation would support a similar process in the human visual system. However, when the texture elements move in opposite directions at the same speed, the letter is almost invisible to the camera (Figure 18-7, *E*), although clearly seen by normally sighted observers. This observation is the basis of a letter-reading test in which the patient is required to read 10 different letters presented in a random fashion; all letters are presented with the same dot speed. The test is repeated at progressively slower dot speeds.[55,56] A psychometric function can then be obtained by plotting the percentage of letters read correctly versus the dot speed. Letter-reading performance can be defined as the dot speed that gives a score halfway between chance (10%) and 100% correct.

The test assesses the visual subsystem for motion-defined form rather than the subsystem for luminance-defined form that is assessed by luminance-defined test patterns such as high- and low-contrast letter charts.

The (motion) contrast sensitivity function for motion-defined form does not extend to such high spatial frequencies as the (luminance) contrast sensitivity function shown in Figure 18-5, *A*; sensitivity falls off as spatial frequency is increased beyond about 0.1 cycle/degree and grating acuity is little higher than 5 cycles/degree.[39] Psychophysical evidence has been reported that the human visual system contains filters sensitive to the spatial frequency of motion-defined form.[28]

Motion-defined bars or rectangles can be created along the lines illustrated in Figure 7, *E*. Vernier step acuity for motion-defined form was reported to be 27 to 45 arcsec,[42] considerably smaller than the 120 arc second dot size, 360 arc second mean dot separation, and 3600 arc second estimated summation field diameter for detectors of motion-defined form.[39,51,68] One proposed explanation for the perceived sharpness and the high acuity for the relative location of a motion-defined boundary is that they are both determined by the pattern of activity among an array of receptive fields that serve different locations along a line perpendicular to the boundary, a neural mechanism that would have an extensive summation field.[42,43] By definition, if a linear system responds strongly to an isolated sharp edge, it follows that the system will respond strongly to a grating of high spatial frequency. Therefore the neural edge-sharpening process that underlies vernier acuity is nonlinear. In this case the nonlinearity manifests itself as a disrup-

tion of edge-sharpening function when more than one motion-defined boundary falls within the summation field of the edge-sharpening mechanism.[46]

Orientation discrimination threshold for a dotted motion-defined bar can be as low as 0.5 degree, and aspect ratio discrimination for a dotted motion-defined rectangle can be as low as 2%, both discriminations being closely similar to the corresponding discrimination for a dotted luminance-defined bar or rectangle.[45,53] A 2% aspect ratio discrimination threshold for a rectangle of area 0.47 degree* implies that the precision of estimating both height and width was about 30 arcsec, close to the foveal cone separation of about 25 arcsec.

The motion-defined letter-reading test can pick up visual dysfunction that is hidden to both high- and low-contrast charts of luminance-defined letters. Brain lesions in the parietotemporal lobe can produce a selective loss of ability to read motion-defined letters, a loss that spares visual acuity and even spares sensitivity to motion per se. Brain lesions in other brain regions have no such effect.[66] A selective loss of ability to read motion-defined letters that spares visual acuity seems to be common in patients with multiple sclerosis and in both the treated and "clinically normal" eyes of unilateral amblyopes.[19,20]

TEXTURE-DEFINED FORM

Figure 18-8, *A* illustrates 1 of 10 texture-defined letters. Its visibility can be reduced by adding 1 randomly placed "noise" dot per texture line (Figure 18-8, *B*) and can still further reduced by adding 2 noise dots per line (Figure 18-8, *C*), and so on, up to 11 noise dots. A psychometric function can be obtained by plotting the percentage of letters read correctly versus the number of noise dots. Letter-reading performance can be defined as the number of noise dots that give a score half way between chance (10% correct) and 100% correct. Reading performance has been described by a physiologically plausible model.[56]

The (texture) contrast sensitivity function is approximately flat from 0.07 to 4 cycles/degree, after which sensitivity declines progressively up to a

---

*Note, however, that this does not necessarily mean "at or beyond" primary visual cortex. Axons conducting from lateral geniculate body to cortex are outnumbered by axons that conduct in the reverse direction. In addition, most corticogeniculate cells receive input from both eyes, even though ascending retinal signals are strictly monocular.[35,73]

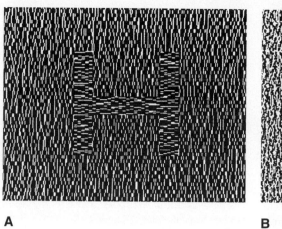

A

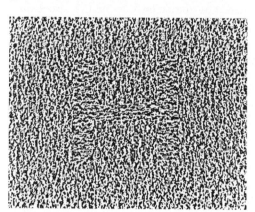

B

C

FIGURE 18-8   Texture-defined letters. **A,** Photograph of a letter whose visibility is created entirely by orientation texture. **B,** The letter's visibility is degraded by adding two randomly located noise dots per texture line. **C,** Letter visibility is further degraded by adding four noise dots per texture line. (From Regan D, Hong XH: *Biological Cybernetics* 72:389, 1995.)

grating acuity of a little beyond 7 cycles/degree. From 0.07 to 4 cycles/degree, spatial frequency discrimination threshold for a texture-defined grating is the same as for a luminance-defined grating of matched spatial sampling; although it is inferior beyond about 4 cycles, discrimination does not fail until beyond 9 cycles/degree.[22] Vernier step acuity and bisection acuity are only a little inferior to the corresponding acuities for luminance-defined form (providing that spatial sampling is matched) up to about 18 texture lines/degree.[21] Psychophysical evidence has been reported that the human visual system contains filters that are selective for the orientation of texture-defined form.[34] Vernier step and bisection acuities are considerably sharper than would be expected from the (texture) contrast sensitivity curve, as is the case for luminance-defined and motion-defined form. Orientation discrimination threshold for a texture-defined bar is approximately 0.6 degree, and aspect ratio discrimination threshold for a texture-defined rectangle can be as low as 2.5%, both thresholds being little, if at all, in-

ferior to the corresponding thresholds for luminance-defined form, providing that spatial sampling is matched.[4,34,48,60,67]

Although texture-defined form recognition tests, such as the texture-defined letter-reading test, have seen little clinical use to date, it has been reported that in patients with multiple sclerosis, the test can detect visual dysfunction that is hidden to high- and low-contrast luminance-defined letter tests and to the motion-defined letter test.[60]

DISPARITY-DEFINED FORM

Julesz[29,30] introduced the random-dot stereogram to vision research. Through the left eye alone, one sees a pattern of random dots. With the right eye alone, one sees a pattern of random dots. However, in binocularly fused vision, camouflage is broken and one sees spatial form (e.g., a square) floating in front of (or behind) the surrounding dot pattern. Because the camouflaged square is not visible through either eye alone, it must be detected at a processing stage after convergence of information from left and right eyes.* This kind of vision has been called *cyclopean*.[29,30]

It remains to be shown, however, that the binocular processing thus isolated provides us with an accurate picture of binocular processing in everyday vision, where spatial forms are usually not camouflaged to monocular vision.[69]

It is sometimes said that random-dot stereograms demonstrate that disparity processing precedes the processing of the camouflaged spatial form. However, this is not necessarily correct. In principle, the camouflaged form can be detected by neurons that are insensitive to disparity and merely sum the signals from the two eyes. (Try superimposing the two images of a stereopair.) Signals from such neurons might simplify the task of extracting the camouflaged form (i.e., the "correspondence problem") faced by disparity-sensitive neurons and would render moot the question of whether form is processed before or after disparity.

Tyler[77] used cyclopean grating to show that the (cyclopean) contrast sensitivity curve is restricted to low spatial frequencies and that cyclopean grating acuity is only 2 to 3 cycles/degree. There is psychophysical evidence that the human visual system contains filters selective for the spatial frequency and orientation of cyclopean form.[31,72,78,79] Morgan[36] showed that vernier step acuity for cyclopean targets is 40 arcsec similar to that for luminance-defined form of matched spatial sampling and considerably better than would be expected from the cyclopean contrast sensitivity curve. In principle, this disagreement can be explained along the same lines as the corresponding problem for motion-defined form discussed earlier.

Aspect ratio discrimination threshold for a cyclopean rectangle can be as low as 3%, little different from that for a luminance-defined rectangle of matched spatial sampling. For a cyclopean rectangle of area 1 degree,* this threshold corresponds to a precision of 1.0 arc minute in encoding the rectangle's width and height, again considerably more precise than would be expected from the (disparity) contrast sensitivity function. Orientation discrimination threshold for a cyclopean bar can be as low as 0.5 degree. This not only is similar to orientation

discrimination threshold for a luminance-defined bar of matched spatial sampling but also compares well with the best threshold reported for luminance-defined form.[24,37]

Although stereoscopic depth perception enables animals to break the camouflage of their otherwise well-camouflaged prey, an absence of this ability seems to have few consequences for modern humans other than, perhaps, a difficulty in judging the time to collision with a rotating nonspherical object.[23] In contrast, inability to achieve binocular single vision (diplopia) can be disabling.

SUMMARY

Perhaps the major role of the human visual system is to support the ability to see an object, that is, to segregate an object from its surroundings by breaking its camouflage. Normally sighted individuals can see an object and process its spatial characteristics if it differs sufficiently from its surroundings in any one of the following five respects: luminance, color, texture, motion, or binocular disparity. In this sense the human visual system contains five distinct subsystems for processing the spatial characteristics of objects. Clinical tests of visual capability are currently almost entirely restricted to the luminance-contrast subsystem. Over the last 20 years it has become clear that retinal and visual pathway disfunction can usefully be distinguished from front-of-the-eye disorders by complementing the use of high-contrast (Snellen charts) with low-contrast charts so as to aid differential diagnosis in a variety of ophthalmologic and neuroophthalmologic disorders. Low-contrast charts are also effective in quantifying the susceptibility to glare of, for example, normally sighted individual drivers as well as patients with early cataract. Although clinical studies are comparatively sparse, evidence has been reported that, in amblyopia and multiple sclerosis, a patient's ability to read motion-defined and texture-defined letters can provide information that complements that provided by the results of luminance-defined letter tests.

ACKNOWLEDGMENTS

I thank Derek Harnanansingh for assistance in the preparation of this manuscript. David Regan holds the NSERC/CAE Industrial Research Chair in Vision and Aviation. This effort is sponsored by the Air Force Office of Science Research, Air Force Material Command, USAF, under grant number F40620-97-1-0051.

---

*Note, however, that this does not necessarily mean "at or beyond" primary visual cortex. Axons conducting from lateral geniculate body to cortex are outnumbered by axons that conduct in the reverse direction. In addition, most corticogeniculate cells receive input from both eyes, even though ascending retinal signals are strictly monocular.[35,73]

REFERENCES

1. Allen MJ, Vos JJ: Ocular scattered light and visual performance as a function of age, *Am J Optom Arch Am Acad Optom* 44;717, 1967.

2. Apkarian P et al: Origin of notches in the CSF: optical or neural? *Invest Ophthalmol Vis Sci* 28:608, 1987.

3. Badcock DR: How do we discriminate relative phase? *Vision Res* 24:1847, 1984.

4. Badcock DR: Spatial phase or luminance profile description? *Vision Res* 24:613, 1984.

5. Bailey IL, Bullimore MA: A new test of disability glare, *Optom Vis Sci* 68:911, 1991.

6. Blakemore C, Campbell FW: On the existence of neurons in the human visual system selectively sensitive to the orientation and size of retinal images, *J Physiol* 203:237, 1969.

7. Bodis-Wollner I: Visual acuity and contrast sensitivity in patients with cerebral lesions, *Science* 178:769, 1972.

8. Bodis-Wollner I, Diamond S: The measurements of spatial contrast sensitivity in cases of blurred vision associated with cerebral lesions, *Brain* 99:695, 1976.

9. Bodis-Wollner I, Regan D: Spatiotemporal contrast vision in Parkinson's disease and MPTP-treated monkeys: the role of dopamine. In Regan D (ed): *Spatial vision,* London, 1991, MacMillan.

10. Burr D: Sensitivity to spatial phase, *Vision Res* 20:391, 1980.

11. Campbell FW, Green DG: Optical and retinal factors affecting visual resolution, *J Physiol* 181:576, 1965.

12. Campbell FW, Nachmias J, Jukes J: Spatial frequency discrimination in human vision, *J Optic Soc Am* 60:555, 1970.

13. Campbell FW, Robson JG: Application of Fourier analysis to the visibility of gratings, *J Physiol* 197:551, 1968.

14. DeWaard PWT et al: Intraocular light scattering in age-related cataracts, *Invest Ophthalmol Vis Sci* 33:618, 1992.

15. Elliott DB, Bullimore MA: Assessing the reliability, discriminative ability and validity of disability glare tests, *Invest Ophthalmol Vis Sci* 34:108, 1993.

16. Elliott DB, Gilchrist J, Whitaker D: Contrast sensitivity and glare sensitivity changes with three types of cataract morphology, *Ophthalmic and Physiological Optics* 9:25, 1989.

17. Elliott DB, Hurst MA, Weatherill J: Comparing clinical tests of visual loss in cataract patients using a quantification of forward light scatter, *Eye* 5:601, 1991.

18. Frisen L, Frisen M: How good is normal visual acuity? *Albrecht v. Graefes Arch Klin Ophthal* 215:149, 1981.

19. Giaschi D et al: Defective processing of motion-defined form in the fellow eye of patients with unilateral amblyopia, *Invest Ophthalmol Vis Sci* 33:2483, 1992.

20. Giaschi D et al: Motion-defined letter detection and recognition in patients with multiple sclerosis, *Ann Neurol* 31:621, 1992.

21. Gray R, Regan D: Vernier step acuity and bisection acuity for texture-defined form, *Vision Res* 37, 1713, 1997.

22. Gary R, Regan D: Spatial frequency discrimination and detection characteristics for gratings defined by orientation texture, *Vision Res* 38:2601, 1998.

23. Gray R, Regan D: Estimating time to collision with a rotating nonspherical object, *Vision Res* 40:49, 2000.

24. Hamstra SJ, Regan D: Orientation discrimination in cyclopean vision, *Vision Res* 35:365, 1995.

25. Hess RF, Plant GJ: The psychophysical loss in optic neuritis: spatial and temporal aspects. In Hess RF, Plant GT, (eds): *Optic neuritis,* Cambridge, Mass, 1986, Cambridge University Press.

26. Hines M: Line-spread function variation near the fovea, *Vision Res* 16:567, 1976.

27. Hirsch J, Hylton R: Limits of spatial frequency discrimination as evidence of neural interpolation, *J Optic Soc Am A* 2, 1170, 1982.

28. Hogervorst MA, Bradshaw MF, Eagle RA: Spatial frequency tuning for 3D corrugations from motion parallax, *Vision Res* 40:2149, 2000.

29. Julesz B: Binocular depth perception of computer-generated patterns, *Bell System Technical Journal* 39:1125, 1960.

30. Julesz B: *Foundations of Cyclopean perception,* Chicago, 1971, University of Chicago Press.

31. Julesz B, Miller JE: Independent spatial-frequency-tuned channels in binocular fusion and rivalry, *Perception* 4:125, 1975.

32. Kelly DH, Magnuski HS. Pattern detection and the two-dimensional Fourier transform: circular targets, *Vision Res* 15:911, 1975.

33. Kulikowski JJ, King-Smith PE: Spatial arrangements of line, edge, and grating detectors revealed by subthreshold summation, *Vision Res* 13:1455, 1973.

34. Kwan L, Regan D: Orientation-tuned spatial filters for texture-defined form, *Vision Res* 38:3849, 1998.

35. Marracco RT, McClurkin JW: Evidence for spatial structure in the cortical input to the monkey lateral geniculate nucleus, *Exp Brain Res* 59:50, 1985.

36. Morgan MJ: Positional acuity without monocular cues, *Perception* 15:157, 1986.

37. Mustillo P et al: Anisotropies in global stereoscopic orientation discrimination, *Vision Res* 28:1315, 1988.

38. Nadler MP, Miller D, Nadler NJ: *Glare and contrast sensitivity for clinicians,* New York, 1990, Springer.

39. Nakayama K, Tyler CW: Psychophysical isolation of movement sensitivity by removal of familiar position cues, *Vision Res* 231:427, 1981.

40. Pelli DG, Robson JG, Wilkins AJ: The design of a new letter chart for measuring contrast sensitivity, *Clin Vis Sci* 2: 187, 1988.

41. Regan D: Visual information channeling in normal and disordered vision, *Psychologic Rev* 89:407, 1982.

42. Regan D: Form from motion parallax and form from luminance contrast: vernier discrimination, *Spatial Vision* 1:305, 1986.

43. Regan D: Visual processing of four kinds of motion, *Vision Res* 26:127, 1986.

44. Regan D: Low contrast letter charts and sinewave grating tests in ophthalmological and neurological disorders, *Clin Vis Sci* 2:235, 1988.

45. Regan D: Orientation discrimination for objects defined by relative motion and objects defined by luminance contrast, *Vision Res* 29:1389, 1989.

46. Regan D: A brief review of some of the stimuli and analysis methods used in spatiotemporal vision research. In Regan D. (ed): *Spatial vision,* London, 1991, MacMillan.

47. Regan D: Specific tests and specific blindness: keys, locks, and parallel processing, *Optom Vis Sci* 68:489, 1991.

48. Regan D: Orientation discrimination threshold for bars defined by orientation texture, *Perception* 24:1131, 1995.

49. Regan D: *Human perception of objects: early visual processing of spatial form defined by luminance, color, texture, motion, and binocular disparity,* Sunderland, Mass, 2000, Sinauer.

50. Regan D, Beverley KI: Spatial frequency discrimination and detection: comparison of postadaption thresholds, *J Optic Soc Am* 73:1684, 1983.

51. Regan D, Beverley KI: Figure-ground segregation by motion contrast and by luminance contrast, *J Optic Soc Am A,* 1, 433, 1984.

52. Regan D, Beverley KI: Postadaptation orientation discrimination, *J Optic Soc Am* 2:147, 1985.

53. Regan D, Hamstra SJ: Shape discrimination for motion-defined and contrast-defined form: squareness is special, *Perception* 20: 315, 1991.

54. Regan D, Hamstra SJ: Shape discrimination and the judgment of perfect symmetry: dissociation of shape from size, *Vision Res* 32: 1845, 1992.

55. Regan D, Hong XH: Visual acuity for optotypes made visible by relative motion, *Optom Vis Sci* 67:49, 1990.

56. Regan D, Hong XH: Two models of the recognition and detection of texture-defined letters compared, *Biological Cybernetics* 72:389, 1995.

57. Regan D, Maxner C: Orientation-selective loss of contrast sensitivity for pattern and flicker in multiple sclerosis, *Clin Vis Sci* 1:1, 1987.

58. Regan D, Neima D: Low-contrast letter charts as a test of visual function, *Ophthalmology* 90:1992, 1983.

59. Regan D, Neima D: Low contrast letter charts in early diabetic retinopathy, ocular hypertension, glaucoma and Parkinson's disease, *Br J Ophthalmol* 68:885, 1984.

60. Regan D, Simpson TL: Multiple sclerosis can cause visual processing deficits specific to texture-defined form, *Neurology* 45:809, 1995.

61. Regan D et al: Measurement of glare sensitivity in cataract patients using low-contrast letter charts, *Ophthalmic and Physiological Optics* 13:115, 1993.

62. Regan D et al: Visual acuity and contrast sensitivity in multiple sclerosis-hidden visual loss: an auxiliary test for diagnostic use, *Brain* 100:563, 1977.

63. Regan D et al: Orientation-specific losses of contrast sensitivity in multiple sclerosis, *Invest Ophthalmol Vis Sci* 19:324, 1980.

64. Regan D et al: Contrast sensitivity, visual acuity and the discrimination of Snellen letters in multiple sclerosis, *Brain* 104:333, 1981.

65. Regan D et al: Spatial frequency discrimination in normal vision and in patients with multiple sclerosis, *Brain* 105:735, 1982.

66. Regan D et al: Visual processing of motion-defined form: selective failure in patients with parieto-temporal lesions, *J Neurosci* 12:2198, 1992.

67. Regan D et al: Two-dimensional aspect ratio discrimination and one-dimensional width and height discrimination for shape defined by orientation texture, *Vision Res* 36:3695, 1996.

68. Richards W: Motion detection in man and other animals, *Brain, Behaviour and Evolution* 4:162, 1975.

69. Richards W: Stereopsis with and without monocular contours, *Vision Res* 17:967, 1977.

70. Robson JG: Spatial and temporal contrast sensitivity functions of the human eye: *J Optic Soc Am* 56:1141, 1966.

71. Robson JG, Graham N: Probability summation and regional variation in contrast sensitivity across the visual field, *Vision Res* 21, 409, 1981.

72. Schumer RA, Ganz L: Independent stereoscopic channels for different extents of spatial pooling, *Vision Res* 19:1303, 1979.

73. Singer W: Control of thalamic transmission by corticofugal and ascending reticular pathways in the visual system, *Physiol Rev* 57:386, 1977.

74. Smallman et al: Fine grain of the neural representation of human spatial vision, *J Neurosci* 16:1852, 1996.

75. Taylor HR: Racial variations in vision, *Am J Epidemiol* 113:62, 1981.

76. Thomas JP, Gille J: Bandwidths of orientation channels in human vision, *J Optic Soc Am* 69, 652, 1979.

77. Tyler CW: Depth perception in disparity gratings, *Nature* 251:140, 1974.

78. Tyler CW: Stereoscopic tile and size aftereffects, *Perception* 4, 187, 1975.

79. Tyler CW: Sensory processing of binocular disparity. In Schor CM, Cuiffreda KJ (eds): *Vergence eye movements*, Boston, 1983, Butterworth.

80. Van den Berg TJTP: Importance of pathological light scatter for visual disability, *Documenta Ophthalmologica* 61:327, 1986.

81. Van den Berg TJTP: On the relation between glare and straylight, *Documenta Ophthalmoligica* 78:177, 1991.

82. Van Nes FL, Bouman M: Spatial modulation transfer in the human eye, *J Optic Soc Am* 57:401, 1967.

83. Westheimer G: Visual acuity and hyperacuity, *Invest Ophthalmol Vis Sci* 14, 570, 1975.

84. Westheimer G: The spatial sense of the eye, *Invest Ophthalmol Vis Sci* 18:893, 1979.

85. Westheimer G, Shimamura K, McKee, SP: Interference with line orientation sensitivity, *J Optic Soc Am* 66:332, 1976.

86. Wilson HR: Quantitative characterization of two types of line-spread function near the fovea, *Vision Res* 18:971, 1978.

87. Wilson HW: Psychophysical models of spatial vision and hyperacuity. In Regan D (ed): *Spatial vision*. London, 1991, MacMillan.

CHAPTER 19

BINOCULAR VISION

RONALD S. HARWERTH AND CLIFTON M. SCHOR

Humans and other animals with frontally located eyes attain binocular vision from the two retinal images through a series of sensory and motor processes that culminate in the perception of singleness and stereoscopic depth. Keen stereopsis is considered the paramount consequence of binocular vision because optimal performance depends on the normal functioning of all of the underlying vision processes, including central fixation with normal visual acuity in each eye, accurate oculomotor control to obtain bifoveal fixation, normal interretinal correspondence of visual directions, sensory mechanisms to produce haplopia (single vision), and neural mechanisms to extract selective depth signals from objects that are nearer or farther than the plane of fixation. Consequently, ordinary binocular vision represents a highly coordinated organization of motor and sensory processes, and if any component in the organization fails, binocular vision and stereopsis must be compromised to some extent. The causes and significance of abnormal binocular vision are the primary clinical emphasis, usually with a goal to alleviate any interference with clear, comfortable, single binocular vision. However, clinical applications must be established from an understanding of normal binocular vision. The topics included in this chapter provide the basic information on normal and abnormal binocular vision that forms the foundation for the clinical science of binocular vision.

TWO EYES ARE BETTER THAN ONE

It is obvious that an organism should gain an advantage by having two eyes rather than one. For example, it may be assumed that binocular vision is an important attribute because 75% to 80% of the neurons in primary visual cortex have inputs from both eyes.[6,74] There are also several functional advantages to having two frontal eyes.

1. The binocular field of view is larger than either monocular field.[57] The normal visual field for each eye extends to approximately 60 degrees superiorly, 60 degrees nasally, 75 degrees inferiorly, and 100 degrees temporally from fixation. Thus, with binocular viewing, the horizontal extent of the visual field is increased from 160 to 200 degrees, with a central 120 degrees of overlap, or superimposition, of the monocular visual fields.

2. Any image distortion caused by optical or pathologic defects in one eye can be masked by a normal image in the other eye. In general, the degree of dysfunction from bilateral eye diseases can be predicted from the performance of the less impaired eye.[96,98]

3. Pragmatically, having two eyes provides a resource to retain functional vision if an accident or disease causes the loss of sight of one eye.

4. Normal binocular vision improves functional vision by binocular summation and stereopsis. Binocular summation, the improvement in visual sensitivity with binocular viewing compared with monocular viewing, provides only a small increase in sensitivity when measured by threshold responses, but it may be a larger factor for performance measured with suprathreshold stimuli.[17,25,62,64] Stereopsis, on the other hand, is the quantitative and qualitative improvement in relative depth perception that occurs with binocular viewing. At its most elementary level, keen stereopsis benefits both the predator, at the point of attack, and the prey, by unmasking the camouflage of predators.[14]

Visual Direction

Ordinarily, a person is not aware that he or she is using two eyes, but rather, the person has an impression of viewing with one eye located about midway between the two eyes (the egocenter, or cyclopean eye). Thus the most basic concept of visual space involves the relationship between the locations of objects in physical space and their perceived (subjective) spatial locations.[101] These concepts are diagrammatically illustrated in Figure 19-1, which presents representations of physical space (see Figure 19-1, A) and subjective space (see Figure 19-1, B). Perceived directions of objects are based on several factors, including the retinal locations of their images. Each retinal image location is associated with a specific visual direction, called its *local sign* or *oculocentric direction*.[73,101] The primary visual direction is the oculocentric direction of an object that is fixated along the primary line of sight and is imaged on the center of the fovea (represented by the *diamond* in Figure 19-1). Secondary lines of sight are the oculocentric directions of other retinal image locations relative to the primary visual direction. As illustrated in Figure 19-1, the perceived visual directions of nonfixated objects (represented by the *circle* and *square*) are relative to the visual direction of a fixated object (represented by the *diamond*). For example, an image located to the left side of the fovea is perceived to the right of the fixated object (e.g., the visual direction of the square). The normal ability to distinguish differences in oculocentric directions is extremely accurate, as demonstrated by vernier alignment thresholds, which are on the order of 5 arcsec for foveal viewing.[86,157]

In a natural, dynamic world, objects are localized with respect to the head and body rather than to the line of sight; therefore retinal image information is not sufficient to define valid relationships between the physical and perceived locations of real objects. The perceived direction of an object in space relative to the body (i.e., its egocentric direction) is derived from the combination of its oculocentric visual direction with information about eye orientation in the head and head position relative to the trunk of the body. Egocentric localization is referenced to a point midway between the two eyes, referred to as the *egocenter,* and allows the individual to distinguish between retinal image motion caused by eye movements or by movement of the object.[73]

From a clinical standpoint, egocentric direction is an important concept for understanding the alterations of normal subjective visual space of patients with a misalignment of the two eyes (strabismus). The general principles of egocentric direction are illustrated in Figure 19-2. With normal binocular vision, the retinal oculocentric directions from the two retinal images of an object at (see Figure 19-2, A) or close to (see Figure 19-2, B, *circle*) the plane of fixation combine to produce a single direction (haplopia) relative to the observer's egocenter. In contrast, for targets outside the range of single vision, either nearer or farther than the plane of fixation, a single target has two separate egocentric directions that correspond to the oculocentric direction of each of the retinal images relative to the egocenter. Therefore single objects appear to have two separate egocentric directions (diplopia) (see Figure 19-2, C).

Binocular eye movements are defined by a combination of version and vergence ocular movements. Versions are yoked or conjugate changes in

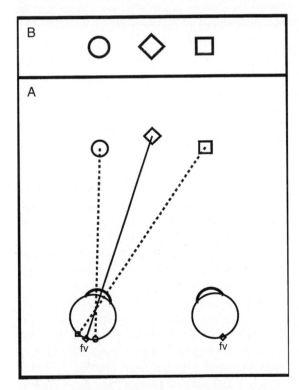

FIGURE 19-1 Perceived visual direction as a function of retinal image location. **A,** The relationships between objects in physical space and their retinal images. The *diamond* represents a fixated object (primary line of sight), and the nonfixated objects *(circle* and *square)* are secondary lines of sight. **B,** The relationships between retinal image locations and their visual directions (oculocentric directions). The perceived visual directions of the nonfixated objects (secondary visual directions of the *circle* and *square)* are relative to the primary visual direction of the fixated diamond. *fv,* Fovea.

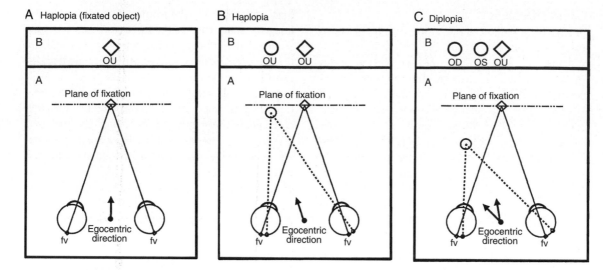

Figure 19-2   Egocentric directions for haplopia and diplopia. **A,** The oculocentric directions of a fixated object are combined to produce a single egocentric direction. **B,** The retinal images of nonfixated objects near the plane of fixation also combine to produce a single egocentric direction. **C,** When the disparity of retinal images is larger than the normal fusion range (Panum's fusional area), the oculocentric directions are not combined and the object has two egocentric directions (physiologic diplopia). *fv,* Fovea.

---

the visual axes of the two eyes in the same direction and amount; vergence movements involve rotations of the visual axes in opposite directions. Only the version component of binocular eye position influences the perception of egocentric direction. Binocular eye position is sensed as the average position of the two eyes. The vergence component is nullified because vergence movements of the two eyes have opposite signs and their correlates cancel one another when the average of right and left eye position is computed. Thus, when the two eyes fixate objects to the left or right of the midline in asymmetric convergence, only the version, or conjugate, component of eye position contributes to perceived direction.[72]

In addition to averaged eye positions, the subjective computation of egocentric directions of nonfixated objects involves a reconciliation of differences in oculocentric visual directions between the two eyes. For example, objects that are small distances in front or behind the plane of fixation are imaged at retinal locations with different angular distances from the visual axis and therefore have different oculocentric directions in each of the two eyes. When the retinal image disparity is small, the target still appears single and the binocular egocentric direction is based on the average oculocentric direction for the two eyes.[133] In other words, the binocular egocentric direction deviates from either

of the monocularly perceived directions by one half of the angular disparity (see Figure 19-2, *B*).

As object distances from the plane of fixation increase, retinal image disparities become large and an object appears to be in two separate egocentric directions (diplopic). Egocentric directions of diplopic images are perceived as though both monocular components had paired images on corresponding points in the contralateral eye (see Figure 19-2, *C*). The relative egocentric direction of each of the diplopic images depends on whether the object is nearer or farther than the plane of fixation. Figure 19-2, *C*, illustrates that, for an object closer than the plane of fixation, the egocentric direction associated with the retinal image of the right eye is to the left of the egocentric direction produced by the image of the left eye. This form of diplopia, produced by near objects, is called *"crossed" diplopia* because of the right-left/left-right relationship between the eyes and perceived locations of the object. Conversely, objects farther than the plane of fixation are perceived with uncrossed diplopia, in which the right eye sees an object located on the right side and the left eye sees an object located on the left side.

In normal binocular vision, diplopia of nonfixated objects, classified as physiologic diplopia, occurs as a natural consequence of the lateral separation of frontally located eyes and the topographic organization of visual directions across the retina. In contrast, patients with strabismus experience pathologic diplopia, wherein objects in the plane of fixation are perceived as doubled.[152] In pathologic diplopia the retinal image location caused by misalignment of the visual axis of the deviating eye causes a fixated target to be seen in different egocentric directions during binocular viewing, yet under monocular conditions, each eye veridically perceives its direction. Under binocular viewing conditions, only one of the two visual directions seen in pathologic diplopia can be veridical at any given moment. In addition to diplopia, a form of visual confusion confounds the space perception of strabismic patients. An object imaged on the fovea of the deviating eye has the same egocentric direction as another object imaged on the fovea of the fixating eye, even though their physical locations are much different. Diplopia and visual confusion create an intolerable visual environment that is typically alleviated during binocular vision by the development of suppression, which is a suspension of the vision in the deviating eye, or anomalous retinal correspondence, which is an alteration of the normal topography of oculocentric directions.[153,154]

NORMAL RETINAL CORRESPONDENCE

The perceptions of haplopia and diplopia arise from the sense of oculocentric visual directions of corresponding or noncorresponding retinal areas that are stimulated during binocular vision. Binocular retinal correspondence is defined by the set of retinal image locations that produces perceptions of identical visual directions when viewing with one eye or with both eyes simultaneously.[101] Identical visual directions associated with corresponding points depend primarily on retinal image locations and their associated oculocentric directions, rather than on eye position and egocentric directions. This fundamental principle was demonstrated by Hering's famous "window experiment" and similarly by the elementary observation that afterimages placed on the fovea of each eye always appear superimposed, regardless of the vergence or version positions of the two eyes.[10,101,154] The identical visual directions of the afterimages show that normally corresponding retinal points are combined physiologically before eye position information is used to compute perceived egocentric direction.

These relationships for binocular visual directions are illustrated in Figure 19-3, in which the two foveal images of a fixated object (see the *diamond*

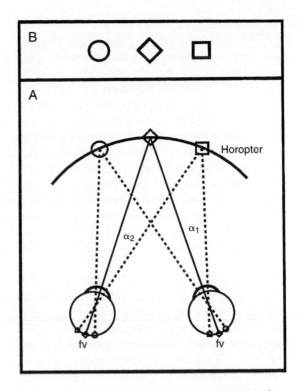

FIGURE 19-3 Corresponding retinal points. Retinal areas in the two eyes with identical oculocentric directions (**B**) are corresponding retinal points. The locations of objects along the horizontal meridian that are imaged on corresponding points (**A**) define the longitudinal horopter. The physical location of an object that is on the horopter is quantified by the longitudinal visual angles, α_1 and α_2. *fv*, Fovea.

in Figure 19-3, *A*) share a common visual direction and are fused to produce the perception of a single haplopic object in subjective space (see Figure 19-3, *B*). The specific pairs of retinal image locations in the two eyes that are perceived to have identical visual directions are called *corresponding retinal points* or *areas*. The foveas represent an important pair of corresponding retinal points, but many other pairs are associated with secondary lines of sight and visual directions. For example, in Figure 19-3 the *square* represents the location of an object in the right visual field that falls on paired retinal areas with a common visual direction for the two eyes, thus defining another set of corresponding retinal areas. Similarly, the *circle* represents a location of an object in the left visual field that is imaged on corresponding retinal points. For an infinite fixation distance, a large number of potential object locations are imaged on corresponding retinal points. These object locations in space that are imaged onto corresponding retinal points can be imagined to define a surface that resembles a cylinder with an infinite radius of curvature. This surface of points stimulates the perception of identical visual directions for the two eyes and is called the *horopter*.[100,101,134] At finite viewing distances, the surface is reduced to a horizontal line and a vertical line that pass through the intersections of the lines of sight when the eyes fixate in symmetric convergence. Points in tertiary locations (elevated and displaced laterally from the lines of sight) are closer to one eye than to the other and subtend larger visual angles at the more proximal eye. As a result, all physical points in tertiary locations at finite viewing distances are imaged with vertical disparities and, by definition, their images do not fall on corresponding points. At finite viewing distances, only points imaged along the horizontal retinal meridian or along the vertical retinal meridian in the midsagittal plane can be formed on corresponding points without vertical disparities. The longitudinal horopter is defined by the locations of object points that are imaged on corresponding points along horizontal meridians through the foveas, shown diagrammatically in Figure 19-3 by the arc passing through the fixated object and the two peripheral objects that stimulate corresponding retinal points. The vertical horopter is defined by the location of object points in the midsagittal plane that are imaged on corresponding points along the vertical meridian.[136,151]

The relationship between object and image space for the longitudinal horopter can be quantified by longitudinal visual angles, defined as the horizontal visual angles subtended by the primary and secondary lines of sight for each eye. The longitudinal visual angles for an object in the right visual field are illustrated by angles α_1 and α_2 in Figure 19-3. Similarly, longitudinal visual angles can be defined for the object in the left visual field. The lateral separation of the eyes in the head results in each eye having a different perspective of objects not on the horopter, and these differences in perspective are used perceptually to reconstruct a three-dimensional space from the two-dimensional retinal images. The objects that are closer or farther than the horopter stimulate noncorresponding points, which is defined as a *binocular disparity, retinal disparity,* or simply, *disparity of the retinal images*.[158] The horizontal component of binocular disparity is the unique stimulus for stereoscopic depth perception, which is quantified by the difference in the longitudinal visual angles, also called *horizontal disparity angles*. The horopter serves as a

zero disparity reference from which the magnitudes of nonzero disparities are computed. In the absence of other depth cues, the curvature and tilt of the horopter influence the perceived shape and orientation of surfaces seen in depth. Optical devices such as spectacle lenses that magnify and distort one of the two eyes' retinal images alter the horopter and produce predictable errors of space perception.[100]

The empiric longitudinal horopter illustrated in Figure 19-3 is a smooth surface that is symmetric about the fixation point, but the actual shape and curvature of the empiric horopter depend on physiologic and optical factors that alter the retinal images and their cortical representation. If the locations of corresponding retinal areas simply are determined by equal angular distances from the primary line of sight, the horopter would be a circle passing through the fixation point and the entrance pupil of each eye[14,101] (geometric or theoretic horopter or Vieth-Muller circle) (Figure 19-4). An analogy of "cover points" has been used to describe corresponding retinal locations determined by retinal distances.[101] If the retina of one eye were to be translated and carefully aligned to cover the retina of the other eye, a pin stuck into the retina would penetrate cover points, or corresponding retinal areas. Cover points, by simple geometry, would become corresponding points because the angles included by lines drawn from two points on the circumference of a circle to any other two points on the circle would be equal. Consequently, the longitudinal visual angles would be equal ($\alpha_1 = \alpha_2$), and the theoretic horopter would be a section of a circle, specified as the Vieth-Muller circle (VMO), as illustrated in Figure 19-4.

Except for rare cases, the empirically defined horopter does not actually coincide with the VMO, but the theoretic longitudinal horopter is an important reference for zero disparity; in fact, clinical tests of stereopsis use the VMO as the zero disparity reference. Another important reference in physical space is the objective frontoparallel plane (OFPP), which is the plane at the fixation distance that is parallel to a line passing through the entrance pupils of the two eyes (see Figure 19-4). Although, both the VMO and the OFPP are used as reference surfaces to describe the empiric horopter, they are predicated on different perceptual correlates. The VMO is based on a physical geometric assumption that identical visual directions are associated with retinal points that are equidistant from their respective foveas. The empiric longitudinal

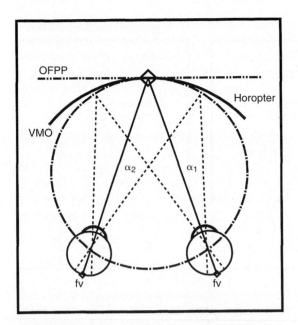

FIGURE 19-4 The empiric horopter in relation to the Vieth-Muller circle (*VMO*), defined by the locations of objects with equal longitudinal visual angles (α_1 and α_2), and the objective frontoparallel plane (*OFPP*), defined by a plane at the fixation distance that is parallel to a line passing through the entrance pupils of the two eyes. *fv,* Fovea.

horopter, which is based primarily on identical visual directions, is the only pure measure of pairs of retinal corresponding points.[134] On the other hand, the OFPP, which is a measure of perceived surface shape and orientation, depends on egocentric directions derived by combining oculocentric directions and information about absolute distance and direction. The OFPP can be used as a frame of reference for adjusting the depth of objects at different retinal eccentricities so that the objects appear to lie in a flat plane parallel to the face (apparent frontoparallel plane [AFPP]). The location and form of the AFPP is based on disparity and absolute distance cues, and the AFPP is used to evaluate how disparity is scaled by absolute distance to enable the organism to estimate the depth of surface shapes and orientations. Both the empiric longitudinal horopter and the AFPP are used to evaluate the influence of optical distortions, such as magnification, on perceived space because they usually yield similar results.

The empiric longitudinal horopter and the AFPP can be measured in several ways, based on different properties of visual directions and stereoscopic depth from objects imaged on corresponding retinal points.[101] The empiric longitudinal horopter can

be determined by identical visual directions for the two eyes, by the highest stereoacuity for points at various eccentricities from fixation, by center of the sensory fusion range known as *Panum's fusional area* (see Figure 19-7), and by object locations eccentric to fixation that result in a zero stimulus for disparity vergence. The vergence criterion assumes that horizontal version movements guide the intersection of the visual axes along the empiric horopter, even if this surface is curved in depth. The AFPP horopter can be measured by positioning eccentric objects so that they all appear to lie in the same plane or by positioning eccentric objects so that they appear to be equidistant from the observer (i.e., equidistant from the egocenter).

ABNORMAL RETINAL CORRESPONDENCE

The properties of corresponding retinal areas underlying normal binocular vision provide a stable sensory organization of the two eyes consistent with the functional properties of neurons in primary visual cortex that are present in infancy.[26,107,143] However, the normal sensory organization of binocular vision can be altered substantively in infantile strabismus by the development of anomalous retinal correspondence and/or suppression.[154] Clinically, the type and extent of sensory adaptation is an important factor to be considered in treatments intended to reestablish functional binocular vision for a strabismic patient.

Sensory adaptations in strabismus are necessary to eliminate the constant diplopia (two egocentric directions for all objects) and common visual directions for fixated and nonfixated objects (visual confusion) that would prevail otherwise[154] (Figure 19-5, *A*). Most strabismic patients do not experience diplopia and visual confusion, but their single vision is a result of suppression or anomalous retinal correspondence.[4,24,53,75] Suppression causes the perception of objects normally visible to the deviating eye to be eliminated during simultaneous binocular viewing to provide single vision.[155] Suppression in some persons with exotropia may involve an entire hemifield, but for persons with esotropia the suppression is limited to a specific area (sometimes called a *suppression scotoma*) bounded by the fovea of the deviating eye and the area stimulated by the object fixated by the nondeviating eye[53,75] (the diplopia point; Figure 19-5, *B*).

Anomalous retinal correspondence (Figure 19-5, *C*) is an adapted shift in the visual directions of the

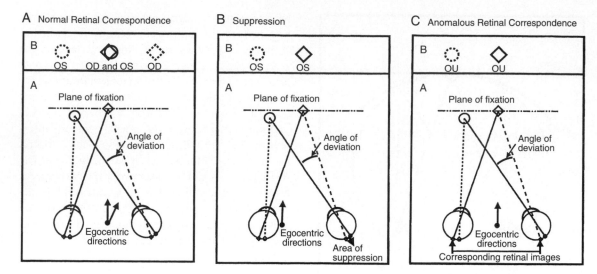

FIGURE 19-5   Retinal correspondence and suppression in strabismus. **A,** A strabismic patient with normal retinal correspondence and without suppression would have diplopia, two egocentric directions of single objects (*solid* and *dashed images* in *B*) and visual confusion, a common visual direction for two separate objects (represented by the superimposition of the images of the fixated diamond and the circle, which is imaged on the fovea of the deviating eye in *B*). **B,** The elimination of diplopia and confusion by suppression of the retinal image of the deviating eye. **C,** The elimination of diplopia and confusion by anomalous retinal correspondence, an adaptation of visual directions of the deviated eye.

deviated eye relative to the normal visual directions of the fixating eye. The result is that during binocular viewing a peripheral retinal area of the deviating eye acquires a common visual direction to that of the fovea of the fixating eye.[4,24,122,154] This shift in retinal correspondence produces a difference in the visual directions between the two eyes for foveally imaged objects, which can be demonstrated clinically with the Hering-Bielschowsky test for anomalous correspondence.[154] For this test, afterimages are formed on the foveas of both eyes. Even with an interocular deviation from strabismus, a patient with normal correspondence perceives the afterimages in a common direction, but a patient with anomalous retinal correspondence perceives the afterimages in different visual directions. The subjective separation of the monocular afterimages is referred to as the *angle of anomaly*, which represents the magnitude of the perceptual shift from the normal corresponding relationship between the two foveas. If the magnitude of the angle of anomaly is equal to the magnitude of the oculomotor misalignment, objects in space can appear single even though the eyes are deviated. On the other hand, when the angle of anomaly is less than the angle of strabismic deviation, the residual disparity causes diplopia unless suppression is also present. The angular separation of the diplopic im-

ages is referred to as the *subjective angle*. In anomalous retinal correspondence the subjective angle is usually smaller than the angle of strabismus (objective angle). The sum of the angle of anomaly and subjective angle equals the magnitude of the angle of strabismus.

A diagnosis of anomalous retinal correspondence for a given strabismic patient is test dependent.[43] Tests for anomalous retinal correspondence either locate the extrafoveal point in the deviating eye that has the same visual direction as the fovea in the fixating eye or quantify the angular separation of the visual directions of the foveas of the two eyes.[154] Tests in the former category, such as Bagolini striated lenses or the Worth four-dot test, have a higher probability of being positive for anomalous retinal correspondence than tests in the latter category, such as the Hering-Bielschowsky afterimage procedure. The dependence of the state of a patient's retinal correspondence on the clinical procedure may be the result of variation in the angle of anomaly across the retina or some other property of the mechanisms underlying anomalous retinal correspondence.[42,79,122,165]

Three main theories on anomalous retinal correspondence have been proposed.[122] The first theory states that, with anomalous correspondence, the two eyes perceive space independently, much like the two hands explore space. Each eye computes egocentric visual direction from its own sense of eye position and oculocentric retinal image location. In effect, there is a lack of correspondence.[22,150] The observation that the separation between foveal after-images changes during spontaneous changes in the magnitude of the angle of strabismus supports this theory. This covariation between the angle of anomaly and objective angle of strabismus results in a stable percept of space, even though the magnitude of the strabismus is unstable and varies in time.[58] The second theory proposes that there is a shift in retinal correspondence.[18,31,154] Normally disparate retinal points are shifted to acquire an anomalous coupling in the striate cortex. The fovea of the fixating eye is anomalously coupled with a peripheral area of the deviating eye. Measures of the identical visual directions horopter in strabismics reveal that correspondence is mainly shifted in the periphery, and the angle of anomaly decreases near the fovea in the region of space that lies between the visual axes that is projected to opposite cortical hemispheres.[20,42] The third theory proposes that patients with strabismus who have no suppression are able to perceive space singly because of enlarged Panum's fusional areas.[2,5,67] These three theories are not mutually exclusive. All of them can be expressed to some degree in the same strabismic patient.

BINOCULAR (RETINAL) DISPARITY

The empiric longitudinal horopter represents the specific locations of objects in physical space that have zero retinal image disparity. Objects not located on the horopter have some amount of lateral binocular (retinal) disparity. With horizontal binocular (retinal) disparity, an object is imaged on laterally separated noncorresponding retinal areas, and as in the case of the empiric horopter, the longitudinal visual angles are not equal. Horizontal retinal disparity is a unique binocular stimulus for stereoscopic depth perception, horizontal disparity vergence eye movements, and diplopia (either physiologic or pathologic). In each case, the perceptual or motor response is a consequence of the relationship between the object's disparate images and the horopter.

The following relationships concerning binocular disparities are important to the understanding of binocular vision.

1. Binocular disparities are classified as uncrossed (distal) or crossed (proximal) based on the relationship between the disparate object and the horopter, as illustrated in Figure

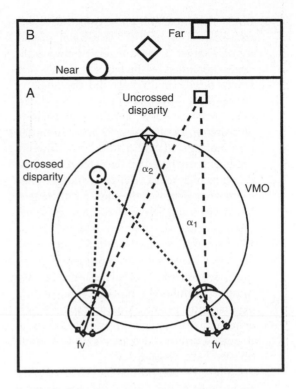

FIGURE 19-6 Binocular disparity and the perception of stereoscopic depth. Objects that are not located on the longitudinal horopter have binocular disparity, which may be crossed disparity (*circle* in **A**) and be perceived as nearer than the fixated object (the relative depth of the *circle* with respect to the *diamond* in **B**) or uncrossed disparity (*square* in **A**) and be perceived as farther than the fixated reference object (**B**). *fv*, Fovea; *VMO*, Vieth-Muller circle.

19-6.[73,158] For example, the square in the right visual field represents an object that is farther than the fixation point (represented by the *diamond*), and the secondary lines of sight for the square intersect behind the horopter. The binocular disparity produced by the square is classified as uncrossed and quantified by the difference between the longitudinal visual angles α_1 and α_2. Perceptually, uncrossed disparities give rise to a sense of relative "far" stereoscopic depth or, if the disparity is large, to uncrossed diplopia (i.e., double vision with the right eye's image seen to the left side of the left eye's image). As oculomotor stimuli, uncrossed disparities evoke divergence eye movements. By a parallel classification, crossed disparities (see the *circle* in the left field in Figure 19-6) give rise to a perception of "near" stereoscopic depth or crossed diplopia and elicit convergence eye movements.

2. Binocular disparities are classified as either relative or absolute.[29,158] The *absolute* disparity of a target is the difference between the angle subtended by the target at the two entrance pupils of the eyes and the angle of convergence. A *relative* disparity is the difference between two absolute disparities. Stereoscopic depth normally arises from discriminating relative disparities, wherein judgments are based on the perception of the depth of one object relative to another (e.g., the relative depth of the square with respect to the diamond, Figure 19-6). Stereopsis with relative disparities, as measured by clinical testing, is fine compared with the perception of depth based solely on absolute disparities.[154] In contrast, an absolute disparity is the optimal stimulus for motor fusion, such as occurs with prism-induced disparity vergence or with changes in fixation distances, because a uniform disparity is present for all objects in the visual field.[77]

3. For a person with normal binocular vision, a finite range of binocular disparities provides a clear perception of relative depth with normal fusion (haplopia) and larger disparities produce diplopia.[97,101] The disparity range for single vision, called *Panum's fusional area* (PFA), is diagrammed in Figure 19-7. Figure 19-7, *A*, illustrates the measurement of Panum's area. A test object is moved along the primary line of sight of the left eye while the two eyes maintain binocular fixation at one point in space. The crossed disparity limit for fusion is the greatest distance that the test object can be moved toward the subject before it appears diplopic. Similarly, the object can be moved away from the subject to establish an uncrossed disparity limit for fusion. Thus, in subjective space (Figure 19-7, *B*), PFA (illustrated by the *dashed oval*) defines the disparity range for fused binocular vision and objects subtending disparities outside this range are diplopic. When the target is intersected by the primary line of sight of the left eye, the image for the right eye is projected to the left visual field in crossed diplopia and to the right visual field in uncrossed diplopia. In addition, a vertical disparity range, which is generally smaller than the horizontal disparity range, is compatible with binocular sensory fusion. Although the size and shape of PFAs depend on retinal ec-

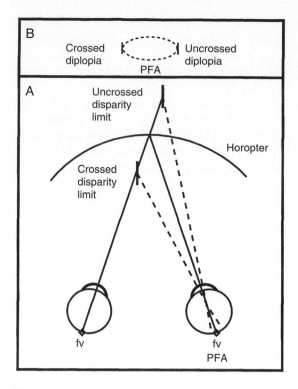

Figure 19-7   The binocular disparity range for single binocular vision (Panum's fusional area [*PFA*]). With constant fixation, an object is moved along the primary line of sight of the left eye until the binocular disparity if the right eye's image exceeds the fusion limit (i.e., appears diplopic) first with crossed disparity and then with uncrossed disparity (**A**). **B,** The dimensions of PFA. *fv,* Fovea.

centricity and spatiotemporal stimulus properties, the classical PFA for foveal vision is a horizontal oval with approximate dimensions of 15 × 6 arcmin.[101,130,148]

4. Most individuals with normal binocular vision have small vergence errors known as *fixation disparities.*[66,103,121] Because the retinal images only need to fall within PFAs for single binocular vision to occur, a small residual misalignment of the visual axes (vergence error) can occur, resulting in a constant retinal disparity of a fixated object (i.e., a fixation disparity) without causing diplopia. This disparity between the fixated object and the intersection of the primary lines of sight is a consequence of the displacement of the longitudinal horopter from the fixated object produced by the vergence error. The example in Figure 19-8 shows a small convergence error (esofixation disparity) for the object of fixation (*diamond*). The convergence error causes

In summary, broad ranges of binocular disparities are present under all conditions of normal seeing and the use of disparity information by the visual sensory and motor systems is the most fundamental process of normal binocular vision. The clinical evaluation of a patient's binocular vision includes tests of several aspects of retinal disparity: relative disparities by measures of stereoacuity, absolute retinal disparities by measures of disparity-induced vergence eye movements, and fixation disparities.[121,122]

STEREOPSIS

Stereopsis is the perception of relative distance, or the depth separation, between objects that occurs as a result of neural processing of the relative horizontal binocular disparities between the monocular retinal images. Binocular disparities are present because the lateral separation of the eyes in the head provides each eye with a slightly disparate view of a given object. Thus, as demonstrated by the seminal research of Wheatstone[161] and Julesz,[78] these horizontal (lateral) retinal image disparities produce stereoscopic depth. By themselves, vertical disparities do not result in depth perception; however, they are used to estimate absolute distance and to scale horizontal disparities into depth magnitudes.[48,52,87,116,160]

Horizontal retinal disparities and therefore clinical measures of the smallest detectable stereoscopic depth (stereoacuities) are quantified by a stereoangle (η), which is equal to the difference in the longitudinal visual angles (α_1 and α_2), or the parallax (convergence) angles (δ_1 and δ_2), as illustrated in Figure 19-9. For a conventional stereogram (see Figure 19-13), η can be derived directly from the angular differences in positions of common objects in the two half-views of the stereogram. The retinal disparity associated with the physical depth of an object in normal vision (see Figure 19-9) can be determined by the following relationship:

$$\eta = [(a \times \Delta b)/d^2] \times c$$

where
    a = Interpupillary distance
    Δb = Depth interval that is equal to the distance between the disparate object and the viewing distance
    d = Viewing distance
    c = A constant to obtain the stereoangle in dimensions of arcmin ($c = 3438$) or arcsec ($c = 206,264$)

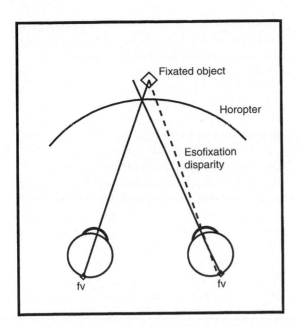

FIGURE 19-8 The displacement of the horopter with an esofixation disparity. Vergence errors cause a displacement of the horopter from the fixation point and retinal disparity of the fixated object. Single binocular vision is maintained if the vergence error is smaller than Panum's fusional area (fixation disparity). *fv*, Fovea.

an inward shift of the horopter (the locations of normal corresponding points); that is, in normal binocular vision, identical primary visual directions result from bifoveal stimulation; therefore the horopter always passes through the intersection of the visual axes. Consequently, the fixated object lies beyond the horopter and, by definition, has an uncrossed retinal disparity, described clinically as an esofixation disparity. Conversely, an exofixation disparity causes a displacement of the horopter beyond the fixation distance and crossed disparity of the object. In any case, the magnitude of a fixation disparity cannot be larger than the width of PFA if the patient is to retain single binocular vision. Because the fixation disparity is absolute or uniform across the visual field, binocular depth perception, which relies on relative disparities, is not affected. Clinically, fixation disparities are considered a sign of stress on the fusional vergence mechanisms. However, more recent data suggest that they provide a steady-state stimulus to maintain ocular alignment during fusion or that they are the result of an imbalance in disparity-selective mechanisms.[121]

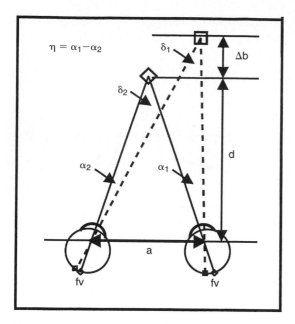

$$\eta = \alpha_1 - \alpha_2$$

FIGURE 19-9   The quantification of binocular disparity. The binocular disparity (η) of an object (represented by the *square*), with respect to a fixated object (*diamond*), is equal to the difference in the longitudinal visual angles (α_1 and α_2) or the parallax angles (δ_1 and δ_2). The magnitude of binocular disparity depends on the fixation distance (*d*), the depth interval (*Δb), and the interpupillary distance (a). fv*, Fovea.

The function shows that, for any given fixation distance, the relationship between depth interval and retinal disparity is linear, but the relationship varies across fixation distances by the square of the distance. For example, if an individual with a 60 mm physical depth (interpupillary distance) can perceive stereoscopic depth from a retinal disparity of 10 arcsec, a depth difference of 0.12 mm can be discriminated at a 40-cm viewing distance. However, the same stereoangle requires a 3-cm depth difference at 6 m, or an 800-m depth difference at a 1000-m viewing distance. The relationships between binocular disparities, linear depth, and observation distance for larger, suprathreshold disparities are shown in Figure 19-10.

To maintain a valid perceptual constancy between depth and disparity, the relationship between stereoangles and viewing distances indicates that an observer must scale the horizontal disparity with viewing distance. Perceptual information about viewing distance may be interpreted from the vertical disparity gradients that occur naturally in tertiary directions of gaze, in which a nearby target subtends a larger visual angle vertically in one eye than in the other.[48,52,87,116,160] If the target is elevated above the visual plane, it has a vertical disparity that increases with horizontal eccentricity and inversely with viewing distance. Other sources of perceptual information about viewing distance include the convergence angle; retinal cues, such as oblique disparities; and nonstereoscopic or perspective cues.[23,44,160]

Quantitative and Qualitative Stereopsis

The perception of stereoscopic depth at a constant viewing distance increases with disparity over a relatively large range.[70,99,127,132,148] The relationship between perceived depth and disparity from the lower (D_{min}) to upper (D_{max}) limits of stereoscopic vision is illustrated by Figure 19-11. A perception of relative depth cannot be detected from disparities below the stereothreshold (D_{min}), but the relationship becomes proportional (quantitative stereopsis) for disparities larger than the stereothreshold. Objects with larger disparities appear in increasing depth even beyond the limit of fusion (Panum's fusional limit), and the maximum perceived stereoscopic depth occurs when the stimulus is clearly diplopic. With larger binocular disparities (qualitative stereopsis), the perception of depth decreases to the upper limit of stereopsis, where the relative depth of diplopic objects cannot be resolved. Qualitative depth has a direction or sign but a vague amplitude.[99]

The specific parameters of the depth-disparity relationship depend on the spatial and temporal properties of the stimulus and on other nonstereoscopic factors. For example, binocular disparities above the stereothreshold produce a vivid quantitative sense of depth and a strong impression of solid three-dimensional structure, but the disparity threshold for the perception of depth is altered by various changes in stimulus parameters, such as contrast, spatial frequency, and viewing duration.* For example, although depth in a stereogram may be perceived with just a spark of illumination, the stereodepth detection threshold decreases with exposure duration for both line and random-dot patterns.[61,104,135] Quantitative stereopsis responds to stimuli that appear fused, the magnitude of perceived depth increases with disparity magnitude up to about 1 degree, and the depth percept improves with exposure duration up to 1 second.[45] A qualitative sense of stereodepth can be seen with even larger disparities, but the magnitude of its range is difficult to specify (i.e., a range of qualitative stere-

---

*References 59, 61, 63, 70, 84, 104, 126, 131, 132, 135.

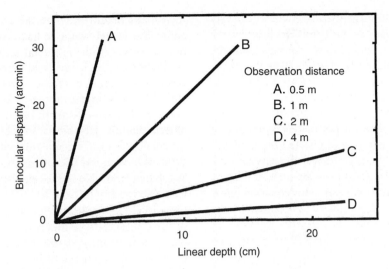

FIGURE 19-10   The relationship between binocular disparity and linear depth for four fixation distances. The disparity-depth relationship is linear for any constant fixation distance, but it is nonlinear across fixation distances.

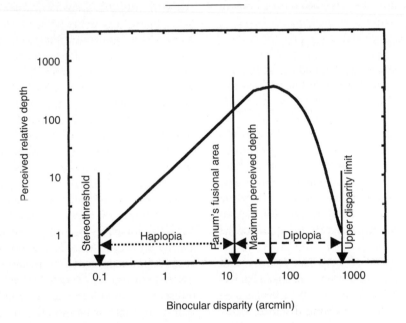

FIGURE 19-11   The relationship between perceived depth and binocular disparity for disparities from the lower to the upper limits of stereoscopic depth perception. (Modified from Tyler CW. Sensory processing of binocular disparity. In Schor CM, Ciuffreda KJ [eds]: *Vergence eye movements: basic and clinical aspects,* Boston, 1983, Butterworths.)

opsis with disparities as large as 10 degrees).[45,99] In addition to the disparity range, qualitative stereopsis and quantitative stereopsis differ in two important ways: Quantitative depth perception improves with exposure duration, whereas qualitative depth perception is optimal with briefly presented stimuli and fades with exposures longer than 0.5 second.[83,104] Thus these two forms of stereopsis can also be classified as sustained-quantitative and transient-qualitative. In addition, the two forms of

stereopsis can be distinguished by the spatial aspects of their stimuli, especially by the similarity between the stimuli for both eyes that is required for quantitative, but not for qualitative, stereopsis.[36,108,124] Qualitative stereopsis arises from briefly presented stimuli even when a difference in size, shape, and/or contrast polarity exists between the two eyes.[36,69,108,124] Transient-qualitative stereopsis is a useful alerting percept for the approximate location of objects that appear suddenly, and it is also a stimulus to initiate vergence alignment of the eyes to transient changes in both for small and large retinal disparities. Quantitative stereopsis, on the other hand, is mainly useful for judging the shape, depth, and orientation of continuously viewed features near the plane of fixation.

The stereoscopic appreciation of either quantitative or qualitative depth is not merely a function of relative retinal disparity. As indicated by the equation for computing retinal image disparity (η), the linear depth interval (Δb) depends on both disparity and viewing distance (d). The equation illustrates that retinal image disparity is scaled by absolute distance to yield stereodepth magnitude in linear units. Both the magnitude of depth and the degree of surface curvature (depth ordering) stimulated by retinal disparity depend on viewing distance. For example, a zero disparity surface can have many different shapes. Because the empiric longitudinal horopter is flatter than the theoretic VMO, its curvature decreases (becomes less concave or more convex) with increasing viewing distance[101] (see Figure 19-3). Nevertheless, flat surfaces appear flat at all viewing distances; thus, without viewing distance information, the pattern of retinal image disparities across the visual field is insufficient to sense either depth ordering (surface curvature) or depth magnitude.[48] Similarly, a given pattern of horizontal disparities can correspond to different slants about a vertical axis presented at various horizontal gaze eccentricities.[101] Convergence distance and direction of gaze are important pieces of information used to interpret slant from the disparity fields associated with slanting surfaces.[7]

Clinical anomalies of both quantitative and qualitative stereopsis have been identified. For example, patients with strabismus or binocular dysfunction demonstrate elevated thresholds for quantitative stereopsis, even when their eyes are aligned by optical or surgical procedures. However, if any residual stereopsis is present, once disparity exceeds the elevated threshold, it stimulates depth perception to the normal upper disparity limit for quantitative stereopsis, with normal qualitative stereopsis at large disparities.[34,123] Interestingly, a normal range for sensory fusion, or PFAs, can also accompany a total loss of stereopsis.[123] However, for strabismic patients with a loss of binocular sensory fusion, stereopsis invariably is lost.[154] For these individuals binocular images appear to wash over one another, with no binocular binding of aligned images. Their vergence is unstable, and their eyes continually shift their fixation disparity.

Nonstrabismic individuals may have subclinical anomalies of stereopsis, as demonstrated by directional biases in their ability to sense transient-qualitative depth from large (greater than 1 degree) crossed and uncrossed disparities. Subjects with these subclinical anomalies generally discriminate the direction of depth better for flashed near objects than for far objects. In subjects with severe stereoanomalies, transient-qualitative stereodepth perception with one or both signs of disparity may be absent.[112,113] Nonstrabismic individuals who have a stereoanomaly can have normal quantitative stereopsis.[76] The selective loss of transient disparity in one direction suggests that the disparity-detecting neurons are grouped into different pools tuned to broad ranges of crossed and uncrossed disparity, and sensitivity to one direction of disparity may be lost without affecting the other. A related motor anomaly of transient vergence has been found in patients with a stereoanomaly, exhibited by a significant reduction or absence of either convergence or divergence responses to large, briefly exposed disparities.[36,76]

Stereoacuity

One of the qualitative aspects of binocular vision commonly evaluated during clinical vision testing is stereoacuity, that is, the smallest relative binocular disparity that can be detected with stereopsis (Figure 19-12). The binocular disparity angles for depth detection normally are smaller than the resolution angles for visual acuity, even for unpracticed clinical patients, and are typically less than 30 arcsec. In practice, the terminology for visual acuity is maintained for stereopsis. A patient's stereo performance is specified as a stereoacuity, rather than stereothreshold. Although the true definition of stereoacuity is the reciprocal of the stereothreshold, stereoacuities are usually specified by arcsec of disparity at threshold; by usage, the terms *stereothreshold* and *stereoacuity* have become clinically interchangeable.

Clinical tests of stereoacuity are designed as screening tools for distinguishing normal from abnormal (e.g., stereoblindness, microstrabismus, monofixation) binocular vision. The stereothreshold of a normal observer is usually lower than the smallest disparity presented by most clinical tests, which use a limited number of stimuli with relatively large disparity increments.[158] Improving the accuracy of clinical stereopsis tests would require a greater number of stimuli with smaller disparity increments, without necessarily improving the detection rate for

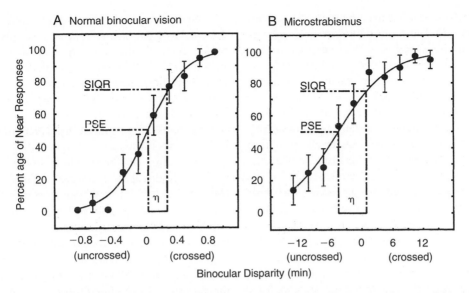

FIGURE 19-12 Psychometric functions for depth discrimination for an observer with normal binocular vision (**A**) and an observer with deficient stereopsis from microstrabismus (**B**). The percentages of responses that a test stimulus appeared to be nearer than the reference stimulus are plotted as a function of the sign (negative values for uncrossed disparities and positive values for crossed disparities) and magnitude of disparity. The subjects' stereoacuities (η) are defined by the disparity range between the point of subject equality (*PSE*) and the semi-intraquartile range (*SIQR*).

abnormal binocular vision. Nevertheless, it is an important concept that for any given patient, the relationship between stereoscopic depth perception and binocular disparity is probabilistic over a range of disparity values, as shown by the psychometric function (see Figure 19-12) for the detection or discrimination of stereoscopic depth.

Consider a stereopsis test in which a test stimulus, with variable disparity direction and magnitude, is located below a zero-disparity reference stimulus.[65] The test stimulus is presented to the observer many times, changing the direction and magnitude of the disparity between presentations, or trials. For each trial the observer judges the relative direction of depth of the test stimulus with respect to the reference stimulus. When the trials are completed, the percentage of near responses is plotted as a function of each disparity magnitude and sign presented (see Figure 19-12). In the range of probabilistic performance the discrimination of near stereoscopic depth with respect to a reference stimulus of zero disparity systematically improves as the sign (direction) of the disparity becomes appropriate for near (i.e., crossed) and as the magnitude of the binocular disparity increases. The disparity between the test and reference stimuli for which the percentage of "near" responses equals

50% denotes the point of subjective equality (PSE) in the depth of the test and reference stimuli. The observer's PSE represents a disparity bias, or constant error, at the specific retinal eccentricity tested. Because this disparity (the PSE) is perceived as having zero depth difference from a foveal reference point, the PSE is, by definition, a point on the longitudinal horopter. The slope of the psychometric function represents the variability of the stereodepth percept and the corresponding stereothreshold. The binocular disparity required to achieve depth discrimination with a given level of accuracy (typically 75%) defines the observer's stereothreshold. Operationally, the stereothreshold (η) is quantified by the semi-intraquartile range (SIQR) of the psychometric function, that is, by the range of disparities from the PSE to the disparity that gives a "near" response rate of 75%.

The fundamental differences between normal and reduced stereoacuities are illustrated in Figure 19-12 by comparison of the psychometric functions for a subject with normal binocular vision and a patient with primary microstrabismus. The subject with normal binocular vision (Figure 19-12, *A*) had nearly perfect (100%) depth discrimination for binocular disparities of 0.6 arcmin, either uncrossed or crossed. Chance performance (PSE) occurred at zero disparity, indicating that the horopter was located at the VMO, and the stereothreshold (η) determined from the SIQR was 12 arcsec. The performance of the microstrabismic subject (Figure 19-12, *B*) showed a similar systematic relationship between discrimination and disparity, although the range of binocular disparities required was 15 times larger. The PSE for the microstrabismic subject was 4.5 arcmin of uncrossed disparity, and the stereothreshold was greater than 320 arcsec. This example shows that the accurate measurement of an abnormal stereoacuity requires the use of a different range and a larger increment of binocular disparities than needed for measuring a normal stereoacuity. Although most clinical tests cover a sufficient range of disparities for evaluating both normal and abnormal subjects, the disparity increments are too large for accurately measuring normal stereothresholds; thus an individual's clinical performance is compared with expected suprathreshold performance levels for patients with normal binocular vision. For the primary purpose of screening for abnormal binocular vision, determining that a patient's stereoacuity is at an expected level of performance is sufficient to demonstrate that the patient's sensory and motor processes are compatible with normal binocular vision.

Stereopsis is not usually evaluated with real-depth stimuli; rather, most clinical tests of stereopsis use stereograms with either contour-defined or disparity-defined forms (examples of the two forms of stereograms are shown in Figure 19-13). In addition, most individuals with normal binocular vision can observe the relative depth in the stereograms with "free fusion" either by overconvergence (crossed-eye viewing) or underconvergence (straight-eye viewing). However, it should be noted that the two viewing strategies produce opposite directions of relative depth. These two configurations of stereograms are often distinguished as being tests of local versus global stereopsis, and each has some desirable attributes for clinical evaluations.[148] For example, stereograms that test local stereopsis use high-contrast test figures that have unambiguous relative disparities that can be detected by all patients with normal binocular vision, and even by some patients with microstrabismus or monofixation.[13,27,106,154] Thus contour-defined stereograms provide valuable information for differentiating between normal and subnormal binocular vision. However, this form of stereogram unavoidably contains monocular cues that are discernible in targets with large disparities. These monocular cues could allow discrimination of depth based on nonstereoscopic information. Such nonstereoscopic cues are illustrated by the stereogram in Figure 19-13, *A*. When properly fused, the contours in this stereogram provide clear stereoscopic depth appreciation from both crossed and uncrossed binocular disparities, but the relative differences in the positions of the stimuli are apparent without fusion or stereopsis.

The design of the random-dot stereogram, which tests global stereopsis, or cyclopean perception, eliminates almost all nonstereoscopic cues.[78] Figure 19-13, *B*, is a random-dot stereogram of the same stimulus pattern as the contour stereogram in Figure 19-13, *A*. Even though the locations, directions, and disparity magnitudes of the stimuli of the random-dot and contour stereograms are identical, the pattern is more difficult to see in the random-dot stereogram. Because of the inherent ambiguity of which element in one half-view is the correct "match" for a given element in the other half-view of random-dot stereograms, global stereopsis is a more complex process than local stereopsis.[78,92]

The correct identification of the disparity-defined form embedded into the random-dot stereogram is definitive evidence that the patient's stereoacuity is higher than the disparity of the form; therefore clinical testing using random-dot stereograms may be preferred. This property is especially useful for children because the identification of a familiar form is cognitively simpler than the discrimination of relative depth. However, clinical testing of global stereopsis requires a relatively long viewing duration to identify the stereoscopic form, and the relative direction of stereoscopic depth in random-dot stereograms can be detected with smaller disparities than what is needed for identification of the disparity-defined form.[21,60,61,117] In addition, an accurate registration of the random-dot patterns on corresponding retinal points is essential for form identification; for that reason, they may not be ideal for assessing the degree of binocularity in patients with subnormal binocular vision from microstrabismus or the monofixation syndrome.[12,154]

Stereoacuity with Refractive Defocus

Occasionally, patients can be stereodeficient or stereoblind even though they have normal eye alignment and visual acuity.[46] More often, stereoacuities are reduced by some factor that has affected the retinal image quality of one or both eyes. For example, optical defocus of the retinal images, as occurs with uncorrected refractive errors, de-

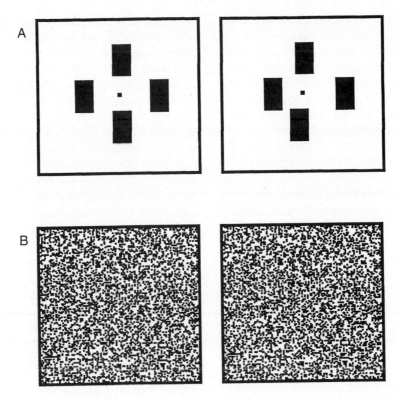

FIGURE 19-13 Examples of stereograms with contour-defined objects (local stereopsis) **(A)** or disparity-defined objects (global stereopsis or cyclopean perception) **(B).** The disparity patterns in the contour and random-dot stereograms are identical in size and disparity magnitude. Most individuals with normal binocular vision can learn to free-fuse the stereograms by either overconvergence or underconvergence and observe the stereoscopic depth in each example. However, it should be noted that the two viewing strategies produce opposite directions of relative depth.

grades stereoacuity in proportion to the magnitude of defocus.[89,118,156] The effect of blurring the retinal images is greater for stereoacuity than for other resolution tasks, such as visual acuity or instantaneous displacement thresholds.[156]

Unilateral optical defocus produces a greater reduction of stereoacuity than does symmetric bilateral defocus, which is consistent with other paradoxic effects on stereoacuity caused by interocular differences in stimulus parameters.[30,49,59,84,126] For example, improving the focus in one eye paradoxically degrades stereopsis more than equal defocus in both eyes does. With unilateral defocus, stereoacuity decreases as the amount of defocus increases until stereopsis is suspended by interocular differences greater than 2 diopters.[49,105] The filtering of high spatial frequencies that occurs in defocused images cannot fully explain the resulting reduction in stereoacuity[161]; hence, foveal suppression may also play a role.[146]

Because of the influence that optical defocus has on stereoacuity, the primary goal of refraction should be to provide an accurate refractive correction for each eye to optimize binocular vision and stereoacuity. However, for one group of patients—those with presbyopia—interocular refractive error corrections are often purposely unbalanced to correct one eye for distance vision and the other eye for near vision. The scheme of providing an ocular correction for distance vision with one eye and a near vision correction for the other eye, either with single vision contact lenses, refractive surgery, or intraocular lens implants, is called *monovision*.[38,128,144] The monovision procedure is successful only for patients with normal binocular vision and usually the dominant (sighting) eye is corrected for distance vision because less disorientation is experienced during perceptual adaptation to the anisometropic refractive correction.[37,95] After adaptation, most patients do not experience symptoms of asthenopia, nor are they aware of blurred vision at far or near viewing distances.[128] Although their binocular field of view and motor fusion ranges are generally normal, many patients with monovision experience diplopia at night or in dim illumination (when their pupils are dilated) or when they view bright targets of high contrast.[128] Some visual functions do not adapt to unilateral optical defocus, resulting in a loss of binocular summation for high spatial frequencies, reduced binocular visual acuity, and degraded stereoacuity with foveal suppression.[35,37,95]

Spatial Frequency and Contrast Effects on Stereopsis

Stereoacuity is influenced by both spatial frequency and contrast. Studies of stereopsis, using narrowly tuned, spatially filtered stimuli, have provided evidence that retinal disparities are processed by independent channels tuned to different spatial frequencies and different types of disparity.* Disparity can be described as either a positional offset of the two retinal images (measured in angular units) or a phase offset, where *phase* describes the disparity as a proportion of the luminance spatial period to which the disparity detector is tuned.[63,131] The neural mechanisms tuned to high spatial frequencies (greater than 2.5 cycles/degree) are sensitive to positional disparity and have higher sensitivities than the mechanisms tuned to lower spatial frequencies, which are sensitive to phase disparity.

Results from early experiments that used small, broadband stimuli suggest that stereoacuity is relatively unaffected by lowering contrast and luminance until their reduction diminishes the monocular visibility of the stereoscopic stimuli.[102] However, more recent investigations, using narrowband stimuli that are more specific for the early spatial filters in the binocular vision pathway, have found that stereoacuity is reduced with decreased binocular contrast and that the reduction is greater for high than low spatial frequency stimuli.[59,84,131] The effects of interocular differences are similar for contrast and optical defocus. Stereoacuity is reduced more with unilateral or asymmetric reductions of contrast than with binocular or symmetric contrast reductions.[59,84,131] In addition, the relative effects of contrast asymmetries are greater for low than for high spatial frequencies.[30] The improvement in stereoacuity with increasing bilateral contrast can be explained by an increased stimulus strength, which either intensifies signals from disparity-selective neurons or recruits signals from more disparity-selective neurons. However, the paradoxic decrease in stereoacuity with unilaterally increased contrast is

not consistent with the improved signal strength explanation, but it requires suppression, or masking, interactions.[146]

For disparities above the stereothreshold, the contrast sensitivity function for depth perception has a unimodal peak when measured with a binocular phase disparity of approximately 90 degrees.[63,137,140] With use of small or narrowband Gabor or difference-of-Gaussian stimuli that have low-range or midrange spatial frequencies, contrast sensitivity falls off as disparity increases, up to the upper disparity limit of stereopsis (D_{max}); however, the upper limit of stereoscopic depth perception also depends on stimulus bandwidth (size).[162]

Spatial Distortions from Aniseikonia

The two retinal images need to be similar in size and shape to support normal binocular vision; nonetheless, the visual system can tolerate small interocular differences without complete disruption of binocular fusion. An inequality in the size and/or shape of the two ocular images (aniseikonia) can occur from differences in the optics of the eyes, in the retinal receptor mosaics, or in cortical magnification.[101] However, the most common cause of aniseikonia is a difference in the refractive errors of the two eyes (anisometropia).[14] In refractive anisometropia, the optical components of the two eyes differ in power. Spherical optical differences produce a relative overall size discrepancy in the two retinal images, and astigmatic optical differences produce a relative meridional size difference in the two retinal images.[101] The most common anisometropia is a result of the natural development of refractive errors, although patients undergoing intraocular lens implantation, refractive surgery, or penetrating keratoplasty can also acquire anisometropia.[11,50,71]

There are large individual differences in symptoms and toleration of aniseikonia. Aniseikonia is usually considered clinically significant when the image size difference is greater than 4%, but many patients experience distortions in spatial perception and/or uncomfortable binocular vision, headaches, and eyestrain with differences as small as 2%.[19,101] The symptoms of eyestrain (asthenopia) are not specific, and the diagnosis of aniseikonia in a patient with fusion and stereopsis must be made from measurements of retinal image size differences or from assessment of the aniseikonic spatial distortions.* The size differences of the retinal images pose problems both for stereopsis and for con-

---

*References 41, 59, 70, 81, 84, 126, 131, 132, 166.

*References 1, 19, 82, 90, 101, 145.

trol of eye alignment. The size discrepancy generated by an anisometropic spectacle correction produces disparities that vary with eye position, causing a noncomitant variation of heterophoria (anisophoria).[125,129] The oculomotor system can adapt tonic vergence to compensate for anisophoria. However, when a person is unable to adapt to the correction, the symptoms of eyestrain occur with attempts to adjust eye alignment as gaze shifts from one direction to another. These motor symptoms can be confused with sensory disorders normally assumed to result from aniseikonia.[47] Anisometropic contact lens corrections do not produce anisophoria because the optical center of the lens remains fixed with respect to the pupil center during eye movements.

The types of spatial distortions perceived from the relative magnification of one retinal image can be understood by the altered perception of the orientation of the frontoparallel plane associated with aniseikonia.[101] Unequal retinal image sizes cause the apparent frontoparallel plane to be tilted around an axis through the fixation point by an amount and direction determined by three components of aniseikonia: the geometric effect, the induced effect, and declination errors. The three components of aniseikonic perceptual distortions are illustrated by stereograms in Figure 19-14, which were constructed for crossed-eye free fusion, and when viewed in a stereoscope or with straight-eye free fusion, the effects are opposite to the descriptions in the text.

The geometric effect, simulated in Figure 19-14, *B*, occurs with retinal image size differences in the horizontal meridian and is a consequence of the horizontal disparity caused by lateral magnification. The frontoparallel plane appears tilted toward the eye with the larger horizontal magnification. The physiologic basis for the altered tilt in the geometric effect is illustrated in Figure 19-15. To simulate a geometric effect, an observer views an objectively flat plane (plane PFQ) through a ×090 size lens or a focal magnifier. A size lens is a small Galilean telescope without refractive power for objects at infinity. In this example, it produces magnification in the horizontal meridian that is in front of the right eye. When the plane is viewed through the size lens, it does not appear parallel to the face, but rather rotated about the fixation point to the plane P'FQ', such that point P is perceived as nearer and point Q is perceived as farther. The amount of perceived rotation is proportional to the magnification difference between the two retinal images produced by the size lens. The direction and magnitude of rotation result from the change in the horizontal disparity gradient produced by the uniocular horizontal magnification. The disparities across the gradient are in opposing directions in the left and right visual fields. In this example the gradient produces crossed disparities for objects in the left visual field and uncrossed disparities for objects in the right visual field. The perceptually tilted plane illustrated in Figure 19-14, *B*, incorporates a perceptual surface rotation and an apparent change in perceived size. Objects in the left visual field appear smaller than those in the right. The size distortion is consistent with learned relationships between size and distance. For example, if one object appears farther than another, but without a correlated difference in retinal image sizes, the cue conflict causes the farther object to be perceived as larger.

The second component of aniseikonia, the induced effect, is caused by a relative magnification difference in the vertical meridians of the two eyes, which can be simulated by a ×180 vertical meridional magnifier. The induced effect is interesting because, as can be observed by the stereogram (Figure 19-14, *C*), vertical binocular disparities, by themselves, do not result in the perception of stereoscopic depth, but vertical meridional aniseikonia in a real-world visual environment causes a perceived rotation of the frontoparallel plane. The induced effect is similar to the geometric effect in that it is perceived as a rotation of the frontoparallel plane about a vertical axis, but the induced effect is in the opposite direction. The OFPP appears tilted away from the eye viewing through the vertical magnifier. Because the phenomenon is similar in form but opposite in direction to the geometric effect, it is called the *induced effect* to convey the notion that the distortion is the same as if it was "induced" by a horizontal meridional magnifier over the fellow eye.

The induced effect results from the magnification of the vertical disparities that are inherently present at relatively near viewing distances because of differences in ocular perspective of the target. Naturally occurring vertical disparities increase as the eccentricity of the target increases and as the viewing distance decreases.[149] If the viewing distance is sensed from convergence, target eccentricity can be derived from the rate of increase of vertical disparity with eccentricity (i.e., from the vertical disparity gradient). Vertical disparity gradients are used to scale disparity to quantify depth and interpret slant information.[3,51] Horizontal dis-

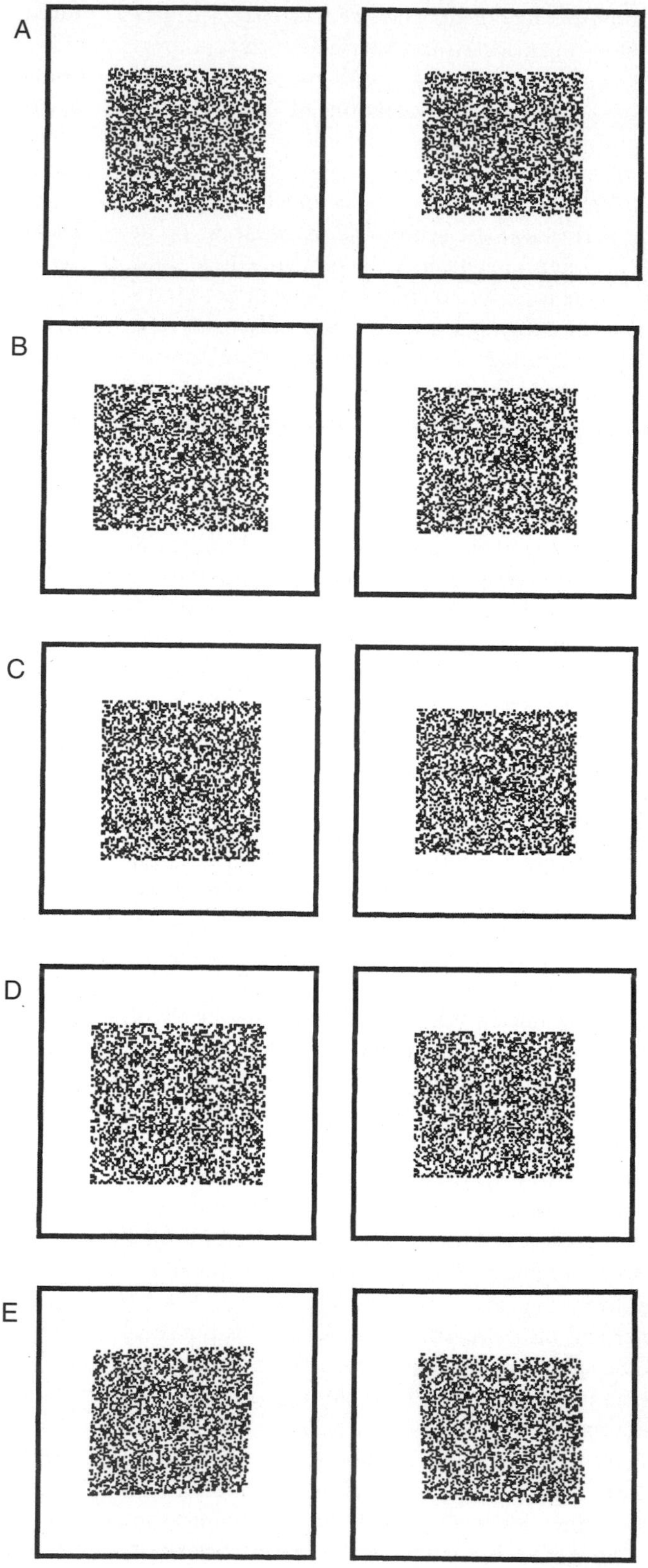

FIGURE 19-14   A series of stereograms to demonstrate the components of relative magnification from aniseikonia to illustrate subjective spatial distortions. The random-dot patterns represent frontoparallel plane stereograms that have been constructed to simulate various components of aniseikonia during binocularly fusion with crossed-eye viewing. (Other viewing strategies produce perceptual effects that are opposite to those described.) **A,** Normal spatial perception with equal-sized images for each eye. For an observer without aniseikonia, the perceived frontoparallel plane should not be distorted. **B,** A stereogram with a relative magnification of 10% in the horizontal meridian to demonstrate the geometric (×090) effect. The observer should perceive a tilt of the frontoparallel plane about a vertical axis with the right edge appearing more remote than the left edge of the plane. **C,** A magnification of 10% in the vertical meridian to simulate the magnification of the induced (×180) effect. For most observers, vertical disparities in a stereogram do not produce the apparent distortion of the frontoparallel plane that can be seen in a natural visual environment. **D,** A combination of horizontal and vertical magnification to produce an overall magnification of 10%. **E,** Relative magnification at oblique meridians (right eye, ×045; left eye, ×135 for crossed-eye fusion) to simulate the declination effect. The fused perception should be a slanted surface with the upper edge appearing more remote than the lower edge.

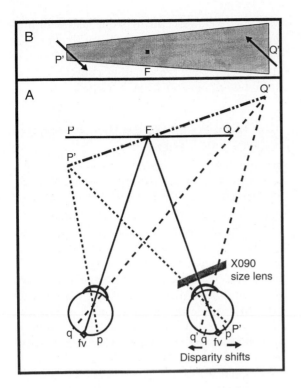

Figure 19-15 The physiologic basis of spatial distortions caused by the aniseikonia from meridional magnification in the horizontal meridian of the right eye. The frontoparallel plane PFQ appears to be rotated to a plane P'FQ' as a result of the binocular disparity produced by meridional magnification. (Adapted from Ogle KN: *Researches in binocular vision,* New York, 1964, Hafner.)

parity alone is an ambiguous stimulus for slant perception. Identical horizontal disparity patterns can correspond to different slant patterns for surfaces seen in symmetric and asymmetric convergence. For example, although a zero disparity pattern describes the VMO, this constant disparity pattern also describes a surface slant that increases with horizontal gaze eccentricity.[100] To interpret slant from horizontal disparity correctly, one needs a knowledge of target distance and gaze eccentricity. Vertical disparity gradients and convergence provide this information. When vertical magnifiers distort vertical disparity gradients, the surface slant is changed to conform to the distorted vertical disparity gradient.[73] This induced effect is weak, or absent, for targets located at an infinite viewing distance because retinal images of remote targets lack a difference in perspective significant enough to produce a vertical disparity gradient. For most observers, induced and geometric effects are about equal in magnitude and opposite in direction[101];

thus overall magnification differences, as opposed to meridional magnification differences, have little effect on the perception of space (see frontoparallel plane stimulus, Figure 19-14, *D*).

The third component of aniseikonia is a declination error (perceived tilt about a horizontal axis) that arises from retinal image shear or magnifications in oblique meridians (Figure 19-14, *E*). The direction of rotation (inclination or declination) of the oblique magnifier is predicted from the combined vertical and horizontal disparity components of the magnified retinal images. For example, the stereogram was constructed to simulate ×045 magnification for the right eye and ×135 magnification for the left eye with crossed-eye viewing, which creates a relative crossed disparity in the lower visual field compared to the upper (Figure 19-14, *E*). The resulting perception is a slanted surface with the bottom part of the surface closer. Oblique magnification can also cause horizontal tilt about a vertical axis if the horizontal and vertical components are unequal. Magnifiers at ×45 and ×135 degrees have equal horizontal and vertical magnification components, so the resulting geometric and induced effects tend to cancel one another. However, oblique magnification along other meridians produces unequal amounts of geometric and induced distortion, and the stronger distortion usually dominates the horizontal tilt percept.

In the final analysis the perceptual distortions from aniseikonia are a combination of the three components, geometric effect, induced effect, and declination error, with individual variability in the degree of tolerance and ability to adapt to stereoscopic misrepresentation of relative depth.

Motion-in-depth

The properties of visual direction and stereoscopic depth perception have been much more extensively studied with static stimuli at a constant fixation distance than under dynamic stimulus conditions. However, providing valid judgments of the trajectories and distances of moving objects, to capture moving objects or avoid collision with them, is a vital function of binocular vision.[54] The mechanisms underlying perception of the distance and the direction of moving objects are not as well understood, but there are at least two possible mechanisms for the perception of motion-in-depth.[33,110] First, the binocular disparity of an object moving in depth changes with time; thus the trajectory and distance could be interpolated from the responses of static disparity-sensitive mechanisms over time.

The second type of mechanism for the perception of motion-in-depth is one that is sensitive to differential velocities of the retinal images. An object that is moving in depth generates movements in the two retinal images that differ in speed and direction.

In natural scenes, as illustrated in Figure 19-7, changes in binocular disparity and differential interocular velocities are correlated. For this example, an object was moved along the visual axis of the left eye until the retinal image of the right eye was displaced outside the retinal region corresponding to Panum's fusional limit. During this measurement, if the test object had been moved from the uncrossed to the crossed disparity limits, it would have appeared to be moving in a depth trajectory toward the observer's left eye. The apparent trajectory is a property of the relative directions and velocities of the retinal images.[109] If in another case, the two retinal images of an object move in the same direction and velocity, the object would not appear to move toward the head; rather, it would be perceived as moving in the frontoparallel plane. If the retinal images move in opposite directions (i.e., temporoward), the object would appear to move toward the observer's head. In each example the object's motion-in-depth may have been detected by mechanisms sensitive to the sign and magnitude of binocular disparity, which have changed with time. On the other hand, for any given time, the direction and velocity of movement of each of the object's retinal images are different; thus the object's motion-in-depth could have been based on differential velocity information.

Some investigations of stereomotion have provided psychophysical and physiologic evidence for velocity-dependent mechanisms, whereas other studies have shown comparable perception of motion-in-depth in the absence of coherent velocity information.[8,9,33,110,111] For example, threshold and adaptation experiments have provided evidence for neural channels that are sensitive to the direction of motion-in-depth, with different channels selectively sensitive to approaching and receding motion. However, stereomotion can also be detected in dynamic random-dot stereograms that produce changes in disparity over time without consistent signals for interocular velocity differences. Regardless of the mechanism, the normal sensitivity to stereomovement requires about 5 to 10 times greater disparity magnitudes than stereoacuity measures with static stimuli.[33,158] Motion-in-depth may be present in patients with stereodeficiencies from early strabismus or amblyopia as a residual form of

stereopsis.[91] However, many individuals with normal visual acuity and stereopsis have areas of the binocular field that are insensitive, or even blind, to motion-in-depth.[114] Currently, clinical tests of stereomotion have not been developed.

SUPPRESSION IN NORMAL BINOCULAR VISION

In complex three-dimensional scenes, several types of binocular information must be combined to produce an integrated percept of depth and distance. Some of the visual information is coherent and unambiguous, such as images formed within the PFA. Coherent information contributes to normal fusion and stereoscopic depth perception. Some binocular information does not stimulate binocular fusion. For example, some regions of space may be clearly visible to only one eye (i.e., partially occluded to other eye), and this fragmented binocular information also contributes to the perceptions of distance and depth. Finally, information from binocular images that are uncorrelated, either because the matches are ambiguous or would conflict with other cues, also influences depth and distance perception. Visual confusion, in which superimposition of separate diplopic images arises from objects seen behind or in front of the plane of fixation, is an example of uncorrelation of binocular images that can be interpreted to suggest depth or distance. The binocular visual system attempts to preserve as much of the depth information as possible from all three sources to make inferences about objective space without introducing ambiguity or confusing space perception. At times, however, conflicts between the two eyes are so great that the conflicting information must be resolved by suppressing or suspending the perception arising from one of the retinal images.

Four classes of stimuli that appear to evoke different interocular suppression mechanisms in normal binocular vision have been identified.

1. Interocular blur suppression occurs when the retinal images have significant differences in blur or contrast.[138] A variety of natural conditions produce unequal contrast of the two ocular images, including naturally occurring anisometropia, unequal amplitudes of accommodation, and asymmetric convergence on targets that are closer to one eye than to the other. The relative differences in blur can be partially eliminated by differential accommodation of the two eyes and by interocular

suppression of the blur.[93,128] The latter mechanism is requisite for adaptation to a monovision correction of presbyopia. Monovision suppression allows clear, nonblurred, binocular percepts and retention of stereopsis, albeit with the stereothreshold elevated by approximately twofold.[35,128]

2. Suspension is the mechanism that eliminates one of the two ocular percepts that arise during physiologic diplopia, in which targets lying in front of or behind the singleness horopter are seen as doubled.[28] Binocular eye alignment optimizes depth information from binocular disparities near the horopter while simultaneously producing large disparities for the objects that are at some distance in front of or behind the plane of fixation. Even with binocular disparities that are well outside the limits of PFAs, the perception of diplopia under normal casual viewing conditions is rare because of the suppression of one image. The suppression of physiologic diplopia is called *suspension* because this form of suppression does not alternate between the two images. Instead, only one image is continually suppressed, favoring visibility of the target imaged on the nasal hemiretina.[32,39,80] However, suspension is not obligatory, and calling attention to the disparate target can evoke physiologic diplopia. It has also been suggested that suspension may be involved in the permanent suppression of pathologic diplopia associated with strabismus.[40,55,119,120]

3. Binocular (retinal) rivalry suppression is a rhythmic alternating perception of each of the retinal images when substantial differences in their sizes or shapes preclude their fusion. The classic demonstration of binocular rivalry arising from nonfusible images formed on or near corresponding retinal points is shown in Figure 19-16, *A*, which presents orthogonal-oriented gratings to the two eyes. In this example, rivalry suppression can take the form of either exclusive domination or mosaic domination. During exclusive domination, each of the two images alternates between dominance and suppression: One set of lines is seen, and after several seconds, the image of the other set of lines appears to wash over the first. In mosaic domination the two monocular images become fragmented, and small interwoven retinal patches from each eye alternate independently of one another. In this case suppression is regional, localized to the vicinity of the contour intersections.

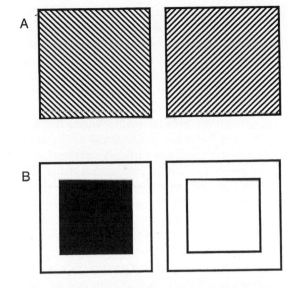

FIGURE 19-16 Stereograms to demonstrate the perceptual consequences of binocular viewing of nonfusible objects or surfaces. **A,** Binocular rivalry. **B,** Binocular luster

dently of one another. In this case suppression is regional, localized to the vicinity of the contour intersections.

The perceived rivalrous patches alternate between the two ocular images approximately once every 4 seconds, but the rate of oscillation and its duty cycle vary with the degree of difference between the two ocular images and with the stimulus strength. The rate of rivalry increases as the orientation difference between the targets increases beyond 22 degrees, indicating that rivalry is not likely to occur within the tuned range for cortical orientation columns.[39,119] Levelt[85] formulated a series of rules describing how the dominance and suppression phases of binocular rivalry vary with the strength of stimulus variables such as brightness, contrast, and motion. He concluded that the duration of the suppression phase of one of the retinal images decreases when its stimulus visibility or strength is increased relative to the retinal image of the fellow eye. If the strengths of the stimuli for both eyes are increased, the suppression phase for each eye decreases and the oscillation rate of rivalry increases. Reducing the stimulus contrast of both eyes also reduces the oscillation rate, until at a low contrast level, rivalry is replaced with a binocular summation of nonfusible targets.[88]

The perception of rivalry has a latency of approximately 200 msec, so briefly presented nonfusible patterns appear superimposed.[68] However, rivalry occurs between dichoptic patterns that are alternated rapidly at 7 Hz or faster, indicating an integration time of at least 150 msec.[163] When rivalrous and fusible stimuli are presented simultaneously, fusion takes precedence over rivalry and the onset of a fusible target can terminate suppression, although the fusion mechanism takes time (150 to 200 msec) to become fully operational.[15,56,164] Suppression and stereofusion appear to be mutually exclusive outcomes of binocular rivalry stimuli presented at a given retinal location, but stereoscopic depth and rivalry can be observed simultaneously when fusible contours are superimposed on rivalrous backgrounds.[16,147]

Because both binocular rivalry suppression and strabismic suppression result in a functional loss of visual information from one eye during binocular viewing, binocular rivalry suppression and strabismic suppression have been hypothesized to be related phenomena.[154] However, the patterns of suppression are different for normal and esotropic subjects, suggesting that strabismic observers do not demonstrate normal binocular rivalry and that strabismic suppression and normal binocular rivalry suppression are mediated by different neural mechanisms.[140-142]

Another form of binocular rivalry occurs when unfusible surface brightnesses (e.g., black and white) or surface colors (e.g., red and green) are dichoptically superimposed. In this form the phenomenon is known as binocular luster or as luminance or color rivalry.[100,161] Figure 19-16, *B*, presents a stereogram that evokes binocular luster, which is usually described as a shimmering, unstable surface percept, as though one surface is being seen through another. The perception of luster requires a certain level of binocular vision, but it does not require fusion ability; therefore testing for binocular luster has been advocated for evaluating binocularity and anomalous retinal correspondence in strabismic patients.

4. Permanent-occlusion suppression is a more stable form of suppression that occurs when one eye views a contoured stimulus while the other eye views a spatially homogenous field.[94] Under these conditions, the image of the eye viewing the contoured field dominates, while the image of the eye viewing the homogeneous field is almost continually suppressed. Because of the stability of the dominance/suppression percept under these viewing conditions, the term *permanent suppression* is used to distinguish this type of suppression from binocular rivalry suppression.

On many occasions the two eyes see dissimilar forms as a result of partial occlusion in the near visual field. Natural partial occlusion occurs when one eye's view of a distal target is partially obstructed by a nearby object, such as the nose, or when distal objects are viewed through a narrow aperture. Under these conditions, the occluding object is normally suppressed to retain a constant view of the background. This phenomenon can be demonstrated by holding a cylindrical tube in front of the right eye and placing the palm of the left hand in front of the left eye near the distal end of the tube. The combined stable percept is that of a hole in the left hand. The hand is seen as the region surrounding the aperture, through which the background is viewed. This ecologically valid example of occlusion gives priority to the background seen through the aperture. The mechanisms underlying stable, permanent suppression are unlike those underlying rivalry suppression because different changes in the increment-threshold spectral sensitivity function are produced by these two phenomena.[115]

SUMMARY

Binocular vision is an intricate organization of biologic and psychologic components to provide haplopia and an accurate subjective representation of the depth and distance of every object in the environment. This chapter has presented some of the basic principles of the normal and clinically abnormal sensory processes, but they are just one part of the system. Equally important are the oculomotor components, which in normal binocular vision interact with sensory mechanisms to place the ocular images on appropriate retinal areas to support fusion and stereopsis or they interact with abnormal oculomotor control, as in strabismus, to enlist adaptive sensory mechanisms of suppression and anomalous retinal correspondence. Furthermore, whether an individual has normal or abnormal binocular vision is a product of environmental influences in infancy. During an early sensitive period, normal visual experience is required to develop the full capacity of the visual system; otherwise, abnormal visual experience produces abnormal monocular or binocular visual processes. Clinical application of the science of binocular vision involves all of these components, with the goal to alleviate any interference with clear, single binocular vision.

REFERENCES

1. Achiron LR et al: The effect of relative spectacle magnification on aniseikonia, *J Am Optom Assoc* 69:591, 1998.
2. Awaya S, von Noorden GK, Romano PE: Sensory adaptations in strabismus: anomalous retinal correspondence in different positions of gaze, *Am Orthopt J* 20:28, 1970.
3. Backus BT et al: Horizontal and vertical disparity, eye position, and stereoscopic slant perception, *Vision Res* 39:1143, 1999.
4. Bagolini B: Anomalous correspondence: definition and diagnostic methods, *Doc Ophthalmol* 23:346, 1967.
5. Bagolini B, Capobianco NM: Subjective space in comitant squint, *Am J Ophthalmol* 59:430, 1965.
6. Baker FH, Grigg P, von Noorden GK: Effects of visual deprivation and strabismus on the response of neurons in the visual cortex of the monkey, including studies on the striate and prestriate cortex in the normal animal, *Brain Res* 66:165, 1974.
7. Banks MS, van Ee R, Backus BT: The computation of binocular visual direction: a re-examination of Manfield and Legge (1996), *Vision Res* 37:1605, 1997.
8. Beverly KI, Regan D: Evidence for the existence of neural mechanisms selectively sensitive to the direction of movement in space, *J Physiol Lond* 235:17, 1973.
9. Beverly KI, Regan D: Selective adaptation in stereoscopic depth perception, *J Physiol Lond* 232:40, 1973.
10. Bielschowsky A: Application of the afterimage test in the investigation of squint, *Am J Ophthalmol* 20:408, 1937.
11. Binder PS: The effect of suture removal on keratoplasty astigmatism, *Am J Ophthalmol* 105:637, 1988.
12. Birch EE, Stager DR: Random dot stereoacuity following surgical correction of infantile esotropia, *J Ped Ophthalmol Strab* 32:231, 1995.
13. Birch EE et al: Prospective assessment of acuity and stereopsis in amblyopic esotropes following early surgery, *Invest Ophthalmol Vis Sci* 31:758, 1990.
14. Bishop PO: Binocular vision. In Moses RA, Hart WM (eds): *Adler's physiology of the eye*, ed 8, St Louis, 1987, Mosby.
15. Blake R, Boothroyd K: The precedence of binocular fusion over binocular rivalry, *Percept Psychophys* 37:114, 1985.
16. Blake R, O'Shea RP: "Abnormal fusion" of stereopsis and binocular rivalry, *Psychol Rev* 95:151, 1988.
17. Blake R, Sloane M, Fox R: Further developments in binocular summation, *Percept Psychophys* 30:266, 1981.
18. Boeder P: The response shift, *Doc Ophthalmol* 23:88, 1967.
19. Borish IM: *Clinical refraction*, ed 3, Chicago, 1975, Professional Press.
20. Boucher JA: Common visual direction horopters in exotropes with anomalous correspondence, *Am J Optom Arch Am Acad Optom* 44:547, 1967.
21. Bradshaw MF, Rogers BJ, De Bruyn B: Perceptual latency and complex random-dot stereograms, *Perception* 24:749, 1995.
22. Brock FW: Projection habits in alternate squints, *Am J Optom* 17:193, 1940.
23. Brown JP, Ogle KN, Reiher L: Stereoscopic acuity and observation distance, *Invest Ophthalmol* 4:894, 1965.
24. Burian HM: Anomalous retinal correspondence: its essence and its significance in diagnosis and treatment, *Am J Ophthalmol* 34:237, 1951.
25. Campbell FW, Green DG: Monocular versus binocular visual acuity, *Nature* 208:191, 1965.
26. Chino YM et al: Postnatal development of binocular disparity sensitivity in neurons of the primate visual cortex, *J Neurosci* 17:296, 1997.
27. Clarke WN, Noel LP: Stereoacuity testing in the monofixation syndrome, *J Pediatr Ophthalmol Strab* 27:161, 1990.
28. Cline D, Hofstetter HW, Griffin JR: *Dictionary of visual science*, ed 4, Radnor, Pa, 1989, Chilton.
29. Collewijn H et al: Binocular fusion, stereopsis and stereoacuity with a moving head. In Regan D (ed): *Vision and visual dysfunction*, vol 9, Boca Raton, Fla, 1991, CRC Press.
30. Cormack LK, Stevenson SB, Landers DD: Interactions of spatial frequency and unequal monocular contrasts in stereopsis, *Perception* 26:1121, 1997.
31. Crone RA: *Diplopia*, Amsterdam, 1973, Excerpta Medica.
32. Crovitz HF, Lipscomb DB: Dominance of the temporal visual fields at a short duration of stimulation, *Am J Psychol* 76:631, 1963.
33. Cumming BG, Parker AJ: Binocular mechanisms for detecting motion-in-depth, *Vision Res* 34:483, 1994.
34. Demanins R, Wang YZ, Hess RF: The neural deficit in strabismic amblyopia: sampling considerations, *Vision Res* 39:3575, 1999.
35. Du Toit R, Ferreira JT, Nel ZJ: Visual and nonvisual variables implicated in monovision wear, *Optom Vis Sci* 75:119, 1998.
36. Edwards M, Pope DR, Schor CM: Luminance contrast and spatial-frequency tuning of the transient-vergence system, *Vision Res* 38:705, 1998.
37. Erickson P, McGill EC: Role of visual acuity, stereoacuity, and ocular dominance in monovision patient success, *Optom Vis Sci* 69:761, 1992.
38. Erickson P, Schor CM: Visual function with presbyopic contact lens correction, *Optom Vis Sci* 67:22, 1990.
39. Fahle M: Binocular rivalry: Suppression depends on orientation and spatial frequency, *Vision Res* 22:787, 1982.
40. Fahle M: Naso-temporal asymmetry of binocular inhibition, *Invest Ophthalmol Vis Sci* 28:1016, 1987.
41. Felton TB, Richards W, Smith RA: Disparity processing of spatial frequencies in man, *J Physiol Lond* 225:349, 1972.
42. Flom MC: Corresponding and disparate retinal points in normal and anomalous correspondence, *Am J Optom Physiol Opt* 57:656, 1980.
43. Flom MC, Kerr KE: Determination of retinal correspondence. Multiple-testing results and the depth of anomaly concept, *Arch Ophthalmol* 77:200, 1967.
44. Foley JM: Binocular distance perception, *Psychol Rev* 87:411, 1980.
45. Foley JM, Applebaum TH, Richards WA: Stereopsis with large disparities: discrimination and depth magnitude, *Vision Res* 15:417, 1975.
46. Fredenburg P, Harwerth RS: The relative sensitivities of sensory and motor fusion to small disparities, *Vision Res* 41:1969, 2001.

47. Friedenwald JS: Diagnosis and treatment of anisophoria, *Arch Ophthalmol* 15:283, 1936.

48. Garding J et al: Stereopsis, vertical disparity and relief transformations, *Vision Res* 35:703, 1995.

49. Geib T, Baumann C: Effect of luminance and contrast on stereoscopic acuity, *Graefe's Arch Clin Exp Ophthalmol* 228:310, 1990.

50. Genvert GI et al: Fitting gas-permeable contact lenses after penetrating keratoplasty, *Am J Ophthalmol* 99:511, 1985.

51. Gillam BJ, Blackburn SG: Surface separation decreases stereoscopic slant but a monocular aperture increases it, *Perception* 27:1267, 1998.

52. Gillam B, Lawergren B: The induced effect, vertical disparity, and stereoscopic theory, *Percept Psycho* 34:121, 1983.

53. Gobin MH: The limitation of suppression to one half of the visual field in the pathogenesis of strabismus, *Br Orthop J* 25:42, 1968.

54. Graham CH: Visual space perception. In Graham CH (ed): *Vision and visual perception,* New York, 1965, Wiley.

55. Harrad R: Psychophysics of suppression, *Eye* 10:270, 1996.

56. Harrad RA et al: Binocular rivalry disrupts stereopsis, *Perception* 23:15, 1994.

57. Harrington DO: *The visual fields,* St Louis, 1964, Mosby.

58. Hallden U: Fusional phenomena in anomalous correspondence, *Acta Ophthalmol* 37:1, 1952.

59. Halpern DL, Blake R: How contrast affects stereoacuity, *Perception* 17:3, 1988.

60. Harwerth RS, Rawlings SC: Pattern and depth discrimination from random dot stereograms, *Am J Optom Physiol Optics* 52:248, 1975.

61. Harwerth RS, Rawlings SC: Viewing time and stereoscopic threshold with random-dot stereograms, *Am J Optom Physiol Optics* 54:452, 1977.

62. Harwerth RS, Smith EL: Binocular summation in man and monkey, *Am J Optom Physiol Optics* 62:439, 1985.

63. Harwerth RS, Smith EL, Crawford MLJ: Motor and sensory fusion in monkeys: psychophysical measurements, *Eye* 10:209, 1996.

64. Harwerth RS, Smith EL, Levi DM: Suprathreshold binocular interactions for grating patterns, *Percept Psychophys* 27:43, 1980.

65. Harwerth RS, Smith EL, Siderov J: Behavioral studies of local stereopsis and disparity vergence in monkeys, *Vision Res* 35:1755, 1995.

66. Hebbard FW: Comparison of subjective and objective measurements of fixation disparity, *J Opt Soc Am* 52:706, 1962.

67. Helveston EM, von Noorden GK, Williams F: Sensory adaptations in strabismus: retinal correspondence in the "A" or "V" pattern, *Am Orthopt J* 20:22, 1970.

68. Hering E: *Beitrage zur Physiologie,* vol 5, Leipzig,1861, Engelmann.

69. Hess RF, Baker CL, Wilcox LM: Comparison of motion and stereopsis: linear and nonlinear performance, *J Opt Soc Am A Opt Image Sci Vis* 16:987, 1999.

70. Hess RF, Wilcox LM: Linear and non-linear filtering in stereopsis, *Vision Res* 34:2431, 1994.

71. Holladay JT et al: Improving the predictability of intraocular lens power calculations, *Arch Ophthalmol* 104:539, 1986.

72. Howard IP: *Human visual orientation,* New York, 1982, Wiley.

73. Howard IP, Rogers BJ: *Binocular vision and stereopsis,* Oxford, 1995, Oxford University Press.

74. Hubel DH, Wiesel TN: Ferrier lecture: functional architecture of macaque monkey visual cortex, *Proc R Soc Lond B Biol Sci* 198:1, 1977.

75. Jampolosky A: Characteristics of suppression in strabismus, *Arch Ophthalmol* 54:683, 1955.

76. Jones R: Anomalies of disparity detection in the human visual system, *J Physiol Lond* 264:621, 1977.

77. Jones R: Horizontal disparity vergence. In Schor CM, Ciuffreda KJ (eds): *Vergence eye movements: basic and clinical aspects,* Boston, 1983, Butterworths.

78. Julesz B: *Foundations of cyclopean perception,* Chicago, 1971, University of Chicago Press.

79. Kerr KE: Anomalous correspondence: the cause or consequence of strabismus? *Optom Vis Sci* 75:17, 1998.

80. Kollner H: Das funktionelle Uberwiegen der nasalen Netzhauthalften im gemeinschaftlichen Schfeld, *Archiv Augenheilkunde* 76:153, 1914.

81. Kontesevich LL, Tyler CW: Analysis of stereothresholds for stimuli below 2.5 c/deg, *Vision Res* 34:2317, 1994.

82. Kramer P et al: A study of aniseikonia and Knapp's law using a projection space eikonometer, *Binocul Vis Strabismus Q* 14:197, 1999.

83. Landers D, Cormack LK: Stereoscopic depth fading is disparity and spatial frequency dependent, *Invest Opthalmol Vis Sci* 40s:416, 1999.

84. Legge GE, Gu Y: Stereopsis and contrast, *Vision Res* 29:989, 1989.

85. Levelt W: *Psychological studies on binocular rivalry,* The Hague, 1968, Mouton.

86. Levi DM, Klein SA, Aitsebaomo P: Vernier acuity, crowding and cortical magnification, *Vision Res* 25:963, 1985.

87. Liu L, Stevenson SB, Schor CM: A polar coordinate system for describing binocular disparity, *Vision Res* 34:1205, 1994.

88. Liu L, Tyler CW, Schor CM: Failure of rivalry at low contrast: evidence of a suprathreshold binocular summation process, *Vision Res* 32:1471, 1992.

89. Lovasik J, Szymkiw M: Effects of aniseikonia, retinal illuminance and pupil size on stereopsis, *Invest Ophthalmol Vis Sci* 26:741, 1985.

90. Lubkin LV et al: Aniseikonia quantification: error rate of rule of thumb estimation, *Binocul Vis Strabismus Q* 14:191, 1999.

91. Maeda M et al: Binocular depth-from-motion in infantile and late-onset esotropia patients with poor stereopsis, *Invest Ophthalmol Vis Sci* 40:3031, 1999.

92. Marr D, Poggio T: A computational theory of human stereo vision, *Proc Royal Soc Lond* 204:301, 1979.

93. Marran L, Schor CM: Lens induced aniso-accommodaton, *Vision Res* 38:3601, 1997.

94. Mauk D, Francis EL, Fox R: The selectivity of permanent suppression, *Invest Ophthalmol Vis Sci* 25s:294, 1984.

95. McGill EC, Erickson P: Sighting dominance and monovision distance binocular fusional ranges, *J Am Optom Assoc* 62:738, 1991.

96. Mills RP: Correlation of quality of life with clinical symptoms and signs at the time of diagnosis, *Trans Am Ophthalmol Soc* 96:753, 1998.

97. Mitchell DE: A review of the concept of "Panum's fusional areas," *Am J Optom Physiol Optics* 43:387, 1966.

98. Musch DC et al: Assessment of health-related quality of life after corneal transplantation, *Am J Ophthalmol* 124:1, 1997.

99. Ogle KN: Disparity limits of stereopsis, *Arch Ophthalmol* 48:50, 1952.

100. Ogle KN: The optical space sense. In Davson H (ed): *The eye,* vol 4, New York, 1962, Academic Press.

101. Ogle KN: *Researches in binocular vision,* New York, 1964, Hafner.

102. Ogle KN, Groch J: Stereopsis and unequal luminosities of the images in the two eyes, *Arch Ophthalmol* 56:878, 1956.

103. Ogle KN, Martens TG, Dyer JA: *Oculomotor imbalance in binocular vision and fixation disparity,* Philadelphia, 1967, Lea Febiger.

104. Ogle KN, Weil MP: Stereoscopic vision and the duration of the stimulus, *Arch Ophthalmol* 59:4, 1958.

105. Ong J, Burley WS: Effect of induced anisometropia on depth perception, *Am J Optom Arch Am Acad Optom* 49:333, 1972.

106. Parks MM: Monofixation syndrome, *Trans Am Ophthalmol Soc* 67:609, 1969.

107. Poggio GF, Gonzalez F, Krause F: Stereoscopic mechanisms in monkey visual cortex: binocular correlation and disparity selectivity, *J Neurosci* 8:4531, 1998.

108. Pope DR, Edwards M, Schor CM: Extraction of depth from opposite-contrast stimuli: transient system can, sustained system can't, *Vision Res* 39:4010, 1999.

109. Regan D: Depth from motion and motion-in-depth. In Regan D (ed): *Vision and visual dysfunction,* vol 9, Boca Raton, Fla, 1991, CRC Press.

110. Regan D: Binocular correlates of the direction of motion in depth, *Vision Res* 33:2359, 1993.

111. Regan D, Beverly KI: Electrophysiological evidence for the existence of neurons sensitive to the direction of depth movement, *Nature* 246:504, 1973.

112. Richards W: Stereopsis and stereoblindness, *Exp Brain Res* 10:380, 1970.

113. Richards W: Anomalous stereoscopic depth perception, *J Opt Soc Am* 61:410, 1971.

114. Richards W, Regan D: A stereo field map with implications for disparity processing, *Invest Ophthalmol* 12:904, 1973.

115. Ridder WH et al: Effects of interocular suppression on spectral sensitivity, *Optom Vis Sci* 69:171, 1992.

116. Rogers BJ, Bradshaw MF: Vertical disparities, differential perspective and binocular stereopsis, *Nature* 361:253, 1993.

117. Saye A, Frisby JP: The role of monocularly conspicuous features in facilitating stereopsis from random-dot stereograms, *Perception* 4:159, 1975.

118. Schmidt PP: Sensitivity of random-dot stereoacuity and Snellen acuity to optical blur, *Optom Vis Sci* 71:466, 1994.

119. Schor CM: Visual stimuli for strabismic suppression, *Perception* 6:583, 1977.

120. Schor CM: Zero retinal image disparity: a stimulus for suppression in small angle strabismus, *Doc Ophthalmol* 46:149, 1978.

121. Schor CM: Fixation disparity and vergence adaptation. In Schor CM, Ciuffreda KJ (eds): *Vergence eye movements: basic and clinical aspects,* Boston, 1983, Butterworths.

122. Schor CM: Binocular sensory disorders. In Regan D (ed): *Vision and visual dysfunction,* vol 9, Boca Raton, Fla, 1991, CRC Press.

123. Schor CM, Bridgeman B, Tyler CW: Spatial characteristics of static and dynamic stereoacuity in strabismus, *Invest Ophthalmol Vis Sci* 24:1572, 1983.

124. Schor CM, Edwards M, Pope D: Spatial-frequency tuning of the transient-stereopsis system, *Vision Res* 38:3057, 1998.

125. Schor CM, Gleason G, Lunn R: Interactions between short-term vertical phoria adaptation and nonconjugate adaptation of vertical pursuits, *Vision Res* 33:55, 1993.

126. Schor CM, Heckman T: Interocular differences in contrast and spatial frequency: effects on stereopsis and fusion, *Vision Res* 29:837, 1989.

127. Schor CM, Heckman T, Tyler CW: Binocular fusion limits are independent of contrast, luminance gradient and component phases, *Vision Res* 29:821, 1989.

128. Schor CM, Landsman L, Erickson P: Ocular dominance and interocular suppression of blur in monovision, *Am J Optom Physiol Optics* 64:723, 1987.

129. Schor CM, McCandless JW: An adaptable association between vertical and horizontal vergence, *Vision Res* 35:3519, 1995.

130. Schor CM, Tyler CW: Spatio-temporal properties of Panum's fusional area, *Vision Res* 21:683, 1981.

131. Schor CM, Wood I: Disparity range for local stereopsis as a function of luminance spatial frequency, *Vision Res* 23:1649, 1983.

132. Schor CM, Wood IC, Ogawa J: Spatial tuning of static and dynamic local stereopsis, *Vision Res* 24:573, 1984.

133. Sheedy JE, Fry GA: The perceived direction of the binocular image, *Vision Res* 19:201, 1979.

134. Shipley T, Rawlings SC: The nonius horopter. I. History and theory, *Vision Res* 10:1255, 1970.

135. Shortess GK, Krauskopf, J: Role of involuntary eye movements in stereoscopic acuity, *J Opt Soc Am* 51:555, 1961.

136. Siderov J, Harwerth RS, Bedell HE: Stereopsis, cyclovergence and the backwards tilt of the vertical horopter, *Vision Res* 39:1347, 1999.

137. Simmons DR, Kingdom FAA: Contrast thresholds for stereoscopic depth identification with isoluminant and isochromatic stimuli, *Vision Res* 34:2971, 1994.

138. Simpson TL, Barbeito R, Bedell HE: The effect of optical blur on visual acuity for targets of different luminances, *Ophthalmic Physiol Opt* 6:279, 1986.

139. Smallman HS, MacLeod DIA: Size-disparity correlation in stereopsis at contrast threshold, *J Opt Soc Am A* 11:2169, 1994.

140. Smith EL et al: Color vision is altered during binocular rivalry, *Science* 218:802, 1982.

141. Smith EL et al: The relationship between binocular rivalry and strabismic suppression, *Invest Ophthalmol Vis Sci* 26:80, 1985.

142. Smith EL et al: Interocular suppression produced by rivalry stimuli: A comparison of normal and abnormal binocular vision, *Optom Vis Sci* 71:479, 1994.

143. Smith EL et al: Binocular spatial phase tuning characteristics of neurons in the macaque striate cortex, *Neurophysiology* 78:351, 1997.

144. Snyder C: Monovision: a clinical review, *Spectrum* 4:30, 1989.

145. Stephens GL, Polasky M: New options for aniseikonia correction: the use of high index materials, *Optom Vis Sci* 68:899, 1991.

146. Stevenson SB, Cormack LK: A contrast paradox in stereopsis, motion detection, and vernier acuity, *Vision Res* 40:2881, 2000.

147. Timney B, Wilcox LM, St. John R: On the evidence for a 'pure' binocular process in human vision, *Spatial Vis* 4:1, 1989.

148. Tyler CW: Sensory processing of binocular disparity. In Schor CM, Ciuffreda KJ (eds): *Vergence eye movements: basic and clinical aspects,* Boston, 1983, Butterworths.

149. Van Ee R, Schor CM: Unconstrained stereoscopic matching of lines, *Vision Res* 40:151, 2000.

150. Verhoeff FH: Anomalous projection and other visual phenomena associated with strabismus, *Arch Ophthalmol* 19:663, 1938.

151. Von Helmholtz H: *Treatise on physiological optics,* vol III, New York 1962, Dover (Translated from the third German edition and edited by Southhall JPC).

152. Von Noorden GK: Infantile esotropia: a continuing riddle, *Am Orthop J* 34:52, 1984.

153. Von Noorden GK: Amblyopia: a multidisciplinary approach. Proctor lecture, *Invest Ophthalmol Vis Sci* 26:1704, 1985.

154. Von Noorden GK: *Binocular vision and ocular motility,* St Louis, 1990, Mosby.

155. Wensveen JM, Harwerth RS, Smith EL: Clinical suppression in monkeys reared with abnormal visual experience, *Vision Res* 41:1593, 2001.

156. Westheimer G: The spatial sense of the eye, *Invest Ophthalmol Vis Sci* 18:893, 1979.

157. Westheimer G: Visual hyperacuity, *Prog Sensory Physiol* 1:1, 1981.

158. Westheimer G: The Ferrier lecture, 1992. Seeing depth with two eyes: stereopsis, *Proc R Soc Lond B Biol Sci* 257:205, 1994.

159. Westheimer G, McKee SP: Stereoscopic acuity with defocused and spatially filtered images, *J Opt Soc Am* 70:772, 1980.

160. Westheimer G, Pettet MW: Detection and processing of vertical disparity by the human observer, *Proc R Soc Lond B Biol Sci* 250:243, 1992.

161. Wheatstone C: Contributions to the physiology of vision: I. On some remarkable, and hitherto unobserved, phenomena of binocular vision, *Phil Trans R Soc Lond* 128:371, 1938.

162. Wilcox LM, Hess RF: Dmax for stereopsis depends on size, not spatial frequency content, *Vision Res* 35:1061, 1995.

163. Wolfe JM: Afterimages, binocular rivalry, and the temporal properties of dominance and suppression, *Perception* 12:439, 1983.

164. Wolfe JM: Stereopsis and binocular rivalry, *Psychol Rev* 93:269, 1986.

165. Wong AM et al: Anomalous retinal correspondence: neuroanatomic mechanism in strabismic monkeys and clinical findings in strabismic children, *J AAPOS* 4:168, 2000.

166. Yang Y, Blake R: Spatial frequency tuning of human stereopsis, *Vision Res* 31:1177, 1991.

CHAPTER 20

TEMPORAL PROPERTIES OF VISION

ALLISON M. MCKENDRICK AND CHRIS A. JOHNSON

Our visual perception arises from the interpretation of light information, which varies in space, wavelength, and time. It is the latter of these attributes that is explored in this chapter. Subjectively, the world appears to be stable despite continuous changes in the visual scene. How does the visual system respond to and interpret light variations that occur as a function of time?

The duration of a light affects how easily we can see it and its subjective appearance. This chapter emphasizes the first of these issues, that is, how sensitive we are to temporal variations in light and which factors influence our sensitivity. Temporal sensitivity cannot be studied in isolation because other stimulus attributes, such as spatial properties, chromaticity, and background and surround characteristics, all influence our ability to detect temporal variations. In the natural world, most temporal variation occurs through image motion. This may arise from motion of the observer, the eyes, or the object itself. Motion is a special form of temporal variation in which the change with time is associated with a change in spatial position.

This chapter summarizes a number of basic phenomena that describe our sensitivity to temporal information. The application of these phenomena to the clinical study of abnormalities of visual processing, such as in disease, is also discussed.

TEMPORAL SUMMATION AND THE CRITICAL DURATION

To detect the presence of something in the visual world, it must be present for a finite period. Although a single quantum of light may be sufficient to generate a neural response, multiple quanta are generally required during a short period before the light is reliably seen, a property known as *temporal summation*. In the human visual system, temporal summation occurs for durations of approximately 40 to 100 milliseconds, depending on the spatial and temporal properties of the object and its background, the adaptation level, and the eccentricity of the stimulus.[29,33,67,103,155] The maximum time over which temporal summation can occur is the *critical duration*.

Let's say we wish to determine how long a light needs to be presented on a dark background to be visible. In general terms, an intense light does not need to be presented for as long as a weak one to reach threshold visibility. The relationship between the luminance of the light and the duration of its exposure to reach visibility is, over a limited range, a linear one. Provided that the light pulse is briefer than the critical duration, it will be at threshold when the product of its duration and its intensity equals a constant. The formula that describes this time-intensity reciprocity is *Bloch's law*[24]:

$$Bt = K$$

where

B = Luminance of the light
t = Duration
K = A constant value

Bloch's law is shown schematically in Figure 20-1, *A*. When plotted on log-log coordinates, as in Figure 20-1, *A*, Bloch's law describes a line with a slope of −1. When the critical duration is reached, the threshold intensity versus duration function is described by a horizontal line; that is, a constant intensity is required to reach threshold. Bloch's law has been shown to be generally valid for a wide range of stimulus and background conditions, including both foveal and peripheral viewing. Once the duration of

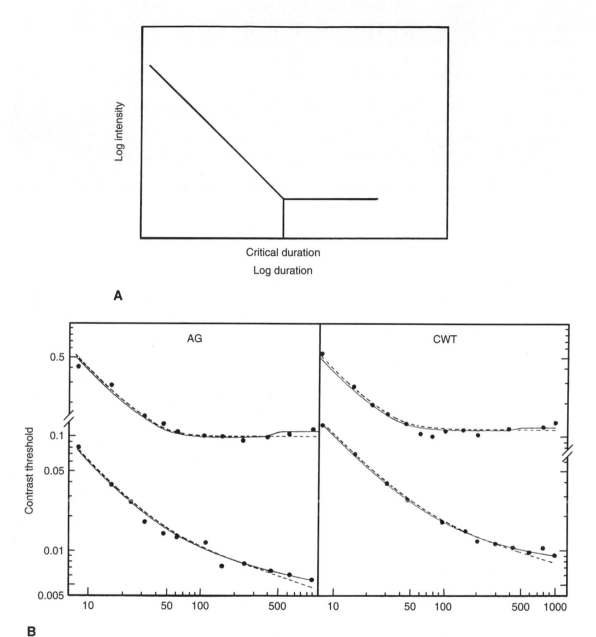

FIGURE 20-1   A, Schematic of the idealized relationship between threshold light intensity and the duration for it to reach visibility. For durations less than the critical duration, the threshold intensity is linearly related to duration, as described by Bloch's law. **B,** The relationship between threshold light intensity and duration for flickering grating stimuli for two observers as measured by Gorea and Tyler.[67] Upper curves represent data from 0.8 cycle per degree gratings, whereas lower curves show data for an 8 degree per cycle grating stimulus. Note that for the higher spatial frequency (lower curve), there is a more gradual transition between the two curves depicted schematically in **A.**

the stimulus exceeds the critical duration, the luminance required for it to reach visibility is classically considered constant.

The preceding discussion assumes that whenever the observer's threshold is exceeded, he or she will respond accurately to the stimulus. This pre-

dicts an abrupt transition between the two curves, as depicted in Figure 20-1, *A,* and is somewhat idealized. In the real world, both visual stimuli and the physiologic mechanisms that we use to detect them are subject to random fluctuations in response. We may consider the length of the stimulus presentation to be divided into a number of discrete time intervals. The signal is detected when the response exceeds threshold in at least one interval in which the probability of detection in each interval is considered independent. This description of the probabilistic nature of visual detection is known as *probability summation over time.*[169] The concept of probability summation is included in many models of temporal visual processing and is thought to be at least partly responsible for the less-than-abrupt transition between the region of temporal summation and constant intensity that occurs under some experimental condtions.[67] One experimental situation in which this arises is when threshold contrast is measured as a function of signal duration for sinusoidal grating stimuli. This is illustrated in Figure 20-1, *B*.[67] In Figure 20-1, *B*, the upper curve shows threshold duration data for a 0.8 cycle per degree grating, and the lower curve shows those for an 8 cycle per degree grating. The upper curve conforms well to the schematic illustrated in Figure 20-1, *A*. For the lower curve depicting results for the 8 cycle per degree grating, however, a gradual transition is observed. In this latter case the actual critical duration (traditionally the point of intercept of the two slopes in Figure 20-1, *A*) is somewhat difficult to define. Data similar to those shown in Figure 20-1, *B*, have been interpreted to indicate that the critical duration increases with increasing spatial frequency.[29,103] Gorea and Tyler[67] use an alternative form of analysis that includes the effects of probability summation; they conclude that the critical duration is minimally affected by spatial frequency.

Factors Affecting the Critical Duration

The time interval defined by the critical duration depends on properties of both the stimulus and the background. The critical duration has been shown to vary with light adaptation level; that is, with brighter backgrounds, the critical duration decreases.[13,99,118,145,158] Conversely, with dark adaptation, the critical duration increases.[119,159] Unless dark adapted, the size of the stimulus also affects the critical duration, with larger stimuli having a decreased critical duration.[13,68,145] Retinal eccentricity also influences the critical duration, as does the visual task.[21,44] Temporal summation is also affected by the spectral composition (wavelength or color) of the light stimuli, with isolated chromatic stimuli having longer temporal integration than achromatic (luminance) stimuli.[46,154] For colored lights, the critical duration decreases with increased chromatic saturation of the background, similar to the decrease in critical duration with increased luminance for achromatic stimuli.[92]

CRITICAL FLICKER FUSION FREQUENCY

When a light is turned on and off repeatedly in rapid succession, the light appears to flicker, provided the on and off intervals are greater than some finite time interval. If the lights are flickered fast enough, we perceive the flashes as a single fused light rather than a series of flashes. In simple terms, when the perception of fusion occurs, we have reached the limit of the temporal-resolving ability of our visual system. The perception of fusion has some everyday advantages; for example, it prevents televisions and computer monitors from appearing to flicker, provided that the refresh rate is fast enough. The transition from the perception of flicker to that of fusion occurs over a range of temporal frequencies; the boundary between the two is called the *critical flicker fusion (CFF) frequency.* The value of the CFF varies, depending on a large number of both stimulus and observer characteristics. Some of the important factors that influence the CFF are discussed in the following sections.

Effect of Stimulus Luminance on CFF

In general, the CFF increases as the luminance of the flashing stimulus increases. This relationship is known as the *Ferry-Porter law,* which states that CFF increases as a linear function of log luminance.[59,131] The Ferry-Porter law is valid for a wide range of stimulus conditions and is illustrated in Figure 20-2.[164] The lower curves (*solid lines* and *symbols*) show data collected in the fovea, and the upper curves show data collected at 35 degrees eccentricity. For both locations the upper curves are for smaller targets (0.05 degree foveally and 0.5 degree eccentrically), and the lower curves are for larger targets (0.5 degree foveally and 5.7 degrees eccentrically). Figure 20-2 demonstrates several interesting observations about the relationship between CFF and luminance. First, the Ferry-Porter law is upheld despite changes in stimulus size. Second, the linear relationship between log luminance and CFF is present for both central and peripheral viewing, although the slope of this relationship increases in the periphery, implying faster processing.[164] The Ferry-Porter law holds not only for spot targets but also for grating stimuli.[164] A practical consequence of the relationship between CFF and log luminance is that visible flicker on a

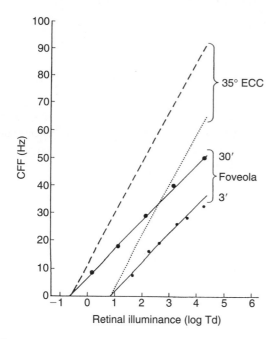

FIGURE 20-2 Photopic critical flicker fusion (*CFF*) versus intensity functions measured in the fovea (*solid symbols* and *lines*) and at 35 degrees eccentricity (*dotted and dashed lines*) from Tyler and Hamer.[164] The test stimulus was 660 nm presented on a equiluminant white surround. Foveal test stimuli were 0.5 degree (*large filled circles*) and 0.05 degree (*small filled circles*). Eccentric stimuli were 5.7 degrees (*dashed line*) and 0.5 degree (*dotted line*). Note the adherence to the Ferry-Porter law for all test conditions. *ECC*, Eccentricity.

---

computer screen can be reduced by decreasing the luminance of the monitor. For scotopic luminance levels, at which rods mediate detection, CFF decreases substantially to approximately 20 Hz and no longer obeys the Ferry-Porter law.[79,88,131]

Effect of Stimulus Chromaticity on CFF

The linear relationship between CFF and log luminance, as described by the Ferry-Porter law, is also valid for purely chromatic stimuli.[65,74,87,130] However, the slope of the relationship has been shown to vary with stimulus wavelength.[74] This relationship is demonstrated in Figure 20-3, which shows CFF versus illuminance functions derived from four separate studies.[65,74,87,130] In all four studies the foveal CFF illuminance functions are well fit by Ferry-Porter lines, and in all cases the functions for green lights were found to be steeper than those for red lights. The steeper slope for green stimuli has been interpreted as evidence of the green cone pathways being inherently faster than the red cone

pathways for the transmission of information near the CFF.[74] The CFF is lowest for blue stimuli detected by the short-wavelength pathways.[30,82]

Effect of Eccentricity on CFF

The CFF varies as a function of eccentricity in the visual field. If the stimulus size and luminance are kept constant, the CFF increases with eccentricity over the central 50 degrees or so of the visual field and then decreases with further increases in eccentricity.[76,142] This is illustrated in Figure 20-4, which plots the CFF as a function of eccentricity in the temporal visual field.

Effect of Stimulus Size on CFF: The Granit-Harper Law

As shown in Figure 20-2, the CFF increases with stimulus size. For a wide range of luminances, CFF increases linearly with the logarithm of the stimulus area. This relationship is known as the *Granit-Harper law*, named after the investigators who first reported it.[70] The Granit-Harper law holds for a wide range of luminances, retinal eccentricities out to 10 degrees, and stimuli as large as almost 50 degrees. However, subsequent investigators have determined that it is not the overall area of the stimulus that is critical, but rather the local retinal area with the best temporal resolution. This was demonstrated by Roehrig,[138,139] who measured the same value for the CFF for a complete 49.6-degree field as for an annulus of the same diameter, with its central 66% not illuminated. Because the midperiphery has better temporal resolution than central vision, an eccentric annulus produced the same CFF as the full 49.6-degree stimulus. The Granit-Harper law does not hold under dim light conditions in which rods mediate performance.

Beyond the fovea, a revised form of the Granit-Harper law is required to fit the changes in CFF with stimulus area. Rovamo and Raninen[143] have shown that the Granit-Harper law can be generalized across the visual field by replacing the retinal stimulus area with the number of ganglion cells stimulated. In this more general case, the CFF increases linearly with the logarithm of the number of ganglion cells stimulated. This is illustrated in Figure 20-5. Figure 20-5, *A*, plots CFF against eccentricity for three different stimulus areas. The CFF decreases with increasing eccentricity irrespective of the stimulus area. Figure 20-5, *B*, plots the same CFF data as a function of the number of retinal ganglion cells stimulated at each eccentricity

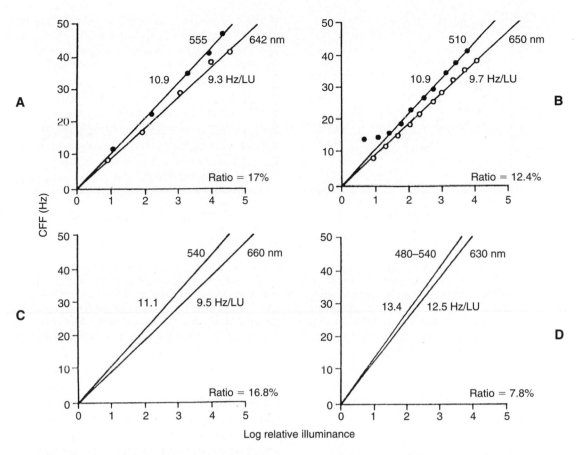

FIGURE 20-3   Critical flicker fusion (*CFF*) versus illuminance functions for red and green flicker measured by Hamer and Tyler.[74] Note that all data are well fit by the Ferry-Porter law, with green lights having a steeper slope than red. **A,** Data for one subject from Hamer and Tyler.[74] The green light function is steeper by 17%. **B,** CFF data from Ives[88] for red (650 nm) and green (510 nm) flicker stimuli viewed foveally. The green light function is steeper by 12.4%. **C,** CFF data for red (660 nm) and green (540 nm) flickering stimuli for a single observer tested by Pokorny and Smith.[130] The green light function is steeper by 16.8%. **D,** CFF data for green light (mean of 480 and 540 nm data) and red light (630 nm) flicker from Giorgi.[65] The green light function is steeper than the red by 7.8%.

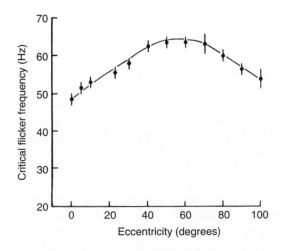

FIGURE 20-4   Critical flicker frequency (mean ± standard deviation) as a function of eccentricity in the temporal visual field of the right eye of one observer, from Rovamo and Raninen.[142] Stimulus area was 88.4 degrees², pupil diameter was 8 mm, and retinal illuminance was 2510 photopic trolands.

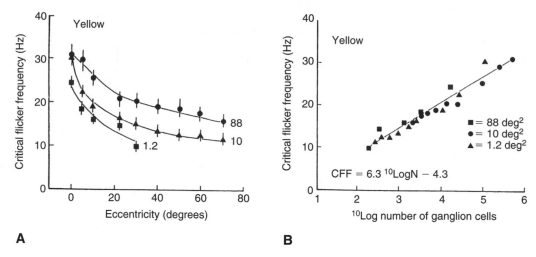

FIGURE 20-5   **A,** Critical flicker frequency (mean ± standard deviation) for targets viewed eccentrically for one observer reported by Rovamo and Raninen.[143] Similar target sizes were used at all eccentricities, but retinal illuminance was F scaled by reducing the average stimulus luminance in inverse proportion to photopic Ricco's area.[144] The numbers on the right of the curves refer to the stimulus area in degrees^2. When eccentricity increased from 0 to 70 degrees, the stimulus luminance nominally decreased from 50 to 0.80 photopic cd/m^2. Note that critical flicker frequency (CFF) decreases with increasing eccentricity irrespective of stimulus area. **B,** CFF data from A plotted as a function of the number of retinal ganglion cells stimulated.

and results in a linear relationship between these two parameters.

TEMPORAL CONTRAST SENSITIVITY

The CFF defines an upper limit for temporal sensitivity, beyond which we can no longer detect that a light is flickering. How sensitive are we to flicker below the CFF, and how does the visual system respond to more complex temporal variations of light than simple flashes or trains of flashes? A general method for predicting and explaining flicker sensitivity for a variety of temporal stimuli was first described by De Lange.[48-50] De Lange evaluated temporal sensitivity to flicker using mathematical analysis of temporal waveforms and linear filter theory. These principles have become the mainstay of research pertaining to temporal sensitivity, so they are briefly discussed here.

The temporal waveform describes the pattern in which a light varies as a function of time. If the temporal waveform is periodic (i.e., it recurs with a regular pattern), it is possible to express the temporal waveform as the sum of elementary sinusoidal oscillations (sine waves, cosine waves, or both). One of these components will have the same periodicity (or repetition rate) as the original waveform and is known as the *fundamental*. All other components, known as *harmonics,* have frequencies that

are integer multiples of the original waveform. The amplitude of a sine wave describes how much it deviates from its average value. The average value of a sine wave is zero, unless a steady nonzero component is added (i.e., the DC component). Light cannot have a negative value, so any temporal waveform describing a series of light flashes has a nonzero DC component. The general mathematical method for determining the sinusoidal and DC components of any given periodic waveform is Fourier analysis.[27]

A system is said to respond in a *linear* fashion if it obeys the principal of superposition. That is, the resultant output from a combination of inputs is the same as if the inputs occurred separately and the individual outputs were summed. For example, when the input to a linear system is a sinusoid, the output is a sinusoid of the same frequency. If the input is a complex waveform that can be broken down to its component sinusoids, the output is the same as the summed output from the individual component sinusoids. However, it does not necessarily follow that the output waveform is the same as the input waveform. The output will be altered if the gain (i.e., the ratio of output amplitude to input amplitude) is not the same for all frequencies. Likewise, the output will also be altered if there is a frequency-dependent time lag between the input and the output. Such a time lag is called a *phase shift*. A linear system with

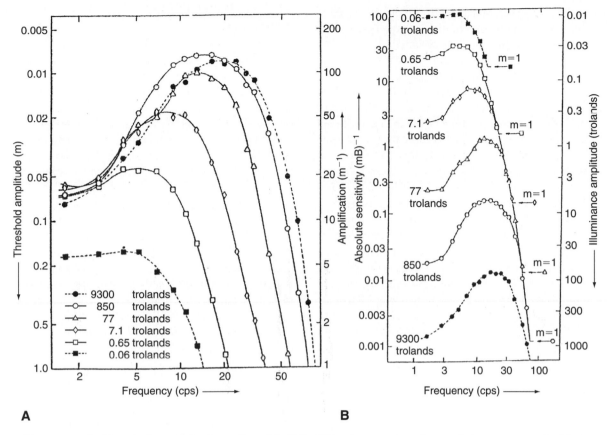

FIGURE 20-6 Temporal sensitivity data collected by Kelly.[94] Visual attenuation characteristics, as measured with sinusoidal variation about different levels of retinal illuminance, are shown. **A,** Threshold modulation ratios for just detectable flicker plotted as a function of temporal frequency. **B,** Absolute amplitudes of retinal illuminance variation for just noticeable flicker plotted as a function of temporal frequency. Absolute sensitivity is the reciprocal of threshold absolute amplitude at each frequency.

a frequency-dependent gain and phase shift is called a *linear filter,* whose characteristics can be completely described by plots of its gain and phase shift, measured as a function of the frequencies of its sinusoidal inputs. A plot of gain versus frequency describes the *attenuation characteristic* of a linear filter. If a system does not behave truly linearly, it may still be appropriate to treat it as linear for low-amplitude stimuli because many nonlinear systems retain some degree of linearity.

De Lange argued that it may be possible to treat the visual system as a combination of linear and nonlinear components. The Talbot-Plateau law, described later, establishes that for stimuli near the CFF, the visual system behaves linearly for the perception of brightness. Hence, De Lange assumed linearity of the visual system for low-signal amplitudes (i.e., for inputs close to threshold) and attempted to determine the attenuation characteris-

tic of the visual system as if it were a linear filter. The input to the filter was a range of sinusoidally flickering lights of different frequencies. The subjective perception of flicker served as the output. Hence, he measured the amplitude of the sinusoidal light stimuli to reach flicker threshold for a range of different sinusoidal frequencies.

Figure 20-6 shows the results from similar flicker-sensitivity experiments by Kelly.[94] The vertical axis plots the flicker sensitivity, which is the reciprocal of the flicker threshold, measured as a "threshold modulation ratio," which is the extent that the sinusoidally modulated light deviates from its DC component. The modulation ratio is calculated as a fraction of its DC value because the amplitude cannot be greater than the DC component (negative values of luminance are not possible). The modulation ratio expresses the amplitude as a percentage deviation of the stimulus from its average value.

The left panel of Figure 20-6 plots the modulation ratio as a function of flicker frequency. A series of curves are shown, each obtained at a different average retinal illumination or adaptation level. The curves define the flicker detection boundary for the particular level of adaptation. For a given level of adaptation, any combination of frequency and modulation amplitude below the curve is seen as flickering, whereas any combination above the curve is perceived as a steady light. The point at which the curve intersects the abscissa (x-axis) corresponds to the CFF. Note that at low adaptation levels, the shape of the curve is low-pass, meaning that modulation sensitivity is similar for low temporal frequencies and then falls off systematically for higher temporal frequencies. At high adaptation levels, the shape of the curve is band-pass, meaning that modulation sensitivity is greatest for a band of temporal frequencies and systematically falls off for lower and higher temporal frequencies.

With increasing retinal illuminance, more conditions are seen as flickering, consistent with the simpler Ferry-Porter law. At low frequencies the curves are similar, indicating that low-frequency flicker reaches threshold at a similar value of modulation ratio for all levels of photopic adaptation. This is not the case for high frequencies, at which the threshold is determined by both adaptation level and frequency. At higher luminance levels the sensitivity for flicker detection peaks at frequencies of approximately 15 to 20 Hz. This is similar to the Brücke brightness enhancement effect, which is discussed later. Because of the linear nature of temporal processing at threshold, De Lange found that the characteristic threshold responses to flickering waveforms, as shown in Figure 20-6, were the same for nonsinusoidal complex waveforms and sinusoids of the same fundamental frequency.

The right panel of Figure 20-6 replots the data of Figure 20-6, *A*, as a function of the absolute amplitude of the high-frequency flicker. This has the effect of reversing the curves so that the amplitude sensitivity is greatest at the lowest adaptation level. It can be seen that the curves of Figure 20-6, *B*, approach a common asymptote at high frequencies. This convergence of curves measured at many different luminance levels implies that at high temporal frequencies, sensitivity is predicted by the absolute amplitude of the signal, independent of adaptation level. This is the behavior expected from a linear system. In the low temporal frequency range, such linear behavior is not apparent because several input amplitudes may be detectable as flicker.

SPATIAL EFFECTS ON TEMPORAL SENSITIVITY

The work of De Lange[49] and Kelly[94] describes our temporal contrast sensitivity, that is, how sensitive we are to temporal sinusoidal variations in stimulus contrast. This does not consider the effect that the spatial characteristics of the light source have on our sensitivity. Human contrast sensitivity depends on both the spatial and temporal characteristics of the stimulus.[96,135] Figure 20-7 shows a surface plot of the human *spatiotemporal contrast sensitivity* function, as derived by Kelly, from a large number of psychophysical measurements.[95,97,98] One axis of the graph shows the temporal frequency of the stimulus; the other shows the spatial frequency. The height represents the observer's contrast sensitivity for the particular spatial and temporal conditions.[96-98] Paths running through the curve parallel to the temporal frequency axis represent the temporal contrast sensitivity functions, and those running parallel to the spatial frequency axis represent the spatial contrast sensitivity functions. The temporal contrast sensitivity function is band-pass at low spatial frequencies, becoming low-pass at high spatial frequencies.

SURROUND EFFECTS ON TEMPORAL SENSITIVITY

Our sensitivity to temporal variations depends not only on the properties of the flickering light but also on those of the background surrounding the light. In the dark (scotopic conditions), detection of light increments is mediated by rods, and in the light (photopic conditions), detection is mediated by cones. For flicker sensitivity, it has been shown that when photopic flickering lights are presented on dark backgrounds, interactions between rods and cones (rod-cone interactions) act to decrease flicker thresholds.* The effects of rod-cone interactions on flicker sensitivity are most significant at high temporal frequencies and in the retinal periphery. Suppressive effects between cone mechanisms of flicker thresholds (e.g., long-wavelength–sensitive cones and medium-wavelength–sensitive cones) have also been demonstrated.[43,54]

At low temporal frequencies, luminance differences between the flickering target and its surround are particularly important in determining temporal contrast sensitivity.[77,93,141,157] This is illustrated in Figure 20-8. The *crosses* represent the temporal

---

*References 3, 7, 42, 43, 63, 66, 102.

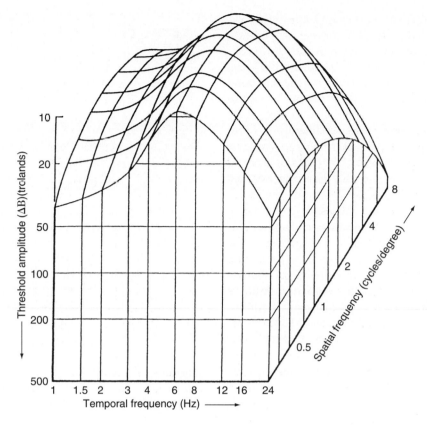

Figure 20-7 Human spatiotemporal amplitude threshold surface obtained with circular gratings of 16 degrees viewed binocularly with natural pupils. (From Kelly D: *Vision Res* 12:89, 1972.)

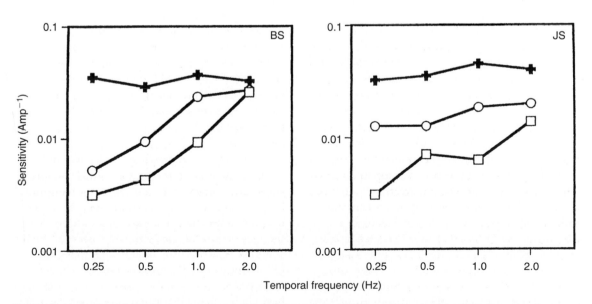

Figure 20-8 Surround effects on temporal sensitivity. Data are from Spehar and Zaidi[157] for two observers. Amplitude sensitivity is plotted as a function of temporal frequency for different surround conditions: *squares*, 0 cd/m² (dark surround); *crosses*, 25.0 cd/m² (equiluminant surround); and *circles*, 50 cd/m² (light surround).

contrast sensitivity for a surround equal to the average luminance of the flickering light (25 cd/m^2), and sensitivity at low temporal frequencies is constant under this condition. For either a dark surround (0 cd/m^2, *squares*) or a light surround (50 cd/m^2, *circles*), the sensitivity drops off at low temporal frequencies.

The presence of a surround differing in luminance from that of the flickering target creates a contrast border at the edge of the target. Spehar and Zaidi[157] have demonstrated that the presence of such a border decreases temporal contrast sensitivity. Whether the background is brighter or dimmer is not important; rather the decrease in temporal contrast sensitivity depends on the magnitude of the contrast at the border, with larger border contrasts resulting in larger decreases in temporal contrast sensitivity at low temporal frequencies. In short, we are most sensitive to temporal changes when the luminance of the background is matched to the average of the flickering target. One experimental paradigm in which such surround effects become important is the case of luminance-pedestal flicker, which is discussed in the following section.[4]

DIFFERENCES BETWEEN MEAN-MODULATED AND LUMINANCE-PEDESTAL FLICKER

Historically, studies of temporal sensitivity have generated flicker using one of two methodologies, which are illustrated schematically in Figure 20-9.[4] The upper panel of Figure 20-9 illustrates mean-modulated flicker, in which flicker is modulated about a mean luminance. Flicker generated in this fashion results in no change in the time-averaged luminance (examples of studies using mean-modulated flicker include those by De Lange[49] and Roufs[141]). The lower panel of Figure 20-9 illustrates luminance-pedestal flicker, in which flicker is generated by modulating a luminance increment over time. This results in both a flickering component and an increase in time-averaged luminance above the background level (examples of studies using luminance-pedestal flicker include those of Alexander and Fishman[3]; Eisner[55]; Eisner, Shapiro, and Middleton[56]; and Anderson and Vingrys[4]). Because both of these methods have been used to assess temporal sensitivity, it is important to understand whether they yield equivalent or differing results.

Luminance-pedestal flicker yields equivalent results to mean-modulated flicker only if the lumi-

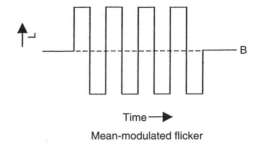

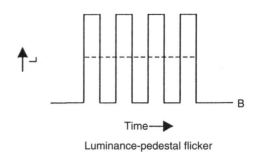

FIGURE 20-9 Schematic of mean-modulated (*upper panel*) and luminance-pedestal (*lower panel*) flicker from Anderson and Vingrys.[4] The time-averaged luminance during the presentation of flicker is represented by the *dashed lines,* and B represents the background luminance. Note that for luminance-pedestal flicker, the time-averaged luminance is greater than the background by an amount that is the luminance pedestal.

nance pedestal has no effect on thresholds, which seems unlikely. In the previous section, we discussed how flicker sensitivity changes with light adaptation (see Figure 20-6); as such, it may be expected that the local increase in luminance created by the luminance pedestal may act to increase thresholds. This is the case and has been reported by Anderson and Vingrys.[4]

Furthermore, the presence of the pedestal causes a difference between the surround and the flickering target. The surround affects temporal sensitivity (see Figure 20-8), so it is likely that the presence of a non–luminance-matched surround, created by the very nature of the luminance-pedestal flicker stimulus, will result in interactions that alter our sensitivity to this type of target.[157] Anderson and Vingrys[5] describe some of these interactions and have shown that the mismatch between the luminance pedestal and its surround creates a contrast border that acts to reduce flicker sensitivity at low temporal frequencies.

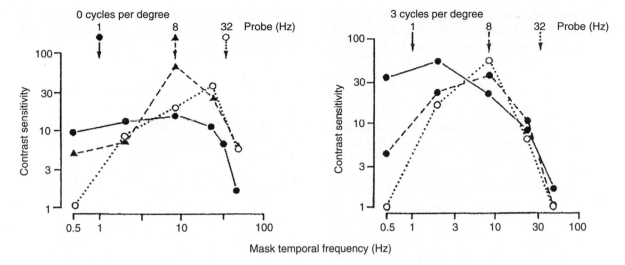

Figure 20-10 Properties of temporal mechanisms identified using a selective adaptation method by Hess and Snowden.[83] Mask contrast sensitivity is plotted against mask temporal frequency for detection of a just suprathreshold probe. Data are for probes of 1, 8, and 32 Hz. The *left panel* shows data for a probe of 0 cycles per degree, for which three mechanisms are revealed: one low-pass and two band-pass. The *right panel* shows data for a 3 cycle per degree probe, and only two mechanisms are revealed.

Mechanisms Underlying Temporal Sensitivity

The shape of the human spatial contrast sensitivity function has been explained in terms of a multiple-channel model in which the total curve is the window of a number of channels, each tuned to a different peak spatial frequency.[23,34,69] Similar to spatial processing, there is evidence for a discrete number of channels for temporal processing, each tuned to a different peak temporal frequency.[83,108,171,176] There appear to be fewer independent temporal frequency filters than there are filters conveying spatial frequency information. The number of temporal mechanisms identified has been shown to be dependent on the spatial frequency of the stimulus, in addition to the retinal location.

How can we determine whether different mechanisms are governing performance? One method relies on the assumption that different mechanisms result in different subjective representations of the stimulus; that is, when separate mechanisms are governing detection, the stimulus looks different. Kelly[96] and Kulikowski[100] report that flickering gratings at threshold produce one of three percepts depending on the spatiotemporal parameters of the grating: slow flicker, apparent motion, or frequency doubling (i.e., the perceived spatial frequency is twice the actual spatial frequency). This is consis-

tent with three mechanisms underlying temporal processing. Watson and Robson[171] measured temporal discrimination, that is, the ability to determine that stimuli are flickering at different rates. For grating patches of 0.25 cycle per degree, there were three temporal frequencies that were uniquely discriminable, which Watson and Robson[171] interpreted as evidence for three unique filters mediating temporal processing. Mandler and Makous[108] modeled temporal discrimination performance and also found evidence for three mechanisms underlying temporal processing.

An alternative method for identifying mechanisms underlying visual processing is that of *selective adaptation*. If a stimulus that activates one mechanism to a greater extent than another mechanism is presented, the sensitivity of the activated mechanism will be selectively depressed if the stimulus is viewed for a prolonged period. This should allow other, less sensitive mechanisms to detect the stimulus and hence allow their profile to be explored. Selective adaptation has been widely used to isolate the mechanisms underlying color vision processing.[160] Hess and Snowden[83] used selective adaptation with temporal stimuli to uncover temporal mechanisms; an example of their data is displayed in Figure 20-10. The first stage of these experiments (not shown in the figure) involved measuring foveal contrast detection thresholds for a wide range of spatial and temporal conditions. These measures were used to set the contrast of the *probe* stimulus, which was set to be just detectable (4 dB above threshold). The detectability of this probe stimulus was then measured in the presence of masking stimuli of the same spatial frequency but different temporal frequency. The contrast of the masking stimulus was varied until the probe was just visible.

Figure 20-10, *A*, presents data for three probes presented foveally with no spatial content (0 cycles per degree) but flickering at either 1, 8, or 32 Hz. The figure shows the contrast sensitivity of the mask plotted against the mask temporal frequency. Three mechanisms are revealed: one low-pass (*solid circles*) and two band-pass (*open circles, solid triangles*). Figure 20-10, *B*, shows data for a probe of 3 cycles per degree, and only two mechanisms are revealed. The band-pass mechanism, centered on higher temporal frequencies in Figure 20-10, *A*, disappears when the spatial frequency content of the stimulus increases.[83] Using a similar method, Snowden and Hess[156] have shown that for retinal eccentricities of 10 degrees, only two mechanisms are found, reducing to a single mechanism at eccentricities of greater than 30 degrees.

The Effects of Flicker on Perception

The presence of flicker can alter both the apparent color and brightness of a light.[10,11,16-20,161] When a light is flickered, its apparent brightness varies depending on the frequency of the flicker, with maximum apparent brightness occurring between 5 and 20 Hz. This phenomenon is known as the *Brücke brightness enhancement effect.*[31] Such brightness enhancement can be demonstrated experimentally by matching the brightness of a flickering light to that of a nonflickering standard.[18] When the light is flickered at rates faster than those that result in brightness enhancement, the apparent brightness of the flickering light decreases. Eventually, the apparent brightness plateaus, and at rates beyond the CFF, the apparent brightness is the same as the apparent brightness of a steady light equal to the time-averaged luminance of the flickering light. This observation was made by Talbot[162] and Plateau[129] and is known as the *Talbot-Plateau law.* Lights flickering above the CFF, at which point flicker is invisible, appear identical to steady lights of the same chromaticity and time-averaged luminance. Under most conditions of adaptation, the Talbot-Plateau law appears to hold. One exception is the case of blue targets presented on bright yellow backgrounds, in which case the target appears more yellow than a steady light, even when it is not visibly flickering.[161]

TEMPORAL PHASE SEGMENTATION

An important task of the visual system is to distinguish objects from their background, a task known as *image segmentation* (see Chapter 18). Useful information for the process of image segmentation includes differences in luminance and color between the image and its background. Differences in temporal phase are also sufficient for image segmentation.[58,62,104,140] For example, if a field of identical dot elements is rapidly flickered from black to white in phase (i.e., all dots appear white simultaneously, then black simultaneously), the field appears to be uniformly flickering. If, however, elements in a subregion flicker in counterphase to the rest (i.e., within the subregion the dots are white when those outside are black), a contour between the subregion and the rest of the display is observed. At high temporal frequencies (greater than approximately 10 Hz), the difference in phase of individual elements cannot be detected; however, the contour between regions is easily visualized provided the gap between regions is less than about 0.4 degree.[62,140] Temporal image segmentation is possible only at low temporal frequencies for chromatic stimuli.[140]

CLINICAL APPLICATIONS OF TEMPORAL SENSITIVITY MEASUREMENTS

Measurements of temporal processing have been used extensively for clinical testing. Visual information from the retina is carried to the visual cortex, via the lateral geniculate nucleus, by two major neural pathways. These pathways are known as the *parvocellular* and *magnocellular pathways* and have been shown to carry largely independent, but sometimes overlapping, visual information. Studies of single-cell neurophysiology, as well behavioral studies in primates subject to selective lesioning, demonstrate that the magnocellular system is preferentially involved in the visual processing of faster flicker and motion.[91,116,147] Hence, clinical assessment of the *functional integrity* of the magnocellular system has used tasks that have flickering or moving components. We concentrate on the use of flickering tasks for clinical visual assessment here and discuss the assessment of motion later in this chapter.

Both measures of CFF and temporal contrast sensitivity have been used to explore visual function in disease. Often, these measures are performed across the visual field, with use of perimetric strategies. There are a number of different perimetric techniques for exploring temporal sensitivity across the visual field: CFF perimetry (which measures the CFF for small spot targets at various field locations), temporal modulation perimetry (which measures temporal contrast sensitivity for small spot targets either about a mean luminance or displayed on a luminance pedestal), and frequency doubling perimetry. Frequency doubling perimetry measures contrast sensitivity for patches of sinusoidal grating of low spatial and high temporal frequency, parameters that result in the grating appearing to have twice its actual spatial frequency.

The development of perimetric methods for measuring temporal sensitivity has been largely directed to the detection of glaucoma or identification of glaucomatous visual field progression.[36,90,101,106,177] Abnormalities in temporal processing have also been identified in a range of other diseases, using perimetric and other strategies, including: Parkinson disease, dyslexia, age-related macular degeneration, multiple sclerosis, optic neuritis, high-risk drusen, central serous chorioretinopathy, and migraine.*

Temporal segmentation stimuli have also been used in a clinical setting to assess the patency of the magnocellular system. Letters created from small rapidly flickering dots are presented, and the subject must then identify the letters. The dots within the letters flicker in opposite phase to the dots external to the letter. Temporal segmentation stimuli have been used to identify abnormalities in temporal sensitivity in dyslexia and glaucoma.[15,61] CFF measures have been used extensively in the field of pharmacology to assess the effect of pharmacotherapy on psychomotor function.[80,84,127]

MOTION PROCESSING

The detection of motion is a special form of temporal processing that forms an extensive area of study. *Motion* is a change in spatial position over time. Indeed, practically everything of visual interest in the world is moving, if not as a result of movement of the object itself, then by movement of the observers head or eyes, causing the image on

the retina to move. As we have already discussed, the ability of the visual system to detect temporal changes in luminance is exquisite. The visual system is also extremely sensitive to changes in spatial position. Hence, it may seem that to extract motion information, all that is needed is a comparison of separate measurements of an object's location at various times. Nevertheless, special visual mechanisms are specifically used for the processing of the linked spatiotemporal information that constitutes motion. This section briefly describes some perceptual and psychophysical data on human motion perception. A brief description of the neurophysiologic substrates underlying motion perception is included because this provides a basis for understanding the applications of motion tasks to the study of functional visual loss in disease. There are a number of detailed reviews of motion processing elsewhere.[120,121,153,168]

Psychophysical and Perceptual Evidence for Unique Motion Processing

A number of perceptual phenomena provide evidence for the existence of mechanisms designed specifically to process motion information. One of these is known as the *motion aftereffect*, which occurs after prolonged viewing of a moving stimulus (this is also known as *motion adaptation*).[85,126,149] After prolonged staring at a moving stimulus, stationary objects appear to move in the opposite direction and the apparent speed of moving objects is distorted. Importantly, the apparent position of such stationary objects does not change, suggesting that motion and position are encoded separately.

Another example demonstrating that the perception of motion is not merely a simple representation of physical motion is that of *apparent motion*. Apparent motion occurs when spatially separate lights are flashed in sequence, giving the perception of movement despite each light remaining stationary. This phenomenon is sometimes used in shop fronts, where the motion induced by sequential flashing of lights is designed to draw attention. Apparent motion can be induced by a single pair of lights flashed in succession. This movement is also known as *phi* and was first described in detail by Wertheimer.[172]

First- and Second-Order Motion. The demonstration of phi was historically interpreted as evidence that a set of sequentially presented stationary images was equivalent to a "pure" motion stimulus. This view is now seen as an oversimplification: The

---

*References 25, 40, 41, 57, 64, 71, 110, 113, 114, 115, 128, 166.

phi mechanism has been shown to be suited to making comparisons over much larger distances and time intervals than the mechanisms involved in the detection of continuous motion.[6] Phi could be attributed to what Braddick[28] would later call the *long-range* motion mechanism. Braddick's experiments used random-dot kinematograms in which a rectangular area with horizontal or vertical orientation was displaced from one frame to the next. This stimulus is illustrated in Figure 20-11. For certain values of spatial displacement and temporal interval between frames, subjects are able to perceive a clear perception of motion. If the spatial displacement was beyond about 0.25 degree, figure-ground separation does not occur. This contrasts with the larger spatial displacement that results in apparent motion for classical sequentially presented lights (e.g., Wertheimer[172]). Braddick[28] suggests that two different processes govern apparent motion: one short range (such as that involved in the random-dot displays) and one long-range (which governs perceived

motion in displays with a small number of clearly defined elements). The limit of spatial displacement over which the short-range process could be activated was termed D_{max}. D_{max} has been shown to depend on the choice of stimulus parameters.[8,37,39]

More recently, it has been argued that the differences between short- and long-range processes are more easily explained by differences in the stimuli used, with stimuli being classified as *first* or *second* order.[22,35,38,73] The motion aspect of first-order stimuli results from variations in image intensity in space and time. For these stimuli, motion can be discriminated by spatially tracking a difference in luminance or color over time. The motion of second-order stimuli is generated by variations of some other stimulus property, such as local contrast or local element size, across space-time.

Models of Motion Perception. There are a variety of different approaches to modeling human motion perception, the details of which fall be-

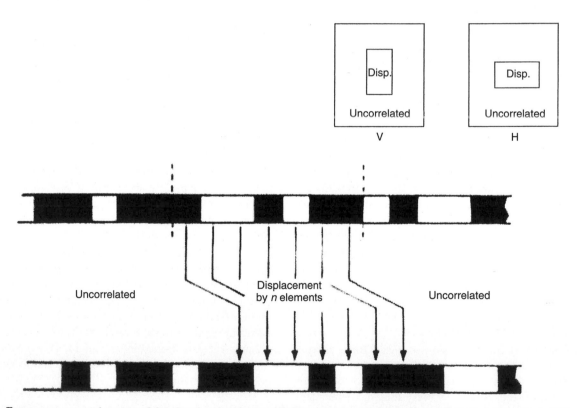

FIGURE 20-11 Schematic of the stimulus used by Braddick[28] to measure the limit of spatial displacement over which the short-range motion process could be activated (D_{max}). The *upper panel* illustrates the size and position of the displaced horizontal (*H*) or vertical (*V*) rectangle within the uncorrelated surround. The overall size of the pattern is 9 × 9 degrees. The *lower panel* illustrates the principle of generation of a single row of each pattern. The dots within the inner rectangle are displaced by *n* elements, and the surround remains uncorrelated. *Disp,* Displaced.

yond the scope of this chapter. Most models fall into one of three categories: correlational models, gradient models, or motion boundary contour system models.*

Correlational models are largely based on Reichardt's motion detector, which combines data separated in both space and time.[14,133,165,175] These models correlate the responses of two or more spatially separated neural elements. Reichardt's motion detector describes two neural elements, with the signal from one element being subject to a delay and then correlated with that from the other element. The difference between these correlated responses is determined and provides information regarding the direction of motion.

Gradient models collect information from a single spatial location and extract motion information by comparing the output of spatially and temporally tuned visual filters.[1,75,109,170] Motion boundary contour system models are more complex neural models of motion perception that incorporate aspects of both gradient and correlational models.[12]

The Neural Encoding of Motion

Further evidence that our visual system detects motion as a primary sensory dimension has arisen from studies of single-cell neurophysiology. Hubel and Wiesel[86] observed that some neurons in cortical area V1 have directionally selective receptive fields. Cells with this property respond well when a stimulus moves in one direction, but they respond in a limited fashion, or not at all, when the stimulus moves in the opposite direction. Direction-selective neurons are not evenly distributed throughout area V1; they are predominantly located in layers 4A, 4B, 4Cα, and 6.[78] Layer 4Cα receives its main input from magnocellular pathways, suggesting that the magnocellular pathway is part of a functional specialization designed to carry information about motion. As discussed earlier, magnocellular neurons are preferentially involved in the visual processing of flicker.[91,116,148] Signals from the magnocellular pathway are passed from 4Cα to layer 4B, from which neurons connect to cortical area MT (medial temporal).[52,105,150,151] In area MT a high proportion of directionally selective cells are present (approximately 80%).[2,112] It should be noted that not all magnocellular neurons follow the path to MT; a number of neurons converge with the parvocellular neurons in area V1.[107,123] Furthermore, a small contribution to

motion processing is made by the parvocellular visual pathways.[51,111,117]

The importance of area MT to motion perception has been demonstrated largely by behavioral studies of primates with selective MT lesions. An MT lesion causes performance deficits in motion tasks, without corresponding losses to visual acuity or color perception.[125,146] Using a dynamic random-dot motion task, Newsome and Paré[125] investigated motion perception in the presence of MT lesions in rhesus monkeys. This task requires the observer to identify the dominant direction of motion within a field of randomly moving dots (Figure 20-12). The proportion of dots moving in a common direction (coherence ratio) is varied to determine the direction identification threshold. Key to this task is that the moving dots be selected randomly for each frame of presentation so that the direction of motion cannot be determined by tracking the location of a single dot. Rather, the local motion signals must be combined over a large area of the visual field to determine the global motion percept. Newsome and Paré[125] found striking elevations in such motion thresholds to be present when selective lesions to area MT were made. Newsome, Britten, and Movshon[124] further demonstrated that the activity in a single MT cell correlated directly with the monkey's trial by trial performance in a motion discrimination task. They also demonstrated that microstimulation of tiny regions of MT can bias a monkey's motion perception in a manner predictable from the response characteristics of cells adjacent to the stimulating electrode.

Zihl, von Cramon, and Mai[178]; Hess, Baker, and Zihl[81]; and Baker, Hess, and Zihl[9] provide a series of reports investigating the motion perception of a human patient with a bilateral loss of the superior temporal cortical region. This patient was found to have a specific deficit to motion processing while other measured forms of visual processing were normal or relatively intact. In particular, the patient performed poorly on a random-dot motion task similar to that used by Newsome and Paré.[125] This pattern of deficit is consistent with that found when area MT is lesioned in primates, providing evidence for a similar specialized area for motion processing in humans.[125,146]

In summary, motion perception appears to be performed largely by the visual pathway leading from the magnocellular layers of the lateral geniculate nucleus through area V1 to area MT. This pathway is not the only carrier of motion information in humans, however; area MT also receives input

---

*References 1, 12, 14, 72, 73, 75, 109, 133, 165, 170, 175.

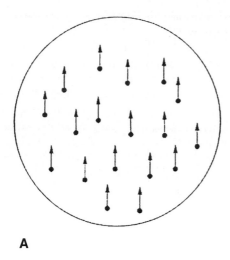

A

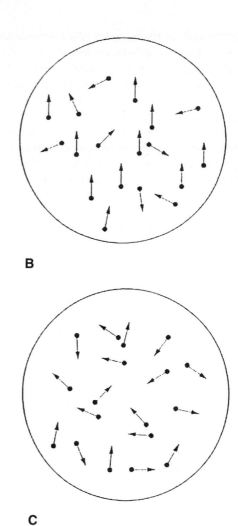

B

C

FIGURE 20-12   Representation of a global-dot motion stimulus reproduced from Edwards and Badcock.[53] The subject is required to identify the global direction of motion of the dots (up/down). The signal strength is varied by changing the number of signal dots moving in that direction in successive frames. The remaining dots, the noise dots, moved in random directions. The dots that comprise the signal dots are chosen at the start of each frame. **A,** One hundred percent signal strength condition. **B,** Fifty percent signal strength condition. **C,** Zero percent signal strength condition; there is no global motion of the dots, only random local motion.

from the superior colliculus.[136,137] In addition, Nawrot and Rizzo[122] have demonstrated that the cerebellum may also play an important role in human motion processing. In their study, motion direction discrimination deficits were found in a group of patients with acute midline cerebellar lesions. These patients were unable to discern the direction of motion in a global motion task, similar to the deficit reported following MT lesions in primates.[125,146] Area V3 also appears to be important to human motion perception, particularly when spatial judgments are required.[45,47]

CLINICAL APPLICATIONS OF MOTION PROCESSING

Because motion is a unique sensory dimension, processed by a relatively well-understood neural pathway, motion perception has been explored ex-

tensively clinically. As discussed in the preceding section, the detection of stimulus motion occurs early in the motion pathway (retina to V1), the ability to discriminate the direction of motion is first present in cortical neurons within V1, and the ability to extract global motion information occurs in the visual association areas (MT or higher). Clinical tasks can be chosen to explore motion processing at these sequential stages. For example, if the ability to detect stimulus motion and discriminate its direction is intact yet global motion perception impaired, this suggests damage at area MT or higher.

The ability to both detect motion and discriminate its direction declines with age.[174] Motion discrimination thresholds have been shown to be affected in Parkinson disease.[163] Global motion processing, as measured using random-dot global motion stimuli (similar to that illustrated in Figure

20-12), has been shown to be affected in people with migraines and Alzheimer disease.[114,134]

Motion processing has also been explored in patients with glaucoma.* Because the visual dysfunction associated with glaucoma is largely in the peripheral visual field, perimetric approaches to testing motion processing have been developed. Random-dot motion perimetry assesses global motion perception at discrete locations across the visual field and has been used to demonstrate motion processing deficits in glaucoma.[26,89,152,167] Because glaucoma is a disease of the optic nerve and results in deficits to flicker perception, the global motion perception deficits demonstrated in glaucoma are most likely caused by disruptions in the early processing of motion information.[36,90,101,106,177] Peripheral motion displacement thresholds (the minimum distance for which a line or random-dot pattern that is laterally displaced appears to move) are also elevated in glaucoma.[32,53,60,173]

The temporal properties of vision thus subserve an important role in the detection and perception of visual stimuli. The visual processing of motion, flicker, and other temporal characteristics is vital for us to effectively interact with and navigate through our environment. Because these visual functions are highly susceptible to pathophysiologic insults to the visual pathways, tests of motion sensitivity, flicker sensitivity, and other temporal visual functions can also serve as sensitive clinical diagnostic procedures.

---

*References 26, 32, 57, 60, 89, 152, 167, 173.

REFERENCES

1. Adelson EH, Bergen JR: Spatiotemporal energy models for the perception of motion, *J Opt Soc Am A* 2:284, 1985.
2. Albright TD: Direction and orientation selectivity of neurons in visual area MT of the macaque, *J Neurophysiol* 52:1106, 1984.
3. Alexander KR, Fishman GA: Rod-cone interaction in flicker perimetry, *Br J Ophthalmol* 68:303, 1984.
4. Anderson AJ, Vingrys AJ: Interactions between flicker thresholds and luminance pedestals, *Vision Res* 40:2579, 2000.
5. Anderson AJ, Vingrys AJ: Multiple processes mediate flicker sensitivity, *Vision Res* 41:2449, 2001.
6. Anstis SM: The perception of apparent movement, *Phil Trans R Soc Lond B* 290:153, 1980.
7. Arden GB, Hogg CR: Rod-cone interactions and analysis of retinal disease, *Br J Ophthalmol* 69:404, 1985.
8. Baker CL, Braddick OJ: Eccentricity-dependent scaling of the limits for short-range apparent motion perception, *Vision Res* 25:803, 1985.
9. Baker CL, Hess RF, Zihl J: Residual motion perception in "a motion-blind" patient, assessed with limited-lifetime random dot stimuli, *J Neurosci* 11:454, 1991.
10. Ball RJ: An investigation of chromatic brightness enhancement tendencies, *Am J Optom Physiol Opt* 41:333, 1964.
11. Ball RJ, Bartley SH: Changes in brightness index, saturation, and hue produced by luminance-wavelength-temporal interactions, *J Opt Soc Am* 66:695, 1966.
12. Baloch AA et al: Neural model of first-order and second-order motion perception and magnocellular dynamics, *J Opt Soc Am A* 16:953, 1999.
13. Barlow HB: Temporal and spatial summation in human vision at different background intensities, *J Physiol Lond* 141:337, 1958.
14. Barlow HB, Levick WR: The mechanism of directionally selective units in the rabbit's retina, *J Physiol* 178:477, 1965.
15. Barnard N, Crewther SG, Crewther DP: Development of a magnocellular function in good and poor primary school-age readers, *Optom Vis Sci* 75:62, 1998.
16. Bartley SH: A central mechanism in brightness enhancement, *Proc Soc Exp Biol Med* 38:535, 1938.
17. Bartley SH: Some effects of intermittent photic stimulation, *J Exp Psychol* 25:462, 1939.
18. Bartley SH: Brightness comparisons when one eye is stimulated intermittently and the other steadily, *J Psychol* 34:165, 1951.
19. Bartley SH: Brightness enhancement in relation to target intensity, *J Psychol* 32:57, 1951.
20. Bartley SH, Nelson TM: Certain chromatic and brightness changes associated with rate of intermittency of photic stimulation, *J Psychol* 50:323, 1960.
21. Baumgardt E, Hillman B: Duration and size as determinants of peripheral retinal response, *J Opt Soc Am* 51:340, 1961.
22. Bischof WF, Di Lollo V: Perception of directional sampled motion in relation to displacement and spatial frequency: evidence for a unitary motion system, *Vision Res* 30:1341, 1990.
23. Blakemore C, Campbell FW: On the existence of neurones in the human visual system selectively sensitive to the orientation and size of retinal images, *J Physiol* 203:237, 1969.
24. Bloch A: Experience sur la vision, *Comptes Rendus de la Societe de Biologie (Paris)* 37:493, 1885.
25. Bodis-Wollner I: Visual deficits related to dopamine deficiency in experimental animals and Parkinson's disease patients, *Trends Neurosci* 13:296, 1990.
26. Bosworth CF et al: Motion automated perimetry identifies early glaucomatous field defects, *Arch Ophthalmol* 116:1153, 1998.
27. Bracewell R: *The Fourier transform and its applications*, ed 2, New York, 1986, McGraw-Hill.
28. Braddick O: A short range process in apparent motion, *Vision Res* 14:519, 1974.
29. Breitmeyer BG, Ganz L: Temporal studies with flashed gratings: inferences about human transient and sustained channels, *Vision Res* 17:861, 1977.
30. Brindley GS, Du Croz JJ, Rushton WAH: The flicker fusion frequency of the blue-sensitive mechanism of colour vision, *J Physiol (Lond)* 183:497, 1966.
31. Brücke E: Uber die Nutzeffect intermitterender Netzhautreizungen. Sitzungsberichte der Mathematisch-Naturwissenschaftlichen, *Classe der Kaiserlichen Akademie der Wissenschaften* 49:128, 1848.
32. Bullimore MA, Wood JM, Swenson K: Motion perception in glaucoma, *Invest Ophthalmol Vis Sci* 34:3526, 1993.
33. Burr DC: Temporal summation of moving images by the human visual system, *Proc R Soc Lond B Biol Sci* 211:321, 1981.
34. Campbell FW, Robson JG: Applications of Fourier analysis to the visibility of gratings, *J Physiol* 197:551, 1968.

35. Cavanagh P, Mather G: Motion: the long and short of it, *Spatial Vis* 4:103, 1989.

36. Cello KE, Nelson-Quigg JM, Johnson CA: Frequency doubling technology perimetry for detection of glaucomatous visual field loss, *Am J Ophthalmol* 129:314, 2000.

37. Chang JJ, Julesz B: Displacement limits for spatial-frequency filtered random-dot cinematograms in apparent motion, *Vision Res* 23:1379, 1983.

38. Chubb C, Sperling G: Drift-balanced random stimuli: a general basis for studying non-Fourier motion perception, *J Opt Soc Am A* 5:1986, 1988.

39. Cleary RF, Braddick OJ: Direction discrimination in narrow-band filtered kinematograms, *Perception* 14:A21, 1985.

40. Coleston DM, Kennard C: Responses to temporal visual stimuli in migraine, the critical flicker fusion test, *Cephalalgia* 15:396, 1995.

41. Coleston DM et al: Precortical dysfunction of spatial and temporal visual processing in migraine, *J Neurol Neurosurg Psychiatry* 57:1208, 1994.

42. Coletta NJ, Adams AJ: Rod-cone interaction in flicker detection, *Vision Res* 24:1333, 1984.

43. Coletta NJ, Adams AJ: Spatial extent of rod-cone and cone-cone interaction for flicker detection, *Vision Res* 26:917, 1986.

44. Connors MM: Luminance requirements for hue perception and identification, for a range of exposure durations, *J Opt Soc Am* 60:958, 1970.

45. Cornette L et al: Human brain regions involved in direction discrimination, *J Neurophysiol* 79:2749, 1998.

46. Dain SJ, King-Smith PE: Visual thresholds in dichromats and normals: the importance of post-receptoral processes, *Vision Res* 21:573, 1981.

47. de Jong BM et al: The cerebral activity related to the visual perception of forward motion in depth, *Brain* 117:1039, 1994.

48. De Lange H: Relationship between critical flicker frequency and a set of low-frequency characteristics of the eye, *J Opt Soc Am* 44:380, 1954.

49. De Lange H: Research into the dynamic nature of the human fovea-cortex systems with intermittent and modulated light: I—attenuation characteristics with white and colored light, *J Opt Soc Am* 48:777, 1958.

50. De Lange H: Research into the dynamic nature of the human fovea-cortex systems with intermittent and modulated light: II. Phase shift in brightness and delay in color perception, *J Opt Soc Am* 48:784, 1958.

51. Derrington AM, Badcock DR: The low level motion system has both chromatic and luminance inputs, *Vision Res* 25:1879, 1985.

52. DeYoe EA, Van Essen DC: Segregation of efferent connections and receptive field properties in visual area V2 of the macaque, *Nature* 317:58, 1985.

53. Edwards M, Badcock DR: Global motion perception: interaction of on and off pathways, *Vision Res* 34:2849, 1994.

54. Eisner A: Non-monotonic effect of test illuminance on flicker detection: a study of foveal light adaptation with annular surrounds, *J Opt Soc Am A* 11:33, 1994.

55. Eisner A: Suppression of flicker response with increasing test illuminance: roles of temporal waveform, modulation depth and frequency, *J Opt Soc Am A* 12:214, 1995.

56. Eisner A, Shapiro AG, Middleton J: Equivalence between temporal frequency and modulation depth for flicker response suppression: analysis of a three-process model of visual adaptation, *J Opt Soc Am A* 15:1987, 1998.

57. Evans BJ, Drasdo N, Richards IL: An investigation of some sensory and refractive visual factors in dyslexia, *Vision Res* 34:1913, 1994.

58. Fahle M: Figure-ground discrimination from temporal information, *Proc Royal Soc Lond B Biol Sci* 254:199, 1993.

59. Ferry E: Persistence of vision, *Am J Sci* 44:192, 1892.

60. Fitzke FW et al: Peripheral displacement thresholds in glaucoma and ocular hypertension. In Heijl A (ed): *Perimetry update 1988/89*, Amsterdam, 1989, Kugler and Ghedini.

61. Flanagan JG et al: The phantom contour illusion letter test: a new psychophysical test for glaucoma? In Mills RP, Wall M (eds): *Perimetry update 1994/1995*, Amsterdam/New York, 1995, Kugler Publications.

62. Forte J, Hogben JH, Ross J: Spatial limitations of temporal segmentation, *Vision Res* 39:4052, 1999.

63. Frumkes TE et al: Influence of rod adaptation upon cone responses to light offset in humans, I, results in normal observers, *Vis Neurosci* 8:83, 1992.

64. Fujimoto N, Adachi-Usami E: Frequency doubling perimetry in resolved optic neuritis, *Invest Ophthalmol Vis Sci* 41:2558, 2000.

65. Giorgi A: Effect of wavelength on the relationship between critical flicker frequency and intensity in foveal vision, *J Opt Soc Am* 53:480, 1963.

66. Goldberg SH, Frumkes TE, Nygaard RW: Inhibitory influence of unstimulated rods in the human retina: evidence provided by examining cone flicker, *Science* 221:180, 1983.

67. Gorea A, Tyler CW: New look at Bloch's law for contrast, *J Opt Soc Am A* 3:52, 1986.

68. Graham CH, Margaria R: Area and intensity-time relation in the peripheral retina, *Am J Physiol* 113:299, 1935.

69. Graham N, Nachmias J: Detection of grating patterns containing two spatial frequencies: a comparison of single channel and multiple-channels models, *Vision Res* 11:251, 1971.

70. Granit R, Harper P: Comparative studies on the peripheral and central retina. II. Synaptic reactions in the eye, *Am J Physiol* 95:211, 1930.

71. Grigsby SS et al: Correlation of chromatic, spatial, and temporal sensitivity in optic nerve disease, *Invest Ophthalmol Vis Sci* 32:3252, 1991.

72. Grossberg S, Mingolla E: Neural dynamics of motion perception: direction fields, apertures and resonant grouping, *Percept Psychophys* 53:243, 1993.

73. Grossberg S, Rudd ME: A neural architecture for visual motion perception: group and element apparent motion, *Neural Networks* 2:421, 1989.

74. Hamer RD, Tyler CW: Analysis of visual modulation sensitivity. V. Faster visual response for G- than R-cone pathway, *J Opt Soc Am A* 9:1889, 1992.

75. Harris MG: The perception of moving stimuli: a model of spatiotemporal coding in human vision, *Vision Res* 26:1281, 1986.

76. Hartmann E, Lachenmayr B, Brettel H: The peripheral critical flicker frequency, *Vision Res* 19:1019, 1979.

77. Harvey LO: Flicker sensitivity and apparent brightness as a function of surround luminance, *J Opt Soc Am* 60:860, 1970.

78. Hawken MJ, Parker AJ, Lund JS: Laminar organisation and contrast sensitivity of direction-selective cells in the striate cortex of the Old World monkey, 10:3541, 1988.

79. Hecht S, Schlaer S: Intermittent stimulation by light. V. The relation between intensity and critical frequency for different parts of the spectrum, *J Gen Physiol* 19:965, 1936.

80. Heine PR et al: Lack of interaction between diazepam and nimodipine during chronic oral administration to healthy elderly subjects, *Br J Clin Pharmacol* 38:39, 1994.

81. Hess RH, Baker CL, Zihl J: The "motion-blind" patient: low-level spatial and temporal filters, *J Neurosci* 9:1628, 1989.

82. Hess RF, Mullen KT, Zrenner E: Human photopic vision with only short wavelength cones: post-receptoral properties, *J Physiol* 417:151, 1989.

83. Hess RF, Snowden RJ: Temporal properties of human visual filters: number, shapes and spatial covariation, *Vision Res* 32:47, 1992.

84. Hindmarch I et al: Pharmacodynamics of milnacipran in young and elderly volunteers, *Br J Clin Pharmacol* 49:118, 2000.

85. Hiris E, Blake R: A new perspective on the visual motion aftereffect, *Proc Nat Acad Sci USA* 89:9025, 1992.

86. Hubel D, Weisel T: Receptive fields and functional architecture of monkey striate cortex, *J Physiol* 195:215, 1968.

87. Ives HE: Studies in the photometry of lights of different colours: II. Spectral luminousity curves by the method of critical frequency, *Philos Mag* 24:352, 1912.

88. Ives HE: A theory of intermittent vision, *J Opt Soc Am Rev Sci Instrum* 6:343, 1922.

89. Joffe KM, Raymond JE, Crichton A: Motion coherence perimetry in glaucoma and suspected glaucoma, *Vision Res* 37:955, 1997.

90. Johnson CA, Samuels SJ: Screening for glaucomatous visual field loss with frequency-doubling perimetry, *Invest Ophthalmol Vis Sci* 38:413, 1997.

91. Kaplan E, Shapley R: The primate retina contains two types of ganglion cells, with high and low contrast sensitivity, *Proc Nat Acad Sci USA* 83:2755, 1986.

92. Kawabata Y: Temporal integration at equiluminance and chromatic adaptation, *Vision Res* 34:1007, 1994.

93. Keesey UT: Variables determining flicker sensitivity in small fields, *J Opt Soc Am* 60:390, 1970.

94. Kelly D: Visual responses to time-dependent stimuli: 1. Amplitude sensitivity measurements, *J Opt Soc Am* 51:422, 1961.

95. Kelly D: Adaptation effects on spatio-temporal sine-wave thresholds, *Vision Res* 12:89, 1972.

96. Kelly DH: Frequency doubling in visual responses, *J Opt Soc Am* 56:1628, 1966.

97. Kelly DH: Motion and vision. I. Stabilized images of stationary gratings, *J Opt Soc Am* 69:1266, 1979.

98. Kelly DH: Motion and vision. II. Stabilized spatio-temporal threshold surfaces *J Opt Soc Am* 69:1340, 1979.

99. Krauskopf J, Mollon JD: The independence of the temporal integration properties of the individual chromatic mechanisms, *J Physiol (Lond)* 219:611, 1971.

100. Kulikowski JJ: Effect of eye movements on the contrast sensitivity of spatio-temporal patterns, *Vision Res* 11:261, 1971.

101. Lachenmayr BJ, Drance SM, Douglas GR: Light-sense, flicker and resolution perimetry in glaucoma: a comparative study, *Graefe's Arch Clin Exp Ophthalmol* 229:246, 1991.

102. Lange G, Denny N, Frumkes TE: Suppressive rod-cone interactions: evidence for separate retinal (temporal) and extraretinal (spatial) mechanisms in achromatic vision, *J Opt Soc Am A* 14:2487, 1997.

103. Legge GE: Sustained and transient mechanisms in human vision: temporal and spatial properties, *Vision Res* 18:69, 1978.

104. Leonards U, Singer W, Fahle M: The influence of temporal phase differences on texture segmentation, *Vision Res* 36:2689, 1996.

105. Livingstone MS, Hubel DH: Connections between layer 4B of area 17 and the thick cytochrome oxidase stripes of area 18 in the squirrel monkey, *J Neurosci* 7:3371, 1987.

106. Maddess T, Henry GH: Performance of nonlinear visual units in ocular hypertension and glaucoma, *Clin Vis Sci* 7:371, 1992.

107. Malpeli JG, Schiller PH, Colby CL: Response properties of single cells in monkey striate cortex during reversible inactivation of individual lateral geniculate laminae, *J Neurophysiol* 46:1102, 1981.

108. Mandler MB, Makous W: A three channel model of temporal frequency perception, *Vision Res* 24:1881, 1984.

109. Marr D, Ullman S: Directional sensitivity and its use in early visual processing, *Proc R Soc Lond B* 211:151, 1981.

110. Mason RJ et al: Abnormalities of chromatic and luminance critical flicker frequency in multiple sclerosis, *Invest Ophthalmol Vis Sci* 23:246, 1982.

111. Maunsell JH, Nealey TA, DePriest DD: Magnocellular and parvocellular contributions to responses in the middle temporal area (MT) of the macaque monkey, *J Neurosci* 10:3323, 1990.

112. Maunsell JH, Van Essen DC: Functional properties of neurons in middle temporal visual area of the macaque monkey. I. Selectivity for stimulus direction, speed, and orientation, *J Neurophysiol* 49:1127, 1983.

113. Mayer MJ et al: Foveal flicker sensitivity discriminates ARM-risk from healthy eyes, *Invest Ophthalmol Vis Sci* 33:3143, 1992.

114. McKendrick AM et al: Visual field losses in subjects with migraine headaches, *Invest Ophthalmol Vis Sc.* 41:1239, 2000.

115. McKendrick AM et al: Visual dysfunction between migraine events, *Invest Ophthalmol Vis Sci* 42:626, 2001.

116. Merigan W, Maunsell J: Macaque vision after magnocellular lateral geniculate lesions, *Vis Neurosci* 5:347, 1990.

117. Metha A, Vingrys AJ, Badcock DR: Detection and discrimination of moving stimuli: the effects of colour, luminance and eccentricity, *J Opt Soc Am A* 11:1697, 1994.

118. Mitsuboshi M, Kawabata Y, Aiba TS: Color-opponent characteristics revealed in temporal integration time, *Vision Res* 27:1197, 1987.

119. Montellese S, Sharpe LT, Brown JL: Changes in critical duration during dark-adaptation, *Vision Res* 19:1147, 1979.

120. Movshon A: Visual processing of moving images. In Barlow H, Blakemore C, Weston-Smith M (eds): *Images and understanding,* Cambridge, 1990, Cambridge University Press.

121. Nakayama K: Biological image motion processing: a review, *Vision Res* 25:625, 1985.

122. Nawrot M, Rizzo M: Motion perception deficits from midline cerebellar lesions in human, *Vision Res* 35:723, 1995.

123. Nealey TA, Maunsell JHR: Magnocellular and parvocellular contributions to the responses of neurons in macaque striate cortex, *J Neurosci* 14:2069, 1994.

124. Newsome WT, Britten KH, Movshon JA: Neuronal correlates of a perceptual decision, *Nature* 341:52, 1989.

125. Newsome WT, Paré EB: A selective impairment of motion perception following lesions of the middle temporal visual area (MT), *J Neurosci* 8:2201, 1988.

126. Nishida S, Sato T: Positive motion after-effect induced by bandpass-filtered random-dot kinematograms, *Vision Res* 32:1635, 1992.

127. Patat A et al: Lack of interaction between two antihistamines, mizolastine and cetirizine, and ethanol in psychomotor and driving performance in healthy subjects, *Eur J Pharmacol* 48:143, 1995.

128. Phipps JA, Guymer RH, Vingrys AJ: Temporal sensitivity deficits in patients with high-risk drusen, *Aust NZ J Ophthalmol* 27:265, 1999.

129. Plateau J: Sur un principle de photometrie, *Bulletins de L'Academie Royale des Sciences et Belles-lettres de Bruxelles* 2:52, 1835.

130. Pokorny J, Smith VC: Luminosity and CFF in deuteranopes and protanopes, *J Opt Soc Am* 62:111, 1972.

131. Porter T: Contributions to the study of flicker, *Proc R Soc A* 62:313, 1902.

132. Regan D: Early visual processing of spatial form: early visual processing of spatial form defined by luminance, color, motion, texture and binocular disparity, Sunderland, Mass, 1999, Sinauer.

133. Reichardt W: Autocorrelation, a principle for the evaluation of sensory information by the central nervous system. In Rosenblith WA (ed): *Sensory communication,* New York, 1961, Wiley.

134. Rizzo M, Nawrot M: Perception of movement and shape in Alzheimer's disease, *Brain* 121:2259, 1998.

135. Robson JG: Spatial and temporal contrast-sensitivity functions of the visual system, *J Opt Soc Am* 56:1141, 1966.

136. Rodman HR, Gross CG, Albright TD: Afferent basis of visual responses in area MT of the macaque. I. Effects of striate cortex removal, *J Neurosci* 9:2033, 1989.

137. Rodman HR, Gross CG, Albright TD: Afferent basis of visual responses in area MT of the macaque, *J Neurosci* 10:1154, 1990.

138. Roehrig W: The influence of area on the critical flicker fusion threshold, *J Psychol* 47:317, 1959.

139. Roehrig W: The influence of the portion of the retina stimulated on the critical flicker-fusion threshold, *J Psychol* 48:57, 1959.

140. Rogers-Ramachandran DC, Ramachandran VS: Psychophysical evidence for boundary and surface systems in human vision, *Vision Res* 38:71, 1998.

141. Roufs JAJ: Dynamic properties of vision. I. Experimental relationships between flicker and flash thresholds, *Vision Res* 12:261, 1972.

142. Rovamo J, Raninen A: Critical flicker frequency and M-scaling of stimulus size and retinal illuminance, *Vision Res* 24:1127, 1984.

143. Rovamo J, Raninen A: Critical flicker frequency as a function of stimulus area and luminance at various eccentricities in human cone vision: a revision of Granit-Harper and Ferry-Porter laws, *Vision Res* 28:785, 1988.

144. Rovamo J, Raninen A, Virsu V: The role of retinal ganglion cell density and receptive-field size in photopic perimetry, *Documenta Ophthal Proc Sec* 42:589, 1985.

145. Saunders RM: The critical duration of temporal summation in the human central fovea, *Vision Res* 15:699, 1975.

146. Schiller PH: The effects of V4 and middle temporal (MT) area lesions on visual performance in the rhesus monkey, *J Neurosci* 10:717, 1993.

147. Schiller PH, Logothetis NK, Charles ER: Role of the color-opponent and broad band channels in vision, *Visual Neurosci* 5:321, 1990.

148. Schiller P, Malpeli J: Functional specificity of lateral geniculate nucleus laminae of the rhesus monkey, *J Neurophysiol* 41:788, 1978.

149. Sekuler RW, Ganz L: Aftereffect of seen motion with a stabilized retinal image, *Science* 139:419, 1963.

150. Shipp S, Zeki S: The organisation of connections between areas V5 and V1 in macaque monkey visual cortex, *Eur J Neurosci* 1:309, 1989.

151. Shipp S, Zeki S: The organisation of connections between areas V5 and V2 in macaque monkey visual cortex, *Eur J Neurosci* 1:333, 1989.

152. Silverman SE, Trick GL, Hart WM: Motion perception is abnormal in primary open-angle glaucoma and ocular hypertension, *Invest Ophthalmol Vis Sci* 31:722, 1990.

153. Smith AT, Snowden RJ: *Visual detection of motion,* San Diego, 1994, Academic Press.

154. Smith VC, Bowen RW, Pokorny J: Threshold temporal integration of chromatic stimuli, *Vision Res* 24:653, 1984.

155. Snowden RJ, Braddick OJ: The temporal integration and resolution of velocity signals, *Vision Res* 31:907, 1991.

156. Snowden RJ, Hess RF: Temporal frequency filters in the human peripheral visual field, *Vision Res* 32:61, 1992.

157. Spehar B, Zaidi Q: Surround effects on the shape of the temporal contrast-sensitivity function, *J Opt Soc Am A* 14:2517, 1997.

158. Sperling HG, Jolliffe CL: Intensity-time relationship at threshold for spectral stimuli in human vision, *J Opt Soc Am* 55:191, 1965.

159. Stewart BR: Temporal summation during dark adaptation, *J Opt Soc Am* 62:449, 1972.

160. Stiles WS: *Separation of the "blue" and "green" mechanisms of foveal vision by measurements of increment thresholds: mechanisms of colour vision,* San Diego, 1978, Academic Press.

161. Stockman A, Plummer DJ: Color from invisible flicker: a failure of the Talbot-Plateau law caused by an early "hard" saturating nonlinearity used to partition the human short-wave cone pathway, *Vision Res* 38:3703, 1998.

162. Talbot HF: Experiments on light, *Philos Mag Ser 3* 5:321, 1834.

163. Trick GL, Kaskie B, Steinman SB: Visual impairment in Parkinson's disease: deficits in orientation and motion discrimination, *Optom Vis Sci* 71:242, 1994.

164. Tyler CW, Hamer RD: Analysis of visual modulation sensitivity. IV. Validity of the Ferry-Porter law, *J Opt Soc Am A* 7:743, 1990.

165. van Santen JPH, Sperling G: Elaborated Reichardt detectors, *J Opt Soc Am A* 2:300, 1985.

166. Vingrys AJ, Pesudovs K: Localised scotomata detected with temporal modulation perimetry in central serous chorioretinopathy, *Aust NZ J Ophthalmol* 27:109, 1999.

167. Wall M, Ketoff KM: Random dot motion perimetry in patients with glaucoma and in normal subjects, *Am J Ophthalmol* 120:587, 1995.

168. Wandell BA: *Foundations of vision,* Sunderland, Mass, 1995, Sinauer.

169. Watson AB: Probability summation over time, *Vision Res* 19:515, 1979.

170. Watson AB, Ahumada AJ: Model of human visual motion sensing, *J Opt Soc Am A* 2:322, 1985.

171. Watson AB, Robson JG: Discrimination at threshold: labelled detectors in human vision, *Vision Res* 21:1115, 1981.

172. Wertheimer M: Experimentelle Studien uber das Sehen von Bewegung, *Zietschrift fur Psychologie* 61:161, 1912.

173. Westcott MC, Fitzke FW, Hitchings RA: Abnormal motion displacement thresholds are associated with fine scale luminance sensitivity loss in glaucoma, *Vision Res* 38:3171, 1998.

174. Willis A, Anderson SJ: Effects of glaucoma and aging on photopic and scotopic motion perception, *Invest Ophthalmol Vis Sci* 41:325, 2000.

175. Wilson HR: A model for direction selectivity in threshold motion detection, *Biol Cybern* 51:213, 1985.

176. Yo C, Wilson HR: Peripheral temporal frequency channels code frequency and speed inaccurately but allow accurate discrimination, *Vision Res* 33:33, 1993.

177. Yoshiyama KK, Johnson CA: Which method of flicker perimetry is most effective for detection of glaucomatous visual field loss? *Invest Ophthalmol Vis Sci* 38:2270, 1997.

178. Zihl J, von Cramon D, Mai N: Selective disturbance of movement vision after bilateral brain damage, *Brain* 106(pt 2):313, 1983.

CHAPTER 21

DEVELOPMENT OF VISION IN INFANCY

ANTHONY M. NORCIA AND RUTH E. MANNY

The limited behavioral repertoire of the infant and the impossibility of instructing the test subject have made it necessary for vision scientists interested in human visual development to adapt the classic methods of psychophysics and electrophysiology for use with infants and preverbal children. First these methodologic adaptations and their interpretation in the context of a hierarchical model of visual processing are considered. Within this framework, the criteria for selecting material for review are discussed.

METHODOLOGIES FOR ASSESSING INFANT VISION AND THEIR INTERPRETATION

Preferential Looking

Infants' spontaneous visual fixation is attracted to certain stimuli more readily than to others.[45,46] In particular, infants prefer to look at patterned stimuli rather than regions of uniform brightness. This spontaneous behavior has served as the basis for a quantitative measure of stimulus visibility known as *forced-choice preferential looking* (FPL).[121] In the FPL task, the infant is confronted with a randomized series of patterns of varying visibility, presented either on the left or the right of a test screen. An observer judges whether the infant's fixation behavior is biased to the left or the right on a trial-by-trial basis. If the observer's judgments agree (or disagree) systematically with the actual position of the stimulus, it can be said that the infant's behavior is under the control of the stimulus. Distributions of the observer's judgments for a series of stimulus

values are used to plot a psychometric function, which relates the observer's percent correct to the stimulus values presented to the infant. Thresholds are estimated by curve fitting and interpolation to a criterion value of percent correct.

Visual Evoked Potentials

Visual Evoked Potentials (VEPs) are electrical brain responses triggered by the presentation of a visual stimulus. VEPs are distinguished from the spontaneous electroencephalogram (EEG) by their consistent time of occurrence (time-locking) after the presentation of the stimulus. For example, the abrupt contrast reversal of a checkerboard pattern consistently produces a positive potential at the surface of the scalp at a latency of approximately 100 milliseconds in adults.[101] Time-locked responses to abrupt presentations are referred to as *transient VEPs*. A second method of recording VEPs, the steady-state method, uses temporally periodic stimuli. For commonly used pattern reversal stimuli, the frequency of the repetition is often specified as the pattern reversal rate in reversals per second. This rate is twice the stimulus fundamental frequency (in Hz), which is more commonly used to describe the temporal frequency of pattern onset-offset stimuli. As the stimulus repetition rate increases, the responses to successive stimuli begin to overlap. At high stimulation rates, the response is composed of only a small number of components that occur at exact integer multiples of the stimulus frequency. Activity at each of the frequency components of the steady-state response is characterized by its amplitude and phase, with phase representing the temporal delay between the stimulus and the evoked response.

The surface-recorded VEP reflects the activity of cortical visual areas, with contributions from subcortical generators being apparent only under highly specialized recording conditions.[5,41,85] The primary adaptations of adult VEP recording techniques for infants involve the control of fixation through the use of fixation toys or superimposed video images and the rejection of trials when the infant's fixation is not centered on the stimulus.

Ocular-Following Movements

Both infants and adults make reflexive eye movements following the presentation of a moving target. Optokinetic nystagmus (OKN) is characterized by a repetitive sawtooth waveform. Rapid displacement of large-fields also elicits short-latency ocular-following movements.[80] Ocular following can also take the form of slower, pursuitlike movements.[55] Reflexive eye movements are controlled by a combination of cortical and subcortical mechanisms.[71] Infrared tracking, electrooculography, and naked-eye observations of the preponderant direction of eye motion (DEM) are the primary assays used in infants and preverbal children.[55,109]

HIERARCHY OF VISUAL PROCESSING

Figure 21-1 presents the schematic framework of visual processing that is used to focus the discussion of empirical studies of visual function in infants and young children. The visual processing hierarchy is divided into three stages: early, middle, and late. The progression from early to late correlates roughly with an ascent from the retina to the cortex and with a functional hierarchy corresponding to the complexity of the information extracted at each level. In this view, early vision begins in the retina and continues through the lateral geniculate and on into the primary visual cortex. By the level of primary visual cortex, stimulus attributes such as orientation, direction of motion, and disparity have been extracted from the retinal images.[13,62,104] Middle vision—the process by which local measurements of image features such as line orientation are integrated across space—begins no sooner than primary visual cortex and no doubt extends through a number of first- and second-tier extrastriate visual areas. The content of the representation at the level of middle vision includes information regarding the shape of extended contours, figure-ground relationships, the symmetry of ob-

jects, and surface depths, but it does not include the identity of the objects in the scene. The identification of objects (object recognition), which involves not only visual perception but also memory, is conceptualized as occurring in higher-order visual and visual association areas functionally associated with "late vision."

Each of the different methods for assessing visual function in the preverbal child has a different relationship to the visual processing hierarchy. The FPL technique depends on the integrity of the early visual system, as well as on additional mechanisms responsible for the spontaneous preference for pattern (labeled "preference generator" in Figure 21-1). Whether middle or late mechanisms are invoked may depend on the discrimination that the infant is called on to perform. Orienting behaviors could be driven from many levels of the cortical hierarchy or from subcortical structures. In any case the output of the preference generator must produce robust fixation behavior that can be detected reliably by the FPL observer. Information regarding the location of the stimulus can be lost at the level of early vision, at the level of the preference generator, or by the observer of the infant's behavior. Given the additional sites for potential information loss after early vision, FPL is a conservative estimator of the function of the early part of the visual pathway.

Like FPL, the VEP depends on the integrity of the retina and an unknown amount of cortical processing. Fixation, in the sense that the stimulus must fall on central retina, is required, but spontaneous orientation to a preferred stimulus is not. Electrical activity in the visual pathway is obscured by non–stimulus-related electrical activity associated with the EEG and muscle activity, as well as with electrode-motion artifacts. The obscuring experimental noise can be reduced effectively, either through time-locked averaging or spectral analysis. At this point relatively little is known about the contribution of extrastriate cortical areas to the VEP. Given this, the VEP likely reflects the capabilities of early vision, but caution must be used in inferring the integrity of later stages of processing, especially if simple stimuli are used.

Ocular-following movements require the integrity of the retina, but given the substantial role of subcortical mechanisms in the control of eye movements, it is difficult to specifically relate eye movement data to the hierarchy of cortical mechanisms in Figure 21-1.[71]

This review emphasizes developmental studies that have used the VEP. The rationale for this

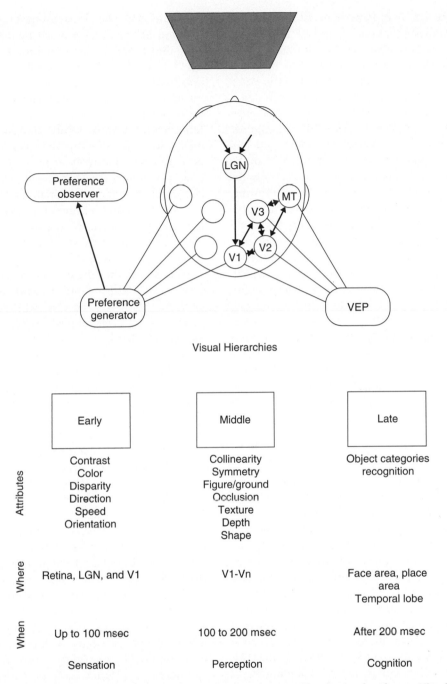

FIGURE 21-1   Visual processing hierarchy. *Top panel,* Schematic diagram of early visual pathways. Visual evoked potential (*VEP*) method picks up activity directly from an unknown complement of early visual areas. Preference-based behavioral measures require an additional "stage," at which preference and spontaneous fixation behavior are generated, as well as a behavioral observation stage. *Bottom panel,* Early, middle, and late stages of the visual processing hierarchy. Different visual attributes become available at different stages of the hierarchy. There is a rough correlation between levels of the hierarchy, anatomic locus, and response timing. *LGN,* Lateral geniculate nucleus.

choice is several fold. First, there is sufficient evidence to indicate that the infant VEP is generated after the site of orientation selectivity, direction selectivity, vernier offset detection, and binocular correlation detection*; all these features are considered the outputs of early vision, as illustrated in the model in Figure 21-1. In adults it has been found that the VEP reflects rivalry and suppression, as well as several aspects of middle vision, including figure-ground segmentation based on either texture or motion.† Second, the VEP does not require visual preference or transfer of information through the observation of spontaneous behavior and is thus less likely to underestimate the capabilities of early vision. Third, the VEP provides a rich source of information regarding the temporal dynamics of the visual response. Finally, there are already excellent reviews that have emphasized FPL and OKN measures of developing visual function.[36,39,55,56,58] In deciding which studies to include, emphasis has been placed, wherever possible, on those results that have been replicated by more than one research group. Data from the other methods are selectively discussed when these data can help fill in gaps or when they illustrate particularly sharp contrasts.

SPATIOTEMPORAL VISION

The retinal images contain a precise spatiotemporal mapping of the visual scene onto two-dimensional surfaces. At the most basic level of processing, the visual system must extract the contrast of the retinal images as a function of time and spatial scale. Visual sensitivity is limited by both spatial and temporal factors. Infant developmental studies have tended to focus on sensitivity along one dimension at a time—by measuring contrast sensitivity as a function of spatial frequency for a fixed temporal frequency or vice versa. Sensitivity depends strongly on both parameters. Although the FPL technique can be used at any combination of spatiotemporal frequency, the eye movement and VEP measures each require temporally modulated stimuli. Given the fundamental importance of contrast sensitivity for subsequent visual processing, contrast sensitivity and the related function grating acuity are among the few visual functions to have been studied extensively with each of the major methods discussed previously.

*References 15, 24, 75, 90, 95, 114, 124.
†References 8, 30, 34, 70, 86, 135.

Figure 21-2 plots peak contrast sensitivity as a function of age as determined by the steady-state VEP, directional eye movements, and FPL methods.[38,57,88,98] Each of these studies obtained peak sensitivity measures at a midrange of temporal frequencies (around 5 to 10 Hz). There is considerable development of contrast sensitivity in each of the techniques, but the absolute contrast sensitivity is higher with the VEP. By 10 weeks of age, infant peak contrast sensitivity over the 0.25 to 1 cpd range is within about a factor of 2 to 4 of adult levels measured on the same apparatus.[66,88] Skoczenski and Norcia[113] found a factor of 4 difference between infant and adult sensitivities at 1 cpd. Shannon, Skoczenski, and Banks[105] found sensitivities at 1.2 cpd that were a factor of 11 lower than adults at 2 months, with the difference decreasing to a factor of 4 at 3 months. Contrast sensitivity measured with the steady-state reversal VEP develops over progressively longer intervals as spatial frequency increases[88] (Figure 21-3).

In contrast to the VEP, several behavioral measures of contrast sensitivity in this age range are much lower than those at adult levels. Rasengane, Allen, and Manny[98] reported that low-spatial-frequency flicker sensitivity of 2-month-old infants was a factor of 45 lower than that of adults, with 3- and 4-month-old infants being a little less than 20 times less sensitive with FPL. Brown et al.[26] used a directional eye movement measure (0.31 cpd/15.5 deg/sec drift) and found that 3-month-old infants were a factor of 100 less sensitive than adults on the same measure. Dobkins and Teller[38] measured both FPL and directional eye movement thresholds in 3-month-old infants. They found that infants were almost 30 times less sensitive on the directional eye movement measure and about 60 times less sensitive when FPL and adults' forced-choice thresholds were compared. FPL and directional eye movement thresholds were within 20% of each other in the infants. In adults DEM thresholds were higher than psychophysical thresholds by a factor of 2 to 3, depending on whether the subjects task was detection of the direction of motion or simple contrast detection.

Hainline and Abramov[57] used directional eye movements recorded by an infrared eye tracker to measure contrast sensitivity. The observer made a forced-choice judgment on the output of the tracker (noise level 0.5 degree) rather than on naked-eye observation. Contrast sensitivity with this method develops to adult levels by 5 months of age (see Figure 21-2). Absolute thresholds are lower than those measured with the VEP by a factor of

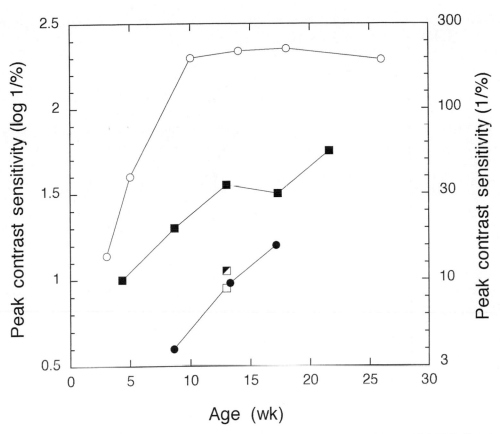

FIGURE 21-2   Peak contrast sensitivity measured with the steady-state visual evoked potential (VEP), direction of eye movement (DEM), and forced-choice preferential looking (FPL) methods. The VEP study (*open circles*, Norcia, Tyler, and Hamer[88]) used grating patterns that were reversed in contrast at 6 Hz (mean luminance of 220 cd/m²). Peak sensitivity was derived from recordings over the 0.25 to 1 cpd range. The DEM studies (*filled squares*, Hainline and Abramov[57]; *half-filled square*, Dobkins and Teller[38]) used 0.07 to 2.4 cpd gratings drifting at a constant velocity of 7 deg/sec or 0.25 cpd gratings drifting at 6 Hz. Dobkins and Teller[38] measured FPL thresholds for 0.25 cpd/6 Hz as well (*open square*). Rasengane, Allen, and Manny,[98] measured contrast sensitivity for 10-degree luminance fields over the range of 1 to 25 Hz (*filled circles*). Peak sensitivity at any temporal frequency is plotted. Contrast sensitivity improves rapidly within each method.

---

about 4. Hainline and Abramov's[57] contrast sensitivities are higher than those observed by Dobkins and Teller[38] or Brown et al.,[26] who used naked-eye observation at substantially higher luminances. The difference in sensitivities obtained with naked-eye and instrumented observation of eye movements suggests that at least some of the lower sensitivity seen in previous behavioral studies may have resulted from information loss in the observer who is judging the infant's behavioral output.

GRATING ACUITY

At the limit of the high-spatial-frequency limb of the contrast sensitivity function lies the observer's grating acuity. Grating acuity is limited by the opti-

cal quality of the eye, the spacing of the photoreceptors, and the spatial pooling properties of the ganglion cells and subsequent receptive field mechanisms.[10,11,133,134] Grating acuity is also limited by temporal factors, being maximal at low temporal frequencies.

VEP grating acuity has been measured most commonly using steady-state, pattern reversal targets in the frequency range of 5 to 10 Hz (10 to 20 contrast reversals per second). The acuity measurement is extrapolated from the high-spatial-frequency portion of the amplitude versus spatial frequency function, an example of which is illustrated in Figure 21-4 for the spatial frequency-sweep technique. In this method, originally developed by Regan,[100] the spatial frequency of a temporally modulated pattern is

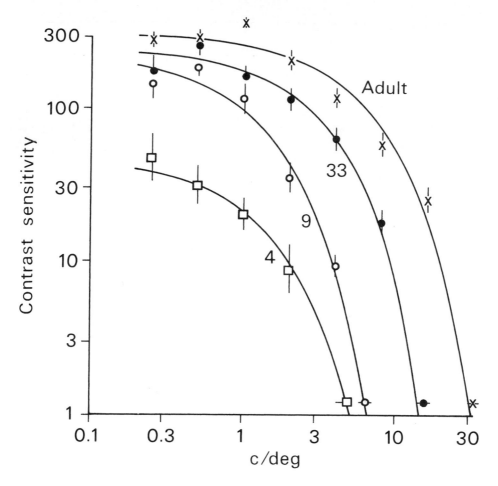

Figure 21-3   Visual evoked potential contrast sensitivity is replotted from Norcia, Tyler, and Hamer[88] as a function of spatial frequency and age (in weeks for infants) for 6-Hz pattern reversal. Sensitivity development is progressively delayed at higher spatial frequencies.

systematically changed (swept) over a large range of spatial frequencies that span the expected acuity limit of the observer. Figure 21-4 plots grating acuity as a function of age for such pattern reversal stimuli. Each study used the swept spatial frequency technique. Acuity growth functions are similar across studies, with acuity increasing from 4 to 6 cpd in 1-month-old infants to around 15 to 20 cpd around 8 months of age.

VEP acuity has also been measured with pattern onset-offset stimuli, in both transient and steady-state paradigms. Two studies of the transient on-off acuity growth function found that acuity improved from approximately 2 cpd at 1 month to 30 cpd by 5 months.[78,93] A third study, which used checks rather than gratings, found an acuity of 2.3 cpd (corrected for Fourier fundamental spatial fre-

quency of the checks) at 8 weeks, with an increase to 8 cpd at 24 weeks.[37] When both transient onset-offset and 6-Hz contrast reversal stimuli were used to measure acuity in the same infants, two different rates of growth were found; transient onset-offset acuity increased 0.63 octaves per month versus 0.28 octaves per month with 6-Hz pattern reversal.[93] The observations that the rate at which acuity increases depends on the response component being measured suggests that different postreceptoral visual mechanisms have different rates of development.

TEMPORAL RESOLUTION

Temporal resolution is highest for coarse stimuli. The highest temporal frequency to which the visual system responds undergoes a somewhat different

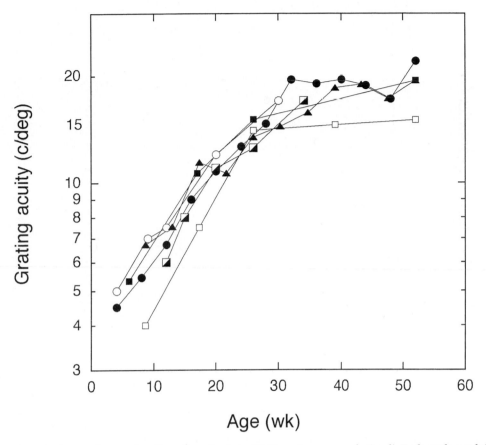

FIGURE 21-4   Grating acuity as a function of age for 5- to 10-Hz pattern reversal stimuli. Each study used the swept spatial frequency technique. Acuity growth functions are similar across studies, with acuity increasing from 4 to 6 cpd in 1-month-old infants to around 15 to 20 cpd around 8 months of age. Data are replotted. *Filled circles,* Norcia and Tyler[87]; *open circles,* Norcia, Tyler and Hamer[88]; *half-filled squares,* Allen, Tyler, and Norcia[1]; *triangles,* Sokol, Moskowitz, and McCormack[118]; *open squares,* Auestad et al[7]; and *filled squares,* Birch et al.[22]

developmental progression than that for spatial resolution at low temporal frequencies. Figure 21-5 shows the development of temporal resolution measured with luminance flicker (a low-spatial-frequency target) in a large group of 130 infants and 6 adults. Temporal resolution was determined from the highest flicker rate from a large series that produced a measurable response. Adult temporal resolutions are approached by 20 to 30 weeks of age, a time at which grating acuity is still significantly lower than that in adults (see Figure 21-4). A psychophysical study in children 4 to 7 years of age found temporal resolution to be fully adult at age 4 years, but grating acuity continued to improve until about 6 years of age.[43]

DEVELOPMENT OF RESPONSE WAVEFORM

Contrast sensitivity and spatial and temporal acuity are all measures of neural activity at visual threshold. Visual processing at suprathreshold levels has been studied most extensively by measuring VEP response waveforms as a function of age and spatial frequency. One of the most striking features of visual development is the very large change in the latency of major response peaks in the VEP that occurs during the first few months of life.

Figure 21-6 shows waveforms for pattern reversal responses recorded between 8 and 24 weeks of age.[82] The pattern was a high-contrast, low-spatial-frequency plaid that square-wave reversed in con-

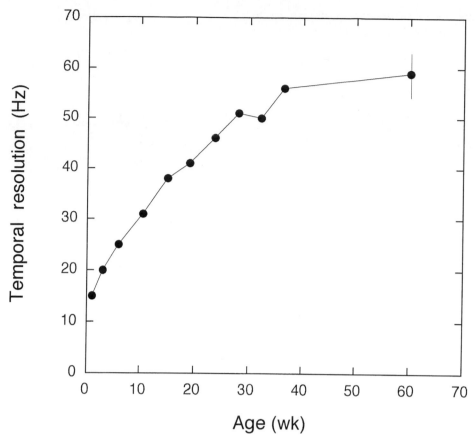

Figure 21-5   Flicker resolution frequency, measured with the steady-state visual evoked potential (replotted from Apkarian[3]). Resolution frequency increased linearly up to age 40 weeks. Adult values are plotted at 60 weeks. Infants in the 20- to 30-week age range have resolution acuities that are nearly adult levels.

trast at 0.75 Hz. At 8 weeks, the response waveform is biphasic, with the time to the first positive peak being 200 milliseconds. The initial positivity decreases in latency and by 17 to 24 weeks; a negative peak at about 70 to 80 milliseconds precedes this initial positive response. Broadly similar waveforms for the transient pattern reversal response have been reported in other studies that have studied this age range.*

A prominent feature of the development of the VEP waveform is the progressive shortening of the latency of major response peaks shown in Figure 21-7 (*left*), which plots data from McCulloch and Skarf.[79] Developmental changes in the latency of the first major positive peak in the transient pattern reversal response have been well-studied, and there is a consistent developmental sequence visible across studies of which the data in Figure 21-6 are repre-

sentative.* The latency of the first positive peak rapidly declines to near-adult levels by approximately 5 months of age for low-spatial-frequency targets. Longer maturational sequences are seen when finer scale patterns are used.[68,79] Small latency decreases continue during childhood and adolescence.[2,138]

The latency of the evoked response is controlled by the neural integration time required in the retina, the conduction velocity through the retinogeniculate pathway, and finally, cortical integration time. Fiorentini and Trimarchi[47] compared latencies of simultaneously recorded pattern ERG and VEP responses (see Figure 21-7, *right panel*). Adults had a 50-millisecond difference in latency between retinal and cortical responses. This difference was 125 millisecond at 5 weeks of age, indicating that much of the change in delay of VEP latency that oc-

*References 6, 35, 47, 68, 79, 83, 97, 117.

*References 6, 35, 47, 68, 79, 97, 117.

curs during the first 5 months is attributable to changes in postretinal mechanisms, most likely in the cortex.

Motion

The detection of motion involves the determination of speed and direction. The presence of direction-selective mechanisms early in development has been demonstrated using each of the three major methods: FPL, VEP, and OKN. Directionally appropriate eye movements can be seen at term or even sooner.[40,55] Uncertainty remains as to whether these early ocular-following responses are controlled by cortical or subcortical pathways. Direction selectivity has been demonstrated behaviorally with the use of FPL and time-habituation methods by 6 to 8 weeks.[125,126] VEP responses associated with changes of direction have been recorded by 10 weeks of age.[15,124]

Motion Asymmetry

On any measure, the adult visual system shows roughly equal sensitivity for all directions of motion (see references in Gros, Blake, and Hiris[53]). Developing infants, on the other hand, show large, systematic biases in their monocular oculomotor and VEP responses. Monocular OKN (MOKN) is robust for nasalward motion but is weak for temporalward motion during the first 3 to 6 months of life,[72,84,103] as shown in Figure 21-8. The time to attain a symmetric MOKN response may depend on the stimulus velocity, with time to maturity being later for higher image velocities.[103]

Young infants also show monocular VEPs response asymmetries suggestive of a nasalward-temporalward bias in cortical responses.[15,63,90,91] These response asymmetries manifest themselves in the monocular steady-state VEP made in response to rapidly oscillating gratings. In adults, oscillating gratings produce responses primarily at twice the stimulus frequency (at the rate that stimulus direction changes, F_2). In young infants, an additional response component is present at the stimulus frequency (first harmonic response, F_1; Figure 21-9). The first harmonic is 180 degrees out of phase in the two eyes. This pattern of response, a significant first harmonic that is of opposite phase in the two eyes, is consistent with a response bias that is in opposite directions in the two eyes. The absolute direction of the bias, nasalward or temporalward, cannot be directly determined from the

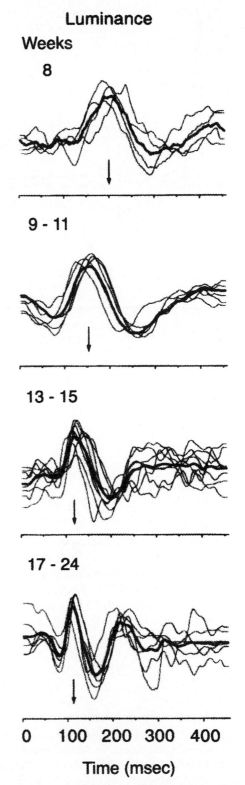

Luminance

Weeks

8

9 - 11

13 - 15

17 - 24

0   100   200   300   400

Time (msec)

Figure 21-6 Development of the transient pattern reversal visual evoked potential waveform. Individual infant data (*thin lines*) and group averages (*thick lines*) are shown for each age. The latency of the major positivity (*arrows*) systematically decreases with age. (Redrawn from Morrone, Fiorentini, and Burr.[82])

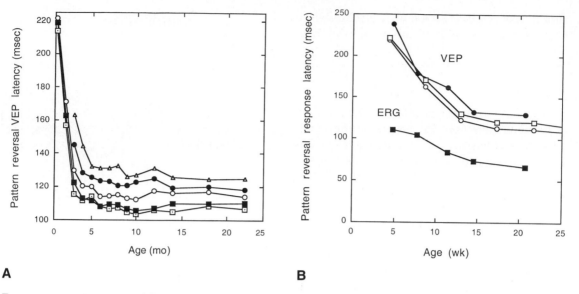

A　　　　　　　　　　　　　　　　　　　　　**B**

Figure 21-7　**A,** Latency of first positive peak in the pattern reversal response as a function of age and check size. (Data replotted from McCulloch and Skarf.[79]) Response latency declines rapidly over the first 6 months of life for all check sizes, although the rate of decline is somewhat slower for finer patterns. **B,** Comparison of the latencies of simultaneously recorded pattern electroretinogram (*ERG*) (*filled squares*) and visual evoked potential (*VEP*) responses (*filled circles*) in infants from Fiorentini and Trimarchi.[47] ERG and VEP latencies were estimated from the steady-state response by converting the measured response phase into an apparent latency. The open symbols plot latency data obtained from the transient pattern reversal VEP using similar-size patterns.

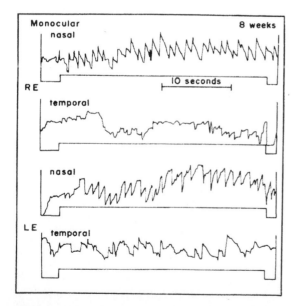

Figure 21-8　Directional asymmetry of monocular optokinetic nystagmus (MOKN). MOKN is robust for nasalward stimulus motion (leftward motion in the right eye [*RE*] and rightward motion in the left eye [*LE*]) but is weak for temporalward motion. This directional asymmetry declines during the first few months of life. (Adapted from Naegele JR, Held R: *Vis Res* 22:341, 1982.)

steady-state response. It is unknown at present whether the cortical motion asymmetry tapped by the VEP causes the oculomotor asymmetry or whether the two phenomena represent immaturities in independent mechanisms with similar developmental sequences.

Symmetric cortical motion responses develop during the first 6 months of life (see Figure 21-9) for 6-Hz oscillatory motion of a low-spatial-frequency gratings. Figure 21-10 plots the ratio of amplitudes at the first harmonic to the sum of amplitudes at the first and second harmonics. This index runs from 1.0 for a completely asymmetric response to 0 for a completely symmetric response. Infants reach adult levels by about 5 months of age for low-spatial-frequency targets oscillating at 6 Hz.

The VEP motion asymmetry has been recorded in infants as young as 2 months of age, suggesting that cortical direction selectivity is present at this time.[15] Interestingly, the motion asymmetry was undetectable in infants younger than 8 weeks at 6 Hz, 1 cpd. Development of motion-specific VEPs over the neonatal period has also been observed in a different stimulation paradigm.[124] Wattam-Bell[124] also found that the age of first direction-specific responses was earlier for lower stimulus velocities.

Normal (10 wk)

Normal (31 wk)

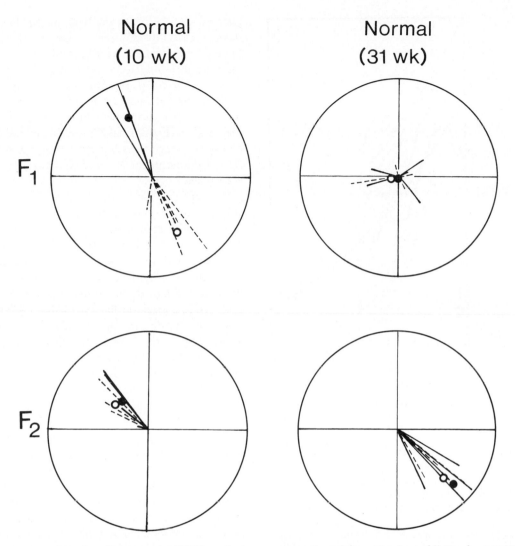

FIGURE 21-9   Visual evoked potential (VEP) motion asymmetry, adapted from Norcia et al.[90] Steady-state VEPs to monocular oscillatory motion contain significant odd harmonics in young infants (F_1). The phase of these components is shifted by 180 degrees between the two eyes in a 10-week-old infant. *Top left plot,* Individual trials are indicated by separate lines radiating from zero. The presence of odd harmonics suggests that the response to left and right motion is asymmetric and that the dominant direction is opposite in the two eyes. The odd-harmonic components decline in amplitude over the first 5 to 6 months of age is indicated by the data from a normal 31-week old (*right panels*). Second harmonic response (F_2) are present at both ages. (Adapted from Norcia AM et al: *Invest Ophthamol Vis Sci* 32:436, 1991.)

VERNIER ACUITY

Vernier acuity refers to a collection of spatial localization tasks requiring the detection of a misalignment relative to a reference. Like stereoacuity, adult vernier thresholds are significantly better than would be predicted on the basis of either the optical or the anatomic properties of the eye. Therefore vernier acuity is considered one of the hyperacuities.[81,127,128] Because cortical processing is believed to be involved, the time course for the development vernier acuity has been investigated with great interest.[12,120,129]

Most investigations of vernier acuity during the first year of life have been cross sectional, employing behavioral responses to moving stimuli.[77,107,108,137] However, two studies used stationary stimuli.[27,76] The results of several of these behavioral studies, plotted over the first 6 months of life, are summarized in Figure 21-11. On average, vernier acuity improves by about a factor of 6 to 8 over the first

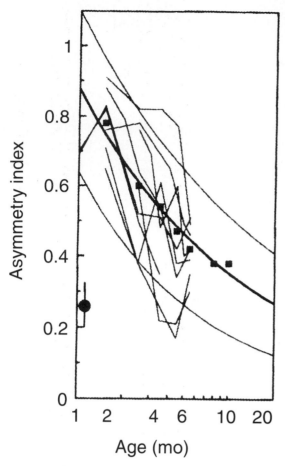

FIGURE 21-10   Developmental sequence for symmetry motion visual evoked potentials (VEPs). The degree of motion asymmetry can be quantified by calculating the fraction of the total response (first plus second harmonic) that is contributed by the first harmonic (asymmetry index). The monocular oscillatory motion VEP is dominated by the first harmonic in early infancy (asymmetry index greater than 0.5), but the degree of asymmetry declines rapidly over the first 6 months for 6-Hz 1-c/deg targets. Filled squares indicate mean responses for infants between 1.5 and 10 months. The thin lines indicate longitudinal recordings. The smooth curves indicate a fit to the mean growth function 1 standard deviation. The filled circle indicates the average asymmetry index for five infants between 0.5 and 1 month of age. (From Birch EE, Fawcett S, Stager D: *Invest Ophthalmol Vis Sci* 41:1719, 2000.)

6 months of life, with the best thresholds recorded to be around 200 seconds, 1.3 to 1.8 log units poorer than adults.

Although Zanker et al.[137] reported that, by 5 years of age, children's performance on the vernier acuity task became comparable to that of adults, others report that vernier development is incom-

plete at age 5.[31,52,67] On the basis of the their data from preschool children, Carkeet, Levi, and Manny[31] calculate that vernier acuity is two times the adult threshold at 5.6 years of age (confidence interval 3.5 to 6.5 years). Thus there is some agreement in the literature that the development of vernier acuity is incomplete during the early school years and reaches normal adult values of 3 to 8 second of arc by age 18 to 20 years.* However, it is not clear if development is complete before 18 to 20 years of age.

As noted previously, most of the behavioral paradigms used to investigate the development of vernier acuity contained motion. Skoczenski and Aslin[112] have demonstrated that temporally modulated stimuli improve the vernier thresholds of 3-month-old infants and suggest that vernier thresholds obtained with moving stimuli may be governed by a local motion mechanism rather than a position-sensitive mechanism. Therefore our understanding of the developmental time course of vernier acuity and its relationship to the development of other visual functions is potentially confounded by some of the stimuli that have been used in behavioral paradigms to gain the infant's attention and interest in the task.

The VEP offers a unique solution to this problem. Norcia, Wesemann, and Manny[89] suggest that through analysis of the separate Fourier components in the steady-state VEP, vernier response components may be isolated from those arising from stimulus motion. The VEP response to the introduction of a vernier offset (alignment/misalignment) differs from the response to the return to alignment (misalignment/alignment). This asymmetric response to the introduction and then removal of a vernier offset is reflected in the odd harmonics of the response to the stimulus modulation. The even harmonics in the evoked potential are produced in response to the symmetric spatial aspects of the stimulus modulation (e.g., local motion of the offset grating) and may be used to examine motion acuity. The results obtained by Skoczenski and Norcia[115] with a sweep VEP technique are shown in Figure 21-12. There is a rapid improvement in vernier acuity over the first 4 months of life. By 6 months of age, vernier acuity has improved by about a factor of 7, reaching a threshold of nearly 70 seconds, approximately 1 log unit poorer than the normal adult values obtained psychophysically. Between 6 months and 7.5 years

*References 14, 69, 73, 92, 102, 122, 130, 131.

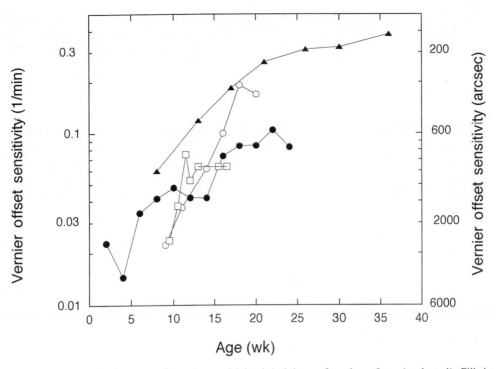

FIGURE 21-11 Behaviorally determined vernier sensitivity (1/min) as a function of age (replotted). *Filled triangles,* Shimojo et al[108]; *open circles,* Shimojo and Held[107]; *filled circles,* Manny and Klein[76]; *open squares,* Brown.[27]

of age, improvement occurs at a slower rate, reaching about 40 seconds, a 1.75 times improvement over the course of about 7 years. After the age of 7.5 years there is another, more rapid improvement in vernier acuity. Although quantitatively better thresholds were obtained psychophysically by Carkeet, Levi, and Manny[31] with stationary stimuli, there is a similar period during the early school years in which no significant change in threshold was found.

Opto-type recognition acuity, as measured with standard eye charts, shows a similar prolonged developmental time course. Improvement has been reported to continue until 25 to 29 years of age, reaching 0.56 minimum angle of resolution (MAR) expressed in minutes of arc to 0.67 to 0.69 MAR.[28,44,51,94] At age 3 to 5 years, chart acuity is 1.25 MAR, about a factor of 1.8 poorer than the most conservative estimate of the adult acuity noted previously.[23,119] At 6.8 years of age, chart acuity has improved to 1.09 MAR, a factor of 1.6 poorer than the most conservative estimate of normal adult recognition acuity.[23]

The developmental time course for vernier acuity appears to occur in at least three phases. There is a rapid development over the first 4 to 6 months of life, then a more gradual improvement up to about 7 to 10 years of age, followed by a more rapid improvement to reach adult levels no later than 18 to 20 years of age. Recognition chart acuity also has a long time course with improvement noted until 25 to 29 years of age.

BINOCULAR VISION

This section explores the development of the sensory aspects of binocular vision, sensory fusion (the neurologic combination of the image from each eye into a single percept), and stereopsis (the perception of depth based on a horizontal disparity between the retinal images in each eye). As with all visual processes, the parameters of the stimulus and the method of measurement may limit the infant's performance, as well as our understanding of the developing visual system. Dichoptic stimulus presentations and the need to eliminate confounding monocular cues present unique challenges to studies of the development of fusion and stereopsis and have guided the selection of the studies reviewed.

Fusion

The most direct approach in determining the onset of sensory fusion in human infants has been to

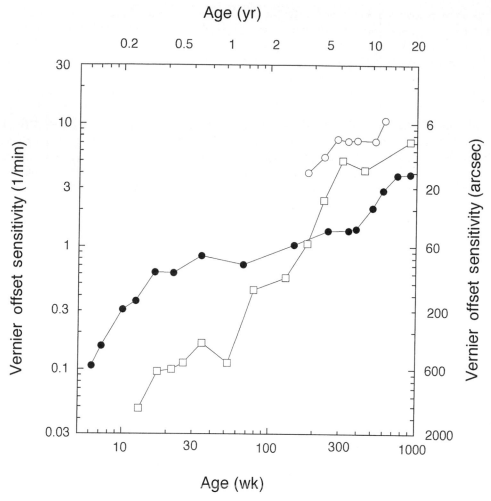

FIGURE 21-12   Vernier sensitivity (1/min) as a function of age determined by the visual evoked potential. *Filled circles,* Skoczenski, Norcia, and Good.[115] Shown for comparison are behavioral data from Carkeet, Levi, and Manny[31] (*open circles,* from Figure 21-4) and Zanker et al.[137] (*open squares,* from Figure 21-2).

record a "cyclopean" VEP using one of two different stimuli. The first approach, popularized by Baitch and Levi[9] and applied to infants by France and Ver Hoeve,[50] presents a uniform field to each eye; this field is then modulated at two different temporal frequencies (e.g., 8 Hz, right eye; 6 Hz, left eye). A cortical response recorded at either the sum (14 Hz) or the difference frequency (2 Hz, also termed the *beat frequency*) suggests the presence of binocular neurons that integrate and respond to the input from both eyes. Using this approach, France and Ver Hoeve[50] reported that a binocular response was present in most normal infants by 2 months of age. The two-frequency approach has also been used to study the development of fusion and rivalry by Brown, Candy, and Norcia.[29] In that

study, beat frequency response was recordable only for stimuli that had the same orientation in the two eyes.

The second approach to identify the integration of information from the two eyes uses dynamic random-dot correlograms.[95] Correlograms consist of a field of random dots presented dichoptically to the two eyes. Correlograms alternate between two different phases: a correlated and anticorrelated phase. In the correlated phase the dot patterns are identical in the two eyes. In the anticorrelated phase a dark dot in the pattern presented to one eye corresponds to a bright dot in the pattern presented to the fellow eye. The cortical response to the alternation between the two phases is recorded. The cyclopean VEP response to these correlated and anticorrelated stimuli has been interpreted as fusion without stereopsis because horizontal disparities are not induced by the stimuli.[42,74,96] With use of this approach, the onset of sensory fusion has been reported to occur between 3 and 5 months of age.[19,25,95]

Stereopsis

Age of Onset. Because of the limited number of reports that have investigated stereopsis in the developing visual system with the VEP, this section emphasizes studies that have applied the behavioral techniques of preferential looking and ocular-following movements. Behaviorally, studies of the onset of stereopsis have used real-depth tests, local or linear stereograms, and global or random-dot stereograms.[64,65] However, real-depth targets and local tests of stereopsis contain monocular cues that can confound a positive response and confuse the interpretation of the results. Because many of the early reports that investigated the onset of stereopsis relied on real-depth tests with multiple cues to depth, these are not reviewed (see Daw[36] for a review). Studies using random-dot stereograms that rely on the detection of a horizontal displacement in the image presented to each eye without monocular cues are emphasized. Results obtained from linear stereograms with adequate controls are also summarized.

There is remarkable consistency among the various laboratories and techniques concerning the onset of global or random-dot stereopsis. Stereopsis emerges between 3 and 5 months of age, whether determined with the VEP or by behavioral methods.*

Several reports from the same laboratory, using disparities ranging from 58 to 32 minutes of arc, have also reported the onset of local or linear stereopsis to be between 3 and 5 months of age.[16,17,21,54]

The age at which at least 75% of infants demonstrate sensory fusion or stereopsis is summarized across studies in Figure 21-13. Details concerning the stimulus and the measurement method for each study are provided in the figure legend.

Stereothreshold. Following the emergence of measurable stereopsis between 3 and 5 months of age, the improvement in local or linear stereoacuity during the first year of life has been reported to be rapid. For a small sample of infants followed longitudinally ($n = 16$), stereoacuity for crossed disparities improved from 58 minutes at 14.8 weeks of age

to 1 minute of arc by 20 weeks of age.[16] A similar time course was noted for uncrossed disparities that emerged slightly later at 16.8 weeks and improved from 58 minutes of arc to 1 minute by 23.2 weeks. Because the five adults tested on the same apparatus averaged 97.6% correct for the 1-minute crossed disparity stimulus and 80.2% for the 0.5-minute crossed disparity stimulus but only 62.6% correct for the 0.5-minute uncrossed disparity target, the authors suggested that the performance of the 5- to 6-month-old infants was adultlike.[16]

However, it is important to recall that stereoacuity belongs to a family of localization tasks known as *hyperacuities.* Hyperacuities provide finer localization than predicted on the basis of either the optic or the anatomic properties of the eye.[81,127] Adult stereothresholds obtained with real-depth stimuli range from about 2 to 5 seconds with the Howard Dolman apparatus.[14,49,99] Similar stereothresholds of about 5 seconds have been reported with the diastereo test.[60,61,136] The diastereo test is another real-depth test of stereopsis that uses three black dots on a translucent background, one of which is physically located in front of the other two, and varies the test distance to obtain threshold. Adult stereothresholds with random-dot stereograms have been reported to range from 5.37 seconds to about 30 seconds, with Simons reporting 15.1 seconds.[99,110,116] Thus a closer look at the time course for the development of stereoacuity appears warranted. On the basis of the number of behavioral studies available from a variety of laboratories covering a large age range, the development of global stereopsis was selected for review. As mentioned previously, global stereopsis has the additional advantage of being based solely on the detection of the horizontal image displacement between the two eyes because the stimulus contains no monocular cues.

Figure 21-14 shows the development of stereoacuity during the first 18 months of life. The filled circles indicate the mean stereoacuity measured behaviorally in response to random-dot stereograms.[21] The open circles are taken from Birch, Gwaizda, and Held[16] and represent the smallest linear disparity at which 50% or more of the infants tested reached criterion. Over the first year of life, global stereoacuity improves by a factor of 8, to about 120 seconds of arc, but it has not yet reached adult levels. This improvement is greater than the factor of 4 or 5 reported for the development of spatial resolution over the same period.

Figure 21-15 illustrates the continued development of global stereopsis during childhood. All

---

*References 4, 19, 20, 48, 95, 106, 111.

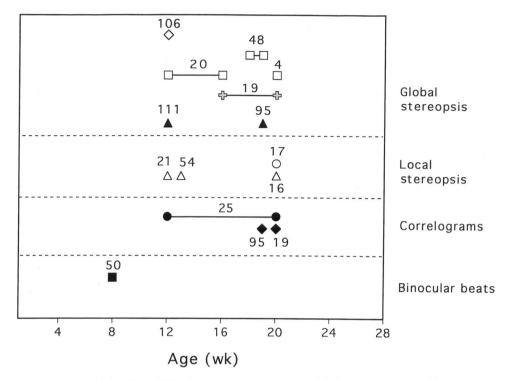

FIGURE 21-13   Age at which at least 75% of those tested demonstrated fusion or stereopsis. Filled symbols represent studies using the visual evoked potential (VEP), open symbols show studies using behavioral paradigms (forced-choice preferential looking [FPL]), and gray symbols indicate both FPL and VEP. The numbers correspond to the numbered reference in the reference section. France and Ver Hoeve,[50] 6- and 8-Hz dichoptic presentation; Birch and Petrig,[19] correlograms 20-minute disparity (FPL) and 30-minute disparity (VEP); Petrig et al.,[95] correlograms 40-minute disparity; Braddick et al.,[25] correlograms; Birch, Shimojo, and Held,[21] 45-minute crossed disparity; Gwiazda, Bauer, and Held,[54] 32-minute crossed disparity; Birch, Gwiazda, and Held,[16] 58-minute crossed and uncrossed disparity; Birch, Gwiazda, and Held,[17] 58-minute disparity; Skarf et al.,[111] alternation of 100-minute crossed to 100-minute uncrossed disparity; Birch and Salomao,[20] less than 1735 arcsec disparity; Archer et al.,[4] 30-minute crossed disparity; Shea et al.,[106] 60-minute disparity; and Fox.[48]

---

show continued improvement during the preschool years. Two studies also report thresholds from normal adults under similar test conditions. Ciner, Schanel-Klitsch, and Scheiman[33] (*filled diamonds*) indicate that at age 5 years, stereoacuity is still about a factor of 3 poorer than that in the adult. Simons[110] (*open circles*) also find stereoacuity is a factor of 3 poorer for 6-year-olds compared with that for adults.

Four studies that measured global stereoacuity with the commercially available TNO test in school-aged children are also illustrated in Figure 21-15. The TNO test is uses anaglyphic separation with six different retinal disparities varying from 480 to 15 seconds of arc. Walraven and Janzen[123]

(*filled circles*) report that the ability to make depth judgments on the basis of random-dot stereograms improves by a factor of 2 between the ages of 4 and 12 years. The data also suggest additional improvement up to 18 years of age, the oldest reported in the study. When the small number (*n* = 4) of 6- to 10-year-olds tested by Sloper and Collins[116] (*filled squares*) are compared with 12 adults with normal vision, stereoacuity remains a factor of 2 poorer than that measured in the adults. However, Heron et al.[59] (*open squares*) report that stereoacuity as measured by the TNO was adultlike at 5 years of age. These investigators also noted that among the four stereotests evaluated in the report, the TNO gave the poorest thresholds and the largest variabil-

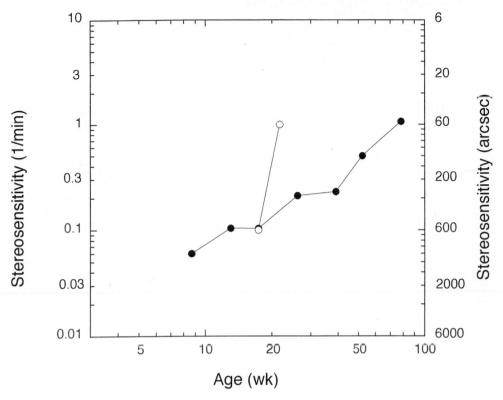

FIGURE 21-14 The development of stereosensitivity (1/min) as a function of age. Global stereoacuity with Polaroid random-dot stereograms from Birch and Salomao[20] (*filled circles*). The smallest linear disparity that 50% or more of the infants tested reached criterion, Birch, Gwiazda, and Held[16] (*open circles*).

ity in their sample. Using a real-depth test, the Frisby stereo test, they found that stereoacuity was not yet adultlike at 7 years of age. Fox, Patterson, and Francis[49] report that with the Howard-Dolman real-depth test, children 3 to 5 years of age were about 2.5 times poorer than adults (12.6 versus 4.9 seconds of arc).

In summary, sensory fusion has been demonstrated as early as 2 months of age, and stereopsis emerges no later than 3 and 5 months of age. Although there is about a factor of 8 improvement in stereoacuity for globally defined targets over the first year of life, stereoacuity does not reach adult levels until some time after age 5. At age 5 or 6, stereoacuity is still about three times poorer than that of the adult.

SUMMARY

Maturation of visual function in humans occurs over different time scales, depending on the partic-

ular aspect of function being measured. Within a particular visual function, development may proceed at different rates during different postnatal periods. In several of the functions reviewed in this chapter, there is an early, rapid period of development that is followed by a long, slow second phase that lasts into childhood or even adolescence. Low-spatial-frequency contrast sensitivity appears to be the most precocious function yet measured. Decreases in the latency of the VEP roughly parallel the increase in contrast sensitivity (see Figure 21-2), and increasing sensitivity may play a substantial role in determining response latency because it is known that response latency decreases as stimulus contrast is increased.[101] A high-contrast stimulus that produces a brisk response in the adult is effectively a lower contrast stimulus to the developing visual system with its lower overall sensitivity to contrast. Thus latency may be prolonged. Flicker sensitivity, another function that is measured with low-spatial-frequency targets, also matures relatively quickly,

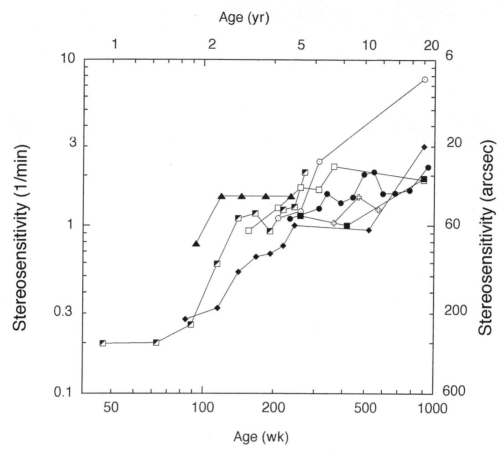

Figure 21-15 The development of stereosensitivity (1/min) as a function of age. All studies are based on a behavioral response to random-dot stereograms. *Filled diamonds,* Ciner, Schanel-Klitsch, and Scheiman[33]; *half-filled squares,* Ciner, Schanel-Klitsch, and Herzberg[32]; *open circles,* Simons[110]; *filled triangles,* Birch and Hale[18]; *open squares,* Heron et al.[59]; *filled squares,* Sloper and Collins[116]; *plus signs,* William, Simpson, and Silva[132]; and *filled circles,* Walraven and Janzen.[123]

---

reaching adult levels during the first 6 months. Grating acuity measured with midfrequency contrast reversal has its initial rapid period of development during the first 8 months, and vernier acuity appears to develop at a different rate over this period and is far from adult levels.

Variations in the developmental sequences across visual functions presumably reflect limitations imposed at different levels of the visual hierarchy shown in Figure 21-1. The critical immaturity limiting contrast sensitivity, grating acuity, and temporal resolution may lie in the early part of the pathway consisting of the retina and early cortical visual areas. Functions such as vernier acuity and stereoacuity are known to be sensitive to contrast in adults; thus some of the immaturity in these functions is likely to be caused by the reduced contrast sensitivity of the infant. However, other factors

must also limit infant vernier acuity and stereoacuity because their developmental sequences are longer than those underlying contrast sensitivity and grating acuity.

References

1. Allen D, Tyler CW, Norcia AM: Development of grating acuity and contrast sensitivity in the central and peripheral visual field of the human infant, *Vis Res* 36:1945, 1996.
2. Allison T, Wood CC, Goff WR: Brain stem auditory, pattern-reversal visual, and short-latency somatosensory evoked potentials: latencies in relation to age, sex, and brain and body size, *Electroencephalogr Clin Neurophysiol* 55:619, 1983.
3. Apkarian P: Temporal frequency responsivity shows multiple maturational phases: state-dependent visual evoked potential luminance flicker fusion from birth to 9 months, *Vis Neurosci* 10:1007, 1993.
4. Archer SM et al: Stereopsis in normal infants and infants with congenital esotropia, *Am J Ophthalmol* 101:591, 1986.

5. Arroyo S et al: Neuronal generators of visual evoked potentials in humans: visual processing in the human cortex, *Epilepsia* 38:600, 1997.

6. Aso K et al: Developmental changes of pattern reversal visual evoked potentials, *Brain Dev* 10:154, 1988.

7. Auestad N et al: Visual acuity, erythrocyte fatty acid composition, and growth in term infants fed formulas with long chain polyunsaturated fatty acids for one year: Ross Pediatric Lipid Study, *Pediatr Res* 41:1, 1997.

8. Bach M, Meigen T: Similar electrophysiological correlates of texture segregation induced by luminance, orientation, motion and stereo, *Vis Res* 37:1409, 1997.

9. Baitch L, Levi D: Evidence for nonlinear binocular interactions in human visual cortex, *Vis Res* 28:1139, 1988.

10. Banks MS, Bennett PJ: Optical and photoreceptor immaturities limit the spatial and chromatic vision of human neonates, *Opt Soc Am A* 5:2059, 1988.

11. Banks MS, Crowell JA: Front-end limitations to infant spatial vision: examination of two analyses. In Simons K (ed): *Early visual development: normal and abnormal,* New York, 1993, Oxford.

12. Barlow HB: Reconstructing the visual image in space and time, *Nature* 279:189, 1979.

13. Barlow HB, Blakemore C, Pettigrew JD: The neural mechanism of binocular depth discrimination, *J Physiol* 193:327, 1967.

14. Berry RN: Quantitative relations among vernier, real depth, and stereoscopic depth acuities, *J Exper Psychol* 38:708, 1948.

15. Birch EE, Fawcett S, Stager D: Co-development of VEP motion response and binocular vision in normal infants and infantile esotropes, *Invest Ophthalmol Vis Sci* 41:1719, 2000.

16. Birch EE, Gwiazda J, Held R: Stereoacuity development for crossed and uncrossed disparities in human infants, *Vis Res* 22:507, 1982.

17. Birch EE, Gwiazda J, Held R: The development of vergence does not account for the onset of stereopsis, *Perception* 12:331, 1983.

18. Birch EE, Hale LA: Operant assessment of stereoacuity, *Clin Vis Sci* 4:295, 1989.

19. Birch EE, Petrig B: FPL and VEP measures of fusion, stereopsis and stereoacuity in normal infants, *Vis Res* 36:1321, 1996.

20. Birch EE, Salomao S: Infant random dot stereoacuity cards, *J Pediatr Ophthalmol Strab* 35:86, 1998.

21. Birch EE, Shimojo S, Held R: Preferential-looking assessment of fusion and stereopsis in infants 1-6 months, *Invest Ophthalmol Vis Sci* 26:366, 1985.

22. Birch EE et al: Visual acuity and the essentiality of docosahexaenoic acid and arachidonic acid in the diet of term infants, *Pediatr Res* 44:201, 1998.

23. Bowman RJC et al: An inner city preschool visual screening programme: long term visual results, *Br J Ophthalmol* 82:543, 1998.

24. Braddick OJ, Wattam-Bell J, Atkinson J: Orientation-specific cortical responses develop in early infancy, *Nature* 320:617, 1986.

25. Braddick OJ et al: Cortical binocularity in infants, *Nature* 288:363, 1980.

26. Brown AB et al: Infant luminance and chromatic contrast sensitivity: optokinetic nystagmus data on 3-month-olds, *Vis Res* 35:3145, 1995.

27. Brown AM: Vernier acuity in human infants: rapid emergence shown in a longitudinal study, *Optom Vis Sci* 74:732, 1997.

28. Brown B, Lovie-Kitchin J: Repeated visual acuity measures: establishing the patient's own criterion for change, *Optom Vis Sci* 70:45, 1993.

29. Brown RJ, Candy TR, Norcia AM: Development of rivalry and dichoptic masking in human infants, *Invest Ophthalmol Vis Sci* 40:3324, 1999.

30. Brown RJ, Norcia AM: A method for investigating binocular rivalry in real-time with the steady-state VEP, *Vis Res* 37:2401, 1997.

31. Carkeet A, Levi DM, Manny RE: Development of vernier acuity in childhood, *Optom Vis Sci* 74:741, 1997.

32. Ciner EB, Schanel-Klitsch E, Herzberg C: Stereoacuity development: 6 months to 5 years: a new tool for testing and screening, *Optom Vis Sci* 73:43, 1996.

33. Ciner EB, Schanel-Klitsch E, Scheiman M: Stereoacuity development in young children, *Optom Vis Sci* 68:533, 1991.

34. Cobb WA, Morton HB, Ettlinger G: Cerebral potentials evoked by pattern reversal and their suppression in visual rivalry, *Nature* 216:1123, 1967.

35. Crognale MA et al: Development of the spatio-chromatic visual evoked potential: a longitudinal study, *Vis Res* 38:3283, 1998.

36. Daw NW: Development of visual capabilities. In *Visual development,* New York, 1995, Plenum Press.

37. DeVries-Khoe LH, Spekreijse H: Maturation of luminance and pattern EPs in man, *Doc Ophthalmol Proc Ser* 31:461, 1982.

38. Dobkins KR, Teller D: Infant motion: detection (M:D) ratios for chromatically defined and luminance-defined moving stimuli, *Vis Res* 36:3293, 1996.

39. Dobson V: The behavioral assessment of visual acuity in human infants. In Berkeley MA, Stebbins WC (eds): *Comparative perception,* Pittsburgh, 1990, Wiley.

40. Dubowitz LM et al: Visual function in the preterm and fullterm newborn infant, *Dev Med Child Neurol* 22:465, 1980.

41. Ducati A, Fava E, Motti ED: Neuronal generators of the visual evoked potentials: intracerebral recording in awake humans, *Electroencephalogr Clin Neurophysiol* 71:89, 1988.

42. Eizenman M et al: Electrophysiological evidence of cortical fusion in children with early-onset esotropia, *Invest Ophthalmol Vis Sci* 40:354, 1999.

43. Ellemberg D et al: Development of spatial and temporal vision during childhood, *Vis Res* 39:2325, 1999.

44. Elliott DB, Yang KCH, Whitaker D: Visual acuity changes through adulthood in normal healthy eyes: seeing beyond 6/6, *Optom Vis Sci* 72:186, 1995.

45. Fantz RL: A method for studying early visual development, *Percept Motor Skills* 6:13, 1956.

46. Fantz RL: Pattern vision in young infants, *Psychol Rec* 8:43, 1958.

47. Fiorentini A, Trimarchi C: Development of temporal properties of pattern electroretinogram and visual evoked potentials in infants, *Vis Res* 32:1609, 1992.

48. Fox R: Stereopsis in animals and human infants: a review of behavioral investigations. In Aslin RN, Alberts JR, Peterson MR (eds): *Development of perception,* vol 2, *The visual system,* New York, 1981, Academic Press.

49. Fox R, Patterson R, Francis EL: Stereoacuity in young children, *Invest Ophthalmol Vis Sci* 7:598, 1986.

50. France FD, Ver Hoeve JN: VECP Evidence for binocular function in infantile esotropia, *J Ped Ophthalmol Strab* 31:225, 1994.

51. Frisén L, Frisén M: How good is normal visual acuity? A study of letter acuity thresholds as a function of age, *Albrecht von Graefes Arch klin Ophthalmol* 215:149, 1981.

52. Gonzalez EG et al: Vernier acuity in monocular and binocular children, *Clin Vis Sci* 7:257, 1992.

53. Gros BL, Blake R, Hiris E: Anisotropies in visual motion perception: a fresh look, *J Opt Soc Am A* 15:2003, 1998.

54. Gwiazda J, Bauer J, Held R: Binocular function in human infants: correlation of stereoptic and fusion-rivalry discriminations, *J Ped Ophthalmol Strab* 26:128, 1989.

55. Hainline L: Conjugate eye movements of infants. In Simons K (ed): *Early visual development, normal and abnormal,* New York, 1993, Oxford University Press.

56. Hainline L: The development of basic visual abilities. In Vital-Durand F, Atkinson J, Braddick O (eds): *Infant vision,* New York, 1996, Oxford University Press.

57. Hainline L, Abramov I: Eye movement based measures of development of contrast sensitivity in infants, *Optom Vis Sci* 74:790, 1997.

58. Hamer R, Mayer L: The development of spatial vision. In Albert DM, Jakobiec FA (eds): *Principles and practice of ophthalmology: basic sciences,* Philadelphia, 1994, WB Saunders.

59. Heron G et al: Stereoscopic threshold in children and adults, *Am J Optom Physiol Opt* 62:505, 1985.

60. Hofstetter HW: Absolute threshold measurements with the diastereo test, *Arch Soc Am Ophthalmol Optom* 6:327, 1968.

61. Hofstetter HW, Bertsch JD: Does stereopsis change with age? *Am J Optom Physiol Opt* 53:664, 1976.

62. Hubel DH, Wiesel TN: Receptive fields, binocular interaction and functional architecture in the cat's visual cortex, *J Physiol* 160:106, 1962.

63. Jampolsky A, Norcia AM, Hamer RD: Preoperative alternate occlusion decreases motion processing abnormalities in infantile esotropia, *J Pediatr Ophthalmol Strab* 31:6, 1994.

64. Julez B: Binocular depth perception of computer-generated patterns, *Bell Syst Tech J* 39:1125, 1960.

65. Julesz B: Binocular depth perception without familiarity cues, *Science* 145:356, 1964.

66. Kelly JP, Borchert K, Teller DY: The development of chromatic and achromatic contrast sensitivity in infancy as tested with the sweep VEP, *Vis Res* 37:2075, 1997.

67. Kim E et al: Performance on the three-point vernier alignment or acuity test as a function of age: measurement extended to ages 5 to 9 years, *Optom Vision Sci* 77:492, 2000.

68. Kos-Pietro S et al: Maturation of human visual evoked potentials: 27 weeks conceptional age to 2 years, *Neuropediatrics* 28:318, 1997.

69. Lakshminarayanan V, Aziz S, Enoch JM: Variation of the hyperacuity gap function with age, *Optom Vision Sci* 69:423, 1992.

70. Lansing RW: Electroencephalographic correlates of binocular rivalry in man, *Science* 146:1325, 1964.

71. Leigh RJ, Zee, DS: *The neurology of eye movements,* ed 2, *Contemporary neurology series,* Philadelphia, 1991, FA Davis.

72. Lewis TL et al: The development of symmetrical OKN in infants: quantification based on OKN acuity for nasalward versus temporalward motion, *Vis Res* 40:445, 2000.

73. Li RWH, Edwards MH, Brown R: Variation in vernier acuity with age, *Vis Res* 40:3665, 2000.

74. Livingstone MS: Differences between stereopsis and interocular correlation and binocularity, *Vis Res* 36:1127, 1996.

75. Manny RE: Orientation selectivity of 3-month-old infants, *Vis Res* 32:1817, 1992.

76. Manny RE, Klein SA: The development of vernier acuity in infants, *Curr Eye Res* 3:453, 1984.

77. Manny RE, Klein SA: A three alternative tracking paradigm to measure vernier acuity of older infants, *Vis Res* 25:1245, 1985.

78. Marg E et al: Visual acuity development in infants: evoked potential measurements, *Invest Ophthalmol* 15:150, 1976.

79. McCulloch DL, Skarf B: Development of the human visual system: monocular and binocular pattern VEP latency, *Invest Ophthalmol Vis Sci* 32:2372, 1991.

80. Miles FA: Short-latency visual stabilization mechanisms that help to compensate for translational disturbances of gaze, *Ann NY Acad Sci* 871:260, 1999.

81. Morgan JM: Hyperacuity. In Regan D (ed): *Spatial vision,* vol 10: *Vision and visual dysfunction,* Boca Raton, Fla, 1991, CRC Press.

82. Morrone MC, Fiorentini A, Burr DC: Development of the temporal properties of visual evoked potentials to luminance and colour contrast in infants, *Vis Res* 36:3141, 1996.

83. Moskowitz A, Sokol S: Developmental changes in the human visual system as reflected by the latency of the pattern reversal VEP, *Electroencephalogr Clin Neurophysiol* 56:1, 1983.

84. Naegele JR, Held R: The postnatal development of monocular optokinetic nystagmus in infants, *Vis Res* 22:341, 1982.

85. Noachtar S, Hashimoto T, Luders H: Pattern visual evoked potentials recorded from human occipital cortex with chronic subdural electrodes, *Electroencephalogr Clin Neurophysiol* 88:435, 1993.

86. Norcia AM, Harrad RA, Brown RJ: Changes in cortical activity during suppression in stereoblindness, *Neuro Report* 11:1007, 2000.

87. Norcia AM, Tyler CW: Spatial frequency sweep VEP: visual acuity during the first year of life, *Vis Res* 25:1399, 1985.

88. Norcia AM, Tyler CW, Hamer RD: Development of contrast sensitivity in the human infant, *Vis Res* 30:1475, 1990.

89. Norcia AM, Wesemann W, Manny RE: Electrophysiological correlates of vernier and relative motion mechanisms in human visual cortex, *Vis Neurosci* 16:1123, 1999.

90. Norcia AM et al: Anomalous motion VEPs in infants and in infantile esotropia, *Invest Ophthalmol Vis Sci* 32:436, 1991.

91. Norcia AM et al: Plasticity of human motion processing mechanisms following surgery for infantile esotropia, *Vis Res* 35:3279, 1995.

92. Odom JV et al: Adult vernier thresholds do not increase with age; vernier bias does, *Invest Ophthalmol Vis Sci* 30:1004, 1989.

93. Orel-Bixler DA, Norcia AM: Differential growth of acuity for steady-state pattern reversal and transient pattern VEPs, *Clin Vis Sci* 2:1, 1987.

94. Owsley C, Sekuler R, Siemsen D: Contrast Sensitivity throughout adulthood, *Vis Res* 23:689, 1983.

95. Petrig B et al: Development of stereopsis and cortical binocularity in human infants: electrophysiological evidence, *Science* 213:1402, 1981.

96. Poggio GF, Gonzalez F, Krause F: Stereoscopic mechanisms in monkey visual cortex: Binocular correlation and disparity selectivity, *J Neurosci* 8:4531, 1988.

97. Porciatti V: Temporal and spatial properties of the pattern-reversal VEPs in infants below 2 months of age, *Hum Neurobiol* 3:97, 1984.

98. Rasengane TA, Allen D, Manny RE: Development of temporal contrast sensitivity in human infants, *Vis Res* 37:1747, 1997.

99. Reading RW, Tanlamai T: Finely graded binocular disparities from random-dot stereograms, *Ophthalmic Physiol Opt* 2:47, 1982.

100. Regan D: Speedy assessment of visual acuity in amblyopia by the evoked potential method, *Ophthalmologica* 175:159, 1977.

101. Regan D: *Human brain electrophysiology: evoked potentials and evoked magnetic fields in science and medicine,* New York, 1989, Elsevier.

102. Reich L, Lakshiminarayanan V, Enoch JM: Analysis of the method of adjustment for testing potential acuity with the hyperacuity gap test: a preliminary report, *Clin Vis Sci* 6:451, 1991.

103. Roy N, Lachapelle P, Lepore F: Maturation of the optokinetic nystagmus as a function of the speed of stimulation in fullterm and preterm infants, *Clin Vis Sci* 4:357, 1989.

104. Schiller PH, Finlay BL, Volman SF: Quantitative studies of single-cell properties in monkey striate cortex. II: Orientation specificity and ocular dominance, *J Neurophysiol* 39:1320, 1976.

105. Shannon E, Skoczenski AM, Banks MS: Retinal illuminance and contrast sensitivity in human infants, *Vis Res* 36:67, 1996.

106. Shea SL et al: Assessment of stereopsis in human infants, *Invest Ophthalmol Vis Sci* 19:1400, 1980.

107. Shimojo S, Held R: Vernier acuity is less than grating acuity in 2- and 3-month-olds, *Vis Res* 27:77, 1987.

108. Shimojo S et al: Development of vernier acuity in infants, *Vis Res* 24:721, 1984.

109. Shupert C, Fuchs AF: Development of conjugate human eye movements, *Vis Res* 28:585, 1988.

110. Simons K: Stereoacuity norms in young children, *Arch Ophthalmol* 99:439, 1981.

111. Skarf B et al: A new VEP system for studying binocular single vision in human infants, *J Pediatr Ophthalmol Strab* 30:237, 1993.

112. Skoczenski AM, Aslin RN: Spatiotemporal factors in infant position sensitivity: single bar stimuli, *Vis Res* 32:1761, 1992.

113. Skoczenski AM, Norcia AM: Neural noise limitations on infant visual sensitivity, *Nature* 391:697, 1998.

114. Skoczenski AM, Norcia AM: Development of VEP vernier acuity and grating acuity in human infants, *Invest Ophthalmol Vis Sci* 40:2411, 1999.

115. Skoczenski AM, Norcia AM: Late maturation of vernier hyperacuity, *Psychol Sci* (in press).

116. Sloper JJ, Collins AD: Reduction in binocular enhancement of the visual-evoked potential during development accompanies increasing stereoacuity, *J Pediatr Ophthalmol Strab* 35:154, 1998.

117. Sokol S, Jones K: Implicit time of pattern evoked potentials in infants, *Vis Res* 19:747, 1979.

118. Sokol S, Moskowitz A, McCormack G: Infant VEP and preferential looking acuity measured with phase alternating gratings, *Invest Ophthalmol Vis Sci* 33:3156, 1992.

119. Sprague JB et al: Study of chart designs and optotypes for preschool vision screening: I. Comparability of chart designs, *J Ped Ophthalmol Strab* 26:189, 1989.

120. Stanley OH: Cortical development and visual function, *Eye* 5:27, 1991.

121. Teller DY: The forced-choice preferential looking procedure: a psychophysical technique for use with human infants, *Infant Behav Develop* 2:135, 1979.

122. Vilar EY et al: Performance on three-point vernier acuity targets as a function of age, *J Opt Soc Am A* 12:2293, 1995.

123. Walraven J, Janzen P: TNO stereopsis test as an aid to the prevention of amblyopia, *Ophthalmic Physiol Opt* 13:350, 1993.

124. Wattam-Bell J: Development of motion-specific cortical responses in infancy, *Vis Res* 31:287, 1991.

125. Wattam-Bell J: Visual motion processing in one-month-old infants: habituation experiments, *Vis Res* 36:1679, 1996.

126. Wattam-Bell J: Visual motion processing in one-month-old infants: preferential looking experiments, *Vis Res* 36:1671, 1996.

127. Westheimer G: Visual acuity and hyperacuity, *Invest Ophthalmol* 14:570, 1975.

128. Westheimer G: The spatial sense of the eye, *Invest Ophthalmol Visual Sci* 18:893, 1979.

129. Westheimer G: The spatial grain of the perifoveal visual field, *Vis Res* 22:157, 1982.

130. Westheimer G, McKee SP: Spatial configurations for visual hyperacuity, *Vis Res* 17:941, 1977.

131. Whitaker D, Elliott DB, MacVeigh D: Variations in hyperacuity performance with age, *Ophthalmic Physiol Opt* 12:29, 1992.

132. William S, Simpsom A, Silva PA: Stereoacuity levels and vision problems in children from 7-11 years, *Ophthalmic Physiol Opt* 8:386, 1988.

133. Wilson HR: Development of spatiotemporal mechanisms in infant vision, *Vis Res* 28:611, 1988.

134. Wilson HR: Theories of infant visual development. In Simons K (ed): *Early visual development: normal and abnormal,* New York, 1993, Oxford.

135. Wright KW et al: Suppression and the pattern visual evoked potential, *J Pediatr Ophthalmol Strab* 23:252, 1986.

136. Woo GC, Sillanpaa V: Absolute stereoscopic thresholds as measured by crossed and uncrossed disparity, *Am J Optom Physiol Opt* 56:350, 1979.

137. Zanker J et al: The development of vernier acuity in human infants, *Vis Res* 8:1557, 1992.

138. Zemon V et al: Contrast-dependent responses in the human visual system: childhood through adulthood, *Int J Neurosci* 80:181, 1995.

PERIMETRY AND VISUAL FIELD TESTING

CHRIS A. JOHNSON AND PAMELA A. SAMPLE

THE PSYCHOPHYSICAL BASIS FOR PERIMETRY

For more than 150 years, perimetry and visual field testing have been used as diagnostic test procedures in ophthalmology. Although these procedures have their limitations, they have withstood the test of time because of their clinical value for revealing previously unknown vision loss, allowing early detection of eye disease, enhancing differential diagnosis of various ocular and neurologic disorders, and monitoring the progression of various eye diseases. New advances in perimetry and visual field testing have furthered their clinical value as diagnostic test procedures. Today, more eye care specialists routinely use perimetry and visual field testing as a part of their evaluation of patients than at any other time. This chapter provides a brief overview of conventional perimetry and visual field testing, as well as some of the more promising new test procedures that have emerged in recent years. Many excellent resources are available for a more comprehensive discussion of perimetry and visual field testing.*

The Increment Threshold (Weber Fraction)

Conventional perimetry involves the detection of a small white light on a uniform background at various locations throughout the visual field. It is based on the increment or differential light threshold, which is the minimum amount of light that is added to a stimulus (ΔL) to make it distinguishable from the background luminance (L). At very low

---

*References 3, 4, 27, 30, 54, 62, 69, 95, 142.

background luminances, the increment threshold is constant ($\Delta L = C$), whereas at higher background luminances, the increment threshold is proportional to the background luminance ($\Delta L/L = C$). This is known as the *Weber fraction*.[154] Pupil size changes, ocular media transmission losses, and other factors that reduce the amount of light reaching the retina equally affect the stimulus and the background. Thus, under conditions in which the Weber fraction pertains, the increment threshold remains stable.

Most of the conventional visual field tests use a background luminance of 31.5 asb (10 cd/m²), which is within the range in which the Weber fraction is valid. At this background luminance, the fovea has the highest sensitivity and is thereby able to detect the dimmest and smallest targets. Sensitivity decreases rapidly from the fovea out to 3 degrees eccentricity, declines more gradually out to 30 degrees eccentricity, and then decreases rapidly from 30 degrees out to the far periphery. Figure 22-1 presents a three-dimensional representation of differential light sensitivity for the right eye of a typical individual. Because of its shape, this profile has often been referred to as the *hill of vision*.

Factors Affecting Sensitivity to Light

The clinical goal for perimetry and visual field testing is to examine the sensitivity of the visual field as a probe for detecting pathologic changes in the visual pathways, as reflected by localized or widespread reductions in differential light sensitivity. However, there are many nonpathologic factors that can also affect differential light sensitivity, and these must be considered carefully.

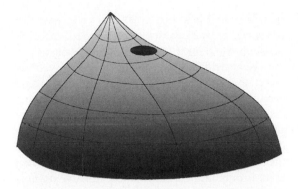

FIGURE 22-1 Three-dimensional representation of the eye's sensitivity to light throughout the visual field.

Testing conditions such as background luminance, stimulus size, stimulus duration, spectral composition of the stimulus, and related factors can all affect differential light sensitivity.* Patient-related characteristics can also affect differential light sensitivity. Physiologic factors such as refractive error, pupil size, ptosis, media opacities, and related properties all affect differential light sensitivity.† In addition, sensitivity can be affected by attentional factors and fatigue[56,65,92] and practice/learning effects.‡ Finally, response errors, fixation instability, and testing artifacts (e.g., lens rim obstruction, misalignment) can influence the sensitivity values obtained through visual field testing.[29,150,166] It is important to account for these influences on differential light sensitivity to properly interpret perimetric test results.

METHODS OF CONDUCTING PERIMETRY

There are numerous methods for conducting visual field tests, the first of which was developed more than 150 years ago. Although each procedure has distinct advantages and disadvantages, no single technique has been developed that provides a comprehensive visual field evaluation for all patients. This section provides a brief overview of the test procedures currently used for visual field testing. A comprehensive description of these procedures is beyond the scope of this chapter. The interested reader can find detailed information pertaining to these procedures in several excellent sources.§

---

*References 5, 39, 47, 70, 71, 84, 117, 142.
†References 7, 19, 31, 45, 96, 107, 109, 116, 149, 163.
‡References 32, 46, 56, 65, 92, 159.
§References 3, 4, 27, 30, 54, 62, 69, 95, 142.

Suprathreshold Screening Procedures

Suprathreshold static perimetric test procedures have been designed to provide a rapid screening of the visual field to determine whether the visual field is within normal limits or whether there are visual field regions with abnormally low sensitivity. Some of the more sophisticated suprathreshold static procedures present multiple stimulus luminances in areas with reduced sensitivity to estimate the severity of the abnormality. However, the time required to perform these more elaborate screening procedures can approach the duration of threshold techniques.

All suprathreshold screening tests present stimuli that are greater than threshold and are thereby readily visible to individuals with normal peripheral vision. The simplest form of suprathreshold testing is the confrontation field, in which the examiner uses various objects (e.g., fingers, medicine bottle caps, pencils) to determine whether they can be seen throughout different regions of the peripheral visual field. This is a quick and convenient procedure capable of detecting areas of significant visual field loss. However, it is not well suited for detecting mild sensitivity loss, it is nonquantitative, and it does not have well-defined standards or norms.

A large number of different screening strategies are available on automated perimeters. The most basic screening procedure uses a single stimulus luminance to evaluate various visual field locations. This procedure can rapidly identify areas of sensitivity loss. However, one of the problems with this approach is that visual field sensitivity varies as a function of visual field location; thus the visibility of a single stimulus luminance is different for various eccentricities and may be subthreshold for far peripheral locations. Other screening procedures adjust the stimulus luminance to conform to the slope of the normal hill of vision, but with the stimulus luminance set to a fixed amount above this level. One method of doing this uses age-adjusted normal population values to establish the suprathreshold stimulus values.[54] Another procedure uses threshold estimates from several visual field locations to estimate the position of the hill of vision to establish suprathreshold stimulus values.[27] Each of these approaches has its own particular advantages and disadvantages. The more elaborate screening procedures obtain additional information for abnormal locations, either by testing with multiple suprathreshold stimulus luminances or by obtaining threshold estimates for these regions. Specific details of these various screening procedures are available in a number of other references. [3,27,30,54]

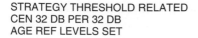

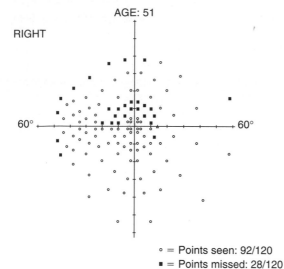

o = Points seen: 92/120
■ = Points missed: 28/120
▲ = Blind spot

Figure 22-2   An example of the two-zone, threshold-related 120-point visual field screening test on the Humphrey Field Analyzer. Results from the right eye of a glaucoma patient with a superior arcuate defect are shown.

Figure 22-2 presents an example of a 120-point two-zone visual field screening test on the Humphrey Field Analyzer (Humphrey Systems, Dublin, California); open circles indicate areas with normal sensitivity, and filled squares represent locations with sensitivity loss.

Threshold Estimation Procedures

Currently, there are three perimetric techniques for determining differential light thresholds: kinetic perimetry, static perimetry using staircase strategies, and maximum likelihood techniques such as Swedish Interactive Threshold Algorithm (SITA). A brief description of each is presented in the following sections.

Kinetic Perimetry. Because of the increasing popularity of automated perimetry, manual kinetic perimetry is becoming less common. However, in some instances, manual kinetic perimetry has advantages over static perimetry. Manual kinetic perimetry is more flexible and interactive than automated static perimetry; therefore it is more suitable for patients who are not able to comply with the more demanding automated test procedures. Manual kinetic perimetry also evaluates the full pe-

ripheral visual field out to 90 degrees eccentricity, whereas most static perimetric test procedures evaluate only the central 24 or 30 degrees. Evaluation of the visual field beyond 30 degrees can sometimes detect abnormalities that would not otherwise have been found or can assist in the interpretation and diagnosis of visual field information. The main disadvantages of manual kinetic perimetry are that the quality of the test results are highly dependent on the skills and knowledge of the perimetrist and that there is only limited information available on normal population characteristics.[3]

Anderson's book[3] provides an excellent description of proper techniques for conducting manual kinetic perimetry. The basic procedure consists of moving a target of a specific size and luminance to map out the boundaries of seeing (isopters) and nonseeing (scotomas). With the patient fixating a central target, the stimulus is moved from the far periphery toward the point of fixation until the patient presses a button to indicate that he or she can detect the stimulus. This is repeated for different meridians around the visual field until a complete contour line (isopter) is generated. Repeating this procedure using different stimulus luminances and sizes allows a series of isopters to be generated, which produces a two-dimensional representation of the hill of vision. Spot checks between isopters are conducted to look for scotomas (localized areas of reduced sensitivity), and if found, they are mapped out. In the normal eye, isopters are egg-shaped because the temporal visual field extends farther than the nasal visual field and the inferior visual field extends farther than the superior visual field. Figure 22-3 presents the results of manual kinetic perimetry for a typical right eye. The scotoma to the right of fixation (filled-in area) represents the location of the blind spot.

Standard Automated Perimetry. With the advent of automated testing, static perimetry using staircase procedures has become the most popular method of visual field testing. The initial threshold estimation procedure implemented for automated perimetry consists of a staircase or bracketing strategy. If the initial target is seen, stimulus luminance is reduced in discrete steps for subsequent presentations until the target is no longer seen. Stimulus luminance is then increased by smaller steps for further presentations until the stimulus is once again seen. If the initial target is not seen, stimulus luminance is increased in discrete steps until it is seen;

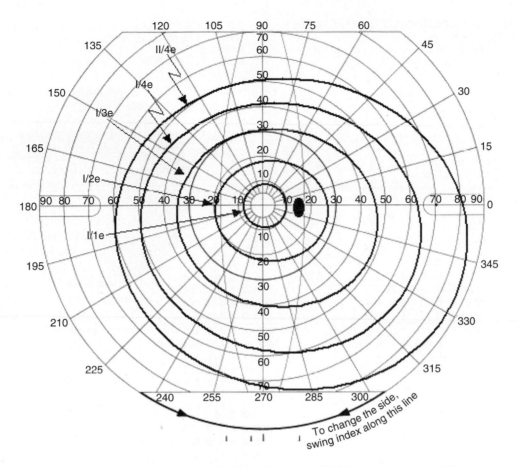

FIGURE 22-3 Representation of a normal visual field for kinetic visual field testing using the Goldmann perimeter.

the stimulus luminance is then reduced in smaller intervals until the target is once again not seen.

Automated static perimetry has a number of advantages: The test strategies are standardized, and the same procedure is therefore conducted from one time to another and from one clinic to another. In addition, a normative database and analysis package make it possible to immediately compare the patient's results against age-corrected normal values and make quantitative, statistical determinations as to whether they are within normal limits. This is done for more global visual field characteristics, as well as on a point-by-point basis. Automated perimetry results can be stored on a disk and retrieved later for comparison with results obtained at different times. Finally, automated static perimetry monitors fixation behavior and response reliability of the patient during the test procedure.

The disadvantage of automated static perimetry is that it is a time-consuming, demanding test procedure. As a consequence, some patients are sus-

ceptible to learning effects, fatigue, attention lapses, and response errors, all of which lead to unreliable test results. These problems can be minimized by instructing the patient properly; administering an initial demonstration of the test procedure; providing appropriate rest breaks; and carefully monitoring the patient for fatigue, drowsiness, misalignment, and related factors.

Most automated static perimetry tests present stimuli at fixed locations that correspond to a grid pattern (bracketing the horizontal and vertical meridians) over the central visual field. Stimuli are presented in a pseudorandom fashion to discourage anticipatory eye movements. The stability of fixation is also monitored using direct visualization of the patient's eye, intermittent stimuli presented to the blind spot, or an eye movement monitor that tracks reflections from the eye. The most common full-threshold static perimetric procedures take about 12 to 20 minutes per eye to perform. Figure 22-4 presents the results of a full-threshold visual

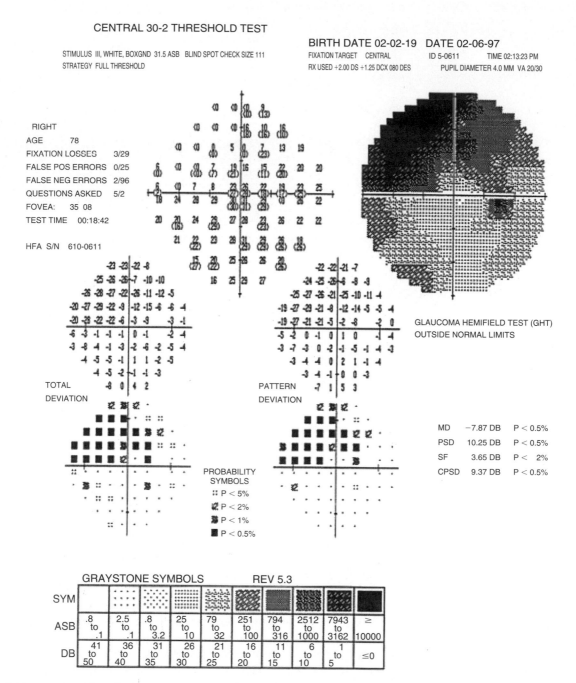

FIGURE 22-4   The full-threshold 30-2 test results (Humphrey Field Analyzer) for the right eye of a glaucoma patient with a superior arcuate scotoma.

field examination performed on the Humphrey Field Analyzer for the right eye of a patient with glaucomatous visual field loss.

Swedish Interactive Threshold Algorithm. The advent of the new threshold algorithm for visual fields, SITA, has lead to an increased interest in stan-

dard visual fields despite evidence that visual function specific subtests are much more sensitive for detection and, in the case of short-wavelength automated perimetry (SWAP), for following progression.[11,12] This new enthusiasm for standard fields is based on two attributes of SITA. The test time for a visual field is reduced by half, and the test-retest variability may also be reduced, which should make the results more reliable for measuring change over time.[8,11,49,161,162] Because SITA is a new threshold procedure that uses information collected during the test to better determine the luminance of the next stimulus at a given location, it easily could be applied to other forms of perimetry, such as SWAP.

A number of factors contribute to the reduction in test time and the success of SITA: (1) detailed visual field modeling, (2) a model that terminates testing at a given field location when a preselected level of certainty is reached, (3) adaptation of the test to more accurately reflect the patient's reaction time, (4) posttest recomputation of the threshold values, and (5) reduction of "catch trials."[4,115]

Studies comparing SITA with the original full-threshold algorithm indicate that SITA shows approximately 1 dB better thresholds than standard full-threshold testing, but with a statistically greater defect on the pattern and total deviation plots in glaucoma patients.[4,9,137,162] The smaller intersubject variance and greater reproducibility in patient eyes may mean shallower defects are needed in SITA fields to detect statistically significant abnormality than are needed for the standard full-threshold algorithm, but this has not been tested.[9,10,50] Finally, when switching from standard full-threshold to the SITA strategy to follow patients, it is desirable to obtain new baseline fields and to make comparisons between the two types of algorithms based on the total and pattern deviation probability plots rather than on absolute threshold values.[50] An example of visual field results obtained with the standard staircase procedures (*left panel*) and SITA (*right panel*) are presented in Figure 22-5. Note that although the results are similar, there is a large difference in testing time.

INTERPRETATION OF VISUAL FIELD INFORMATION

Visual field information is used for several clinical purposes: (1) early detection of ocular and neurologic disorders by looking for sensitivity losses throughout the visual field; (2) differential diagnosis of specific ocular and neurologic diseases by evaluating the pattern and location of visual field deficits; and (3) monitoring of the status of the visual field over time to determine whether a condition is improving, progressing, or remaining stable. It is therefore important to interpret the visual field information properly. A large number of patterns and locations of visual field loss associated with various ocular and neurologic disorders are useful for differential diagnosis. A thorough discussion of the different patterns of visual field loss is beyond the scope of this chapter, but several excellent resources are available for the reader interested in obtaining this information.* The following sections concentrate on single and multiple visual field interpretation. Because of its widespread use, our comments are specifically directed to threshold results obtained using a Humphrey Field Analyzer.

Single Visual Field Analysis

All aspects of the visual field output are important. It is not advisable to concentrate on a single portion of the data output or to exclude some portions of the output. There are four or five sections of information, depending on whether the results were obtained with the older HFA I or the currently available HFA II. Figure 22-6 presents representative results for the right eye of a patient with glaucoma who was evaluated with a full-threshold test procedure and a 24-2 stimulus presentation pattern on an HFA II.

Demographic Data, Test Information, and Reliability Indices. Figure 22-6 contains information pertaining to the patient, the test conditions used, and the reliability indices. This information should be examined routinely. It is important to determine whether proper test conditions were maintained, whether appropriate stimulus sizes were used, and whether other test parameters were appropriate. It is also important to determine whether the patient's birth date is correct because results are compared against age-matched normal values; an incorrect birth date can result in spurious analyses. Examination of the refractive correction used, pupil size, and visual acuity should also be performed. Small pupils and inappropriate refractive corrections can significantly influence test results. Examination of the foveal threshold in relation to the patient's visual acuity can also be helpful in the interpretation of test results.

Reliability indices consist of false-positive errors, false-negative errors, and fixation losses. False-positive errors denote the percentage of times that the patient pressed the response button when no stimulus was presented. It can be a useful indicator of an unreliable patient who is "trigger happy" or uncooperative. False-negative errors represent the percentage of times a patient failed to respond to a

---

*References 3, 4, 27, 62, 69, 142.

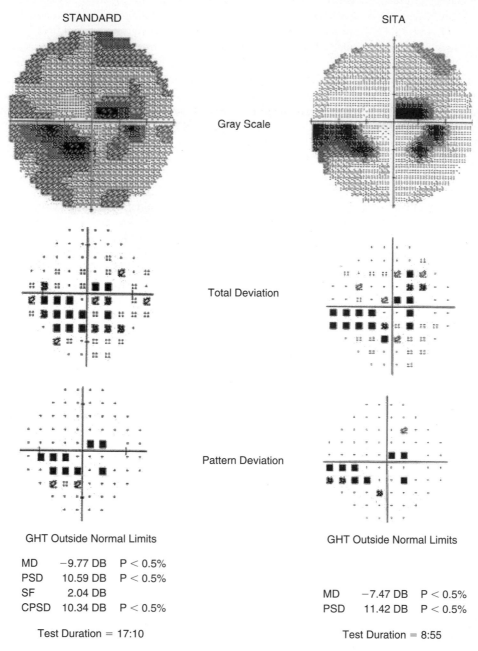

FIGURE 22-5 A comparison of visual field results obtained with standard automated perimetry and Swedish Interactive Threshold Algorithm (SITA) using the Humphrey Field Analyzer. Results from the right eye of a glaucoma patient with superior and inferior visual field loss are shown. Note that the test results are similar, especially for the probability plots, but the test duration for SITA is nearly half as long as for the standard (full-threshold) test. *GHT,* Glaucoma hemifield test.

stimulus that is substantially brighter than a previously determined threshold value at that location. Many false-negative errors can be an indicator of inattention, fatigue, or malingering. However, patients with significant visual field loss demonstrate

high variability in damaged visual field areas and can therefore generate many false-negative errors. Fixation losses are determined by presenting a stimulus in the location of the blind spot and determining whether the patient responds to the blind spot

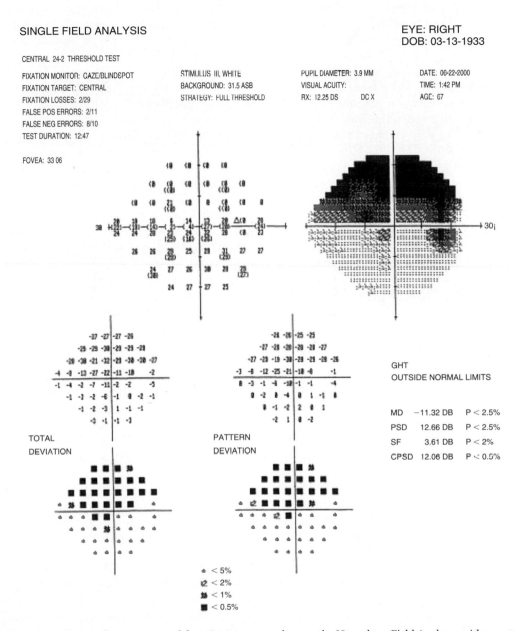

FIGURE 22-6   Test results are presented for a 24-2 test procedure on the Humphrey Field Analyzer with gaze tracking enabled. Note on the gaze tracking that there is an increasing number of downward deflections as the test progresses, indicating that the upper lid was obstructing the pupillary light reflex with greater frequency as the patient became drowsier.

stimulus. Although high fixation losses can indicate poor fixation, they can also result from mislocalizing the blind spot. To avoid this problem, one should carefully monitor the patient during the first minute or two of the test; if the patient exhibits high fixation losses, it is best to pause the test and replot the blind spot. For all of the reliability indices, comparisons are made to typical population characteristics. If greater than 33% false-positive errors, greater than 33% false-negative errors, or greater than 20%

fixation losses are present, a "Low Patient Reliability" warning is printed. It should be noted that the new SITA strategy does not perform blind-spot trials and false-positive and false-negative errors are calculated using a different algorithm.

Numeric, Gray Scale, and Deviation Values. Below the demographic, test procedure, and reliability information, there is a printout of the numeric sensitivity values (in dB) for each visual field location and a gray scale graphical representation of visual field sensitivity. The gray scale representation provides a topographic indication of the hill of vision, with lighter areas depicting areas of higher sensitivity and darker areas depicting areas of lower sensitivity. Thus the gray scale representation provides a good "Gestalt" of the overall sensitivity characteristics and patterns of sensitivity loss for the visual field; however, it is not as accurate as the total or pattern deviation plots. The gray scale interpolates values for areas between actually measured test points.

Visual Field Indices. Located below the gray scale, the visual field indices are summary statistics to describe the general characteristics of the visual field. Each of the indices are compared with age-matched normative values; values that are worse than the normal 5%, 2%, 1%, and 0.5% probability levels are indicated on the output. The mean deviation (MD) is calculated by determining the average deviation from average normal values for each point in the visual field. Positive values for MD indicate that the patient's overall visual field sensitivity is above that of the average normal, whereas negative values indicate that the patient's overall visual field sensitivity is lower than normal.

The pattern standard deviation (PSD) is a measure of the irregularity of the slope of the visual field. The PSD index first adjusts the patient's visual field by MD to account for any diffuse loss. It then determines the degree of departure of each location from the smooth slope of the average normal visual field. If there is no irregularity, PSD is zero. The greater the amount of irregularity or perterbation in the visual field slope, the higher the PSD value. PSD is intended to be a general indicator of the degree of localized visual field loss because the borders of scotomas produce steep departures from the normal slope.

Short-term fluctuation (SF) is intended to be an indication of the amount of variability exhibited by the patient during the test procedure. Double threshold determinations are performed at 10 predetermined visual field locations, and the average variation in repeated measures then constitutes the SF value. The corrected pattern standard deviation (CPSD) is the PSD value that has been corrected for the patient's SF during the test. It should be noted that the new SITA test procedure provides only the MD and PSD indices. Double determinations are not performed with SITA, and the SF and CPSD indices are therefore not calculated.

The final visual field index is the glaucoma hemifield test (GHT), which was particularly designed to detect early glaucomatous visual field loss. The GHT groups individual visual field locations into clusters that are based on nerve fiber bundle patterns. As shown in Figure 22-7, the GHT has five mirror-image clusters for the superior and inferior hemifields. For each pair of mirror-image clusters, the asymmetry in sensitivity across the horizontal midline is determined and compared with normal population characteristics. Depending on the outcome of this analysis, one of four messages is generated. "Outside Normal Limits" is printed if one or more of the hemifield cluster asymmetries is worse than the normal 1% probability level. If all hemifield cluster asymmetries are equal to or better than the 1% probability level but one or more is worse than the 3% probability level, "Borderline" is printed. Otherwise, the message "Within Normal Limits" is printed, unless the overall visual field sensitivity is considerably higher than the average normal sensitivity, in which case "Abnormally High Sensitivity" is printed. "Outside Normal Limits" also occurs if the individual zone scores in both members of any zone pair exceed that found in 99.5% of normal individuals.

Total and Pattern Deviation Probability Plots. The total and pattern deviation probability plots provide some of the most useful visual field information. The total deviation values are derived by comparing the patient's sensitivity at each location to the average sensitivity of a normal individual of the same age. Positive values indicate that the patient's sensitivity is higher than the average normal, whereas negative values indicate that the patient's sensitivity is lower than the average normal. The probability plot presents a single dot for locations that have sensitivities equal to or better than the lower 5% of age-corrected normal values. Squares with progressively denser stippling are used to indicate locations that are worse than the normal 5% (light stippling), 2% (medium stippling), 1% (heavy

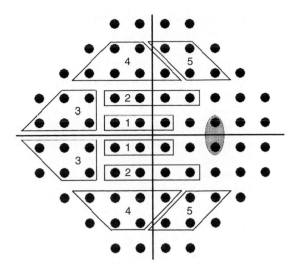

FIGURE 22-7 The clusters of visual field locations used to evaluate superior and inferior hemifield asymmetry as part of the glaucoma hemifield test. The clusters were selected to generally correspond to the pattern of nerve fiber bundles entering the optic nerve head.

stippling), and 0.5% (solid black) probability levels, respectively. This provides a direct indication of the locations that have abnormally low sensitivity and an indication of its severity.

The pattern deviation probability plot is similar to the total deviation plot, except that the overall height of the visual field is adjusted to "correct" for diffuse visual field loss. The visual field sensitivity corresponding to the 85th percentile (seventh highest sensitivity) is determined and compared with average normal values. The entire visual field is then either adjusted up or down to compensate for this difference. Probability values are then derived and probability levels assessed. The pattern deviation probability plot thus provides an indication of localized visual field loss.

Comparing the total and pattern deviation probability plots allows the amount of diffuse and localized visual field loss to be determined. Completely diffuse loss produces abnormal sensitivity symbols on the total deviation plot, but they are not present on the pattern deviation plot. For completely localized loss the symbols on the total and pattern deviation plots are essentially identical. Examining the degrees of similarity between the total and pattern deviation probability plots makes it possible to gain an appreciation of how much of the visual field loss is diffuse and how much is localized. For small shallow defects, it is sometimes possible for the total de-

viation plot to be normal and the pattern deviation plot to show a small number of locations that are abnormal. However, if the total deviation plot is normal and there are a large number of abnormal points on the pattern deviation plot, this is usually indicative of a trigger happy patient who has generated numerous false-positive responses (pressing the button when no target should have been detected), thereby producing artificial, unphysiologically high sensitivity values.

Gaze Tracking. On the new HFA II models, the output of the eye movement monitor (gaze tracker) is presented at the bottom of the visual field output. This is intended to present a timeline of fixation behavior during the test. A horizontal or nearly horizontal line indicates that the patient maintained good fixation and alignment throughout the test procedure. Upward deflections represent eye movements or misalignment of the eye, whereas downward deflections denote blinks or droopy lids. This information can be useful. Because fixation lapses occur more frequently with fatigue, this can be detected by a change from a horizontal line early in the test to more frequent upward deflections toward the end of the test. Continual upward deflections are often an indicator that the patient's eye or head position has shifted during the test. Continual downward deflects are an indicator of a droopy lid and drowsiness. A "noisy" tracking (erratic deflections) suggests that the patient has been unreliable or uncooperative during the test. Again, it is important that the gaze tracking be properly initialized at the start of the test. Mistakes in this procedure are the most common source of gaze monitor malfunction.

Assessing Multiple Visual Fields to Determine Progression

Following the course of vision loss continues to be a major problem as more is learned about current testing techniques and the nature of the disease. There is no agreed-upon standard for identifying progression in glaucomatous visual fields. Visual fields may appear worse on one visit, but they may improve on subsequent visits. For example, the National Eye Institute–sponsored Advanced Glaucoma Intervention Study reports that more than 30% of the fields originally classified as progressed on two follow-up visits later failed to maintain this classification.[58] Similarly, more than 85% of initial glaucomatous visual field deficits in the Ocular Hypertension Treatment Study were not confirmed on retest.[83]

Sample et al.[131] also found that progressed fields recovered in 33% of eyes for standard fields and 29% for SWAP. Demirel and Johnson[28] found that normal fields converting to abnormal were stable in only 45% to 56% of standard fields but were more stable using SWAP (69% to 80%).

Separating true progression from fluctuations in field results because of learning effects, fatigue, and the long-term fluctuation inherent in the test is extremely difficult.[38,160] Each visual field is influenced by a variety of factors, including patient performance, fixation losses, pupil size, refractive correction, and changes in degree of lens opacity. These factors combine with underlying physiologic changes in visual sensitivity to produce significant long-term fluctuation, even in healthy eyes.[14,38,51,81,160] In addition, the rate of progression in visual fields is slow in treated glaucoma eyes, and it is also influenced by age and initial severity of visual field loss. Changes less than 1 dB per year are difficult to detect, even over a series of fields covering 6 years.[114,141]

So, what is *visual field progression* and how is it measured? Most would agree on a general definition that visual field progression is a worsening in sensitivity that is repeatable and consistent with true glaucomatous progression, either a change from a normal field to an abnormal field or progression of an existing defect. It is more difficult to decide what is meant by *worsening of sensitivity* and what is *repeatable*.

Approaches for Identifying Progression

Two general approaches have been used to judge visual field progression: One is to analyze a series of visual fields, and the other is to compare a single field against a baseline.

Series analyses include the various follow-up displays provided with automated perimeters and assorted forms of linear regression. Linear regression techniques require a minimum of five and preferably seven or more visual fields to determine if progression is present.[81,106,114,141] Smith, Katz, and Quigley[139] concluded that progression rates between 1 and 5 dB per year could be detected with a minimum of 5 years of data. These methods have also shown that the noise (variability) is greater for certain visual field locations and that change in noisy locations must be of a greater magnitude than a change in a more stable location to be called *true progression*.[48,52] The commercially available PROGRESSOR program uses pointwise linear regression analysis for each location in the visual field from several visual fields against time of follow-up for all of the individual patient's available visual

field data.[37] This technique is also most useful with a series of seven visual fields.

Clinical Trials and Progression. Because it is often necessary in clinical trials to determine whether progression is occurring before a series of five to seven fields can be obtained, linear regression has not been the method of choice. Instead different methods have been adopted by each of several clinical trials. The reader may see published reports from each study for more detail on the methods described later.

Normal Tension Glaucoma Study. The Normal Tension Glaucoma Study was developed to assess the effect of lowering intraocular pressure on the progression rate of normal tension glaucoma.[134] To be eligible for this study, patient eyes had to have glaucomatous excavation of the optic disc and a field defect on standard achromatic perimetry, consisting of a cluster of three nonedge points depressed by 5 dB, with one of the points also depressed by 10 dB. This defect had to be confirmed by two of three follow-up fields performed within a 4-week window.

Progression was suspected when (1) at least two contiguous points within or adjacent to a baseline defect showed a reduction in sensitivity from baseline of at least 10 dB, or three times the average baseline short-term fluctuation for that patient, whichever was greater; (2) the sensitivity of each suspected point was outside the range of values observed during baseline testing; or (3) a defect occurred in a previously normal part of the field. To reach a definitive decision of progression, four confirmatory tests were required. This large number of confirmatory fields was necessary to be able to reliably distinguish smaller glaucomatous visual field changes from long-term fluctuation.[134]

Early Manifest Glaucoma Trial. The Early Manifest Glaucoma Trial (EMGT) was developed to assess the effectiveness of reducing intraocular pressure in early, previously untreated, open-angle glaucoma. Because EMGT uses field progression as a study end point, a progression algorithm was developed using the glaucoma change probability (GCP) analysis, included in Statpac II of the Humphrey Visual Field Analyzer.[94]

To look for change, the GCP uses a pointwise comparison of the standard visual field against the average of the first two reliable baseline visual fields (Figure 22-8). The commercially available version of the GCP currently evaluates change based on the

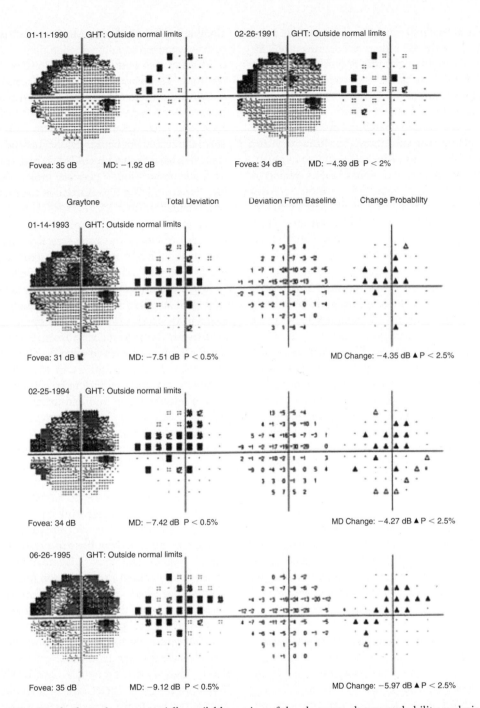

Figure 22-8 Results from the commercially available version of the glaucoma change probability analysis based on total deviation. The two baseline fields (gray scales and total deviation plots) are shown at the top. Below these are three consecutive follow-up fields showing points with significant change for the worse (*filled triangles*) and points with significant improvement (*open triangles*). Points that deteriorate but are too defective at baseline to judge progression are marked with an *x*. The change is repeatable on all follow-ups for this individual. *GHT*, Glaucoma hemifield test.

total deviation probability map. The EMGT study uses a modified version based on the pattern deviation probability map. The change in pattern deviation is thought to provide a more accurate assessment of visual field progression of early defects because this plot is less influenced by shifts in the global hill of vision because of cataract, pupil size changes, or refractive errors.[13]

The GCP flags a change in sensitivity greater than the long-term fluctuation found in a group of stable glaucoma patients at each particular location.[53] Because the GCP does not define cutoffs for visual field progression, the EMGT investigators had to develop criteria for what constitutes significant progression. For the EMGT, there is an initial screening, two preintervention field tests, and two baseline visits. The two baseline visits must have a GHT "Outside Normal Limits" resulting from the same sectors or a borderline GHT on two consecutive field examinations with obvious localized change to the optic disc.[94] Progression requires three or more points flagged by the pattern deviation version of the GCP analysis. Only if these same points are confirmed on two subsequent visual fields is progression verified.

Advanced Glaucoma Intervention Study. The Advanced Glaucoma Intervention Study (AGIS) algorithm was developed to determine eligibility for the AGIS and to evaluate disease progression in patients with more advanced glaucomatous visual fields. The AGIS scoring system is based on the concepts that (1) multiple defects can occur in the upper, lower, and nasal hemifields; (2) a defect requires two or more adjacent defective points; (3) the severity of depression must be greater than changes resulting from variability; and (4) the defect must be caused by glaucoma. The AGIS score is calculated by totaling the number of adjacent depressed test points in the upper, lower, and nasal hemifields compared with age-matched normal eyes in the total deviation printout of Statpac II. The score becomes larger with increases in the number of depressed test sites and with increasing depth of defect.[58] The final AGIS score ranges from 0 to 20. Progression is quantified as an increase in score from baseline reference by four or more points on three consecutive reliable fields.

Collaborative Initial Glaucoma Treatment Study. The Collaborative Initial Glaucoma Treatment Study (CIGTS) is a scoring system modified from AGIS. In brief, scoring is based on the total deviation probability plot. Each abnormal test location must then be accompanied by at least two adjacent abnormal points, and each abnormal point is given a score from 1 to 4 based on the probability level (5% to 0.5%) of the three contiguous depressed points. The value for each of the 52 locations within the visual field is combined to get a maximum possible score of 208. The total score is then divided by a conversion factor (10.4) to get a final score, ranging from 0 to 20. Progression is quantified as an increase in score from baseline reference by 3 points or more on three consecutive reliable fields.[111]

Comparing the Methods. Many specialists in glaucoma were involved in the development of the methods used in each of these studies. However, few studies have compared the different methods for identifying progression on the same series of visual fields. Comparing AGIS, CIGTS, and EMGT criteria, Katz[79] and Katz, Congdon, and Friedman[80] have evaluated the agreement between these methods and two glaucoma specialists who graded the patient fields as "definite progression," "possible progression," "stable," "improved," or "too unreliable to assess." Their results indicated that EMGT, CIGTS, and the glaucoma specialists produced similar percentages of progression, but not in the same eyes. Furthermore, the EMGT and CIGTS methods produced rates of apparent progression that were twice those of AGIS.

These studies indicate the difficulties when there is no gold standard for progression independent of visual fields. Until a nonfield gold standard is established, only the agreement between different methods for grading progression can be determined and the sensitivity and specificity of the various techniques for determining progression will remain unknown. Identification and confirmation of change in visual fields remain important aspects for identifying true glaucoma progression, but there is as yet no agreed-upon set of methods to do so.

NEW PERIMETRIC TEST PROCEDURES

Recent developments in perimetry have incorporated the evaluation of specific visual functions believed to be mediated by distinct subpopulations of retinal ganglion cells.[93,97,98,135] There are several major groups of retinal ganglion cells that project to different portions of the lateral geniculate nucleus. One group of cells that project to the parvocellular layers of the lateral geniculate (P cells) are concentrated in central vision, have slower conduction velocities, have thinner axons, and are most responsive to high spatial frequencies and low temporal frequencies.[93,97,98,135] P cells are believed to be primarily involved in the processing of color information, spatial resolution, and form vision. About 80% of all retinal ganglion cells are P cells. It has recently been reported that blue-sensitive retinal ganglion cells project to the koniocellular layers of the lateral geniculate nucleus (K cells).[103] These cells are believed to be involved in the processing of blue-yellow color opponent information and comprise about 5% of the retinal ganglion cell population. A third group projects to the magnocellular layers of the lateral geniculate (M cells), are distributed rather uniformly throughout the visual field, have fast conduction velocities, have thicker axons, and are most responsive to low spatial frequencies and high temporal frequencies.[93,97,98,135] M cells are believed to be primarily involved in the processing of rapid flicker, motion, and related temporal visual functions. They comprise about 15% of the total number of retinal ganglion cells. This section briefly discusses five new perimetric test procedures that are based on the premise of selectively evaluating specific retinal ganglion cell subpopulations.

Short-Wavelength Automated Perimetry

SWAP isolates and measures the sensitivity of the short-wavelength–sensitive (blue-sensitive) visual pathways by presenting large blue stimuli on a bright yellow background. The bright yellow background significantly depresses the sensitivity of the middle (green) and long (red) wavelength mechanisms and thereby permits the sensitivity of the short-wavelength–sensitive mechanisms to be evaluated. Felius et al.,[34] Sample and Weinreb,[124] and Sample et al.[130] have shown that for SWAP, detection of the short-wavelength stimulus at threshold is mediated by the blue-yellow opponent chromatic mechanisms. Moreover, their results and those of Demirel and Johnson[28] indicate that the blue-yellow opponent chromatic pathways are responsible for detecting the blue stimulus, even in areas with extensive glaucomatous visual field loss.

The optimal stimulus conditions for SWAP consist of a 100 cd/m² yellow background (Schott OG 530 filter), a Goldmann size V stimulus, a 200-millisecond stimulus duration, and a narrow-band blue stimulus (Omega 440-nm filter, 27-nm bandwidth).[130] With use of the optimal stimulus conditions for SWAP, approximately 17 dB of isolation can be achieved.[130] These conditions provide the best isolation of short-wavelength–sensitive pathways, the greatest dynamic range, and the least amount of influence by age-related lens yellowing.

A substantial part of the initial development and validation of SWAP was conducted independently in the laboratory of Sample[122-125,129,130,156] at the University of California, San Diego and in the laboratory of Johnson[1,63,64,74-77] at the University of California, Davis. Prospective longitudinal evaluations conducted at both laboratories and cross-sectional evaluations performed by other investigators have shown that (1) SWAP deficits are more prevalent in high-risk ocular hypertensives and are progressively less prevalent in medium- and low-risk ocular hypertensives, as would be expected; (2) SWAP deficits precede visual field loss for standard automated perimetry (SAP) and are

predictive of future deficits for SAP; (3) SWAP deficits are more extensive than those found for SAP; (4) SWAP deficits progress at a higher rate than for SAP losses; and (5) SWAP deficits are correlated with structural abnormalities of the optic disc and retinal nerve fiber layer in glaucoma.* In addition, SWAP has been shown to be useful in detecting the earliest signs of visual function loss in retinal diseases and neuroophthalmologic disorders.[43,55,68,82,99]

An example of SWAP's earlier detection of glaucomatous visual field loss is shown in Figure 22-9, which presents a comparison of SAP (*left column*) and SWAP (*right column*) in the right eye of a patient over 5 years. For both tests, locations with normal sensitivity are indicated by open circles, locations with sensitivity lower than the normal 5% probability level are shaded gray, and locations with sensitivity below the normal 1% probability level are solid black circles. A SWAP deficit in the form of a superior nasal step begins to appear in year 1 and then progresses over the next 4 years. SAP results begin to show a superior nasal step about 4 years after it appears for SWAP.

Some disadvantages are associated with SWAP. Age-related lens yellowing, macular pigment, cataract, and other ocular media opacities can reduce short-wavelength sensitivity.[110,127,158] These confounding factors can be accounted for by measuring the short-wavelength transmission losses produced by the ocular media, although this is not practical in a clinical setting.[74,127] However, it is possible to determine localized SWAP deficits without having to measure ocular media transmission losses.[123] Another disadvantage of SWAP is that it has a greater amount of interindividual and intraindividual variation than SAP, and this must be accounted for in normative databases and statistical analysis procedures for SWAP.

However, even with these disadvantages, SWAP is more sensitive to change than standard perimetry, identifying progression 1 to 3 years earlier.[76,125] The SWAP results indicating progression were more likely to be repeatable than those for SAP.[28,131]

Frequency Doubling Technology Perimetry

A low spatial frequency sinusoidal grating (less than 1 cycle per degree) that undergoes high temporal frequency counterphase flicker (greater than 15 Hz) appears to have twice as many light and dark bars than are physically present; that is, the grating's spa-

---

*References 44, 86, 101, 102, 143, 144, 146, 164, 167.

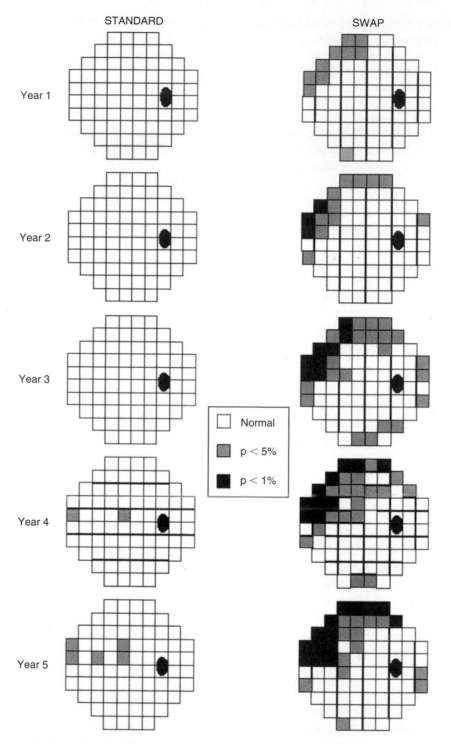

Figure 22-9 A longitudinal comparison of standard automated perimetry and short-wavelength automated perimetry (*SWAP*) in the right eye of a glaucoma suspect. *Open squares* are within normal limits, *gray squares* represent locations that are worse than the normal 5% probability level, and *black squares* indicate locations that are worse than the normal 1% probability level. In year 1, SWAP results show a nasal step, which progresses over the 5-year period. Standard automated perimetry results are within normal limits for the first 3 years, with the nasal step beginning to be detected in years 4 and 5.

tial frequency appears to be doubled and hence it has been referred to as the *frequency doubling effect.* Maddess and Henry[100] report that the frequency doubling effect is mediated by a subset of M cells with nonlinear response properties (M*y* cells). Recently, the frequency doubling effect has been adapted for perimetric testing, and it is referred to as *frequency doubling technology* (FDT) *perimetry.*[73,78] Contrast sensitivity for detection of the frequency-doubled stimulus is determined at various locations throughout the central visual field. The most common form of FDT perimetry uses large targets (10 degrees × 10 degrees) to evaluate the central visual field at 19 locations, although a 24-2 stimulus presentation pattern (54 target locations throughout the central 30-degree visual field) using smaller targets has also been used.[67,78]

FDT perimetry has a number of desirable characteristics as a clinical diagnostic test procedure. A number of studies have now demonstrated that FDT perimetry has high sensitivity and specificity for detection of glaucomatous visual field loss, as well as deficits from neuroophthalmologic disorders.* FDT perimetry has low test-retest variability, which increases by only about 30% in moderately damaged visual field regions, in contrast to SAP, which shows a 300% to 400% increase in variability for moderately damaged visual field locations.[25] The commercially available version of FDT perimetry includes an extensive normative database and statistical analysis package with reliability indices (false-positive and false-negative errors and fixation losses), visual field indices (MD and PSD) and total and pattern deviation probability plots.[78] FDT perimetry is also relatively unaffected by blur of up to 6 diopters or variations in pupil size, provided that the pupil is at least 2 mm in diameter.[61] FDT perimetry is easy to administer, is simple for patients to perform, and has minimal learning and fatigue effects.[57] In addition, FDT perimetry is a relatively fast test procedure. The full-threshold test procedure requires approximately 5 minutes per eye, and recent investigations of maximum likelihood procedures and optimized modified binary search strategies have reduced the threshold test time to approximately 2.5 minutes per eye.[148] Two rapid suprathreshold screening procedures, requiring approximately 45 to 60 seconds per eye, have also been developed and validated.[66,119] The disadvantages of FDT perimetry are that it is affected by ocular media opacities and that there is currently

little information concerning its ability to monitor progressive visual field loss. Also, FDT perimetry has limited spatial resolution because of the small number of large targets that are used. Studies have demonstrated that it is possible to implement a 24-2 stimulus presentation pattern for FDT perimetry using smaller targets and that this improves its sensitivity and provides better characterization of localized visual field loss.[67]

Figure 22-10 presents results for the right eye of a patient with early glaucomatous visual field loss. FDT perimetry results are presented on the left, with corresponding SAP results presented for comparison on the right. Note that there is a remarkable similarity in the location and extent of damage indicated by each of the test procedures. Studies have reported a good correlation between visual field indices and individual threshold values for FDT and SAP.[23,140]

Motion-Automated Perimetry and Displacement Perimetry

Some histologic evidence has suggested that damage to larger diameter retinal ganglion cell axons occurs first in the course of glaucoma, but these results have been questioned.[60,120] Many have used these histologic results to assume that "larger axons" means magnocellular axons are most at risk. This interpretation has also been questioned.[155] However, tests that target visual functions associated with this axon population are promising.

Various forms of motion testing have been developed to assess the responses of the magnocellular ganglion cells.[17,138,145,152] Motion testing uses video displays to generate stimuli, usually random-dot displays in which many dots move in random directions while a percentage move coherently (in the same direction). An example of this type of display is presented in Figure 22-11.

The patient's task is to determine the direction of motion in the coherent dots, with the percentage of coherent dots increasing until there is a correct response. This is the patient's motion coherence threshold.[16,20,138,145] An alternative approach is for the percentage of dots to be held constant and the size of the moving area to increase until the patient can correctly discern the direction of motion.[152] Turano, Huang, and Quigley[147] also used drifting sinusoidal patterns embedded in dynamic spatial noise and showed that glaucoma patients discern a reduced range of spatial frequencies compared with normals. Although motion tests are structured to test magnocellular ganglion cells, their designs were based on

---

*References 23, 66, 68, 73, 78, 85, 91, 113, 119, 132, 140.

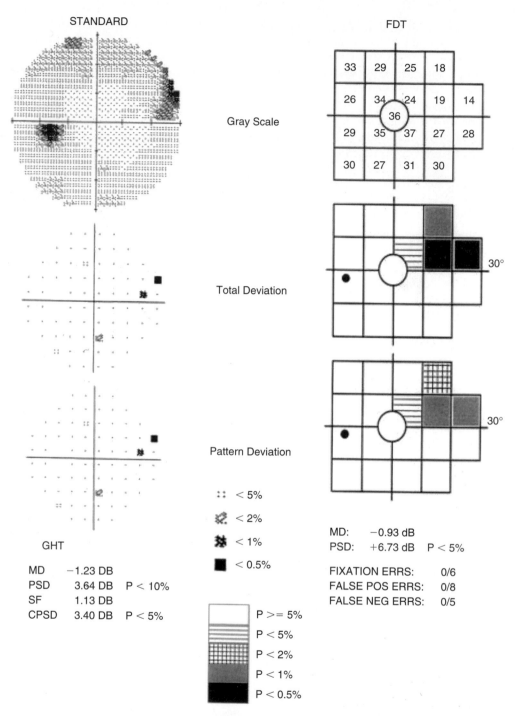

STANDARD

Gray Scale

Total Deviation

Pattern Deviation

:: < 5%

< 2%

< 1%

■ < 0.5%

GHT

MD   −1.23 DB
PSD   3.64 DB   P < 10%
SF   1.13 DB
CPSD   3.40 DB   P < 5%

P >= 5%
P < 5%
P < 2%
P < 1%
P < 0.5%

FDT

33	29	25	18	
26	34	24	19	14
		36		
29	35	37	27	28
30	27	31	30	

30°

30°

MD: −0.93 dB
PSD: +6.73 dB   P < 5%

FIXATION ERRS: 0/6
FALSE POS ERRS: 0/8
FALSE NEG ERRS: 0/5

FIGURE 22-10   A comparison of results obtained for standard automated perimetry and frequency doubling technology (*FDT*) perimetry for the right eye of a glaucoma patient with a small superior nasal step. Note that the extent of the area with reduced sensitivity is much greater for FDT than for standard automated perimetry. *GHT,* Glaucoma hemifield test.

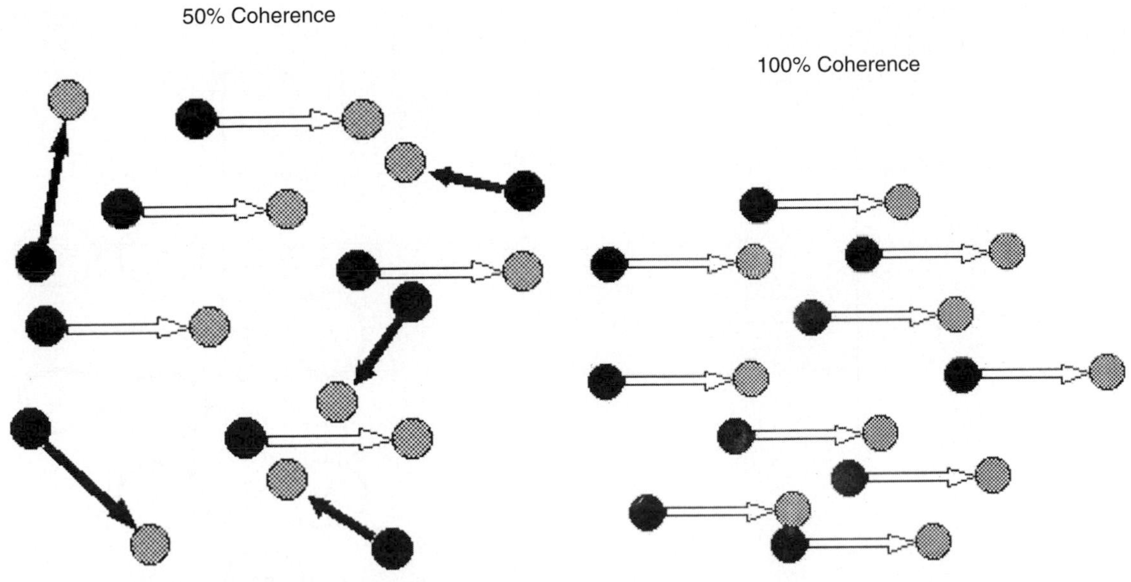

50% Coherence

100% Coherence

FIGURE 22-11 Schematic representation of the display used to measure motion coherence thresholds. Examples of 50% and 100% motion coherence are presented.

what is known about normal visual processing and from electrophysiologic and lesion studies in cat and monkey. The actual amount of isolation before another retinal ganglion cell type begins processing the signal is not yet known. Results should therefore be interpreted with this in mind.

Testing motion perception with random-dot displays reduces the influence of other visual cues, such as form perception, and limits the observer's ability to make displacement judgments of directional decisions based on positional or orientational cues.[112] There is good evidence that these types of random-dot displays are processed through the magnocellular pathways.[98,133,136] Motion testing more successfully differentiates glaucomatous from nonglaucomatous eyes when stimulus exposure durations were shorter (less than 1 second), stimulus patches were smaller, a larger number of locations were tested, and sensitivity was analyzed by quadrants instead of by the whole field.[16,59] Foveal stimuli are less effective in identifying glaucomatous damage.[17,59] In addition, motion thresholds with these displays are not associated with short-term changes in ocular pressure, pupil size, or age.[16,20,138] However, intersubject variability in coherence thresholds is high, indicating that a motion threshold has to be more defective to be identified as abnormal than it would with smaller intersubject variability.[17,59]

Patients with primary open-angle glaucoma consistently show deficits in motion processing compared with normal controls.* An example of motion-automated perimetry results in a glaucomatous eye are presented in Figure 22-12, along with the results from SAP using the Humphrey Field Analyzer. Bosworth, Sample, and Weinreb[16] showed that motion coherence thresholds for a given individual were significantly elevated in areas of the visual field with glaucomatous defect compared with areas in the same eye with relative sparing. This group also showed that results on MAP, using several small stimuli in a perimetric format, showed early glaucomatous defects in more than 90% of patients with primary open-angle glaucoma, 28% of patients with ocular hypertension, and 39% of patients with glaucomatous optic neuropathy and normal standard visual fields. This perimetric test was superior to testing with only one large motion target.[17] Focal defects on MAP also correlate well with focal damage at the optic nerve head.[18] Using motion size thresholds and a perimetric technique, Wall, Jennisch, and Munden[151] and Wall and Ketoff[152] found similar results for both glaucoma and ocular hypertensive patients.

Fitzke and others have used a different approach.[35,36,72,118,157] Their procedure involves the determination of a minimum displacement threshold

---

*References 16, 17, 20, 59, 138, 152.

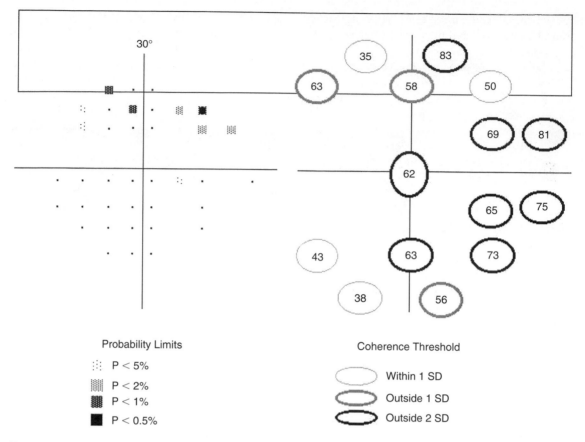

FIGURE 22-12   A comparison of pattern deviation plots results obtained for standard automated perimetry (*left*) and motion-automated perimetry (MAP) results (*right*) for the left eye of a glaucoma patient. Note that the extent of the area with reduced sensitivity is much greater for MAP than for standard automated perimetry.

for a single moving line stimulus. Thresholds are measured at a variety of visual field locations in a manner similar to conventional automated perimetry. Results of these investigations indicate that this form of displacement perimetry is also effective in detecting glaucomatous visual field loss and appears to be more sensitive than conventional automated perimetry for detecting the earliest functional deficits in glaucoma.

In summary, perimetric measures of motion and displacement sensitivity show great promise for early detection of glaucoma-related vision loss. More studies are needed to evaluate the predictive ability of the test and to determine its usefulness for following glaucoma over time.

Flicker Perimetry (Temporal Modulation Perimetry and Critical Flicker Fusion)

The ability to detect rapidly flickering stimuli is believed to be mediated by magnocellular (M cell) mechanisms. Flicker perimetry has several advan-

tages over conventional automated perimetry. Normal aging effects appear to be more gradual than for conventional automated perimetry, especially for older ages, and flicker perimetry is more resistant to optical degradation (e.g., blur, cataract) than conventional automated perimetry.[87,90] In addition, it has been reported that flicker perimetry is more sensitive than SAP for detecting glaucomatous visual field loss and other optic neuropathies and that flicker perimetry deficits are predictive of future glaucomatous visual field defects for SAP.*

Several methods of flicker perimetry have been used, each with their advantages and disadvantages. One procedure developed by Lachenmayr measures the maximum flicker rate (critical flicker fusion [CFF]) that can be distinguished from a steady light.[87,89,90] The stimuli are matched in luminance to the background and are then briefly flickered at

---

*References 6, 21, 22, 33, 89, 165, 168.

100% contrast (above and below the average background luminance), and the patient is instructed to press a button when flicker is detected. The temporal frequency or rate of flicker is varied until the CFF (highest frequency at which flicker can be detected) is determined. In addition to being more sensitive for detection of early glaucomatous visual field loss, Lachenmayr et al.[88] have also reported that this form of flicker perimetry is more highly correlated with optic nerve fiber layer and neuroretinal rim measurements than SAP.

Another form of flicker perimetry uses a fixed rate of flicker and varies stimulus contrast to determine the minimum amount of contrast needed to detect flicker.[21,22,165] This procedure is referred to as *temporal modulation perimetry* (TMP). Stimuli are matched in luminance to the background, and the stimulus luminance is modulated above and below the background luminance for a fixed rate of flicker. It has been reported that this form of flicker perimetry is effective in detecting early glaucomatous visual field loss and may be predictive of future visual field loss for SAP.[21,22] Although both forms of flicker perimetry are effective, an investigation by Yoshiyama and Johnson[165] indicated that the TMP procedure performed moderately better than CFF. An example of CFF and TMP perimetry results in a glaucomatous eye are presented in Figure 22-13, along with the results from SAP using the Humphrey Field Analyzer.

A third form of flicker perimetry is available on the Medmont perimeter (Medmont Pty Ltd., Camberwell, Victoria, Australia).[168] It presents a flickering target on a luminance pedestal. The flicker rate and contrast are fixed, and the height of the luminance pedestal is varied to determine the patient's threshold for detecting flicker. Finally, flicker perimetry is commercially available on newer Octopus perimeters (Interzeag, Inc., Switzerland). Matsumoto et al.[105] have shown that flicker sensitivity is reduced in patients with glaucoma in field areas correlating to locations of nerve fiber layer defects. All four forms of flicker perimetry have been shown to be effective in detecting early glaucomatous visual field loss.

High-Pass Resolution Perimetry

Frisen[40] developed high-pass resolution perimetry (HRP), which consists of a series of ring targets of varying size that are presented on a computer monitor by performing a "high-pass" spatial frequency filtering of a target incorporating a light circular center and a dark annular surround. The contrast and spatial frequency characteristics were selected so that the target's detection and resolution thresholds were equivalent; that is, the target could be detected and its fine details could be resolved at the same threshold target size. The stimulus was designed to correspond to the center-surround arrangement of retinal ganglion cell receptive fields, and Frisen has proposed that HRP thresholds provide an estimate of the density of P cells throughout the central visual field. In this view, he provides a visual field index of "neural capacity" or "functional channels" that is proposed to reflect the proportion of remaining ganglion cell receptive fields that are functioning properly within the central visual field.[41,42]

A number of investigators have reported that HRP has good sensitivity and specificity for detection of glaucomatous visual field loss and deficits produced by various neuroophthalmologic disorders.* It is also a rapid test (approximately 5 minutes per eye), simple to administer, easy for patients to perform, and interactive in that it provides feedback to the patient. Several studies have reported that HRP has excellent test-retest reliability and that there are only minimal increases in variability for moderate and extensively damaged visual field areas.[24,153] The low test-retest variability exhibited by HRP makes it possible to detect progressive visual field loss earlier than with SAP. Chauhan et al.[26] found that, in most glaucoma patients exhibiting progressive glaucomatous visual field loss, HRP was able to determine the progressive changes an average of 18 months earlier than SAP. HRP results have also been reported to be highly correlated with optic disc characteristics and retinal nerve fiber layer measurements in patients with glaucoma.[2]

The biggest disadvantage of HRP at present is its limited commercial distribution and representation, particularly in North America. Another minor disadvantage is the need to use a high near-correction and a special trial lens set for testing. An example of the results of HRP are presented in Figure 22-14.

Comparing Tests

Although the newer perimetric procedures have all been compared with SAP, there are few studies comparing the new tests to each other in the same patient population. Sample et al.[132] began with a comparison of SWAP and MAP and found that

---

*References 15, 41, 42, 104, 108, 128, 153.

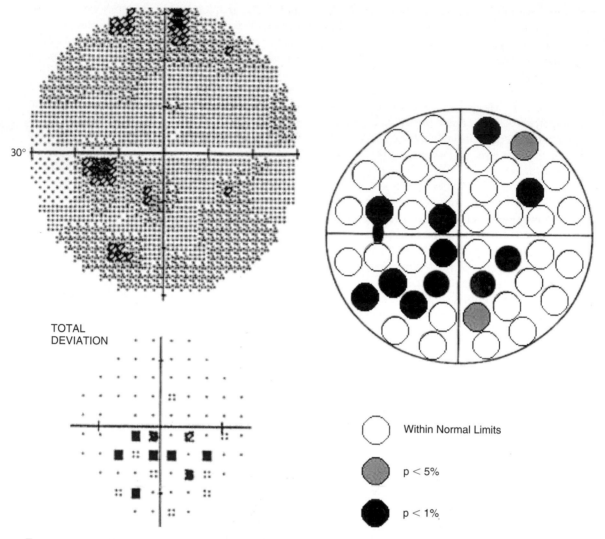

Figure 22-13   A comparison of standard automated perimetry and temporal modulation perimetry for the left eye of a patient with early glaucoma. For the temporal modulation perimetry results, *filled gray circles* indicate locations that have sensitivity below the normal 5% probability level and *filled black circles* indicate locations with sensitivity below the normal 1% probability level.

both tests successfully identified eyes with glaucoma and a percentage of the suspect eyes. Location of visual field defect overlapped in 94% of the glaucoma eyes, and suspect eyes may have had a defect in only one or the other test.[121] This group has recently added FDT to the comparison of SAP, SWAP, and MAP and found again that in a given individual, the same retinal location is damaged for all affected tests. All visual function specific tests were superior to standard visual fields.[132] Ninety percent of the eyes with glaucomatous optic neuropathy were identified by one of the visual function specific tests. SAP missed 54% of these eyes. SWAP,

FDT, and MAP each identified a subset of the ocular hypertensive eyes. Casson, Johnson, and Shapiro[22] also found considerable overlap between flicker and SWAP deficits in ocular hypertensive and glaucomatous eyes.

Summary

A number of innovations have occurred for perimetry and visual field testing in recent years, which have resulted in a greater degree of standardization through automation and the development of new test procedures that are more effi-

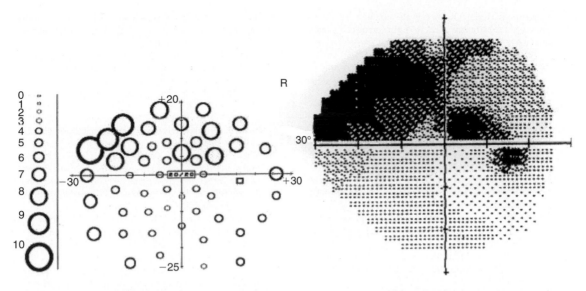

FIGURE 22-14 Comparison of high-pass resolution perimetry (*left*) and standard automated perimetry conducted on the Humphrey Field Analyzer (*right*) for the right eye of a patient with glaucoma. (Reprinted from Birt CM et al: *J Glaucoma* 7:111, 1998.)

cient, more reliable, and more sensitive. Advances in quantitative analysis methods have also enhanced the ability to detect early, subtle deficits and to monitor progressive visual field loss. However, there are still significant limitations that need to be addressed by future research and development. Perimetry remains a subjective test procedure and depends on the cooperation and attentiveness of the patient. Existing analysis procedures require many visual field tests to accurately distinguish progression from intertest variability. The development of new nonconventional analysis methods may reveal markers for visual field progression with fewer tests. Finally, the relationship between ocular structural changes and sensitivity loss is still not well understood for many eye diseases. The development of techniques for measuring the functional properties of nerve fiber bundles and other structural features will significantly enhance the ability to understand the underlying basis of pathologic changes. If progress in perimetry and visual field testing continues at its current pace or faster, we will not have long to wait for these innovations.

ACKNOWLEDGMENTS

This work is supported in part by National Eye Institute Research Grants #EY-03424 (to Chris A. Johnson) and #EY-08208 (to Pamela A. Sample).

REFERENCES

1. Adams AJ, Johnson CA, Lewis RA: S cone pathway sensitivity loss in ocular hypertension and early glaucoma has nerve fiber bundle pattern. In Drum B, Moreland J, Serra A (eds): *Proceedings of the 10th symposium of the International Research Group on Colour Vision Deficiencies*, Dordrecht, The Netherlands, 1991, Kluwer Academic Publishers.
2. Airaksinen PJ et al: Retinal nerve fiber layer abnormalities and high-pass resolution perimetry, *Acta Ophthalmol* 68:687, 1990.
3. Anderson DR: *Perimetry with and without automation*, St Louis, 1987, Mosby.
4. Anderson DR, Patella VM: *Automated static perimetry*, St Louis, 1999, Mosby.
5. Aulhorn E, Harms H: Visual perimetry. In Jameson D, Hurvich LM (eds): *Visual psychophysics: handbook of sensory physiology*, vol VII/4, New York, 1972, Springer-Verlag.
6. Austin MW, O'Brien CJ, Wishart PK: Flicker perimetry using a luminance threshold strategy at frequencies from 5-25 Hz in glaucoma, ocular hypertension and normal controls, *Curr Eye Res* 13:717, 1994.
7. Benedetto M, Cyrlin MN: The effect of blur upon static perimetric thresholds, *Doc Ophthalmol Proc Ser* 42:563, 1985.
8. Bengtsson B, Heijl A: Evaluation of a new perimetric threshold strategy, SITA, in patients with manifest and suspect glaucoma, *Acta Ophthalmol* 76:268, 1998.
9. Bengtsson B, Heijl A: Comparing significance and magnitude of glaucomatous visual field defects using the SITA and full threshold strategies, *Acta Ophthalmol* 77:143, 1999.
10. Bengtsson B, Heijl A: Inter-subject variability and normal limits of the SITA standard, SITA fast, and the Humphrey full threshold computerized perimetry strategies, SITA STATPAC, *Acta Ophthalmol* 77:125, 1999.

11. Bengtsson B, Heijl A, Olsson J: Evaluation of a new threshold visual field strategy, SITA, in normal subjects: Swedish interactive thresholding algorithm, *Acta Ophthalmol Scand* 76:165, 1998.

12. Bengtsson B et al: A new generation of algorithms for computerized threshold perimetry, SITA, *Acta Ophthalmol Scand* 75:368, 1997.

13. Bengtsson B et al: Perimetric probability maps to separate change caused by glaucoma from that caused by cataract, *Acta Ophthalmol Scand* 75:184, 1997.

14. Birch MK, Wishart PK, O'Donnell NP: Determining progressive visual field loss in serial Humphrey visual fields, *Ophthalmology* 102:1227, 1995.

15. Birt CM et al: Comparison between high-pass resolution perimetry and differential light sensitivity perimetry in patients with glaucoma, *J Glaucoma* 7:111, 1998.

16. Bosworth C, Sample P, Weinreb R: Motion perception thresholds in areas of glaucomatous visual field loss, *Vis Res* 37:355, 1997.

17. Bosworth C et al: Motion automated perimetry (MAP) identifies early glaucomatous field defects, *Arch Ophthalmol* 116:1153, 1998.

18. Bosworth CF et al: Spatial relationship of motion automated perimetry and optic disc topography in patients with glaucomatous optic neuropathy, *J Glaucoma* 8:281, 1999.

19. Budenz DL, Feuer WJ, Anderson DR: The effect of simulated cataract on the glaucomatous visual field, *Ophthalmology* 100:511, 1993.

20. Bullimore MA, Wood JM, Swenson K: Motion perception in glaucoma, *Invest Ophthalmol Vis Sci* 34:3526, 1993.

21. Casson EJ, Johnson CA: Temporal modulation perimetry in glaucoma and ocular hypertension. In Mills RP (ed): *Perimetry update 1992/1993,* Amsterdam, 1993, Kugler Publications.

22. Casson EJ, Johnson CA, Shapiro LR: Longitudinal comparison of temporal-modulation perimetry with white-on-white and blue-on-yellow perimetry in ocular hypertension and early glaucoma, *J Opt Soc Am A* 10:1792, 1993.

23. Cello KE, Nelson-Quigg JM, Johnson CA: Frequency doubling technology (FDT) perimetry as a means of detecting glaucomatous visual field loss, *Am J Ophthalmol* 129:314, 2000.

24. Chauhan BC, House PH: Intratest variability in conventional and high-pass resolution perimetry, *Ophthalmology* 98:79, 1991.

25. Chauhan BC, Johnson CA: Test-retest variability characteristics of frequency doubling perimetry and conventional perimetry in glaucoma patients and normal controls, *Invest Ophthalmol Vis Sci* 40:648, 1999.

26. Chauhan BC et al: Comparison of conventional and high-pass resolution perimetry in a prospective study of patients with glaucoma and healthy controls, *Arch Ophthalmol* 117:24, 1999.

27. Choplin NT, Edwards RP: *Visual field testing with the Humphrey Field Analyzer,* Thoroughfare, NJ, 1995, Slack.

28. Demirel S, Johnson CA: Incidence and prevalence of short wavelength automated perimetry (SWAP) deficits in ocular hypertensive patients, *Am J Ophthalmol* 131:709, 2001.

29. Demirel S, Vingrys AJ: Fixational instability during perimetry and the blindspot monitor. In Mills RP (ed): *Perimetry update 1992/93,* Amsterdam, 1993, Kugler Publications.

30. Drance SM, Anderson DL: *Automated perimetry in glaucoma: a practical guide,* New York, 1985, Grune & Stratton.

31. Fankhauser F, Enoch JM: The effects of blur on perimetric thresholds, *Arch Ophthalmol* 68:120, 1962.

32. Fazio P et al: Effect of patient experience on the results of automated perimetry in glaucoma suspect patients, *Ophthalmology* 97:44, 1990.

33. Feghall JG et al: Static flicker perimetry in glaucoma and ocular hypertension, *Curr Eye Res* 10:205, 1991.

34. Felius J et al: Functional characteristics of blue-on-yellow perimetric thresholds in glaucoma, *Invest Ophthalmol Vis Sci* 36:1665, 1995.

35. Fitzke FW et al: Peripheral displacement thresholds in normals, ocular hypertensives and glaucoma, *Doc Ophthalmol Proc Ser* 49:447, 1987.

36. Fitzke FW et al: Peripheral displacement thresholds in glaucoma and ocular hypertension. In Heijl A (ed): *Perimetry update 1988/1989,* Amsterdam, 1989, Kugler Publications.

37. Fitzke FW et al: Analysis of visual field progression in glaucoma, *Br J Ophthalmol* 80:40, 1996.

38. Flammer J, Drance SM, Zulauf M: Differential light threshold: short- and long-term fluctuation in patients with glaucoma, normal controls, and patients with suspected glaucoma, *Arch Ophthalmol* 102:704, 1984.

39. Flanagan JG, Hovis JK: Colored targets in the assessment of differential light sensitivity. In Heijl A (ed): *Perimetry update 1988/89,* Amsterdam, 1989, Kugler Publications.

40. Frisen L: A computer-graphics visual field screener using high-pass spatial frequency resolution targets and multiple feedback devices, *Doc Ophthalmol Proc Ser* 49:441, 1987.

41. Frisen L: Acuity perimetry: estimation of neural channels, *Int Ophthalmol* 12:169, 1988.

42. Frisen L: High-pass resolution perimetry: a clinical review, *Doc Ophthalmol* 83:1, 1993.

43. Fujimoto N, Adachi-Usami E: Use of blue-on-yellow perimetry to demonstrate quadrantanopia in multiple sclerosis, *Arch Ophthalmol* 116:828, 1998.

44. Girkin CA et al: Comparison of short-wavelength automated perimetry and conventional white-on-white perimetry in patients with progressive optic disc cupping, *Arch Ophthalmol* 118:1231, 2000.

45. Greve EL: *Single and multiple stimulus static perimetry: the two phases of perimetry,* The Hague, The Netherlands, 1973, Dr W Junk Publishers.

46. Guttridge NM et al: Influence of learning on the peripheral field as assessed by automated perimetry. In Mills RP, Heijl A (eds): *Perimetry update 1990/91,* Amsterdam, 1991, Kugler & Ghedini.

47. Hedin A, Verriest G: Is clinical color perimetry useful? *Doc Ophthalmol Proc Ser* 26:161, 1980.

48. Heijl A, Asman P: A clinical study of perimetric probability maps, *Arch Ophthalmol* 107:199, 1989.

49. Heijl A, Bengtsson B: Third generation rapid algorithms for static computerized perimetry, SITA. In Kriglestein G (ed): *Glaucoma update VI,* Berlin, 2000, Springer-Verlag.

50. Heijl A, Bengtsson B, Patella VM: Glaucoma follow-up when converting from long to short perimetric threshold tests, *Arch Ophthalmol* 118:489, 2000.

51. Heijl A, Lindgren A, Lindgren G: Test-retest variability in glaucomatous visual fields, *Am J Ophthalmol* 108:130, 1989.

52. Heijl A, Lindgren G, Olsson J: Normal variability of static perimetric threshold values across the central visual field, *Arch Ophthalmol* 105:1544, 1987.

53. Heijl A et al: Extended empirical statistical package for evaluation of single and multiple fields in glaucoma: Statpac 2. In Mills RP, Heijl A (eds): *Perimetry update,* Amsterdam, 1991, Kugler & Ghedini.

54. Henson DB: *Visual fields,* New York, 1993, Oxford University Press.

55. Hudson C et al: Short-wavelength sensitive visual field loss in patients with clinically significant diabetic macular oedema, *Diabetologia* 41:918, 1998.

56. Hudson C et al: The magnitude and locus of perimetric fatigue in normals and ocular hypertensives. In Mills RP (ed): *Perimetry update 1992/93,* Amsterdam, 1993, Kugler Publications.

57. Iester M et al: Learning effect, short-term fluctuation and long term fluctuation in frequency doubling technique, *Am J Ophthalmol* 130:160, 2000.

58. Investigators: The Advanced Glaucoma Intervention Study (AGIS): 2. Visual field scoring and reliability, *Ophthalmology* 101:1445, 1994.

59. Joffe KM, Raymond JE, Crichton A: Motion coherence perimetry in glaucoma and suspected glaucoma, *Vis Res* 37:955, 1997.

60. Johnson CA: Selective versus non-selective losses in glaucoma, *J Glaucoma* 3(suppl):S32, 1994.

61. Johnson CA: Frequency doubling perimetry as a means of screening for glaucomatous visual field loss, *Invest Ophthalmol Vis Sci* 36(suppl):S335, 1995 (ARVO abstract).

62. Johnson CA: Perimetry and visual field testing. In Zadnik K (ed): *The optometric examination: measurements and findings,* Philadelphia, 1996, WB Saunders.

63. Johnson CA, Adams AJ, Casson: Blue-on-yellow perimetry: a five year overview. In Mills RP (ed): *Perimetry update 1992/93,* New York, 1993, Kugler Publications.

64. Johnson CA, Adams, AJ, Lewis RA: Automated perimetry of short-wavelength sensitive mechanisms in glaucoma and ocular hypertension: preliminary findings. In Heijl A (ed): *Perimetry update 1988/89,* New York, 1989, Kugler & Ghedini.

65. Johnson CA, Adams CW, Lewis RA: Fatigue effects in automated perimetry, *Appl Opt* 27:1030, 1988.

66. Johnson CA, Cioffi GA, Van Buskirk EM: Evaluation of two screening tests for frequency doubling technology perimetry. In Wall M, Wild J (eds): *Perimetry update 1998/1999,* Amsterdam, 1998, Kugler Publications.

67. Johnson, CA, Cioffi GA, Van Buskirk EM: Frequency doubling technology perimetry using a 24-2 stimulus presentation pattern, *Optom Vis Sci* 76:571, 1999.

68. Johnson CA, Keltner JL: Short-wavelength automated perimetry (SWAP) in optic neuritis. In Mills RP, Wall M (eds): *Perimetry update 94/95,* Amsterdam, 1995, Kugler Publications.

69. Johnson CA, Keltner JL: Principles and techniques of the examination of the visual sensory system. In Miller NR, Newman NJ (eds): *Walsh and Hoyt's clinical neuro-ophthalmology,* Philadelphia, 1998, Lippincott Williams & Wilkins.

70. Johnson CA, Keltner JL, Balestrery F: Effects of target size and eccentricity on visual detection and resolution, *Vis Res* 18:1217, 1978.

71. Johnson CA, Keltner JL, Balestrery FG: Static and acuity profile perimetry at various adaptation levels, *Doc Ophthalmol* 50:371, 1981.

72. Johnson CA, Marshall D, Eng K: Displacement threshold perimetry in glaucoma using a Macintosh computer system and a 21 inch monitor. In Mills RP, Wall M (eds): *Perimetry update 1994/95,* Amsterdam, 1995, Kugler Publications.

73. Johnson CA, Samuels SJ: Screening for glaucomatous visual field loss with frequency doubling perimetry, *Invest Ophthalmol Vis Sci* 28:413, 1997.

74. Johnson CA et al: Age-related changes in the central visual field for short-wavelength-sensitive pathways, *J Opt Soc Am A* 5:2131, 1988.

75. Johnson CA et al: Blue-on-yellow perimetry can predict the development of glaucomatous visual field loss, *Arch Ophthalmol* 111:645, 1993.

76. Johnson CA et al: Progression of early glaucomatous visual field loss for blue-on-yellow and standard white-on-white automated perimetry, *Arch Ophthalmol* 111:651, 1993.

77. Johnson CA et al: Short-wavelength automated perimetry in low-, medium- and high-risk ocular hypertensives: initial baseline results, *Arch Ophthalmol* 113:70, 1995.

78. Johnson CA et al: *A primer for frequency doubling technology perimetry,* Dublin, Calif, 1998, Humphrey Systems.

79. Katz J: Scoring systems for measuring progression of visual field loss in clinical trials of glaucoma treatment, *Ophthalmology* 106:391, 1999.

80. Katz J, Congdon N, Friedman D: Methodological variations in estimating apparent progressive visual field loss in clinical trials of glaucoma treatment, *Arch Ophthalmol* 117:1137, 1999.

81. Katz J et al: Estimating progression of visual field loss in glaucoma, *Ophthalmology* 104:1017, 1997.

82. Keltner JL, Johnson CA: Short-wavelength automated perimetry in neuro-ophthalmologic disorders, *Arch Ophthalmol* 113:475, 1995.

83. Keltner JL et al, and the Ocular Hypertension Study Group: Confirmation of visual field abnormalities in the ocular hypertension treatment study (OHTS), *Arch Ophthalmol* 118:1187, 2000.

84. Kitahara K et al: Spectral sensitivities on a white background as a function of retinal eccentricity, *Doc Ophthalmol Proc Ser* 49:651, 1987.

85. Kondo Y et al: A frequency-doubling perimetric study in normal-tension glaucoma with hemifield defect, *J Glaucoma* 7:261, 1998.

86. Kono Y et al: Relationship between parapapillary atrophy and visual field abnormality in primary open angle glaucoma, *Am J Ophthalmol* 127:674, 1999.

87. Lachenmayr BJ, Gleissner M: Flicker perimetry resists retinal image degradation, *Invest Ophthalmol Vis Sci* 33:3539, 1992.

88. Lachenmayr BJ et al: Correlation of retinal nerve-fiber-layer loss, changes at the optic nerve head and various psychophysical criteria in glaucoma, *Graefes Arch Clin Exp Ophthalmol* 229:133, 1991.

89. Lachenmayr BJ et al: Diffuse and localized glaucomatous field loss in light-sense, flicker and resolution perimetry, *Graefes Arch Clin Exp Ophthalmol* 229:267, 1991.

90. Lachenmayr BJ et al: The different effects of aging on normal sensitivity in flicker and light-sense perimetry, *Invest Ophthalmol Vis Sci* 35:2741, 1994.

91. Landers J, Goldberg I, Graham S: A comparison of short wavelength automated perimetry with frequency doubling perimetry for the early detection of visual field loss in ocular hypertension, *Clin Exp Ophthalmol* 28:248, 2000.

92. Langerhorst CT et al: Population study of global and local fatigue with prolonged threshold testing in automated perimetry, *Doc Ophthalmol Proc Ser* 49:657, 1987.

93. Lennie P: Parallel visual pathways: a review, *Vis Res* 20:561, 1980.

94. Leske C et al, and The EMGT Group: Early manifest glaucoma trial, *Ophthalmology* 106:2144, 1999.

95. Lieberman, MF, Drake, MV: *Computerized perimetry: a simplified guide,* Thoroughfare, NJ, 1992, Slack.

96. Lindemuth KA et al: Effects of pupillary constriction on automated perimetry in normal eyes, *Ophthalmology* 96:1298, 1989.

97. Livingstone M, Hubel D. Psychophysical evidence for separate channels for the perception of form, color, movement and depth, *J Neurosci* 7:3416, 1987.

98. Livingstone M, Hubel D: Segregation of form, color, movement and depth: anatomy, physiology and perception, *Science* 240:740, 1988.

99. Lobefalo L et al: Blue-on-yellow and achromatic perimetry in diabetic children without retinopathy, *Diabetes Care* 21:2003, 1998.

100. Maddess T, Henry GH: Performance of nonlinear visual units in ocular hypertension and glaucoma, *Clin Vis Sci* 7:371, 1992.

101. Mansberger SL et al: Achromatic and short-wavelength automated perimetry in patients with glaucomatous large cups, *Arch Ophthalmol* 117:1473, 1999.

102. Mansberger SL et al: Confocal scanning laser ophthalmoscopy in patients with large cup to disc ratios and normal or abnormal functional testing, *Invest Ophthalmol Vis Sci* 40:S675, 1999 (ARVO abstract).

103. Martin PR et al: Evidence that blue-on cells are part of the third geniculocortical pathway in primates, *Eur J Neurosci* 9:1536, 1997.

104. Martinez GA, Sample PA, Weinreb RN: Comparison of high-pass resolution perimetry and standard automated perimetry in glaucoma, *Am J Ophthalmol* 119:195, 1995.

105. Matsumoto C et al: Automated flicker perimetry in glaucoma and retinal detachment patients. In Wall M, Wild J (eds): *Perimetry update 1998/1999*, Amsterdam, 1999, Kugler Publications.

106. McNaught AI et al: Visual field progression: comparison of Humphrey Statpac2 and pointwise linear regression analysis, *Graefes Arch Clin Exp Ophthalmol* 234:411, 1996.

107. Meyer DR et al: Evaluating the visual field effects of blepharoptosis using automated static perimetry, *Ophthalmology* 100:651, 1993.

108. Meyer JH, Funk J: High-pass resolution perimetry and light-sense perimetry in open angle glaucoma, *Ger J Glaucoma* 4:222, 1995.

109. Mikelberg FS et al: The effect of miosis on visual field indices, *Doc Ophthalmol Proc Ser* 49:645, 1987.

110. Moss ID, Wild JM, Whitaker DJ: The influence of age-related cataract on blue-on-yellow perimetry, *Invest Ophthalmol Vis Sci* 36:764, 1995.

111. Musch DC et al: The collaborative initial glaucoma treatment study: study design, methods, and baseline characteristics of enrolled patients, *Ophthalmology* 106:653, 1999.

112. Nakayama K, Tyler CW: Psychophysical isolation of movement sensitivity by removal of familiar position cues, *Vis Res* 21:427, 1981.

113. Nearhing RK, Wall M, Withrow K: Sensitivity and specificity of frequency doubling perimetry in neuro-ophthalmologic disorders, *Invest Ophthalmol Vis Sci* 38(suppl): S390, 1999 (ARVO abstract).

114. O'Brien C, Schwartz B: The visual field in chronic open angle glaucoma: the rate of change in different regions of the field, *Eye* 4:557, 1990.

115. Olsson J, Rootzen H: An image model for quantal response analysis in perimetry, *Scand J Stat* 21:375, 1994.

116. Patipa M: Visual field loss in primary gaze and reading gaze due to acquired blepharoptosis and visual field improvement following ptosis surgery, *Arch Ophthalmol* 110:63, 1992.

117. Pennebacker GE et al: The effect of stimulus duration upon the components of fluctuation in static automated perimetry, *Eye* 6:353, 1992.

118. Poinoosawmy D et al: Discrimination between progression and non-progression visual field loss in low tension glaucoma using MDT. In Mills RP (ed): *Perimetry update 1992/93*, Amsterdam, 1993, Kugler Publications.

119. Quigley HA: Identification of glaucoma-related visual field abnormality with the screening protocol of frequency doubling technology, *Am J Ophthalmol* 125:819, 1998.

120. Quigley HA et al: Chronic glaucoma selectively damages large optic nerve fibers, *Invest Ophthalmol Vis Sci* 28:913, 1987.

121. Sample PA, Bosworth CF, Weinreb RN: Short wavelength automated perimetry and motion automated perimetry in patients with glaucoma, *Arch Ophthalmol* 115:1129, 1997.

122. Sample PA, Martinez GA, Weinreb RN: Color visual fields: A 5 year prospective study in eyes with primary open angle glaucoma. In Mills RP (ed): *Perimetry update 1992/93*, New York, 1993, Kugler Publications.

123. Sample PA, Martinez GA, Weinreb RN: Short-wavelength automated perimetry without lens density testing, *Am J Ophthalmol* 118:632, 1994.

124. Sample PA, Weinreb RN: Color perimetry for assessment of primary open angle glaucoma, *Invest Ophthalmol Vis Sci* 31:1869, 1990.

125. Sample PA, Weinreb RN: Progressive color visual field loss in glaucoma, *Invest Ophthalmol Vis Sci* 33:240, 1992.

126. Sample PA, Weinreb RN, Boynton RM: Isolating color vision loss of primary open angle glaucoma, *Am J Ophthalmol* 106:686, 1988.

127. Sample PA et al: The aging lens: in vivo assessment of light absorption in 84 human eyes, *Invest Ophthalmol Vis Sci* 29:1306, 1988.

128. Sample PA et al: High-pass resolution perimetry in eyes with ocular hypertension and primary open-angle glaucoma, *Am J Ophthalmol* 113:309, 1992.

129. Sample PA et al: Short wavelength color visual fields in glaucoma suspects at risk, *Am J Ophthalmol* 115:225, 1993.

130. Sample PA et al: The optimum parameters for short-wavelength automated perimetry, *J Glaucoma* 5:375, 1996.

131. Sample PA et al: Repeatability of abnormality and progression in glaucomatous standard and SWAP visual fields. In Wall M, Heijl A (eds): *Perimetry update 1997/98*, Amsterdam, 1998, Kugler Publishers.

132. Sample PA et al: Visual function-specific perimetry for indirect comparison of different ganglion cell populations in glaucoma, *Invest Ophthalmol Vis Sci* 41:1783, 2000.

133. Schiller PH, Malpeli JG: Functional specificity of lateral geniculate nucleus laminae of the rhesus monkey, *J Neurophysiol* 41:788, 1978.

134. Schulzer M: Errors in the diagnosis of visual field progression in normal-tension glaucoma, *Ophthalmology* 101: 1589, 1994.

135. Shapley R: Visual sensitivity and parallel retinocortical channels, *Ann Rev Psychol* 41:635, 1990.

136. Shapley R, Kaplan E, Soodak R: Spatial summation and contrast sensitivity of X and Y cells in the lateral geniculate nucleus of the macaque, *Nature* 292:543, 1981.

137. Sharma AK et al: Comparison of the Humphrey Swedish interactive thresholding algorithm (SITA) and full threshold strategies, *J Glaucoma* 9:20, 2000.

138. Silverman SE, Trick GL, Hart WM Jr: Motion perception is abnormal in primary open-angle glaucoma and ocular hypertension, *Invest Ophthalmol Vis Sci* 31:722, 1990.

139. Smith S, Katz J, Quigley H: Analysis of progressive change in automated visual fields in glaucoma, *Invest Ophthalmol Vis Sci* 37:1419, 1996.

140. Sponsel WE et al: Clinical classification of glaucomatous visual field loss by frequency doubling perimetry, *Am J Ophthalmol* 125:830, 1998.

141. Spry PGD et al: Evaluation of pointwise linear regression for detection of glaucomatous visual field defect progression using computer simulation, *Invest Ophthalmol Vis Sci* 41:2192, 2000.

142. Tate GW, Lynn JR: *Principles of quantitative perimetry: testing and interpreting the visual field,* New York, 1977, Grune & Stratton.

143. Teesalu P, Airaksinen P, Tuulonen A: Blue-on-yellow visual field and retinal nerve fiber layer in ocular hypertension and glaucoma, *Ophthalmology* 105:2077, 1998.

144. Teesalu P et al: Correlation of blue-on-yellow visual fields with scanning confocal laser optic disc measurements, *Invest Ophthalmol Vis Sci* 38:2452, 1997.

145. Trick GL, Steinman SB, Amyot M: Motion perception deficits in glaucomatous optic neuropathy, *Vis Res* 35:2225, 1995.

146. Tsai C et al: Correlation of peripapillary retinal height and visual field in glaucoma and normal subjects, *J Glaucoma* 4:110, 1995.

147. Turano KA, Huang AS, Quigley HA: Temporal filter of the motion sensor in glaucoma, *Vis Res* 37:2315, 1997.

148. Turpin A et al: Development of efficient threshold strategies for frequency doubling technology perimetry using computer simulation, *Invest Ophthalmol Vis Sci* 43:322, 2002.

149. van den Berg TJTP: Relation between media disturbances and the visual field, *Doc Ophthalmol Proc Ser* 49:33, 1987.

150. Vingrys AJ, Demirel S: Performance of unreliable patients on repeat perimetry. In Mills RP (ed): *Perimetry update 1992/93,* Amsterdam, 1993 Kugler Publications.

151. Wall M, Jennisch CS, Munden PM: Motion perimetry identifies nerve fiber bundlelike defects in ocular hypertension, *Arch Ophthalmol* 115:26, 1991.

152. Wall M, Ketoff KM: Random dot motion perimetry in patients with glaucoma and in normal subjects, *Am J Ophthalmol* 120:587, 1995.

153. Wall M, LeFante J, Conway M: Variability of high-pass resolution perimetry in normals and patients with idiopathic intracranial hypertension, *Invest Ophthalmol Vis Sci* 32:3091, 1991.

154. Weber EH: Quoted in Boring EG: *A history of experimental psychology,* New York, 1950, Appleton-Century-Crofts.

155. Weinreb R, Lindsey J, Sample P: Lateral geniculate nucleus in glaucoma, *Am J Ophthalmol* 118:126, 1994 (letter to editor).

156. Weinreb RN, Sample PA: Short-wavelength visual field testing in eyes with primary open angle glaucoma. In Krigelstein GK (ed): *Glaucoma update IV,* Berlin, 1991, Springer-Verlag.

157. Westcott MC, Fitzke FW, Hitchings RA: Abnormal motion displacement thresholds are associated with fine scale luminance sensitivity loss in glaucoma, *Vis Res* 38:3171, 1998.

158. Wild JM, Hudson C: The attenuation of blue-on-yellow perimetry by the macular pigment, *Ophthalmology* 102:911, 1995.

159. Wild JM et al: The influence of the learning effect on automated perimetry in patients with suspected glaucoma, *Acta Ophthalmol* 67:537, 1989.

160. Wild JM et al: Long-term follow-up of baseline learning and fatigue effects in automated perimetry of glaucoma and ocular hypertensive patients, *Acta Ophthalmol* 69:210, 1991.

161. Wild JM et al: Between-algorithm, between-individual differences in normal perimetric sensitivity: full threshold, FASTPAC, and SITA. Swedish interactive threshold algorithm, *Invest Ophthalmol Vis Sci* 40:1152, 1999.

162. Wild JM et al: The SITA perimetric threshold algorithms in glaucoma, *Invest Ophthalmol Vis Sci* 40:1998, 1999.

163. Wood JM et al: Alterations in the shape of the automated perimetric profile arising from cataract, *Graefes Arch Clin Exp Ophthalmol* 227:157, 1989.

164. Yamagishi N et al: Mapping structural damage of the optic disc to visual field defect in glaucoma, *Am J Ophthalmol* 123:667, 1997.

165. Yoshiyama KK, Johnson CA: Which method of flicker perimetry is most effective for detection of glaucomatous visual field loss? *Invest Ophthalmol Vis Sci* 38:2270, 1997.

166. Zalta AH: Lens rim artifact in automated threshold perimetry, *Ophthalmology* 96:1302, 1989.

167. Zangwill L, de Suasa Lima M, Weinreb R: Confocal scanning laser ophthalmoscopy to detect glaucomatous optic neuropathy. In Schuman J (ed): *Imaging in glaucoma,* Thoroughfare, NJ, 1997, Slack.

168. Zhang L, Drance SM, Douglas GR: The ability of Medmont M600 automated perimetry to detect threats to fixation, *J Glaucoma* 6:259, 1997.

CHAPTER 23

COLOR VISION

THOMAS P. SAKMAR

Color vision is the ability to discriminate a light stimulus as a function of its wavelength. Various sensory and cognitive processes combine to result in the sense of color. The cooperative physical effects of light and object, the physiologic reaction of the visual organ to light, and the psychologic context of color perception together produce the picture of our surroundings, thus influencing our relationship and attitude toward our environment. This chapter focuses specifically on the reaction of the retina to light stimulus. The details of physical events outside of the body known as *optical physics,* theories of color, and the higher-order processing of the visual signal in the brain to produce visual experience are beyond the scope of this chapter.

COLOR AND LIGHT

Electromagnetic energy is wavelengths between approximately 380 and 760 nm and causes photoreactions on the human retina, which leads to the experience of vision. Although the perceptions caused by light waves cannot be directly measured, optical physics describes the origin of colors as a breaking down of light into its spectral constituents.[1] A *prism,* a transparent solid body with a triangular cross section, causes white, or neutral, light to be refracted so that it is divided into the spectrum of rainbow colors. Short-wavelength visible light causes the sensation of violet, and in an uneven transition, the colors blue, blue-green, green, yellow-green, yellow, orange, and red are perceived. For example, red does not noticeably change in perception from approximately 680 nm onward. *Monochromatic light* is colored light of a single wavelength. The remixing of all colors of light created by a prism, for example with a convex lens, will create the sensation of white. The sensation of white can also be created from the monochromatic light rays from the short-, middle-, and long-wavelength zones of the spectrum. For example, mixing blue (435 nm), green (545 nm), and red (700 nm) light produces white. These three light rays can also be combined to create any other color by changing the relative intensities of the individual components. Thus violet-blue, green, and red are called the *additive primary colors.*

The light rays from the mixing of any two thirds of the spectrum cause the sensations of yellow, magenta-red, and cyan-blue. These three colors are the so-called subtractive primary colors. Magenta-red, the mixing of rays of the short- and long-wavelength ends of the spectrum, does not itself exist in the natural spectrum. Any two colors are called *complementary colors* if their additive mixing forms white. Therefore it follows that blending any one additive primary color with the corresponding subtractive primary color forms the whole spectrum. The mixing of color pigments or dyes is an example of subtractive color mixing. The mixing of a cyan-blue dye and a yellow dye produces green. The cyan-blue dye absorbs, or subtracts, the long-wavelength part of the spectrum; the yellow dye absorbs the short-wavelength part. Because both dyes reflect the middle-wavelength light, green color is appreciated.

Color mixing (subtractive, additive, or proportional mixing of pairs of the six primary colors) produces the nearly limitless range of color hues that can be perceived. In addition to additive or subtractive mixing, color can be produced through the scatter of white light. One example is the deep blue–colored sky that is apparent at midday in the summer when the air is clean and dry. The sun's rays pass vertically through the earth's atmosphere and the longer wavelengths are scattered. However, at sunrise and sunset the sun's rays fall on an acute angle and their pathlength is longer, giving rise to intense red color depending on prevailing atmospheric conditions. Finally, color can result from interference on thin films. Color perception changes with slight changes in the thickness of a film or with the angle of vision. The mother-of-pearl color of soap bubbles or the feathers of iridescent birds are examples of so-called interference colors.

The human eye differentiates colors according to the color itself (its wavelength), the brightness, and the saturation. Therefore a systematic organization of all colors would be possible only in the three-dimensional system. There is no perceptual basis for a hierarchy of colors, but color wheels generally are used to organize and group chromatic colors according to their appearance.

The existence of color is at some level a topic that is equally relevant to philosophy and science. Throughout recorded history, great philosophers and scientists have written on theories of color and color sense and have provided a rich literature on the subject. Isaac Newton (1642-1727) carried out experiments with a prism that transformed the science of color from the study of objects to the study of light. Johann Wolfgang von Goethe (1749-1832) wrote extensively on the experience of color. Thomas Young (1773-1829) proposed a theory of color vision based on three receptors in the retina that are sensitive to different spectral regions. David Brewster (1781-1868) introduced the term *color blindness,* which was formerly known as *daltonism,* after John Dalton (1766-1844), who described in detail his own inability to distinguish red. The genetic basis of Dalton's color blindness was recently determined, by polymerase chain reaction analysis of DNA extracted from his preserved postmortem eye, to be deuteranopia (see following discussion).[5] Arthur Schopenhauer (1788-1860) expanded on the work of Goethe and Immanuel Kant (1724-1804). Joseph Antoine Ferdinand Plateau (1801-1883) studied afterimages and color mixing and proposed the Talbot-Plateau law of color intensity perception. Hermann Ludwig Ferdinand von Helmholtz (1821-1894) extended Young's hypothesis, henceforth called the *Young-Helmholtz hypothesis,* and devised spectral absorption curves for three visual photoreceptors. Herman Rudolf Aubert (1826-1892) was one of the key contributors to physiologic optics in addition to measuring absolute visual sensitivity and light and dark adaptation. He demonstrated that color perception was largely restricted to the foveal region and depended on context in other parts of the retina. James Clerk Maxwell (1831-1879) was largely responsible for making the study of color vision a quantitative science. He devised methods to study additive and subtractive color mixing and color-defective subjects and developed many of the classifications that are still used today.

BIOCHEMISTRY OF COLOR VISION

All human visual pigments share a common chromophore, which is chemically related to vitamin A_1. The 11-*cis*-structural isomer of the aldehyde of vitamin A_1 reacts with an opsin protein to form a photoreceptor-pigment complex. The rod and cone cell pigments are all complexes of the same chromophore with different, but related, opsin proteins. Interestingly, the genes encoding the opsin proteins are members of a superfamily of related receptors called *G protein–coupled receptors.* These receptors are involved in different sensory and intercellular signaling pathways across a wide range of organisms. The receptors are integral membrane proteins that all share a common structural motif—seven-transmembrane segments—and they all communicate with cellular biochemical signal-transducer proteins in the cellular cytoplasm called *heterotrimeric G proteins.* In the case of rod and cone cells, the G proteins are called *transducins.* Specific forms of transducins are found in rods and cones, although the three cone cell types share a common form of transducin.

The unique properties of the chromophore in its opsin-bound state contribute to the key physiologic properties of vision, including color vision. Spectral tuning at a molecular level is related to the so-called opsin-shift. The *opsin-shift* refers to the change in the absorption of the chromophore when it becomes bound to a particular opsin. The magnitude of the opsin-shift varies with each particular visual pigment.

In the biochemical amplification cascade of the photoreceptor cells of the vertebrate visual system, the capture of a photon causes irreversible photochemical isomerization of the chromophore in the visual pigment. A series of protein conformational changes ensues, and the active pigment becomes a catalyst that converts transducin into its active form. Active transducin modulates cyclic guanosine monophosphate (GMP) phosphodiesterase, cGMP levels drop, and plasma membrane–cation conductance through a cGMP-gated membrane channel protein decreases. The resulting hyperpolarization of the photoreceptor cell causes synaptic modulation, and downstream retinal signal processing can occur. Thus the basic elements of the biochemical transduction cascade are pigment, G protein, phosphodiesterase, and channel. However, numerous other regulatory proteins participate in various modulations of the signal, including signal turn-off, dark adaptation, and light adaptation.

Much of the biochemistry of visual signal transduction has been elucidated through the study of rod cells. One of the most salient and striking results of biophysical studies is that through coupled amplification cycles, the absorption of a single photon by the photopigment in a rod cell, rhodopsin, prevents approximately 10^7 ions from crossing the plasma membrane. However, despite their histologic and physiologic differences, the gains of transduction in rods and cones appear to be similar. Whereas rods are specialized for sensitivity, cone physiology is specialized for rapid temporal response, rapid recovery after exposure to intense light, and nonsaturable function over a wide range of luminosity.

The electrophysiology of cone photoreceptors and their associated retinal circuitry in the primate and human retinas are of considerable interest. One key component for future study is to elucidate the mechanism of photopic desensitization with background illumination. For example, because the magnitude of desensitization cannot be accounted for by the observed reduction of cone photocurrent or voltage, adaptation might somehow affect cone cell synaptic signaling.

Photoreceptor Cells and the Concept of Trichromacy

The retina can be thought of as the point of contact between radiated energy, light, and the human nervous system. In the initial step of color perception, light must be converted into a neurochemical signal by photoreceptor cells. As detailed in other chapters of this text, the photoreceptor cell layer is the innermost layer of the retinal neuronal cells. The two main classes of photoreceptor cells are rods and cones. Rod cells primarily mediate scotopic (dim-light) vision. Rods differentiate light intensity with a maximum response at approximately 510 nm. Cone photoreceptor cells are responsible for photopic (bright-light) color vision. Cones are significantly less sensitive than rods, but they can mediate differentiation of colors. Humans can distinguish two monochromatic light rays as close as approximately 2 nm apart, giving an effective color palette of up to 300 distinct spectral colors. The human retinal fovea contains a high density of cones but essentially no rods.

The part of the electromagnetic spectrum that makes up the sensory visible spectrum varies among organisms and species. For example, insects generally possess ultraviolet perception but lack long-wavelength sensitivity. The mammalian retina is actually highly evolved for scotopic vision as opposed to color vision. Among land mammals, only humans and old-world primates possess true trichromatic vision. Relatively recent gene duplication and unequal homologous recombination most likely produced the potential for trichromatic color vision in humans and certain nonhuman primates. The topics of ecology and evolution of visual pigment sensitivity are of considerable interest but are not discussed further here.

The most salient feature of normal human color vision is that it is trichromatic. Trichromacy results from the physiology of the retina—it is not a physical property of light. The three physiologic detection systems are the three classes of photoreceptor cells—each class containing a different photoreceptor pigment molecule—those being blue or short (S)-sensitive, green or middle (M)-sensitive, and red or long (L)-sensitive cones.[2,9] The three human cone types represent the three additive primary colors: blue, green, and red. Each pigment has a distinct absorption spectrum where absorbance is plotted as a function of the wavelength (λ) of incident light (see Color Plate 12). The peaks of absorbance vary for the three cone cell pigments, but their absorbance spectra overlap considerably so that a combination of one, two, or three cone types reacts more or less strongly to a given light stimulus.

A key fact is that the response of a particular cone cell is the same no matter what the energy is of the photon that it captures. Only the efficiency of photon capture varies with photon energy, and the dynamic output relates only to the rate of photon capture. For example, in the simplest case of a retina with only three individual cone cells, one of each class, chromatic lights would be perceived to be identical if they produce the same absorptions in all three cells, and different if they did not. Thus trichromatic vision is the result of three independent comparisons of rates of photon absorption by the three cone types.

Luminosity curves can be constructed as a function of wavelength for both scotopic and photopic vision. The entire visible spectrum ranges from approximately 400 to 700 nm. However, the peak of the photopic curve (555 nm) is red-shifted relative to that of the scotopic curve (505 nm). The scotopic curve essentially represents the photosensitivity of a single pigment, rhodopsin, whereas the photopic curve is a composite (essentially a weighted average of overlapping cone sensitivities). The boundaries of color sensitivity as projected on the retina depend on the distribution of the cone types, which are not uniform (see Color Plate 13). Of course, because the distribution of cone types varies, the photopic luminosity curve varies depending on the experimental conditions.

Signal Processing in the Retina

In development, the retina arises from an evagination of neural tube to form the optic vesicle, which subsequently invaginates to form the optic cup. The optic cup thus consists of two juxtaposed layers: The inner layer differentiates into the neural retina (rods, cones, bipolar cells, ganglion cells, horizontal cells, amacrine cells, glial cells) and the outer layer differentiates into the pigment epithelium. The neural retina is extensively laminated, but three main layers are easily appreciated. The deepest layer contains the photoreceptors. The inner nuclear layer (in the middle) contains perikarya of bipolar cells and interneurons (horizontal and amacrine cells) and glial cell nuclei. The most superficial layer is the ganglion cell layer, containing cell bodies of ganglion cells whose axons form the optic nerve.

These three layers are relatively easy to identify because they contain mainly cell bodies and are separated by thin neuropil layers: the outer plexiform layer between photoreceptors and inner nuclear layer and the inner plexiform layer between the inner nuclear and ganglion cell layers. The proportion, distribution, and patterning of rods and cones over the retina vary among species. In humans, cones are concentrated in the central retina. The unique biochemistry and ultrastructural anatomy of photoreceptor cells accounts for their unusual physiology: They are neurons that do not generate all-or-none action potentials. Rather, light causes a graded response, a membrane hyperpolarization that is detected by ganglion cells that do produce action potentials. The most simplified linear axis of retinal signaling is photoreceptor cell to bipolar cell to ganglion cell.

In addition to the response of threshold of an individual photoreceptor cell to light, the phenomena of convergence and divergence are functionally important neural mechanisms for determining acuity and spectral sensitivity. *Convergence,* or pooling, refers to the projection of multiple photoreceptor cells on a lesser number of bipolar cells. *Divergence* refers to the projection of a single photoreceptor cell on multiple cells in the next layer. For example, one cone may form functional synapses to three bipolar cells. One key difference between rod and cone systems is their respective degrees of convergence. Foveal cone cells tend to have so-called private-line communication—no divergence. In the retinal periphery, the photoreceptor cells, including mostly rods but also some cones, greatly outnumber the ganglion cells. Convergence is the rule in the periphery; the result is high sensitivity but low acuity.

The amacrine and horizontal cells are interneurons that permit lateral interactions within the retina. Although amacrine and horizontal cells are separate and distinct cell types, it should be noted that a wide range of distinctly different morphologic cell types exists in the primate interneuron layer. For example, there may be 20 to 50 types of amacrine cells, and the physiology of only a few of these cell types has been studied in any detail. A presentation of the precise topographic organization of the retina, the central visual pathways, and the subcortical and cortical visual center is beyond the intended scope of this chapter.

An understanding of the connections between retinal physiology and peripheral mechanisms in general and the associated central mechanisms to color perception is incomplete in any case. Color perception does, of course, require photon absorption by the three classes of receptors with different spectral responses. The chemical results of the photon capture are then transmitted to so-called opponent processes. A great deal is known about the process of proton absorption and subsequent signaling in the retina. Significant signal processing related to color perception occurs in the neuronal cell layers of the retina, and the peripheral mechanisms underlying color perception, in contrast with the central mechanisms, are generally well understood. Although a number of significant questions remain to be answered, psychophysical studies have provided a well-defined framework. Retinal neurons respond reliably to chromatic stimuli. Neurons of a particular class tend to behave reproducibly, and if not linearly, they at least display straightforward nonlinearities. However, understanding color perception requires the study of higher-order color mechanisms, primarily through psychophysical experiments.

The Young-Helmholtz theory of color vision emphasizes trichromacy and was essentially confirmed by the discovery of three cone photoreceptor systems as described previously. Historically, however, another theory was proposed to describe the process of color perception. Karl Hering (1834-1918) developed the opponent theory of color vision based on the hypothetical existence of three oppositional color pigment pairs.[4] These oppositional pairs are now known not to exist, but Hering's theory was correct in the sense that the signals from the three cone types are combined, not at the pigment level as he had suggested, but at the level of neurons to produce opposing pairs of red-green, blue-yellow, and black-white. Later work confirmed the role of opposing excitatory and inhibitory interactions in color perception.

Hering's proposals concerning opponent processes arose from relatively simple observations, but more recently, detailed definitions of a variety of concepts have advanced the study of second-stage mechanisms of color perception (i.e., mechanisms subsequent to activation of the cone cell biochemical signal-transduction pathway). The concepts relevant to second-stage mechanisms include definitions of color space useful for both psychophysical and electrophysiologic experiments and the identification of neural mechanisms that essentially transform in some way the retinal image (e.g., edge enhancement, spectral differencing, contrast induction, adaptation to steady background or temporally varying illumination, interference of motion and three-dimensional shape, perceptual constancy). If the most important task of visual perception is to segregate different objects from each other and from background, it follows that any visual process that enhances the perception of a difference between two contiguous fields will be beneficial. In this regard, color cues provide useful information in the perception of both shape and motion.

Opponent processes refer to apparently antagonistic responses within the retina that can be best understood by considering the concepts of neuronal excitation and inhibition. In the retina, opposing positive excitatory and negative inhibitory effects are organized in a clear, concentric spatial format. Kuffler[7] first mapped the organization of receptive fields in the retina in 1953.[7] In the retina the receptive field of a single ganglion cell can be defined by mapping the area of a stimulus that affects its rate of discharge in electrophysiologic recordings. A typical ganglion cell responds to an achromatic (dark-light) stimulus of its receptive field according to a pattern termed *center-surround.* The examples of two particular center-surround neurons (ON-center and OFF-center) demonstrate the concept of balanced antagonistic mechanisms in the retina. Ambient light produces a background rate of discharge. In ON-center neurons, a tiny spot of white light focused at the center of the receptive field produces a burst of discharge. When the center stimulus is terminated, a transient decrease in the rate of background discharge is observed. This temporal pattern of discharge is called an *ON-response.* If the light is focused as a discrete annulus surrounding a dark center of the field, the background discharge is inhibited. When the ring-shaped surround stimulus is terminated, a burst of discharge is noted. This temporal pattern of discharge is called an *OFF-response.* In OFF-center neurons, stimulation of the receptive field center causes an OFF-response and stimulation of the surround causes an ON-response. For achromatic stimuli the sizes of receptive field centers vary. Receptive field centers may be approximately 2 minutes of arc in the fovea and 2 degrees in the periphery. The size of the surround region is similar (approximately 2 degrees) throughout the retina.

For color vision, these opponent processes are also significant because antagonistic color responses are found at each level of the visual pathway, including the retina. In animals with high proportions of cone photoreceptors, center-surround mechanisms generally exhibit spectral sensitivities. For example, the center mechanism, which may be "ON" or "OFF," might display the spectral sensitivity curve of M-wavelength–sensing cones. The surround mechanism, which is antagonistic to the center mechanism, might display an L-wavelength–sensing cone sensitivity. Such receptive fields are classified according to whether they are ON-center or OFF-center and whether the center and surround show a spectral sensitivity approximating M-, L-, or S-wavelength–sensing cones. Less common are fields with center and surround mechanisms with the same, or similar, spectral sensitivities. Rarely, a receptive field shows no evidence of center-surround organization: A stimulus by light of one wavelength anywhere in the field causes an ON response, whereas a stimulus by light of a different wavelength produces an OFF response. In general, the range of color opponency displayed by M- and L-wavelength–sensing cones is greater than that of S-wavelength–sensing cones. Color Plate 14 represents schematically how the three cone systems might contribute to three types of receptive field neurons.

Several additional phenomena occur at the level of the retina and influence color perception, including optical mixing of small surfaces. For example, a color photographic print consists of three layers of color in a so-called gray screen of small dots of yellow, magenta-red, and cyan-blue. All other colors arc created at the level of the retina through optical mixing. Black is created where all three dots overlap, and gray is created when the proportion and distribution of the three-color dots is equal. Subtractive mixing of overlapping transparent color dots in the retina creates violet-blue, green, and red. Optical mixing is also exploited in glowing television or computer screens that consist of points of blue, green, and red light that mix to form a gray background. As the intensities of the points change, all other colors are created.

Another example of optical mixing is easily demonstrated by using a colored disc on a spinning top, often called *Maxwell's disc* after James Clerk Maxwell. If the disc is colored half red and half blue, the perceived color of the spinning disc resembles magenta, a color that is not present on the object at all. The spinning disc stimulates red and blue sectors of the same point of the retina in rapid succession.

Color sensation can be caused by colored light rays and also by the activity of cone cells, principally by the phenomenon known as *negative afterimage,* in which an unchanging (adapted) image impressed on the retina moves when the eyes move and refocus. Afterimages can influence color perception, but generally not consciously.

Discussions of color adaptation and the influence of the appearance of color by its surroundings, or so-called simultaneous alternating effects of colors, are beyond the scope of this chapter.[8] However, the key point to be made is that the appearance of a color depends on its relationship to its surroundings.

MOLECULAR GENETICS OF COLOR VISION

Because human trichromatic color vision requires three classes of pigments with overlapping relative spectral sensitivities, but not necessarily any one particular pigment color, it is common to refer to the photopigment classes as short (S)-, middle (M)-, and long (L)-wavelength sensitive, rather than blue, green, and red sensitive. The molecular genetics of human color vision is complex because one of three distinct genes has to be expressed in a particular cone cell that is otherwise identical to its neighboring cones. The complexity arises in part because of M- and L-sensitive genes, which are approximately 98% identical, are juxtaposed on the X chromosome. Individual X chromosomes contain variable numbers of M- and L-sensitive genes arranged linearly in a tandem repeat array. Gene rearrangements including duplication and recombination have caused a great deal of variability in these gene arrays in the human population.

Recent advances in molecular biology have allowed remarkable parallel advances in understanding the molecular basis for color perception, especially at the level of the photoreceptor molecules.[5] However, variations in red-green color perception vary widely even within a particular broad genetic classification. The most reasonable hypothesis that links genotype to clinical phenotype may be the so-called spectral proximity hypothesis, which states that red-green color discrimination is a function of the difference between the wavelengths of maximal absorption of the M- and L-sensitive pigments. A normal separation of approximately 30 nm (approximately 560 nm versus 530 nm) might be optimal.

COLOR VISION DEFECTS AND COLOR VISION TESTING

Red-green color vision deficiency may result from the loss of an M- or L-wavelength gene, called *deuteranopia* and *protanopia,* respectively.[10,11,14] Loss of the S-sensitive wavelength gene would result in *tritanopia.* Inherited color vision defects that affect one pigment class are not generally associated with other visual dysfunction. However, severe loss of visual acuity may be associated with the absence of multiple cone types, as in various incomplete or complete achromatopsias.[3]

A short discussion of inherited defects in red-green, or X-linked, color perception is relevant because up to 10% of males in the United States are affected. The most severely affected individuals are called *dichromats* because the sensitivity of one cone type is absent—L-sensing cones in protanopes and M-sensing cones in deuteranopes. The cones' sensitivities are absent because the corresponding pigment gene has been deleted from the X chromosome. Although anomalous trichromacy produces a milder form of color vision defect, which is still based on the presence of three spectral classes of functional cone cells, the underlying molecular genetics is much more complicated. In the case of *protanomaly* the presence of an L-wavelength–

sensitive pigment with an anomalous absorption spectrum, the normal L-wavelength–sensing gene is absent but its function is partially replaced by the presence of a second M-wavelength–sensing gene with a shift in its spectral peak relative to the normal M-sensing gene. The presence of anomalous M-wavelength–sensing pigment genes can be explained in terms of the mechanism of genetic rearrangements and the observation that a high degree of genetic polymorphism exists within both the M- and L-wavelength–sensing genes in humans.

Deuteranomaly, which is the most common type of color vision defect, may affect 1 in 20 males and 3 in 1000 females in the United States. In analogy with protanomaly, three functional cone classes exist—normal S- and L-wavelength–sensing cones and a spectrally anomalous second L-wavelength pigment. What are the consequences of a defect in red-green color perception, if any? Dichromacy and severe anomalous trichromacy result in significant perceptual disabilities. The normal visual perception of more than 100 different fully saturated hues may be reduced to one or two. Many of the activities of daily life are based on color images and color cues designed on a presumption of universal capacity for trichromatic color vision. Thus early diagnosis of color vision defects might allow for early modifications in educational and other activities.

Patients with severe cases of protanopia or deuteranopia confuse red and green, and those with tritanopia confuse yellow and blue or orange and violet. A variety of methods to screen for color defects, particularly protan and deutan defects, have been devised.[1,13] These include pseudoisochromatic color confusion charts (e.g., Dvorine, Ishihara, Stilling, Neitz), hue arrangement tasks (e.g., Farnsworth-Munsell 100-hue test, Farnsworth Panel D15, Lanthony Desaturated D-15), and lantern detection tests (e.g., Edridge-Green, Holmes-Wright). Despite the variety of testing methods available, or perhaps partly because of it, diagnostic testing for detecting color vision defects is not straightforward. Any test should ideally distinguish between patients with normal and abnormal color vision, between protan and deutan defects, and between congenital and acquired defects. In addition, tests should be easy to administer and should not require significant active cooperation on the part of the patient. The most widely used diagnostic tool is the Ishihara test, a collection of printed pseudoisochromatic plates. The Ishihara test is one of the best screening tests available, but it is not ideal because it is difficult to stan-

dardize and insensitive. Many patients with normal color vision make errors, and the test cannot reliably characterize a defect as protan versus deutan. Furthermore, the test cannot distinguish mild from severe defects or congenital from acquired defects. Color vision defects identified by a variety of screening tests, including the Ishihara test, generally require additional genetic and psychophysical testing by an experienced practitioner.

Precise follow-up testing is usually carried out using an instrument called an *anomaloscope* (Nagel Type I anomaloscope) to characterize so-called Rayleigh matches.[1] In a Rayleigh matching experiment the subject is simply asked to match a primary light that is spectral yellow (589 nm) to a mixture of primary light comprised of spectral red (679 nm) and spectral green (544 nm). The two variables are the intensity of the primary yellow light and the relative intensities of red and green lights that make up the mix. The rods and S-sensitive cones are excluded by limiting the viewing field to approximately 2 degrees of the fovea. The Rayleigh match is the intersection on a plot of the yellow intensity and the green–red mix ratio, and most normal trichromats choose a unique match reproducibly. Patients with defects may choose a match outside of the normal range, or they may allow more than one matching green–red ratio, depending on the type of defect. In summary, the precise phenotypes of color vision defects broadly called *protanopia* and *deuteranopia* are complex and variable, as are the underlying genotypes.

Disease or exposure to drugs or toxins also can affect color perception. Acquired disturbances of color vision are highly variable, and the clinical nomenclature tends to be somewhat confusing. Although the term *dyschromatopsia* refers to any disturbance of color perception, it is more commonly used in connection with acquired rather than congenital defects. *Chromatopsia,* which refers to the perception of color into a normally white or achromatic scene, is a particularly important symptom of many types of acquired defects. For example, xanthopsia is associated with the use of cardiac glycosides, and cyanopsia has been associated with the use of sildenafil citrate. Both of these adverse drug effects probably occur at the level of the retina. Dyschromatopsia is often a sensitive early symptom or diagnostic sign of an associated disease such as macular degeneration, glaucoma, or diabetic retinopathy. As such, color vision testing may be appropriate as a single noninvasive diagnostic screening test for a variety of disorders.

REFERENCES

1. Birch J: *Diagnosis of defective colour vision*, Oxford, UK, 1993, Oxford University Press.
2. Fasick JI, Lee N, Oprian DD: Spectral tuning in the human blue cone pigment, *Biochemistry* 38:11593, 1999.
3. Fletcher R, Voke J: *Defective colour vision: fundamentals, diagnosis and management*, Bristol, UK, 1985, Adam Hilger.
4. Hering E: *Outline of a theory of the light sense*, Cambridge, Mass, 1964, Harvard University Press (Translated by L Hurvich, D Jameson; originally published in 1874).
5. Hunt DM et al: The chemistry of John Dalton's color blindness, *Science* 267:984, 1995.
6. Krauskopf J: Higher order color mechanisms. In Gegenfurtner KR, Sharpe LT (eds): *Color vision: from genes to perception*, Cambridge, UK, 1999, Cambridge University Press.
7. Kuffler SW: Discharge patterns and functional organisation of mammalian retina, *J Neurophysiol* 16:37, 1953.
8. Lennie P: Color coding in the cortex. In Gegenfurtner KR, Sharpe LT (eds): *Color vision: from genes to perception*, Cambridge, UK, 1999, Cambridge University Press.
9. Merbs SL, Nathans J: Absorption spectra of human cone pigments, *Nature* 34:433, 1992.
10. Nathans J et al: Molecular genetics of inherited variations in human color vision, *Science* 232:203, 1986.
11. Neitz M, Neitz J: Molecular genetics of color vision and color vision defects, *Arch Ophthalmol* 118:691, 2000.
12. Oprian DD et al: Design, chemical synthesis, and expression of genes for the three human color vision pigments, *Biochemistry* 30:11367, 1991.
13. Regan BC, Reffin JP, Mollon JD: Luminance noise and the rapid determination of discrimination ellipses in color deficiency, *Vision Res* 34:1279, 1994.
14. Sharpe LT et al: Opsin genes, cone photopigments, color vision, and color blindness. In Gegenfurtner KR, Sharpe LT (eds): *Color vision: from genes to perception*, Cambridge, UK, 1999, Cambridge University Press.
15. Zaidi Q: Color and brightness induction: from Mach bands to three-dimensional configurations. In Gegenfurtner KR, Sharpe LT (eds): *Color vision: from genes to perception*, Cambridge, UK, 1999, Cambridge University Press.
16. Zwimpfer M: *Color: light sight, sense—an elementary theory of color in pictures*, West Chester, Pa, 1988, Schiffer.

CHAPTER 24

VISUAL ADAPTATION

DAVID G. BIRCH

The range of illuminances to which humans are exposed daily is enormous. Although it may be less important today than for our ancestors, we can see on dim moonless nights when only a few quanta reach the eye from an object. At the other extreme, we must be able to see at midday on the beach, when millions of quanta may be entering the eye each second. These ambient light levels vary over a range of 1 billion-fold. Because of the magnitude of these numbers, it is traditional in visual science to deal with the $\log_{10}$ of the illuminances involved, so one says, for example, that light levels range over 9 logarithmic (log) units. Of course, it is not the illuminance falling on objects that is of primary concern, but rather the light reflected from objects, or their luminance. At different times of day (and year), the visual environment has a different mean luminance, and around this average, particular objects may be brighter or darker than the mean. Because these differences define the shapes and ultimately the identification of objects within the visual world, the task of the visual system is to detect small differences around the mean luminance. Over millions of years, mammalian visual systems have evolved to maximize the ability to detect these slight increments and decrements in luminance.

The output of the retina is the axon potentials transmitted to the lateral geniculate nucleus and visual cortex by ganglion cells. Axons have a range of firing rates, varying roughly from 1 to 100 spikes per second (with bursts to 1000 per second). This 2- to 3-log unit variation is considered the operating range of the cell. It is clear that a major task of the retina is to adjust the operating range of the ganglion cells to the ambient light level in the environment. The retinal origin of mechanisms underlying light and dark adaptation has been under-

stood for many years. Light and dark adaptation proceeded normally in a human subject when the eye was pressure-blinded during the light-adaptation period.[32] The adapting light was not seen because ganglion cell output from the retina was blocked. Nevertheless, visual sensitivity measured in that eye when the pressure was relieved was decreased to the same extent as that in a non–pressure-blinded eye, and the subsequent time course of dark adaptation was perfectly normal. Moreover, many aspects of adaptation can be studied in both humans and animals with the electroretinogram (ERG). The ERG is a record of the diffuse electrical activity generated by the retina in response to light stimulation. With appropriate stimulation and recording techniques, it is possible to derive responses that can be localized to different cell types and layers within the retina.

The speed with which the retina must make the adjustment depends on the rapidity of the change in the environment. Some mechanisms of adaptation are extremely slow and involve structural modifications of the visual apparatus. This plasticity in structure allows humans to adjust to slow changes in ambient light level as a result of changes in latitude, season, or habitat. More rapid, primarily photochemical, adjustments are needed to match sensitivity to the daily light cycle. Extremely rapid neural adjustments constantly fine-tune the match to mean luminance during daily activity. These mechanisms for adjusting the operating range of the visual system are not only interesting in their own right, representing as they do one of the primary functions of the retina, but are also becoming increasingly important for understanding, and in some cases diagnosing, retinal disease. The number of mapped chromosomal loci encoding genes active primarily in the retina presently stands at 124, and 62 of these genes have been cloned.[90] Because of the exponential growth in gene mapping, it is likely that all retinal genes will be cloned within a few years. What is emerging is a molecular biologic understanding of the phototransduction cycle and the visual cycle. It is already clear that patients with mutations in certain specific genes have predictable deficits in adapting to variations in ambient lighting. An understanding of the phenomena and predominant theories of light and dark adaptation is therefore also important for understanding certain symptoms of genetic eye disease.

STRUCTURAL MECHANISMS OF ADAPTATION

The most obvious structural adaptation to the problem of detection over an enormous range of illumination is the evolution of two overlapping systems. Just as a photographer may switch the speed of the film, most mammals switch from "fine-grain" color detection in bright light to highly sensitive, "coarse-grain" achromatic detection at low light levels. It seems reasonable that the mechanisms of dark and light adaptation evolved to meet the needs of the environment. It takes a long time to become accustomed to the dark. In fact, the time course of dark adaptation is well matched to slow onset of dusk and darkness when the sun sets. There was probably little evolutionary pressure to evolve a faster mechanism. However, the slow time course is often a hindrance in the modern world of artificial lighting and darkness. When entering the dark from a brightly lit environment, this switch to rod-mediated vision appears to take an inordinate amount of time. At first one is severely handicapped, unable to distinguish any detail. One quickly reaches a level at which one can maneuver with the help of a flashlight. In these initial moments, one is functioning with cone-mediated vision alone. However, it may take 15 or 20 minutes before it is possible to move around without stumbling over objects. This length of time is required for the rods to reach their maximum efficiency. The reverse process, adaptation to a high level of illumination, is more rapid. When one ventures outside on a bright day, there may be a brief period of being dazzled by bright sunlight. Within a few minutes, however, the discomfort that might have been experienced disappears and one can comfortably negotiate the environment.

The rod system in most mammals is ideally adapted for optimal detection of visible quanta (i.e., those within the spectral range of rod visual pigment). It has become apparent in recent years, however, that there are trade-offs involved in maximizing sensitivity. Rods that are more sensitive to light appear to also be more susceptible to light damage. Thus mechanisms for long-term structural adaptation exist to match the sensitivity of rods to the photic environment. For example, rats reared in cyclic light had shorter rod outer segments than did animals reared for at least 2 weeks in total darkness.[5,77] In addition, the phospholipid/opsin ratio was 20% to 25% higher in the cyclic-light animals, and the total rod outer segment phospholipid weight was reduced.[77] Taken together, these results suggest that sizable differences in photopigment concentration result from variations in ambient light environment. Consistent with this suggestion, Figure 24-1 shows axial absorbance in rats raised in lighting regimens with a 12 hour on/12 hour off cycle at different levels of illumination. For rats raised under each intensity, axial absorbance varies with retinal position. The higher axial absorbance in rats maintained in darkness leads to lower rod ERG thresholds than in cyclic-reared rats.[15] These animals are also more susceptible to retinal light damage than are animals maintained in a daily regimen of 12 hours of dim light and 12 hours of darkness.[16,76,78] The area of the retina of a dim-light–reared rat containing the highest rhodopsin concentration (the superior central region in Figure 24-1) is that which sustains the greatest loss in photoreceptors on exposure to bright light. It has been proposed that retinal changes induced by bright light may also be viewed as adaptive,[79] in that they are part of the mechanism whereby the photon-catching ability of the retina can be adjusted up or down to compensate for a long-term change in environmental lighting.[108] The plasticity in the retina that is necessary to achieve this regulation despite variations in day length, average light intensities, and preretinal filtering has been termed *photostasis*.[80] Subsequent work has shown that a photostasis number of about 10^6 absorbed photons per eye per day is maintained by varying rhodopsin levels and numbers of rod cells in response to habitat light intensity.[109]

Photostasis requires a mechanism for adjusting mammalian rod light-absorbing properties in response to the demands of the photic environment. One such mechanism may involve light regulation of rod outer segment renewal. Histologic studies have documented a burst of disc shedding from the rod outer segment tip between 1 and 2 hours after daily light onset.[66] The renewal process can be docu-

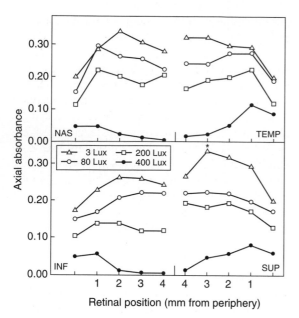

FIGURE 24-1   Axial absorbance versus retinal position for 10 locations each in the horizontal and vertical meridians. Axial absorbance is the absorbance at 500 nm per micron, multiplied by the average length of rod outer segments in that area. Animals maintained under dim lighting conditions have the greatest axial absorbance. The region between 1 and 2 mm superior to the optic nerve has the highest absorbance and is the most susceptible to light damage. (From Penn JS, Williams TP: *Exp Eye Res* 43:915, 1986.)

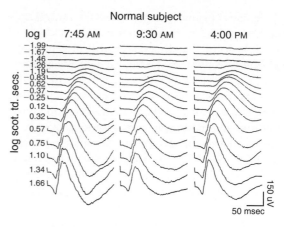

FIGURE 24-2   Rod responses over a series of retinal illuminances at three times of day in an entrained normal subject. Responses at each retinal illuminance were smaller at 9:30 AM than at other times of day. (From Birch DG: *Invest Ophthalmol Vis Sci* 28:2042, 1987.)

mented in humans maintained under strictly controlled diurnal lighting. As shown in Figure 24-2, rod ERGs are visibly smaller to all flash intensities at a time 90 minutes after the sudden onset of light than at other times of day. These ERG correlates of renewal have been obtained with a strict regimen of light exposure controlled by light-tight occluders.[13,18] Psychophysical methods have not been used with the same control over light onset. Available studies do suggest, however, that there is modest diurnal rhythmicity for visual sensitivity in humans.[104] During the course of the day, new outer segment discs are synthesized at the base of the rod.[12] The entire outer segment is renewed every 10 days.[114] One function of this renewal may be to create the plasticity that allows for adaptation by photoreceptors to the environment across a wide range of ambient lighting conditions.[80] Thus animals living in dim light conditions, where ambient photons are scarce, would have retinas with greater photon-catching ability than would animals living in a brighter light environment, where photons are abundant. Rod outer seg-

ment renewal would be partly responsible for these adjustments. Synthesis of membrane components in the inner segment and their subsequent incorporation into the outer segment would control both the number of discs produced per day and the rhodopsin concentration per disc, whereas shedding at the tip, combined with synthesis, would determine the outer segment length.

RECEPTORAL MECHANISMS OF ADAPTATION

An important achievement of the science of visual psychophysics has been the establishment of techniques that make the response from a human subject observable. Whereas the goal is often to understand visual experience and sensations, psychophysical techniques render these experiences objective and observable. Psychophysical techniques have been used since the 1930s to probe the underlying physiologic basis of visual adaptation.[50,100] These techniques have revealed extremely rapid adjustments in sensitivity in response to moderate changes in background intensity (light adaptation) and prolonged recovery of sensitivity after exposure to extremely intense light (dark adaptation). Historically, it has also been clear that adaptive mechanisms exists at receptoral, postreceptoral, and cortical levels of visual processing, in part because light adaptation begins at background levels well below those that cause measurable decreases in photoreceptor sensitivity.[6,42,46,93] In fact, the rod system is desensitized by backgrounds in which less than 1 quantum is absorbed per rod. Nevertheless, postreceptoral processes are dependent on photoreceptor activity, so it seems clear that the adaptational state of the visual system will ultimately be determined by events in the photoreceptors.[105]

Processes underlying activation and inactivation in vertebrate rods are now understood in great detail[39] (Figure 24-3). During the excitation phase of the rod photoresponse, light stimulates an enzymatic cascade that culminates in the hydrolysis of cyclic guanosine monophosphate (cGMP).[60,101] The interaction of excited rhodopsin (R*) with many G protein molecules (transducin [T]) causes each of them to release guanosine diphosphate (GDP) and bind guanosine triphosphate (GTP). T-GTP then activates cGMP phosphodiesterase (PDE) that hydrolyses cGMP to 5′-GMP. The drop in cGMP caused by PDE activation causes closure of plasma membrane channels held open by cGMP in darkness, which halts the continuous entry of Na^+ and Ca^{2+} ions and results in a transient hyperpolarization of the cell. Several processes contribute to the recovery phase of the photoresponse. First, activated rhodopsin is phosphorylated by rhodopsin kinase, which decreases the ability of R* to stimulate T. It also stimulates the binding of Arrestin to rhodopsin, further reducing its ability to activate T. Activated transducin α-subunits (Tα) already formed by the activated rhodopsin deactivate when their bound GTP is hydrolyzed to GDP. GTP hydrolysis appears to be modulated by the newly discovered RGS-9 protein.[25,49] Tα-GDP then reassociates with transducin βγ-subunits (Tβγ) and releases the phosphodiesterase γ-subunit (PDEγ), which reinhibits PDE activity. Light-stimulated hydrolysis of cGMP within rod photoreceptors leads to the closure of cGMP-gated cation channels in the photoreceptor plasma membrane. Because the cGMP channels are the major route by which Ca^{2+} enters the photoreceptor, this light-stimulated closure of these channels causes the intracellular concentration of Ca^{2+} to fall. Lowered Ca^{2+} levels stimulate the activity of guanylate cyclase, which then accelerates cGMP resynthesis and the restoration of the dark conductance.

Only recently has it become clear that in many warm-blooded animals, including rats, cats, rabbits, cows, monkeys, and humans, rod photoreceptors show the same kind of background adaptation once thought to be characteristic of lower vertebrates.[54,58,73,103] It may be relatively less important in warm-blooded animals because it is evident only at

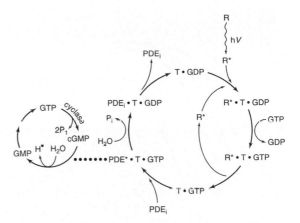

FIGURE 24-3 The cyclic guanosine monophosphate cascade of phototransduction. Activation of rhodopsin (*R*) by light leads to the activation of phosphodiesterase (*PDE*) and hydrolysis of cyclic guanosine monophosphate (*cGMP*). *GDP*, Guanosine diphosphate; *T-GTP*, transducin bound to guanosine triphosphate. (From Falk G: Retinal physiology. In Heckenlively J, Arden G (eds): *Principles and practice of clinical electrophysiology of vision*, St Louis, 1991, Mosby.)

high background levels. Responses to flashes superimposed on a steady background become smaller and more rapid than responses to flashes in the dark, with a pronounced shortening in the time to peak photoresponse.[8,38,74] Characteristic data obtained from intracellular microelectrode recording techniques are shown in Figure 24-4.[38] Responses were obtained from a single rod photoreceptor after stimulation by test flashes superimposed on full-field adapting backgrounds. With increasing levels of adaptation, a family of curves is produced that is shifted progressively toward the right. The flash sensitivity, defined as the change in current per photon absorbed, declines linearly with log increases in background intensity. During recovery in the dark after bright exposure, sensitivity remains low (bleaching adaptation) as long as unregenerated rhodopsin is still present. Recent evidence suggests that the underlying mechanism may be similar to background adaptation.[30,31] At this time it is unclear where in the photoreceptor enzymatic cascade adaptation occurs, but there is evidence that it may occur at multiple stages. Although still controversial, the preponderance of evidence suggests that it probably does not occur in the initial kinetics of T activation.* However, adaptation could influence

*References 7, 54, 61, 63, 75, 83.

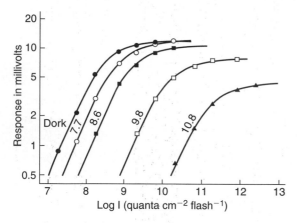

FIGURE 24-4   Shifting of rod intensity–response curves with variations in adapting background illumination. Photoresponse amplitudes are plotted against log stimulus intensity for five different levels of background illumination. Background intensities are given at left of each curve in same units as stimulus intensities (log quanta cm^{-2} flash^{-1}). (From Fain GL: *J Physiol Lond* 261:71, 1976.)

the duration of T activation, the turnoff of activated PDE, or channel sensitivity. A large body of evidence suggests that the drop in cytoplasmic Ca^{2+} caused by channel closing activates a negative feedback loop by stimulating guanylate cyclase and cGMP recovery.[102,113] Thus the decrease in cytoplasmic calcium may be crucial in regulating the adaptation of the photoresponse.[70,85]

Although the effects of background light on photoreceptor activation and inactivation have been worked out primarily in vitro, new techniques developed in the past decade seek to establish a bridge to human vision and ultimately to retinal disease. It has become evident that the leading edge of the a wave of the ERG, which has long been known to reflect photoreceptor activity, can in fact provide a precise measure of the massed response of the photoreceptors.[53,54] Moreover, it is possible to fit the computational model of Lamb and Pugh[64] to families of rod a-wave responses to derive parameters reflecting the activation stages of phototransduction.[23,28,54,98] However, the b wave and other postreceptor components begin to dominate the human ERG at approximately 10 to 20 milliseconds and thus obscure the subsequent response of the rods. Photocurrent data obtained from mammalian rods in vitro predict a time scale of several hundred milliseconds or more, depending on flash intensity, for the rod response in vivo.[9,26,58,73,103] Thus, in the human ERG, the period of develop-

ment of the leading edge of the rod a wave represents only a tiny fraction of the duration of the rod flash response and special procedures are necessary to measure the entire rod photoresponse from the ERG in human patients. These procedures use the paired-flash method used in recent studies of the human ERG and in similar in vivo studies of the mouse ERG to analyze the recovery kinetics of the rod a wave after a saturating test flash.* In this method the amplitude of the rod response at a given time after the test flash is determined from the a-wave response to a bright probe flash that rapidly drives the rods to saturation. Properties of the derived response from the human ERG (time course, sensitivity, and adaptation) are comparable to those of in vitro rod photocurrent responses obtained in previous studies.[81] For flashes of increasing intensities above amplitude saturation, there is a progressively delayed onset of the falling (recovery) phase of the response with increasing flash intensity.[19] Thus ERG recordings in normal humans and patients with retinal disease can be used to study photoreceptor background adaptation directly. Moreover, these same techniques can be used in animals, in which intracellular recordings are also available for comparison and in which powerful molecular and biochemical techniques can be used to probe mechanisms of phototransduction and adaptation.

The leading edge of the a wave can also be used to study the time course of rod photoreceptor adaptation after a bleaching light exposure. Representative recovery functions derived from the rod ERG in human subjects and mice are shown in Figure 24-5. The left panel shows rod-isolated a-wave responses obtained from a normal human subject at various times after exposure to a full-field adapting light that resulted in an approximately 30% photobleach.[53] The superimposed responses are to bright flashes that saturate the photoresponse (i.e., produce a maximal photoresponse amplitude). The amplitude of the underlying photoresponse can be determined by fitting the phototransduction activation model, an example of which is shown by the dashed curve fit to the dark-adapted response. It can be seen that the rod photoresponse is barely detectable 1 minute after the bleaching exposure and that it grows in amplitude over a 20-minute period. A recovery function from a human subject based on the amplitude of the photoresponse at a fixed time interval following the flash is shown in Figure 24-5, *B*.

---

*References 14, 17, 20, 45, 51, 68, 81, 82.

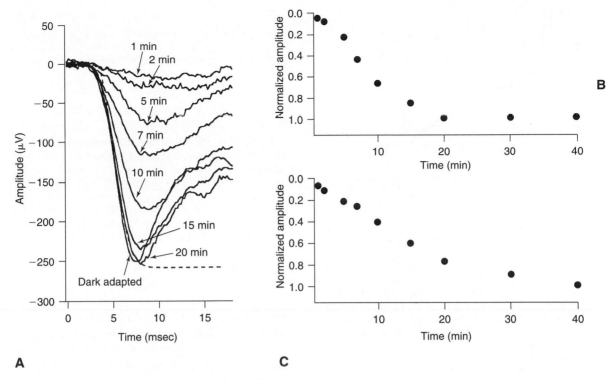

FIGURE 24-5 Recovery of responses to a bright flash after a bleach. **A,** Superimposed rod-only responses (after subtracting cone components) to bright flashes (4.0 log scot td-sec) at times indicated in a human subject. *Dashed line* is fit of phototransduction model to leading edge of dark-adapted response. **B,** Time course of recovery after a 30% bleach in a human subject. Normalized amplitudes at a fixed time interval after the flash are based on data similar to that in **A. C,** Time course of recovery after a 45% bleach in a pigmented mouse.

There is an obvious overall similarity to the a-wave–derived curve from a pigmented mouse shown following an approximately 45% photobleach (Figure 24-5, *C*).

The rod-isolated components of the ERG provide a measure of the time course of recovery for the rod system in isolation. In contrast, the psychophysically determined dark-adaptation function in the human is more complex, representing as it does the sensitivity of the most sensitive mechanism at any given time. As shown in Figure 24-6, sensitivity immediately after a full bleach is mediated by cones over the initial several minutes. The cone-mediated threshold falls relatively rapidly during dark adaptation and reaches a plateau within about 5 minutes. After approximately 10 minutes, the rod system takes over and rod thresholds fall gradually over the next 20 minutes to reach maximum sensitivity, that, is, the absolute threshold. Dark-adaptation functions such as these can readily be obtained in the clinic with the Goldmann-Weekers (G-W) Dark Adaptometer (Haag-Streit). Traditional testing with the G-W involves repeated presentation of an 11-degree achromatic stimulus to a retinal locus in the parafovea. The luminosity of the G-W stimulus is continuously adjustable over an 8 log unit range. After a patient has been exposed to a bleaching adaptation field, the examiner traces the ever-decreasing threshold of the patient for approximately 30 minutes, when dark adaptation is normal; however, dark adaptation can last several hours in certain retinal disorders.

The focus of the early work for the key determinant in the rise of visual threshold after exposure to a prolonged adapting light is the amount of visual pigment (rhodopsin) bleached. For the case in which the duration is well below the regeneration time constant, the fraction p_o of unbleached rhodopsin remaining immediately after bleaching by a light of intensity (I) and duration t_o is given by the following formula[92]

$$\log(\log 1/p_o) = \log(It_o) - 7.3$$

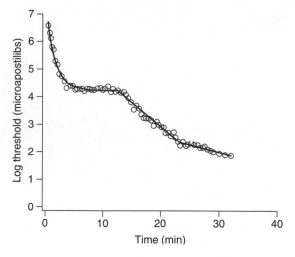

FIGURE 24-6 Psychophysical dark adaptation function from a normal human subject. An exponential decay function is fit to the cone component of recovery. Following Lamb,[62] three rate constants are fit to the rod limb. The first component of the rod-mediated dark adaptation is obscured by the cone limb. The second limb (here between approximately 11 and 22 minutes) has a time constant of about 100 seconds. The third component (here after 22 minutes) has a time constant of about 7 minutes.

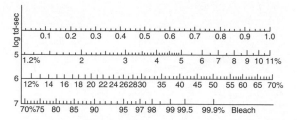

FIGURE 24-7 Scales to show the relation between log (It_o), the bleaching energy in log td-sec, and the percentage of pigment bleached by it. Lower three scales show figures of percentage of bleaching from 1% to 99.9%. The number at the left of the scale containing a specific percentage followed by the decimal on the top scale is the log td-sec that bleached the selected percentage of rhodopsin. (From Rushton WAH, Powell DS: *Vis Res* 12:1073, 1972.)

If this equation seems intimidating, there are useful scales provided by Rushton and Powell[95] and reproduced in Figure 24-7. The lower three scales show the percentage of bleaching from 1% to 99.9%. Simply place a vertical edge through any value of percent bleach. Read off the number at the left of the scale containing the value followed by the decimal on the top scale indicated by the vertical edge. For cxample, a 30% bleach of rhodopsin is produced by an exposure of about 6.5 log scotopic troland-sec. A troland-sec is a measure of retinal illuminance and is equal to the luminance in cd/m² × the pupil area × the duration of the flash. Thus a light of 1600 scotopic cd/m² (3.2 log) with a dilated pupil area of 50 mm² (1.7 log) for 40 seconds (1.6 log) would equal an exposure of 6.5 log scotopic troland-sec.

The regeneration of rhodopsin after bleaching follows a fixed exponential course regardless of how large the fraction ($1-p_o$) bleached. When ($1-p$) is the fraction of rhodopsin in the bleached state after t (minutes) in the dark

$$(1-p) = (1 - p_o) \, 10^{-t/14}$$

For bleaches of greater than 10%, there is excellent correspondence between visual thresholds and the amount of pigment still bleached at various times in the dark. This direct, although not proportional, relationship between the extent of photopigment depletion by bleaching and the degree of threshold elevation after exposure to bright light suggests a relationship to the stable levels of neural activity resulting from steady-state concentrations of photopigment products in the presence of a background. Thus similarities in behavior during light adaptation and dark adaptation have led to suggestions that the underlying mechanisms may be similar. This concept of an equivalent background, first proposed by Crawford,[33] is illustrated in Figure 24-8. Note that when measured with psychophysical techniques, both light- and dark-adaptation functions typically contain two segments reflecting adaptation of the rod and cone systems. To study the behavior of the rod system in isolation, it is advantageous to measure thresholds in a rod monochromat. Rod monochromacy is a recessively inherited genetic defect in which there is no detectable cone photoreceptor function from birth. The rod system governs dim light vision, so these patients see normally in dim light but are severely impaired and photophobic under moderate to high levels of lighting. The left half of Figure 24-8 shows the recovery of rod threshold in a rod monochromat following a bright-light adaptation period.[21] The right half of Figure 24-8 shows the effect of increasing illuminance on visual threshold. In this kind of typical light-adaptation experiment, most of the rise in log threshold occurs very rapidly, typically within a few seconds, when the background light is turned on. Thus the light-adaptation curve reflects the

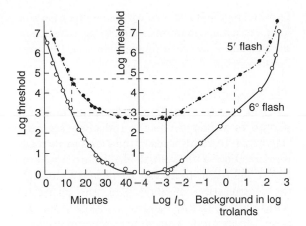

Figure 24-8 Equivalent background experiment in a rod monochromat. Curves on the left are dark-adaptation curves, plotting log threshold against time in dark. Curves on the right show log increment threshold against log intensity of steady adapting background light. *Open circles,* Test flash size of 6 degrees. *Closed circles,* Test flash size of 5 minutes. (From Blakemore CB, Rushton WAH: *J Physiol Lond* 181:612, 1965.)

steady-state threshold as a function of adapting intensity as opposed to the slow decrease in visual threshold as a function of time.[99] In Figure 24-8 the principle of the equivalent background was found to apply over a range of more than 7 log units of rod sensitivity. Furthermore, the equivalence applies over a range of stimulus conditions. For example, the curves on the left show recovery of threshold during dark adaptation for spots of two different sizes. The larger test targets had the lower thresholds because of spatial summation within rod receptive fields. The curves shown to the right show thresholds for incremental detection of the same sizes of test flash after steady-state adaptation to constant background levels. At any given time during the course of dark adaptation, the log threshold for either of the two sizes of test flashes can be compared with the log threshold for the same sizes of test flashes measured under conditions of steady-state adaptation. The dotted lines show that the equivalent background for a given time of dark adaptation may be read from the abscissa at the bottom right by dropping a vertical line from the corresponding points on the threshold curves on the right side of the figure. This yields an experimental determination of the equivalent background luminance reached after a given time of dark adaptation. The vertical solid line indicates the equivalent background level in the fully dark-

adapted retina. With certain qualifications, this may correspond to the residual level of neural activity ("noise") in the retinal circuitry in the absence of light.

Several other adaptational characteristics of the rod system are apparent in Figure 24-8. First is the characteristic behavior by which the rod system loses sensitivity as background illumination is increased. Over much of the range, the increase in threshold is linearly proportional to the adapting illuminance. This is described by the Weber-Fechner relationship in which $\Delta I/I = c$, where ΔI is the increment threshold (threshold measured against background illumination), I is the background intensity, and c is a constant value of 1.0 when the size and duration of the stimulus is optimally adjusted.

Second is the way in which the equivalent background corresponding to a given time of dark adaptation is a constant that is independent of the size or duration of the test flashes used to determine the equivalent background. This can be seen from a comparison of the thresholds to the two different spot sizes, in which the change in equivalent background with time is identical for the two different spot sizes used to determine visual thresholds during the course of dark adaptation.

As described previously, a strong candidate for the mechanism limiting recovery after a bleach and thereby setting the equivalent background is the amount of rhodopsin in the bleached state. However, there are many situations in which thresholds are clearly limited by something other than rhodopsin level. In contrast to the gradual recovery of dark adaptation that follows an extensive and prolonged exposure to light, recovery after a brief exposure can be rapid. A car's headlights at night, for example, can be dazzling and temporarily blinding, but they leave nothing more than a temporary deficit for a few seconds. Similarly, we have all experienced temporary night blindness after turning on the lights briefly to find something at night. This phenomenon was appreciated in the pioneering studies of dark adaptation.[50,94] After substantial bleaching, rod recovery curves all exhibited the same exponential shape but were shifted to earlier recovery times because the bleaching was less. However, the rod curves were found to change shape when bleaching was less than 10%. As shown in Figure 24-9, the initial elevation in threshold after a bleach of less than 10% is considerably greater than predicted by the amount of rhodopsin in the bleached state. For several minutes after the termination of the adapting light, thresholds are considerably above that predicted by the amount of bleached rhodopsin. Another situation in which the amount of bleached rhodopsin does not seem to be limiting thresholds has become known as *Rushton's paradox.* Rushton's paradox involves adaptation to a bright flash. A brief flash, regardless of the intensity, is incapable of bleaching more than half the available visual pigment.[47] Stages within the rhodopsin cycle are photoreversible, so a sufficiently brief, intense flash causes one or more of the early photoproducts to enter into a momentary photoequilibrium with the parent species rhodopsin. Despite the differences in the level of bleach, the rod dark-adaptation curve after a photoregenerating flash bleach is indistinguishable from that after a 30-second full bleach.[91] A similar paradox can be measured in a rod monochromat, demonstrating that the paradox has nothing to do with the presence or absence of cones.[2] The findings are paradoxic because they violate what has come to be known as the *Dowling-Rushton relationship;* that is, log visual sensitivity during dark adaptation is a linear function of unregenerated photopigment. The agreement between rod dark-adaptation curves after a flash bleach and after a 30-second full bleach is not coincidental; rather, it points to a common mechanism.[84] Something other than the amount of bleached pigment has been equated in the flash and long exposure conditions. Something other than the amount of bleached pigment must be the rate-limiting step in dark adaptation.

The Rhodopsin Visual Cycle

The first step in rod vision is the absorption of a photon by rhodopsin in the rod outer segment (Figure 24-10). This leads to the 11-*cis* to all-*trans* isomerization of the retinaldehyde chromophore. Before light sensitivity can be regained through the regeneration of rhodopsin, the all-*trans*-retinaldehyde (atRAL) must dissociate from the opsin apoprotein and a molecule of 11-*cis*-retinaldehyde must combine with opsin at the chromophore binding site. This process, known as the *visual cycle,* is well understood in the rods.[22,35,86] After photoisomerization and reduction by all-*trans*-retinal dehydrogenase (atRDH), the resulting all-*trans*-retinol (atROL) is translocated across the extracellular space from the rod outer segment to the retinal pigment epithelium (RPE). It is re-isomerized to 11-*cis*-retinol (11cROL) in a two-step process involving synthesis of a fatty acyl ester by lecithin-retinol acyltransferase (LRAT) and ester hydrolysis coupled energetically to *trans*-to-*cis* isomerization by isomerohydrolase (IMH). Finally, 11cROL is oxidized to 11-*cis*-retinal (11cRAL) by 11-*cis*-retinol dehydrogenase (11cRDH5) in RPE cells. The 11-*cis*-retinal moves back to the rod outer segments, where it combines with opsin to form rhodopsin.

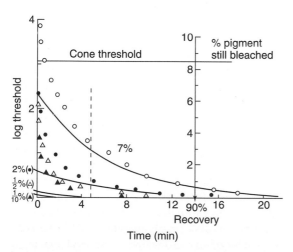

FIGURE 24-9 Continuous curves show expected rhodopsin levels after bleaches of less than 10%. *Circles* and *triangles* represent psychophysical thresholds during dark adaptation. *Black triangles* follow a 0.1% bleach, and the other symbols follow bleaching that was 4, 16, and 64 times as strong. Thresholds are considerably higher than predicted by the amount of bleached rhodopsin, for example, *white triangles* (0.5% bleached) at time zero should lie at 0.2 but instead lie at 2.2—100 times too high. (From Rushton WAH, Powell DS: *Vis Res* 12:1073, 1972.)

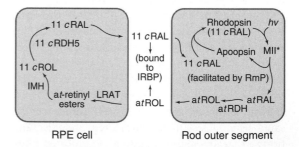

FIGURE 24-10 The visual cycle in rods. *atRAL,* All-*trans*-retinaldehyde; *atRDH,* all-*trans*-retinal dehydrogenase; *atROL,* all-*trans*-retinal; *11cRAL,* 11-*cis*-retinal; *11cRDH5,* 11-*cis*-retinol dehydrogenase; *11cROL,* 11-*cis*-retinol; *IMH,* isomerohydrolase; *LRAT,* lecithin-retinol acyltransferase; *RPE,* retinal pigment epithelium. (Courtesy Gabriel H. Travis.)

As noted previously, there are numerous situations in which visual thresholds do not appear to be logarithmically related to the concentration of pigment remaining in the bleached state. The equivalent background hypothesis provides an alternative scheme, based on the biochemistry of phototransduction and the visual cycle. As first elaborated by Lamb,[62] threshold elevation during dark adaptation is directly proportional to the equivalent background intensity, which is itself directly proportional to photoproduct concentration. Stated another way, the threshold elevation measured during dark adaptation should be directly proportional to photoproduct concentration.

When the removal of a photoproduct is first order, its concentration decays exponentially over time and, to the extent that its removal is rate limiting, desensitization also declines exponentially. In a typical dark-adaptation plot of log threshold versus time (see Figure 24-6), such an exponential decay appears as a straight line. Decay through two removal steps with different exponential time constants give rise to two straight lines with different slopes. Recently, attempts have been made to relate thresholds during recovery from a bleach to the biochemical steps involved through a quantitative model.[65,67] Lamb's model contains two rate constants for the cone limb of dark adaptation and three rate constants for the rod limb. The first component of rod-mediated dark adaptation is obscured by the cone-mediated phase in normal subjects. The rate-limiting step for this first component is thought to be the deactivation of activated proteins (Rh*, T*, and PDE*) within the phototransduction cascade. The time constant for this step is on the order of 2 seconds.[67] The second and third components of the rod-mediated phase can be derived from nonlinear regression techniques.[69] The solid line fit to the second component in Figure 24-6 has a slope of 0.24 decades min$-$1, which corresponds to an exponential time constant of about 100 seconds (i.e., 0.43 times the reciprocal of the slope in $\log_{10}$ units). The rate-limiting mechanism for the second component in the Lamb model is believed to be the hydrolysis of metarhodopsin-II-arrestin.[67] Also shown in Figure 24-6 is a third component that appears to dominate over the second component at times greater than about 22 minutes. The rate-limiting mechanism for the third component appears to be the regeneration of rhodopsin, and the time constant for this component is approximately 7 minutes. In addition, bleaching products and unregenerated rhodopsin are able to activate the transduction cascade weakly.[57] Under normal conditions, when 11-*cis*-retinal is readily available from the RPE, photoproduct activation of the cascade may be negligible. However, when the rate of translocation or the availability of 11-*cis*-retinal from the RPE to the rod outer segment is diminished, opsin may play a considerable role. Thus, for example, unregenerated rhodopsin in conditions such as vitamin A deficiency and Sorsby fundus dystrophy may lead to slow dark adaptation because the opsin presumably contributes to generating a persistent equivalent intensity.[29]

POSTRECEPTORAL MECHANISMS OF ADAPTATION

Although many of the elements of the rapid and slow processes of adaptation are present at the level of the photoreceptor, it is evident that there is extensive integration of information by subsequent neural elements within the retina. An important feature that results from neural convergence is the formation of a spatial distribution of visual sensitivity for a retinal cell. This distribution of sensitivity in space is known as the *receptive field* of the cell. In many cases the information fed to a cell from surrounding regions is antagonistic to that fed to the center, and the cell is said to have a center-surround organization. Because of their large-field characteristics, horizontal cells are well suited to provide the antagonistic surround to bipolar cells. Horizontal cells make synaptic contact with bipolar cells and also feed back synaptically onto cones in such a way as to oppose the light-induced center response of the bipolar cells. The antagonistic center-surround organization of the bipolar cell receptive field is illustrated in Figure 24-11. Responses are shown to spots of light of varying diameter positioned over the center of the receptive field.[107] The response first increased in amplitude as the diameter of the circular stimulus was increased from an initial size of 200 m to a diameter of 400 m, above which the maximum amplitude decreased slightly. There was a more dramatic decrease in the plateau response measured approximately 150 milliseconds after the initiation of the stimulus. The level of the plateau continued to decrease for larger stimulus sizes, up to the maximum diameter of 2000 m. This pattern of responses suggests a receptive field center of 400 m in diameter, surrounded by an annular zone of antagonism extending out to a diameter of 2000 m (2 mm on the retinal surface).

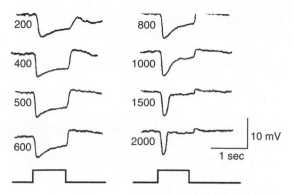

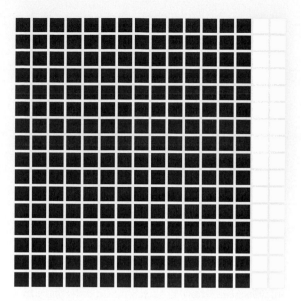

FIGURE 24-11   Center-surround organization of bipolar cell receptive field. Graded potential responses of bipolar cell to stimulation by spots of light of increasing diameter. Numbers by each tracing specify stimulus diameter in micrometers. Initial peak response is greatest at 400 mm; increasing spot sizes inhibit response up to diameter of 2000 mm. Diameter of receptive field excitatory center is 400 mm; inhibitory surround, 2000 mm. (From Werblin FS: Synaptic interactions mediating bipolar responses in the retina of the tiger salamander. In Barlow HB, Fatt P [eds]: *Vertebrate photoreception*, New York, 1977, Academic Press.)

FIGURE 24-12   The Hermann grid illusion, demonstrating illusory gray areas at the intersections of the white grid lines.

The center-surround organization of receptive fields is widespread throughout the retina, being found in many cell types, including ganglion cells.[3,4,48,59] The antagonistic organization of receptive field center and surround provides a plausible explanation for illusory phenomena such as Mach bands and the Hermann grid illusion (Figure 24-12). Mach bands are apparent in uniform solid gray rectangles of differing brightness placed adjacent to each other. Because of lateral inhibition, a dark band is seen on the dark side of each contrast border and a light band is evident on each light side.[88] The Hermann grid illusion also reflects lateral inhibition. Receptive fields with their centers falling at the intersections of lines are subjected to more inhibition in the surround than cells with receptive fields away from the intersections. As a result, there is the illusory appearance of a dark spot at each intersection.

Inhibitory surrounds of bipolar cells and ganglion cells provide a rapid form of neural adaptation. Variations in light falling on the inhibitory surround cause the response curve of the cell to be shifted or repositioned to different parts of the range of stimulus intensities covered by the receptors. The extensive literature on the relationship between ganglion cell behavior and the dynamics of light adaptation is beyond the scope of this chapter.

Models exist that produce good predictions of the outputs of M and P ganglion cells for a wide range of spatiotemporal variations in stimuli.[55,96,110] In turn, with simplifying assumptions about cortical processing, investigators are close to producing a comprehensive model that will predict the data of human psychophysics from emerging knowledge of lower-level retinal processing.[52]

ABNORMAL ADAPTATION IN RETINAL DISEASE

Gene mutations affecting phototransduction or the visual cycle can have specific effects on mechanisms of visual adaptation. In some cases the resulting defect is stationary night blindness; in others the defect is subtler, involving a change in the dynamics of dark adaptation. Certain mutations within the rhodopsin molecule (i.e., Ala292Glu or Gly90Asp) block inactivation completely.[36,87] Rods in these patients are apparently active continuously as if a background light were on even when the patient is in darkness.[97] Surprisingly, this constitutive activation and continuous depolarization of the rods produces only a stationary disorder, with minimal retinal pigmentary disturbance and little field constriction. Thus these rhodopsin mutations blocking inactivation are fundamentally different from other rhodopsin mutations that cause autosomal dominant forms of the progressive retinal degeneration retinitis pigmentosa.

The Nougaret form of stationary night blindness has recently been linked to a Gly38Asp mutation within the gene for T.[37] In these patients the cone limb of the dark-adaptation function is slowed and there is no evidence whatsoever of a rod limb. A similar complete absence of rod function is seen in patients with a particular mutation in the β-subunit of PDE.[44] Two other forms of stationary night blindness are inherited in an X-linked manner. Males with the incomplete form retain some residual rod function, although rod thresholds are greatly elevated and rod ERGs are barely detectable. The incomplete form is caused by mutations within a gene for the L-type voltage-gated calcium channel.[10] Males with the complete form of X-linked stationary blindness show virtually no evidence of rod-mediated vision.[71] Recently, mutations in the gene for a novel protein, nyctalopin, were discovered to cause the disruption in retinal circuitry.[11]

Patients with recessively inherited Oguchi disease show a profound slowing of the time course of dark adaptation after a bleach.[24] Mutations involving rhodopsin kinase have been found in some patients[112]; in others, mutations have been found in the Arrestin gene.[43] In either case, there is a dramatic slowing in the inactivation of activated rhodopsin. Even after 2 hours in the dark, these patients apparently still have a subset of active rhodopsin molecules activating the phototransduction cascade and elevating the visual threshold in much the same way as a real background.

Defects in adaptation can also be caused by mutations that produce defects within the visual cycle. In these patients, however, the loss of vision may be profound, involving both the rod and cone systems. Leber congenital amaurosis is a profound infantile form of blindness. Mutations in the *RPE65* gene can be found in approximately 15% of patients with this recessive disease.[72] The gene product of *RPE65* is thought to act at or near the isomerohydrolase in the RPE for the *trans*-to-*cis* isomerization.[27,56,89] The enzyme 11*c*RDH5 also plays a crucial role in this pathway. Mutations in the *RDH5* gene for 11*c*RDH5 cause fundus albipunctatus, a rare form of stationary night blindness characterized by slowed dark adaptation resulting from an extreme delay in the regeneration of rod and cone photopigments.[111]

Slowed dark adaptation can also be present in progressive retinal degenerations such as retinitis

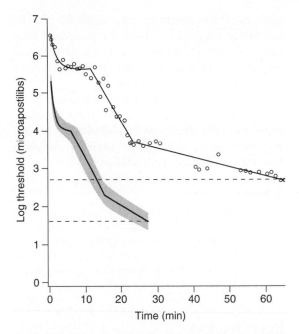

FIGURE 24-13 Slowed dark adaptation (*open symbols*) in a patient with cone-rod dystrophy and associated *ABCR* mutation. Normal mean and 95% confidence limits (*shaded area*) are shown for comparison. Both the second and third components have shallower slopes (slower time constants) than normal.

---

pigmentosa, Stargardt disease, and cone-rod dystrophy (CRD).[1,40,41] Shown in Figure 24-13 is the time course of dark adaptation for a patient with CRD, which is a progressive retinal degeneration characterized by loss of visual acuity at an early age, peripheral field loss, and loss of cone function that is greater than or equal to the loss of rod function. Approximately 30% of patients with CRD have an associated mutation in the *ABCR* gene, which encodes a large glycoprotein found only in the rim of the photoreceptor outer-segment discs.[34] The slowed time course of dark adaptation compared with normal in patients with CRD and associated *ABCR* mutations is clearly evident. These findings are consistent with the proposed role of the *ABCR* rim protein as an outwardly directed flippase for protonated *N*-retinylidene-PE. The current model for the function of rim protein suggests that it may accelerate dark adaptation by speeding the transfer of all-*trans*-retinaldehyde from the disc interior to the cytoplasmic surface after a photobleach.[106] Patients with defective rim protein may not be able to efficiently clear this photoproduct, which if it persists, can form a complex that activates the transduction pathway with approximately 100-fold greater efficiency than opsin alone and nearly 10% the efficiency of photoactivated rhodopsin.[57] Thus the prolonged time course of dark adaptation in some forms of retinal disease may be a direct result of an inability to rapidly clear residual photoproducts.

Although the story of visual adaptation is far from complete, the recent convergence of disciplines from the clinical to the molecular guarantee ever-accelerating insights into some of the most fundamental of all visual processes.

Acknowledgments

Eileen Birch, Don Hood, and David Pepperberg provided invaluable comments and suggestions. I also borrowed liberally from the excellent chapter by William M. Hart in the previous edition of Adler's *Physiology of the Eye*. This work was supported by the Foundation Fighting Blindness and the National Institutes of Health.

References

1. Alexander KR, Fishman GA: Prolonged dark adaptation in retinitis pigmentosa, *Br J Ophthalmol* 68:561, 1984.
2. Alpern M: The effect of a bright light flash on dark adaptation of human rods, *Nat Lond* 230:394, 1971.
3. Barlow HB: Action potentials from the frog's retina, *J Physiol Lond* 207:77, 1953.
4. Barlow HB: Summation and inhibition in the frog's retina, *J Physiol Lond* 119:68, 1953.
5. Battelle BA, LaVail MM: Rhodopsin content and rod outer segment length in albino rat eyes: modification by dark adaptation, *Exp Eye Res* 26:487, 1978.
6. Baylor DA: Photoreceptor signals and vision, *Invest Ophthalmol Vis Sci* 28:34, 1987.
7. Baylor DA, Hodgkin AL: Changes in time scale and sensitivity in turtle photoreceptors, *J Physiol Lond* 242:729, 1974.
8. Baylor DA, Lamb TD, Yau K-W: Two components of electrical dark noise in toad retinal rod outer segments, *J Physiol Lond* 309:591, 1980.
9. Baylor DA, Nunn BJ, Schnapf JL: The photocurrent, noise and spectral sensitivity of rods of the monkey *Macaca fascicularis*, *J Physiol* 357:575, 1984.
10. Bech-Hansen NT et al: Loss-of-function mutations in a calcium-channel alpha1-subunit gene in Xp11.23 cause incomplete X-linked congenital stationary night blindness, *Nat Genet* 19:264, 1998.
11. Bech-Hansen NT et al: Mutations in the gene for a novel leucine-rich protein, nyctalopin, cause the developmental retinal-circuitry abnormality of x-linked complete congenital stationary night blindness, *Nat Genet* 26:319, 2000.
12. Besharse JC, Hollyfield JG, Rayborn ME: Photoreceptor outer segments: accelerated membrane renewal in rods after exposure to light, *Science* 196:536, 1977.
13. Birch DG: Diurnal rhythm in the human rod ERG: retinitis pigmentosa, *Invest Ophthalmol Vis Sci* 28:2042, 1987.
14. Birch DG: ERG measures of photoreceptor deactivation in retinitis pigmentosa, *Digital J Ophthalmol* 5:1, 1999.
15. Birch DG, Jacobs GH: The effects of prolonged dark exposure on visual thresholds in young and adult rats, *Invest Ophthalmol Vis Sci* 18:752, 1979.
16. Birch DG, Jacobs GH: Light-induced damage to photopic and scotopic mechanisms in the rat depends upon rearing conditions, *Exp Neurol* 68:269, 1980.
17. Birch DG, Pepperberg DR, Hood DC: The effects of light adaptation on recovery kinetics of the human rod photoresponse: vision science and its applications, *OSA Tech Digest Ser* 1:60, 1996.
18. Birch DG, Sandberg MA, Berson EL: Diurnal rhythm in the human rod ERG: relationship to cyclic lighting, *Invest Ophthalmol Vis Sci* 27:268, 1986.
19. Birch DG et al: Abnormal activation and inactivation mechanisms of rod transduction in patients with autosomal dominant retinitis pigmentosa and the pro-23-his mutation, *Invest Ophthalmol Vis Sci* 36:1603, 1995.
20. Birch DG et al: ERGs in mice with rds/peripherin and rom1 mutations, *Invest Ophthalmol Vis Sci* 38:S316, 1997.
21. Blakemore CB, Rushton WAH: Dark adaptation and increment threshold in a rod monochromat, *J Physiol Lond* 181:612, 1965.
22. Bok D: Processing and transport of retinoids by the retinal pigment epithelium, *Eye* 4:326, 1990.
23. Breton ME et al: Analysis of ERG a-wave amplification and kinetics in terms of the G-protein cascade of phototransduction, *Invest Ophthalmol Vis Sci* 35:295, 1994.
24. Carr RE, Ripps H: Rhodopsin kinetics and rod adaptation in Oguchi disease, *Invest Ophthalmol* 6:426, 1991.
25. Chen CK et al: Slowed recovery of rod photoresponse in mice lacking the GTPase accelerating protein RGS9-1, *Nature* 403:557, 2000.
26. Chen J et al: Mechanisms of rhodopsin inactivation in vivo as revealed by a COOH-terminal truncation mutant, *Science* 267:374, 1995.
27. **Choo DW, Cheung E, Rando RR: Lack of effect of RPE65 removal on the enzymatic processing of all-*trans*-retinal in vitro, *FABS Lett* 440:195, 1998.**
28. Cideciyan AV, Jacobson SG: An alternative phototransduction model for human rod and cone ERG a-waves: normal parameters and variation with age, *Vis Res* 36:2609, 1996.
29. Cideciyan AV et al: Rod plateaux during dark adaptation in Sorsby's fundus dystrophy and vitamin A deficiency, *Invest Ophthalmol Vis Sci* 38:1786, 1997.
30. Clack JW, Pepperberg DR: Desensitization of skate photoreceptor by bleaching and background light, *J Gen Physiol* 80:863, 1982.
31. Cornwall MC, Fain GL: Bleaching of rhodopsin in isolated rods causes a sustained activation of PDE and cyclase which is reversed by pigment regeneration, *Invest Ophthalmol Vis Sci* 33:1103, 1992.
32. Craik KJW, Vernon MD: The nature of dark adaptation, *Br J Psychol* 32:62, 1941.
33. Crawford BH: Visual adaptation in relation to brief conditioning stimuli, *Proc R Soc Lond Biol* 134:283, 1947.
34. Cremers FPM et al: Autosomal recessive retinitis pigmentosa and cone-rod dystrophy caused by splice site mutations in the Stargardt's disease gene ABCR, *Hum Mol Genet* 7:355, 1998.
35. Crouch RK et al: Retinoids and the visual process, *Photochem Photobiol* 64:613, 1996.
36. Dryja T et al: Heterozygous missense mutation in the rhodopsin gene as a cause of congenital stationary night blindness, *Nat Genet* 4:280, 1993.
37. Dryja TP et al: Missense mutation in the gene encoding the alpha subunit of rod transducin in the Nougaret form of congenital stationary night blindness, *Nat Genet* 13:358, 1996.
38. Fain GL: Sensitivity of toad rods: dependence on wavelength and background illumination, *J Physiol Lond* 261:71, 1976.
39. Falk G: Retinal physiology. In Heckenlively J, Arden G (eds): *Principles and practice of clinical electrophysiology of vision,* St Louis, 1991, Mosby.

40. Fishman GA, Farbman JS, Alexander KR: Delayed rod dark adaptation in patients with Stargardt's disease, *Ophthalmology* 98:957, 1991.

41. Fishman GA et al: Prolonged rod dark adaptation in patients with cone-rod dystrophy, *Am J Ophthalmol* 118:362, 1994.

42. Frishman LJ, Sieving PA: Evidence for two sites of adaptation affecting the dark-adapted ERG of cats and primates, *Vis Res* 35:435, 1995.

43. Fuchs S et al: A homozygous 1-base pair deletion in the Arrestin gene is a frequent cause of Oguchi disease in Japanese, *Nat Genet* 10:360, 1995.

44. Gal A et al: Heterozygous missense mutation in the rod cGMP phosphodiesterase beta-subunit gene in autosomal dominant stationary night blindness, *Nat Genet* 7:64, 1994.

45. Goto Y et al: Rod phototransduction in transgenic mice expressing a mutant opsin gene, *J Opt Soc Am A* 13:577, 1996.

46. Green DG et al: Retinal mechanisms of visual adaptation in the skate, *J Gen Physiol* 65:483, 1975.

47. Hagins WA: Flash photolysis of rhodopsin in the retina, *Nat Lond* 177:989, 1956.

48. Hartline HK: The receptive fields of optic nerve fibers, *Am J Physiol* 130:690, 1940.

49. He W, Cowan CW, Wensel TG: RGS9, a GTPase accelerator for phototransduction, *Neuron* 20:95, 1998.

50. Hecht S, Haig C, Chase AM: The influence of light adaptation on subsequent dark adaptation of the eye, *J Gen Physiol* 20:831, 1937.

51. Hetling JR, Pepperberg DR: Sensitivity and kinetics of mouse rod flash responses determined in vivo from paired-flash electroretinograms, *J Physiol Lond* 516(pt 2): 593, 1999.

52. Hood DC: Lower-level visual processing and models of light adaptation, *Annu Rev Psychol* 49:503, 1998.

53. Hood DC, Birch DG: A quantitative measure of the electrical activity of human rod photoreceptors using electroretinography, *Vis Neurosci* 5:379, 1990.

54. Hood DC, Birch DG: Light adaptation of human rod receptors: the leading edge of the human a-wave and models of rod receptor activity, *Vis Res* 33:1605, 1993.

55. Hood DC, Graham N: Threshold fluctuations on temporally modulated backgrounds; a possible physiological explanation based upon a recent computational model, *Vis Neurosci* 15:957, 1998.

56. Hooser JPV et al: Rapid restoration of visual pigment and function with oral retinoid in a mouse model of childhood blindness, *Proc Natl Acad Sci USA* 18:8623, 2000.

57. Jager S, Palczewski K, Hofmann KP: Opsin/all-trans-retinal complex activates transducin by different mechanisms than photolyzed rhodopsin, *Biochemistry* 35:2901, 1996.

58. Kraft TW, Schneeweis DM, Schnapf JL: Visual transduction in human rod photoreceptors, *J Physiol* 464:747, 1993.

59. Kuffler SW: Discharge patterns and functional organization of mammalian retina, *J Neurophysiol* 16:37, 1953.

60. Lagnado L, Baylor D: Signal flow in visual transduction, *Neuron* 8:995, 1992.

61. Lagnado L, Baylor D: Calcium controls light-triggered formation of catalytically active rhodopsin, *Nature* 367:273, 1994.

62. Lamb TD: The involvement of rod photoreceptors in dark adaptation, *Vis Res* 21:1773, 1981.

63. Lamb TD: Effects of temperature changes on toad rod photocurrents, *J Physiol Lond* 346:557, 1984.

64. Lamb TD, Pugh EN: A quantitative account of the activation steps involved in phototransduction in amphibian photoreceptors, *J Physiol* 499:719, 1992.

65. Lamb TD et al: Towards a molecular description of human dark adaptation, *J Physiol* 506:88P, 1998.

66. LaVail MM: Rod outer segment disk shedding in rat retina: relationship to cyclic lighting, *Science* 194:1071, 1976.

67. Leibrock CS, Reuter T, Lamb TD: Molecular basis of dark adaptation in rod photoreceptors, *Eye* 12:511, 1998.

68. Lyubarsky AL, Pugh EN: Recovery phase of the murine rod photoresponse reconstructed from electroretinographic recordings, *J Neurosci* 16:563, 1996.

69. McGwin G, Jackson GR, Owsley C: Using nonlinear regression to estimate parameters of dark adaptation, *Behav Res Methods Instrum Comput* 31:712, 1999.

70. McNaughton PA: Light response of vertebrate photoreceptors, *Physiol Rev* 70:847, 1990.

71. Miyake Y et al: Congenital stationary night blindness with negative electroretinogram, *Arch Ophthalmol* 104:1013, 1986.

72. Morimura H et al: Mutations in the RPE65 gene in patients with autosomal recessive retinitis pigmentosa or Leber congenital amaurosis, *Proc Natl Acad Sci USA* 95:3088, 1998.

73. Nakatani K, Tamura T, Yau K-W: Light adaptation in retinal rods of the rabbit and two other nonprimate mammals, *J Gen Physiol* 97:413, 1991.

74. Nicol GD, Bownds MD: Calcium regulates some, but not all, aspects of light adaptation in rod photoreceptors, *J Gen Physiol* 94:233, 1989.

75. Nikonov S, Lamb TD, Pugh EN: The role of steady phosphodiesterase activity in the kinetics and sensitivity of the light-adapted salamander rod photoresponse, *J Gen Physiol* 116:795, 2000.

76. Noell WK, Albrecht R: Irreversible effects of visible light on the retina: role of vitamin A, *Science* 172:76, 1971.

77. Organisciak DT, Noell WK: The rod outer segment phospholipid/opsin ratio of rats maintained in darkness or cyclic light, *Invest Ophthalmol Vis Sci* 16:188, 1977.

78. Organisciak DT et al: Light history and age-related changes in retinal light damage, *Invest Ophthalmol Vis Sci* 39:1107, 1998.

79. Penn JS, Thum LA: A comparison of the retinal effects of light damage and high illuminance light history. In Hollyfield JG, Anderson RE, LaVail MM (eds): *Degenerative retinal disorders: clinical and laboratory investigations*, New York, 1987, Alan R Hiss.

80. Penn JS, Williams TP: Photostasis: regulation of daily photon-catch by rat retinas in response to various cyclic illuminances, *Exp Eye Res* 43:915, 1986.

81. Pepperberg DR, Birch DG, Hood DC: Photoresponses of human rods *in vivo* derived from paired-flash electroretinograms, *Vis Neurosci* 14:73, 1997.

82. Pepperberg DR, Birch DG, Hood DC: Electroretinographic determination of the human rod flash response in vivo, *Methods Enzymol* 316:202, 2000.

83. Pepperberg DR et al: Light-dependent delay in the falling phase of the retinal rod response, *Vis Neurosci* 8:9, 1992.

84. Pugh EN: Rhodopsin flash photolysis in man, *J Physiol* 248:393, 1975.

85. Pugh EN Jr, Lamb TD: Cyclic GMP and calcium: the internal messengers of excitation and adaptation in vertebrate photoreceptors, *Vis Res* 30:1923, 1990.

86. Rando RR: Molecular mechanisms in visual pigment regeneration, *Photochem Photobiol* 56:1145, 1992.

87. Rao V, Cohen G, Oprian D: Rhodopsin mutation G90D and a molecular mechanism for congenital night blindness, *Nature* 367:639, 1994.

88. Ratliff F: *Mach bands: quantitative studies on neural networks in the retina*, San Francisco, 1965, Holden Day.

89. Redmond TM et al: Rpe65 is necessary for production of 11-*cis*-vitamin A in the retinal visual cycle, *Nat Genet* 20:344, 1998.

90. RetNet: www.sph.uth.tmc.edu/retnet.

91. Rushton WAH: Effects of instantaneous flashes on adaptation of the eye, *Nat Lond* 199:971, 1963.

92. Rushton WAH: The difference spectrum and photosensitivity of rhodopsin in the living human eye, *J Physiol Lond* 134:11, 1965.

93. Rushton WAH: The Ferrier lecture, 1962. Visual adaptation, *Proc R Soc B* 162:20, 1965.

94. Rushton WAH, Powell DS: The early phase of dark adaptation, *Vis Res* 12:1083, 1972.

95. Rushton WAH, Powell DS: The rhodopsin content and the visual threshold of human rods, *Vis Res* 12:1073, 1972.

96. Shah S, Levine M: Visual information processing in primate cone pathways: part I. A model, *IEEE Trans Syst Man Cyber* 26:259, 1996.

97. Sieving PA, Richards JE, Naarendorp FEA: Dark-light-model for nightblindness from the human rhodopsin Gly-90-Asp mutation, *Proc Natl Acad Sci USA* 92:880, 1995.

98. Smith NP, Lamb TD: The a-wave of the human electroretinogram recorded with a minimally invasive technique, *Vis Res* 37:2943, 1997.

99. Stiles WS: Increment thresholds and the mechanisms of colour vision, *Doc Ophthalmol* 3:138, 1949.

100. Stiles WS, Crawford BH: *Equivalent adaptational levels in localized retinal areas. Report of a joint discussion on vision, Physical Society of London,* Cambridge, England, 1932, Cambridge University Press.

101. Stryer L: Cyclic GMP cascade of vision, *Annu Rev Neurosci* 9:87, 1986.

102. Stryer L: Visual excitation and recovery, *J Biol Chem* 266:10711, 1991.

103. Tamura T, Nakatani K, Yau K-W: Light adaptation in cat retinal rods, *Science* 245:755, 1989.

104. Tassi P, Pins D: Diurnal rhythmicity for visual sensitivity in humans, *Chronobiol Int* 14:35, 1997.

105. Thomas MM, Lamb TD: Light adaptation and dark adaptation of human rod photoreceptors measured from the a-wave of the electroretinogram, *J Physiol Lond* 518(pt 2): 479, 1999.

106. Weng J et al: Insights into the function of Rim protein in photoreceptors and etiology of Stargardt's disease from the phenotype in abcr knockout mice, *Cell* 98:13, 1999.

107. Werblin FS: Synaptic interactions mediating bipolar responses in the retina of the tiger salamander. In Barlow HB, Fatt P (eds): *Vertebrate photoreception,* New York, 1977, Academic Press.

108. Williams TP: Regulation of retinal light damage, *Proc Int Soc Eye Res* VI:145, 1990.

109. Williams TP, Baker BN, Dodge J: Regulation of light absorption in the pigmented rat retina. In Hollyfield JG, Anderson RE, LaVail MM (eds): *Retinal degenerative disease and experimental therapy,* New York, 1999, Kluver Academic/Plenum Publishers.

110. Wilson HR: A neural model of foveal light adaptation and afterimage formation, *Vis Neurosci* 14:403, 1997.

111. Yamamoto H et al: Mutations in the gene encoding 11-*cis* retinol dehydrogenase cause delayed dark adaptation and fundus albipunctatus, *Nat Genet* 22:188, 1999.

112. Yamamoto S et al: Defects in the rhodopsin kinase gene in the Oguchi form of stationary night blindness, *Nat Genet* 15:175, 1997.

113. Yau K-W: Phototransduction mechanism in retinal rods and cones, *Invest Ophthalmol Vis Sci* 35:9, 1994.

114. Young RW: The renewal of rod and cone outer segments in the rhesus monkey, *J Cell Biol* 49:303, 1971.

SECTION 10

OPTIC NERVE

LEONARD A. LEVIN

CHAPTER 25

OPTIC NERVE*

LEONARD A. LEVIN

The optic nerve is not a peripheral nerve, but rather it is a white matter tract of the central nervous system (CNS), projecting outside the confines of the cranium. There are two optic nerves, each connecting the retinas within each globe to target areas within the brain. Because most of our sensory perception is based on vision, the optic nerves carry most sensory information into the brain, and thence to consciousness. Diseases that affect the optic nerve are therefore common causes of blindness. Because the CNS does not generally respond to injury by producing new cells or repairing axons, the blindness from optic nerve disease is typically irreversible. This chapter covers the principal aspects of optic nerve anatomy, physiology, and response to pathologic changes in the context of clinical disease. When possible, references to review articles are used, as well as primary sources of special interest for those interested in more detailed knowledge about particular topics.

TOPOGRAPHIC ANATOMY

Retinal Ganglion Cell Axons within the Nerve Fiber Layer

The optic nerve begins with the retinal ganglion cell, which is located in the innermost layer of the retina, within the ganglion cell layer. Although most neurons in this layer are retinal ganglion cells, in humans approximately 3% of cells in the central retina and up to 80% in the peripheral retina may be other cell types, primarily amacrine cells.[98] In addition, studies in mammals have demonstrated a few displaced retinal ganglion cells located in the inner nuclear layer.[245] As discussed in Chapter 14, the retinal ganglion cells receive input from bipolar

cells and amacrine cells and project their axon toward the vitreous, whereupon it makes an approximately 90-degree turn and projects toward the optic nerve head in the *nerve fiber layer*. Contrary to expectation, the nerve fiber layer is not radially arranged in a starburst pattern around the optic nerve head (optic disc), but instead it follows a particular course whereby the fibers in the temporal part of the retina (corresponding to the nasal visual field) course away from the fovea, and then once in the nasal retina, turn back toward the optic disc, entering in the superior and inferior portions of the disc (Figure 25-1). The retinal ganglion cell axons arising from retinal ganglion cells in the nasal retina project more directly to the disc, as follows: The fibers from the nasal half of the macula, forming the papillomacular bundle (or more properly, the maculopapillary bundle), enter at the temporal disc, while the fibers arising from ganglion cells nasal to the disc enter at the nasal part of the disc. The vertical distribution of ganglion cell axons within the primate nerve fiber layer is as follows: The axons from more peripheral retinal ganglion cells are more superficial (vitread) to those arising from less peripheral ganglion cells[306] (Figure 25-2).

In addition, those fibers arising from retinal ganglion cells located superior to the temporal horizontal meridian (temporal raphe) and those fibers arising from retinal ganglion cells located inferior to the horizontal raphe are strictly segregated. Because of

*Portions of this chapter were adapted from Levin LA: Biology of the optic nerve. In Albert DM, Jakobiec FA (eds): *Principles and practice of ophthalmology.* Philadelphia, 2000, WB Saunders; and Levin LA: Physiology of the optic nerve. In Tasman W, Jaeger EA (eds): *Duane's foundations of ophthalmology,* Philadelphia, 2001, Lippincott.

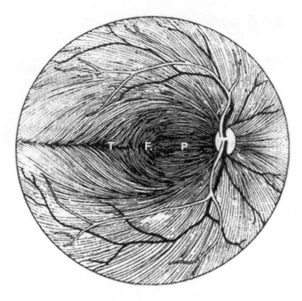

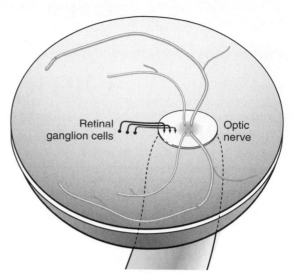

FIGURE 25-1 Course of the retinal ganglion cell axons within the nerve fiber layer of the retina. *F,* Fovea; *P,* papillomacular bundle; *T,* temporal raphe. (Redrawn from Kline LB: *Am Acad Ophthalmol* 4:4, 1996.)

FIGURE 25-2 Simplification of the topographic relations between retinal ganglion axons arising from different locations within the retina. More peripheral retinal ganglion cells send axons more vitread within the nerve fiber layer and more peripherally within the optic nerve.

this segregation, visual field defects corresponding to the injury to the retinal ganglion cell axons typically have stereotyped patterns such as superior or inferior nasal steps, temporal wedges, or the arcuate scotomas. These are called *nerve fiber bundle defects* and are covered in more detail in Chapter 22.

Once at the optic disc, the ganglion cell axons take a 90-degree turn away from the vitreous, toward the brain. Axons arising from more peripheral retinal ganglion cells are peripheral within the optic nerve head, whereas those arising from proximal retinal ganglion cells are more central within the nerve head.[282] That part of the disc corresponding to the projection of the nerve fibers into the optic nerve corresponds to the neuroretinal rim of the disc. That part of the disc that does not contain retinal ganglion cell axons is called the cup. Depending on the size of the disc and whether any developmental or acquired injury is present, the cup-to-disc ratio may range from 0 to 1.0, the former representing a congenitally full disc, and the latter representing a disc that is completely "cupped out," most commonly as a result of glaucomatous optic neuropathy.

Intraorbital Optic Nerve

Although the retinal ganglion cell axon begins in the inner retina and continues along the nerve fiber layer of the retina, the optic nerve itself is considered to begin at the optic nerve head. An approximately 1-mm component of optic nerve is within the intrascleral part of the globe (which includes the lamina cribrosa), and approximately a 30-mm length of optic nerve extends from the globe to the optic canal.[468] The straight-line distance from the back of the globe to the optic canal is much less (the exact amount depending on individual orbital depth), with the relative excess optic nerve being necessary for free movement of the globe during eye movements. In some cases excessive proptosis can exhaust the surplus length of optic nerve, resulting in tethering of the globe by the nerve.

The retinotopic (topographic correspondence of optic nerve fibers to retinal location) segregation of retinal ganglion cell axons, particularly the segregation between axons arising from the superior retina and inferior retina, is gradually lost as the axons enter the nerve. There is only moderate retinotopy in the initial segment of the optic nerve.[126] The retinotopy decreases distally and then becomes ordered for eventual nasal decussation near the chiasm.[75,194,359] The loss of retinotopy is not absolute because the fibers from the nasal (but not temporal) macula continue to be located centrally within the nerve over a considerable distance.[296] Fibers from large retinal ganglion cells are less retinotopically organized than those from smaller ganglion cells.[296] Although studies in humans are difficult to do antemortem, postmortem studies of nerves with specific visual field defects demonstrate similar findings, and postmortem studies of developing fetuses and adult eyes also show loss of retinotopy within the transition from the optic nerve head to the nerve.[125,126] Within the orbit, the optic nerve travels within the muscle cone formed by the superior rectus, lateral rectus, inferior rectus, and medial rectus muscles. Tumors within the cone are common sources of compression of the optic nerve, or *compressive optic neuropathy.* Examples of these tumors include cavernous hemangioma, hemangiopericytoma, fibrous histiocytoma, lymphoma, and schwannoma. In addition, enlargement of the muscles themselves, particularly the inferior rectus and/or the medial rectus muscle in Grave's (dysthyroid) ophthalmopathy, may also compress the optic nerve.

The Optic Canal

The optic nerve enters the cranium by way of the optic canal, a 5- to 12-mm passage that lies immediately superonasal to the superior orbital fissure.[260] The optic canal contains some axons of sympathetic neurons destined for the orbit, as well as the ophthalmic artery. The latter lies immediately inferolateral to the optic nerve itself, covered in dura. At the distal end of the canal is a half-moon–shaped segment of dura that overhangs the optic nerve superiorly and thereby lengthens the canal by a few millimeters. Within the canal, and immediately posterior to the optic canal, meningeal tissue is adjacent to the optic nerve. Benign tumors of the meninges, or meningiomas, are common causes of compressive optic neuropathies in these locations. Small tumors within the canal itself, where free space is minimal, may lead to compressive optic neuropathy without a radiographically visible tumor.

Intracranial Optic Nerve and the Chiasm

Once the nerve has entered the cranium, there is a highly variable (8 to 19 mm, mean of 12 mm) length of nerve until the chiasm is reached.[362] The length of the chiasm itself is approximately 8 mm. The intracranial optic nerve and chiasm are immediately above the planum sphenoidale and sella turcica, the latter of which contains pituitary gland. There is approximately 10 mm between the inferior part of the nerve and the superior part of the pituitary. Therefore tumors of the pituitary, which increase in size enough to compress the chiasm, may cause compressive optic neuropathy. The chiasm is prefixed (anteriorly displaced) in approximately 10% of subjects, postfixed in approximately 15%, and normal in 75%.[362]

The nature of the retinotopic segregation changes as the fibers approach the chiasm, with temporal fibers destined to remain ipsilateral while nasal fibers cross. The developmental ordering of the axons as they pass through the chiasm and go on to innervate the lateral geniculate primarily reflects their time of arrival and is dependent on the presence of pathfinder neurons generated at the chiasm early on.[74,358,408] The percentage of fibers that cross versus those that do not is anatomically 53:47 and functionally 52:48.[219,385] This small difference between the number of crossing and noncrossing fibers is unlikely to be responsible for the relative afferent pupillary defect seen in disorders of the optic tract, in which an afferent pupillary defect is seen contralateral to the injured tract (see also Chapter 32). Instead, it may reflect the fact that some fibers from specialized cells within the retinal responsible for the pupillary reflex may cross from the temporal retina into the contralateral optic tract.[385]

The Optic Tract and Lateral Geniculate Nucleus

Although the optic nerve anatomically ends at the chiasm, the retinal ganglion cell axons continue within the optic tract until the lateral geniculate nucleus (LGN), superior colliculus, pretectal nuclei, or hypothalamus (see following discussion). Circuitry and processing by these targets are discussed in Chapters 26 and 28.

OPTIC NERVE AXON COUNTS AND DIMENSIONS

Approximately 1 million retinal ganglion cells are in each retina, with each cell sending a single axon down the optic nerve. Therefore approximately 1 million axons are within the optic nerve. Studies in animals suggest that during development, approximately 50% to 100% excess retinal ganglion cells are produced, and the number of retinal ganglion cells decreases by programmed cell death, in many cases because not all of the axons reach their target regions within the brain. Likewise, in human development excess retinal ganglion cells die, presumably by programmed cell death during development. Up to two thirds are subsequently lost, predominantly during the second trimester.[335] Several groups have used various techniques to count adult human optic nerve axons. In the normal adult human optic nerve, manual techniques have been used to count approximately 1.2 million ganglion cell axons per nerve, whereas automated techniques give figures of 700,000 to 1.4 million axons.[23,278,279] These differences are presumably the result of variations in autolysis, age, or systematic undercounting of small axons. There is a strong correlation between the size of the neuroretinal rim and the number of axons and between the number of axons and the size of the scleral canal in primates, although the degree of correlation is controversial.[119,279,342,348]

Many factors affect the number of axons within the optic nerve. Animal studies reveal that there are clearly inherited differences in axon counts. Damage to axons from disease (e.g., optic neuropathy) is common and is discussed in a later section in this chapter. Finally, there is a gradual loss of retinal ganglion cells during normal human aging, with an approximate 5000-axon loss per year of life[23,278] In rhesus monkeys the number of ganglion cell axons is also variable, with a probable loss of approximately 0.45% of axons per year of life.[292] These changes are similar to the aging-related loss of retinal ganglion cells and parallel the loss of rod (but not cone) photoreceptors with age.[143] For unclear reasons, there is a smaller degree of loss of macular retinal ganglion cells with age, compared with peripheral retinal ganglion cells, and this may reflect contraction of the macula with time.[167]

The diameter of the optic nerve varies. At the disc itself, where the fibers are completely unmyelinated, the mean vertical diameter of the disc is 1.9 mm (range, 1.0 to 3.0 mm) and the mean horizontal diameter is 1.7 to 1.8 mm (range, 0.9 to 2.6 mm).[200,348] The mean area of the disc is 2.7 mm^2 (range, 0.8 to 5.5 mm^2). The mean area of the neuroretinal rim (not including the cup) is 2.0 mm^2 (range, 0.8 to 4.7 mm^2). The diameter of the optic nerve approximately doubles posterior to the globe as a result of myelination of the axons.

MICROSCOPIC ANATOMY AND CYTOLOGY

Axons

The most important components of the optic nerve are the axons of the retinal ganglion cells. Although the retinal ganglion cell bodies themselves are situated within the retina, the axons are all located within the optic nerve. No other neuronal cell bodies are within the optic nerve, making it a pure white matter tract. Although the optic nerve itself may contain other small nerves, particularly tiny peripheral nerves (branches of the trigeminal sys-

tem), that carry pain sensation or control vascular tone, most of the optic nerve is composed of the approximately 1 million axons of the retinal ganglion cells.

Optic nerve axons are collected in fascicles, which are separated by pia-derived septa. The number of fascicles ranges from approximately 50 to 300, being maximal immediately retrobulbar and at the optic canal.[195] The mean axon diameter is slightly less than 1 m, with a unimodal distribution skewed to the left. The mean diameter may decrease during aging, possibly through loss of large-diameter axons.[364] Compared with the optic tract, there is relatively little segregation of axons by size within the optic nerve, except for a tendency for finer axons to be located inferocentrotemporally.[359,379] Axonal diameter and myelin thickness from the retina to the brain are variable. Studies in the ferret show that the diameters of the largest axons increase as the distance from the retina increases.[22] The diameter of individual axons is regulated by multiple factors, including oligodendrocytes and activity, and correlates with local accumulation of specifically phosphorylated neurofilament proteins.[88,121,303]

Oligodendrocytes and Myelin

Axonal conduction in the optic nerve depends on the presence of myelin, a fatty multilaminated structure that insulates each axon and greatly increases the speed and efficiency of conduction. This is discussed at length in the section on axonal conduction. The retrolaminar optic nerve is completely myelinated under nonpathologic circumstances. Nonmyelinated axons of the peripheral nervous systems are within the adventitia of the central retinal artery, and nonmyelinated and myelinated Schwann cells are found around peripheral axons of the outer dura. Each axon is myelinated with several lamellae of myelin bilayers, with the number of lamellae varying from axon to axon.[17,136,417] Injections of individual oligodendrocytes have shown an average of 20 to 30 processes per cell, each of which myelinates 150 to 200 m of axon.[270]

Oligodendrocytes develop from O-2A progenitor cells. O-2A cells migrate from the brain into the optic nerve, perhaps from the base of the preoptic recess, and this migration may continue during adult life.[247] The O-2A progenitor has a complex regulatory mechanism, with in vitro studies implicating platelet-derived growth factor (PDGF) and ciliary neurotrophic factor (CNTF). Other factors in the differential control of differentiation, division, and renewal of the stem cell population, such as basic fibroblast growth factor, are likewise involved.[99,110] An intrinsic developmental clock controls the differentiation of O-2A progenitor cells into oligodendrocytes, after which the cell is mitotically unresponsive to PDGF. In normal development, some O-2A cells are thought to divide, then differentiate, into oligodendrocytes and form myelin. Transplanted O-2A progenitor cells are capable of remyelinating.*

The developmental regulation of myelination of the optic nerve and tract occurs earliest at the brain end of the optic nerve, then travels distally toward the eye (i.e., proximally with respect to the ganglion cell axon.) This is in contradistinction to myelination elsewhere in the CNS, which usually occurs from the neuron cell body outward along the axon. The brain-to-eye direction of myelination correlates with animal studies demonstrating migration and differientiation of dividing O-2A progenitor cells outward along the optic nerve, as well as their differentiation.[89,332] In humans, oligodendrocytes are not seen in the optic nerve before 18 weeks of gestation.[332] Later, optic tract and intracranial nerve axons begin myelination at 32 weeks of gestation, with the process virtually complete at term. The axons adjacent to the globe begin myelination only at birth; all are myelinated by about 7 months of age.[259] Further myelination continues, however, and thickening of axonal myelin may continue for 2 years or longer. Size of the optic nerve follows a similar patter.[367] The diameter of myelinated axons varies greatly; in longitudinal studies of rat optic nerve development, axons that become myelinated increased in diameter, whereas those that are not myelinated maintained a similar diameter.[230] The signal for change in caliber is generated by the oligodendrocyte.[88,378] Although unmyelinated and not yet myelinated axons can conduct electrical impulses in developing optic nerve, there is a surprising increase in conduction velocity during development, independent of diameter or myelination status, the reasons for which are unclear.[130]

The nature of the interaction between the axon and the oligodendrocyte is the subject of much research. The presence of axons modulates the production of myelin proteins by oligodendrocytes, probably through their electrical activity.[101,206] Oligodendrocytes do not survive in the absence of live axons in young animals but can survive in adult, axotomized animals, albeit in a shrunken, quiescent form.[254] There is also a reciprocal control

of oligodendrocyte number based on the number of retinal ganglion cells.[54] Regulation of oligodendrocyte number appears to be caused by axonal electrical activity.[28] In the presence of demyelination, cells antigenically and functionally resembling oligodendrocytes may reconstitute themselves and remyelinate axons, although the nature of the inducing chemical signals has not been well characterized.[68,410] Reciprocally, oligodendrocytes and myelin are partially responsible for inhibition of neurite outgrowth (see previous discussion).[380,394] Ionic channels for potassium, of which there are several types in cultured rat optic nerve oligodendrocytes, may help regulate extracellular potassium concentrations or contribute to activity-dependent changes in myelin chemistry.[28,41,295]

A peculiarity of the relationship between the oligodendrocyte and the optic nerve axon is that the intraretinal ganglion cell axons are not normally myelinated in most species. This is because of the absence of oligodendrocytes in the retina, and it has been hypothesized that the lamina cribrosa prevents migration of those cells, or their precursors, in development. Studies of rat optic nerve head and anterior optic nerve demonstrate an abnormal transition zone from unmyelinated axons to myelinated axons, with varying lengths and thicknesses of myelin, unusual nodal region morphology, and few normal oligodendrocytes.[180] Studies of rat optic nerve suggest a barrier to the migration of the O-2A progenitor cells into the retina.[123] This barrier is possibly caused by the presence of type 1 astrocytes, serum factors from a focally deficient blood-nerve barrier, or the adhesion substrate tenascin.[32,247,328,440] In rabbits, which have no lamina cribrosa, axons are myelinated by oligodendrocytes in the retina and intraretinal O-2A cells can be identified.[123] Furthermore, the retinal portion of the ganglion cell axon has no constitutive barrier to myelination because ganglion cell axons of retina transplanted into rat midbrain can be myelinated, whereas oligodendrocyte precursors injected intraretinally can myelinate retinal ganglion cell axons.[221,328] Myelination may also be artifactually induced by injuring the retina from the scleral side. This trauma leads to migration of Schwann cells and subsequent intraretinal myelination.[327] In human eyes, myelination of part of the nerve fiber layer is occasionally seen; it is assumed that this results because of ectopic oligodendrocytes, although there are reports of Schwann cells myelinating intraretinal axons in normal cat and rat.[55,201] Although oligodendrogliomas within other parts of the CNS are sometimes seen,

---

*References 31, 45, 142, 156, 225, 404.

neoplasms of oligodendrocytes within the optic nerve are rare.

Astrocytes

A major supporting cell of the optic nerve is the astrocyte. Astrocytes, named for their stellate appearance, are ubiquitous components of the CNS. Although the Schwann cell alone performs both support and insulating functions to the enveloped axon in the peripheral nervous system, in the CNS the two roles are divided between the astrocyte and the oligodendrocyte, respectively. Astrocytes have several functions, the most important of which are maintaining ionic homeostasis and serving as an energy source. Astrocytes are highly efficient at transporting potassium, and increases in the level of extracellular potassium as a result of repolarization are buffered by the presence of astrocytes. Their ability to accumulate glycogen may allow them to serve as an energy source for the optic nerve in the absence of glucose (e.g., ischemia) by shuttling lactate to adjacent axons.[464] Like oligodendrocytes, astrocytes are cells of glial lineage.

Astrocytes and their processes not only make up large portions of the optic nerve parenchyma in positions adjacent to neurons and vessels but also are present wherever neuroectodermal structures are adjacent to connective tissues, such as the pial septa, the adventitia of the central retinal artery and vein, and the pia in a layer named the *glial mantle of Fuchs.*[17] Developmental regulation of astrocyte number is determined by the retinal ganglion cell through several mechanisms.[53]

Normal optic nerve contains the so-called type 1 astrocyte, which subserves multiple functions.[58,62,63] It is typically flat in culture, resembling in morphology a fibroblast; contains few fibrils; and divides frequently in vitro. It is thought to arise from a unipotential neuroepithelial precursor. The astrocyte, the processes of which are orthogonal to the longitudinal axis of the optic nerve, forms the glial-limiting membrane, is responsible for inducing endothelial cells to form the blood-brain barrier, and may serve as a substrate for gliosis.[122,192,280,354]

Astrocytes, whether from optic nerve or from other CNS structures, may be immunohistochemically identified by the presence of intracellular glial fibrillary acidic protein (GFAP), an intermediate filament protein akin to the cytokeratins of epithelial cells. GFAP is probably important in maintaining the structure of the astrocyte cell body, in contrast to microtubules, which are critical to development of the astrocyte's stellate morphology processes.[438]

Transgenic mice devoid of GFAP have abnormal myelination and blood-brain barriers.[241]

In the retina, two types of astrocytes are seen: the Müller cell and the retinal astrocyte. Müller cells are oriented perpendicular to the retinal plane, spanning it radially, and originate from neuroepithelium during retinal development.[442] Retinal astrocytes are found in the nerve fiber layer, codistributed with retinal blood vessels.[389] These cells almost certainly migrate from the optic nerve, where they may be targeted by basal lamina from vessel precursor cells.[76,247,248,453] The retinal astrocyte, like that of the optic nerve, is probably a supporting cell for the ganglion cell axon.[56]

Initially thought to serve solely as the "glue" that held the axons together, astrocytes are now thought to play significant functional roles, including serving as a glycogen storehouse, taking up and inactivating neurotransmitters, aiding in immune responses, and developmentally regulating axonal extension from the retina to the LGN. Perhaps the most important function of the astrocyte in the optic nerve is its ability to help regulate the extracellular concentration of certain ions, particularly potassium.

Astrocyte processes are concentrated at the nodes of Ranvier, and freeze-fracture electron microscopy demonstrates orthogonal arrays of particles within the membrane at the node as well as gap junctions between astrocytes and between astrocytes and adjacent oligodendrocytes.[455] They typically have endfeet in contact with nearby capillaries, presumably to allow transportation of substances between the local circulation and the axons. At least two types of endfeet are seen in the astrocytic processes contacting the subpial glial limitans.[40] Lucifer yellow injections of rat astrocytes demonstrate an average of 50 to 60 processes per astrocyte, with endfeet in the nerve parenchyma, on blood vessels, or at the pial surface.[61,63]

Although neurons are classically considered the only electrically active cell population in the CNS, astrocytes also have ionic channels. For example, multiple voltage-sensitive sodium channels have been demonstrated in rat optic nerve astrocytes.[41,42,307] Both sodium and potassium channels have been studied electrophysiologically in cultured type 1 and type 2 astrocytes.[38] With the use of electrophysiologic techniques in serum-cultured rat optic nerve astrocytes, at least six ionic currents appear to be in type 2 astrocytes: a voltage-sensitive sodium current (of the neuronal type), a delayed potassium current and a calcium-sensitive potassium current, two calcium currents, and a chloride current.[26] Different electrophysiologic properties are seen in recordings from O-2A cells in culture.[29] In type 1 astrocytes, there appear to be a voltage-sensitive sodium current (of the glial type), a delayed rectifier potassium current, and an inward rectifier potassium current, with a calcium current being seen only in cyclic adenosine monophosphate (cAMP)–treated cells.[27] Other experiments have revealed the presence of glutamate-activated currents in both the O-2A progenitor cells and the type 2 astrocyte, as well as effects of the neurotransmitter γ-aminobutyric acid (GABA) on O-2A progenitor cells and astrocytes.[29,48,59] Within the intact optic nerve, nonvesicularly released glutamate from the axon may induce glial cell spiking and possibly other effects.[196,216] Whether ionic channels or neurotransmitter receptors on optic nerve glia is physiologically important in vivo has yet to be demonstrated, but their presence suggests that optic nerve astrocytes may be more functionally specialized than previously recognized.

Astrocytes may be critical for optic nerve development in that they may serve as the substrate over which extending ganglion cell axons grow.[253] The particular cell surface molecules or released substances responsible for this are the subject of great dispute; the extracellular matrix glycoprotein laminin has been studied as a mediator for neuronal-glial adhesion in the developing optic nerve and can induce ganglion cell outgrowth in vitro and in vivo when gliosis is inhibited with cytosine arabinoside.[270,275,291,332] Arguing against the importance of laminin is the observation that leptomeningeal cells, which are rich in laminin, do not support neurite extension as well as astrocytes do.[99] Astrocytes isolated from cerebral cortex bear a putative receptor for the Thy-1 glycoprotein, which is expressed on retinal ganglion cells and appears to modulate ganglion cell neurite extension in vitro.[110,225] The adhesion molecules L1, neural cell adhesion molecule, and myelin-associated glycoprotein have been immunohistochemically localized to contacts between axons, growth cones, astrocytes, and oligodendrocytes in developing and adult mouse optic nerve but are not necessarily equivalent in function. The cadherins have recently been shown to regulate axonal outgrowth.*

The role of optic nerve astrocytes in the pathologic processes of gliosis is complex.[57,60] As a reaction either to local injury or to remote death of ad-

jacent axons, astrocytes are observed to divide and extend processes, without the formation of collagen that typifies the classic fibroblastic response to injury. Astrocytic gliosis presumably occurs partly to replace neural tissue—as a type of scar formation—but may also relate to astrocyte secretion of cytokines, which may recruit or modulate other cell types. The cells responsible for gliosis are predominantly type 1 astrocytes.[247,389] There are several other lines of evidence for astrocyte activation during gliosis. During wallerian degeneration caused by optic nerve transection, both fibrous astrocytes and reactive astrocytes divide, as demonstrated by 3H-thymidine incorporation.[404] Similar increases in cell number are seen in glioblasts and microglia. During antibody-induced demyelination of the optic nerve, cells morphologically resembling astrocytes are observed to express both GFAP and the oligodendrocyte surface-marker galactocerebroside, suggesting that a dedifferentiation is taking place.[67] Quantification of the astrocytic enzyme glutamine synthetase reveals increased activity distal to optic nerve crush injury.[333] Immunohistochemistry of axotomized rat optic nerves reveals increased amounts of GFAP, whereas there is no significant increase in laminin.[269] Expression of the intermediate filament protein nestin is associated with reactive gliosis after optic nerve crush, and one or more of these processes may explain the failure of ganglion cell axons to regenerate after injury.[137,394] The density of small intramembranous particles, a normal plasma membrane component of astrocytes, increases after enucleation; this is hypothesized to correlate with the reactive astrocyte's inability to support axonal outgrowth.[469] Although CNS astrocytes normally express a variety of neuropeptide receptors, they are not commonly seen in the normal optic nerve.[262] After nerve transection, however, glial scars appear to express large numbers of receptors for substance P, a neuropeptide associated with inflammatory and immune response modulation.[262] Similarly, the constitutively low levels of endothelin-B receptor levels increase greatly after optic nerve injury.[372]

In recent years the ability of CNS cells not normally considered part of the immune system to function immunologically has been studied intensively. Although most work has focused on cells of cerebral origin, the virtually identical phenotypes of cells from the optic nerve with those elsewhere in the CNS suggest that similar cell biology can be assumed in both groups. Studies with cerebral astrocytes have shown that they can express Ia antigens

---

*References 31, 37, 166, 325, 357, 366.

when induced with γ-interferon and can present antigen to T lymphocytes.[128]

The most common intrinsic tumor of the optic nerve is an astrocytoma, or optic nerve glioma. This is usually a low-grade tumor of well-differentiated astrocytic cells that appear hairlike, or "pilocytic." Pilocytic astrocytomas are usually seen in childhood and have a favorable prognosis. They are also commonly seen in association with neurofibromatosis. Rarely, more malignant neoplasms of astrocytic origin develop in adults. These resemble the higher-grade astrocytic neoplasms found elsewhere in the CNS and are usually fatal.

Microglia

Microglia, a type of resident macrophage, are an important cellular component of the optic nerve. Although their origin was debated for decades, they have been shown experimentally to be of bone marrow origin.[177] Microglia share several markers with macrophages, with both having Fc receptors (for immunoglobulin), C3 receptors (for complement), binding of Griffonia isolectin B4, and antigenicity for F4/80 and ED1 monoclonal antibodies.[413] In the human optic nerve, microglia can be seen at 8 weeks after conception, when they are relatively undifferentiated. Microglia become more differentiated during fetal development, going from tuberous to amoeboid to a ramified morphology.[416] They are associated with axon bundles, but not necessarily with blood vessels, and they are found in both the nerve parenchyma and its meninges. Nerve and meningeal microglia are similar ultrastructurally except for vacuoles and endoplasmic reticulum in the former. This may be because of the phagocytosis of dying axons during development.[420] Microglia share several characteristics of immune capacities of macrophages. By phagocytosing extracellular material, degradation within intracellular compartments can occur. This may be followed by antigen presentation on the cell surface. In combination with certain histocompatibility antigens, this presented antigen can cause stimulation of T lymphocytes and subsequent immune system activation.

CNS microglia can spontaneously express histocompatibility class I antigens and can be induced to express class II (Ia) antigens, for example after enucleation-induced wallerian degeneration.[214,473] This may be of pathophysiologic importance in autoimmune diseases because foci of inflammatory lesions may be found at the sites of Ia-positive microglia when experimental allergic encephalomyelitis, an animal model for multiple sclerosis, is induced through adoptive transfer.[214]

Meninges

The optic nerve is covered with three layers of meninges: dura, arachnoid, and pia. The meninges can also be divided up into *pachymeninges* (dura) and *leptomeninges* (arachnoid and pia). The outermost meningeal layer is the dura. This is a thick fibrovascular tissue, which is a direct extension of the sclera and is in immediate contiguity with the periorbita and the dural layer of the lining of the cranial contents. The dura also continues within the optic canal. The arachnoid is the middle meningeal layer. It is a fairly loose, thin, fibrovascular tissue. The innermost meningeal layer is the pia, a tightly adherent layer that is extremely thin. Extensions of the pia continue within the nerve itself as the pial septa and provide the blood supply to the intraorbital and intracranial optic nerve, as discussed in the section on vasculature. The fibroblastic cells of the pial septa also form a matrix through which the fascicles of ganglion cell axons course.[195] In the optic canal there are numerous trabeculae connecting the dura through the arachnoid to the pia, which reduce the free space of the nerve sheath in this area.[168] The pia extends collagenous septa into the optic nerve parenchyma, containing blood vessels that nourish the nerve. These septa, which partially separate bundles of optic nerve axons, increase in size during aging.[293] Experimental tracer studies in rabbits and humans have revealed a pathway for particulate matter from the optic nerve subarachnoid space through the dura to fine epidural lymphatics; arachnoid villi not related to venous outflow channels are seen projecting into the subdural space of the optic nerve, presumably serving as an outflow channel for cerebrospinal fluid.[100,193,207]

The space between the dura and arachnoid is the subdural space, whereas the space between the arachnoid and pia is the subarachnoid space. The subdural space around the optic nerve is small and is not in communication with the intracranial subdural space. The subarachnoid space, on the other hand, is in communication with the intracranial subarachnoid space. The optic nerve subarachnoid space ends anteriorly within a blind pouch just before the disc (see Color Plate 15). As discussed in the section on increased intracranial pressure, the extension of the subarachnoid space from the brain into the orbit implies that elevated intracranial pressure has the potential to cause compression of the optic nerve by elevating the hydraulic pressure. There is an appreciable pressure within the subarachnoid space, measuring from 4 to 14 mm Hg.[249]

Although all three layers of meninges are present in the intraorbital and intracanalicular optic nerve, only the pia continues along the intracranial optic nerve. The clinical relevance of this is that a tumor arising from the optic nerve meninges themselves (i.e., an optic nerve sheath meningioma) normally continues through the optic canal but then extends along the sphenoid bone, and not along the course of the intracranial optic nerve. This means that it is extremely rare for an optic nerve sheath tumor to extend toward the chiasm and thereby affect the other side. The more common way for optic nerve sheath meningiomas to become bilateral is by directly extending along the sphenoid bone meninges.

Meningothelial Cells

Meningothelial cells may have several functions, including that of wound repair and scarring, phagocytosis, and collagen production; when transformed, these cells are the proliferating component of optic nerve meningiomas.[11] The meninges are vascularized, with component cells similar to those found in other vessels, including pericytes and endothelial cells. The latter have tight junctions from 8 weeks of development on, except in the outer dura.[417] Although the pial endothelial cells have tight junctions, they are not continuous because horseradish peroxidase injected into the optic nerve subarachnoid space in rats diffuses into the nerve.[441] Tumors of meningeal vascular elements are not uncommon, with meningeal hemangioblastoma and hemangiopericytoma making up a category otherwise known as *angioblastic meningiomas.*[46] The dura is innervated by peripheral nerves, which are accompanied by Schwann cells, the latter being capable of malignant transformation. Macrophages and mast cells are also found in the meninges.[231,418] The role of these and other resident cells in meningeal inflammations is only speculative. Fluorescent granular perithelial cells found in human meninges may act as scavenger cells for lipids and other substances.[421]

The cytoskeleton of optic nerve meningeal cells varies greatly across species.[1] Ultrastructural and immunohistochemical studies have revealed the presence of desmosomes in amphibian, chicken, bovine, and human arachnoid cells but not in rat. Intermediate filament proteins of the cytokeratin type are found in amphibian, chicken, and bovine arachnoid but not in human or rat, whereas vimentin is found in chicken, bovine, and human arachnoid but not in amphibian or rat arachnoid.

The anatomy and development of the optic nerve meninges have been well described.[11,417] All three meningeal layers are formed from fibroblast-like cells, which vary in ultrastructural appearance from typical process-bearing fibroblasts to mesothelial cells lining the subdural and subarachnoid space. The meningeal layers are particularly rich in collagen and elastin. Trabeculae between the arachnoid and pia are formed from collagen and are lined with the same mesothelial cells that line the subarachnoid space. The most rapid proliferation of human meningeal cells during development occurs within 8 to 18 weeks of conception, with centrally located fibroblasts and peripherally located cells containing glycogen that increase during this time.[417,418] By 14 weeks the three layers of the meninges can be distinguished. These glycogen-rich cells go on to produce large amounts of collagen, which is deposited in the dura after 14 or 15 weeks.

Mast Cells

Mast cells, the tissue equivalent of circulating basophils, are responsible for immediate hypersensitivity (allergic) responses. They contain cytoplasmic granules of histamine, serotonin, and other inflammatory and vasoactive compounds. These granules are released when molecules of immunoglobulin E bound to high-affinity receptors on the mast cell surface contact particular target antigens. The products of degranulation are responsible for a local acute inflammatory response, with vasodilation and increased permeability of capillaries causing consequent edema. Cytokines released by mast cells may activate local inflammatory cells or may act as chemoattractants to recruit cells from the circulation.

Mast cells are found in the meninges surrounding the brain and in certain brain subregions, particularly the thalamus.[112,113,312] Mast cells have been histochemically identified in the meninges of human optic nerve, and histamine of mast cell origin has been described in rabbit and bovine optic nerve.[231,304] Although in situ activation of mast cells has not yet been demonstrated in optic nerve, parallel studies in the brain suggest that mast cells may have a role in autoimmune diseases of the CNS.[436] Mast cells surrounding vasa nervorum may be increased in rats with experimentally induced diabetes mellitus; this has not been established in human optic nerve.[102]

Other Cells

Blood vessels within the optic nerve contain a variety of cell types. These are discussed further in the section on vascular supply to the optic nerve. Fibroblastic cells within the optic nerve are usually extensions of the meninges, and these are discussed in that section. The lamina cribrosa contains specialized fibroblastic cells.

Targets of Retinal Ganglion Cell Axons

There are four main targets of retinal ganglion cells axons contained within the optic nerve: (1) LGN, (2) pretectal nucleus, (3) superior colliculus, and (4) suprachiasmatic nucleus. Most axons are unbranched, but studies in many animals, including primates, have demonstrated the existence of axon collaterals, suggesting that the same may be true for human optic nerves.[50,213] This section discusses each of the synaptic targets of retinal ganglion cells axons.

Lateral Geniculate Nucleus

The main function of the optic nerve is for vision, and this is primarily subsumed by projections to the LGN (discussed at length in Chapter 28). The primate LGN is a six-layered structure, with layers 1 and 2 consisting of large (magnocellular) cells and layers 3, 4, 5, and 6 consisting of small (parvocellular) cells. The magnocellular layers receive input from the midget retinal ganglion cells, and the parvocellular layers receive input from the parasol retinal ganglion cells. Layers 2, 3, and 5 receive input from the ipsilateral retina, and layers 1, 4, and 6 receive input from the contralateral retina. In addition, interlaminar cells form the koniocellular layers. These cells are smaller than those of the parvocellular layers and receive synaptic input from blue-yellow retinal ganglion cells.[173] The first (and only) synapse of most axons within the optic nerve takes place at the LGN. These postsynaptic neurons then project to area V1 of the occipital cortex (i.e., the striate cortex). Details of this projection and the functional anatomy of the part of the cerebral cortex that is devoted to vision are discussed at length in Chapters 29 and 30.

Pretectal Nuclei

A second function of the optic nerve is for the afferent portion of the pupillary response.[24,189] These fibers project to the pretectal nuclei within the midbrain. Although the exact number is not known in humans, retrograde labeling studies in pigeons and rats indicate that only a small percentage of retinal ganglion cell axons are responsible for the pupillary reflex.[141,477]

Animal studies suggest that W-like retinal ganglion cells with large receptive fields (see also Chapter 32) originate most of the axons destined for the pretectal nuclei.[104,371,477] It has been proposed that there are differences between the myelin-surrounding axons destined for the LGN and those responsible for the pupillomotor reflex because of the existence, albeit rare, of patients with demyelinative optic neuropathies and monocular blindness with preserved pupillary reflexes.[237] These patients do not have apparent conduction toward the LGN but do have conduction toward the pretectal areas responsible for the pupillary reflex.

The pretectal projection is bilateral; in addition, fibers from each pretectal nucleus project both ipsilaterally and contralaterally to the Edinger-Westphal subnuclei of the third nerve nucleus. The latter then projects parasympathetic axons along the course of the third nerve to the ciliary ganglion within the orbit, where a synapse is made. Postsynaptic parasympathetic fibers continue to the pupilloconstrictor muscle, constriction of which is visible as the pupillary light reflex.

The combined ipsilateral and contralateral projections from the retina to the pretectal nuclei, and from the pretectal nuclei to the Edinger-Westphal subnuclei necessitate that a light stimulus causing impulses along either optic nerve will cause equal constriction of both pupils. This is the physiologic basis for detecting an afferent pupillary defect (also called the *swinging flashlight test* or *Marcus Gunn pupil*). If there is a functional difference in the number of optic nerve axons carrying impulses from each retina, then light shined into the eye with fewer axons will cause a lesser amount of (bilaterally symmetric) pupillary constriction than light shined into the other eye. By alternating the light between the two eyes and observing the difference in pupil size dependent on which eye the light is shined into, one can detect which optic nerve is functionally conducting less than the other. This measure is highly correlated with differences in the number of surviving retinal ganglion cells.[222] Detection of the afferent pupillary defect is discussed at length in Chapter 32.

Superior Colliculus

A third set of optic nerve axons project to the superior colliculus, a paired structure of the dorsal midbrain. In lower animals, such as rodents, most fibers of the optic nerve project to the superior colliculus. In primates, including humans, only a minority does so, with most axons destined instead for the

LGN. These fibers arise from most of the retina, except for the central 10 degrees.[52] The superior colliculus has a laminar organization and is retinotopically mapped.[470] Most studies of superior colliculus architecture have been done in animals, although the human superior colliculus appears to have similar anatomy.[179] The function of the superior colliculus is to coordinate retinal and cortical control of saccades and fixation.[470] Fibers branching to midbrain terminal nuclei stabilize the retinal image during movement of the eye, head, or body.[135] Control of extraocular movements is covered in detail in Chapter 36.

Hypothalamus
A fourth projection of optic nerve axons is through the retinohypothalamic tract to the suprachiasmatic nucleus and the paraventricular nucleus within the hypothalamus. These fibers are responsible for circadian control of the sleep-wake cycle, temperature, and other systemic functions.[199,376,384]

Retinopetal Projections
Optic nerve axons carry impulses *toward* the retina from CNS structures in animals; sources of these fibers include the suprachiasmatic nucleus of the hypothalamus, the dorsal raphe nucleus, and other midbrain areas.[47,220,393,448] This has not been confirmed in humans.

OPTIC NERVE ELECTROPHYSIOLOGY
Retinal Ganglion Cell Electrophysiology and Synaptic Transmission
Retinal ganglion cells receive synaptic input from bipolar and amacrine cells. The bipolar inputs are the results of graded potentials, as of all retinal neurons, only retinal ganglion cells exclusively use action potentials (amacrine cells have features of both).[39] The synapses from bipolar and amacrine cells primarily use glutamate as the major excitatory neurotransmitter, and retinal ganglion cells have both *N*-methyl-D-aspartate (NMDA) and non-NMDA ionotropic receptors, as well as metabotropic receptors.* Other neurotransmitters modulating retinal ganglion cells include GABA, acetylcholine (which may be of particular importance during development), and aspartate (acting on NMDA receptors).[120,205,217,373] Within the retina itself the levels of glutamate are controlled by Müller cells, which have glutamate transporters

and contain the enzyme glutamine synthetase, converting glutamate to the amino acid glutamine. Glutamate reuptake within the retina is necessary for maintaining appropriate retinal ganglion cell function.[25,178,265,334] The electrophysiology of retinal ganglion cells is complex and is discussed at length in Chapter 14.[157,386-388,428,429] Electrophysiology of retinal ganglion cell dendrites is also not discussed here but is reviewed in a recent communication.[445] The retinal ganglion cell synapse on its targets, primarily the LGN in higher animals, is glutamate, but other neurotransmitters are also used, including substance P and serotonin.[69,70,115,116,330]

Excitotoxicity
Retinal ganglion cells are particularly susceptible to high levels of glutamate in the extracellular space.[252,311,402,403] This causes cell death mediated by overexcitation, or excitotoxicity.[165] It has been proposed that excitotoxic retinal ganglion cell death may explain pathologic conditions, such as glaucoma, in which an excess of retina ganglion cells die akin to what occurs with cerebral infarct or other diseases.[392] The evidence supporting this is that antagonists of glutamate excitotoxicity mediated by NMDA receptors generally decrease retinal ganglion cell death after optic nerve injury and that glutamate levels may be elevated within the eye after optic nerve injury or experimental or human glaucoma.[111,375,474,475] Changes in NMDA receptor subunit expression follow axonal injury and may underlie changes in susceptibility to excitotoxicity.[215]

Axonal Conduction
Action Potentials. The primary function of the optic nerve is to carry information from the retina to target areas within the brain. Individual retinal ganglion cell axons transmit information through action potentials, which are all-or-nothing spikes of electrical activity. This is in contrast with intercellular communication within the retina, where *graded potentials* are used to transmit information. In other words, the retinal ganglion cells and their axons are the first neurons in the transmission of visual information from the eye to use action potentials as the mechanism for transmission. With action potentials, the actual amount of voltage change (i.e., depolarization) is the same, and the number of impulses per second and the distribution of impulses within various axons is the mechanism by which visual information is carried down the optic nerve. Conduction down individual axons occurs through the same biophysical mechanisms that occur in any myelinated

---

*References 238, 264, 308, 373, 374, 402.

axon (see later section on myelin). Variations in conduction velocity of individual axons probably helps coordinate conduction time between retinal ganglion cells located at differing distances between their retinal location and the optic nerve.[409]

In physiologic culture studies of rat optic nerve, conduction can be blocked either by replacing the sodium ions in the bath media or by applying the voltage-dependent sodium channel blocker tetrodotoxin. This implies that sodium is a major ion in axonal conduction.[130] In adult rats, optic nerve sodium channels in high density have been localized with immunoultrastructural techniques to the nodes of Ranvier; these channels presumably play a role in extracellular ionic homeostasis and are induced by oligodendrocytes.[41,202] Neonatal axons, which are unmyelinated, have a low density of sodium channels. This decreased density suffices, however, for axonal conduction.[456] It is possible that the low density of internodal sodium channels in adult optic nerve may allow conduction when diseased or demyelinated, supplanting the physiologic conduction that occurs through the densely populated nodal sodium channels.[456] Astrocytic processes extending into the nodal region have a high density of sodium channels. The physiologic relevance of this is uncertain but may relate to their role as a source for neuronal sodium.[41] Non-inactivating sodium channels may underlie the pathologic response to anoxia.[425]

Voltage-sensitive potassium channels allow positively charged potassium ions to exit the cell, where they are in relatively higher concentration than the extracellular fluid. The membrane potential thereby becomes relatively more negative, and this can contribute to the end of the action potential. In rat optic nerve, this fast potassium channel has been extensively studied. It is sensitive to the potassium channel blocker 4-aminopyridine (4-AP) and is electrophysiologically similar to the potassium channel that accounts for postaction potential hyperpolarization seen in other axons. Blockade of this channel by incubation with 4-AP causes impulse slowing. In addition, a second type of potassium channel has been described. This slow potassium channel is tetraethylammonium (TEA) sensitive and appears to modulate repetitive axonal action potentials by hyperpolarizing the axon after a train of firings.[152-154,212] There is a differential anatomic distribution of the two potassium channels with respect to axonal diameter; both are present at nodes of Ranvier in large, fast-conducting axons, but with the TEA-sensitive channel present alone in the internode region in slower-conducting

axons.[132] In addition, neonatal optic nerve axons have GABA-A receptors, which modulate axonal transmission, only partly through extracellular potassium changes.[377]

The mechanism of axonal conduction is straightforward. At rest, the inside of an axon is at a negative voltage with respect to the outside of the axon. This *resting potential* is negative and primarily results from the fact that the concentration of potassium is much higher within the axon compared with its extracellular concentration. As a small number of potassium ions flow down their concentration gradient from the inside of the axon to the outside, this movement of positive charge out of the axon results in a negative potential within the axon. Outward flux of potassium continues until the charge separation becomes too great and can no longer be driven by the concentration difference between inside and outside the axon. The point at which the gradient for potassium concentration is balanced by the gradient for separation of charge results in an equilibrium potential for potassium. Although the resting potential is primarily determined by potassium, there is also a smaller contribution from sodium flowing down its concentration gradient. In the case of sodium the concentration in the extracellular space is high, compared with a low concentration within the axon. This concentration gradient would induce sodium to enter the axon, and movement of a small number of sodium ions results in a positive sodium equilibrium potential. However, in a resting (nondepolarizing) axon the conductance for sodium is much smaller than that for potassium; therefore the final resting potential is weighted much more by the equilibrium potential for potassium than for sodium.

The situation changes during axonal conduction. Partial axon depolarization (resulting from an adjacent section of membrane that is already depolarized) induces opening of voltage-sensitive sodium channels located within the membrane. These allow much greater amounts of sodium to enter the axon, and the positive sodium ions cause the axon to become more positive, that is, *depolarized*. In this case the potential across the membrane is now weighted far more by the sodium equilibrium potential than by the potassium equilibrium potential. Why do the sodium channels open? These channels are voltage sensitive, and a relatively small depolarization of the membrane causes them to open transiently. Increased potential within the axon rapidly affects adjacent sections of the axon and causes sodium channels in these adjacent areas of axonal membrane to likewise become partially depolarized. These then completely open and cause a compete depolarization. This chain of events continues down the axon, resulting in a transmission of action potential.

Repolarization is the return of the axonal membrane potential to the original (negative resting potential) state and is necessary for more than a single action potential to be transmitted down the axon. Repolarization is caused by the closure of the voltage-sensitive sodium channels and a transient opening of voltage-sensitive potassium channels. Once the latter occurs, the membrane resting potential is weighted more by the potassium equilibrium potential than by the sodium equilibrium potential. This results in a restoration of membrane potential to the resting state.

In the process of transmission of an action potential, there is movement of sodium and potassium ions along their concentration gradients. If action potentials continued indefinitely, the sodium and potassium concentrations would reach equilibrium across the axonal membrane, resulting in loss of their concentration gradients and blocking conduction. Therefore, to reestablish their concentration gradients, a relatively slow redistribution process of these ions takes place through Na^+-K^+-ATPase. This process is highly energy dependent and fails to happen if axonal metabolism is disturbed.

Glia. Although neurons are classically considered the only electrically active cell population in the CNS, astrocytes also have ionic channels. For example, multiple voltage-sensitive sodium channels have been demonstrated in rat optic nerve astrocytes.[41,42,307] Both sodium and potassium channels have been studied electrophysiologically in cultured astrocytes.[38] In type 1 astrocytes, there appear to be a voltage-sensitive sodium current (of the glial type), a delayed rectifier potassium current, and an inward rectifier potassium current, with a calcium current being seen only in cAMP-treated cells.[27] Within the intact optic nerve, nonvesicularly released glutamate from the axon may induce glial cell spiking and possibly other effects.[196,216] Whether ionic channels or neurotransmitter receptors on optic nerve glia are physiologically important in vivo has yet to be demonstrated, but their presence suggests that optic nerve astrocytes may be more functionally specialized than previously recognized.

Role of Myelin. An additional complexity is added by the presence of myelin. Myelin has two physiologic properties: It increases the resistance and decreases the capacitance of the axon. The decreased capacitance means fewer sodium ions (less positive charge) are needed to enter the axon in order to depolarize the membrane to a given voltage. The increased resistance means that there is less leakage of charge across the membrane. Together, these properties decrease the amount of ionic flux needed to achieve changes in voltage across the membrane. If conduction can be achieved with less ionic flux, then less energy is needed to maintain ionic homeostasis after conduction and therefore less Na^+-K^+-ATPase activity is necessary. Therefore myelinated conduction is more efficient. In accord with this degree of energy conservation, there is a relatively higher density of axonal mitochondria just anterior to where axonal myelination in the nerve begins and a greater amount of enzymes for oxidative metabolism in the nonmyelinated portion.[229,285] These changes may also be caused by a physiologic relative block to axonal transport.[285]

Ionic channels are not distributed uniformly along a myelinated axon. Instead, the channels are segregated into patches located within the small areas where the axon is unmyelinated. These are called *nodes of Ranvier* (see Color Plate 16). Therefore conduction in a myelinated axon becomes much faster because the depolarization of the axon at one node leads to depolarization at the next node by the intrinsic conduction within the axon (the "cable properties" of the axon), instead of by sequential opening of channels along the axon. The depolarization thus "jumps" from one node to another; this is therefore called *saltatory conduction*. The prior section on action potentials discusses the electrophysiology of ion channels in more detail.

In cases of acquired loss of myelin, for example, in idiopathic optic neuritis (a common inflammatory optic neuropathy), conduction is abnormal because of the changes in resistive and capacitive properties of the membrane brought about by demyelination. This can happen through loss of the compact morphology of the myelin alone (i.e., without frank demyelination).[158] Axonal conduction becomes slowed and in some cases may be blocked ("conduction block"), both resulting in decreased visual function. Even in a completely demyelinated axon, a low density of internodal sodium channels in demyelinated optic nerve may still allow conduction.[456] Another phenomenon peculiar to demyelination is worsening of vision with heat or exercise, or *Uhthoff's phenomenon.* Increased temperature and exercise are thought to decrease the sodium channel open-time during depolarization, resulting in less charge entering the axon and a decreased likelihood that an adjacent section of demyelinated axon can depolarize enough to cause opening of its own voltage-sensitive sodium channels. This leads to temperature-sensitive conduction block.

Axonal Transport

The entire length of the retinal ganglion cell axon must be maintained by transporting proteins and other subcellular constituents several centimeters from the cell body, where the nucleus and virtually all of the protein synthetic machinery resides. These axons are several centimeters long; thus the health of the nerve relies on axonal transport of a multitude of substances over a distance many times the size of the ganglion cell body itself. The processes underlying axonal transport have been well studied, both in the optic nerve and in other nerves, and several important features can be identified.

Axonal transport occurs in two directions: orthograde (away from the cell body and toward the brain) and retrograde (toward the cell body and away from the brain). With injection of radioactive, fluorescent, or enzymatically active macromolecular tracers into either the eye or the terminal fields of the axons, the course and timing of orthograde and retrograde transport can be determined. Through analysis of the individual intraaxonal substances that become labeled, the differentiation of transport into several classes becomes possible. Depending on the fineness of the separation, two to five groups of substances appear to be axonally transported, each with their own characteristic velocity. Studies have generally been performed in experimental mammals, with findings generally consistent across species.[235] The rates of transport of specific moieties may vary as a function of stage of optic nerve development, suggesting a developmental role and regulation for axonal transport.[465] Different rates of axonal transport may be related to differences in the motor proteins interacting with microtubules, such as kinesin for fast transport and dynein for slow transport.[9,103]

Fast axonal transport carries several subcellular organelles, such as the vesicles of neurotransmitter used in synaptic transmission, as well as other particulate matter, toward the axon terminal.[290] Proteins carried by this process are usually membrane associated.[251] This process has been measured at 90 to 350 mm/day in the rat and chick optic nerve.[19,96] Fast axonal transport is sensitive to metabolic inhibitors and to agents such as colchicine, suggesting, respectively, an energy- and microtubule-dependent mechanism for transport.[267] This class of transport continues despite transection of the axon distal to the cell body, suggesting that intraaxonal components are sufficient for the process to occur.

Slow axonal transport carries several types of proteins, many of which are as yet unidentified. Most components carried by slow axonal transport end up within the axon itself. There are two classes of slow transport. The slower class of slow axonal transport (SCa) occurs at 0.2 to 1 mm/day and carries cytoskeletal proteins, primarily tubulins, which make up microtubules, and neurofilament proteins, a member of the intermediate filament group. These are the major skeleton proteins for the neuron.[43] The process of microtubule-associated transport is complex.[272] It is possible that the microtubules are transported as intact elements, based on the finding of cotransport of some microtubule-associated proteins in this slow component.[443] The more rapid class of slow axonal transport (SCb) occurs at 2 to 8 mm/day and carries proteins such as actin and myosin, as well as the enzymes of intermediate metabolism and myelin-associated proteins.[43,150,466] Mitochondria are transported by this process. However, the physiology of slow axonal transport is complex and even closely related proteins such as tau, tubulins, and other microtubule-associated proteins may be transported at different rates.[272,302] Slow axonal transport does not continue after transection of the axon distal to the cell body, unlike fast axonal transport.[138] Similarly, interruption of circulation to the proximal axon, for example by cutting of the short posterior ciliary arteries, causes interruption of slow transport.[236]

Retrograde transport occurs at about half the velocity of fast orthograde transport and is the means by which endocytosed substances from the synapse, such as released neurotransmitter, may be returned to the cell body. Likewise, wear and breakdown products from the axon and its terminal are similarly returned to the cell soma. Retrograde transport of neurotrophic molecules during development may signal the cell body regarding the presence of a growth target.

Axonal transport may be affected in disease, possibly potentiating nerve injury, such as in experimental allergic encephalomyelitis or glaucoma.[351]

Axonal transport within the optic nerve may have important clinical implications. For example, increased intraocular pressure can perturb rapid axonal transport at the lamina cribrosa, experimentally demonstrated by focal accumulation of labeled proteins after injection of radiolabeled precursors into the vitreous.[15,344,351] The same is true for retrograde axonal transport, demonstrated by injecting a marker into the LGN or optic tracts.[284] These data suggest a role for interruption of axonal transport in the pathophysiology of axonal loss in glaucoma. Accumulation of labeled proteins also occurs at physiologic intraocular pressures, implying that a qualititatively greater disturbance of axonal transport must be necessary for damage to occur through this mechanism.[286] Other important clinical correlations of altered axonal transport are in disc edema, in which blockage of axonal transport has been observed to occur, for example, with ocular hypotony or increased intracranial pressure, with diabetes, and in optic neuritis.[160,188,287,439]

BLOOD SUPPLY

The blood supply to the optic nerve is complex and changes qualitatively along its course. Because of the varying nature of the vascular supply to the optic nerve, a variety of clinical syndromes may result from ischemia or infarction at each location. This section discusses the vascular supply to the retinal ganglion cell axons as a function of location, starting at the retina, then the optic nerve head, the intraorbital optic nerve, the optic canal, the intracranial optic nerve, and the chiasm and optic tract. This material is covered in greater depth in Chapter 33 and in recent reviews.[315,317] The vascular biology of the optic nerve is discussed in the following sections.

Retina

Although the retina has two circulations, the retinal vascular circulation (derived from the central retinal artery) and the choroidal circulation (derived from the short posterior ciliary arteries), only the former is relevant to perfusion of the retinal ganglion cells and their axons within the nerve fiber layer. The retinal ganglion cells are located within the inner retina, in the ganglion cell layer, and the nerve fiber layer is vitread to the ganglion cell layer and is the innermost neuronal layer of the retina. Both derive their blood supply from capillary branches of the retinal circulation, although presumably some small amount of oxygen is exchanged with the vitreous itself. The clinical relevance of the retinal circulation perfusing the retinal ganglion cells and their axons is that an inner retinal infarction (e.g., from a central retinal artery occlusion) results in an optic neuropathy, with a pale disc and loss of axons within the optic nerve itself.

Optic Nerve Head

The circulation of the optic nerve head is complex and varies depending on which particular layer is studied. Our understanding of this circulation has been greatly enhanced by studies of histologic sections and of corrosion casting of the vessels themselves. Differences between circulations of rodents, subhuman primates, and humans necessitates focusing on the human optic nerve head circulation.[14] Although the nerve head circulation is derived from two sources, the central retinal artery and the posterior ciliary arteries, the latter provides the most important contribution. The central retinal artery is a branch of the intraorbital ophthalmic artery, and enters the optic nerve during its intraorbital course, approximately 12 mm behind the globe. As it heads toward the disc, it provides minimal perfusion of the nerve through which it courses.[240] As it branches on the disc into the retinal arterioles, it provides partial perfusion of the superficial disc through small capillaries.

In contrast, branches of the short posterior ciliary arteries provide the major blood supply to the optic nerve head. There are usually two posterior ciliary arteries, a medial and a lateral, which originate from the ophthalmic artery and form several branches. One set of branches becomes the major perfusion of the choroid, forming the choriocapillaris. Another set of branches perfuses the optic nerve, both anteriorly through direct branches and posteriorly through a retrograde arteriolar investiture of the optic nerve (see following discussion). Anastomoses of posterior ciliary artery branches form the circle of Zinn-Haller, which contributes significant perfusion to the optic nerve head.[313,314] In addition, there are contributions from recurrent choroidal arterioles to the prelaminar and laminar optic nerve head and contributions from recurrent pial arterioles to the laminar and retrolaminar optic nerve head. A clinical implication of the common posterior ciliary arterial source of the choroid and deep optic nerve head is that they fluoresce simultaneously during the earliest phase of fluorescein angiography before the retinal arterioles transit dye.

Although the choroid and the optic nerve head both receive blood supply from the posterior ciliary circulation, the histologic characteristics of the capillaries of each differ tremendously. Choroidal vessels have fenestrated endothelial cells, whereas optic nerve vessels have nonfenestrated endothelial cells with tight junctions surrounded by pericytes. Therefore optic nerve vessels share the same blood-nerve barrier characteristics as the blood-brain barrier. The clinical implication is that only a restricted number of molecules can cross the blood-nerve barrier. For example, gadolinium enhancement on magnetic resonance imaging is not seen unless some pathologic process within the optic nerve (e.g., inflammation) disrupts the blood-nerve barrier.[162,163]

Another major difference between choroidal and optic nerve head vessels is that only the latter can autoregulate (i.e., maintain approximately constant blood flow despite most changes in intraocular pressure).[148,368,462] The clinical implication is that there is compensation of perfusion for a wide range of intraocular pressures in normal individuals. Studies of oxygen tension in the cat optic nerve head support this, with relative preservation of a mean PO_2 of 10 to 20 mm Hg despite raising the intraocular pressure to 40 to 60 mm Hg.[4]

Intraorbital Optic Nerve and Optic Canal

The intraorbital optic nerve is perfused by the pial circulation. Branches of the ophthalmic artery either directly perfuse the pia or indirectly perfuse it anteriorly through recurrent branches of the short posterior ciliary arteries or a branch of the central retinal artery. The pia then sends penetrating (centripetal) vessels into the intraorbital optic nerve along the fibrovascular pial septa, from which a capillary network extends into neural tissue (axons and glia). Similarly, the intracanalicular optic nerve is perfused by up to three branches of the ophthalmic artery, namely a medial collateral, lateral collateral, and ventral branch.[80,133] These also perfuse the pial surface and then penetrate the nerve.

An important clinical implication of the pia supplying the intraorbital and intracanalicular optic nerve relates to optic nerve sheath meningiomas. If a surgeon strips the meningioma away from the nerve, the pia is removed as well, resulting in loss of the blood supply to the nerve, infarction, and blindness. Another clinical correlation is related to the small amount of free space within the canal, which when occupied by hematoma from shearing of the delicate vessels there, may result in a sight-threatening hematoma.[80]

Intracranial Optic Nerve, Chiasm, and Optic Tract

The intracranial optic nerve and chiasm are perfused by the internal carotid artery and its branches, primarily the anterior cerebral, anterior communicating, and superior hypophyseal artery. The posterior chiasm may also be perfused by branches of the posterior communicating artery. The optic tract is predominantly perfused by branches of the posterior communicating and anterior choroidal arteries. Similar to the intraorbital and intracanalicular optic nerve, the blood supply occurs through small pial penetrating vessels. However, no dura or arachnoid surrounds the optic nerve posterior to the optic canal; thus the risk of infarction is not from stripping a tumor off the nerve, but rather from inadvertent detachment of the fine vessels during surgical manipulation.

Vascular Biology

Vessels of the human optic nerve contain endothelial cells separated from pericytes by a basement membrane, with endfeet of astrocytes making up a surrounding coat. These features are all present early in development.[419] The tight junctions between endothelial cells make up the blood-nerve barrier, which is present in normal optic nerve throughout its length. The anterior part of the optic nerve, however, shares a distinctive feature with the area postrema, choroid plexus, and median eminence in that there is local disturbance of the blood-brain barrier. Although the optic nerve capillary endothelial cells in the anterior optic nerve have tight junctions, leakage can occur from adjacent choriocapillaris through the border tissue of Elschnig at the level of the lamina choroidalis.[127,355] Further leakage from this area into the subretinal space may be prevented by tight junctions between the glia making up the intermediary tissue of Kuhnt.[355,441] The blood-nerve barrier may be incompetent in focal inflammatory disorders, such as optic neuritis.[159]

The optic nerve differs from almost all other areas of the CNS in that there is connective tissue around vessels. Elsewhere, astrocytes alone are present.[17] In the human nerve parenchyma, pial septa containing the vessels that supply the optic nerve penetrate and interdigitate within the parenchyma. The vessels are closely surrounded by morphologically specialized collagen and pial fibroblasts, beyond which are astrocytic foot processes.[17,87,381,419] These pial septa are not a constant factor of mammalian optic nerves; rats, for example, do not have septa.

The vessels within the nerve have their own innervation. These nervi vasorum contain multiple neurotransmitters.[244] Because of the importance of the central retinal artery, its innervation has been well studied. Within the optic nerve, the central retinal artery is supplied by a plexus of nerve fibers that use a multitude of neurotransmitters. These have been studied in the rhesus monkey and include adrenergic, cholinergic, and calcitonin gene-related peptide; neuropeptide Y; substance P; and vasoactive intestinal peptide.[472] Human posterior ciliary arteries respond to the potent vasoconstrictor angiotensin II.[305]

AXONAL INJURY
Clinical Implications
The optic nerve is commonly involved in disease, resulting in optic neuropathy. Optic neuropathies are major causes of visual loss. The most common optic neuropathy is that associated with glaucoma, that is, glaucomatous optic neuropathy. A variety of other optic neuropathies also cause visual loss. The inflammatory optic neuropathies are most commonly seen in young or middle-aged adults, and the most common is optic neuritis associated with the demyelinating disease multiple sclerosis. Ischemic optic neuropathy usually affects older adults. The most common type is nonarteritic anterior ischemic optic neuropathy, a disorder of unknown cause that results in sudden visual loss associated with disc edema; arteritic anterior ischemic optic neuropathy has a similar clinical presentation but is caused by a vasculitic process, usually from giant cell arteritis. Compressive optic neuropathy, in which the optic nerve is compressed by a mass lesion, commonly a tumor or aneurysm, results in slowly progressive loss of visual function as the mass increases in size. Although not proven, some researchers believe that Leber's hereditary optic neuropathy and some of the toxic optic neuropathies may reflect damage to the retinal ganglion cell body within the retina. Except for these, most optic neuropathies result from direct damage to the optic nerve.

Therefore most optic neuropathies involve axonal injury. This section discusses how axonal damage results in death of the retinal ganglion cell. For example, glaucomatous optic neuropathy likely results from axonal injury at the optic nerve head, particularly at the lamina cribrosa. Nonarteritic anterior ischemic optic neuropathy also results from damage at the optic nerve head, in many cases just posterior to the lamina cribrosa. The locus of injury for compressive optic nerve injury is usually obvious and may range from within the orbit (e.g., with Graves' ophthalmopathy) to the chiasm (e.g., from a pituitary adenoma or craniopharyngioma).

Retinal Ganglion Cell Death after Axonal Injury
Death of retinal ganglion cells is the final common pathway underlying virtually all diseases of the optic nerve, including glaucomatous optic neuropathy, anterior ischemic optic neuropathy, optic neuritis, and compressive optic neuropathy. These disorders all cause injury to the axon of the retinal ganglion cell within the bulbar, orbital, intracanalicular, or intracranial optic nerve, yet the pathology at the level of the retina is primarily loss of retinal ganglion cells. In many diseases affecting the retinal ganglion cell axons (e.g., glaucoma, arteritic ischemia), the visual loss is permanent, reflecting the fact that retinal ganglion cell loss is irreversible. In some cases (e.g., chronic compressive optic neuropathy, acute optic neuritis, papilledema), the visual loss can be reversed when the axonal damage is relieved, presumably because retinal ganglion cell death has not yet occurred. However, if allowed to continue, even these disorders eventually can result in permanent retinal ganglion cell death.

Most research on optic neuropathies has focused on the pathophysiology specific to the particular disorder, such as elevated intraocular pressure for glaucoma, inflammation for optic neuritis, and ischemia for anterior ischemic optic neuropathy. However, optic neuropathies all share in common retinal ganglion cell axonal injury, except for the few disorders for which the locus of injury is unknown, such as Leber's hereditary optic neuropathy. Therefore an understanding of the molecular response of the retinal ganglion cell to axonal injury is applicable to a variety of diseases of the optic nerve, independent of the mechanism by which the nerve is injured. It should be understood that not all axonal injuries cause similar processes in retinal ganglion cells. For example, even transection of the optic nerve is not the same as a crush injury.[289] Nonetheless, for the purpose of simplification, the next sections group together axonal injuries with respect to their effect on retinal ganglion cells.

Time Course. When axons contained within the optic nerve are transected or crushed, the associated retinal ganglion cells usually die. However, depending on the age and species of the animal, the cell body size, and the distance from the site of injury to the retinal ganglion cell, up to 70% may survive. In lower animals, such as goldfish and frogs, ganglion cells do not die, but hypertrophy and regenerate axons within 1 to 2 months.[185,186,294] The fact that ganglion cell death is not a necessary consequence of axotomy suggests that regulatory mechanisms underlie retinal ganglion cell survival after axonal injury.

Studies of the time course of retinal ganglion cell death in rodents after optic nerve injury demonstrate a partial (20% to 40%) loss within the first 3 to 7 days, the remainder (50% to 90%) taking weeks to sometimes months.* Ganglion cells from squirrel and owl monkeys die approximately 4 to 6 weeks after axotomy.[341,352] In humans with chiasmal compression for at least 6 months, loss of ganglion cells from the nasal hemiretinas is extensive; yet even 35 days after transection of the ipsilateral optic tract, some temporal ganglion cells are spared.[218]

In general, neonatal retinal ganglion cells are far more sensitive to axotomy than adults, perhaps because naturally occurring developmental cell death is taking place at the same time.[7,151,414] Whether the response of ganglion cells to axotomy depends on the distance between the lesion and the cell body is controversial. Some studies have shown that the shorter that distance, the more rapid the degeneration and the more severe the effect.† This could be caused by the lack of a trophic factor or transmission of a signal mediating cell death, either mechanism possibly mediated through retrograde axonal transport.[12,30,341] Others have suggested that the timing of ganglion cell degeneration is not correlated with the distance to the lesion.[341,352] Axotomized fibers from the macula degenerate later than those more peripheral, suggesting that the distance from the site of axotomy to the retina does not affect timing of retinal ganglion cell death.[341] Differences in ganglion cell survival also depend on the site of optic nerve transection in relation to the vascular supply of the retina. If the ophthalmic or central retinal arteries are transected, the inner retina, including the ganglion cell layer, is infarcted, confusing interpretation of retinal ganglion cell survival.[257]

Loss of retinal ganglion cells results in anterograde (wallerian) degeneration of their axons and consequential loss of optic nerve fibers. This can be studied as an isolated phenomenon by experimental enucleation. Studies in rodents demonstrate an exponential loss of fibers over time, with loss of 50% within the first 2 days and 90% by 4 days.[446] Loss of larger axons is preferentially faster.[446] Unlike the programmed cell death process occurring in the cell bodies of retinal ganglion cells (see next section), wallerian axonal degeneration does not depend on caspase activation, a hallmark of apoptosis.[124]

Apoptosis. The mode of death of retinal ganglion cells after axonal injury is complex and appears to involve a programmed cell death process called *apoptosis.* At the beginning of this century, Ramon-y-Cajal described "*massues terminales*" that resembled pyknotic nuclei in the ganglion cells of retinas 40 days after optic nerve transection. Pathologic studies in the modern era demonstrated condensation of the nucleus, formation of nuclear dense bodies, and dislocation of the nucleus.[30,434] These features are now recognized to be those of apoptosis, a form of programmed cell death characterized by condensation of the nucleus and cytoplasm, budding of the cytoplasmic membrane, cleavage of deoxyribonucleic acid (DNA) into 180- to 200-bp fragments, fragmentation of the cell into membrane-bound bodies, and heterophagy of these bodies.[147,203] A subset of retinal ganglion cells undergoes apoptosis during developmental cell death, as shown by morphologic changes and DNA fragmentation and pressure-induced ischemia.[51,187,323] Various techniques have been used to show that the death of retinal ganglion cells after axotomy occurs by apoptosis.* It is likely that neurotrophin deprivation or some other signal may induce a death program in these cells (see following discussion).[435]

Unlike the cell death associated with a cytotoxic injury to the cell body, resulting in *necrosis,* apoptosis is a form of cell suicide in which the steps of cell death are primarily cell autonomous. The apoptosis program is an intricate and sequential activation of multiple intracellular enzymes, including cysteine-dependent aspartate-directed proteases (caspases) and endonucleases. Although apoptosis is an active area of cell biology research, it is evident that many of the earliest steps that take place during apoptosis are at the mitochondrial level. Early in apoptosis the mitochondria release cytochrome c, procaspase-9, and other apoptosis-inducing factors. In addition, either sequentially or in parallel, the mitochondrial membrane potential (formed from the pumping of protons into the intermembrane space) is lost. It is

---

*References 7, 8, 30, 155, 288, 321, 449.
†References 155, 226, 239, 288, 434, 454.

*References 36, 73, 145, 233, 349, 360.

thought that this mitochondrial depolarization might play a role in the signaling of apoptosis. Once the *apoptosome* is formed from the factors released from the mitochondria, the activation of caspases takes place. These in turn activate other caspases, and this cascade of events results in the activation of other enzymes within the cell, which results in the breakdown of DNA and other macromolecules, compartmentalization of cell components, and eventual dissolution of the cell into small membrane-bound compartments, which are then phagocytosed by adjacent cells.

Besides axonal injury, several other modes of cell death may induce the apoptosis mechanism. For example, the binding of tumor necrosis factor to tumor necrosis factor receptors may induce apoptosis by way of death domain signaling and subsequent activation of caspase-8, initially bypassing the caspase-9 activation by the mitochondria. Also, glutamate excitoxicity may also induce apoptosis if the cell survives the early stimulus to necrosis, and antibodies to heat shock protein 27 (hsp27) can induce apoptosis of retinal ganglion cells.[18,430]

Signaling of Axonal Injury. Several theories are proposed to explain the mechanism by which axonal injury results in induction of apoptosis. Retinal ganglion cell death after optic nerve injury or target removal appears to take place through several mechanisms, including lack of neurotrophic factors from the target tissue, excitotoxicity from physiologic or pathologic levels of glutamate, free radical formation, leakage of cellular constituents out the end of the axon, proliferation of macroglia, activation of microglia, buildup of excess retrogradely transported macromolecules, and breakdown of the blood-brain barrier.* Even the contralateral retina may be affected by a unilateral optic nerve injury, suggesting the involvement of intrachiasmal signaling or retinopetal fibers.[44] Of greatest interest is neurotrophic factor deprivation from blocked retrograde transport of neurotrophic factors (neurotrophins) or decreased levels of endogenous ocular neurotrophins, analogous to the loss of a target during development.[3,435] The subject has recently been reviewed.[450]

Retinal ganglion cells are known to be highly dependent on neurotrophic factors during development, and the normal developmental loss of retinal ganglion cells is partly the result of competition for target-derived molecules, such as neurotrophins, while attempting to extend their axons and form

connections in target areas of the CNS. In the adult human CNS, the predominant targets of the axons contained within the optic nerve are the LGN, the superior colliculus, the pretectal nuclei, and the suprachiasmatic nucleus of the hypothalamus. It is thought that adult retinal ganglion cells, like other neurons, are partly dependent on neurotrophic agents for their survival.[365] First shown in sympathetic neurons with respect to nerve growth factor (NGF), support for the role of neurotrophin dependence comes from experiments using identified neurotrophic factors to rescue axotomized neurons, including retinal ganglion cells, and intraocular administration of certain neurotrophins (particularly brain-derived neurotrophic factor [BDNF]) delays retinal ganglion cell death after axotomy in adult animals.* Historically, the survival of ganglion cells in adult animals has also been facilitated by acidic and basic fibroblast growth factor, CNTF, NGF, and conditioned medium from transected sciatic nerve.† Purified neonatal retinal ganglion cells (which are axotomized during dissociation) can be kept alive for significant periods beyond the normal time of developmental death with a cocktail of factors, including BDNF, CNTF, forskolin, and insulin.[276] Supplying neurotrophin alone is insufficient because responsiveness to neurotrophin also appears to require a cAMP elevation signal.[277,399] Microglia may play a subsidiary role in ganglion cell death, based on experiments using macrophage inhibitory factor (MIF) to inhibit microglial activation and enhance ganglion cell survival after axotomy.[432]

Our understanding of how deprivation of neurotrophic agents causes neuronal cell death relates to the signal transduction cascades by which these factors normally maintain viability. The most well characterized are the tyrosine receptor kinases for the neurotrophic factors. TrkB functions as a receptor for BDNF and NT-4/5, trkA for NGF, and trkC for NT-3. TrkB itself is regulated by activity or cAMP levels.[277] TrkB and its ligand BDNF are expressed in retinal ganglion cells during postnatal development.[324] TrkB occupancy causes autophosphorylation, inducing binding of the Shc PTB domain, Shc phosphorylation, and association with Grb2-SOS1.[397] Subsequently, guanosine diphosphate (GDP) is exchanged for guanosine triphosphate (GTP) on Ras, following which Raf is activated, and then the MAP kinase cascade, eventually leading to transcription factor-mediated changes in

---

*References 93, 97, 155, 261, 390, 434, 454, 474.

*References 72, 208-211, 258, 261, 273, 321, 460.
†References 21, 65, 84, 273, 401, 433.

gene expression. Although this pathway is the best characterized, there are presumably multiple other signal transduction pathways for neurotrophic factors. For example, Ras GTPase activity also leads to activation of PI3-kinase activity, which transduces a separate set of signals through activation of Akt (protein kinase B).[114,172] Although these pathways have not been completely unraveled in retinal ganglion cells, evidence suggests that a single pathway does not explain the signal transduction of BDNF, their role in survival of these cells and other neurons is well established.[211]

If the optic nerve is injured and BDNF or other neurotrophins are introduced into the vitreous or retina, survival of retinal ganglion cells, compared with control eyes, is increased.* However, no direct evidence indicates that adult retinal ganglion cells are normally dependent on BDNF or other neurotrophic factors, and it is possible that the increased survival seen after neurotrophin administration is not a *specific* rescue effect from neurotrophin deprivation, but rather a generalized prosurvival effect. Furthermore, retrograde axonal transport is rapid, and the subacute time course by which retinal ganglion cells die after axonal injury does not reflect the time course of interrupted retrograde axonal transport. This probably explains why damage to the retinal ganglion cell axon in several different places results in similar rates of death after axonal injury.

Another mechanism by which axonal injury may induce retinal ganglion cell death is through the induction of an *injury signal*. Although this area is relatively unexplored for the optic nerve, findings in other nerves (e.g., peripheral nerves) suggest that there may be transduction of signals within cell bodies targeted by axons that result from injury to the axon itself. Multiple genes appear to be induced or inhibited in expression by axonal injury (e.g., BDNF, PDGF B-chain, ceruloplasmin, bcl-X_L, tubulin, c-Jun, GAP-43, activated transcription factor-3).† Furthermore, there may also be role for anterogradely transported and paracrine neurotrophic factors in retinal ganglion cell survival.[450,451]

Therapies of Axonal Injury. Neuroprotection, first proposed for other CNS diseases, has been considered in recent years as a possible treatment for optic neuropathies.[396,461] Neuroprotective strategies include blocking retinal excitotoxicity mediated by glutamate (which binds to NMDA receptors and induces retinal ganglion cell death); administering neurotrophic factors (e.g., BDNF), which maintain retinal ganglion cell survival; activating small molecule receptors, which may enhance neuronal resistance to insult; inhibiting nitric oxide synthase-2, which may prevent axonal injury at the lamina cribrosa; and providing immunization with certain synthetic polypeptides.* Not one of these strategies has yet been successfully proven in randomized controlled clinical trials in human patients with glaucoma. However, there is a variety of laboratory evidence using cell culture or animal models of optic nerve disease to suggest that one or more neuroprotective methodologies eventually may be successful in clinical disease.

Phagocytosis and Immune Activation

An example of microglial phagocytosis occurs during wallerian degeneration. In this pathologic process, resident microglia and circulating monocytes are thought to be the primary cells responsible for phagocytosis of myelin debris, although there may be a contribution from oligodendrocytes and astrocytes.[255,412,441] Probably, most phagocytes in degenerating optic nerve are derived from the circulation and relatively fewer from intrinsic cells, although not all studies are in agreement.[246,411] During wallerian degeneration, the number of microglia increases, presumably as a result of activation or invasion from as yet unidentified chemical or electrical signals.[223] Microglia can be observed to invade the myelin sheath and disrupt the myelin lamellae; the fragments are then phagocytosed.[250] However, deficiencies in the activation of microglia may lead to decreased clearance of myelin debris and subsequent inhibition of axonal regeneration.[361] Increasing macrophage-mediated clearance of debris can increase regeneration.[224]

Ia antigen expression does not necessarily occur as part of an immunologic process because wallerian degeneration induced by optic nerve transection in rats can increase Ia expression on microglia/macrophages, perhaps through targeting of activated cells to the degenerating nerve or induction in situ.[12,441] In addition, enucleation can induce astrocytes in terminal regions of optic nerve to express both class I and class II histocompatibility antigens.[355]

Although the predominant cells for phagocytosis after injury in optic nerve are probably microglia, the contribution of other cell types to this

---

*References 72, 258, 261, 273, 321, 460.
†References 106, 131, 144, 184, 232, 234, 271, 427.

*References 72, 109, 261, 299, 321, 391, 463, 476.

process is controversial. It has been suggested that both astrocytes and oligodendrocytes can contribute to the phagocytosis of myelin and axonal debris resulting from wallerian degeneration.[91,201,472] Other studies in crushed rat optic nerve have revealed initial loss of apolipoprotein from astrocyte cell bodies, followed by appearance after several weeks of a phagocytic morphology and appearance of the macrophage marker ED1 on these GFAP-positive cells—consistent with the hypothesis that reactive optic nerve astrocytes can share several features with microglia.[305] A partial answer to the contradictory reports of phagocytic cells after optic nerve injury may come from a study in which several zones of the monkey nerve were examined after transection behind the globe.[92] Under these conditions, phagocytosis by macrophages of presumed hematogenous origin were seen focally, whereas endogenous cells, perhaps oligodendrocytes, phagocytosed at distant sites of wallerian degeneration. This is supported by the findings of ED1-positive macrophages in regions of GFAP-negative crushed optic nerve.[331]

Gliosis

The role of optic nerve astrocytes in the pathologic processes of gliosis is complex.[57,60] As a reaction either to local injury or to remote death of adjacent axons, astrocytes are observed to divide and extend processes, without the formation of collagen that typifies the classic fibroblastic response to injury. Astrocytic gliosis presumably occurs partly to replace neural tissue—as a type of scar formation—but may also relate to astrocyte secretion of cytokines, which may recruit or modulate other cell types. The cells responsible for gliosis are predominantly type 1 astrocytes.[247,389] There are several other lines of evidence for astrocyte activation during gliosis. During wallerian degeneration caused by optic nerve transection, both fibrous astrocytes and reactive astrocytes divide, as demonstrated by 3H-thymidine incorporation.[404] Similar increases in cell number are seen in glioblasts and microglia. During antibody-induced demyelination of the optic nerve, cells morphologically resembling astrocytes are observed to express both GFAP and the oligodendrocyte surface-marker galactocerebroside, suggesting that a dedifferentiation is taking place.[67] Quantification of the astrocytic enzyme glutamine synthetase reveals increased activity distal to optic nerve crush injury.[333] Immunohistochemistry of axotomized rat optic nerves reveals increased amounts of GFAP, whereas the increase

in laminin is not significant.[269] Unlike transection, crush injury may locally inhibit GFAP expression but increase the recruitment of macrophages (see also previous discussion).[331] Expression of the intermediate filament protein nestin is associated with reactive gliosis after optic nerve crush, and one or more of these processes may explain the failure of ganglion cell axons to regenerate after injury.[137,394] The density of small intramembranous particles, a normal plasma membrane component of astrocytes, increases after enucleation; this is hypothesized to correlate with the reactive astrocyte's inability to support axonal outgrowth.[469] Although CNS astrocytes normally express a variety of neuropeptide receptors, they are not commonly seen in the normal optic nerve.[262] After nerve transection, however, glial scars appear to express large numbers of receptors for substance P, a neuropeptide associated with inflammatory and immune response modulation.[262] Similarly, the constitutively low levels of endothelin ETB receptor levels increase greatly after optic nerve injury.[372]

Types of Optic Nerve Injury

As previously discussed, injury to the axons contained within the optic nerve results in retinal ganglion cell death. However, axonal injuries differ substantially, especially with respect to clinical disease. This section mentions some of the major types of axonal injuries in the context of local pathology.

Transection. Transection of optic nerve axons results in a discontinuity of the axonal membrane and its contents. It is relatively uncommon for the human optic nerve to undergo an acute partial or complete transection, with the most common examples being direct traumatic optic neuropathy (e.g., from a bullet or knife) and iatrogenic transection during surgical resection of an adjacent or intrinsic tumor. Although many animal models that are used to study the effects of optic nerve injury involve transection of axons, this is therefore not reflected by clinical disease. This disparity means that the large number of experimental studies of the pathways of retinal ganglion cell death after axonal injury do not necessarily reflect most diseases of the optic nerve because of the great difference in time course of the initial insults. Animal studies relating to the pathophysiology of optic nerve are discussed in an earlier section.

Ischemia. The evidence backing ischemia as a cause of human optic neuropathies varies, depending on the disease. For example, there is little doubt that arteritic anterior ischemic optic neuropathy resulting from giant cell arteritis is associated with histopathologically verifiable vasculitic occlusion of posterior ciliary arteries. On the other hand, whether the effects of intraocular pressure causing axonal damage in glaucomatous optic neuropathy is primarily an ischemic or compressive process is highly controversial. Even nonarteritic anterior ischemic optic neuropathy has features that make it unlike many other ischemic diseases.[228] Perhaps the least dispute relates to ischemia from hypotension or severe blood loss, although even in these cases the pathophysiology may vary.[90,198]

Ischemic optic nerve injury can be modeled in experimental animals through various approaches. A powerful method is to occlude the posterior ciliary arteries, best done in primate animals; however, this method has the disadvantage of also affecting the choroidal circulation.[169,170] Infusion of the vasoconstrictor endothelin-1 into the perineural space is a good model of subacute to chronic ischemia and can be performed in various species.[81-83,301,310,318,319] Perhaps one of the best methods to model ischemia is in the isolated optic nerve contained in a bath of buffer, the chemical and gaseous content of which can be controlled by the experimenter.[424]

The pathophysiology of myelinated axonal ischemia is complex and has recently been reviewed.[329,422] The presence of myelination affects the metabolism of the axon. Because less current is necessary for depolarization to occur, less adenosine triphosphate (ATP) is needed for transmission of action potentials. At the same time, the myelinated axon is more sensitive to anoxic damage. Although neonatal optic nerve, which is not myelinated, does not easily suffer irreversible damage from anoxia, more mature nerves from animals that have just undergone myelination are highly sensitive to anoxia. Similarly, optic nerves from *md* rats, a myelin-deficient rat strain, are sensitive to anoxia.[457] Nonetheless, even myelinated axons (white matter) are relatively less sensitive to ischemia than neuronal cell bodies (gray matter).[263] Direct ischemic injury to the optic nerve probably occurs as a result of an increase in intracellular Ca_2^+ caused by a reversal of the Na^+-Ca_2^+ exchanger.[423,424] Other evidence for the crucial role of sodium entry (primarily through voltage-sensitive sodium channels) in the deleterious effects of axonal ischemia is the ability of sodium channel blockers to ameliorate anoxic injury.[146,423] Glial cells play an important role in the response to ischemia,

with adjacent astrocytes helping buffer the decrease in glucose by shuttling lactate produced from their glycogen stores.[464]

Inflammation. Inflammation of the optic nerve, or optic neuritis, is the most common form of acute optic neuropathy in young and middle-aged adults and is a common harbinger of multiple sclerosis.[316,369] Demyelination is the most common pathologic accompaniment of optic nerve inflammation, and conduction block resulting from this or other effects of inflammation is responsible for the usually temporary loss of visual function seen in patients with optic neuritis.[471] This is discussed at length in the previous section on axonal conduction. Demyelination itself would not necessarily cause loss of retinal ganglion cells, highlighting the importance of the recognition that CNS inflammation in multiple sclerosis is also associated with axonal loss.[118,326,437] Axonal loss in optic neuritis has been long appreciated clinically as optic atrophy and loss of the nerve fiber layer, and experimental models of optic nerve inflammation can be used to elucidate how this axonal damage occurs.[171,256,398,481] Although it is not completely clear, it is likely that one major effect of inflammation is on the axonal cytoskeleton, as witnessed by changes in microtubule and neurofilament organization in experimentally optic neuritis.[481] This would also explain changes in axonal transport in experimental optic nerve inflammation.[160,161,356] In addition, changes in the blood-nerve barrier consequent to the inflammatory process and generation of reactive oxygen species may also affect axonal function.[163]

Compression. Compression of the optic nerve is a common clinical correlate of a large number of optic neuropathies. Besides the obvious causes such as neoplasms and aneurysms, the optic nerve can also be compressed by enlarged extraocular muscles (as in Graves' ophthalmopathy), edema (as seen with indirect traumatic optic neuropathy, in which the nerve is contused within the optic canal), or optic disc Drusen. Compression intrinsic to the nerve itself can occur in some forms of glaucomatous optic neuropathy in which increased intraocular pressure causes bowing out and shifting of the lamina cribrosa, constricting the bundles of optic nerve axons within the cribrosal pores.[129]

The effects of chronic experimental compression of the intraorbital optic nerve were delineated at the microscopic and ultrastructural level in a classic series of experiments by Clifford-Jones et al.[85,86] They found demyelination initially, followed by remyelination, even while the axons were still compressed. Findings of direct axonal loss were relatively minor. Demyelinated axons or the direct effects of pressure might be expected to lead to conduction block, which would be reversible. This could therefore explain the remarkable return of visual function after removal of tumors compressing the optic nerve.[164]

Glaucoma. The most common optic neuropathy is glaucomatous optic neuropathy, distinguished by a distinct morphology of progressive excavation of the nerve head without significant pallor of the remaining neuroretinal rim.

Clinical and histologic evidence show changes in several locations along the course of the retinal ganglion cell axon and its targets. The number of retinal ganglion cell bodies are decreased in glaucoma, and this likely reflects death by the cell-autonomous process of apoptosis.* The number of retinal ganglion cells lost correlates with the visual field deficit.[343] In addition to the retinal ganglion cell body loss, there is loss of the ganglion cell axons, manifested by segmental loss of the nerve fiber layer, increased cup-to-disc ratio, thinning of the optic nerve and chiasm, changes in postsynaptic cell counts within the LGN (the main target of retinal ganglion cell axons in higher animals), and even the cerebral cortex.† Clinically, a cup-to-disc ratio increase of 0.1 corresponds to approximately 10% loss in the number of retinal ganglion cell axons.[444]

Even though every point along the axon is eventually involved in the disc cupping of glaucomatous optic neuropathy, the site of injury being the optic disc is consistent with a variety of evidence demonstrating pathologic conditions at the level of the disc, particularly the lamina cribrosa, as well as the occurrence of splinter hemorrhages and focal notching at the disc.‡ Studies of tissue from human patients with glaucoma and nonhuman primates with experimental glaucoma confirm changes at the optic nerve head, such as with respect to bowing out of the lamina cribrosa, intraaxonal accumulation of organelles (consistent with blocked axonal transport), and wallerian degeneration distal to the lamina cribrosa.[129,339,346] Whether because of mechanical trauma of axons, ischemia, generation of nitric oxide, or other causes, axonal injury is

known to cause changes in retinal ganglion cells, eventually resulting in death.*

What is the mechanism by which increased intraocular pressure induces retinal ganglion cell death? As mentioned, increased intraocular pressure perturbs rapid anterograde and retrograde axonal transport at the lamina cribrosa.[15,284,344,351] This probably causes retinal ganglion cells to be deprived of neurotrophic factors produced by brain targets. Studies in experimental animals have shown that injury to the optic nerve, for example, from increased intraocular pressure in experimental glaucoma, blocks the retrograde transport of BDNF along with its associated receptor, trkB[197,320,350] (see Color Plate 17). Although not proven in adult mammals, it is likely that deprivation of neurotrophic factors induces retinal ganglion cell death (the "neurotrophin hypothesis").[338]

The most typical glaucomatous visual field defect spreads in an arcuate pattern or as an altitudinal nasal step. In clinical practice the spread of the field defect usually appears to stop at the horizontal meridian in the nasal field. This site corresponds to the temporal raphe of the nerve fibers within the retina. When defects are seen on both sides of the horizontal meridian, it can be seen that spread has occurred in both the superior and inferior visual fields, but not directly across the meridian.

What is the implication of the spread of glaucomatous injury taking place at the disc? This would result in a visual field defect that respects the nasal horizontal meridian. The nasal horizontal meridian corresponds to the temporal raphe of the retina, and from the preceding discussion, it should be apparent that spread of injury along the disc would inexorably affect fibers in an altitudinal hemiretina but should not cross into the other hemiretina. The reason for this is that although there is a small distance between adjacent retinal ganglion cells across the temporal raphe, the axons that correspond to these retinal ganglion cells are separated by a large distance at the optic disc.

Papilledema. *Papilledema* is optic disc edema resulting from elevated intracranial pressure. Despite the apparent etymology, it is not a term that should be used nonspecifically to denote disc edema. Pathologic examination of optic nerve heads with papilledema reveals intraaxonal edema, consistent with abnormalities of axonal transport. However, the pathogenesis of papilledema is controversial. Although primate experiments show definite ab-

*References 105, 149, 204, 282, 309, 337, 349.
†References 6, 77, 94, 95, 107, 183, 190, 191, 345, 415, 447, 458, 478.
‡References 5, 13, 108, 117, 139, 140, 175, 176, 182, 322, 336, 337, 340, 347, 407, 426, 431.

*References 7, 8, 30, 36, 81, 297, 298.

normalities of slow axonal transport, evidence for abnormalities of fast axonal transport (which would include retrograde transport) is less clear and, in part, depends on experimental paradigms where papilledema is simulated by ocular hypotony.[16,283,287,353,439] It is also unclear whether the visual loss associated with chronic papilledema results from disturbances of axonal transport, or from ischemia caused by congestion of the optic nerve head.

OPTIC NERVE REGENERATION

Failure of Central Nervous System Axonal Regeneration

Differences between lower animals and mammals with respect to retinal ganglion cell responses after axonal damage are numerous. For example, not only do goldfish retinal ganglion cells survive after their axons are transected, but they are also able to extend neurites and establish ultimately correct connections with their targets.[266,452] Our understanding of the mechanisms preventing higher animals from regenerating their axons continues to advance, particularly with respect to the role of inflammation, subcellular mechanisms, and myelin-associated inhibitory signals.

Research by Ramon-y-Cajal in the early twentieth century showed that central neurons make abortive attempts to regenerate their axons. This implies that the defect is not always the initiation of neurite extension within the CNS but also elongation of an initiated neurite. It is unclear whether it is the failure of retinal ganglion cell axon initiation, or of elongation, that ultimately becomes the major limiting factor for effective neurorepair. Even when conditions permit axonal extension, only a small minority of retinal ganglion cells eventually extend their axons, suggesting that those that do not have an initiation failure. Axotomy of rat retinal ganglion cells produces complex changes in the pattern of proteins that undergo fast axonal transport, but eventually the apoptosis program supervenes, effectively terminating the regenerative response.[467] Research into what determines initiation of neurite extension has been far less than what prevents elongation and has focused on markers at the cellular level (e.g., GAP-43) and is not discussed further here.[49,383]

When initiation of axonal regeneration occurs, it is insufficient to provide functional connections in the mammalian CNS without experimental intervention. For example, rodent retinal ganglion cell axons approach the optic nerve head but then reverse direction and meander in another direction.[382] This is evidence that regeneration may occur naturally but that it may be incomplete or inaccurate. Analysis of the proximal stump of the transected optic nerve just posterior to the optic nerve head shows early regenerating axons, which then die off.[480] Multiple hypotheses have been advanced to account for the failure of neurite extension in the regenerating mammalian CNS. In most cases it seems that either molecules in the milieu of the growth cones of regenerating axons inhibit neurite extension or a lack of molecules is able to attract the growth cone.

Inhibition of Neurite Extension

Since the early experiments of Aguayo et al.,[3] it has long been known that retinal ganglion cells and other CNS neurons regenerate axons into peripheral nervous system (PNS) grafts (e.g., sciatic nerve) but not into CNS tissue.[406] The nonpermissive nature of the CNS (but not PNS) substrate for axonal elongation is therefore of great interest and has resulted in a large number of candidate molecules. The most studied inhibitory molecules are components of CNS myelin, and this has recently been reviewed in detail.[395] One of the early motivations for these studies was the fact that regeneration can take place in nonmyelinated, but not myelinated, regions of the rodent retina.[268] Efforts to isolate the inhibitory substances focused on isolation of myelin or oligodendrocyte fractions that were able to inhibit neurite outgrowth in biologic assays.[66] IN-1, a monoclonal antibody developed against one of these components, was able to neutralize their inhibitory effect in lesioned spinal cord or optic nerve axons.[394,459] An in vitro system for assaying the ability of human myelin to inhibit regeneration has been defined.[300]

The locus at which axonal injury occurs may therefore serve as a focal point for blocked axonal extension. Histologic analyses demonstrate dramatic changes in the cellular milieu. A key variable is the nature of the proliferating resident microglia and/or macrophages recruited to the site of injury. The response of the latter differs quantitatively from that observed in the PNS, possibly because of the inability of the endothelium to recruit these cells.[71] Although macrophages/microglia do increase in number, they may not be appropriately activated for support of axonal extension and may differ from other macrophages in fundamental ways.[71,134,224,331] For example, CNS optic nerve may inadequately activate macrophages, whereas sciatic nerve from the PNS may appropriately activate them.[479] If activated macrophages/microglia are poorly able to phagocytose degraded myelin, the previously described extension-inhibitory signals found in myelin components may prevent axonal regeneration.[361]

Substrates for Neurite Extension

The presence of inhibitors of neurite extension within myelinated tissue should not be taken to mean that this is the only mechanism for modulating regenerative abilities of CNS tissue. For example, topographic pathfinding of regenerating axons depends on cues independent of these inhibitory substances, as demonstrated by the ability of retinal ganglion cell axons to correctly sort themselves in the presence of IN-1 antibody, as they grew toward artificial superior colliculus stripes.[20] Similarly, goldfish retinal ganglion cell axons, which regenerate in a retinotopic distribution, do not even contain myelin-associated inhibitors of extension neutralizable by IN-1.[452]

A large number of molecules have been shown to be conducive of CNS neurite extension in general and for retinal ganglion cell axonal extension in particular. Perhaps the most studied are the neurotrophins, or growth factors for neurons. Some of these support not only axonal extension of retinal ganglion cells but also their survival. An in-depth review of this subject has recently been published and is not discussed here further.[450] Some are molecules contained in the extracellular matrix, including laminin, fibronectin, certain collagens, thrombospondin, and tenascin-C.[35,64,181,405] Because some of these may be secreted by astrocytes, this may explain why retinal ganglion cells preferentially extend neurites over astrocytes in cell culture.[242,243] Other candidates for growth permissibility may be cell surface receptors or other surface molecules. For example, retinal ganglion cells express Thy-1, and astrocytes have a Thy-1–binding molecule, which would account for the proregenerative activity of antibodies to Thy-1.[110,225]

Interest has also focused on the possibility that failure of regeneration reflects a specific inability of a *postnatal* retinal ganglion cell to extend its axon because embryonic axons are able to do so when transplanted into adult tissue. To support a difference in extension of embryonic and adult axons, it was demonstrated that while both extend well on laminin substrates, only the embryonic axon appears to bind to the primary extension domain of laminin, whereas the adult presumably binds to a

different domain.[34] Another variation on this theme, that the PNS graft actively supports regeneration by releasing a diffusable factor, was supported by studies showing that intravitreal injection of sciatic nerve exudate induced sprouting of axotomized retinal ganglion cells.[79,274]

Finally, different methods of producing optic nerve crush can result in either increases or decreases in reactive astrocytes at the injury site.[134,331] This is important because having the right kind of astrocyte at the injury site may increase the likelihood of axonal regeneration.[10,224,253]

Other Signals for Optic Nerve Regeneration

Overexpression of the antiapoptotic gene *bcl-2* appears to increase retinal ganglion cell survival under certain circumstances. Surprisingly, it also appears to promote regeneration of retinal ganglion cell axons in coculture of mouse retina and superior colliculus and in vivo, beyond that determined by increased survival.[78] Even more dramatically, young mice overexpressing *bcl-2* can regenerate transected retinal ganglion cell axons a short distance. The nature of the signal transduction pathway for regeneration is unclear, however, but could involve nitric oxide, the Eph family of receptor tyrosine kinases, G proteins, bZip family transcription factors, or other mechanisms.[363] Finally, lens injury induces regeneration of rat optic nerve.[33,174,227,363,370]

ACKNOWLEDGMENTS

Supported by NIH EY12492, the Retina Research Foundation, the Glaucoma Foundation, and an unrestricted departmental grant from Research to Prevent Blindness, Inc. Leonard A. Levin is a Research to Prevent Blindness Dolly Green scholar.

REFERENCES

1. Achtsätter T et al: Cytokeratin filaments and desmosomes in the epithelioid cells of the perineurial and arachnoidal sheaths of some vertebrate species, *Differentiation* 40:129, 1989.
2. Aguayo AJ, David S, Bray GM: Influences of the glial environment on the elongation of axons after injury: transplantation studies in adult rodents, *J Exp Biol* 95:231, 1981.
3. Aguayo AJ et al: Effects of neurotrophins on the survival and regrowth of injured retinal neurons, *Ciba Foundation Symp* 196:135, 1996.
4. Ahmed J, Linsenmeier RA, Dunn R Jr: The oxygen distribution in the prelaminar optic nerve head of the cat, *Exp Eye Res* 59:457, 1994.
5. Airaksinen PJ, Mustonen E, Alanko HI: Optic disc haemorrhages precede retinal nerve fibre layer defects in ocular hypertension, *Acta Ophthalmol (Copenh)* 59:627, 1981.

6. Airaksinen PJ et al: Diffuse and localized nerve fiber loss in glaucoma, *Am J Ophthalmol* 98:566, 1984.

7. Allcutt D, Berry M, Sievers J: A qualitative comparison of the reactions of retinal ganglion cell axons to optic nerve crush in neonatal and adult mice, *Brain Res* 318:231, 1984.

8. Allcutt D, Berry M, Sievers J: A quantitative comparison of the reactions of retinal ganglion cells to optic nerve crush in neonatal and adult mice, *Brain Res* 318:219, 1984.

9. Amaratunga A et al: Inhibition of kinesin synthesis and rapid anterograde axonal transport in vivo by an antisense oligonucleotide, *J Biol Chem* 268:17427, 1993.

10. Anders JJ, Hurlock JA: Transplanted glial scar impedes olfactory bulb reinnervation, *Exp Neurol* 142:144, 1996.

11. Anderson DR: Ultrastructure of meningeal sheaths: normal human and monkey optic nerves, *Arch Ophthalmol* 82:659, 1969.

12. Anderson DR: Ascending and descending optic atrophy produced experimentally in squirrel monkeys, *Am J Ophthalmol* 76:693, 1973.

13. Anderson DR: What happens to the optic disc and retina in glaucoma? *Ophthalmology* 90:766, 1983.

14. Anderson DR, Braverman S: Reevaluation of the optic disk vasculature, *Am J Ophthalmol* 82:165, 1976.

15. Anderson DR, Hendrickson A: Effect of intraocular pressure on rapid axoplasmic transport in monkey optic nerve, *Invest Ophthalmol* 13:771, 1974.

16. Anderson DR, Hendrickson AE: Failure of increased intracranial pressure to affect rapid axonal transport at the optic nerve head, *Invest Ophthalmol Vis Sci* 16:423, 1977.

17. Anderson DR, Hoyt WF: Ultrastructure of intraorbital portion of human and monkey optic nerve, *Arch Ophthalmol* 82:506, 1969.

18. Ankarcrona M et al: Glutamate-induced neuronal death: a succession of necrosis or apoptosis depending on mitochondrial function, *Neuron* 15:961, 1995.

19. Aschner M, Rodier PM, Finkelstein JN: Increased axonal transport in the rat optic system after systemic exposure to methylmercury: differential effects in local vs systemic exposure conditions, *Brain Res* 401:132, 1987.

20. Bahr M, Schwab ME: Antibody that neutralizes myelin-associated inhibitors of axon growth does not interfere with recognition of target-specific guidance information by rat retinal axons, *J Neurobiol* 30:281, 1996.

21. Bahr M, Vanselow J, Thanos S: Ability of adult rat ganglion cells to regrow axons in vitro can be confluenced by fibroblast growth factor and gangliosides, *Neurosci Lett* 96:197, 1989.

22. Baker GE, Stryker MP: Retinofugal fibres change conduction velocity and diameter between the optic nerve and tract in ferrets, *Nature* 344:342, 1990.

23. Balazsi AG et al: The effect of age on the nerve fiber population of the human optic nerve, *Am J Ophthalmol* 97:760, 1984.

24. Baleydier C, Magnin M, Cooper HM: Macaque accessory optic system: II: Connections with the pretectum, *J Comp Neurol* 302:405, 1990.

25. Barnett NL, Pow DV: Antisense knockdown of GLAST, a glial glutamate transporter, compromises retinal function, *Invest Ophthalmol Vis Sci* 41:585, 2000.

26. Barres BA, Chun LL, Corey DP: Ion channel expression by white matter glia: I. Type 2 astrocytes and oligodendrocytes, *Glia* 1:10, 1988.

27. Barres BA, Chun LLY, Corey DP: Ion channels in vertebrate glia, *Annu Rev Neurosci* 13:441, 1990.

28. Barres BA, Raff MC: Proliferation of oligodendrocyte precursor cells depends on electrical activity in axons, *Nature* 361:258, 1993.

29. Barres BA et al: Ion channel expression by white matter glia: the O-2A glial progenitor cell, *Neuron* 4:507, 1990.

30. Barron KD et al: Qualitative and quantitative ultrastructural observations on retinal ganglion cell layer of rat after intraorbital optic nerve crush, *J Neurocytol* 15:345, 1986.

31. Bartsch U, Kirchhoff F, Schachner M: Immunohistological localization of the adhesion molecules L1, N-CAM, and MAG in the developing and adult optic nerve of mice, *J Comp Neurol* 284:451, 1989.

32. Bartsch U et al: Tenascin demarcates the boundary between the myelinated and nonmyelinated part of retinal ganglion cell axons in the developing and adult mouse, *J Neurosci* 14:4756, 1994.

33. Bates CA, Meyer RL: Heterotrimeric G protein activation rapidly inhibits outgrowth of optic axons from adult and embryonic mouse, and goldfish retinal explants, *Brain Res* 714:65, 1996.

34. Bates CA, Meyer RL: The neurite-promoting effect of laminin is mediated by different mechanisms in embryonic and adult regenerating mouse optic axons in vitro, *Dev Biol* 181:91, 1997.

35. Becker T et al: Immunohistological localization of tenascin-C in the developing and regenerating retinotectal system of two amphibian species, *J Comp Neurol* 360:643, 1995.

36. Berkelaar M et al: Axotomy results in delayed death and apoptosis of retinal ganglion cells in adult rats, *J Neurosci* 14:4368, 1994.

37. Bernhardt RR et al: Increased expression of specific recognition molecules by retinal ganglion cells and by optic pathway glia accompanies the successful regeneration of retinal axons in adult zebrafish, *J Comp Neurol* 376:253, 1996.

38. Bevan S et al: Voltage gated ionic channels in rat cultured astrocytes, reactive astrocytes and an astrocyte-oligodendrocyte progenitor cell, *J Physiol (Paris)* 82:327, 1987.

39. Bieda MC, Copenhagen DR: Sodium action potentials are not required for light-evoked release of GABA or glycine from retinal amacrine cells, *J Neurophysiol* 81:3092, 1999.

40. Black JA, Waxman SG: Specialization of astrocytic membrane at glia limitans in rat optic nerve: freeze-fracture observations, *Neurosci Lett* 55:371, 1985.

41. Black JA et al: Immuno-ultrastructural localization of sodium channels at nodes of Ranvier and perinodal astrocytes in rat optic nerve, *Proc R Soc Lond (Biol)* 238:39, 1989.

42. Black JA et al: Sodium channels in astrocytes of rat optic nerve in situ: immuno-electron microscopic studies, *Glia* 2:353, 1989.

43. Black MM, Lasek RJ: Axonal transport of actin: Slow component b is the principal source of actin for the axon, *Brain Res* 171:401, 1979.

44. Bodeutsch N et al: Unilateral injury to the adult rat optic nerve causes multiple cellular responses in the contralateral site, *J Neurobiol* 38:116, 1999.

45. Bogler O, Noble M: Measurement of time in oligodendrocyte-type-2 astrocyte (O-2A) progenitors is a cellular process distinct from differentiation or division, *Dev Biol* 162:525, 1994.

46. Boniuk M, Messmer EP, Font RL: Hemangiopericytoma of the meninges of the optic nerve: a clinicopathologic report including electron microscopic observations, *Ophthalmology* 92:1780, 1985.

47. Bons N: Demonstration of centrifugal fibers in the optic chiasma and optic nerves in the rat after lesions of the suprachiasmatic nucleus, *CR Soc Biol (Paris)* 181:274, 1987.

48. Borges K et al: Adult rat optic nerve oligodendrocyte progenitor cells express a distinct repertoire of voltage- and ligand-gated ion channels, *J Neurosci* Res 40:591, 1995.

49. Bormann P et al: Target contact regulates GAP-43 and alpha-tubulin mRNA levels in regenerating retinal ganglion cells, *J Neurosci Res* 52:405, 1998.

50. Bowling DB, Michael CR: Projection patterns of single physiologically characterized optic tract fibres in cat, *Nature* 286:899, 1980.

51. Buchi ER: Cell death in the rat retina after a pressure-induced ischaemia-reperfusion insult: an electron microscopic study: I. Ganglion cell layer and inner nuclear layer, *Exp Eye Res* 55:605, 1992.

52. Bunt AH et al: Monkey retinal ganglion cells: morphometric analysis and tracing of axonal projections, with a consideration of the peroxidase technique, *J Comp Neurol* 164:265, 1975.

53. Burne JF, Raff MC: Retinal ganglion cell axons drive the proliferation of astrocytes in the developing rodent optic nerve, *Neuron* 18:223, 1997.

54. Burne JF, Staple JK, Raff MC: Glial cells are increased proportionally in transgenic optic nerves with increased numbers of axons, *J Neurosci* 16:2064, 1996.

55. Bussow H: Schwann cell myelin ensheathing CNS axons in the nerve fibre layer of the cat retina, *J Neurocytol* 7:207, 1978.

56. Bussow H: The astrocytes in the retina and optic nerve head of mammals: a special glia for the ganglion cell axons, *Cell Tissue Res* 206:367, 1980.

57. Butt AM, Colquhoun K: Glial cells in transected optic nerves of immature rats. I. An analysis of individual cells by intracellular dye-injection, *J Neurocytol* 25:365, 1996.

58. Butt AM, Colquhoun K, Berry M: Confocal imaging of glial cells in the intact rat optic nerve, *Glia* 10:315, 1994.

59. Butt AM, Jennings J: Response of astrocytes to gamma-aminobutyric acid in the neonatal rat optic nerve, *Neurosci Lett* 168:53, 1994.

60. Butt AM, Kirvell S: Glial cells in transected optic nerves of immature rats. II. An immunohistochemical study, *J Neurocytol* 25:381, 1996.

61. Butt AM, Ransom BR: Visualization of oligodendrocytes and astrocytes in the intact rat optic nerve by intracellular injection of Lucifer yellow and horseradish peroxidase, *Glia* 2:470, 1989.

62. Butt AM, Ransom BR: Morphology of astrocytes and oligodendrocytes during development in the intact rat optic nerve, *J Comp Neurol* 338:141, 1993.

63. Butt AM et al: Three-dimensional morphology of astrocytes and oligodendrocytes in the intact mouse optic nerve, *J Neurocytol* 23:469, 1994.

64. Carbonetto S, Cochard P: In vitro studies on the control of nerve fiber growth by the extracellular matrix of the nervous system, *J Physiologie* 82:258, 1987.

65. Carmignoto G et al: Effect of NGF on the survival of rat retinal ganglion cells following optic nerve section, *J Neurosci* 9:1263, 1989.

66. Caroni P, Schwab ME: Two membrane protein fractions from rat central myelin with inhibitory properties for neurite growth and fibroblast spreading, *J Cell Biol* 106:1281, 1988.

67. Carroll WM, Jennings AR, Mastaglia FL: Reactive glial cells in CNS demyelination contain both GC and GFAP, *Brain Res* 411:364, 1987.

68. Carroll WM, Jennings AR, Mastaglia FL: The origin of re-myelinating oligodendrocytes in antiserum-mediated demyelinative optic neuropathy, *Brain* 113:953, 1990.

69. Caruso DM, Owczarzak MT, Pourcho RG: Colocalization of substance P and GABA in retinal ganglion cells: a computer-assisted visualization, *Vis Neurosci* 5:389, 1990.

70. Caruso DM et al: GABA-immunoreactivity in ganglion cells of the rat retina, *Brain Res* 476:129, 1989.

71. Castano A, Bell MD, Perry VH: Unusual aspects of inflammation in the nervous system: wallerian degeneration, *Neurobiol Aging* 17:745, 1996.

72. Castillo BJ et al: Retinal ganglion cell survival is promoted by genetically modified astrocytes designed to secrete brain-derived neurotrophic factor (BDNF), *Brain Res* 647:30, 1994.

73. Cellerino A, Galli-Resta L, Colombaioni L: The dynamics of neuronal death: a time-lapse study in the retina, *J Neurosci* 20:RC92, 2000.

74. Chalupa LM, Meissirel C, Lia B: Specificity of retinal ganglion cell projections in the embryonic rhesus monkey, *Perspect Dev Biol* 3:223, 1996.

75. Chan SO, Guillery RW: Changes in fiber order in the optic nerve and tract of rat embryos, *J Comp Neurol* 344:20, 1994.

76. Chan-Ling T, Stone J: Factors determining the migration of astrocytes into the developing retina: migration does not depend on intact axons or patent vessels, *J Comp Neurol* 303:375, 1991.

77. Chaturvedi N, Hedley-Whyte ET, Dreyer EB: Lateral geniculate nucleus in glaucoma, *Am J Ophthalmol* 116:182, 1993.

78. Chen DF et al: Bcl-2 promotes regeneration of severed axons in mammalian CNS, *Nature* 385:434, 1997.

79. Cho KS, So KF, Chung SK: Induction of axon-like processes from axotomized retinal ganglion cells of adult hamsters after intravitreal injection of sciatic nerve exudates, *Neuroreport* 7:2879, 1996.

80. Chou PI, Sadun AA, Lee H: Vasculature and morphometry of the optic canal and intracanalicular optic nerve, *J Neuroophthalmol* 15:186, 1995.

81. Cioffi GA, Sullivan P: The effect of chronic ischemia on the primate optic nerve, *Eur J Ophthalmol* 9(suppl 1):S34, 1999.

82. Cioffi GA, Van Buskirk EM: Microvasculature of the anterior optic nerve, *Surv Ophthalmol* 38(suppl):S107, 1994.

83. Cioffi GA et al: An in vivo model of chronic optic nerve ischemia: the dose-dependent effects of endothelin-1 on the optic nerve microvasculature, *Curr Eye Res* 14:1147, 1995.

84. Clarke DB et al: Effect of neurotrophin-4 administration on the survival of axotomized retinal ganglion cells in adult rats, *Soc Neurosci Abstr* 19:1104, 1993.

85. Clifford-Jones RE, Landon DN, McDonald WI: Remyelination during optic nerve compression, *J Neurol Sci* 46:239, 1980.

86. Clifford-Jones RE, McDonald WI, Landon DN: Chronic optic nerve compression. An experimental study, *Brain* 108:241, 1985.

87. Cohen AI: Ultrastructural aspects of the human optic nerve, *Invest Ophthalmol* 6:294, 1967.

88. Colello RJ, Pott U, Schwab ME: The role of oligodendrocytes and myelin on axon maturation in the developing rat retinofugal pathway, *J Neurosci* 14:2594, 1994.

89. Colello RJ et al: The chronology of oligodendrocyte differentiation in the rat optic nerve: evidence for a signaling step initiating myelination in the CNS, *J Neurosci* 15:7665, 1995.

90. Connolly SE, Gordon KB, Horton JC: Salvage of vision after hypotension-induced ischemic optic neuropathy, *Am J Ophthalmol* 117:235, 1994.

91. Cook RD, Wisniewski HM: The role of oligodendroglia and astroglia in wallerian degeneration of the optic nerve, *Brain Res* 61:191, 1973.

92. Cook RD, Wisniewski HM: The spatio-temporal pattern of wallerian degeneration in the rhesus monkey optic nerve, *Acta Neuropathol (Berl)* 72:261, 1987.

93. Cragg BG: What is the signal for chromatolysis? *Brain Res* 23:1, 1970.

94. Crawford ML et al: Glaucoma in primates: cytochrome oxidase reactivity in parvo- and magnocellular pathways, *Invest Ophthalmol Vis Sci* 41:1791, 2000.

95. Crawford ML et al: Experimental glaucoma in primates: changes in cytochrome oxidase blobs in V1 cortex, *Invest Ophthalmol Vis Sci* 42:358, 2001.

96. Crossland WJ: Fast axonal transport in the visual pathway of the chick and rat, *Brain Res* 340:373, 1985.

97. Cui Q, Harvey AR: At least two mechanisms are involved in the death of retinal ganglion cells following target ablation in neonatal rats, *J Neurosci* 15:8143, 1995.

98. Curcio CA, Allen KA: Topography of ganglion cells in human retina, *J Comp Neurol* 300:5, 1990.

99. David S: Neurite outgrowth from mammalian CNS neurons on astrocytes in vitro may not be mediated primarily by laminin, *J Neurocytol* 17:131, 1988.

100. De La Motte DJ: Removal of horseradish peroxidase and fluorescein-labelled dextran from CSF spaces of rabbit optic nerve: a light and electron microscope study, *Exp Eye Res* 27:585, 1978.

101. Demerens C et al: Induction of myelination in the central nervous system by electrical activity, *Proc Natl Acad Sci USA* 93:9887, 1996.

102. Dhital K et al: Adrenergic innervation of vasa and nervi nervorum of optic, sciatic, vagus and sympathetic nerve trunks in normal and streptozotocin-diabetic rats, *Brain Res* 367:39, 1986.

103. Dillman JFI, Dabney LP, Pfister KK: Cytoplasmic dynein is associated with slow axonal transport, *Proc Natl Acad Sci USA* 93:141, 1996.

104. Distler C, Hoffmann KP: The pupillary light reflex in normal and innate microstrabismic cats, II: Retinal and cortical input to the nucleus praetectalis olivaris, *Vis Neurosci* 3:139, 1989.

105. Dkhissi O et al: Retinal TUNEL-positive cells and high glutamate levels in vitreous humor of mutant quail with a glaucoma-like disorder, *Invest Ophthalmol Vis Sci* 40:990, 1999.

106. Doster SK et al: Expression of the growth-associated protein GAP-43 in adult rat retinal ganglion cells following axon injury, *Neuron* 6:635, 1991.

107. Drance SM: The early structural and functional disturbances of chronic open-angle glaucoma. Robert N. Shaffer lecture, *Ophthalmology* 92:853, 1985.

108. Drance SM et al: The importance of disc hemorrhage in the prognosis of chronic open angle glaucoma, *Arch Ophthalmol* 95:226, 1977.

109. Dreyer EB: A proposed role for excitotoxicity in glaucoma, *J Glaucoma* 7:62, 1998.

110. Dreyer EB et al: An astrocytic binding site for neuronal Thy-1 and its effect on neurite outgrowth, *Proc Natl Acad Sci USA* 92:11195, 1995.

111. Dreyer EB et al: Elevated glutamate levels in the vitreous body of humans and monkeys with glaucoma, *Arch Ophthalmol* 114:299, 1996.

112. Dropp JJ: Mast cells in mammalian brain, *Acta Anat (Basel)* 94:1, 1976.

113. Dropp JJ: Mast cells in the human brain, *Acta Anat (Basel)* 105:505, 1979.

114. Dudek H et al: Regulation of neuronal survival by the serine-threonine protein kinase Akt, *Science* 275:661, 1997.

115. Ehrlich D, Keyser KT, Karten HJ: Distribution of substance P-like immunoreactive retinal ganglion cells and their pattern of termination in the optic tectum of chick (*Gallus gallus*), *J Comp Neurol* 266:220, 1987.

116. Ehrlich D et al: Differential effects of axotomy on substance P-containing and nicotinic acetylcholine receptor-containing retinal ganglion cells: time course of degeneration and effects of nerve growth factor, *Neuroscience* 36:699, 1990.

117. Emery JM et al: The lamina cribrosa in normal and glaucomatous human eyes, *Trans Am Acad Ophthalmol Otolaryngol* 78:OP290, 1974.

118. Evangelou N et al: Quantitative pathological evidence for axonal loss in normal appearing white matter in multiple sclerosis, *Ann Neurol* 47:391, 2000.

119. Falck FY, Klein TB, Higginbotham EJ: Larger optic nerve heads have more nerve fibers in normal monkey eyes, *Arch Ophthalmol* 110:1042, 1992.

120. Feller MB et al: Requirement for cholinergic synaptic transmission in the propagation of spontaneous retinal waves, *Science* 272:1182, 1996.

121. Fernandez E et al: Visual experience during postnatal development determines the size of optic nerve axons, *Neuroreport* 5:365, 1993.

122. ffrench-Constant C, Raff MC: The oligodendrocyte-type-2 astrocyte cell lineage is specialized for myelination, *Nature* 323:335, 1986.

123. ffrench-Constant C et al: Evidence that migratory oligodendrocyte-type-2 astrocyte (O-2A) progenitor cells are kept out of the rat retina by a barrier at the eye-end of the optic nerve, *J Neurocytol* 17:13, 1988.

124. Finn JT et al: Evidence that wallerian degeneration and localized axon degeneration induced by local neurotrophin deprivation do not involve caspases, *J Neurosci* 20:1333, 2000.

125. FitzGibbon T: The human fetal retinal nerve fiber layer and optic nerve head: a DiI and DiA tracing study, *Vis Neurosci* 14:433, 1997.

126. Fitzgibbon T, Taylor SF: Retinotopy of the human retinal nerve fibre layer and optic nerve head, *J Comp Neurol* 375:238, 1996.

127. Flage T: Permeability properties of the tissues in the optic nerve head region in the rabbit and the monkey: an ultrastructural study, *Acta Ophthalmol* 55:652, 1977.

128. Fontana A, Fierz W, Wekerle H: Astrocytes present myelin basic protein to encephalitogenic T cell lines, *Nature* 307:273, 1984.

129. Fontana L et al: In vivo morphometry of the lamina cribrosa and its relation to visual field loss in glaucoma, *Curr Eye Res* 17:363, 1998.

130. Foster RE, Connors BW, Waxman SG: Rat optic nerve: electrophysiological, pharmacological and anatomical studies during development, *Brain Res* 255:371, 1982.

131. Fournier AE, McKerracher L: Expression of specific tubulin isotypes increases during regeneration of injured CNS neurons, but not after the application of brain-derived neurotrophic factor (BDNF), *J Neurosci* 17:4623, 1997.

132. Fox DA, Ruan DY: Time- and frequency-dependent effects of potassium channel blockers on large and medium diameter optic tract axons, *Brain Res* 498:229, 1989.

133. Francois J, Fryczkowski A: The blood supply of the optic nerve, *Adv Ophthalmol* 36:164, 1978.

134. Frank M, Wolburg H: Cellular reactions at the lesion site after crushing of the rat optic nerve, *Glia* 16:227, 1996.

135. Fredericks CA et al: The human accessory optic system, *Brain Res* 454:116, 1988.

136. Friedrich VL, Mugnaini E: Myelin sheath thickness in the CNS is regulated near the axon, *Brain Res* 274:329, 1983.

137. Frisen J et al: Rapid, widespread, and longlasting induction of nestin contributes to the generation of glial scar tissue after CNS injury, *J Cell Biol* 131:453, 1995.

138. Frizell M, McLean WG, Sjostrand J: Slow axonal transport of proteins: blockade by interruption of contact between cell body and axon, *Brain Res* 86:67, 1975.

139. Fukuchi T et al: Extracellular matrix changes of the optic nerve lamina cribrosa in monkey eyes with experimentally chronic glaucoma, *Graefes Arch Clin Exp Ophthalmol* 230:421, 1992.

140. Fukuchi T et al: Sulfated proteoglycans in the lamina cribrosa of normal monkey eyes and monkey eyes with laser-induced glaucoma, *Exp Eye Res* 58:231, 1994.

141. Gamlin PD et al: The neural substrate for the pupillary light reflex in the pigeon (*Columba livia*), *J Comp Neurol* 226:523, 1984.

142. Gao FB, Durand B, Raff M: Oligodendrocyte precursor cells count time but not cell divisions before differentiation, *Curr Biol* 7:152, 1997.

143. Gao H, Hollyfield JG: Aging of the human retina. Differential loss of neurons and retinal pigment epithelial cells, *Invest Ophthalmol Vis Sci* 33:1, 1992.

144. Gao H et al: Elevated mRNA expression of brain-derived neurotrophic factor in retinal ganglion cell layer after optic nerve injury, *Invest Ophthalmol Vis Sci* 38:1840, 1997.

145. Garcia-Valenzuela E et al: Apoptosis in adult retinal ganglion cells after axotomy, *J Neurobiol* 25:431, 1994.

146. Garthwaite G et al: Mechanisms of ischaemic damage to central white matter axons: a quantitative histological analysis using rat optic nerve, *Neuroscience* 94:1219, 1999.

147. Gavrieli Y, Sherman Y, Ben-Sasson SA: Identification of programmed cell death in situ via specific labeling of nuclear DNA fragmentation, *J Cell Biol* 119:493, 1992.

148. Geijer C, Bill A: Effects of raised intraocular pressure on retinal, prelaminar, laminar, and retrolaminar optic nerve blood flow in monkeys, *Invest Ophthalmol Vis Sci* 18:1030, 1979.

149. Giles CL, Soble AR: Intracranial hypertension and tetracycline therapy, *Am J Ophthalmol* 72:981, 1971.

150. Giorgi PP, DuBois H: Labelling by axonal transport of myelin-associated proteins in the rabbit visual pathway, *Biochem J* 196:537, 1981.

151. Goldberg S, Frank B: Do young axons regenerate better than old axons? *Exp Neurol* 74:245, 1981.

152. Gordon TR, Kocsis JD, Waxman SG: Evidence for the presence of two types of potassium channels in the rat optic nerve, *Brain Res* 447:1, 1988.

153. Gordon TR, Kocsis JD, Waxman SG: Pharmacological sensitivities of two afterhyperpolarizations in rat optic nerve, *Brain Res* 502:252, 1989.

154. Gordon TR, Kocsis JD, Waxman SG: Electrogenic pump (Na+/K+-ATPase) activity in rat optic nerve, *Neuroscience* 37:829, 1990.

155. Grafstein B, Ingoglia NA: Intracranial transection of the optic nerve in adult mice: preliminary observations, *Exp Neurol* 76:318, 1982.

156. Groves AK et al: Repair of demyelinated lesions by transplantation of purified O-2A progenitor cells, *Nature* 362:453, 1993.

157. Guenther E et al: Maturation of intrinsic membrane properties in rat retinal ganglion cells, *Vision Res* 39:2477, 1999.

158. Gutierrez R et al: Decompaction of CNS myelin leads to a reduction of the conduction velocity of action potentials in optic nerve, *Neurosci Lett* 195:93, 1995.

159. Guy J, Rao NA: Acute and chronic experimental optic neuritis: alteration in the blood-optic nerve barrier, *Arch Ophthalmol* 102:450, 1984.

160. Guy J et al: Axonal transport reductions in acute experimental allergic encephalomyelitis: qualitative analysis of the optic nerve, *Curr Eye Res* 8:261, 1989.

161. Guy J et al: Quantitative analysis of labelled inner retinal proteins in experimental optic neuritis, *Curr Eye Res* 8:253, 1989.

162. Guy J et al: Intraorbital optic nerve and experimental optic neuritis. Correlation of fat suppression magnetic resonance imaging and electron microscopy, *Ophthalmology* 99:720, 1992.

163. Guy J et al: Disruption of the blood-brain barrier in experimental optic neuritis: immunocytochemical co-localization of H_2O_2 and extravasated serum albumin, *Invest Ophthalmol Vis Sci* 35:1114, 1994.

164. Guyer DR et al: Visual function following optic canal decompression via craniotomy, *J Neurosurg* 62:631, 1985.

165. Hahn JS, Aizenman E, Lipton SA: Central mammalian neurons normally resistant to glutamate toxicity are made sensitive by elevated extracellular Ca2+: Toxicity is blocked by the N-methyl-D-aspartate antagonist MK-801, *Proc Natl Acad Sci USA* 85:6556, 1988.

166. Hankin MH, Lagenaur CF: Cell adhesion molecules in the early developing mouse retina: retinal neurons show preferential outgrowth in vitro on L1 but not N-CAM, *J Neurobiol* 25:472, 1994.

167. Harman A et al: Neuronal density in the human retinal ganglion cell layer from 16-77 years, *Anat Rec* 260:124, 2000.

168. Hayreh SS: The sheath of the optic nerve, *Ophthalmologica* 189:54, 1984.

169. Hayreh SS, Baines JA: Occlusion of the posterior ciliary artery. I. Effects on choroidal circulation, *Br J Ophthalmol* 56:719, 1972.

170. Hayreh SS, Baines JA: Occlusion of the posterior ciliary artery: 3. Effects on the optic nerve head, *Br J Ophthalmol* 56:754, 1972.

171. Hayreh SS et al: Experimental allergic encephalomyelitis: I. Optic nerve and central nervous system manifestations, *Invest Ophthalmol Vis Sci* 21:256, 1981.

172. Hemmings BA: Akt signaling: linking membrane events to life and death decisions, *Science* 275:628, 1997.

173. Hendry SH, Reid RC: The koniocellular pathway in primate vision, *Annu Rev Neurosci* 23:127, 2000.

174. Henkemeyer M et al: Nuk controls pathfinding of commissural axons in the mammalian central nervous system, *Cell* 86:35, 1996.

175. Hernandez MR: Ultrastructural immunocytochemical analysis of elastin in the human lamina cribrosa. Changes in elastic fibers in primary open-angle glaucoma, *Invest Ophthalmol Vis Sci* 33:2891, 1992.

176. Hernandez MR, Pena JD: The optic nerve head in glaucomatous optic neuropathy, *Arch Ophthalmol* 115:389, 1997.

177. Hickey WF, Kimura H: Perivascular microglial cells of the CNS are bone marrow-derived and present antigen in vivo, *Science* 239:290, 1988.

178. Higgs MH, Lukasiewicz PD: Glutamate uptake limits synaptic excitation of retinal ganglion cells, *J Neurosci* 19:3691, 1999.

179. Hilbig H et al: Neuronal and glial structures of the superficial layers of the human superior colliculus, *Anat Embryol (Berl)* 200:103, 1999.

180. Hildebrand C, Remahl S, Waxman SG: Axo-glial relations in the retina-optic nerve junction of the adult rat: electron-microscopic observations, *J Neurocytol* 14:597, 1985.

181. Hoffman JR, Dixit VM, O'Shea KS: Expression of thrombospondin in the adult nervous system, *J Comp Neurol* 340:126, 1994.

182. Hollander H et al: Evidence of constriction of optic nerve axons at the lamina cribrosa in the normotensive eye in humans and other mammals, *Ophthalmic Res* 27:296, 1995.

183. Hoyt WF, Frisen L, Newman NM: Fundoscopy of nerve fiber layer defects in glaucoma, *Invest Ophthalmol* 12:814, 1973.

184. Hull M, Bahr M: Differential regulation of c-JUN expression in rat retinal ganglion cells after proximal and distal optic nerve transection, *Neurosci Lett* 178:39, 1994.

185. Humphrey MF: A morphometric study of the retinal ganglion cell response to optic nerve severance in the frog Rana pipiens, *J Neurocytol* 17:293, 1988.

186. Humphrey MF, Beazley LD: Retinal ganglion cell death during optic nerve regeneration in the frog Hyla moorei, *J Comp Neurol* 263:382, 1985.

187. Ilschner SU, Waring P: Fragmentation of DNA in the retina of chicken embryos coincides with retinal ganglion cell death, *Biochem Biophys Res Comm* 183:1056, 1992.

188. Ino-Ue M et al: Polyol metabolism of retrograde axonal transport in diabetic rat large optic nerve fiber, *Invest Ophthalmol Vis Sci* 41:4055, 2000.

189. Itoh K et al: A pretectofacial projection in the cat: a possible link in the visually-triggered blink reflex pathways, *Brain Res* 275:332, 1983.

190. Iwata F et al: Association of visual field, cup-disc ratio, and magnetic resonance imaging of optic chiasm, *Arch Ophthalmol* 115:729, 1997.

191. Iwata K, Kurosawa A, Sawaguchi S: Wedge-shaped retinal nerve fiber layer defects in experimental glaucoma preliminary report, *Graefes Arch Clin Exp Ophthalmol* 223:184, 1985.

192. Janzer RC, Raff MC: Astrocytes induce blood-brain barrier properties in endothelial cells, *Nature* 325:253, 1987.

193. Jayatilaka AD: A note on arachnoid villi in relation to human optic nerves, *J Anat* 101:171, 1967.

194. Jeffery G: Distribution and trajectory of uncrossed axons in the optic nerves of pigmented and albino rats, *J Comp Neurol* 289:462, 1989.

195. Jeffery G et al: The human optic nerve: fascicular organisation and connective tissue types along the extra-fascicular matrix, *Anat Embryol* 191:491, 1995.

196. Jeffery G et al: Cellular localisation of metabotropic glutamate receptors in the mammalian optic nerve: a mechanism for axon-glia communication, *Brain Res* 741:75, 1996.

197. Johnson EC et al: Chronology of optic nerve head and retinal responses to elevated intraocular pressure, *Invest Ophthalmol Vis Sci* 41:431, 2000.

198. Johnson MW, Kincaid MC, Trobe JD: Bilateral retrobulbar optic nerve infarctions after blood loss and hypotension. A clinicopathologic case study, *Ophthalmology* 94:1577, 1987.

199. Johnson RF, Morin LP, Moore RY: Retinohypothalamic projections in the hamster and rat demonstrated using cholera toxin, *Brain Res* 462:301, 1988.

200. Jonas JB, Gusek GC, Naumann GO: Optic disc, cup and neuroretinal rim size, configuration and correlations in normal eyes, *Invest Ophthalmol Vis Sci* 29:1151, 1988.

201. Jung HJ, Raine CS, Suzuki K: Schwann cells and peripheral nervous system myelin in the rat retina, *Acta Neuropathol (Berl)* 44:245, 1978.

202. Kaplan MR et al: Induction of sodium channel clustering by oligodendrocytes, *Nature* 386:724, 1997.

203. Kerr JF, Wyllie AH, Currie AR: Apoptosis: a basic biological phenomenon with wide-ranging implications in tissue kinetics, *Br J Cancer* 26:239, 1972.

204. Kerrigan LA et al: TUNEL-positive ganglion cells in human primary open-angle glaucoma, *Arch Ophthalmol* 115:1031, 1997.

205. Keyser KT et al: Amacrine, ganglion, and displaced amacrine cells in the rabbit retina express nicotinic acetylcholine receptors, *Vis Neurosci* 17:743, 2000.

206. Kidd GJ, Hauer PE, Trapp BD: Axons modulate myelin protein messenger RNA levels during central nervous system myelination in vivo, *J Neurosci Res* 26:409, 1990.

207. Killer HE, Laeng HR, Groscurth P: Lymphatic capillaries in the meninges of the human optic nerve, *J Neuroophthalmol* 19:222, 1999.

208. Klocker N, Cellerino A, Bahr M: Free radical scavenging and inhibition of nitric oxide synthase potentiates the neurotrophic effects of brain-derived neurotrophic factor on axotomized retinal ganglion cells in vivo, *J Neurosci* 18:1038, 1998.

209. Klocker N et al: In vivo neurotrophic effects of GDNF on axotomized retinal ganglion cells, *Neuroreport* 8:3439, 1997.

210. Klocker N et al: Both the neuronal and inducible isoforms contribute to upregulation of retinal nitric oxide synthase activity by brain-derived neurotrophic factor, *J Neurosci* 19:8517, 1999.

211. Klocker N et al: Brain-derived neurotrophic factor-mediated neuroprotection of adult rat retinal ganglion cells in vivo does not exclusively depend on phosphatidyl-inositol-3'-kinase/protein kinase B signaling, *J Neurosci* 20:6962, 2000.

212. Kocsis JD, Gordon TR, Waxman SG: Mammalian optic nerve fibers display two pharmacologically distinct potassium channels, *Brain Res* 383:357, 1986.

213. Kondo Y et al: Single retinal ganglion cells sending axon collaterals to the bilateral superior colliculi: a fluorescent retrograde double-labeling study in the Japanese monkey (*Macaca fuscata*), *Brain Res* 597:155, 1992.

214. Konno H et al: Targeting of adoptively transferred experimental allergic encephalitis lesion at the sites of wallerian degeneration, *Acta Neuropathol (Berl)* 80:521, 1990.

215. Kreutz MR et al: Axonal injury alters alternative splicing of the retinal NR1 receptor: the preferential expression of the NR1b isoforms is crucial for retinal ganglion cell survival, *J Neurosci* 18:8278, 1998.

216. Kriegler S, Chiu SY: Calcium signaling of glial cells along mammalian axons, *J Neurosci* 13:4229, 1993.

217. Kubrusly RC, de Mello MC, de Mello FG: Aspartate as a selective NMDA receptor agonist in cultured cells from the avian retina, *Neurochem Int* 32:47, 1998.

218. Kupfer C: Retinal ganglion cell degeneration following chiasmal lesions in man, *Arch Ophthalmol* 70:256, 1963.

219. Kupfer C, Chumbley L, Downer JC: Quantitative histology of optic nerve, optic tract and lateral geniculate nucleus of man, *J Anat* 101:393, 1967.

220. Labandeira-Garcia JL et al: Location of neurons projecting to the retina in mammals, *Neurosci Res* 8:291, 1990.

221. Laeng P et al: Transplantation of oligodendrocyte progenitor cells into the rat retina: extensive myelination of retinal ganglion cell axons, *Glia* 18:200, 1996.

222. Lagrèze WA, Kardon RH: Correlation of relative afferent pupillary defect and estimated retinal ganglion cell loss, *Graefes Arch Clin Exp Ophthalmol* 236:401, 1998.

223. Lawson LJ et al: Quantification of the mononuclear phagocyte response to wallerian degeneration of the optic nerve, *J Neurocytol* 23:729, 1994.

224. Lazarov-Spiegler O et al: Transplantation of activated macrophages overcomes central nervous system regrowth failure, *FASEB Journal* 10:1296, 1996.

225. Leifer D et al: Monoclonal antibody to Thy-1 enhances regeneration of processes by rat retinal ganglion cells in culture, *Science* 224:303, 1984.

226. Leinfelder PJ: Retrograde degeneration in the optic nerves and tracts, *Am J Ophthalmol* 23:796, 1940.

227. Leon S et al: Lens injury stimulates axon regeneration in the mature rat optic nerve, *J Neurosci* 20:4615, 2000.

228. Lessell S: Nonarteritic anterior ischemic optic neuropathy: enigma variations, *Arch Ophthalmol* 117:386, 1999.

229. Lessell S, Horovitz B: Histochemical study of enzymes of optic nerve of monkey and rat, *Am J Ophthalmol* 74:118, 1972.

230. Lev-Ram V, Grinvald A: Ca2+- and K+-dependent communication between central nervous system myelinated axons and oligodendrocytes revealed by voltage-sensitive dyes, *Proc Natl Acad Sci USA* 83:6651, 1986.

231. Levin LA, Albert DM, Johnson D: Mast cells in human optic nerve, *Invest Ophthalmol Vis Sci* 34:3147, 1993.

232. Levin LA, Geszvain KM: Expression of ceruloplasmin in the retina: Induction after retinal ganglion cell axotomy, *Invest Ophthalmol Vis Sci* 39:157, 1998.

233. Levin LA, Louhab A: Apoptosis of retinal ganglion cells in anterior ischemic optic neuropathy, *Arch Ophthalmol* 114:488, 1996.

234. Levin LA et al: Identification of bcl-2 family genes in the rat retina, *Invest Ophthalmol Vis Sci* 38, 1997.

235. Levine J, Willard M: The composition and organization of axonally transported proteins in the retinal ganglion cells of the guinea pig, *Brain Res* 194:137, 1980.

236. Levy NS: The effect of interruption of the short posterior ciliary arteries on slow axoplasmic transport and histology within the optic nerve of the rhesus monkey, *Invest Ophthalmol* 15:495, 1976.

237. Lhermitte F, Guillaumat L, Lyon CO: Monocular blindness with preserved direct and consensual pupillary reflex in multiple sclerosis, *Arch Neurol* 41:993, 1984.

238. Li X et al: Studies on the identity of the rat optic nerve transmitter, *Brain Res* 706:89, 1996.

239. Lieberman AR: A review of the principal features of perikaryal responses to axon injury, *Int Rev Neurobiol* 14:49, 1971.

240. Lieberman MF, Maumenee AE, Green WR: Histologic studies of the vasculature of the anterior optic nerve, *Am J Ophthalmol* 82:405, 1976.

241. Liedtke W et al: GFAP is necessary for the integrity of CNS white matter architecture and long-term maintenance of myelination, *Neuron* 17:607, 1996.

242. Liesi P: Laminin-immunoreactive glia distinguish regenerative adult CNS systems from non-regenerative ones, *EMBO J* 4:2505, 1985.

243. Liesi P, Silver J: Is astrocyte laminin involved in axon guidance in the mammalian CNS? *Dev Biol* 130:774, 1988.

244. Lincoln J et al: Innervation of normal human sural and optic nerves by noradrenaline- and peptide-containing nervi vasorum and nervorum: effect of diabetes and alcoholism, *Brain Res* 632:48, 1993.

245. Linden R: Displaced ganglion cells in the retina of the rat, *J Comp Neurol* 258:138, 1987.

246. Ling EA: Electron microscopic studies of macrophages in wallerian degeneration of rat optic nerve after intravenous injection of colloidal carbon, *J Anat* 126:111, 1978.

247. Ling TL, Mitrofanis J, Stone J: Origin of retinal astrocytes in the rat: evidence of migration from the optic nerve, *J Comp Neurol* 286:345, 1989.

248. Ling TL, Stone J: The development of astrocytes in the cat retina: evidence of migration from the optic nerve, *Brain Res Dev Brain Res* 44:73, 1988.

249. Liu D, Michon J: Measurement of the subarachnoid pressure of the optic nerve in human subjects, *Am J Ophthalmol* 119:81, 1995.

250. Liu KM, Shen CL: Ultrastructural sequence of myelin breakdown during wallerian degeneration in the rat optic nerve, *Cell Tissue Res* 242:245, 1985.

251. Lorenz T, Willard M: Subcellular fractionation of intra-axonally transport polypeptides in the rabbit visual system, *Proc Natl Acad Sci USA* 75:505, 1978.

252. Lucas M, Solano F, Sanz A: Induction of programmed cell death (apoptosis) in mature lymphocytes, *FEBS Letters* 279:19, 1991.

253. Lucius R et al: Growth stimulation and chemotropic attraction of rat retinal ganglion cell axons in vitro by co-cultured optic nerves, astrocytes and astrocyte conditioned medium, *Int J Develop Neurosci* 14:387, 1996.

254. Ludwin SK: Oligodendrocyte survival in wallerian degeneration, *Acta Neuropathol (Berl)* 80:184, 1990.

255. Ludwin SK: Phagocytosis in the rat optic nerve following wallerian degeneration, *Acta Neuropathol (Berl)* 80:266, 1990.

256. MacFadyen DJ et al: The retinal nerve fiber layer, neuroretinal rim area, and visual evoked potentials in MS, *Neurology* 38:1353, 1988.

257. Madison R, Moore MR, Sidman RL: Retinal ganglion cells and axons survive optic nerve transection, *Int J Neurosci* 23:15, 1984.

258. Maffei L et al: Schwann cells promote the survival of rat retinal ganglion cells after optic nerve section, *Proc Natl Acad Sci USA* 87:1855, 1990.

259. Magoon EH, Robb RM: Development of myelin in human optic nerve and tract: a light and electron microscopic study, *Arch Ophthalmol* 99:655, 1981.

260. Maniscalco JE, Habal MB: Microanatomy of the optic canal, *J Neurosurg* 48:402, 1978.

261. Mansour-Robaey S et al: Effects of ocular injury and administration of brain-derived neurotrophic factor on survival and regrowth of axotomized retinal ganglion cells, *Proc Natl Acad Sci USA* 91:1632, 1994.

262. Mantyh PW et al: Substance P receptor binding sites are expressed by glia in vivo after neuronal injury, *Proc Natl Acad Sci USA* 86:5193, 1989.

263. Marcoux FW et al: Differential regional vulnerability in transient focal cerebral ischemia, *Stroke* 13:339, 1982.

264. Matsui K, Hosoi N, Tachibana M: Excitatory synaptic transmission in the inner retina: paired recordings of bipolar cells and neurons of the ganglion cell layer, *J Neurosci* 18:4500, 1998.

265. Matsui K, Hosoi N, Tachibana M: Active role of glutamate uptake in the synaptic transmission from retinal nonspiking neurons, *J Neurosci* 19:6755, 1999.

266. Matsumoto N, Kometani M, Nagano K: Regenerating retinal fibers of the goldfish make temporary and unspecific but functional synapses before forming the final retinotopic projection, *Neuroscience* 22:1103, 1987.

267. Matthews MA, Cornell WJ, Alchediak T: Inhibition of axoplasmic transport in the developing visual system of the rat: I: Structural changes in the retina and optic nerve with graded doses of intraocular colchicines, *Neuroscience* 7:365, 1982.

268. McConnell P, Berry M: Regeneration of ganglion cell axons in the adult mouse retina, *Brain Res* 241:362, 1982.

269. McLoon SC: Response of astrocytes in the visual system to wallerian degeneration: an immunohistochemical analysis of laminin and glial fibrillary acidic protein (GFAP), *Exp Neurol* 91:613, 1986.

270. McLoon SC et al: Transient expression of laminin in the optic nerve of the developing rat, *J Neurosci* 8:1981, 1988.

271. Mekada A et al: Platelet-derived growth factor B-chain expression in the rat retina and optic nerve: distribution and changes after transection of the optic nerve, *Vision Res* 38:3031, 1998.

272. Mercken M et al: Three distinct axonal transport rates for tau, tubulin, and other microtubule-associated proteins: evidence for dynamic interactions of tau with microtubules in vivo, *J Neuroscience* 15:8259, 1995.

273. Mey J, Thanos S: Intravitreal injections of neurotrophic factors support the survival of axotomized retinal ganglion cells in adult rats in vivo, *Brain Res* 602:304, 1993.

274. Mey J, Thanos S: Functional and biochemical analysis of CNS-relevant neurotrophic activity in the lesioned sciatic nerve of adult rats, *J Hirnforsch* 37:25, 1996.

275. Meyer RL, Miotke J: Rapid initiation of neurite outgrowth onto laminin from explants of adult mouse retina induced by optic nerve crush, *Exp Neurol* 107:214, 1990.

276. Meyer-Franke A et al: Characterization of the signaling interactions that promote the survival and growth of developing retinal ganglion cells in culture, *Neuron* 15:805, 1995.

277. Meyer-Franke A et al: Depolarization and cAMP elevation rapidly recruit TrkB to the plasma membrane of CNS neurons, *Neuron* 21:681, 1998.

278. Mikelberg FS et al: The normal human optic nerve: axon count and axon diameter distribution, *Ophthalmology* 96:1325, 1989.

279. Mikelberg FS et al: Relation between optic nerve axon number and axon diameter to scleral canal area, *Ophthalmology* 98:60, 1991.

280. Miller RH et al: Is reactive gliosis a property of a distinct subpopulation of astrocytes? *J Neurosci* 6:22, 1986.

281. Minckler DS: The organization of nerve fiber bundles in the primate optic nerve head, *Arch Ophthalmol* 98:1630, 1980.

282. Minckler DS: Histology of optic nerve damage in ocular hypertension and early glaucoma, *Surv Ophthalmol* 33(suppl):401, 1989.

283. Minckler DS, Bunt AH: Axoplasmic transport in ocular hypotony and papilledema in the monkey, *Arch Ophthalmol* 95:1430, 1977.

284. Minckler DS, Bunt AH, Johanson GW: Orthograde and retrograde axoplasmic transport during acute ocular hypertension in the monkey, *Invest Ophthalmol Vis Sci* 16:426, 1977.

285. Minckler DS, McLean IW, Tso MO: Distribution of axonal and glial elements in the rhesus optic nerve head studied by electron microscopy, *Am J Ophthalmol* 82:179, 1976.

286. Minckler DS, Tso MO: A light microscopic, autoradiographic study of axoplasmic transport in the normal rhesus optic nerve head, *Am J Ophthalmol* 82:1, 1976.

287. Minckler DS, Tso MO, Zimmerman LE: A light microscopic, autoradiographic study of axoplasmic transport in the optic nerve head during ocular hypotony, increased intraocular pressure, and papilledema, *Am J Ophthalmol* 82:741, 1976.

288. Misantone LJ, Gershenbaum M, Murray M: Viability of retinal ganglion cells after optic nerve crush in adult rats, *J Neurocytol* 13:449, 1984.

289. Moore S, Thanos S: Differential increases in rat retinal ganglion cell size with various methods of optic nerve lesion, *Neurosci Lett* 207:117, 1996.

290. Morin PJ et al: Isolation and characterization of rapid transport vesicle subtypes from rabbit optic nerve, *J Neurochem* 56:415, 1991.

291. Morissette N, Carbonetto S: Laminin alpha 2 chain (M chain) is found within the pathway of avian and murine retinal projections, *J Neurosci* 15:8067, 1995.

292. Morrison JC et al: Aging changes of the rhesus monkey optic nerve, *Invest Ophthalmol Vis Sci* 31:1623, 1990.

293. Munari PF, De CR, Colletti D: Anatomy of the optic nerve in elderly men, *Metab Pediatr Syst Ophthalmol* 12:13, 1989.

294. Murray M, Grafstein B: Changes in the morphology and amino acid incorporation of regenerating goldfish optic neurons, *Exp Neurol* 23:544, 1969.

295. Murray N, Steck AJ: Impulse conduction regulates myelin basic protein phosphorylation in rat optic nerve, *J Neurochem* 43:243, 1984.

296. Naito J: Retinogeniculate projection fibers in the monkey optic nerve: a demonstration of the fiber pathways by retrograde axonal transport of WGA-HRP, *J Comp Neurol* 284:174, 1989.

297. Neufeld AH: Nitric oxide: a potential mediator of retinal ganglion cell damage in glaucoma, *Surv Ophthalmol* 43(suppl 1):S129, 1999.

298. Neufeld AH, Hernandez MR, Gonzalez M: Nitric oxide synthase in the human glaucomatous optic nerve head, *Arch Ophthalmol* 115:497, 1997.

299. Neufeld AH, Sawada A, Becker B: Inhibition of nitric-oxide synthase 2 by aminoguanidine provides neuroprotection of retinal ganglion cells in a rat model of chronic glaucoma, *Proc Natl Acad Sci USA* 96:9944, 1999.

300. Ng WP et al: Human central nervous system myelin inhibits neurite outgrowth, *Brain Res* 720:17, 1996.

301. Nishimura K et al: Effects of endothelin-1 on optic nerve head blood flow in cats, *J Ocul Pharmacol Ther* 12:75, 1996.

302. Nixon RA, Fischer I, Lewis SE: Synthesis, axonal transport, and turnover of the high molecular weight microtubule-associated protein MAP 1A in mouse retinal ganglion cells: tubulin and MAP 1A display distinct transport kinetics, *J Cell Biol* 110:437, 1990.

303. Nixon RA et al: Phosphorylation on carboxyl terminus domains of neurofilament proteins in retinal ganglion cell neurons in vivo: influences on regional neurofilament accumulation, interneurofilament spacing, and axon caliber, *J Cell Biol* 126:1031, 1994.

304. Nowak JZ, Nawrocki J, Maslinski C: Distribution and localization of histamine in bovine and rabbit eye, *Agents Actions* 14:335, 1984.

305. Nyborg NC, Nielsen PJ: Angiotensin-II contracts isolated human posterior ciliary arteries, *Invest Ophthalmol Vis Sci* 31:2471, 1990.

306. Ogden TE: Nerve fiber layer of the macaque retina: retinotopic organization, *Invest Ophthalmol Vis Sci* 24:85, 1983.

307. Oh Y, Black JA, Waxman SG: The expression of rat brain voltage-sensitive Na+ channel mRNAs in astrocytes, *Molec Brain Res* 23:57, 1994.

308. Ohishi H et al: Distribution of the messenger RNA for a metabotropic glutamate receptor, mGluR2, in the central nervous system of the rat, *Neuroscience* 53:1009, 1993.

309. Okisaka S et al: Apoptosis in retinal ganglion cell decrease in human glaucomatous eyes, *Jpn J Ophthalmol* 41:84, 1997.

310. Oku H et al: Experimental optic cup enlargement caused by endothelin-1-induced chronic optic nerve head ischemia, *Surv Ophthalmol* 44(suppl 1):S74, 1999.

311. Olney JW: The toxic effects of glutamate and related compounds in the retina and the brain, *Retina* 2:341, 1982.

312. Olsson Y: Mast cells in the nervous system, *Int Rev Cytol* 24:27, 1968.

313. Olver JM: Functional anatomy of the choroidal circulation: methyl methacrylate casting of human choroids, *Eye* 4:262, 1990.

314. Olver JM, Spalton DJ, McCartney AC: Microvascular study of the retrolaminar optic nerve in man: the possible significance in anterior ischaemic optic neuropathy, *Eye* 4:7, 1990.

315. Olver JM, Spalton DJ, McCartney AC: Quantitative morphology of human retrolaminar optic nerve vasculature, *Invest Ophthalmol Vis Sci* 35:3858, 1994.

316. Optic Neuritis Study Group: The 5-year risk of MS after optic neuritis. Experience of the optic neuritis treatment trial, *Neurology* 49:1404, 1997.

317. Orgul S, Cioffi GA: Embryology, anatomy, and histology of the optic nerve vasculature, *J Glaucoma* 5:285, 1996.

318. Orgul S et al: An endothelin-1-induced model of chronic optic nerve ischemia in rhesus monkeys, *J Glaucoma* 5:135, 1996.

319. Orgul S et al: An endothelin-1 induced model of optic nerve ischemia in the rabbit, *Invest Ophthalmol Vis Sci* 37:1860, 1996.

320. Pease ME et al: Obstructed axonal transport of BDNF and its receptor TrkB in experimental glaucoma, *Invest Ophthalmol Vis Sci* 41:764, 2000.

321. Peinado-Ramon P et al: Effects of axotomy and intraocular administration of NT-4, NT-3, and brain-derived neurotrophic factor on the survival of adult rat retinal ganglion cells. A quantitative in vivo study, *Invest Ophthalmol Vis Sci* 37:489, 1996.

322. Pena JD et al: Elastosis of the lamina cribrosa in glaucomatous optic neuropathy, *Exp Eye Res* 67:517, 1998.

323. Penfold PL, Provis JM: Cell death in the development of the human retina: phagocytosis of pyknotic and apoptotic bodies by retinal cells, *Graefes Arch Clin Exp Ophthalmol* 224:549, 1986.

324. Perez MT, Caminos E: Expression of brain-derived neurotrophic factor and of its functional receptor in neonatal and adult rat retina, *Neurosci Lett* 183:96, 1995.

325. Perez RG, Halfter W: Tenascin in the developing chick visual system: distribution and potential role as a modulator of retinal axon growth, *Dev Biol* 156:278, 1993.

326. Perry VH, Anthony DC: Axon damage and repair in multiple sclerosis, *Philos Trans R Soc Lond B Biol Sci* 354:1641, 1999.

327. Perry VH, Hayes L: Lesion-induced myelin formation in the retina, *J Neurocytol* 14:297, 1985.

328. Perry VH, Lund RD: Evidence that the lamina cribrosa prevents intraretinal myelination of retinal ganglion cell axons, *J Neurocytol* 19:265, 1990.

329. Petty MA, Wettstein JG: White matter ischaemia, *Brain Res Brain Res Rev* 31:58, 1999.

330. Pickard GE, Rea MA: Serotonergic innervation of the hypothalamic suprachiasmatic nucleus and photic regulation of circadian rhythms, *Biol Cell* 89:513, 1997.

331. Podhajsky RJ et al: A quantitative immunohistochemical study of the cellular response to crush injury in optic nerve, *Exp Neurol* 143:153, 1997.

332. Politis MJ: Exogenous laminin induces regenerative changes in traumatized sciatic and optic nerve, *Plast Reconstr Surg* 83:228, 1989.

333. Politis MJ, Miller JE: Post-traumatic alterations in glutamine synthetase activity in peripheral and central nerves, *Brain Res* 359:183, 1985.

334. Pow DV, Barnett NL, Penfold P: Are neuronal transporters relevant in retinal glutamate homeostasis? *Neurochem Int* 37:191, 2000.

335. Provis JM et al: Human fetal optic nerve: overproduction and elimination of retinal axons during development, *J Comp Neurol* 238:92, 1985.

336. Quigley H, Pease ME, Thibault D: Change in the appearance of elastin in the lamina cribrosa of glaucomatous optic nerve heads, *Graefes Arch Clin Exp Ophthalmol* 232:257, 1994.

337. Quigley HA: Ganglion cell death in glaucoma: pathology recapitulates ontogeny, *Aust NZ J Ophthalmol* 23:85, 1995.

338. Quigley HA: Neuronal death in glaucoma, *Prog Retin Eye Res* 18:39, 1999.

339. Quigley HA, Addicks EM: Chronic experimental glaucoma in primates: II. Effect of extended intraocular pressure elevation on optic nerve head and axonal transport, *Invest Ophthalmol Vis Sci* 19:137, 1980.

340. Quigley HA, Addicks EM: Regional differences in the structure of the lamina cribrosa and their relation to glaucomatous optic nerve damage, *Arch Ophthalmol* 99:137, 1981.

341. Quigley HA, Anderson DR: Descending optic nerve degeneration in primates, *Invest Ophthalmol Vis Sci* 16:841, 1977.

342. Quigley HA, Coleman AL, Dorman-Pease ME: Larger optic nerve heads have more nerve fibers in normal monkey eyes, *Arch Ophthalmol* 109:1441, 1991.

343. Quigley HA, Dunkelberger GR, Green WR: Retinal ganglion cell atrophy correlated with automated perimetry in human eyes with glaucoma, *Am J Ophthalmol* 107:453, 1989.

344. Quigley HA, Guy J, Anderson DR: Blockade of rapid axonal transport. Effect of intraocular pressure elevation in primate optic nerve, *Arch Ophthalmol* 97:525, 1979.

345. Quigley HA, Miller NR, George T: Clinical evaluation of nerve fiber layer atrophy as an indicator of glaucomatous optic nerve damage, *Arch Ophthalmol* 98:1564, 1980.

346. Quigley HA et al: Optic nerve damage in human glaucoma: II. The site of injury and susceptibility to damage, *Arch Ophthalmol* 99:635, 1981.

347. Quigley HA et al: Morphologic changes in the lamina cribrosa correlated with neural loss in open-angle glaucoma, *Am J Ophthalmol* 95:673, 1983.

348. Quigley HA et al: The size and shape of the optic disc in normal human eyes, *Arch Ophthalmol* 108:51, 1990.

349. Quigley HA et al: Retinal ganglion cell death in experimental glaucoma and after axotomy occurs by apoptosis, *Invest Ophthalmol Vis Sci* 36:774, 1995.

350. Quigley HA et al: Retrograde axonal transport of BDNF in retinal ganglion cells is blocked by acute IOP elevation in rats, *Invest Ophthalmol Vis Sci* 41:3460, 2000.

351. Radius RL: Pressure-induced fast axonal transport abnormalities and the anatomy at the lamina cribrosa in primate eyes, *Invest Ophthalmol Vis Sci* 24:343, 1983.

352. Radius RL, Anderson DR: Retinal ganglion cell degeneration in experimental optic atrophy, *Am J Ophthalmol* 86:673, 1978.

353. Radius RL, Anderson DR: Fast axonal transport in early experimental disc edema, *Invest Ophthalmol Vis Sci* 19:158, 1980.

354. Raff MC, ffrench-Constant C, Miller RH: Glial cells in the rat optic nerve and some thoughts on remyelination in the mammalian CNS, *J Exp Biol* 132:35, 1987.

355. Rao K, Lund RD: Degeneration of optic axons induces the expression of major histocompatibility antigens, *Brain Res* 488:332, 1989.

356. Rao NA, Guy J, Sheffield PS: Effects of chronic demyelination on axonal transport in experimental allergic optic neuritis, *Invest Ophthalmol Vis Sci* 21:606, 1981.

357. Redies C, Takeichi M: N- and R-cadherin expression in the optic nerve of the chicken embryo, *Glia* 8:161, 1993.

358. Reese BE: The chronotopic reordering of optic axons, *Perspect Dev Biol* 3:233, 1996.

359. Reese BE, Ho KY: Axon diameter distributions across the monkey's optic nerve, *Neuroscience* 27:205, 1988.

360. Rehen SK, Linden R: Apoptosis in the developing retina: paradoxical effects of protein synthesis inhibition, *Braz J Med Biol Res* 27:1647, 1994.

361. Reichert F, Rotshenker S: Deficient activation of microglia during optic nerve degeneration, *J Neuroimmunol* 70:153, 1996.

362. Renn WH, Rhoton AL Jr: Microsurgical anatomy of the sellar region, *J Neurosurg* 43:288, 1975.

363. Renteria RC, Constantine-Paton M: Exogenous nitric oxide causes collapse of retinal ganglion cell axonal growth cones in vitro, *J Neurobiol* 29:415, 1996.

364. Repka MX, Quigley HA: The effect of age on normal human optic nerve fiber number and diameter, *Ophthalmology* 96:26, 1989.

365. Reynolds AJ, Bartlett SE, Hendry IA: Molecular mechanisms regulating the retrograde axonal transport of neurotrophins, *Brain Res Brain Res Rev* 33:169, 2000.

366. Riehl R et al: Cadherin function is required for axon outgrowth in retinal ganglion cells in vivo, *Neuron* 17:837, 1996.

367. Rimmer S et al: Growth of the human optic disk and nerve during gestation, childhood, and early adulthood, *Am J Ophthalmol* 116:748, 1993.

368. Riva CE, Grunwald JE, Petrig BL: Autoregulation of human retinal blood flow: an investigation with laser Doppler velocimetry, *Invest Ophthalmol Vis Sci* 27:1706, 1986.

369. Rizzo JFd, Lessell S: Risk of developing multiple sclerosis after uncomplicated optic neuritis: a long-term prospective study, *Neurology* 38:185, 1988.

370. Robinson GA: Changes in the expression of transcription factors ATF-2 and Fra-2 after axotomy and during regeneration in rat retinal ganglion cells, *Molec Brain Res* 41:57, 1996.

371. Rodieck RW, Watanabe M: Survey of the morphology of macaque retinal ganglion cells that project to the pretectum, superior colliculus, and parvicellular laminae of the lateral geniculate nucleus, *J Comp Neurol* 338:289, 1993.

372. Rogers SD et al: Expression of endothelin-B receptors by glia in vivo is increased after CNS injury in rats, rabbits, and humans, *Exp Neurol* 145:180, 1997.

373. Rorig B, Grantyn R: Rat retinal ganglion cells express Ca(2+)-permeable non-NMDA glutamate receptors during the period of histogenetic cell death, *Neurosci Lett* 153:32, 1993.

374. Rothe T, Bigl V, Grantyn R: Potentiating and depressant effects of metabotropic glutamate receptor agonists on high-voltage-activated calcium currents in cultured retinal ganglion neurons from postnatal mice, *Pflugers Arch* 426:161, 1994.

375. Russelakis-Carneiro M, Silveira LC, Perry VH: Factors affecting the survival of cat retinal ganglion cells after optic nerve injury, *J Neurocytol* 25:393, 1996.

376. Sadun AA, Schaechter JD, Smith LE: A retinohypothalamic pathway in man: light mediation of circadian rhythms, *Brain Res* 302:371, 1984.

377. Sakatani K, Hassan AZ, Chesler M: Effects of GABA on axonal conduction and extracellular potassium activity in the neonatal rat optic nerve, *Exp Neurol* 127:291, 1994.

378. Sanchez I et al: Oligodendroglia regulate the regional expansion of axon caliber and local accumulation of neurofilaments during development independently of myelin formation, *J Neuroscience* 16:5095, 1996.

379. Sanchez RM, Dunkelberger GR, Quigley HA: The number and diameter distribution of axons in the monkey optic nerve, *Invest Ophthalmol Vis Sci* 27:1342, 1986.

380. Savio T, Schwab ME: Rat CNS white matter, but not gray matter, is nonpermissive for neuronal cell adhesion and fiber outgrowth, *J Neurosci* 9:1126, 1989.

381. Sawaguchi S et al: The collagen fibrillar network in the human pial septa, *Curr Eye Res* 13:819, 1994.

382. Sawai H et al: Brain-derived neurotrophic factor and neurotrophin-4/5 stimulate growth of axonal branches from regenerating retinal ganglion cells, *J Neurosci* 16:3887, 1996.

383. Schaden H, Stuermer CA, Bahr M: GAP-43 immunoreactivity and axon regeneration in retinal ganglion cells of the rat, *J Neurobiol* 25:1570, 1994.

384. Schaecter JD, Sadun AA: A second hypothalamic nucleus receiving retinal input in man: the paraventricular nucleus, *Brain Res* 340:243, 1985.

385. Schmid R, Wilhelm B, Wilhelm H: Naso-temporal asymmetry and contraction anisocoria in the pupillomotor system, *Graefes Arch Clin Exp Ophthalmol* 238:123, 2000.

386. Schmid S, Guenther E: Developmental regulation of voltage-activated Na+ and Ca2+ currents in rat retinal ganglion cells, *Neuroreport* 7:677, 1996.

387. Schmid S, Guenther E: Alterations in channel density and kinetic properties of the sodium current in retinal ganglion cells of the rat during in vivo differentiation, *Neuroscience* 85:249, 1998.

388. Schmid S, Guenther E: Voltage-activated calcium currents in rat retinal ganglion cells in situ: changes during prenatal and postnatal development, *J Neurosci* 19:3486, 1999.

389. Schnitzer J: Astrocytes in the guinea pig, horse, and monkey retina: Their occurrence coincides with the presence of blood vessels, *Glia* 1:74, 1988.

390. Schnitzer J, Scherer J: Microglial cell responses in the rabbit retina following transection of the optic nerve, *J Comp Neurol* 302:779, 1990.

391. Schori H et al: Vaccination for protection of retinal ganglion cells against death from glutamate cytotoxicity and ocular hypertension: Implications for glaucoma, *Proc Natl Acad Sci USA* 98:3398, 2001.

392. Schumer RA, Podos SM: The nerve of glaucoma! *Arch Ophthalmol* 112:37, 1994.

393. Schutte M: Centrifugal innervation of the rat retina, *Vis Neurosci* 12:1083, 1995.

394. Schwab ME: Myelin-associated inhibitors of neurite growth, *Exp Neurol* 109:2, 1990.

395. Schwab ME: Structural plasticity of the adult CNS. Negative control by neurite growth inhibitory signals, *Int J Dev Neurosci* 14:379, 1996.

396. Schwartz M et al: Potential treatment modalities for glaucomatous neuropathy: neuroprotection and neuroregeneration, *J Glaucoma* 5:427, 1996.

397. Segal RA, Greenberg ME: Intracellular signaling pathways activated by neurotrophic factors, *Ann Rev Neurosci* 19:463, 1996.

398. Sergott RC et al: Antigalactocerebroside serum demyelinates optic nerve in vivo, *J Neurol Sci* 64:297, 1984.

399. Shen S et al: Retinal ganglion cells lose trophic responsiveness after axotomy, *Neuron* 23:285, 1999.

400. Shihab ZM, Lee PF, Hay P: The significance of disc hemorrhage in open-angle glaucoma, *Ophthalmology* 89:211, 1982.

401. Sievers J et al: Fibroblast growth factors promote the survival of adult rat retinal ganglion cells after transection of the optic nerve, *Neurosci Lett* 76:157, 1987.

402. Siliprandi R et al: N-methyl-D-aspartate-induced neurotoxicity in the adult rat retina, *Vis Neurosci* 8:567, 1992.

403. Sisk DR, Kuwabara T: Histologic changes in the inner retina of albino rats following intravitreal injection of monosodium L-glutamate, *Graefes Arch Clin Exp Ophthalmol* 223:250, 1985.

404. Skoff RP: The fine structure of pulse labeled (3H-thymidine cells) in degenerating rat optic nerve, *J Comp Neurol* 161:595, 1975.

405. Smalheiser NR, Crain SM, Reid LM: Laminin as a substrate for retinal axons in vitro, *Brain Res* 314:136, 1984.

406. So KF, Aguayo AJ: Lengthy regrowth of cut axons from ganglion cells after peripheral nerve transplantation into the retina of adult rats, *Brain Res* 328:349, 1985.

407. Spileers W, Goethals M: Structural changes of the lamina cribrosa and of the trabeculum in primary open angle glaucoma (POAG), *Bull Soc Belge Ophtalmol* 244:27, 1992.

408. Sretavan DW et al: Disruption of retinal axon ingrowth by ablation of embryonic mouse optic chiasm neurons, *Science* 269:98, 1995.

409. Stanford LR: Conduction velocity variations minimize conduction time differences among retinal ganglion cell axons, *Science* 238:358, 1987.

410. Stanhope GB, Billings-Gagliardi S, Wolf MK: Myelination requirements of central nervous system glia in vitro: statistical validation of differences between glia from adult and immature mice, *Glia* 3:125, 1990.

411. Stevens A, Bahr M: Origin of macrophages in central nervous tissue: a study using intraperitoneal transplants contained in Millipore diffusion chambers, *J Neurol Sci* 118:117, 1993.

412. Stoll G, Mueller HW: Lesion-induced changes of astrocyte morphology and protein expression in rat optic nerve, *Ann NY Acad Sci* 540:461, 1988.

413. Stoll G, Trapp BD, Griffin JW: Macrophage function during wallerian degeneration of rat optic nerve: clearance of degenerating myelin and Ia expression, *J Neurosci* 9:2327, 1989.

414. Stone J: The naso-temporal division of the cat's retina, *J Comp Neurol* 126:585, 1966.

415. Stroman GA et al: Magnetic resonance imaging in patients with low-tension glaucoma, *Arch Ophthalmol* 113:168, 1995.

416. Sturrock RR: Microglia in the human embryonic optic nerve, *J Anat* 139:81, 1984.

417. Sturrock RR: Development of the meninges of the human embryonic optic nerve, *J Hirnforsch* 28:603, 1987.

418. Sturrock RR: A quantitative histological study of cell division and changes in cell number in the meningeal sheath of the embryonic human optic nerve, *J Anat* 155:133, 1987.

419. Sturrock RR: Vascularization of the human embryonic optic nerve, *J Hirnforsch* 28:615, 1987.

420. Sturrock RR: An electron microscopic study of macrophages in the meninges of the human embryonic optic nerve, *J Anat* 157:145, 1988.

421. Sturrock RR: Fluorescent granular perithelial cells in the meninges and optic nerve of the human embryo, *Anat Anz* 166:323, 1988.

422. Stys PK: Anoxic and ischemic injury of myelinated axons in CNS white matter: from mechanistic concepts to therapeutics, *J Cereb Blood Flow Metab* 18:2, 1998.

423. Stys PK, Lesiuk H: Correlation between electrophysiological effects of mexiletine and ischemic protection in central nervous system white matter, *Neuroscience* 71:27, 1996.

424. Stys PK et al: Role of extracellular calcium in anoxic injury of mammalian central white matter, *Proc Natl Acad Sci USA* 87:4212, 1990.

425. Stys PK et al: Noninactivating, tetrodotoxin-sensitive Na+ conductance in rat optic nerve axons, *Proc Natl Acad Sci USA* 90:6976, 1993.

426. Susanna R Jr: The lamina cribrosa and visual field defects in open-angle glaucoma, *Can J Ophthalmol* 18:124, 1983.

427. Takeda M et al: Injury-specific expression of activating transcription factor-3 in retinal ganglion cells and its colocalized expression with phosphorylated c-Jun, *Invest Ophthalmol Vis Sci* 41:2412, 2000.

428. Taschenberger H, Grantyn R: Several types of Ca2+ channels mediate glutamatergic synaptic responses to activation of single Thy-1-immunolabeled rat retinal ganglion neurons, *J Neurosci* 15:2240, 1995.

429. Taschenberger H, Juttner R, Grantyn R: Ca2+-permeable P2X receptor channels in cultured rat retinal ganglion cells, *J Neurosci* 19:3353, 1999.

430. Tezel G, Wax MB: The mechanisms of hsp27 antibody-mediated apoptosis in retinal neuronal cells, *J Neurosci* 20:3552, 2000.

431. Thale A, Tillmann B, Rochels R: SEM studies of the collagen architecture of the human lamina cribrosa: normal and pathological findings, *Ophthalmologica* 210:142, 1996.

432. Thanos S, Mey J, Wild M: Treatment of the adult retina with microglia-suppressing factors retards axotomy-induced neuronal degradation and enhances axonal regeneration in vivo and in vitro, *J Neurosci* 13:455, 1993.

433. Thanos S et al: Survival and axonal elongation of adult rat retinal ganglion cells: In vitro effects of lesioned sciatic nerve and brain derived neurotrophic factor, *Eur J Neurosci* 1:19, 1989.

434. Thanos S et al: Specific transcellular staining of microglia in the adult rat after traumatic degeneration of carbocyanine-filled retinal ganglion cells, *Exp Eye Res* 55:101, 1992.

435. Thoenen H: The changing scene of neurotrophic factors, *Trends Neurosci* 14:165, 1991.

436. Toms R, Weiner HL, Johnson D: Identification of IgE-positive cells and mast cells in frozen sections of multiple sclerosis brains, *J Neuroimmunol* 30:169, 1990.

437. Trapp BD et al: Axonal transection in the lesions of multiple sclerosis, *N Engl J Med* 338:278, 1998.

438. Trimmer PA et al: An ultrastructural and immunocytochemical study of astrocytic differentiation in vitro: changes in the composition and distribution of the cellular cytoskeleton, *J Neuroimmunol* 2:235, 1982.

439. Tso MO, Hayreh SS: Optic disc edema in raised intracranial pressure. IV. Axoplasmic transport in experimental papilledema, *Arch Ophthalmol* 95:1458, 1977.

440. Tso MO, Shih CV, McLean IW: Is there a blood brain barrier at the optic nerve head? *Arch Ophthalmol* 93:815, 1975.

441. Tsukahara I, Yamashita H: An electron microscopic study on the blood-optic nerve and fluid-optic nerve barrier, *Graefes Arch Clin Exp Ophthalmol* 196:239, 1975.

442. Turner DL, Cepko CL: A common progenitor for neurons and glia persists in rat retina late in development, *Nature* 328:131, 1987.

443. Tytell M, Brady ST, Lasek RJ: Axonal transport of a subclass of tau proteins: evidence for the regional differentiation of microtubules in neurons, *Proc Natl Acad Sci USA* 81:1570, 1984.

444. Varma R, Quigley HA, Pease ME: Changes in optic disk characteristics and number of nerve fibers in experimental glaucoma, *Am J Ophthalmol* 114:554, 1992.

445. Velte TJ, Masland RH: Action potentials in the dendrites of retinal ganglion cells, *J Neurophysiol* 81:1412, 1999.

446. Veronesi B, Boyes WK: Morphometric and electrophysiological evidence for a diameter-based rate of degeneration in the optic nerve of the rat, *Exp Neurol* 101:176, 1988.

447. Vickers JC et al: Magnocellular and parvocellular visual pathways are both affected in a macaque monkey model of glaucoma, *Aust NZ J Ophthalmol* 25:239, 1997.

448. Villar MJ, Vitale ML, Parisi MN: Dorsal raphe serotonergic projection to the retina: a combined peroxidase tracing-neurochemical/high-performance liquid chromatography study in the rat, *Neuroscience* 22:681, 1987.

449. Villegas-Perez MP et al: Rapid and protracted phases of retinal ganglion cell loss follow axotomy in the optic nerve of adult rats, *J Neurobiol* 24:23, 1993.

450. von Bartheld CS: Neurotrophins in the developing and regenerating visual system, *Histol Histopath* 13:437, 1998.

451. von Bartheld CS et al: Anterograde transport of neurotrophins and axodendritic transfer in the developing visual system, *Nature* 379:830, 1996.

452. Wanner M et al: Reevaluation of the growth-permissive substrate properties of goldfish optic nerve myelin and myelin proteins, *J Neurosci* 15:7500, 1995.

453. Watanabe T, Raff MC: Retinal astrocytes are immigrants from the optic nerve, *Nature* 332:834, 1988.

454. Watson WE: Cellular responses to axotomy and to related procedures, *Br Med Bull* 30:112, 1974.

455. Waxman SG, Black JA: Freeze-fracture ultrastructure of the perinodal astrocyte and associated glial junctions, *Brain Res* 308:77, 1984.

456. Waxman SG et al: Low density of sodium channels supports action potential conduction in axons of neonatal rat optic nerve, *Proc Natl Acad Sci USA* 86:1406, 1989.

457. Waxman SG et al: Anoxic injury of mammalian central white matter: decreased susceptibility in myelin-deficient optic nerve, *Ann Neurol* 28:335, 1990.

458. Weber AJ et al: Experimental glaucoma and cell size, density, and number in the primate lateral geniculate nucleus, *Invest Ophthalmol Vis Sci* 41:1370, 2000.

459. Weibel D, Cadelli D, Schwab ME: Regeneration of lesioned rat optic nerve fibers is improved after neutralization of myelin-associated neurite growth inhibitors, *Brain Res* 642:259, 1994.

460. Weibel D, Kreutzberg GW, Schwab ME: Brain-derived neurotrophic factor (BDNF) prevents lesion-induced axonal die-back in young rat optic nerve, *Brain Res* 679:249, 1995.

461. Weinreb RN, Levin LA: Is neuroprotection a viable therapy for glaucoma? *Arch Ophthalmol* 117:1540, 1999.

462. Weinstein JM et al: Regional optic nerve blood flow and its autoregulation, *Invest Ophthalmol Vis Sci* 24:1559, 1983.

463. Wen R et al: Alpha 2-adrenergic agonists induce basic fibroblast growth factor expression in photoreceptors in vivo and ameliorate light damage, *J Neurosci* 16:5986, 1996.

464. Wender R et al: Astrocytic glycogen influences axon function and survival during glucose deprivation in central white matter, *J Neurosci* 20:6804, 2000.

465. Willard M, Simon C: Modulations of neurofilament axonal transport during the development of rabbit retinal ganglion cells, *Cell* 35:551, 1983.

466. Willard M et al: Axonal transport of actin in rabbit retinal ganglion cells, *J Cell Biol* 81:581, 1979.

467. Wodarczyk L, Merrill VK, Perry GW: Differential regulation of fast axonally transported proteins during the early response of rat retinal ganglion cells to axotomy, *J Neurochem* 68:1114, 1997.

468. Wolff E: *The anatomy of the eye and orbit,* Philadelphia, 1948, Blakiston.

469. Wujek JR, Reier PJ: Astrocytic membrane morphology: differences between mammalian and amphibian astrocytes after axotomy, *J Comp Neurol* 222:607, 1984.

470. Wurtz RH: Vision for the control of movement: the Friedenwald lecture, *Invest Ophthalmol Vis Sci* 37:2130, 1996.

471. Yarom Y et al: Immunospecific inhibition of nerve conduction by T lymphocytes reactive to basic protein of myelin, *Nature* 303:246, 1983.

472. Ye XD, Laties AM, Stone RA: Peptidergic innervation of the retinal vasculature and optic nerve head, *Invest Ophthalmol Vis Sci* 31:1731, 1990.

473. Yee KT et al: Differential expression of class I and class II major histocompatibility complex antigen in early postnatal rats, *Brain Res* 530:121, 1990.

474. Yoles E, Muller S, Schwartz M: NMDA-receptor antagonist protects neurons from secondary degeneration after partial optic nerve crush, *J Neurotrauma* 14:665, 1997.

475. Yoles E, Schwartz M: Elevation of intraocular glutamate levels in rats with partial lesion of the optic nerve, *Arch Ophthalmol* 116:906, 1998.

476. Yoles E, Wheeler LA, Schwartz M: Alpha2-adrenoreceptor agonists are neuroprotective in a rat model of optic nerve degeneration, *Invest Ophthalmol Vis Sci* 40:65, 1999.

477. Young MJ, Lund RD: The retinal ganglion cells that drive the pupilloconstrictor response in rats, *Brain Res* 787:191, 1998.

478. Yücel YH et al: Loss of neurons in magnocellular and parvocellular layers of the lateral geniculate nucleus in glaucoma, *Arch Ophthalmol* 118:378, 2000.

479. Zeev-Brann AB et al: Differential effects of central and peripheral nerves on macrophages and microglia, *Glia* 23:181, 1998.

480. Zeng BY et al: Regenerative and other responses to injury in the retinal stump of the optic nerve in adult albino rats: transection of the intraorbital optic nerve, *J Anat* 185:643, 1994.

481. Zhu B et al: Axonal cytoskeleton changes in experimental optic neuritis, *Brain Res* 824:204, 1999.

SECTION 11

CENTRAL VISUAL PATHWAYS

JOANNE A. MATSUBARA

CHAPTER 26

OVERVIEW OF THE CENTRAL VISUAL PATHWAYS

JAMIE D. BOYD, QIANG GU, AND JOANNE A. MATSUBARA

The role of the central visual pathways is to process and integrate visual information that travels to the brain by means of the optic nerves. Although the eye is responsible for transducing patterns of light energy into neuronal signals, it is the brain that is ultimately responsible for visual perception and cognition. Vision at the level of the central nervous system is perhaps the best understood of all the sensory systems, partly because there is a wealth of information on its neuroanatomic and functional organization. In this chapter an overview of the central visual pathways is given, beginning with a brief description of the retinal projections and their putative functional roles and ending with an overview of the consequences of lesions along the visual pathway. Schematic views of the central nuclei that receive a retinal projection are shown in Figures 26-1 and 26-2. The most significant, in terms of the number of optic nerve fibers, is the projection to the lateral geniculate nucleus (LGN) in the thalamus. The LGN, described in detail in Chapter 28, is an important relay in the visual pathway involved with form vision. The precision and specificity of the retinogeniculate connections are crucial to form vision, and Chapter 27 describes the role of spontaneous retinal activity during development in shaping this specificity. From the LGN, the visual pathway proceeds to the primary visual cortex, V1. It is at the level of V1 that visual signals take on complex processing, which is detailed in Chapter 29. Visual processing of a combination of stimulus features such as color, contrast, motion, texture, depth, and object recognition is further enhanced by more than 30 extrastriate cortical areas, some of which are described in Chapter 30. Finally, the de-velopmental role of experience and visual deprivation on the central visual pathways is discussed in Chapter 31.

TARGETS OF THE RETINAL PROJECTIONS

The major targets of the retinal ganglion cell axons are the LGN, superior colliculus (SC), pretectum, and pulvinar. There is a weaker projection to several small hypothalamic nuclei (including suprachiasmatic, supraoptic, and paraventricular nuclei) and the accessory optic system (AOS) (including the nucleus of the optic tract [NOT] and the dorsal, medial, and terminal nuclei).

The LGN of the thalamus is the major termination site of the retinal ganglion cells and plays an important role in the visual pathway leading to the primary visual cortex. Approximately 90% of all retinal ganglion cells project to the LGN, which is laminated and displays retinotopic organization. Each layer receives input from a specific eye and class of ganglion cell. Although electrophysiologic studies have determined that the neuronal signals coming into and leaving the LGN are not appreciably different, the processing that takes place in the LGN appears to be involved in regulating the flow of information to the primary visual cortex (V1), the major projection target of the LGN (see Chapter 28).

The SC is a midbrain structure, which in conjunction with the cortical frontal eye fields and the brainstem reticular formation, is involved in the generation of visually guided saccadic eye movements[7,11] (see Chapter 36). The SC is a laminated, retinotopically organized nucleus, and as seen in

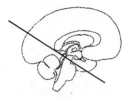

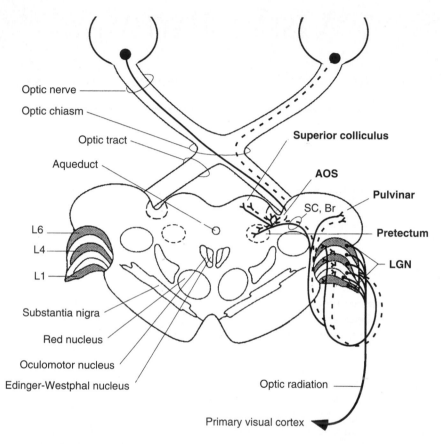

Optic nerve

Optic chiasm

Optic tract

Aqueduct

Superior colliculus

AOS

Pulvinar

SC, Br

Pretectum

L6

L4

L1

LGN

Substantia nigra

Red nucleus

Oculomotor nucleus

Edinger-Westphal nucleus

Optic radiation

Primary visual cortex

FIGURE 26-1   Schematic drawing of a section through the human brain at the level of the midbrain-diencephalon transition (*top left inset*). Several of the target sites of the retinal projection are present at this level and labeled in bold on the right: the superior colliculus, pretectum, accessory optic system (*AOS*), pulvinar, and lateral geniculate nucleus (*LGN*). Optic nerve fibers originating from ganglion cells of the contralateral nasal retina cross at the optic chiasm and join the uncrossed optic nerve fibers from the ipsilateral temporal retina to form the optic tract. The layers of the LGN, the major termination site of the optic nerve fibers, receive contralateral eye (layers 1, 4, 6; *shaded*) or ipsilateral eye (layers 2, 3, 5; *unshaded*) inputs. Cells in all six layers of the LGN project to the primary visual cortex via the optic radiation. *SC, Br,* Brachium of the superior colliculus.

the LGN, the retinal projection retains eye segregation with alternating columns of left and right eye terminals forming a banded pattern throughout the superficial layers. Approximately 10% of all retinal ganglion cells project to the SC. Most retinal axons that terminate in the SC are small caliber, originate from ganglion cells with small dendritic fields, and do not project to other retinal targets.[10]

The pretectal complex, a group of small midbrain nuclei, is just rostral to the SC. It receives sig-

nals from a group of small diameter retinal ganglion cells with large receptive fields and is involved with the control of the pupillary light reflex by means of a projection to the Edinger-Westphal nucleus of the oculomotor complex. The pupillary light reflex demonstrates a consensual response primarily resulting from crossed and uncrossed optic nerve fibers that enter each pretectal complex, which in turn sends a bilateral projection to the Edinger-Westphal nucleus (see Chapter 32).

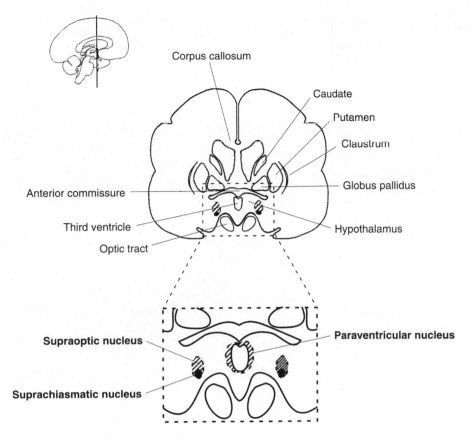

FIGURE 26-2 Schematic drawing of a section through the human brain at the level of the anterior commissure (*top left inset*). Retinal target in the hypothalamic area are labeled in bold (*bottom enlargement*). A small number of fibers branch off the optic tract, forming the retinohypothalamic tract, and terminate in the supraoptic, suprachiasmatic, and paraventricular nuclei of the hypothalamus. Visual input to the hypothalamus drives the light-dark entrainment of neuroendocrine function and other circadian rhythms.

The retinal ganglion cells also project to three of four major subdivisions of the pulvinar nucleus of the thalamus.[5] The pulvinar is the largest nuclear mass in the primate thalamus and receives a projection from the small-caliber fibers from the optic nerve and the SC. It projects to several visual cortical areas, including V1, and extrastriate, parietal areas. Thus the pulvinar represents a second pathway that can bypass the LGN to get to V1 and may play a role in processing form vision. More recent studies point to a role for the pulvinar in the coding of the "importance" of visual stimuli (i.e., visual salience or attention).[9] It has been shown that the pulvinar integrates neural signals associated with eye and hand and arm movements and may receive signals associated with saccadic eye movements, which suggests its role is also one of formulating reference frames for hand-eye coordination.[1,2,8]

Several small hypothalamic nuclei receive a direct retinal projection. The suprachiasmatic nucleus receives a sparse projection from fibers that leave the dorsal surface of the optic chiasma and has been implicated in the synchronization of circadian rhythms.[6] The paraventricular and supraoptic nuclei are likely also involved with the regulation of the light-dark cycle for neuroendocrine functions.

The AOS consists of several small nuclei, the lateral terminal nucleus (LTN), the medial terminal nucleus (MTN), and the dorsal terminal nucleus (DTN), as well as the NOT in the midbrain.[4] The AOS plays an important role in optokinetic nystagmus (OKN) in which slow compensatory and pursuit-type eye movements alternate with fast saccadic-type eye movements in response to viewing prolonged large field motion (see Chapter 36). In primates, lesions of the NOT and the DTN have been shown to modify the OKN and reduce or abolish optokinetic afternystagmus (OKAN).[12]

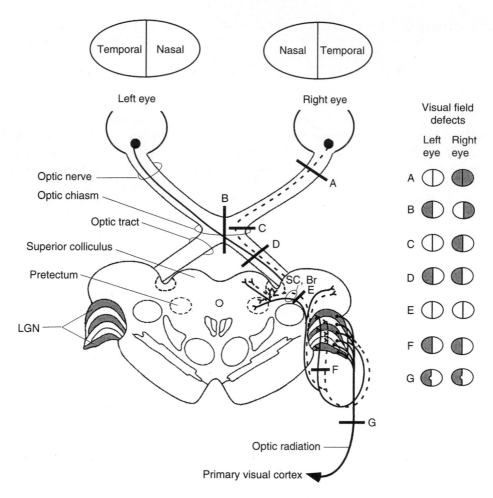

FIGURE 26-3   Visual field defects associated with lesions of the visual pathway. The bars (*A-G*) depict the location of lesions, and the associated visual field defect is shown at the right (*shaded area* represents visual field loss). *A,* Lesion of the right optic nerve causes blindness in the right eye. *B,* Optic chiasm lesion results in a bitemporal hemianopsia, a loss of vision in the temporal visual field of both eyes. *C,* Lesion affecting only the uncrossed fibers of the optic chiasm results in a loss of vision in the nasal field of the ipsilateral eye. *D,* Lesion of the optic tract causes homonymous hemianopsia, or complete loss of vision in the contralateral visual field. An afferent pupillary defect also arises from a lesion at this level. *E,* Lesion affecting the fibers in the brachium of the superior colliculus (*SC, Br*) results in an afferent pupillary defect, but with intact visual fields because the projection to the lateral geniculate nucleus (*LGN*) remains intact. *F,* Lesions at the level of the LGN are similar to lesions at *D* and result in homonymous hemianopsia, but with an intact, normal pupillary reflex. *G,* Lesions at the level of the optic radiation also result in a homonymous hemianopsia, but with sparing of macular vision.

VISUAL FIELD LESIONS

Much of our knowledge of the retinotopic organization of the central visual nuclei arises from the visual field defects associated with lesions along the major pathway leading to form vision, the retino-geniculocortical pathway. Figure 26-3 illustrates several known anatomic lesions of the visual pathway, from the retina to the occipital lobes, and their subsequent effect on the visual fields. In the example shown in Figure 26-3, *A,* complete interruption of one optic nerve, which may occur with severe degenerative disease or injury, results in permanent blindness in the affected eye. Partial interruption of the nerve fiber layer results in a partial loss of the visual field and can occur with glaucoma, optic disc drusen, pits, infarcts, or optic neuritis.

Slightly further along the visual pathway, interruption of the decussating optic nerve fibers in the optic chiasm (Figure 26-3, *B*) results in loss of vision in the temporal visual hemifields of both eyes, called *bitemporal hemianopsia*. Damage of this type may occur with pituitary tumors as they grow and compress the overlying optic chiasm. If, instead, pressure is exerted on the lateral edge of the optic chiasma (Figure 26-3, *C*), damage arises primarily in the uncrossed fibers, resulting in loss of vision in the nasal hemifield, or *nasal hemianopsia,* ipsilateral to the compression.

Lesions that occur after the chiasm are characterized by visual field defects that involve the temporal hemifield of the contralateral eye and the nasal hemifield of the ipsilateral eye; this is because of the partial decussation of optic nerve fibers at the optic chiasm. In this type of lesion, visual field loss occurs on the side contralateral to the lesion. Complete interruption at the level of the optic tract (Figure 26-3, *D*) or beyond results in loss of vision in the contralateral visual field, called *homonymous hemianopsia.* It is usually difficult to determine whether the site of the lesion is at the level of the optic tract, LGN, or visual cortex for most homonymous hemianopsias. In cases in which the lesion is in the optic tract, the homonymous hemianopsia may be accompanied by an afferent pupillary defect in the contralateral eye. The reason for this is likely because ganglion cells in the nasal retina outnumber those in the temporal retina, thus causing a greater loss of fibers for the pupillary response of the contralateral eye (however, also see reference 13).[3] Lesions at the level of the brachium of the SC (Figure 26-3, *E*) may result in an afferent pupillary defect in the contralateral eye, but with intact, normal visual fields because lesions at this level spare the retinogeniculate fibers.

Lesions involving the LGN (Figure 26-3, *F*) are often difficult to distinguish from other optic tract lesions, but they usually present with a visual field defect and an intact contralateral afferent pupillary reflex because lesions at this level normally spare the retinal fibers terminating in the pretectum responsible for the afferent pupillary reflex.

Lesions involving the optic radiation (Figure 26-3, *G*) or the visual cortex result in homonymous hemianopsia, but with sparing of the central, macular field. Several hypotheses have been put forward to explain macular sparing, but in many patients, macular sparing is likely more apparent than real because it is likely an artifact of visual field testing caused by poor foveal fixation or eye movements. In other patients in whom macular sparing is not artifactual, the most likely explanation is the immense areal dimension of the cortical representation of the retinal fovea. The posterior cerebral artery supplies the occipital poles, but in some individuals the occipital poles are supplied by both the posterior and middle cerebral arteries. Thus infarcts of the posterior cerebral artery would affect only part of the occipital poles, sparing portions of the foveal representation and sparing macular vision.

REFERENCES

1. Acuna C, Gonzalez F, Dominguez R: Sensorimotor unit activity related to intention in the pulvinar of behaving *Cebus apella* monkeys, *Exp Brain Res* 52:411, 1983.
2. Cudeiro J et al: Does the pulvinar-LP complex contribute to motor programming? *Brain Res* 484:367, 1989.
3. Curcio CA, Allen KA: Topography of ganglion cells in human retina, *J Comp Neurol* 300:5, 1990.
4. Fredericks CA et al: The human accessory optic system, *Brain Res* 454:116, 1988.
5. Grieve KL, Acuna C, Cudeiro J: The primate pulvinar nuclei: vision and action, *Trends Neurosci* 23:35, 2000.
6. Moore RY: Organization of the primate circadian system, *J Biol Rhythms* 8:S3, 1993.
7. Munoz DP et al: On your mark, get set: brainstem circuitry underlying saccadic initiation, *Can J Physiol Pharmacol* 78:934, 2000.
8. Robinson DL, McClurkin JW, Kertzman C: Orbital position and eye movement influences on visual responses in the pulvinar nuclei of the behaving macaque, *Exp Brain Res* 82:235, 1990.
9. Robinson DL, Petersen SE: The pulvinar and visual salience, *Trends Neurosci* 15:127, 1992.
10. Rodieck RW, Watanabe M: Survey of the morphology of macaque retinal ganglion cells that project to the pretectum, superior colliculus, and parvicellular laminae of the lateral geniculate nucleus, *J Comp Neurol* 338:289, 1993.
11. Schall JD: Neural basis of saccade target selection, *Rev Neurosci* 6:63, 1995.
12. Schiff D et al: Effects of lesions of the nucleus of the optic tract on optokinetic nystagmus and after-nystagmus in the monkey, *Exp Brain Res* 79:225, 1990.
13. Schmid R, Wilhelm B, Wilhelm H: Naso-temporal asymmetry and contraction anisocoria in the pupillomotor system, *Grafes Arch Clin Exp Ophthalmol* 238:123, 2000.

ACTIVITY-DEPENDENT DEVELOPMENT OF RETINOGENICULATE PROJECTIONS

RACHEL O. WONG AND REBECCA C. STACY

The projection patterns of retinal ganglion cells in the mature visual system are highly precise and organized into several stereotypic patterns.[21,42,62] One arrangement that is common among higher vertebrates is that ganglion cells from each eye project to separate layers within their primary target, the dorsal lateral geniculate nucleus (dLGN). As a result, each mature dLGN neuron is monocularly driven. Another common organization of retinogeniculate projections across species is the retinotopic map.[43] Projections from each retina are arranged such that neighboring ganglion cells project topographically to neighboring cells in the dLGN. Finally, although many distinct functional classes of retinal ganglion cells exist, adult dLGN neurons receive inputs from only one class of ganglion cell.[42,62] However, these precise patterns of connectivity between retinal ganglion cells and their central targets are initially less well defined.[3,15,16,49] The refinement of the early retinogeniculate projection patterns occurs before vision.[15,16,49] Many studies now show that, despite such absence of visual stimulation, spontaneous neuronal activity from the retina is important for ensuring that the retinal projections are established appropriately.[16,36,67]

RETINOGENICULATE PROJECTIONS ARE REFINED DURING DEVELOPMENT

Neurons in the developing dLGN receive binocular input, but after maturation, connections from only one eye remain.[48] Monocular innervation is achieved before birth, indicating that the development of eye-specific inputs to dLGN neurons does not require visual experience. Structurally, neurons in the dLGN that are innervated by the same eye are organized into layers within this nucleus (see Color Plate 18). These "eye-specific" layers are formed as the axon terminals from the left and right eye become progressively confined to a single layer.[54,55] The segregation into eye-specific layers involves both the elimination of aberrant synapses and the addition of synapses from the appropriate presynaptic terminals.[23,49]

During the period when eye-specific laminas are sculpted, the retinotopic map also appears to undergo refinement. In the tectum of lower vertebrates (e.g., fish, amphibians), the retinotopic map is fairly precise from the outset.[43,60] However, in higher vertebrates (e.g., chicks, mammals), the topographic map is progressively refined with maturation.[33,51,52] Because retinotopic maps undergo fine-tuning before vision onset, it is difficult to assess their level of precision functionally. However, dye labeling of retinal ganglion cells in neonatal rats demonstrates that, early on, retinal axons form many side branches that terminate in inappropriate regions of their target nucleus[51,52] (Figure 27-1). With age, the axon terminals become highly localized and the side branches are eliminated. Although these observations were obtained for the superior colliculus, another major central target of retinal ganglion cells, they may also reflect a similar process in the dLGN. Recently, physiologic mapping of the shape and sizes of receptive fields of dLGN neurons in the neonatal ferret demonstrated that the number of ganglion cells that remain connected to a single dLGN is further reduced after eye

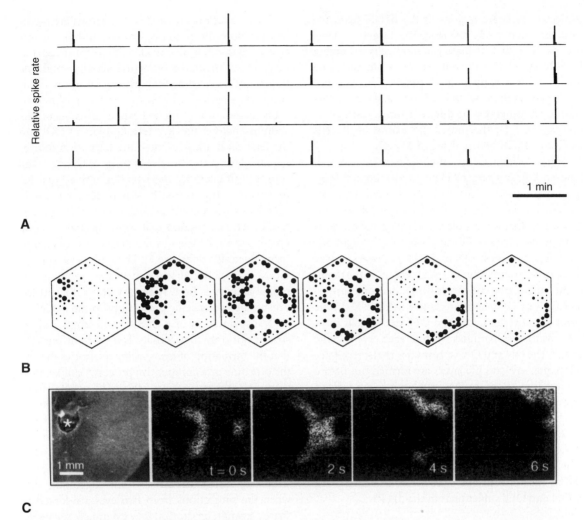

FIGURE 27-1 The immature retina generates a pattern of synchronized bursting activity before vision. **A,** Multielectrode recording of the spike activity from many cells in the isolated but intact ferret retina reveals the presence of rhythmic bursting in individual cells (*each line*). The bursts of four neighboring cells (shown by the *vertical histograms*) are correlated in time. **B,** During a burst of activity, retinal ganglion cells are activated sequentially as a wave propagates across the recording electrodes. Shown here is an example of such a wave propagating across the hexagonal multielectrode array. *Left to right*, Sequential "snapshots" of the activity recorded every 0.5 second. Each dot is a cell, and the size of the dot is proportional to the spike rate. **C,** Retinal waves are easily observed using calcium imaging. Changes in fluorescence intensity over time detected using a low-light camera show two waves that collide in a neonatal mouse retina. First panel shows the fluorescence labeling by fura-2, and white regions in the subsequent images show elevations in intracellular calcium. *Asterisk*, Optic nerve head.

opening.[59] Reduction in the degree of convergence of retinal ganglion cell input to dLGN neurons would result in a sharper retinotopic map. The number of cells connected to each dLGN may be reduced by naturally occurring cell death or by the elimination of synaptic inputs.[23,35]

Apart from the overall organization into eye-specific laminas and retinotopic maps, adult dLGN neurons receive inputs from only one of many

functionally distinct classes of retinal ganglion cell. For example, the cat and ferret dLGN receive projections from ganglion cells that process movement (Y ganglion cells), cells that are high acuity detectors (X ganglion cells), and a heterogeneous population of W cells.[15,66] Whether synaptic inputs from these different classes of ganglion cells initially converge onto individual dLGN neurons is unclear.[15] In primates, however, M and P retinal ganglion cells project to separate regions of the dLGN from the time that their axons first reach this target.[26,53] Thus it is possible that primate ganglion cells belonging to different classes do not synapse onto the same dLGN cell even early in development. This may not be surprising because different retinal ganglion cell classes are generated at different times during development.[39] Furthermore, the axons of P cells reach the dLGN before those of M cells.[26]

Some evidence for the refinement of cell type–specific retinogeniculate inputs comes from studies of another functionally defined pathway. Each major class of ganglion cell consists of two subtypes: cells that are depolarized (ON ganglion cells) or hyperpolarized (OFF ganglion cells) by light onset.[34] Together, these ON and OFF pathways convey changes in illumination to visual centers in the brain. In the cat and primate, single dLGN neurons have either ON- or OFF-center receptive fields.[15,42,62] In the ferret visual system, ON and OFF dLGN cells form two distinct sublaminas within each eye-specific layer.[58] The ON and OFF sublaminas in the ferret develop after eye-specific layers are formed but before eye opening.[7] Because these sublaminas are present before vision occurs, it is not possible to assess physiologically whether dLGN neurons transiently receive converging ON and OFF synaptic inputs. However, this is likely because retinal ganglion cell axon terminals are not confined to the inner or outer half of each eye-specific layer before the emergence of ON and OFF sublaminas in the dLGN.[7]

ACTIVITY HELPS REFINE RETINOGENICULATE PROJECTIONS

Over the last two to three decades, there has been a wealth of evidence implicating neuronal activity in the refinement of many aspects of retinogeniculate connectivity.[15,16,49,67] Perhaps the best studied thus far is the role of activity in the formation of eye-specific inputs. The seminal work of Hubel and Wiesel[19,20] first demonstrated a role for visual experience in the separation of inputs from the two eyes in layer IV of the visual cortex. Following this work, many studies have examined the role of retinal afferents in the establishment of dLGN structure using a variety of manipulations, including monocular or binocular visual deprivation, fetal or neonatal enucleation, and induction of strabismus.[15] Together, these studies suggest that both interocular and intraocular interactions are needed for the normal development of the overall size and laminar organization of the dLGN.

Because retinogeniculate connections are established before the retina is sensitive to light, it was suspected that retinogeniculate interactions, particularly those mediated by neural activity, might be important for refining the early organization of this subcortical pathway. Evidence for a role of neurotransmission was provided when infusion of the sodium channel blocker tetrodotoxin (TTX) into the fetal cat brain prevented the formation of eye-specific layers in the developing dLGN.[50,56] The source of this activity was later determined to originate from the retina.[38] When pharmacologic agents that prevent the generation of action potentials in retinal ganglion cells were injected into one eye, eye-specific layers in the dLGN again failed to form[38] (see also reference 5). These observations indicate that in the absence of vision, spontaneous retinal activity is both necessary and sufficient for organizing eye-specific projections to the dLGN.

Transplantation of a third eye in frogs demonstrated not only that activity is important but also that the formation of eye-specific territories may be the outcome of a competitive process.[4] Unlike most mammals, the retinal projections in normal frogs are completely crossed such that there is no intermingling of axons from the two eyes. In this classic three-eyed frog experiment, the third eye was forced to innervate a tectum that already received projections from another eye. Amazingly, eye-specific stripes appeared in the tectum, suggesting that when the projections from two eyes are forced to share common territories, they eventually segregate. However, stripes failed to form in the three-eyed frog when retinal activity was blocked, strongly implying that retinal activity drives the competitive process.[40]

The refinement of retinotopic maps also appears to rely on neural activity. Blockade of postsynaptic cells in the superior colliculus in rats prevents the elimination of "misplaced" axonal branches.[52] To date, it is unknown how retinotopic maps develop in the dLGN, but they too may follow a course similar to that of the maps in the colliculus. Moreover, experiments in the ferret visual system also show that both blockade of retinal activity or postsynaptic activation of LGN neurons prevents the formation of ON and OFF sublaminas.[6,17] Thus communication from the retina is important for ensuring that the different patterns of retinal ganglion cell projections are established appropriately with maturation.

Interestingly, retinogeniculate projections are not only organized by retinal activity during development; activity is also needed for maintaining the precision established during development. For example, blockade of retinal activity after eye-specific layers have formed in the ferret causes the silenced projections to lose the territory that they had previously occupied.[2] Physiologic recordings also show that individual dLGN neurons in the neonatal cat develop mixed inputs (such as ON and OFF, X and Y) if retinal activity is blocked after birth.[8] However activity blockade is effective only if performed within an early period of development, suggesting that, like the visual cortex, there is a critical period after which blockade of retinal activity does not alter the precision of retinogeniculate connections.

RETINAL ACTIVITY BEFORE VISION IS SPATIALLY AND TEMPORALLY PATTERNED

Theoretic studies have long suggested that activity alone may not be sufficient to reshape connectivity patterns. Instead, activity that is patterned in a distinct way is likely to be important. In the visual system, patterned activity is easily produced by visual stimulation of the diverse functional types of retinal neurons. Surprisingly, even before vision is possible, the retina produces action potential (spike) activity that is temporally and spatially organized.

Recordings from the isolated retina first showed that before eye opening, retinal ganglion cells periodically fire action potentials in short bursts.[25] In vivo recordings from fetal rats later showed that the bursts of spikes from neighboring retinal ganglion cells are temporally synchronized.[14,24] Subsequently, simultaneous recording from hundreds of cells in vitro revealed the presence of correlated bursting activity between large numbers of neighboring ganglion cells. Both multielectrode array recording and calcium imaging demonstrated that the bursting activity in ganglion cells is correlated in the form of propagating waves[10,27,68,70] (see Figure 27-1). Retinal waves have now been observed in many vertebrate species. Generally, waves travel with an average speed of 100 to 300 m per second and involve many ganglion cells and amacrine cells (retinal interneurons).

Waves sweep across a region of retina approximately once every minute and originate and propagate in any direction. The region that is recently activated, however, remains silent during the refractory period before becoming excited again. The refractory period appears to be governed primarily by the network of cells rather than the inability of retinal ganglion cells to fire spikes repetitively because retinal ganglion cells can be stimulated during the refractory period of the waves.[10,11] As photoreceptors mature, waves disappear. Thus retinal waves are a feature of early retinal development and are present throughout the period when retinogeniculate connectivity becomes refined. After eye opening, retinal ganglion cells remain spontaneously active, even though waves are absent.[68]

What information or cues might waves carry that can help refine the early connectivity of retinal ganglion cells? As in other parts of the nervous system, retinal ganglion cells appear to compete to retain their connections with their target neurons.[23] This competition is fueled by neural activity, but how? Both theoretic and experimental studies in other systems suggest that Hebbian mechanisms may eliminate synaptic inputs over time* (see Color Plate 19). If the action potentials from two ganglion cells reach a common target dLGN neuron within a narrow time window, both their synaptic inputs are strengthened. Conversely, if one ganglion cell is silent when spikes from the other cell activate the LGN neuron, the silent connections are weakened. This "Hebbian-like" model of synaptic competition predicts that ganglion cells that "fire together, wire together." Such coincident firing can be a consequence of wave propagation.

Retinal waves appear to contain several cues that are suitable for the refinement of retinogeniculate connectivity patterns through Hebbian mechanisms. First, propagating waves of activity ensure that neighboring, but not distant, retinal ganglion cells are more synchronized in their activity. Thus wave propagation could be useful for helping refine the retinotopic map because connections from neighboring ganglion cells are costrengthened, whereas connections from distant cells are weakened. Second, the random nature of wave initiation and the relatively long refractory period would result in a low probability of coincident firing of ganglion cells in separate eyes. This favors the segregation of input from different eyes. However, wave activity itself does not seem necessary for the segregation of eye-specific input; asynchronous firing between inputs from the two eyes could occur even if all cells within each retina were coactivated. However, the presence of periodically generated waves could simultaneously remodel the connectivity between the two eyes and refine the retinotopic map.

The mechanism by which waves refine the projection patterns of subtypes of retinal ganglion cells is not as easily apparent. For example, ON and OFF

---

*References 1, 9, 18, 28, 29, 64, 65.

retinal ganglion cells are distributed next to each other in the retina; thus their activity is likely to be synchronized by propagating waves. However, the segregation of ON and OFF projection patterns in the LGN is clearly activity dependent.[6,17] Further analysis of the activity patterns of identified subsets of retinal ganglion cells revealed that, in fact, during the period of ON and OFF segregation in the dLGN, ON and OFF ganglion cells adopt distinct patterns of rhythmic bursting activity.[69] Although the bursts of neighboring ON and OFF ganglion cells remain synchronized, ON cells are spontaneously active for only about one third of the time that OFF cells fire action potentials. The result is a reduction in the degree to which the spikes of ON and OFF ganglion cells are correlated. The spikes of cells with the same center sign (ON:ON, OFF:OFF) appear better synchronized then those of opposite sign (ON:OFF). Modeling studies based on Hebbian mechanisms suggest that the change in the relative correlation in the spike activity of ON and OFF ganglion cells could lead to the segregation of their inputs in the LGN.[22]

Although retinal waves appear to bear information suitable for the refinement of retinogeniculate connections, their role in vivo has not been determined. It is known, however, that rhythmic activity in the retina is relayed to the developing dLGN and that synaptic strengths of the retinal inputs are strengthened only when these cells fire in periodic bursts.[30,31] To obtain evidence for such a role, it would be necessary to perturb the pattern of activity without abolishing it altogether. This requires knowledge of the mechanisms that generate and regulate the spatiotemporal properties of the waves.

EARLY RETINAL ACTIVITY INVOLVES A NETWORK OF CELLS

Retinal waves are generated within a network of neurons and require synaptic transmission for their generation and propagation.[10] The waves are present during the period when the retinal circuitry itself is being assembled. Two major excitatory drives, cholinergic and glutamatergic transmission, are responsible for generating bursting activity in the retinal ganglion cells.[10,46,71] However, these forms of neurotransmission are important at distinct periods of development.

The first synaptic connections in the inner retina are formed between ganglion cells and amacrine cells[41] (see Color Plate 20). At this stage of development, cholinergic transmission provides the primary excitatory drive onto ganglion cells. The cholinergic drive is likely to arise from starburst amacrine cells, which are the only known cholinergic cells in the developing and adult retina. These starburst amacrine cells themselves participate in the rhythmic bursting activity, and their activity is synchronized with that of the ganglion cells.[73] Whether starburst amacrine cells are sole initiators of the bursting activity in ganglion cells is still unknown, although their participation appears necessary. Interestingly, there is no inhibition present in this early network. GABA-ergic (γ-aminobutyric acid) transmission from other amacrine cells depolarizes ganglion cells early in development.[12] Whole-cell patch clamp recordings demonstrate that both cholinergic and GABA-ergic inputs are activated during a burst of spontaneous activity in the ganglion cells.[10] Although cholinergic transmission is essential for the generation of spontaneous activity in the ganglion cells, GABA-ergic transmission plays a modulatory role.[12] The network that forms a substrate for the waves becomes more complex with maturation. In the latter phase of development, the vertical pathway matures—in the inner retina, bipolar cell synaptogenesis takes place[41] (see Plate 27-3). At this stage, but before photoreceptors mature, correlated spontaneous bursting activity becomes dependent on glutamatergic transmission and loses its dependence on nicotinic cholinergic transmission.[71]

The mechanisms that underlie bursting activity itself may differ from those required for wave propagation. At early ages, local stimulation of the retina fails to generate a wave in the absence of cholinergic transmission.[10] Thus the network of cholinergic cells may provide a substrate for the lateral propagation of activity. At older ages, when glutamatergic inputs are present, glutamatergic transmission regulates the speed of the waves but may not be directly involved in wave propagation itself.[46] It is likely that at this later stage, glutamatergic bipolar cells induce the lateral spread of activity through amacrine cells. An obvious mechanism that can mediate the propagation of activity between cells is gap-junctional coupling. In the retina, gap-junctional coupling is present both during development and in the adult.[37,61] Although it is not known whether ganglion cells form direct connections with each other, injection of small-molecular-weight tracers into one ganglion cell results in the spread of the tracer to neighboring ganglion cells and to a subset of amacrine cells.[37,61] Not all ganglion cell classes are tracer-coupled, however, although all classes participate in the waves. Thus, although gap-junctional coupling could account in part for the propagation of the waves, it does not appear to be the only mechanism involved. Much work remains before scientists fully understand how the activity spreads from cell to cell—the most important of which is to determine the interconnections between ganglion cells, amacrine cells, and bipolar cells throughout the developmental period when waves are present.

Perhaps even more challenging is determining what factors regulate the spatiotemporal properties of the waves. These properties are important, for example, in regulating how precisely activity can refine the retinotopic map. If, for example, waves become broader or travel more quickly, ganglion cells that are located relatively far apart would become better synchronized in their bursting activity. This could lead to a reduction in the precision of the retinotopic map. An increase in the frequency of waves also increases the probability of coincident firing between the two eyes, making it difficult to segregate their inputs. Several neurotransmitters and neuromodulators are known to regulate the spatial and temporal properties of the waves. At more mature stages, inhibitory GABA-ergic transmission reduces the frequency of bursting.[12] Adenosine, also found in starburst amacrine cells, regulates the width, speed, and frequency of the waves.[57] Activation of adenosine receptors results in changes in intracellular levels of cyclic adenosine monophosphate (cAMP). When cAMP levels are raised above normal, waves cover a much larger area of retina, travel faster, and occur more frequently. Future experiments that use such information to pharmacologically manipulate wave dynamics may help scientists dissect how waves affect retinogeniculate development in vivo.

As indicated earlier, the bursting rhythms of ON and OFF ganglion cells are altered when glutamatergic bipolar cells form contacts with the ganglion cells and amacrine cells.[71] Electrophysiologic studies show that this is partly because of the development of different intrinsic membrane properties of ON and OFF retinal ganglion cells.[32] For a given amount of input, OFF ganglion cells are more likely to fire spikes compared with ON ganglion cells. The developmental increase in spiking in OFF ganglion cells is also caused by the generation of action potentials during the period between their major bursts. Overall, it appears that in addition to the presence of waves that continue to synchronize the activity of ON and OFF ganglion cells, OFF ganglion cells fire spikes at times between consecutive

waves. This is not surprising because OFF bipolar cells are relatively more active compared with ON bipolar cells in the dark.[63]

Taken together, the mechanisms that could underlie changes in the spontaneous activity patterns of retinal ganglion cells during development seem well orchestrated. In the beginning, all ganglion cell types that are neighbors are well synchronized in their bursting activity, facilitating the asynchronous firing of cells from the two eyes. Then, as eye-specific lamination becomes established and ON and OFF segregation is required, "noise" is introduced into the OFF ganglion cells to decrease the degree of coincident firing between ON and OFF cells. Although it may be more efficient if ON and OFF activity becomes asynchronous, wave activity may be maintained during this latter phase of development to ensure that eye inputs remain separated and that the retinotopic map is refined. Amazingly, the retina has to produce activity patterns suitable for the refinement of each set of axonal projections while working to assemble the retinal circuitry itself.

If waves persist to adulthood, however, they interfere with patterned vision. Although it is not currently known what leads to the disappearance of waves with maturation, several observations suggest that signaling from photoreceptors might be important. For example, taurine deficiency can cause photoreceptor degeneration over time. In regions depleted of photoreceptors in the adult animal, retinal ganglion cells resume a rhythmic burst-like firing pattern that resembles that observed in immature retina (Levick WR, personal communication, 1999). Children who develop cone-rod dystrophy and patients with Charles Bonnet syndrome often perceive moving objects shortly after loss of vision.[45] Whether waves reemerge in the absence of photoreceptor activation is unknown, but if so, such activity could contribute to the visual hallucinations. It remains possible that the anatomic circuitry that underlies the waves may not be dismantled with maturation, but rather masked by photoreceptor signaling. Interestingly, when animals are raised in the dark, spontaneous rhythmic bursting in retinal ganglion cells persists even after photoreceptors mature.[47] Thus visual experience itself may trigger a loss in the pattern of rhythmic bursting and, possibly, the waves.

ACTIVITY ALONE IS NOT SUFFICIENT

Even though retinal activity is required for the formation of specific dLGN sublaminas in some species, activity alone cannot account for their stereotypic organization across animals. For instance, layer A in the ferret always receives contralateral eye input, whereas layer A1 is innervated by the ipsilateral eye. This pattern is reproducible from animal to animal. It is likely that molecular cues initially guide retinal axons to the correct regions within their visual targets and that errors are then eliminated by activity-dependent competition.[13,72] The recruitment of activity to refine connectivity is useful and enables the pathways to be more plastic and amenable to reorganization.

In addition, as discussed earlier, the M and P projections in the primate may be highly specific on reaching their targets, and unlike the cat and ferret visual system, M and P retinal axons early in fetal development have few, if any, side branches.[26,53] Thus elimination of inappropriate terminals may take place by cell death (see also reference 34) rather than by elimination of misplaced branches.

SUMMARY

The retinogeniculate pathway is highly organized in structure and function. Although a great deal of precision is present early in development, in many species, retinal activity is required to fine-tune the retinogeniculate projections. Although scientists now understand what retinal activity patterns are relayed to the dLGN, it is not yet shown how these activity patterns guide the segregation of eye input, ON and OFF input, and the refinement of retinotopic maps. In addition, it is important to note that the topographic maps from each eye must be aligned by maturity. Whether coordinated activity within the dLGN is needed for such a process has yet to be determined. Nevertheless, the immature retina appears not only to generate a pattern of activity to help refine the retinogeniculate pathway but also to possess mechanisms to regulate these activity patterns. Future studies that allow investigators to monitor changes in axonal and dendritic structure in the living animal over time will no doubt provide greater insight into how retinal ganglion cells become wired up during development. With rapid advances in live-imaging technology, investigators' ability to visualize the early development of the visual system in vivo is likely to be realized in the near future.

ACKNOWLEDGMENT
This work is supported by the National Institutes of Health.

REFERENCES

1. Bi GQ, Poo MM: Synaptic modifications in cultured hippocampal neurons: dependence on spike timing, synaptic strength, and postsynaptic cell type, *J Neurosci* 15:10464, 1998.
2. Chapman B: Necessity for afferent activity to maintain eye-specific segregation in ferret lateral geniculate nucleus, *Science* 287:2479, 2000.
3. Constantine-Paton M, Cline HT, Debski E: Patterned activity, synaptic convergence, and the NMDA receptor in developing visual pathways, *Annu Rev Neurosci* 13:129, 1990.
4. Constantine-Paton M, Law MI: Eye-specific termination bands in tecta of three-eyed frogs, *Science* 202:639, 1978.
5. Cook PM, Prusky G, Ramoa AS: The role of spontaneous retinal activity before eye opening in the maturation of form and function in the retinogeniculate pathway of the ferret, *Vis Neurosci* 16:491, 1999.
6. Cramer KS, Sur M: Blockade of afferent impulse activity disrupts on/off sublamination in the ferret lateral geniculate nucleus, *Dev Brain Res* 98:287, 1997.
7. Cucchiaro J, Guillery RW: The development of the retinogeniculate pathways in normal and albino ferrets, *Proc R Soc Lond B* 223:141, 1984.
8. Dubin MW, Stark LA, Archer SM: A role for action potential activity in the development of neuronal connections in the kitten retinogeniculate pathway, *J Neurosci* 6:1021, 1986.
9. Eglen SJ: The role of retinal waves and synaptic normalization in retinogeniculate development, *Philos Trans R Soc Lond B Biol Sci* 354:497, 1999.
10. Feller MB et al: Requirement for cholinergic synaptic transmission in the propagation of spontaneous retinal waves, *Science* 272:1182, 1996.
11. Feller MB et al: Dynamic processes shape spatiotemporal properties of retinal waves, *Neuron* 19:293, 1997.
12. Fischer KF, Lukasiewicz PD, Wong ROL: Age-dependent and cell-specific modulation of retinal ganglion cell bursting activity by GABA, *J Neurosci* 18:3767, 1998.
13. Friedman GC, O'Leary DDM: Eph receptor tyrosine kinases and their ligands in neural development, *Curr Opin Neurobiol* 6:127, 1996.
14. Galli L, Maffei L: Spontaneous impulse activity of rat retinal ganglion cells in prenatal life, *Science* 24:90, 1988.
15. Garraghty PE, Sur M: Competitive interactions influencing the development of retinal axonal arbors in cat lateral geniculate nucleus, *Physiol Rev* 73:529, 1993.
16. Goodman CS, Shatz CJ: Developmental mechanisms that generate precise patterns of neuronal connectivity, *Cell* 72/Neuron Suppl 10:77, 1993.
17. Hahm JO, Langdon RB, Sur M: Disruption of retinogeniculate afferent segregation by antagonists to NMDA receptors, *Nature* 351:568, 1991.
18. Hebb DO: *The organization of behaviour,* New York, 1949, John Wiley & Sons.
19. Hubel DH, Wiesel TN: The period of susceptibility to the physiological effects of unilateral eye closure in kittens, *J Physiol* 206:419, 1970.
20. Hubel DH, Wiesel TN, LeVay S: Plasticity of ocular dominance columns in monkey striate cortex, *Phil Trans R Soc Lond B* 278:377, 1977.
21. Kaas JH, Guillery RW, Allman JM: Some principles of organization in the dorsal lateral geniculate nucleus, *Brain Behav Evol* 6:253, 1972.
22. Lee CW, Wong, ROL: Developmental patterns of on/off retinal ganglion cell activity lead to segregation of their afferents under a Hebbian synaptic rule, *Soc Neurosci* 22:1202, 1996.

23. Lichtman JW et al: Synapse formation and elimination. In Zigmond MJ et al (eds): *Fundamental neuroscience,* San Diego, 1998, Academic Press.

24. Maffei L, Galli-Resta L: Correlation in the discharges of neighboring rat retinal ganglion cells during prenatal life, *Proc Natl Acad Sci USA* 87:2861, 1990.

25. Masland RH: Maturation of function in the developing rabbit retina, *J Comp Neurol* 175:275, 1977.

26. Meissirel C et al: Early divergence of magnocellular and parvocellular functional subsystems in the embryonic primate visual system, *Proc Natl Acad Sci USA* 94:5900, 1997.

27. Meister M et al: Synchronous bursts of action potentials in ganglion cells of the developing mammalian retina, *Science* 252:939, 1991.

28. Miller KD: Models of activity-dependent neural development, *Semin Neurosci* 4:61, 1992.

29. Miller KD: Synaptic economics: competition and cooperation in synaptic plasticity, *Neuron* 17:371, 1996.

30. Mooney R, Madison DV, Shatz CJ: Enhancement of transmission at the developing retinogeniculate synapse, *Neuron* 10:815, 1993.

31. Mooney R et al: Thalamic relay of spontaneous retinal activity prior to vision, *Neuron* 17:863, 1996.

32. Myhr KL, Lukasiewicz PD, Wong ROL: Mechanisms underlying developmental changes in the firing patterns of ON and OFF retinal ganglion cells during refinement of their central projections, *J Neurosci* 21:8664, 2001.

33. Nakamura H, O'Leary DDM: Inaccuracies in initial growth and arborization of chick retinotectal axons followed by course corrections and axon remodeling to develop topographic order, *J Neurosci* 9:3776, 1989.

34. Nelson R, Famiglietti EV, Kolb H: Intracellular staining reveals different levels of stratification for on and off-center ganglion cells in cat retina, *J Neurophysiol* 41:472, 1978.

35. O'Leary DDM, Fawcett JW, Cowan WM: Topographic targeting errors in the retinocollicular projection and their elimination by selective ganglion cell death, *J Neurosci* 6:3692, 1986.

36. Penn AA, Shatz CJ: Brain waves and brain wiring: the role of endogenous and sensory-driven neural activity in development, *Pediatr Res* 45:447, 1999.

37. Penn AA, Wong ROL, Shatz CJ: Neuronal coupling in the developing mammalian retina, *J Neurosci* 14:3805, 1994.

38. Penn AA et al: Competition in retinogeniculate patterning driven by spontaneous activity, *Science* 279:2108, 1998.

39. Rapaport DH et al: Genesis of neurons in the retinal ganglion cell layer of the monkey, *J Comp Neurol* 322:577, 1992.

40. Reh TA, Constantine-Paton M: Eye-specific segregation requires neural activity in three-eyed *Rana pipiens, J Neurosci* 15:1132, 1985.

41. Robinson SR: Development of the mammalian retina. In Dreher B, Robinson SR (section eds), Cronly-Dillon JR (series ed): *Neuroanatomy of the visual pathways and their development, vision and visual dysfunction,* vol 3, Boca Raton, Fla, 1991, CRC Press.

42. Rodieck RW: Visual pathways, *Annu Rev Neurosci* 2:193, 1979.

43. Roskies A, Friedman GC, O'Leary DDM: Mechanisms and molecules controlling the development of retinal maps, *Persp Dev Neurobiol* 3:63, 1995.

44. Sanderson KJ: The projection of the visual field to the lateral geniculate and medial interlaminar nuclei in the cat, *J Comp Neurol* 143:101, 1971.

45. Schwartz TL, Vahgei L: Charles Bonnet syndrome in children, *J Am Assoc Ped Ophthalmol* 2:310, 1998.

46. Sernagor E, Eglen SJ, O'Donovan MJ: Differential effects of acetylcholine and glutamate blockade on the spatiotemporal dynamics of retinal waves, *J Neurosci* 20:RC 56, 2000.

47. Sernagor E, Grzywacz NM: Influence of spontaneous activity and visual experience on developing retinal receptive fields, *Curr Biol* 6:1503, 1996.

48. Shatz CJ, Kirkwood PA: Prenatal development of functional connections in the cat's retinogeniculate pathway, *J Neurosci* 4:1378, 1984.

49. Shatz CJ, Sretavan DW: Interactions between retinal ganglion cells during the development of the mammalian visual system, *Annu Rev Neurosci* 9:171, 1986.

50. Shatz CJ, Stryker MP: Prenatal tetrodotoxin infusion blocks segregation of retinogeniculate afferents, *Science* 242:87, 1988.

51. Simon DK, O'Leary DDM: Development of topographic order in the mammalian retinocollicular projection, *J Neurosci* 12:1212, 1992.

52. Simon DK et al: N-methyl-D-asparate receptor antagonists disrupts the formation of a mammalian neural map, *Proc Natl Acad Sci USA* 89:10593, 1992.

53. Snider CJ et al: Prenatal development of retinogeniculate axons in the macaque monkey during segregation of binocular inputs, *J Neurosci* 19:220, 1999.

54. Sretavan DW, Shatz CJ: Prenatal development of retinal ganglion cell axons: segregation into eye-specific layers within the cat's lateral geniculate nucleus, *J Neurosci* 6:234, 1986.

55. Sretavan DW, Shatz CJ: Axon trajectories and pattern of terminal arborization during the prenatal development of the cat's retinogeniculate pathway, *J Comp Neurol* 255:386, 1987.

56. Sretavan DW, Shatz CJ, Stryker MP: Modification of retinal ganglion cell axon morphology by prenatal infusion of tetrodotoxin, *Nature* 336:468, 1988.

57. Stellwagen D, Shatz CJ, Feller MB: Dynamics of retinal waves are controlled by cyclic AMP, *Neuron* 24:673, 1999.

58. Stryker MP, Zahs KR: ON and OFF sublaminae in the lateral geniculate nucleus of the ferret, *J Neurosci* 3:1943, 1983.

59. Tavazoie SF, Reid RC: Diverse receptive fields in the lateral geniculate nucleus during thalamocortical development, *Nat Neurosci* 3:608, 2000.

60. Udin SB, Fawcett JW: Formation of topographic maps, *Annu Rev Neurosci* 11:289, 1988.

61. Vaney DI: Patterns of neuronal coupling in the retina, *Prog Ret Eye Res* 13:301, 1994.

62. Wässle H: Morphological types and central projections of ganglion cells in the cat retina. In Osborne N, Chader G (eds): *Progress in retinal research,* Oxford, England, 1982, Pergamon.

63. Wässle H, Boycott BB: Functional architecture of the mammalian retina, *Physiol Rev* 71:447, 1991.

64. Wigstrom DJ, Gustaffson B: On long-lasting potentiation in the hippocampus: a proposed mechanism for its dependence on coincident pre- and post-synaptic activity, *Acta Physiol Scand* 123:519, 1985.

65. Willshaw DJ, von der Malsberg C: How patterned neural connections can be set up by self-organization, *Proc R Soc Lond B* 194:431, 1976.

66. Wingate RJT, Fitzgibbon T, Thompson ID: Lucifer yellow, retrograde tracers, and fractal analysis characterise adult ferret retinal ganglion cells, *J Comp Neurol* 323:449, 1992.

67. Wong ROL: Retinal waves and visual system development, *Annu Rev Neurosci* 22:29, 1999.

68. Wong ROL, Meister M, Shatz CJ: Transient period of correlated bursting activity during development of the mammalian retina, *Neuron* 11:923, 1993.

69. Wong ROL, Oakley DM: Changing patterns of spontaneous bursting activity of on and off retinal ganglion cells during development, *Neuron* 16:1087, 1996.
70. Wong ROL et al: Early functional neural networks in the developing retina, *Nature* 374:716, 1995.
71. Wong WT et al: Developmental changes in the neurotransmitter regulation of correlated spontaneous retinal activity, *J Neurosci* 20:351, 2000.

72. Yamagata M, Sanes JR: Lamina-specific cues guide outgrowth and arborization of retinal axons in the optic tectum, *Development* 121:189, 1995.
73. Zhou ZJ: Direct participation of starburst amacrine cells in spontaneous rhythmic activities in the developing mammalian retina, *J Neurosci* 18:4155, 1998.

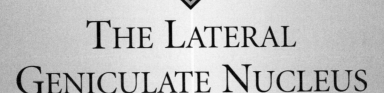

CHAPTER 28

THE LATERAL GENICULATE NUCLEUS

VIVIEN A. CASAGRANDE AND JENNIFER M. ICHIDA

OVERVIEW: LATERAL GENICULATE NUCLEUS REGULATES FLOW OF VISUAL SIGNALS TO CORTEX

In primates all visual information from the retina critical to conscious perception travels through the dorsal lateral geniculate nucleus (LGN). The LGN is a distinctively layered structure in primates and is located at the posterior lateral margin of the dorsal thalamus (Figure 28-1). Although there is general agreement that the LGN provides the key gateway to visual signals entering the cortex, there is less agreement concerning the role of this structure in vision.[5,9,47] The main reason that it has been difficult to understand the functions of this nucleus is that the receptive field properties of LGN cells are similar to those of their retinal ganglion cell inputs. Given that visual signals are transformed as they pass from one cell to the next in the retina and from cell to cell in the visual cortex, it seemed puzzling that a similar transformation could not be identified within the structure connecting the retina to the visual cortex. The most reasonable current explanation for the lack of transformation of visual signals within the LGN is that the main role of this nucleus is to regulate the flow and strength of visual signals sent to cortex. Evidence now indicates that this regulation is much more complex than simply opening and closing a single gate. The parallel processing of visual information, elaborate circuitry, and many extraretinal inputs to the LGN all suggest that visual signals can be regulated in a variety of ways within this nucleus.

This chapter is divided into four sections. The first section describes the anatomic organization of the nucleus. We begin with a general description of the laminar organization and topography of the nucleus. Next we show how retinal and extraretinal information is mapped onto the different layers of the LGN. We also consider the different classes of LGN cells and the organization of their output connections to primary visual cortex. The next section describes the circuits within the LGN and shows how visual signals are regulated by means of feedforward and feedback pathways involving inhibitory neurons. In addition, we consider how intrinsic cell properties and the timing of action potentials in different LGN cells affect the manner in which visual signals are transmitted to cortex. The third section describes the parallel processing of visual signals within the LGN and considers the functional meaning of this type of organization. The final section summarizes key points about LGN organization.

STRUCTURAL ORGANIZATION: ANATOMIC TOUR WITHIN THE LATERAL GENICULATE NUCLEUS

Knowledge about the structural organization and the microcircuitry of the LGN comes mainly from work in animals, especially the cat. Although the organization of the LGN in cats is distinct from that seen in primates, similarities between primates and cats allow us to draw general conclusions. Except for some basic histologic observations, we know relatively little about the human LGN, but histologic similarities between humans and primates, as well as the similarities among or between primates, provide justification for generalization.

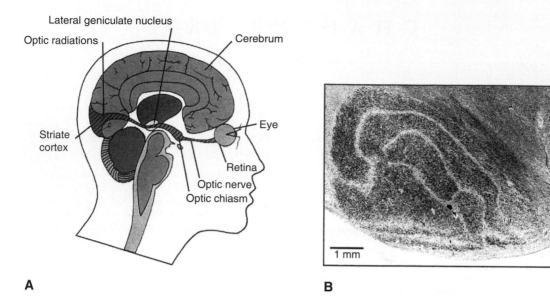

A   **B**

FIGURE 28-1   **A,** Diagrammatic section through the head showing principal features of the major visual pathways linking the eyes to the cerebrum. **B,** Histologically stained section through the human lateral geniculate nucleus showing the laminar organization. *Arrow* indicates the optic disc representation. (**A** from Frisby JP: *Seeing: illusion brain and mind,* New York, 1979, Oxford University Press. **B** from Hickey TL, Guillery RW: *J Comp Neurol* 183:221, 1979.)

Layers and Maps

The LGN is an elongated layered structure, with each layer representing the opposite visual hemifield (Figure 28-2). One can imagine the structure as a stack of pancakes longer in the anteroposterior direction, with the smallest pancakes or layers located ventrally and the largest pancakes or layers located dorsally. Continuing with this analogy, one can imagine that because pancakes are flexible, the larger ones drape over the smaller ones in the stack. Within each pancake or layer, the opposite hemifield is represented such that the superior and inferior visual fields are located toward the lateral and medial zones of the layer, respectively, and the central (toward the fovea) and peripheral visual fields are located at the posterior and anterior zones of the layer, respectively. Each layer receives monocular input from the retina, and only those layers receiving input from the contralateral eye (nasal retina) represent the entire contralateral visual hemifield; this is because LGN layers receiving input from the ipsilateral eye (temporal retina) cannot represent the monocular portion of the hemifield. In structural terms this means that the ipsilateral layers are always shorter in all dimensions than the corresponding contralateral layers (see Figure 28-2). The maps in each layer are retinotopically aligned such that each point in visual space is represented along a line perpendicular

to the layers. One can imagine such a line as a toothpick stuck through our imaginary stack of pancakes. The alignment of the maps is so precise that a cell-free gap representing the optic disc (see *arrows* in Figures 28-1, *B,* and 28-2.) exists in all contralaterally innervated layers to maintain retinotopic alignment with the ipsilaterally innervated layers.

Three types of cell layers can be defined in primate LGN: those with large cells (the magnocellular [M] layers), those with medium size cells (the parvocellular [P] layers), and those with small cells (the koniocellular [K] layers). All primates have at least two P and two M layers, with K layers lying below each M and P layer. In humans and some other primates, each P layer can split into two or sometimes more layers in some parts of the nucleus; thus the normal human LGN can contain as few as two or as many as six P layers.[19]

Among primates the laminar organization and topography of the LGN has been studied in the most detail in the macaque monkey. In this species Malpeli and Baker[31] and Malpeli, Lee, and Baker[32] have performed careful reconstructions of the entire LGN, documenting the retinotopic organization and number of M and P cells within each LGN layer (K cells were not counted). These studies have shown that, in macaque monkeys, the representa-

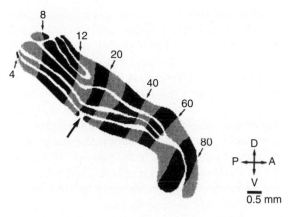

FIGURE 28-2 An example of a reconstructed sagittal section through the lateral geniculate nucleus of a macaque monkey. *Light* and *dark bands* represent eccentricity hemizones that have been mapped onto layers. *Numbers* refer to the eccentricity at the border between two adjacent eccentric hemizones. The gap in layer 1 represents the optic disc (*arrow*). Note also that the ipsilaterally innervated layers are shorter than those that are contralaterally innervated (see text for details). The *cluster of arrows* indicates anatomic orientation (*A*, Anterior; *D*, dorsal; *P*, posterior; *V*, ventral). (From Malpeli JG, Lee D, Baker FH: *J Comp Neurol* 375:363, 1996.)

tion of the central visual field is magnified in the LGN and the number of layers varies with eccentricity (see Figure 28-2 and reference 32). The magnified representation of the central few degrees in the LGN is easy to understand given that each LGN cell receives input from approximately one to three retinal ganglion cells and that ganglion cell density is much higher in the central retina. Only within the portion of the nucleus representing eccentricities from 2 to 17 degrees do the two P layers split to represent four or more P layers, an arrangement that may reflect an increase in the diversity of retinal ganglion cells representing this portion of visual space. Classical textbook sections of the LGN typically are taken from this region of the LGN, which shows four P layers and two M layers; we now know that K layers lie below each P and M layer (Figure 28-3).

Cell Classes

When one divides cells into classes, the assumption is made that the criteria that are used identify meaningful differences that translate into functionally distinct populations. Because biologic populations are inherently variable and can vary along a continuum and still belong to one population, we emphasize here only cell classes that have been de-

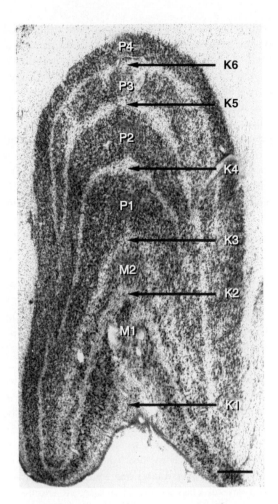

FIGURE 28-3 A coronal section through the lateral geniculate nucleus of a macaque monkey showing the parvocellular (*P*), magnocellular (*M*), and koniocellular (*K*) layers. At this plane there are four P layers, two M layers, and six K layers. Scale bar = 500 μm.

fined parametrically (see references 42, 43, and 48 for discussion). Within this context, LGN cells can be grouped into two principal cell classes: *relay* cells that send an axon to visual cortex and *interneurons* whose axons remain within the LGN. LGN relay cells use the transmitter glutamic acid (glutamate), whereas interneurons use the transmitter γ-aminobutyric acid (GABA). Relay cells and interneurons occur in a ratio of approximately 4:1 throughout the LGN and exhibit distinct dendritic morphologies. As mentioned earlier, distinct relay cell classes also exist within the LGN. These different classes are segregated into different layers and can be distinguished by cell size and input from the retina. In addition, each of the three main LGN relay cell classes (M, P, and K) can be distinguished on the basis of the morphology of their dendrites, their calcium-binding protein content, their physiologic properties, and their axonal projection patterns within visual cortex.[4,5,16] The dendrites of P cells are oriented perpendicular to the cell layers in which they maintain a compact profile as might be predicted from a cell class with small receptive field centers concerned with transmitting information about spatial detail. In contrast, the larger M cells, with their larger receptive fields, have complex radially branching dendrites that sample more widely within the M layers. The small K cells have only a few long dendrites that are often oriented parallel to the LGN layers; such a parallel orientation fits with the larger receptive fields reported for some K cells.[21,35,55] K relay cells also can be distinguished from the other classes on the basis of their calcium-binding protein content. K cells contain calbindin D 28K, whereas P and M cells contain parvalbumin.[18,22,23] The functional reason for this difference in calcium-binding protein content is unknown, but this distinction between M/P and K is seen in the LGNs of all primates studied, suggesting that it is a conserved feature and may be physiologically important (see also later discussion).

Afferent Axons

LGN neurons in primates receive their main drive from several classes of retinal afferent axons. In macaque monkeys and probably also humans, approximately 80% of the input comes from small midget (P-type) ganglion cells, which innervate the P LGN layers.[29,37] Between 7% and 9% of the retinal input to the LGN comes from parasol (M-type) ganglion cells that send axons to the LGN M layers.[29,37] Less is known about retinal input to the K class of LGN cells, and some investigators have even argued against such input.[36] However, studies in the bush baby, a prosimian primate, have demonstrated that at least two classes of retinal axons distinct from the P and M classes innervate LGN K cells based on terminal morphology.[28] Moreover, Rodieck and Watanabe[40] identified at least six distinct classes of retinal ganglion cells whose axons end in the LGN in macaque monkeys. Of these six classes of retinal ganglion cells, the strongest evidence suggests that the small bistratified ganglion cells carrying signals from short-wavelength cones (S cones) provide input to at least some K cells in diurnal primates.[16]

In addition to retinal input, LGN cells receive input from a variety of both visual and nonvisual extraretinal sources. This extraretinal afferent source provides a much larger input to the LGN in terms of synapse number than does the retina. (For review, see reference 45.) These extraretinal inputs also regulate the flow of information in the LGN in a variety of ways given the different transmitters they contain and the number of transmitter receptors that exist on LGN neurons (Figures 28-4 and 28-5). In studies of cat LGN that have numerically compared these inputs, it was found that extraretinal input outnumbers retinal input by at least 5 to 1.[34,50] The extraretinal input from visual sources maintains retinotopic fidelity. In other words, regions representing a common point in visual space are connected. Extraretinal visual input to the LGN has been documented from the following areas in primates with their transmitter type in parentheses: primary visual cortex (glutamate), some extrastriate areas (possibly glutamate), superior colliculus (glutamate), pretectum (GABA), parabigeminal nucleus (acetylcholine [ACh]), and the visual sector of the thalamic reticular nucleus (TRN; GABA). Of these extraretinal sources, feedback from the primary visual cortex provides the largest number of synapses to the LGN. It is beyond the scope of this chapter to describe the projection patterns of each of these inputs. Suffice it to say that laminar differences exist in the termination patterns of these inputs, suggesting that visual signals may be regulated in different ways in the different layers of the LGN (see references 2, 5, and 47). Extraretinal input to the LGN also arrives from several nonvisual sources. The most well studied of these afferents are the cholinergic afferents from the pons that innervate all LGN layers and also contain the transmitter nitric oxide at least in the cat.[1] Other afferent sources include a serotonergic input from the dorsal raphe nucleus and a histaminergic input from the hypothalamus.[6,11,26,49]

Efferent Axons

In primates the bulk of the efferent axonal output from the LGN terminates within the primary visual cortex and the visual sector of the TRN (Figure 28-6). Although not documented in primates, in cats the projection to the equivalent of the visual sector of the TRN comes from collateral branches of relay cell axons, not from a separate projection that goes solely to this thalamic nucleus. A minor efferent projection from the LGN also has been reported to terminate in several extrastriate areas. The latter appears to originate from K LGN cells based on double-labeling studies using retrograde tracers and

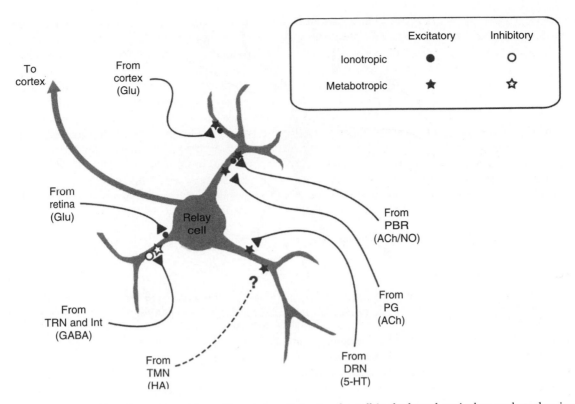

FIGURE 28-4 Schematic representation of inputs to a thalamic relay cell in the lateral geniculate nucleus showing neurotransmitters (in parentheses) and ionotropic or metabotropic types of postsynaptic receptors. The *question mark* indicates uncertainty about the synaptic relationships of the histaminergic input. *ACh,* Acetylcholine; *DRN,* dorsal raphe nucleus; *Glu,* glutamate; *HA,* histamine; *5-HT,* serotonin; *Int,* interneuron; *NA,* noradrenaline; *NO,* nitric oxide; *PBR,* parabrachial region; *PG,* parabigeminal nucleus; *TMN,* tuberomamillary nucleus; *TRN,* thalamic reticular nucleus. (From Sherman SM, Guillery RW: *Exploring the thalamus,* San Diego, 2001, Academic Press.)

immunocytochemistry for calbindin.[41] Although minor, this LGN extrastriate projection has been implicated in the residual vision referred to as *blind sight* in patients who have lost their primary visual cortex.[16] In macaque monkeys, some K cells, identified by immunolabeling for calbindin, clearly survive when all of primary visual cortex is removed, further supporting the existence of this pathway. Nevertheless, most K cells and all P and M cells send axons to primary visual cortex. In primates, studies have shown that P cells send axons principally to the lower tier of layer IVC of primary visual cortex (using the nomenclature of Brodmann[3]). In addition, some P cells in macaque monkeys send axons to IVA and sparsely to layer VI. The projection to layer IVA appears to be a specialization of only certain primates because it is absent in chimpanzees and likely also absent in humans. M cells send their efferent axons to the upper tier of layer IVC of primary visual cortex, as well as more sparsely to cortical layer VI. Finally, K cells send their axons to cortical layer IIIB,

where they terminate in patches of cells whose mitochondria contain high amounts of cytochrome oxidase (CO), the "CO blobs."[8,27] Some K cells also send axons to cortical layer I. In the owl monkey, there is evidence that K cells in different K layers send axons either preferentially to cortical layer I (LGN K layer 1) or to the CO blobs (LGN K layer 3).[8]

LGN CIRCUITS: HOW ARE VISUAL SIGNALS REGULATED BY LGN SYNAPTIC CIRCUITRY?

This section presents the essential features of the functional circuitry of the LGN. Because the LGN and its connections often have served as a model to explain the general role of the thalamus and the specific roles of sensory nuclei in regulating information used by the cortex, the literature is enormous. (For recent review, see reference 47.) Here we begin by outlining the key elements of the physiology, anatomy, and neuropharmacology of the

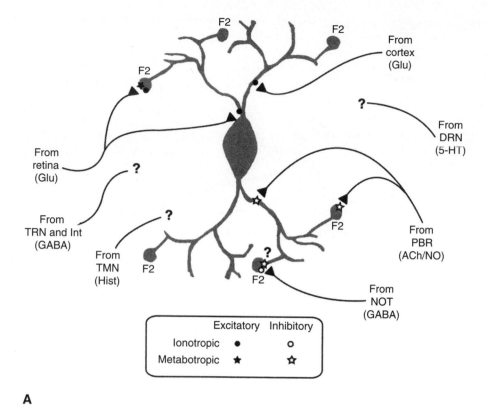

A

B

FIGURE 28-5 Schematic representation of inputs to an interneuron in the lateral geniculate nucleus (**A**) and a cell of the thalamic reticular nucleus (**B**) shown with the same conventions as in Figure 28-4. The *question marks* indicate uncertainty about the postsynaptic receptors involved because of the lack of information; in some cases we know so little that no synaptic site is drawn, and in others, we have limited information about these sites and associated receptors. Note that the F2 terminals of the interneuron receive synaptic inputs. *ACh,* Acetylcholine; *BF,* basal forebrain; *DRN,* dorsal raphe nucleus; *Glu,* glutamate; *HA,* histamine; *5-HT,* serotonin; *Int,* interneuron; *NA,* noradrenaline; *NO,* nitric oxide; *NOT,* nucleus of the optic tract; *PBR,* parabrachial region; *PG,* parabigeminal nucleus; *TMN,* tuberomamillary nucleus; *TRN,* thalamic reticular nucleus. (From Sherman SM, Guillery RW: *Exploring the thalamus,* San Diego, 2001, Academic Press.)

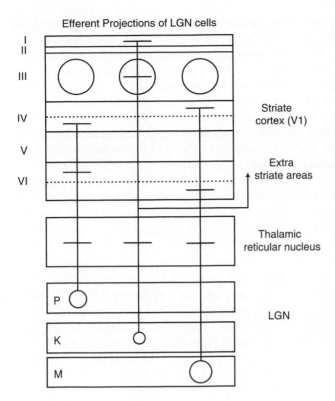

Efferent Projections of LGN cells

FIGURE 28-6 Simplified schematic diagram of the efferent projections of lateral geniculate nucleus (*LGN*) cells. Parvocellular (*P*), magnocellular (*M*) and koniocellular (*K*) LGN cells have different projections to striate cortex. P cells mainly terminate in lower layer IV, with sparse projections to upper layer VI. M cells have the bulk of their terminations in upper layer IV, with a sparse projection to lower layer VI. K cells terminate within the cytochrome oxidase blobs in layer III and in layer I. K cell projections to layer I and the blobs in layer III usually arise from populations of K cells that lie in different layers. In addition, K cells have been shown to have some projections to extrastriate areas. In primates, it is unknown whether all cells have collateral efferents in the thalamic reticular nucleus (see text for details).

LGN that are at the heart of most models designed to understand the function of the LGN. In these models, extraretinal inputs from the cortex and the TRN are often highlighted, so these inputs are emphasized here as well. We describe the circuits within the LGN and show how visual signals are regulated by means of feed-forward and feedback pathways involving both local inhibitory interneurons and inhibitory neurons within the TRN. This section also considers how the intrinsic cell properties and the timing of action potentials in different LGN cells affect the manner in which visual signals are transmitted to cortex.

Receptive Field Properties

With some exceptions, the receptive field properties of LGN cells are inherited from retinal ganglion cells even though the synaptic inputs from other sources outnumber those of retinal axons within the LGN. It has been argued that retinal axons are "drivers" for LGN cells and that the other inputs are "modulators" based on the effect each source has on LGN relay cell output. Retinal axons probably are drivers because these axons terminate closer than other excitatory inputs to the axon hillock of relay cells, have much larger terminals, and signal through fast ionotropic glutamate channels located at these synaptic sites on LGN relay cell dendrites[46] (see Figure 28-4).

As in the retina, most primate LGN cells have receptive fields defined as ON- or OFF-center, with opposing surrounds. However, some K LGN relay cells appear to have nonstandard visual receptive fields that have been difficult to characterize. Included in this category are cells with large diffuse fields, cells with no clear surround, and cells with more complex properties such as direction selectivity. Because some nonstandard cells have also been identified in the primate retina, these unusual LGN cells also may reflect their retinal inputs. (For review, see reference 5.)

Whether the visual receptive field structure of the majority of LGN relay cells is altered compared with retinal inputs has been the subject of some debate. (For discussion, see reference 5.). Nevertheless, it is evident that all retinal action potentials do not lead to action potentials within target LGN relay cells and that, as shown later, there is ample opportunity to alter receptive field properties based on circuits within the LGN itself. The changes seen in receptive field structure between retina and LGN are subtle and are best thought of as adjustments necessary to efficiently transfer relevant information to cortex. When the input from the retina is measured within an LGN relay cell in the form of synaptic or S-potentials and these S-potentials are compared with the output of that same cell recorded as action potentials, the *ratio* of S potentials that result in action potentials (the *transfer ratio*) is less than 1.0, typically around 0.3 to 0.5 in an anesthetized preparation.[25] This would seem, ostensibly, to be a wasteful loss of important visual information. Kaplan, Purpura, and Shapley,[25] however, argue that such a decrease in the transfer ratio of signals between retina and LGN is nonlinear and is largest when higher stimulus contrasts are used. They argue that this nonlinear transfer of signals from retina to LGN protects the cortex from response saturation under conditions of high stimulus contrast and thus preserves the dynamic range of cortical cells. Others argue that relevant visual signals, such as information about stimulus contrast, also may be enhanced at the level of the LGN. For example, Hubel and Wiesel[20] suggested that LGN cells recorded in the cat exhibit a stronger surround mechanism than their retinal inputs and concluded from these data that the role of the LGN was to sharpen contrast differences and reduce responses to diffuse illumination (see also references 20 and 53). Although other interpretations of Hubel and Wiesel's original data exist (see reference 5), it is evident that the LGN can act as both a spatial and temporal filter for the visual signals that it receives from the retina. These filtering mechanisms are further discussed later, but to appreciate how the LGN can filter or gate retinal signals, it is first necessary to describe the basic LGN circuitry.

Feedback and Feed-Forward Pathways

Visual signals within the LGN are regulated by circuits involving two groups of inhibitory neurons: local inhibitory neurons and TRN inhibitory neurons. These inhibitory neurons are connected in feed-forward and feedback circuits to LGN relay cells involving retinal input to local inhibitory cells and relay cell input to TRN neurons, respectively, as shown schematically in Figure 28-7, *A*. Details of the synaptic arrangements made in the LGN involving these and other pathways have been described, especially in the cat, beginning with the classic studies of Guillery.[12,13] (For review, see reference 14.) The latter studies were able to show that retinal terminals can be identified on the basis of vesicle shape (round [R]), size (large [L]), and appearance of their mitochondria (pale [P]). These RLP terminals can be contrasted with other presumed excitatory terminals on the basis of their size (small [S]) and from inhibitory terminals on the basis of the shape of vesicles (flattened [F]) and the type of synapse that they make. The excitatory synapses made by RLP and RS terminals tend to

have larger synaptic clefts and thicker postsynaptic densities compared with presynaptic densities (i.e., asymmetric), making these synapses appear more striking at the ultrastructural level than the inhibitory F-type synapses, with their narrower clefts and symmetric weakly stained presynaptic and postsynaptic densities. The feed-forward pathway involves a unique synaptic arrangement referred to as a *triad,* in which an RLP terminal terminates on both a relay cell dendrite and the dendrite of an inhibitory interneuron. The dendrite of the inhibitory interneuron, in turn, makes an F2 synapse (dendrodendritic synapse) on the same relay cell dendrite as shown in Figure 28-7, *B*. In contrast, in feedback inhibition the relay cell synapses on the dendrite of a TRN neuron that then sends an inhibitory F1 axon back to terminate on the dendrite of the same relay cell (see Figure 28-7, *A*). In cats, it has been shown that feed-forward circuitry is found mainly on one relay cell class (X) and feedback circuitry involves another class (Y). Because F1 and F2 terminals have been identified within both P and M layers and triadic arrangements are reported to be more common in the M layers of primates, the differences reported in cats do not appear to translate directly to primates.[54] Nevertheless, given that feed-forward and feedback circuits can influence the transfer ratio of visual signals in different ways, further documentation of ultrastructural differences in the circuits within the different layers of the primate LGN will become critical to the development of accurate physiologic models.

Circuit Neurochemistry

Although the feedback and feed-forward circuits to LGN relay cells form the basic architecture for controlling visual signals, the final information that is sent to the visual cortex depends in complex ways on all of the inputs that can impinge on this circuitry and the variety of transmitter receptors that are activated by these inputs. The transmitters and transmitter receptor types used by the different inputs to the cat LGN are shown in Figures 28-4 and 28-5. In a number of cases, similar transmitters, receptors, and circuitry have been confirmed in primates, but details are still lacking. Many of the same inputs that contact LGN relay cells are known to also contact inhibitory interneurons within the LGN or within the TRN, although the transmitter receptors in some cases differ (see Figure 28-5). Two examples can illustrate the complexity of these arrangements. The visual cortex is known to provide the most massive extraretinal input to the

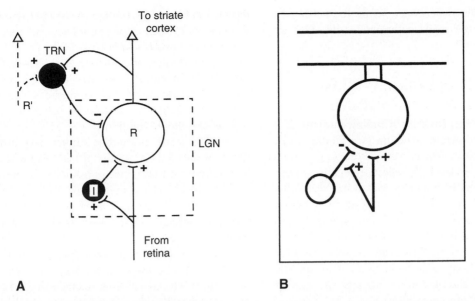

A   **B**

FIGURE 28-7   A, Simplified schematic diagram of visual thalamic circuitry concentrating on the synaptic contacts between retinal afferents, lateral geniculate nucleus (*LGN*) relay cells (*R*), feed-forward interneurons (*I*), and feedback cells in the thalamic reticular nucleus (*TRN*). In this figure, no distinction is made as to the location of synapses with respect to the soma. GABA-ergic inhibitory neurons are indicated in black. The *dashed line* making a synapse onto the TRN cell represents collateral inputs from other relay cells (*R'*) adjacent to the relay cell that is shown. **B,** Schematic diagram showing the spine triad circuit within the LGN. Within a triad a retinal afferent synapses on a relay cell dendrite and an interneuron dendrite, which in turn synapses onto the same relay cell dendrite. (From Norton TT, Casagrande VA: *J Neurophysiol* 47:715, 1982.)

LGN. This glutamatergic input arriving from cells in layer VI of cortex activates both ionotropic and a specific class (group 1) of metabotropic glutamate receptors, both of which can directly depolarize relay cells, although with different time courses and potentially different effects on the firing pattern of LGN relay cells[10] (see also reference 47). Because cortical axons also synapse with inhibitory interneurons and TRN neurons that themselves have both types of receptors, the net output from the relay cell cannot easily be predicted, even from a simple circuit involving feedback from the visual cortex. A second major input to the LGN comes from cholinergic neurons in the pons (the parabrachial region in the cat). These cholinergic fibers innervating the interneurons and relay cells of the LGN and the TRN also are capable of releasing a second transmitter, nitric oxide.[1] The impact of this input on the output of visual signals to the cortex is complicated by the fact that the ACh released can activate both fast ionotropic nicotinic receptors and slower metabotropic M_1 receptors on relay cells; both result in relay cell depolarization. These same ACh-containing pontine axons activate M_2 receptors on interneurons and TRN cells, resulting in hy-

perpolarization of these cells. Therefore the net impact of this ACh input on LGN relay cells would be predicted to be excitatory because relay cells would be directly depolarized and feedback and feed-forward inhibition blocked (for details, see reference 47). Under this condition, one would predict an increased transfer ratio of retinal signals to the cortex. In contrast, activation of the inhibitory circuitry would lower the transfer ratio and, under some circumstances, could change the temporal structure of signals arriving from the retina. The cortical and pontine inputs and their receptors in the LGN just described are but two examples of several that have been worked out for the cat LGN. Obviously, the number of axonal inputs to the LGN and the variety of effects that each can have, depending on which receptor is activated (see Figures 28-4 and 28-5), argue strongly that LGN gating is not equivalent to simply opening or closing down a water hose connecting the retina to the cortex. In fact, evidence suggests that LGN activity can be modulated not only by level of arousal but also by input from other sensory systems, eye movements, eye position, and stimulus relevance. Further research examining the responses of the LGN in awake primates is necessary before the behavioral relevance of the many pathways to the LGN are fully understood.

Parallel Processing: Why Is the LGN Layered in Primates?

The LGN in all primates, including humans, is a beautifully laminated structure (see Figure 28-3). As in other areas of the nervous system (e.g., retina, cortex), layers in the LGN reflect segregation of cell types that have distinct properties. It has been difficult to decide why nature has gone to so much trouble to create layers in the LGN. Lamination is not required for information segregation; pathways from the retina to the cortex can remain separate at the LGN without lamination as long as specific ganglion cell classes connect to separate sets of LGN cells without cross talk.

Physiology of M, P, and K Cells

Regardless of the reasons, the layers of the LGN do appear to segregate relay cells that are morphologically, neurochemically, and physiologically distinct. A number of ideas have been proposed to explain the functional basis of lamination within the LGN beginning in the 1940s when Le Gros Clark (see reference 51) proposed that the six LGN layers separated input coming from the two eyes and the three cone types. On the basis of comparative studies of the proportionate development of LGN layers in different primate species, Hässler[15] proposed that the P layers served daylight vision and the M layers served night vision. Although neither of these theories has withstood the test of time, it is noteworthy that most physiologic studies of the LGN find that cells within the P layers exhibit color opponent center-surround receptive fields and cells within the M layers show little evidence of such color opponency and are often referred to as *broad band* because of the broad selectivity of the centers and surrounds of these cells to different wavelengths.[5] Moreover, although rod input has been demonstrated within both P and M cells, there is evidence that M cells may be more active under scotopic conditions.[38]

Over the years, numerous studies have investigated the detailed physiology of LGN P and M cells in different primate species.[5] Although most of these studies used anesthetized paralyzed preparations, a few have also used awake behaving macaque monkeys. In addition, there is now more information on the K class of LGN cells from recordings in several primate species (see reference 55). Table 28-1 summarizes the key differences between these cell classes. From the table, it can be appreciated that P cells are sensitive to the highest spatial frequencies and M cells are most sensitive to the highest temporal frequencies and to the lowest stimulus contrast. Many K cells fall between the two other classes in terms of spatial and temporal resolution, suggesting that the visual resolution of the whole system may reflect a combined contribution of all of these cell classes under some conditions. In terms of wavelength selectivity, there is evidence that both P and K cells contribute to this function, at least in some diurnal primates such as the marmoset and macaque monkey.[17,33,52] In the latter species, some K cells have been shown to respond to S cone input.[33,52] Because the K pathway is well developed in nocturnal primates that lack S cones, it is clear that the K pathway must do more than simply contribute chromatic signals to cortex.[4]

Typically, studies designed to examine the physiology of M, P, or K cells have examined the average

Table 28-1

Properties of Magnocellular (M), Parvocellular (P), and Koniocellular (K) Cells in the Primate Lateral Geniculate Nucleus

Property	M Cell	P Cell	K Cell
Soma size	Large	Medium	Small
Receptive field organization	Center/surround	Center/surround	Variable
Dendritic field size	Medium	Small	Large (on average)
Wavelength selective	No	Yes	Some blue-on
Preferred spatial frequency	Low	High	Low
Contrast sensitivity	High	Low	Intermediate
Preferred temporal frequency	High	Low	Intermediate/variable
Sustained/transient response	Transient	Sustained	Both types
Axon speed	High (2.0 msec)	Medium (4.0 msec)	Low (>5.0 msec)

firing rate of cells in response to different stimuli. The assumption, of course, is that information is coded in the rate of production of action potentials over some period in relationship to the stimulus. There also is evidence that information is contained in the pattern of action potentials. For example, in sleeping cats, cells within the LGN tend to exhibit a regular bursting pattern of action potentials. Whether bursting is capable of transmitting information in awake animals has been the subject of some debate.[44] Nevertheless, the pattern has been seen in awake monkeys.[39] Godwin, Vaughan, and Sherman[10] and Sherman and Guillery[45,47] have argued that bursting performs a nonlinear amplification of the visual signal, sacrificing signal discrimination for signal detectability in the awake animal. According to this hypothesis, bursting is more efficient at alerting an animal to novel stimuli, whereas tonic firing is more efficient for transferring information about stimulus quality. Whether these two modes of firing are found more in one class of LGN cell than in another remains to be investigated.

Behavioral Results of M and P Lesions: Linking Physiology to Behavior

It has been popular to link the properties of cells in specific visual pathways such as the M and P pathways to perceptual attributes. For example, it is of-ten said that the P pathway contributes to the discrimination of visual forms and their colors, whereas the M pathway contributes to visual motion.[7,30] The problem with this approach is that it assumes that there are direct links between the behavior of single cells and the behavior of the whole animal. Direct tests of the contributions of P and M cells to visual behavior have been attempted by examining visual losses after making lesions within either the P or M layers of the LGN in macaque monkeys[24] (Figure 28-8). The monkeys were then trained to look at a fixation spot with one eye only while the other eye was covered. Stimuli to be discriminated were presented in various locations, including that part of the visual field that corresponds to the damaged portion of the M or P layers. As can be seen from Figure 28-8, each lesion extended into adjacent layers and therefore included some of the K layers. The behavioral tests demonstrated that monkeys *can discriminate form and motion with either pathway.* Therefore it is incorrect to say that P cells are necessary for form discrimination and M cells are necessary for motion discrimination. Instead, the behavioral tests revealed that after P layer lesions (including the associated K layers 4 through 6), monkeys lost the ability to discriminate high spatial frequencies (and any forms made up solely of these frequencies) and

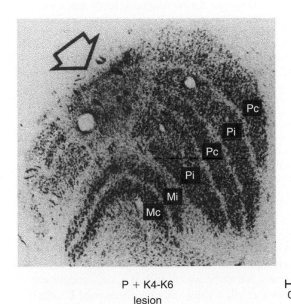

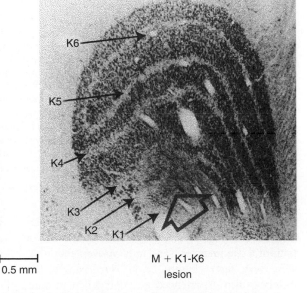

FIGURE 28-8 Lesions (*arrows*) in the lateral geniculate nucleus of a monkey that selectively alter visual function. Lesions were made with an excitotoxin (ibotenic acid). Coronal sections were stained with cresyl violet. *c,* Contra; *i,* ipsi; *K,* koniocellular; *M,* magnocellular; *P,* parvocellular. (From Kandel ER, Schwartz JH, Jessell TM: *Principles of neural science,* New York, 2000, McGraw-Hill.)

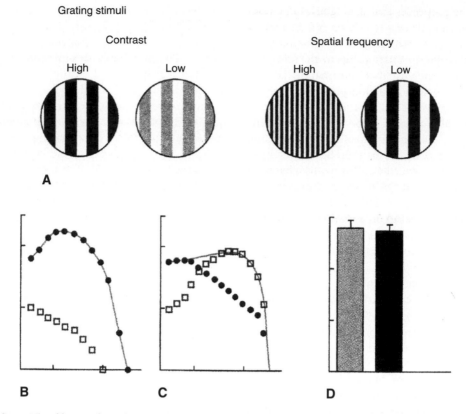

FIGURE 28-9   Visual losses after selective ablation of the magnocellular, parvocellular, and associated koniocellular layers of the lateral geniculate nucleus (LGN) in macaque monkeys. The monkeys were trained to look at a fixation spot on a TV monitor, and stimuli were then presented at one location in the visual field. The location was selected to coincide with the part of the visual field affected by a lesion in the LGN (such as those shown in Figure 28-8). Each lesion was centered on one layer that received information from one eye; therefore, in the test, the eye unaffected by the lesion was covered. On each presentation the monkeys indicated whether the gratings were vertical or horizontal, and this distinction became more difficult as the luminance contrast of the gratings became very low or the spatial frequency became very high. **A,** Luminance contrast is the difference between the brightest and darkest parts of the grating. Spatial frequency is the number of *light* and *dark bars* (cycles) in the grating per degree of visual angle. Temporal frequency (not shown) is how fast the stationary grating is turned on and off per second (Hz). **B,** Contrast sensitivity is the inverse of the lowest stimulus contrast that can be detected. Contrast sensitivity for all spatial frequencies is reduced when only the magnocellular (*M*) and koniocellular (*K*) layers 1 through 3 remain intact after the lesioning parvocellular (*P*) layers and the koniocellular (*K*) layers 4 through 6. The *solid gray line* in **B** and **C** shows sensitivity of the normal monkey; *filled circles* show the contribution of the P pathway (after M lesions), and *open squares* the contribution of the M pathway (after P lesions). **C,** Contrast sensitivity to a grating with low spatial frequency is reduced at lower temporal frequencies when only P cells remain. **D,** Color contrast is measured the same way as luminance contrast except that bars of different colors are used instead of light and dark bars. Color contrast sensitivity is lost when only the M cells remain. (From Kandel ER, Schwartz JH, Jessell TM: *Principles of neural science,* New York, 2000, McGraw-Hill.)

colors, whereas after M and associate K layer lesions, monkeys lost the ability to discriminate high temporal frequencies (and any movements that were very fast) (Figure 28-9). Surprisingly, the monkeys also experienced a major deficit in contrast sensitivity following a loss of P cells (see Figure 28-9). The latter was unexpected given that individual M LGN cells show much higher contrast sensitivity than individual P cells. From M-cell be-

havior alone, one would have expected a significant loss in contrast sensitivity following M layer lesions, but none was found. If K cells contribute to color at all, it must only be a subset of K cells because M layer lesions also destroyed layers K1 through K3, where most K cells are located in macaque monkeys, and the monkeys with M cell + K1 through K3 lesions showed no deficits in color discrimination. Taken together, these results suggest that the properties that distinguish cell classes at the retina and LGN provide basic information about contrast, size, wavelength, and speed and that higher-level analysis, such as that necessary for the discrimination of complex shapes and the movement of these shapes in space, is performed in the cortex.

SUMMARY OF KEY POINTS

- LGN layers contain maps of the contralateral visual hemifield that lie in topographic register with each other.
- Each layer receives input from one eye and from one class of ganglion cells.
- There are three main classes of LGN relay cells in primates, the M, P, and K cells, and one class of inhibitory interneurons.
- LGN cell receptive fields reflect their retinal inputs. LGN signals to the cortex, however, are modulated by a variety of nonretinal inputs that interact with the feedback and feed-forward inhibitory circuitry of the LGN.
- The M, P, and K cells can be distinguished from each other on the basis of their morphology, anatomic connections, neurochemistry, spatial and temporal resolution, and sensitivity to wavelength (color properties).
- The main role of the LGN is to regulate the flow of visual information to the cortex and to maintain the segregation of stimulus properties for efficient use by cortical neurons.

REFERENCES

1. Bickford ME et al: Evidence that cholinergic axons from the parabrachial region of the brainstem are the exclusive source of nitric oxide in the lateral geniculate nucleus of the cat, *J Comp Neurol* 334:410, 1993.
2. Bickford ME et al: Neurotransmitters contained in the subcortical extraretinal inputs to the monkey lateral geniculate nucleus, *J Comp Neurol* 424:701, 2000.
3. Brodmann K: *Vergleichende lokalisationlehre der grosshirnrinde in ihren prinzipien dargestellt auf grund des zellenbaues*, Leipzig, Germany, 1909, JA Barth.
4. Casagrande VA: A third parallel visual pathway to primate area V1, *Trends Neurosci* 17:305, 1994.
5. Casagrande VA, Norton TT: Lateral geniculate nucleus: a review of its physiology and function. In Leventhal AG (ed): *Vision and visual dysfunction*, London, 1991, Macmillan.
6. de Lima AD, Singer W: The brainstem projection to the lateral geniculate nucleus of the cat: identification of cholinergic and monoaminergic elements, *J Comp Neurol* 259:92, 1987.
7. DeYoe EA, Van Essen DC: Concurrent processing streams in monkey visual cortex, *Trends Neurosci* 11:219, 1988.
8. Ding Y, Casagrande VA: The distribution and morphology of LGN K pathway axons within the layers and CO blobs of owl monkey V1, *Vis Neurosci* 14:691, 1997.
9. Frisby JP: *Seeing: illusion brain and mind,* New York, 1979, Oxford University Press.
10. Godwin DW, Vaughan JW, Sherman SM: Metabotropic glutamate receptors switch visual response mode of lateral geniculate nucleus cells from burst to tonic, *J Neurophysiol* 76:1800, 1996.
11. Gonzalo-Ruiz A, Lieberman AR, Sanz-Anquela JM: Organization of serotonergic projections from the raphe nuclei to the anterior thalamic nuclei in the rat: a combined retrograde tracing and 5-HT immunohistochemical study, *J Chem Neuroanat* 8:103, 1995.
12. Guillery RW: The organization of synaptic interconnections in the laminae of the dorsal lateral geniculate nucleus of the cat, *Z Zellforsch* 96:1, 1969.
13. Guillery RW: A quantitative study of the synaptic interconnections in the dorsal lateral geniculate nucleus of the cat, *Z Zellforsch* 96:39, 1969.
14. Guillery RW: Patterns of synaptic interconnections in the dorsal lateral geniculate nucleus of the cat and monkey: a brief review, *Vision Res* 11:211, 1971.
15. Hässler R: Comparative anatomy of the central visual system in day and night-active primates. In Hässler R, Stephan H (eds): *Evolution of the forebrain*, Stuttgart, Germany, 1966, Thieme.
16. Hendry SH, Reid C: The koniocellular pathway in primate vision, *Annu Rev Neurosci* 23:127, 2000.
17. Hendry SHC, Calkins D: Ganglion cell innervation of K layers in macaque LGN, *Soc Neurosci Abs* 29, 1999.
18. Hendry SHC, Yoshioka T: A neurochemically distinct third channel in the macaque dorsal lateral geniculate nucleus, *Science* 264:575, 1994.
19. Hickey TL, Guillery RW: Variability of laminar patterns in the human lateral geniculate nucleus, *J Comp Neurol* 183:221, 1979.
20. Hubel DH, Wiesel TN: Integrative action in the cat's lateral geniculate body, *J Physiol* 155:385, 1961.
21. Irvin GE, Casagrande VA, Norton TT: Center/surround relationships of magnocellular, parvocellular, and koniocellular relay cells in primate lateral geniculate nucleus, *Vis Neurosci* 10:363, 1993.
22. Johnson JK, Casagrande VA: Distribution of calcium-binding proteins within the parallel visual pathways of a primate (*Galago crassicaudatus*), *J Comp Neurol* 356:238, 1995.
23. Jones EG, Hendry SHC: Differential calcium binding protein immunoreactivity distinguishes classes of relay neurons in monkey thalamic nuclei of primates, *J Comp Neurol* 182:517, 1989.
24. Kandel ER, Schwartz JH, Jessell TM: *Principles of neural science*, New York, 2000, McGraw-Hill.
25. Kaplan E, Purpura K, Shapley RM: Contrast affects the transmission of visual information through the mammalian lateral geniculate nucleus, *J Physiol* 391:267, 1987.
26. Kayama Y et al: Effects of stimulating the dorsal raphe nucleus of the rat on neuronal activity in the dorsal lateral geniculate nucleus, *Brain Res* 489:1, 1989.
27. Lachica EA, Beck PD, Casagrande VA: Parallel pathways in macaque monkey striate cortex: anatomically defined columns in layer III, *Proc Natl Acad Sci USA* 89:3566, 1992.
28. Lachica EA, Casagrande VA: The morphology of collicular and retinal axons ending on small relay (W-like) cells of the primate lateral geniculate nucleus, *Vis Neurosci* 10:403, 1993.
29. Leventhal AG, Rodieck RW, Dreher B: Retinal ganglion cell classes in the Old World monkey: morphology and central projections, *Science* 213:1139, 1981.

30. Livingstone MS, Hubel DH: Segregation of form, color, movement and depth: anatomy, physiology, and perception, *Science* 240:740, 1988.

31. Malpeli JG, Baker FH: The representation of the visual field in the lateral geniculate nucleus of *Macaca mulatta, J Comp Neurol* 161:569, 1975.

32. Malpeli JG, Lee D, Baker FH: Laminar and retinotopic organization of the macaque lateral geniculate nucleus: magnocellular and parvocellular magnification functions, *J Comp Neurol* 375:363, 1996.

33. Martin PR et al: Evidence that blue-on cells are part of the third geniculocortical pathway in primates, *Eur J Neurosci* 9:1536, 1997.

34. Montero VM: A quantitative study of synaptic contacts on interneurons and relay cells of the cat lateral geniculate nucleus, *Exp Brain Res* 86:257, 1991.

35. Norton TT, Casagrande VA: Laminar organization of receptive-field properties in lateral geniculate nucleus of bush baby (*Galago crassicaudatus*), *J Neurophysiol* 47:715, 1982.

36. Perry VH, Cowey A: Retinal ganglion cells that project to the superior colliculus and pretectum in the macaque monkey, *Neuroscience* 12:1125, 1984.

37. Perry VH, Oehler R, Cowey A: Retinal ganglion cells that project to the dorsal geniculate nucleus in the macaque monkey, *Neuroscience* 12:1101, 1984.

38. Purpura K, Kaplan E, Shapley RM: Background light and the contrast gain of primate P and M retinal ganglion cells, *Proc Natl Acad Sci USA* 85:4534, 1988.

39. Ramcharan EJ, Gnadt JW, Sherman SM: Burst and tonic firing in thalamic cells of unanesthetized, behaving monkeys, *Vis Neurosci* 17:55, 2000.

40. Rodieck RW, Watanabe M: Survey of the morphology of macaque retinal ganglion cells that project to the pretectum, superior colliculus, and parvocellular laminae of the lateral geniculate nucleus, *J Comp Neurol* 338:289, 1993.

41. Rodman HR et al: Calbindin immunoreactivity in the geniculo-extrastriate system of the macaque: implications for heterogeneity in the koniocellular pathway and recovery from cortical damage, *J Comp Neurol* 431:168, 2001.

42. Rowe MH, Stone J: The interpretation of variation in the classification of nerve cells, *Brain Behav Evol* 17:123, 1980.

43. Rowe MH, Stone J: Parametric and feature extraction analyses of the receptive fields of visual neurons, *Brain Behav Evol* 17:103, 1980.

44. Sherman SM: Tonic and burst firing: dual modes of thalamocortical relay, *Trends Neurosci* 24:122, 2001.

45. Sherman SM, Guillery RW: The functional organization of thalamocortical relays, *J Neurophysiol* 76:1367, 1996.

46. Sherman SM, Guillery RW: On the actions that one nerve cell can have on another: Distinguishing "drivers" from "modulators," *Proc Natl Acad Sci USA* 95:7121, 1998.

47. Sherman SM, Guillery RW: *Exploring the thalamus,* San Diego, 2001, Academic Press.

48. Stone J: *Parallel processing in the visual system,* New York, 1983, Plenum Press.

49. Uhlrich DJ, Manning KA, Pienkowski TP: The histaminergic innervation of the lateral geniculate complex in the cat, *Vis Neurosci* 10:225, 1993.

50. Van Horn SC, Erisir A, Sherman SM: Relative distribution of synapses in the A-laminae of the lateral geniculate nucleus of the cat, *J Comp Neurol* 416:509, 2000.

51. Walls GL: The lateral geniculate nucleus and visual histophysiology, *Univ Calif Publ Physiol* 1:1, 1953.

52. White AJ et al: Segregation of receptive field properties in the lateral geniculate nucleus of a New-World monkey, the marmoset *Callithrix jacchus, J Neurophysiol* 80:2063, 1998.

53. Wiesel TN, Hubel DH: Spatial and chromatic interactions in the lateral geniculate body of the rhesus monkey, *J Neurophysiol* 29:1115, 1966.

54. Wilson JR: Synaptic organization of individual neurons in the macaque lateral geniculate nucleus, *J Neurosci* 9:2931, 1989.

55. Xu X et al: A comparison of koniocellular, magnocellular, and parvocellular receptive field properties in the lateral geniculate nucleus of the owl monkey (*Aotus trivirgatus*), *J Physiol* 531:203, 2001.

CHAPTER 29

THE PRIMARY VISUAL CORTEX

VIVIEN A. CASAGRANDE AND JENNIFER M. ICHIDA

OVERVIEW: PRIMARY VISUAL CORTEX CONSTRUCTS LOCAL IMAGE FEATURES

The visual system is designed to provide a description of the location and identification of objects that have survival value to the species. These descriptions must be made accurately not in a static world but in a dynamic one in which gaze is constantly shifting and in which objects move. Beginning in the retina the visual system selects what is needed to accomplish this goal. The retina contributes to this selection process by throwing away information about absolute light intensity, emphasizing local image contours, and compressing the visual signal information into a manageable size during a manageable time period to be transmitted to the lateral geniculate nucleus (LGN). The LGN contributes by regulating the flow of visual signals so that only the most relevant signals reach cortex. Primary visual cortex (also called *V1* or *striate cortex*), as described in this section, contributes by coding important aspects of local image features, including their size, orientation, local direction of movement, and binocular disparity. All of these local descriptions of stimulus quality are critical for the more global and complex identification of objects ("what") and spatial relations ("where") that will take place in extrastriate areas. At one level, one can think of V1 as an area where information provided by the separate channels within the LGN is combined in different ways before it is sent to extrastriate visual areas for further processing. To do its job, V1 must solve the geometry puzzle of representing all stimulus qualities necessary for the subsequent steps of analyses within the different parts of the visual field map. V1 accom-

plishes this goal by a division of labor between different layers and different iterated modules within each layer. The following sections describe how visual signals are put together in V1 by first providing a review of the gross anatomy and laminar structure of V1 and illustrating how the visual world is mapped onto the layers. The next two subsections delineate the connections, cell types, and basic receptive field properties of V1 cells. Later in this chapter we consider how microcircuits within V1 have been proposed to work together and how parallel inputs to V1 relate to the output channels that are constructed in V1. The final section of this chapter summarizes key points.

OVERVIEW OF CORTICAL ORGANIZATION: GENERAL ROAD MAP

The primary visual cortex in humans is an area the size of a large index card, is about 2 mm thick, and, is located within the occipital lobe extending from the posterior pole along the medial wall of the hemisphere[16] (Figure 29-1). (Also see Figure 28-1.) Like the rest of the cerebral cortex, primary visual cortex contains six principle layers. This area is often called *striate cortex* in recognition of its original identification by the Italian medical student Francesco Gennari more than 200 years ago. Gennari observed that at the posterior pole, the cortex contains a striking white stripe visible in both raw and fixed brain tissue, which is known as the *stria of Gennari*. The stria of Gennari actually marks one heavily myelinated layer in the middle of the gray matter of this area of cortex. Primary visual cortex also is referred to by several other names, including, most commonly, *area 17 of*

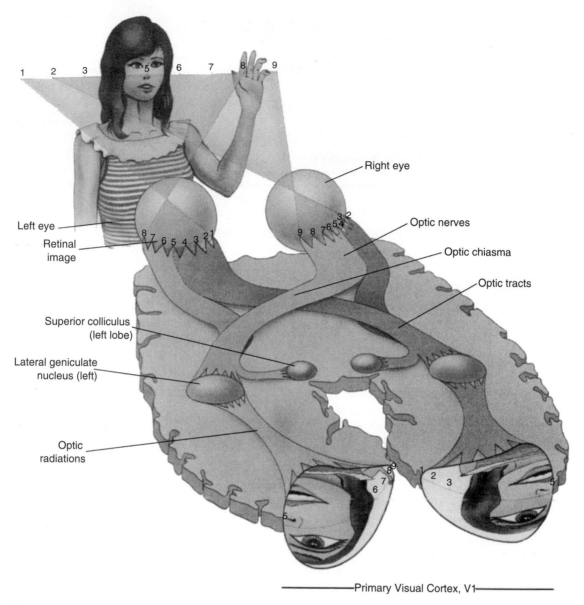

Right eye

Left eye

Optic nerves

Retinal image

Optic chiasma

Optic tracts

Superior colliculus (left lobe)

Lateral geniculate nucleus (left)

Optic radiations

Primary Visual Cortex, V1

FIGURE 29-1   Schematic illustration of two important visual pathways, one from the eyes to V1 and one from the eyes to the superior colliculus. The messages in the first pathway begin in the retina of each eye, travel from each eye via an optic nerve, pass through structures called the *optic chiasm* and the *lateral geniculate nuclei*, proceed on their way via the optic radiations, and finally arrive in a region of the cerebrum at the back of the head called the *primary visual cortex* or *V1*. (From Frisby JP: *Seeing: illusion brain and mind,* New York, 1979, Oxford University Press.)

Brodmann or *area V1.* For convenience, we use the latter term for the remainder of this section.

As discussed in Chapter 26, damage to V1 results in a hole (scotoma) or blind spot in one visual hemifield. Also, as in the LGN, the location of damage to V1 can be predicted based on the topographic map of the opposite visual hemifield that is known to exist in this region in all mammalian species. In humans, detailed knowledge about the manner in which the visual field is mapped onto V1 has been

obtained from a variety of sources, including clinical assessments of damage, results of electrical stimulation, and more recently, functional maps using magnetic resonance imaging (MRI) and positron emission tomography (PET).[11,15,20] Knowledge about the retinotopic organization of V1 in humans is relevant not only to the clinical evaluation of damage but also to research efforts designed to develop visual prosthetic devices involving visual cortical electrical stimulation for individuals with incurable retinal

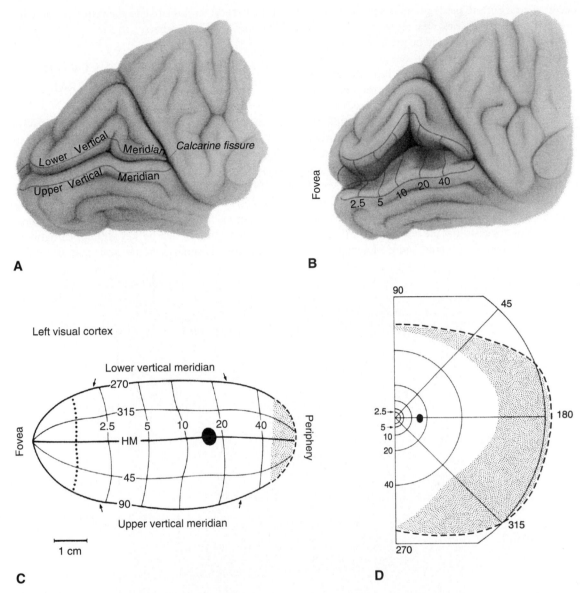

FIGURE 29-2 **A,** Left occipital lobe showing the location of V1 within the calcarine fissure. **B,** View of V1 after opening the lips of the calcarine fissure. The lines indicate the coordinates of the visual field map. The representation of the horizontal meridian runs approximately along the base of the calcarine fissure. The vertical lines mark the isoeccentricity contours from 2.5 to 40 degrees. V1 wraps around the occipital pole to extend about 1 cm onto the lateral convexity, where the fovea is represented. **C,** Schematic map showing the projection of the right visual hemifield on the left visual cortex by transposing the map illustrated in B onto a flat surface. The row of dots indicates approximately where V1 folds around the occipital tip. The black ovals mark the region of V1 corresponding to the contralateral eye's blind spot. It is important to note that considerable variation occurs among individuals in the exact dimensions and location of V1. *HM,* Horizontal meridian. **D,** Right visual hemifield plotted with a Goldmann perimeter. The stippled region corresponds to the monocular temporal crescent, which is mapped within the most anterior 8% to 10% of V1. (From Horton JC, Hoyt WF: *Arch Ophthalmol* 109:816, 1991.)

---

diseases. All of the methods used to understand the map of the visual field in V1 are in general agreement, showing, as illustrated in Figure 29-2, that the fovea is represented in the occipital pole and the far periphery is represented in the anterior margin of the calcarine fissure with the upper and lower visual fields being mapped onto the lower (lingual gyrus) and upper (cuneus gyrus) banks, respectively.[20] As in the LGN, the visual field map in human cortex is distorted such that the representation of central vision occupies much more tissue than does peripheral vision. Whether or not the foveal representation in V1 is expanded over what would be predicted simply by assigning each retinal ganglion cell or LGN cell the same amount of cortical tissue has been the subject of considerable debate. Some investigators[3] have argued that foveal ganglion cells are allocated between three to six times more space than are peripheral ganglion cells; others[43] argue that there is no further magnification over that predicted by ganglion cell number alone. One explanation for these differences of opinion is that the proportion of cortex devoted to central vision has been shown to be highly individually variable at least in macaque monkeys.[41] The latter finding suggests that the relative amount of tissue devoted to the fovea could, indeed, be magnified at the cortical level relative to the retina in some individuals but not in others.

LAYERS AND CONNECTIONS OF V1: INPUTS, OUTPUTS, AND GENERAL WIRING

As in other cortical areas, V1 has six main layers that can be identified in a cell stain as shown in Figure 29-3. The layers and sublayers of V1 have been named in different ways depending on investigator interpretation. The most common laminar scheme is the one adopted by Brodmann,[6] whose designations for the V1 layers are shown in parenthesis in Figure 29-3. The key difference between Brodmann's laminar scheme and that of others

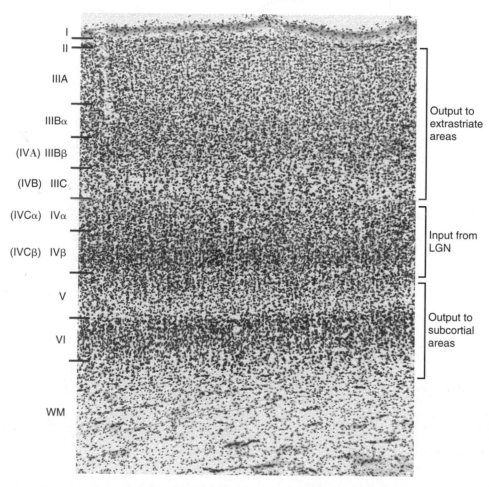

FIGURE 29-3   Nissl-stained section through V1 of macaque monkey. The layers are numbered according to a modification of Hässler's nomenclature with Brodmann's nomenclature in parentheses (see text for details). As indicated by the brackets, layer IV receives the main input from the lateral geniculate nucleus (*LGN*), the layers above IV send projections to other cortical areas, and the layers below IV send projections to subcortical areas (see text for details). *WM,* White matter.

concerns what is included as part of layer IV. Brodmann's definition of layer IV included subdivisions that are interpreted by others as part of layer III (for review, see reference 9). The latter scheme, originally suggested by Hässler,[18] is more in keeping with the laminar schemes used in all other areas of sensory cortex. Hence, as in other cortical areas, the bulk of the input from the thalamus (LGN) to V1 terminates within layer IV (IVC of Brodmann); the main output to other cortical areas exits from the layers above layer IV, mainly layer III (IVB, IVA, and III of Brodmann); and the main output to subcortical areas exits from layers V and VI (Figure 29-3).

Lateral Geniculate Nucleus Inputs

Studies done in anesthetized monkeys have shown that activation of V1 neurons depends completely on input from the LGN because if the LGN is inactivated, visually evoked potentials in V1 are blocked.[33] As discussed in the last section, LGN axons carrying signals from the left and right eyes and from koniocellular (K), magnocellular (M), and parvocellular (P) layers remain segregated at the first synapse in V1 in primates. As shown in Figure 28-6, K, M, and P axons terminate within layers IVα, IVβ, and layers III and I, respectively. In some primates, such as macaque monkeys, the P layers send additional input to layer IIIBβ (IVA of Brodmann), but data suggest that this input does not exist in other primates, such as humans.[19] KLGN axons are somewhat different in their termination pattern from M and P axons in that they terminate within segregated patches of high cytochrome oxidase (CO) density known as the *CO blobs* located within layer IIIB, as well as within layer I.

In addition, input arriving from left and right eye LGN layers remains segregated in the form of *ocular dominance columns* both in humans and in other primates, although the degree of segregation varies greatly between primate species.[13,14] Figure 29-4 shows the complete pattern of ocular dominance columns on a flattened reconstruction through layer IV of V1 in a macaque monkey. In this case the pattern of eye input was revealed by using a histochemical stain to show the downregulation of CO mitochondrial enzyme activity associated with the loss of one eye. CO staining is normally dark in all layers of V1 that receive input from the LGN; therefore loss of one eye results in lighter staining in areas connected to that eye. The result is shown in Figure 29-4 in tangential sections through layer IV of V1 following flattening of the tissue. Black re-

gions depict CO-dense areas in cortex. As can be seen in Figure 29-4, ocular input is segregated into bands within V1 that are less regular in the portions of V1 representing central vision.

The fact that input from the left and right eye remains segregated at the first synapse in V1 raises an interesting question concerning the retinotopic map. Recall that in the LGN, each layer contains a continuous map of the opposite visual hemifield. This means that in the cortex, there must be two topographic maps, one for each eye, within the *same* layer, at least at the first synapse from the LGN. This is exactly what was found in layer IV of the macaque monkey using detailed electrophysiologic recordings.[24] Tangential recordings made

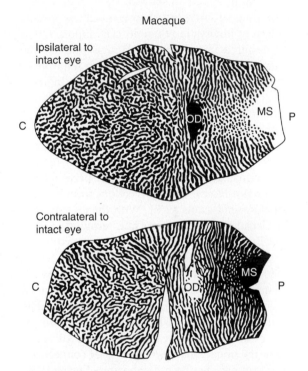

FIGURE 29-4 Distributions of ocular dominance columns in a macaque monkey ipsilateral and contralateral to the intact eye. These drawings were made from photographic montages. Black regions depict cytochrome oxidase (CO)–dense reactivity related to the intact eye. The ocular dominance patterns in the two hemispheres are highly similar, although not identical. Splits that occurred during the flattening process are shown. The visual field is represented from central (*C*) to the peripheral (*P*) as indicated. The representation of the optic disc (*OD*) of the nasal retina is centered 17 degrees from the fovea. The unbanded segments to the right correspond to the monocular temporal segment (*MS*) of the visual field. (Scale bar = 5 mm.) (From Florence SL, Kaas JH: *Vis Neurosci* 8:449, 1992.)

within layer IV revealed that the segments of the visual field mapped in one ocular dominance column for one eye were also represented in the adjacent column that received input from the other eye. As shown later, information from the two eyes and from K, M, and P cells is combined in different ways within other layers of V1 so that most cells in V1 receive a combination of many extrinsic and intrinsic inputs.

Other Inputs to V1

Besides the LGN, V1 receives a variety of other modulatory inputs both from subcortical and cortical areas. These inputs include serotonergic, noradrenergic, and cholinergic inputs from the brainstem and basal forebrain nuclei, respectively.[26] The latter inputs appear to show differences in density within the V1 layers but show a much less specific pattern of innervation than do LGN inputs. Other input sources include the intralaminar nuclei of the thalamus and pulvinar, both of which send broad projections most heavily to layer I of V1. In addition, there are retinotopically more specific sources of input to V1, many of which also receive projections from V1, including the claustrum and visual areas 2, 3, 4, and 5 (V4 and V5 are also commonly referred to as areas *DL* and *MT*).[9,31] Many higher-order visual areas in the temporal and parietal lobes that do not receive direct projections from V1 nevertheless send axons to V1. With the exception of the claustrum, whose axons also terminate within layer IV of V1, all of the other extrastriate visual inputs to V1 terminate outside of layer IV.

So why are there so many other inputs to V1 if the main drive comes from the LGN? As described earlier with the LGN, the numerous nongeniculate inputs to V1 regulate which visual signals will be transmitted to higher-order visual areas. An example of the impact that these non-LGN connections to V1 can have has been demonstrated using fMRI methods. With use of these imaging methods in humans, it has been shown that topographic regions of V1 can be activated simply by asking normal subjects to imagine (with eyes closed) visual objects within particular areas of the visual field (i.e., in the *absence* of any direct stimulus to the retina).[10] These findings argue that non-LGN inputs can have a strong effect on activity in V1.

Output Pathways from V1

As mentioned previously, many cells in the layers that lie outside of layer IV (IVC of Brodmann) send axons to other areas of the brain (for review, see reference 9). The lower layers, V and VI, send axons back to the thalamus and to the midbrain and pons. Layer VI is unique in that cells in this layer provide direct feedback to the LGN and, as discussed in Chapter 28, provide a major pathway for V1 to regulate its own input. Cells in layer VI also send axons to the visual sectors of the thalamic reticular nucleus (see Chapter 28) and the claustrum. Cells in layer V provide the major driving input to many cells in the pulvinar nucleus of the thalamus in monkeys; the pulvinar in turn provides input to a number of extrastriate areas that also feed signals back to V1. In addition, cells in layer V send a major projection to the superficial layers of the superior colliculus and other midbrain areas such as the pretectum, as well as nuclei in the pons that are concerned with eye movements. Thus V1 is in a position to inform these structures of its activities and be informed by them indirectly through connections with the LGN that were discussed earlier or through feedback from extrastriate areas.

As listed earlier, the superficial cortical layers of V1 provide output connections to a number of extrastriate cortical areas (Figure 29-5). These connections emerge from different layers or modules within layers, suggesting that they carry different messages. In macaque monkeys the largest output connection is to visual area 2 (V2). Connections to V2 emerge from three populations of cells. Cells within the CO-rich blobs of layer IIIA and IIIB send a major input to thin CO-rich bands in V2 (Figure 29-6), and the cells between the CO blobs (the interblobs) send projections to CO pale bands of cells (the interbands) in V2.[28] Finally, cells in layer IIIC (also called the *stria of Gennari* or *layer IVB of Brodmann*) send axons to the thick CO bands in V2.

In addition to these connections, there are direct connections from layer IIIB to the dorsal medial visual area (DM) and from patches of cells that lie below the CO blobs in layer IIIC directly to extrastriate area MT.[5] Other output connections of layer III of V1 include projections to areas V3 and V4 (for review, see reference 9).

CELL TYPES AND RECEPTIVE FIELD PROPERTIES: HOW IS V1 DIFFERENT FROM THE LGN?

Examination of the receptive field properties of V1 neurons suggests that visual signals are transformed from those seen in the retina and LGN. In other words, new properties emerge in V1, such as

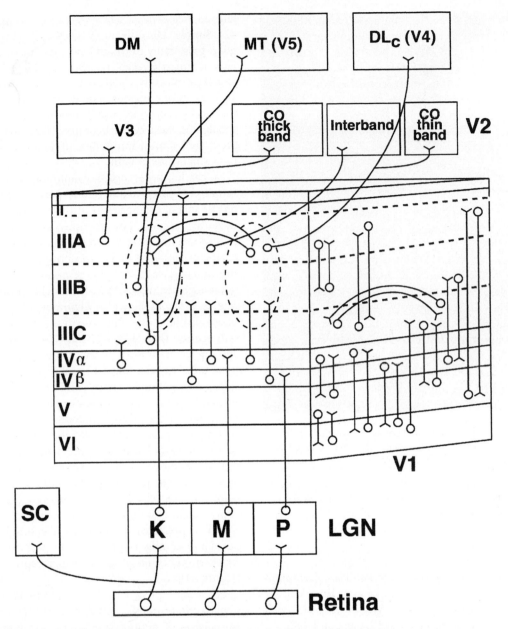

FIGURE 29-5 Schematic indicating some of the main intrinsic and extrinsic connections of V1 in primates, as described in the text. No effort is made to define the strength of connections or to indicate true axon collaterals or species-unique features. Feedback connections to V1 and the lateral geniculate nucleus (*LGN*), as well as connections between extrastriate areas, are not shown. The major input to VI is from the LGN, which arrives via three pathways: the koniocellular (*K*), magnocellular (*M*), and parvocellular (*P*) pathways. The retina also projects to other targets, one of which, the superior colliculus (*SC*), is shown. Within VI, cell layers are heavily interconnected, not only by some of the axonal pathways shown but also by dendritic arbors (not shown). The main ipsilateral connections to extrastriate cortex exit from layer III. In layer IIIA, the cells within cytochrome oxidase (*CO*)–rich blobs, indicated by dotted ovals, and CO-poor interblobs send information to different target cells within bands in V2. In layer IIIB, cells within the CO blobs send projections to the dorsomedial area (*DM*). Cells that lie under the CO blobs in layer IIIC send information to the middle temporal area (*MT*), also called *V5*. Although the connection between V1 and V3 has been documented, it is not known from which layer/module this connection arises. *DLc* (*V4*), Dorsolateral caudal. (Modified from Casagrande VA, Kaas JH: The afferent, intrinsic and efferent connections of primary visual cortex in primates. In Peters A, Rockland KS [eds]: *Cerebral cortex,* vol 10, New York, 1994, Plenum Press.)

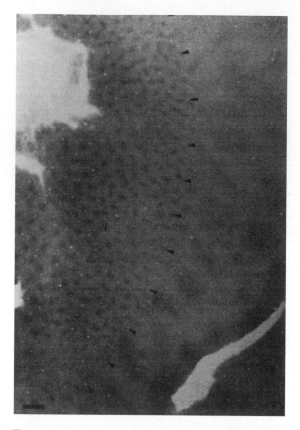

Figure 29-6   Tangential section through layer III of squirrel monkey V1. This section has been stained with cytochrome oxidase (CO) to reveal the CO blobs in V1 and the CO stripes in V2 (see text for details). The boundary between V1 and V2 is indicated by *arrowheads.* (Scale bar = 500 μm.) (From Lachica EA, Beck PD, Casagrande VA: *J Comp Neurol* 329:163, 1993.)

binocularity and sensitivity to stimulus orientation and movement direction. At the same time, V1 cells retain the retinotopic selectivity of their LGN cell inputs, although receptive fields are a bit larger.

In the late 1950s and early 1960s, Hubel and Wiesel[22,23] began to characterize the properties of V1 receptive fields in cats and monkeys using a variety of patterns, including line segments and spots of light displayed at discrete locations on a screen. In these seminal studies, they showed that V1 cells could be subdivided on the basis of their responses to light. Hubel and Wiesel[25] proposed that the cell types in V1 were arranged in serial order of complexity, beginning with those that receive input directly from the LGN, which they termed *simple cells.* They originally proposed that simple cell responses could best be explained by assuming that the receptive fields of a number of LGN cells were

aligned as shown in Figure 29-7 (see also reference 42). Simple cells differ from LGN and retinal ganglion cells, many of which have more or less circularly symmetric receptive fields. Simple cells have elongated receptive fields with adjacent excitatory and inhibitory regions. Hubel and Wiesel called these cells *simple* because it appeared that the responses of these cells to complex shapes could be predicted by linear summation of their responses to individual spots of light.

As can be appreciated by examining Figure 29-7, simple cells can give different responses depending on the spatial arrangement of their inhibitory and excitatory regions. For example, although all the cells shown in Figure 29-7 respond to the same orientation, cells with longer receptive fields, such as shown in Figure 29-7, *C,* will respond to a narrower range of orientations than those with shorter receptive fields, as shown in Figure 29-7, *A.* As this figure also illustrates, the receptive fields of simple cells require that LGN ON- and OFF-center cells are aligned because it is the center responses of these cells that dominate the subfield response of simple cells within V1. Hubel and Wiesel also identified other cell classes with more complex response properties. These cells, generally called *complex cells,* are different from simple cells in that their responses to stimuli cannot be predicted on the basis of linear addition of the cell's response to spots of light presented in different parts of the receptive field; complex cells do not have discrete regions of excitation and inhibition. Instead, complex cells respond to preferred orientations like simple cells, but complex cells respond equally well to a preferred stimulus anywhere in their receptive field[21] (Figure 29-8).

A special type of V1 cell, referred to as an *end-stopped cell,* responds only if the correctly oriented stimulus is of appropriate length. Extending the length of a bar beyond the field into an inhibitory zone of an end-stopped cell diminishes the cell's responses, suggesting that these cells may signal more complex shapes. Hubel and Wiesel originally proposed that the receptive fields of each cell class (namely, LGN, simple, complex, and end-stopped cells) built on the properties of their predecessors in serial order. Scientists know now that connections are more complex, that complex cells can receive input directly from the LGN, and that end-stopped cells can either be simple or complex cells.

Other receptive field properties that emerge within area V1 are direction selectivity and binocularity. Although in some mammals, such as rabbits,

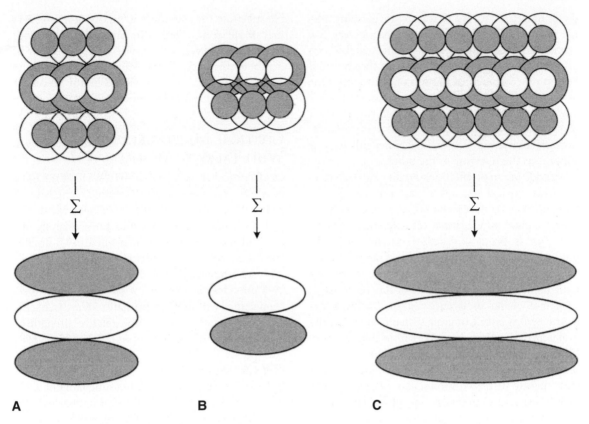

A   B   C

Figure 29-7 Orientation-selective receptive fields can be created by summing the responses of neurons with nonoriented, circularly symmetric receptive fields. The receptive fields of three hypothetical neurons are shown. Each hypothetical receptive field has adjacent excitatory and inhibitory regions. A comparison of **A, B,** and **C** illustrates that the degree of orientation selectivity can vary depending on the number of neurons combined along the main axis. (From Wandell B: *Foundations of vision,* Sunderland, Mass, 1995, Sinauer Associates.)

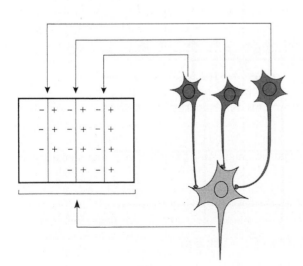

Figure 29-8 The complex cell in this diagram receives input from three simple cells. Each simple cell responds optimally to a vertically oriented edge of light. The receptive fields are scattered in overlapping fashion throughout the rectangle, which represents the receptive field of the complex cell. An edge falling anywhere within the rectangle evokes a response from a few simple cells; this in turn evokes a response in the complex cell. Because there is adaptation at the synapses, only a moving stimulus will keep up a steady bombardment of the complex cell. (From Hubel DH: *Eye, brain and vision,* New York, 1988, Scientific American Library.)

direction selectivity is a characteristic of many retinal ganglion cells, in primates there are very few retinal ganglion and LGN cells that exhibit this property.[2] In V1 there are many cells that respond best to one direction of motion of a stimulus. One explanation for how this property is constructed is that there is a temporal delay between two adjacent connected cortical neurons with the same orientation selectivity, such that one cell either enhances or suppresses the response of the other.

In addition to orientation and direction selectivity, many cortical neurons in cats and monkeys are binocular (i.e., receive signals from both eyes). V1 is the first place where visual information from the two eyes is brought together (Figure 29-9). In binocular V1 neurons, there exists a range of cells, with many responding somewhat more to one eye than to the other. The bias in ocular response is such that ocular preference within a column extending from layer I to layer VI tends to reflect the preference of cells in layer IV within that column. This is because cortical cells tend to be connected preferentially in vertical columns. Binocular cells with slightly displaced monocular fields (i.e., cells with a disparity between the receptive fields of the left and right eye) have been proposed as the possible substrate for stereoscopic vision. Some readers may recall seeing three-dimensional images with small stereoviewers as a child. The impression of depth requires that each view of the image be slightly different, just as it would be for binocular V1 cells with disparate monocular fields.

CORTICAL MICROCIRCUITRY: WHO TALKS TO WHOM IN V1?

Of all cortical areas, V1 has been studied in the most detail. The numbers of cell classes and complexity of connections of this area that have been identified, and the controversies over the functional significance of the many circuits identified in V1 are beyond the scope of this short chapter (for recent review, see reference 7). The diagram shown in Figure 29-5 provides an overview of some of the intrinsic connections within V1 in primates. What such a diagram does not convey is the relative strength of connections and which types of cells are involved.

Cell Classes in V1

In V1, as in the LGN, cells containing glutamate account for the vast majority (approximately 80%) with the remaining cells containing γ-aminobutyric

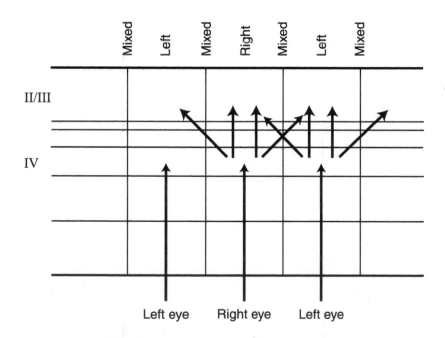

FIGURE 29-9   Information from the two eyes remains segregated until it reaches V1. Within layer IV, information from the right and left eye are still segregated, but connections between layers IV and III combine inputs from both eyes through horizontal and diagonal connections. This combination of inputs results in cells in V1 that respond to input from both eyes (see text for details). (From Hubel DH: *Eye, brain and vision,* New York, 1988, Scientific American Library.)

acid (GABA).[12] These two main cell classes are morphologically distinct[27,40] (Figure 29-10). Two types of cells contain glutamate: the spiny stellate cells that occur mainly in layer IV and the pyramidal cells that occur in all of the layers. Both of these glutamate-containing neurons have a high density of dendritic spines. Although pyramidal cells are the only class of cell that sends axons outside of V1, many pyramidal cells have only local axons within V1. In contrast to the pyramidal cells, the inhibitory GABA-ergic cells have few to no spines on their dendrites. The latter are multipolar neurons whose dendritic arbors come in a variety of shapes. Many subclasses of GABA-ergic interneurons have been

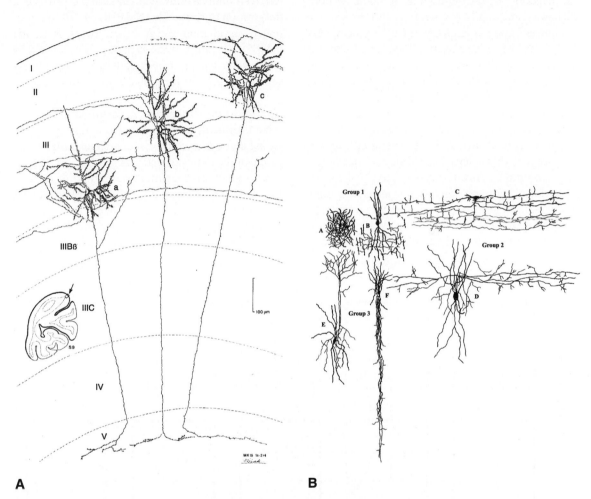

A **B**

FIGURE 29-10 **A,** Camera lucida drawings of three examples of pyramidal cells in primary visual cortex of rhesus monkey. Note that examples *a* and *b* are in layer III, and *c* (*far right*) is in layer II. The diagram of the coronal section on the left denotes the portion of primary visual cortex from which the material was taken. All three have the relatively classic morphology of a pronounced apical dendrite, an axon that exits from the cortical gray matter, and several recurrent collaterals that extend for a millimeter or more in the horizontal plane (*a, b*). The drawings are based on a Golgi stain. **B,** Major classes of aspiny nonpyramidal cells in the primate cerebral cortex as seen in Golgi preparation. Group 1 cells, represented by a neurogliaform cell (*A*) and chandelier cell (*B*), form local connections. Cells in Group 2 have long horizontal axon collaterals and include Cajal-Retzius neurons (*C*) and large basket cells (*D*). Group 3 neurons form vertical connections and are represented by a Martinotti cell with an ascending axonal arbor (*E*) and a double bouquet cell with both ascending and descending axonal arbor that can extend for up to a mm or more in the radial domain (*F*). All of these neurons use GABA as their neurotransmitter, as well as several peptides; in addition, calcium-binding proteins are colocalized in different combinations of these morphologic classes. (**A** from Valverde F: The organizing principles of the primary visual cortex in the monkey. In Peters A, Jones EG [eds]: *Cerebral cortex,* vol 3, New York, 1985, Plenum Press; **B** from Jones EG et al: GABA neurons ans their role in activity-dependent plasticity of adult primate visual cortex. In Peters A, Rockland KS [eds]: *Cerebral cortex,* vol 10, New York, 1994, Plenum Press.)

identified on the basis of morphology, the presence of different calcium-binding proteins such as calbindin and parvalbumin, or various peptides (see Figure 29-10, *B*). The proportion of glutamate/GABA cells remains fairly constant across layers, at least in macaque monkeys.[12]

Connections within V1

Connections between layers can be made by both excitatory and inhibitory neurons (for review, see references 7 and 32). Efforts to trace the general flow of information using pharmacologic manipulations have suggested that layer IV becomes active first and after this the upper layers followed by the lower layers.[4] Circuits that connect layers III and V are especially robust, as are circuits that connect layers IV and VI (at least from VI to IV, see reference 7).

Most of the connections between V1 cells are local, either within a layer or within a vertically defined column of cortex approximately 350 to 500 μm wide. There are, however, longer connections of up to 3 mm in macaque monkeys that occur typically between cells with similar properties (e.g., selectivity for the same orientation or ocular prefer-

ence). These long tangential connections are found most commonly in layers I, III, and V.[38] The effect of these longer connections has been noted in the responses of V1 cells when areas beyond the classical receptive field are stimulated. Studies have shown that although V1 cells do not respond directly to stimuli presented outside of their receptive fields, if these cells are actively responding to a preferred stimulus within their classical receptive field, this response can be modulated by stimuli presented simultaneously at other locations in the field.[29] Such interactions suggest a means whereby responses to local features might begin to be put together to represent the global features of objects.[17]

Comment on Processing Dynamics

What is difficult to appreciate from descriptions of wiring alone is that the visual system is highly dynamic in the living animal. The problem is that the visual system must maintain stability while animals are constantly looking around and often moving through their environments. Therefore the receptive fields of V1 neurons can provide only useful snapshots within short windows of time. A good

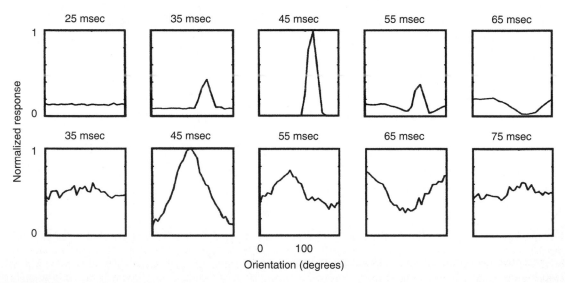

FIGURE 29-11 Reverse correlation measurements of the time evolution of orientation tuning in macaque V1 neurons (Ringach, Hawken, and Shapley, unpublished results). Here the results are obtained by reverse correlation in the orientation domain. To study the dynamics of orientation tuning, they used as stimuli the set of sine gratings of optimal spatial frequency at many orientations (around the clock in 10-degree steps). The dynamic stimuli used consisted of a rapidly changing sequence of sinusoidal gratings. The responses of the neurons are the cross-correlations of their spike trains with the sequence of images; this gives the neurons' orientation-tuning functions as functions of time. In each graph the horizontal axis goes from 0- to 180-degree orientation. This figure displays orientation-tuning functions for two neurons in macaque V1 layer IIIC. Results for each cell occupy a different row. The five different panels for each neuron correspond to give different delays between neural response and stimulus onset. Note that the response to orientation has a dynamic nature; the same cell responds differently to the same orientation at different times (see text for details). (From Shapley R: The receptive fields of visual neurons. In De Valois KK [ed]: *Seeing,* New York, 2000, Academic Press.)

example showing that receptive fields are highly dynamic can be appreciated by examining the evolution of orientation tuning in a single V1 cell in a macaque monkey (Figure 29-11). (See reference 39.) Two cells located in layer IIIC were stimulated with rapidly changing sequences of differently oriented sinusoidal gratings. The horizontal axis represents orientation preference from 0 to 180 degrees, and the vertical axis represents the normalized response of the cells. The responses of the cells are measured as the cross-correlations of their spike train outputs against the sequence of images. These cross-correlations show the orientation preference of the cell as a function of time. Each panel represents a period (in milliseconds) after stimulus onset. The main point is that averaging responses over long periods (i.e., 500 milliseconds), as is typically done in most experiments, masks the complex dynamics that take place over time. The cell in the top row shows clear evidence of a peak excitatory response at 45 milliseconds at one orientation but inhibition at that same orientation 20 milliseconds later. The second cell (*bottom row*) not only shows similar evidence of inhibition but also appears to show a shift in orientation preference at 65 milliseconds after stimulus onset compared with the peak shown 10 milliseconds earlier. As techniques for sampling from many neurons over time in awake monkeys become more sophisticated, it is clear from this example that the concept of how V1 cells contribute to vision will have to move from static pictures of single simple cell receptive fields to a more dynamic view involving network relations between many cells.

COLUMNS AND MODULES: OUTLINING THE FUNCTIONAL ARCHITECTURE OF V1

As shown, V1, like the LGN, is arranged in layers containing cells of different types. Unlike the LGN, new receptive field properties such as selectivity for stimulus orientation, movement direction, and binocularity are constructed at the level of V1. In addition, information about spatial frequency, temporal frequency, brightness, and color contrast, sent by cells of the LGN, must be either preserved or incorporated into the coding of V1 cells. Given the precision of the visuotopic map in V1, this means that critical stimulus attributes must be coded in an iterated manner to cover each location in visual space so that form and movement can be appreciated equally well without holes or gaps at different locations.

How is this accomplished? Hubel and Wiesel[25] were cognizant of the problem that local stimulus attributes would need to be represented again and again at each locale. What they noticed early on in their studies was that orientation preference in cat and monkey V1 changes regularly as one moves an electrode tangentially within any layer (Figure 29-12). An advance of 1 to 2 mm was usually found to be sufficient to rotate twice through 180 degrees of orientation preference. This distance was also found to be sufficient to include at least one left and right eye ocular dominance column. From this information, Hubel and Wiesel constructed a model in which they proposed that the cortex is composed of repeating modules called *hypercolumns*. They argued that each hypercolumn, whose exact boundaries were not fixed, should contain all of the machinery necessary to analyze one portion of visual space. More recently, Livingstone and Hubel[30] argued that CO blobs should be added to this modular organization as zones uniquely equipped to transmit color signals to

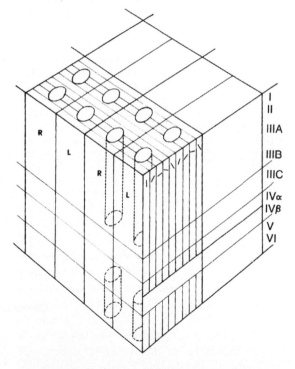

FIGURE 29-12 Schematic diagram of the modular organization of V1. Each module (or hypercolumn; see text for details) consists of two ocular dominance columns (representing right [R] and left [L] eyes), a series of orientation columns (representing 180 degrees of rotation), and cytochrome oxidase blobs (*dotted columns;* representing color information). (From Livingstone MS, Hubel DH: *J Neurosci* 4:309, 1984.)

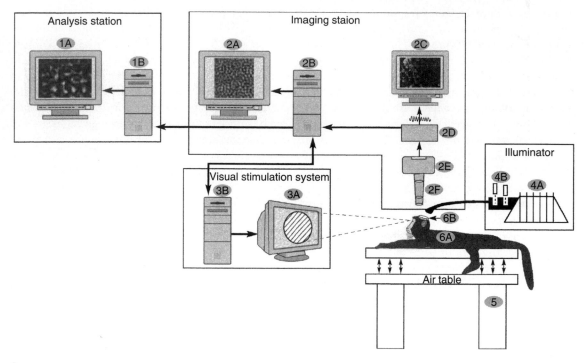

A

FIGURE 29-13   **A,** Computer-generated stimuli presented on a display monitor (*3A*) activate functionally specific regions of monkey (*6A*) cortex. Stimulus-evoked activity in regions near the brain surface modulates reflectance of light (from [*4A, 4B*]) off the brain, a phenomenon mediated by an increase in the oxyhemoglobin/deoxyhemoglobin ratio in regions of greater metabolic activity. The illuminated brain surface is imaged through a cranial window chamber (*6B*) by a magnifying lens (*2F*) onto the charge coupled device (CCD) of a low-noise camera (*2E*), which converts the optical image of the brain to an analog video electrical signal. A video-enhancement amplifier (*2D*) boosts image contrast (*2C*). Images sampled on repeated trials are stored and averaged by the imaging computer (*2B*), and the results are presented pictorially on a monitor (*2A*). Subsequent analyses of averaged data are performed on the analysis station (*1A, 1B*). Because images are averaged over repeated trials, the images must be aligned and the camera must not move with respect to the brain. A mechanically isolating air table (*5*) reduces movement induced by floor vibration.

Continued

the next level (see Figure 29-5). Although there is considerable debate as to whether CO blobs are actually uniquely designed for color processing because they appear to exist in all primates, even nocturnal species with only a single cone type, the fact that these modules are the targets of LGN input from a separate class of cells, the K cells, suggests that CO blobs do something special.[8] Moreover, there appear to be enough CO blobs so that whatever is processed within these modules can clearly be represented across all topographic areas. Because CO blobs are positioned in the centers of ocular dominance columns in macaque monkeys, they were added as another dimension to be included within a V1 hypercolumn (Figure 29-12). The geometric problem is not so difficult for the cortex to solve when only three stimulus properties—orientation, ocular dominance, and color—must be constrained by topography, but

when more properties, such as spatial frequency, direction selectivity, and binocular disparity are added, the task becomes more challenging.

Recently, optical imaging of intrinsic signals has been used to try to determine the relationship between maps of different stimulus properties in single animals. Figure 29-13, *A*, shows the basic set up and procedures used.[36] The signals imaged using this technique are tiny differences in the reflected light from cortex based on dynamic differences in oxygenated and deoxygenated blood that occur as a result of the relative activity of cells. This technique has several advantages, including excellent spatial resolution (approximately 50 μm) and the ability to image several different stimulus properties in one experiment, as well as the ability to be combined with anatomic and single-unit electrophysiologic methods. Of course, the disadvantages are

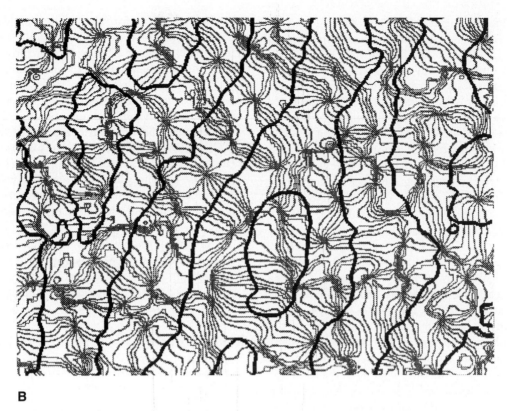

B

FIGURE 29-13, CONT'D   B, Example of a contour plot of orientation preferences in overlay with the borders of ocular dominance bands imaged from macaque monkey V1. Isoorientation lines (*gray*) are drawn in intervals of 11.25 degrees. *Black lines* indicate the border of ocular dominance bands. (From Obermayer K, Blasdel GG: *J Neurosci* 13:4114,

that it is invasive, has poor temporal resolution, and is limited to surface structure. With use of this technique, it has been found that changes in orientation selectivity are represented mainly in pinwheel formation, with some regions also showing more gradual linear or abrupt fractures in the orientation map. The structure of orientation maps in different primates and in other species shows a great deal of similarity, suggesting that orientation-selective cells are organized the same way in humans. Maps of different stimulus qualities also suggest that, although not organized exactly as originally envisioned in the hypercolumn model of Hubel and Wiesel,[25] maps of stimulus attributes are nevertheless iterated in such a manner that there are no "holes" in the map across space (Figure 29-13, *B*).

HOW DO PARALLEL INPUTS RELATE TO PARALLEL OUTPUTS?

It has been popular to suggest that there is a direct link between the input and output pathways of V1. There is considerable support for the idea that two hierarchies of extrastriate visual areas exist: one de-

voted to object vision or *what* something is and one to support spatial vision or complex tasks related to *where* items are in space relative to ourselves. The "what" and "where" pathways, also called the *ventral* and *dorsal streams,* consist of projections through V2 to V4 and into areas of temporal cortex and projections through area MT to regions in the parietal cortex, respectively.[34] It is less clear whether they are directly linked to the K, M, and P LGN pathways. The best evidence for such a direct link comes from studies in which input from the M and P pathways and associated K cells were temporarily blocked in macaque monkeys with microinjections of GABA.[35] These studies clearly demonstrated that the majority of input to area MT comes either from M cells or M and neighboring K cells; K and M cells could not be inactivated separately in these studies. Despite these results, some MT cells could still be driven by the remaining P and/or K cells within the LGN. The importance of M input to area MT is not surprising given the importance of the ability to detect rapidly moving stimuli. A fairly direct pathway for signals from M LGN cells to area MT has also been demonstrated anatomically given that cells in layer IVα, the target layer for LGN M cells, send axons directly to cells in layer IIIC, which, in turn, can send signals to area MT. Nevertheless, cells in layer IIIC that project to MT do not reflect the receptive field properties of M cells; instead, most are complex direction selective cells whose receptive fields are constructed through circuits within cortex.[37]

Even more opportunity for integration between pathways seems to exist before signals enter the ventral stream ("what" pathway). Blockade of the P layers and surrounding K layers does not silence cells within output layers IIIA and IIIB, both of which respond well with either M or P layers blocked.[1] Moreover, anatomically, much of the output to the ventral stream leaves from layer IIIA, which gets no direct input from layer IV but receives signals only after they have passed to other layers. Thus both the wiring and physiology suggest that considerable integration of signals takes place in V1 before they are transmitted into the ventral stream for further analysis of object identity. Finally, as discussed in Chapter 28, the fact that lesions of either M or P layers in the LGN (together with associated K layers) do not eliminate either form or motion vision reinforces the view that it is inappropriate to equate complex visual behavior with the threshold properties of retinal and LGN cells.

SUMMARY OF KEY POINTS

- All visual signals necessary for conscious visual perception are processed in V1 before being sent to other visual areas.
- Primate V1 contains a complete map of the opposite hemifield, in which the representation of central vision is greatly magnified.
- As in the LGN, inputs from K, M, and P and left and right eye remain separate at the first synapse. M and P axons terminate within the upper and lower tier of layer IV, where left and right eye input is segregated into ocular dominance columns. K axons terminate within the CO blobs of layer IIIB and layer I.
- Activation of V1 neurons depends completely on LGN input, but V1 also receives many other cortical and subcortical modulatory inputs.
- V1 subcortical output axons originate within the lower two layers. Layer VI provides the main feedback to the LGN, and layer V axons provide the main drive to cells of the pulvinar, which, in turn, sends axons to extrastriate areas. Each layer also sends axons to other subcortical visual targets.

- V1 cortical output axons originate mainly from layer III; each extrastriate area receives input from different layer III sublayers and from CO blob and interblob compartments within layer III. V1 projects to extrastriate areas concerned with both the "what" (portions of V2 and V4) and "where" (V3 and V5) components of vision.
- New receptive field properties are created within the complex circuitry of V1 and involve both excitatory spiny pyramidal cells and a variety of nonspiny inhibitory interneurons. The new receptive fields code for local image features, including orientation, direction of motion, and binocular disparity.
- The functional geometry of V1 is organized such that each stimulus property is mapped in an iterated fashion to provide each point in the visual field with all necessary stimulus information.

REFERENCES

1. Allison JD et al: Differential contributions of magnocellular and parvocellular pathways to the contrast response of neurons in bush baby primary visual cortex (V1), *Vis Neurosci* 17:71, 2000.
2. Amthor FR, Grzywacz NM: Directional selectivity in vertebrate retinal ganglion cells, *Rev Oculomot Res* 5:79, 1993.
3. Azzopardi P, Cowey A: Preferential representation of the fovea in the primary visual cortex, *Nature* 361:719, 1993.
4. Bolz J, Gilbert CD, Wiesel TN: Pharmacological analysis of cortical circuitry, *Trends Neurosci* 12:292, 1989.
5. Boyd JD, Casagrande VA: Relationships between cytochrome oxidase (CO) blobs in primate primary visual cortex (V1) and the distribution of neurons projecting to the middle temporal area (MT), *J Comp Neurol* 409:573, 1999.
6. Brodmann K: *Localization in the cerebral cortex*, London, 1994, Smith-Gordon and Co Ltd (Translated and edited by LJ Garey from *Vergleichen lokalisationslehre der grosshirnrinde in ihren prinzipien dargestellt auf grund des zellenbaues*, Leipzig, 1909, Johann Ambrosius Barth).
7. Callaway EM: Local circuits in primary visual cortex of the macaque monkey, *Annu Rev Neurosci* 21:47, 1998.
8. Casagrande VA: A third parallel visual pathway to primate area V1, *Trends Neurosci* 17:305, 1994.
9. Casagrande VA, Kaas JH: The afferent, intrinsic and efferent connections of primary visual cortex in primates. In Peters A, Rockland KS (eds): *Cerebral cortex*, vol 10, New York, 1994, Plenum Press.
10. Chen W et al: Human primary visual cortex and lateral geniculate nucleus activation during visual imagery, *Neuroreport* 9:3669, 1998.
11. Engel SA et al: fMRI of human visual cortex, *Nature* 369:525, 1994.
12. Fitzpatrick D et al: Distribution of GABAergic neurons and axon terminals in the macaque striate cortex, *J Comp Neurol* 264:73, 1987.
13. Florence SL, Casagrande VA: Changes in the distribution of geniculocortical projections following monocular deprivation in tree shrews, *Brain Res* 374:179, 1986.

14. Florence SL, Kaas JH: Ocular dominance columns in area 17 of Old World macaque and talapoin monkeys: complete reconstructions and quantitative analyses, *Vis Neurosci* 8:449, 1992.

15. Fox PT et al: Retinotopic organization of human visual cortex mapped with positron-emission tomography, *J Neurosci* 7:913, 1987.

16. Frisby JP: *Seeing: illusion brain and mind,* New York, 1979, Oxford University Press.

17. Gilbert C et al: Interactions between attention, context and learning in primary visual cortex, *Vis Res* 40:1217, 2000.

18. Hässler R: Comparative anatomy of the central visual systems in day- and night-active primates. In Hässler R, Stephen S (eds): *Evolution of the forebrain,* Stuttgart, Germany, 1967, Thieme.

19. Horton JC, Hedley-Whyte ET: Mapping of cytochrome oxidase patches and ocular dominance columns in human visual cortex, *Phil Trans R Soc Lond B* 304:255, 1984.

20. Horton JC, Hoyt WF: Quadrantic visual field defects: a hallmark of lesions in extrastriate (V2/V3) cortex, *Brain* 114:1703, 1991.

21. Hubel DH: *Eye, brain and vision,* New York, 1988, Scientific American Library.

22. Hubel DH, Wiesel TN: Receptive fields, binocular interaction and functional architecture in the cat's striate cortex, *J Physiol* 154:572, 1962.

23. Hubel DH, Wiesel TN: Receptive fields and functional architecture of monkey striate cortex, *J Physiol* 195:215, 1968.

24. Hubel DH, Wiesel TN: Laminar and columnar distribution of geniculo-cortical fibers in the macaque monkey, *J Comp Neurol* 146:421, 1972.

25. Hubel DH, Wiesel TN: Ferrier lecture. Functional architecture of macaque monkey visual cortex, *Proc R Soc Lond B* 198:1, 1977.

26. Jones EG: The thalamus of primates. In Björklund A, Hökfelt T (eds): *Handbook of chemical neuroanatomy,* vol 14, New York, 1998, Elsevier.

27. Jones EG et al: GABA neurons ans their role in activity-dependent plasticity of adult primate visual cortex. In Peters A, Rockland KS (eds): *Cerebral cortex,* vol 10, New York, 1994, Plenum Press.

28. Lachica EA, Beck PD, Casagrande VA: Intrinsic connections of layer III of striate cortex in squirrel monkey and bush baby: correlations with patterns of cytochrome oxidase, *J Comp Neurol* 329:163, 1993.

29. Levitt JB, Lund JS: Contrast dependence of contextual effects in primate visual cortex, *Nature* 387:73, 1997.

30. Livingstone MS, Hubel DH: Anatomy and physiology of a color system in the primate visual cortex, *J Neurosci* 4:309, 1984.

31. Lyon DC, Kaas JH: Connectional and architectonic evidence for dorsal and ventral V3, and dorsomedial area in marmoset monkeys, *J Neurosci* 21: 249, 2001.

32. Lund JS: Anatomical organization of macaque monkey striate visual cortex, *Annu Rev Neurosci* 11:253, 1988.

33. Malpeli JG, Schiller PH, Colby CL: Response properties of single cells in monkey striate cortex during reversible inactivation of individual lateral geniculate laminae, *J Neurophysiol* 46:1102, 1981.

34. Merigan WH, Maunsell JH: How parallel are the primate visual pathways? *Annu Rev Neurosci* 16:369, 1993.

35. Nealey TA, Maunsell JH: Magnocellular and parvocellular contributions to the responses of neurons in macaque striate cortex, *J Neurosci* 14:2069, 1994.

36. Obermayer K, Blasdel GG: Geometry of orientation and ocular dominance columns in monkey striate cortex, *J Neurosci* 13:4114, 1993.

37. Recanzone GH, Wurtz RH, Schwarz U: Responses of MT and MST neurons to one and two moving objects in the receptive field, *J Neurophysiol* 78:2904, 1997.

38. Rockland KS, Lund JS: Widespread periodic intrinsic connections in the tree shrew visual cortex, *Science* 215:1532, 1982.

39. Shapley R: The receptive fields of visual neurons. In De Valois KK (ed): *Seeing,* New York, 2000, Academic Press.

40. Valverde F: The organizing principles of the primary visual cortex in the monkey. In Peters A, Jones EG (eds): *Cerebral cortex,* vol 3, New York, 1985, Plenum Press.

41. Van Essen DC, Newsome WT, Maunsell JH: The visual field representation in striate cortex of the macaque monkey: asymmetries, anisotropies, and individual variability, *Vis Res* 24:429, 1984.

42. Wandell B: *Foundations of vision,* Sunderland, Mass, 1995, Sinauer Associates.

43. Wassle H et al: Retinal ganglion cell density and cortical magnification factor in the primate, *Vis Res* 30:1897, 1990.

CHAPTER 30

EXTRASTRIATE VISUAL CORTEX

JAMIE D. BOYD AND JOANNE A. MATSUBARA

DEFINING VISUAL AREAS

More than half of the neocortex in nonhuman primates is responsive to visual stimulation. Dividing this large heterogeneous expanse of cortex into functional areas is neither straightforward nor completely resolved.[41] Several criteria are used, and cortical areas are defined by a combination of these characteristics.[28]

Histology

Cortical areas can be expected to have a uniform and distinct histology, such that borders can be recognized by changes in the laminar organization, density, or size of neurons, myelinated fibers, enzyme activity, and so forth. However, not all borders can be recognized with all stains. Based on Nissl staining of neuronal cell bodies, Brodmann[6] divided most of extrastriate occipital cortex, in both human and nonhuman primates, into only two areas: 18 and 19. This missed some important divisions. Other histologic stains not available to Brodmann, such as cytochrome oxidase (CO) histochemistry, reveal the borders of some of the many different visual areas within the cortical territory occupied by Brodmann's areas 18 and 19. CO is a metabolic enzyme that serves as a marker for activity levels of neurons. Immunocytochemistry, visualizing specific tissue components with targeted and labeled antibodies, is another technique important to modern neuroanatomy. For example, the CAT-301 antibody, which recognizes a cell surface glycoprotein, can be used to immunocytochemically stain neurons in the magnocellular layers of the lateral geniculate nucleus (LGN) and in the magnocellular-recipient layers of V1. Even with improved staining techniques, however, it is possible that some areas defined by other criteria may be indistinguishable by any histologic methods.

Retinotopographic Mapping

Each visual area comprises a single map of receptive field locations. These maps can be studied with electrophysiologic recordings in nonhuman primates and with functional magnetic resonance imaging (fMRI) or positron emission tomography (PET) in humans. However, in no extrastriate area is the map as regular as in striate cortex (V1). Extrastriate areas have larger receptive fields and more scattering of receptive field positions, giving "cruder" maps. There is generally a smooth transition of receptive field locations from one area to the next. Visual areas can have "mirror-image" representations of the visual field, where the topography of the visual field map is reversed relative to the visual field itself, as if it were reflected across the vertical meridian of the visual field. When a mirror-image area like V1 borders a non–mirror-image representation like V2, the vertical meridian representation forms the border of the two areas and allows continuity of receptive field locations across the border. Extrastriate maps also tend to show breaks in the retinotopy (split representations) along the horizontal meridian representation. These breaks often form the borders of visual areas, allowing smooth transitions of receptive field locations from one area to the next, at the expense, in this case, of splitting the receptive field map within a single area. The splitting of maps within a single area and the continuity of receptive field positions at the borders of different areas make it difficult to decide areal boundaries on the basis of receptive field maps alone.

Connection Patterns

Each visual area is interconnected with a particular subset of the other visual areas and subcortical visual structures, giving it a unique connectional signature. Neuroanatomic tracing methods in nonhuman primates involve injecting tracers into one area either to label cells projecting to the injected area or to label axons projecting from the injected area to other areas. Tracing connectivity in humans is limited to staining for degenerating axons in cases in which patients have died subsequent to cortical lesions. It is important to note that connections are between retinotopically corresponding points in the visual field representation of the interconnected areas. Thus connectivity information has been used to infer receptive field maps.

Functional Specificity

The functional properties of neurons in extrastriate areas are often different. A range of visual stimuli, selected to emphasize, for example, motion versus form and color information, can be used to selectively activate different areas. These studies can be performed in humans using functional imaging techniques (fMRI, PET) or in nonhuman primates using imaging or electrophysiologic techniques. In humans, specific with use of imaging techniques, deficits have been found after cortical lesions caused by strokes, and the damage can be localized postmortem.

With use of the aforementioned methods, at least 25 cortical areas predominately or exclusively engaged in vision have been described in Old World primates, such as macaque monkeys (Figure 30-1). New World primates, such as owl monkeys, have a similar number. As discussed previously, extrastriate cortical areas can be difficult to distinguish unambiguously, and different investigators have their own diverging schemata for parceling cortical areas. Moreover, there are differences in the layout of extrastriate visual areas between different primate species. The following discussion focuses on those areas that have been studied closely enough that some consensus has emerged and that seem to be common to at least humans and Old World primates, if not to all primate species.

PROCESSING STREAMS IN EXTRASTRIATE CORTEX

Nearly all of the projections from the main visual thalamic relay in the lateral geniculate nucleus (LGN) terminate in striate cortex, so the extrastriate areas receive their driving inputs through area 17, either directly or indirectly. (Some extrastriate areas do receive minor thalamic inputs from the lateral geniculate body and the pulvinar, which may contribute to blindsight.[15,79,80]) The main extrastriate projections of V1 are to V2, V3, V4, and V5. As mentioned earlier (see Chapter 29), these projections arise from different subsets of neurons in V1 with different laminar and columnar distributions and likely different functional properties. Zeki[90] first pointed out that striate cortex thus acts to initially segregate and then recombine the information coming over the parallel retinogeniculocortical pathways, such that information is parceled out to different cortical areas for further analysis. As described in Chapter 29, two main streams of extrastriate cortical processing can be defined: a dorsal stream devoted to spatial and a ventral stream devoted to object vision. As in V1, there is often a tangential segregation of the inputs and outputs of the two processing streams, forming a mosaic pattern when viewed from the cortical surface. This columnar organization of connectivity is often marked by differences in histochemical, particularly CO, staining.

V2

The segregation of inputs and outputs within area V2 is as dramatic as within V1 and, as in V1, is associated with a special pattern of CO staining. CO staining in V2 shows a series of parallel stripes of alternating dark and light staining that are oriented perpendicularly to the V1/V2 border.[55,69] The stripes, which are larger than the blobs in V1, extend across the whole width of the area, allowing its borders to be demarcated histologically. The darker staining stripes differ in thickness, with thin and thick stripes alternating, thus defining three compartments within V2. Other stains, such as myelin and immunocytochemistry for CAT-301, also show the stripes.[39] Each of these CO compartments has a different set of connections. The thin stripes receive input from layer-3B CO blobs within V1, whereas the pale-staining interstripes receive input from layer-3B interblobs.[45] The thick stripes receive input from cells in layer 3C of V1, directly above the input layer of the magnocellular LGN inputs.[46] Thus the thick stripes are driven by a more direct pathway through V1, dominated by the fast magnocellular stream. CAT-301 immunostaining, which is strong in parts of the LGN and V1 that contain magnocellular or magnocellular-recipient neurons, preferentially stains the thick stripes, marking them as part of the magnocellular pathway. The thin stripes and

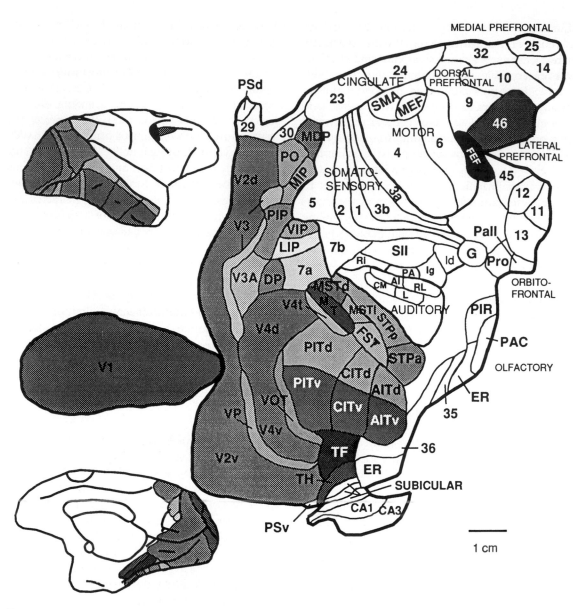

FIGURE 30-1   One interpretation of cortical areas in the macaque monkey. The areas are shown on a flat map, as if cuts were made around the borders of V1 and the cortex was removed from the brainstem and unfolded. Areas involved in vision are shaded. In the occipital cortex, there are the second visual area (*V2*) and its ventral (*V2v*) and dorsal (*V2d*) subdivisions, the third visual area (*V3*), the ventral posterior area (*VP*), V3 anterior (*V3A*), the fourth visual area (*V4*) and its transitional zone (*V4t*), the ventral (*V4v*) and dorsal (*V4d*) subdivisions of V4, the ventral occipital temporal area (*VOT*), and the middle temporal area (*MT*). In the temporal lobe are the posterior inferotemporal area, with dorsal (*PITd*) and ventral (*PITv*) subdivisions; the central inferotemporal area, with dorsal (*CITd*) and ventral (*CITv*) subdivisions; the anterior inferotemporal area, with dorsal (*AITd*) and ventral (*AITv*) subdivisions; the superior temporal polysensory area, with anterior (*STPa*) and posterior (*STPp*) subdivisions; the floor of the superior temporal sulcus (*FST*); and temporal areas F (*TF*) and H (*TH*). In the parietal lobe are the medial and superior temporal area, with dorsal (*MSTd*) and lateral (*MSTl*) subdivisions; the parietooccipital area (*PO*); the posterior intraparietal area (*PIP*); the lateral intraparietal area (*LIP*); the ventral intraparietal area (*VIP*); the medial intraparietal area (*MIP*); the medial dorsal parietal area (*MDP*); the dorsal prelunate area (*DP*); and Brodmann's area 7a (*7a*). In the frontal lobe, Brodmann's area 46 (*46*) and the frontal eye field (*FEF*) are also involved in vision. (From Felleman DJ, Van Essen DC: *Cereb Cortex* 1:1, 1991.)

interstripes are driven by a more indirect pathway through V1, dominated by the slower parvocellular stream, although also reflecting contributions from the magnocellular pathway.

The differences in inputs are reflected in the distribution of latencies of neuronal response to visual stimulation within the three compartments, with cells in the thick stripes responding 20 milliseconds earlier than those in the thin stripes and interstripes.[7,51] According to Hässler's layering scheme for V1 (with Brodmann's in parentheses), the order of visual activation for layers and compartments in V1 and V2 is as follows: V1 layer 4α (4Cα); V1 layer 3C (4B); V2 thick bands; V2 pale bands; V1 layer 4β4Cβ; V1 supragranular layers; and V2 thick bands.[7] Thus the faster magnocellular pathway activates V2 by connection in layers 4α and 3C in less time than it takes the slower parvocellular pathway to activate V1, let alone V2. There are also differences in the receptive field properties of cells in V2 that correlate with CO activity, although the degree of segregation of receptive field types within and between CO compartments is debated. Studies reporting segregation of receptive field properties generally agree that thin stripes contain proportionately more cells with receptive fields that are unoriented and color opponent, whereas the interstripes contain more oriented cells and fewer color-coded units. Clustered in the thick stripes are a class of cells that are oriented and sensitive for retinal disparity, which is important for generating depth perception. Within an individual CO compartment, there is also a columnar organization according to preferred orientation, disparity tuning, or color selectivity, depending on the stripe type.

The visual topography of V2 is interesting in that the CO stripes are oriented perpendicular to lines of isopolarity in V2, but parallel to the isoeccentricity lines. If V2 had a fine-grained continuous map of the visual field, submodalities of visual function associated with each stripe type would be restricted to parts of the visual field mapped onto that stripe. In fact, the visual map in V2 consists of three distinct, interleaved maps.[56,84] Each region of visual space is represented three times, once for each stripe type. The regular progression of receptive field positions seen when traversing across a single stripe are interrupted by jumps in receptive field location at stripe borders. This ensures that visual space is represented completely in all of the stripe types of V2.

The corticocortically and subcortically projecting cells of V2 are also segregated into CO com-

partments. The thin stripes and interstripes project to V4, thought to be involved in form processing, whereas the thick stripes project to regions of the brain associated with motion processing, such as middle temporal area (MT)/V5. Cells projecting subcortically to the superior colliculus are also preferentially clustered in the thick stripes, as are cells involved with disparity tuning, both of which play a role in the generation of eye movements. However, not all connections are segregated by stripe type. Feedback connections from higher-order visual areas tend not to be stripe specific. In addition, the local pathways within V2 interconnect stripes of all types. Thus there is a substrate for binding different attributes of a visual stimulus into a coherent perceptual whole, even at relatively early levels of visual processing.

Areas of the Dorsal Stream

The dorsal stream of visual processing deals with the general problem of where objects are in visual space and how to manipulate them. Dorsal stream–bound outputs from V1 and V2 funnel through MT and V3 to reach areas of the parietal cortex.

MT/V5 and Related Areas. A group of visual areas exists in the superior temporal sulcus (STS) of the macaque monkey, with likely homologs in other primate species, including humans. These areas are recognized by their interconnections and by the fact that many of their neurons are direction selective. The largest of these areas, V5, also known as *MT*, is probably the most easily identified visual area outside of V1. In addition to direction selectivity, MT is marked by heavy myelination, strong immunoreactivity for the CAT-301 antibody, a complete representation of the contralateral visual field, and strong direct input from V1. Thus MT can be identified by all of the accepted criteria for identifying discrete visual areas.

MT receives projections from direction-selective cells in layers 3C (4B) and 6 of V1 and from the thick stripes of area V2.[50] As discussed previously, both of these sources of afferents are dominated by the magnocellular pathway. Blocking the magnocellular layers of the LGN greatly affects the responses in MT, whereas blocking the parvocellular layers has much smaller effects on responses in MT, confirming the dominance of the magnocellular pathway to MT.[48] MT is one of two major recipients of magnocellular-dominated outputs from V1 and V2 (the other being V3) and thus serves as an important gateway for magnocellular information into other areas important for motion processing in the STS, the parietal lobe, and the frontal eye fields. Not surprisingly, lesions of MT in monkeys lead to deficits in motion processing, assessed behaviorally. Monkeys with lesions in MT have elevated detection thresholds of a motion signal in the midst of masking motion noise.[53] The detection threshold for contrast of a visual stimulus was not affected by the MT lesion, showing that the MT lesion effect was selective for motion perception. Deficits for eye movements made to moving targets are also impaired by MT lesion, whereas eye movements made to stationary targets are unaffected by the MT lesions, suggesting that monkeys with MT lesions have more difficulty responding to moving than to stationary stimuli.[54]

Several forms of columnar organization are found within MT. These include organizations for direction tuning, disparity tuning, and selectivity for wide-field versus local motion contrast.[1,5,19] The tangential organization of direction selectivity in MT resembles the organization of orientation selectivity in V1 (see Chapter 29); regions of gradual change in preference are interrupted by sudden shifts of approximately 180 degrees. Approximately 180 degrees of axis of motion are represented in 400 to 500 μm of cortex, similar to the size of orientation columns in V1. This organization of direction-selective neurons made possible an elegant experiment using cortical microstimulation in awake behaving monkeys, showing how the stimulus selectivity of neurons in visual cortex underlies the perception of visual stimuli.[59] A microelectrode in MT in the middle of a cluster of neurons that shared a common preferred direction of motion was used to stimulate those neurons while the monkey performed a motion-discrimination task. Monkeys were required to discriminate between motion shown either in the direction preferred by the neurons or in the opposite direction, and noise was added to make the difficulty of discrimination near the monkeys' threshold for being able to perform the task. When electrical microstimulation was applied, the monkeys indicated that the motion was in the stimulated neurons' preferred direction more frequently than without stimulation. Thus a functional link was established between the activity of direction-selective neurons and perceptual judgments of motion direction.[59]

Within MT, patches of disparity-selective neurons alternate with neurons not selective for disparity. Within disparity-selective patches in MT, there is a smooth progression of preferred disparity across the cortical surface and neurons in the same column have similar disparity tuning. The presence of disparity-tuned neurons in MT is not surprising, given the disparity tuning found in the thick stripes of V2 and the connections between the thick stripes and MT. Microstimulation experiments on disparity-tuned columns in MT similar to the previously described experiment for the direction columns show that electrical stimulation of clusters of disparity-selective MT neurons bias perceptual judgments of depth in a way that is predictable from the disparity preference of neurons at the stimulation site.[18] Thus MT is also important in the perception of depth, as well as motion. Moreover, the two certainly interact, as image movement is an important cue for depth perception.

The receptive fields of some MT neurons have antagonistic surrounds which, when stimulated with moving stimuli, reduce the response to motion in the receptive field center, providing information about local motion contrast that may be used to detect motion boundaries or to indicate retinal slip during visual tracking. Other neurons have surrounds that reinforce the center response and thus integrate motion cues over large areas of the visual field, providing information about global motion that might be useful for orienting the animal in its environment. These two classes of cells are arranged in columns in MT.[5] The columns containing cells with reinforcing surrounds can be selectively activated by large-field random-dot patterns and visualized with an activity marker such as 2-deoxyglucose.

The wide-field and local motion contrast columns are interesting because they have been shown to make connections to different sets of MT's neighboring areas within the STS.[3] MT projects to the medial superior temporal area (MST), where cells have larger receptive fields than in MT, and to an area in the fundus of the STS (abbreviated FST), which has a lower incidence of direction-selective cells than MT or MST. MST can be divided into dorsal and ventral areas by the presence of cells preferring small moving stimuli in MSTv and cells responding to rotation and expansion/contraction in MSTd. Wide-field motion columns project to FST and ventral MST, whereas local motion columns project to dorsal MST. Thus MT may act to distribute different submodalities of motion information into extrastriate areas, much the same way as V1 segregates different submodalities of visual information in general.

V3 and V3A. V3 consists of a narrow belt of cortex immediately adjacent to V2. Much less is known about the structure and function of V3 compared with that of V2 or MT. The original conception of V3 was of a single visual area, a mirror representation of V2, with the representation of the horizontal meridian forming the border between V2 and V3, and the vertical meridian representation forming the outer border.[87,88,91] V3 is thus divided into dorsal and ventral halves that wrap around V2, with the lower (dorsal cortex) and upper (ventral cortex) visual field quadrants being discontinuous across the representation of the horizontal meridian. In addition to the physical separation, evidence has accumulated that the upper and lower visual field representations are anatomically and physiologically distinguishable.[9,10,27,73] This has led to the renaming of the upper visual field representation as the *ventral posterior area* (VP), and the lower visual field representation as the *dorsal V3, or V3 proper.*

Dorsal V3 is heavily myelinated; VP is not. In addition, dorsal V3 stains with the magnocellular-related marker CAT-301, whereas VP does not.[23] Although both dorsal V3 and VP are interconnected with V2, MT, and areas in the parietal lobe, only the dorsal V3 receives projections from V1.[27] The V2 projections to dorsal V3 originate from the magnocellular-dominated layer 4B. Physiologic responses in dorsal V3 and VP also differ. In VP, most cells are selective for stimulus color and orientation but are not direction selective. In dorsal V3, in keeping with the magnocellular-dominated input from V1, color selectivity is less common than in VP, whereas direction-selective cells are more common. The columnar organization of receptive field properties and anatomic connections has not been determined for V3 or VP. However, CO staining does not reveal a mosaic organization within dorsal V3 or VP.

If dorsal V3 and VP are really parts of the same area, or if they are distinct areas with each containing only part of the visual field, it would suggest that upper and lower visual fields are processed differently in the visual system. Another possibility is that dorsal V3 and VP are distinct areas but the "missing" visual field representations are to be found in adjoining cortical territories.[41] This controversy highlights the difficulty of assigning areal borders in extrastriate cortex, where none of the criteria is as clear as for striate cortex, and shows that the possibility exists for multiple partitioning schemes of the same cortical territory.

V3A is a visual area located between dorsal V3 and V4.[92,93] Although originally thought to function as an "accessory" to V3, this area is not especially tied to V3 functionally.[34] Unlike V3/VP, V3A contains representations of both upper and lower visual fields. Physiologically, the neurons of V3A differ from those of neighboring dorsal V3 in being less selective to the speed and direction of stimulus motion.[31] Anatomically, V3A receives projections from V1, V2, and V3/VP. V3A projects to both temporal lobe and parietal lobe areas.[4,25]

Parietal Lobe Areas

The dorsal stream of visual processing terminates in areas of the parietal lobe. In the macaque monkey, these areas are known as the *lateral intraparietal area* (LIP) and *area 7a*. LIP receives input from MT and MST and, in turn, project to area 7.[61] Area 7a sends ascending projections to frontal cortex, including the frontal eye fields, which are important in programming eye movements, as well as cingulate and parahippocampal cortices.[11] Area 7a is also interconnected with subcortical structures related to ocular and vestibuloocular function.[26,74] As the apex of the "where" pathway, area 7a integrates multiple sources of information necessary to represent space.[49]

Receptive fields of neurons in area 7a are large, as much as 60 degrees across, and often extend across the midline.[47] Neurons display selectivity for different classes of optic flow stimuli, that is, stimuli caused by the motion of the observer in the environment from which the direction of heading and the layout of the visual environment can be extracted.[58] Neurons in area 7a also receive extraretinal oculomotor inputs, and their firing may be modulated by the horizontal and vertical position of the eyes in the orbits.[2] The combined eye position and visual signal in area 7a is sufficient to determine the spatial location of an object. Accordingly, lesions in this area lead to deficits in reaching for an object in three dimensions using visual guidance.[43]

Areas of the Ventral Stream

The ventral stream of visual processing deals with the general problem of object recognition. Ventral stream–bound outputs from V1 and V2 funnel through V4 to reach areas of the temporal lobe.

V4. V4 was first described in the macaque monkey as a target field of projections from V2 and V3 in the lunate sulcus.[88] V4 is sandwiched between ventral V3 and MT, with the lower visual quadrant represented dorsally and the upper visual quadrant represented ventrally.[32] A transitional area, V4t, is often described as separating V4 proper from MT. The upper visual quadrant apparently extends into the temporal lobe, although the border of V4 here is unclear, and V4 as defined by some researchers may encroach on other areas in the temporal lobe.[66] V4 is not distinct histologically in Nissl or myelin stains.

V4 receives ascending projections from V1 and V2. The neurons of origin of the V1 projection are concentrated in the foveal part of V1 and arise from neurons in layers 2 and 3, and from both CO blobs and interblobs.[52,81] Inactivation studies show that V4 depends on both the parvocellular and magnocellular LGN channels.[29] From V2, projections arise from cells in thin stripes and interstripes, so neurons projecting from V2 to V4 interdigitate with those projecting to MT.[24,52,64] Although no mosaic organization is present in CO staining in V4, the projections from thin stripes and interstripes appear to be segregated within V4, suggesting that the separation of blob/interblob-related information may continue in V4, although not seen in the histology.[77,85] The size and arrangement of these columns are not well characterized, although they are larger than the modules in V2. The main outputs of V4, to the inferotemporal areas in the temporal lobe, also show this segregation, because injection sites in V4 labeling thin stripes tended to receive more restricted feedback from temporal cortex than injection sites labeling interstripes.[77]

Physiologically, cells in V4 were originally described as being predominantly tuned for color.[89] However, later studies have shown that not all cells in V4 are color selective and that neurons in V4 also show selectivity for orientation, size, and binocular disparity.[20,21,60] Only a small proportion of cells in V4 show direction selectivity.[20] Thus V4 is sensitive to many parameters that might be involved in object recognition. Optical imaging experiments have demonstrated a tangential organization of functional properties in V4. As in other cortical areas with orientation selectivity, orientation-selective cells are clustered into regions of isoorientation preference, although these regions are larger in V4.[33] In addition, regions of V4 selective for small stimuli are segregated from regions inhibited by larger stimuli.[33] The spacing of these regions, like the spacing shown by the cortical connectivity, is larger than in other areas, but the relationship between the functional and anatomic compartments is not yet known.

Inferotemporal Cortex. The areas of the inferotemporal cortex form the final stage of the ventral visual pathway for the recognition of visual objects. The inferotemporal cortex receives projections from V2 and V4, and projects to many multimodal brain sites including the perirhinal cortex, prefrontal cortex, amygdala, and the striatum.[52,62,65,78] Inferotemporal cortex consists of several different areas, but the borders of these areas are unclear, and several different naming schemes are used.[57]

Many cells in the inferotemporal cortex are selective for certain combinations of stimulus features, more complex than orientation, size, color, or simple texture, yet not complex enough to fully describe an object by the activity of a single cell.[42,67] Tanaka et al.[67] presented a series of complex images to inferotemporal cells, found the image that gave maximal response, and systematically simplified the image to find the minimal requirements for activation. A cell that responded to a picture of a water bottle, for example, also responded to a simpler stimulus composed of a vertical ellipse with a downward projection, but it did not respond to the ellipse alone. Some neurons in the inferotemporal cortex respond selectively to faces. There is a columnar organization to the selectivity for critical features in inferotemporal cortex, such that cells within the same cortical column respond to similar, although not identical, features.[30,75]

Evidence for Extrastriate Cortical Areas in Humans

Compared with nonhuman primates, fewer visual areas have been identified (so far) in humans, although it seems likely that humans will be found to have at least as many visual areas as nonhuman primates. Information on extrastriate cortical areas in humans has been amassed from nearly all of the same types of evidence as for nonhuman primates. The presence and locations of V2 and MT/V5 are well established in humans, and less solid evidence exists for the presence of V3 and the V4 region.[40] One of the problems in comparing human visual areas with those of nonhuman primates is the difference in positions in sulci and gyri and the relationship of cortical areas to sulcal landmarks. For instance, there is no human analog of the macaque monkey's lunate sulcus, in which lie visual areas V2, V3, and V4. In addition, human V1 does not extend onto the external aspect of the hemisphere as much as in monkeys. However, extrastriate areas maintain their approximate relative positions on the cortical surface, and accordingly, all of the human extrastriate areas appear displaced posteriorly relative to their positions in primates. Thus MT in humans is usually located in the inferior temporal sulcus rather than in the STS as in other primates. Borders of cortical areas relative to sulcal landmarks also tend to vary more among individuals in humans than in nonhuman primates.

Retinotopy from Callosal Degeneration and Functional Imaging

Early attempts at identifying the borders of extrastriate areas in humans examined the pattern of axonal degeneration following large lesions in the opposite hemisphere.[13] As has been shown previously in animal experiments, callosal connections connect vertical meridian representations, which are often areal borders. In addition to the expected band of callosal afferents on the 17/18 border, patches of callosal afferents were found to alternate with callosal-free regions more laterally in areas 18 and 19. V2 was located within Brodmann's area 18, horseshoe-shaped around area 17, contained within an acallosal stripe adjacent to the callosal band along the 17/18 border. The third visual area was located to the outer part of this acallosal stripe, placing the lower part of the second and third visual area on the fusiform gyrus.

These results have been confirmed and extended by functional magnetic resonance imaging (fMRI) combined with stimuli designed to reveal retinotopic organization.[24,71,72] Color Plate 21 shows maps of the visuotopic organization of V1, V2, V3, and V3A.[72] These maps were made with an annular stimulus that expanded and contracted from the center of the visual field to the periphery. For easier visualization, the two-dimensional MRI slices were stacked into a three-dimensional model and the cortical convolutions of the model were flattened using special software, giving flattened maps. Responses were encoded in polar coordinates as a function of the position of the annulus, giving a map of polar angle (see Color Plate 21, *A*), and isoeccentricity contours (see Color Plate 21, *B*). These maps were then analyzed for local changes in the direction of the gradients of receptive field locations (visual field sign, i.e., mirror image or non–mirror image). Because mirror-image representations usually neighbor non–mirror-image representations, maps of visual field sign (see Color Plate 21, *C*) can be used to objectively parcel complex maps into areas of constant visual field sign. Areas of mirror-image representation that correspond to V1 and V3 can be seen, whereas areas of non–mirror-image representation identify V2 and V3A. Color Plate 21, *D*, shows the borders of the cortical areas thus determined on the

three-dimensional reconstruction of the brain, showing the relationship of the cortical areas to the sulci and gyri. Only some of the areas were imaged in this study. Other studies have imaged areas such as MT that are not shown here.

The visuotopic arrangement of many of the areas in human visual cortex is similar to that of other primates. The dorsal flank of V2 contains the lower visual field representation, and the ventral flank contains the upper field representation. The vertical meridian runs along the border of V1 and V2, and the horizontal meridian runs along the border between V2 and V3. As in other primates, it may be that the upper and lower field representations in V3 are not confluent but are separated into dorsal area, V3d, and a ventral area, VP. Area V3A has a complete representation of the visual field, with a representation of the fovea that is separate from the confluent foveal representations of V1, V2, and V3. Retinotopic mapping identifies human MT, although it has only a crude retinotopy, as well as several areas that may correspond to the V4 complex.[63,68,71]

Histology of Human Extrastriate Cortex

Several areas in human extrastriate cortex can be identified histologically and compared with their counterparts in nonhuman primates.[95] Histologic studies of myeloarchitecture and cytoarchitecture recognize V2 because it is relatively heavily myelinated and its layer III contains relatively large pyramidal cells.[13] Tangential sections through human V2 reveal a striped organization when stained for cytochrome oxidase, myelin, and the CAT-301 antibody.[8,12,38,72] In the cytochrome oxidase stain, the stripes are more disordered and patchy than in most primates and cannot reliably be distinguished into thick and thin stripes. However, they appear more orderly in the myelin and CAT-301 stains. The width of the stripes is larger than in monkeys. The presence of stripes in human V2 suggests that it may have the same intricate functional and connectional organization as shown in other primates. As in nonhuman primates, the extent of the stripes shows the extent of V2, the outer border of which is hard to delimit in Nissl or myelin stains, especially for the upper visual field representation that borders V3d, which has similar architecture. The area bordering the upper field representation, VP, has less myelination and lacks the large pyramidal cells in layer 3 characteristic of V2.[13]

MT can also be recognized in histologic preparations of human cortex.[8,12,38,72] MT corresponds to a heavily myelinated area near the occipitotemporal junction, in the dorsal part of the inferior temporal sulcus. In addition to its dense myelination, human MT shows the same dark, patchy CO staining seen in other primates. The CAT-301 antibody, which marks MT in other primates, also stains heavily in human MT.

Functional Specificity in Human Extrastriate Cortex. Functional specificity in human visual cortex has been investigated by two methods. The first involves using functional imaging techniques, in conjunction with carefully chosen visual stimuli, and the second involves the examination of patients with lesions in different parts of the cortex. Motion selectivity in MT/V5 in humans has been shown with imaging studies comparing activation with moving versus stationary stimuli.[76,86] With use of functional imaging techniques, human MT has also been shown to have higher contrast sensitivity than surrounding cortex and to respond poorly to contours demarcated solely by wavelength.[71] Patients with lesions that include MT have difficulty with motion perception, a condition known as *akinetopsia*.[83,94] One such patient complained that she could not cross the street because of her inability to judge the speed of a car, although she could identify the car itself without difficulty, showing the specificity of the deficit.[94]

The dorsal visual stream areas in the parietal are likely also to be present in humans. Optic flow stimuli have been shown to activate a region on the posterior surface of the precuneus, part of the superior parietal lobule, the same area where similar optic flow responses were found in single cells of macaque monkeys.[17] Such stimuli do not evoke significant activation of V1/V2, nor of MT, showing the specificity of the activation. Furthermore, the presence of extraretinal signals to human parietal cortex, as in monkey cortex, has been shown by functional imaging studies involving subjects making eye movements in the dark.[44] Function deficits resulting from lesions of this area in humans include deficits in visually guided behaviors, as has been noted in monkeys with parietal lesions.[36,43]

Another strikingly specific deficit is cerebral achromatopsia, an inability to discriminate color; this condition arises as a result of damage to a specific area of ventromedial occipital cortex in the region of the lingual and fusiform gyri.[82,83] Given the wavelength selectivity associated with V4, it was originally proposed that the area damaged in human achromatopsia was homologous to primate V4, although it was not in a similar location.[83]

However, when V4 was ablated in monkeys they showed only a mild color discrimination impairment.[14] In contrast, monkeys with lesions in a medial occipitotemporal area roughly corresponding in cranial location to the lesion that produces human cerebral achromatopsia did show a severe impairment in color vision, suggesting that the area producing achromatopsia in humans does have a homologue in monkeys, but it is separate from V4.[37]

The complex selectivity of cells in the inferotemporal cortex of nonhuman primates also has a functional counterpart in human cortex. Comparison of activation of cortex with face versus nonface stimuli shows a fusiform face area in humans, in an area that may be roughly homologous in location to temporal area F (TF) or central inferotemporal area, ventral division (CITv), in the inferotemporal cortex of monkeys.[35] Patients with lesions in inferotemporal cortex display difficulty in object recognition, including prosopagnosia, a specific inability to recognize individual faces.[16]

SUMMARY OF KEY POINTS

- Extrastriate visual areas are identified by a combination of features including receptive field mapping, histology, patterns of connections with other brain regions, and functional specificity.
- In all primates, including humans, a dorsal visual pathway dealing with object location extends through V2, V3, MT, and into parietal cortex.
- In all primates, including humans, a ventral pathway dealing with object recognition extends through V2, V4, and into temporal cortex.

REFERENCES

1. Albright TD, Desimone R, Gross CG: Columnar organization of directionally selective cells in visual area MT of the macaque, *J Neurophysiol* 51:16, 1984.
2. Andersen RA, Essick GK, Siegel RM: Encoding of spatial location by posterior parietal neurons, *Science* 230:456, 1985.
3. Berezovskii VK, Born RT: Specificity of projections from wide-field and local motion-processing regions within the middle temporal visual area of the owl monkey, *J Neurosci* 20:1157, 2000.
4. Blatt GJ, Andersen RA, Stoner GR: Visual receptive field organization and cortico-cortical connections of the lateral intraparietal area (area LIP) in the macaque, *J Comp Neurol* 299:421, 1990.
5. Born RT, Tootell RB: Segregation of global and local motion processing in primate middle temporal visual area, *Nature* 357:497, 1992.
6. Brodmann K: *Vergleichende lokalisationlehre der grosshirnrinde in ihren prinzipien dargestellt auf grund in zellenbaues,* Leipzig, 1909, Barth.

7. Bullier J, Nowak LG: Parallel versus serial processing: new vistas on the distributed organization of the visual system, *Curr Opin Neurobiol* 5:497, 1995.

8. Burkhalter A, Bernardo KL: Organization of corticocortical connections in human visual cortex, *Proc Natl Acad Sci USA* 86:1071, 1989.

9. Burkhalter A, Van Essen DC: Processing of color, form and disparity information in visual areas VP and V2 of ventral extrastriate cortex in the macaque monkey, *J Neurosci* 6:2327, 1986.

10. Burkhalter A et al: Anatomical and physiological asymmetries related to visual areas V3 and VP in macaque extrastriate cortex *Vision Res* 26:63, 1986.

11. Cavada C, Goldman-Rakic PS: Posterior parietal cortex in rhesus monkey: II. Evidence for segregated corticocortical networks linking sensory and limbic areas with the frontal lobe, *J Comp Neurol* 287:422, 1989.

12. Clarke S: Modular organization of human extrastriate visual cortex: evidence from cytochrome oxidase pattern in normal and macular degeneration cases, *Eur J Neurosci* 6:725, 1994.

13. Clarke S, Miklossy J: Occipital cortex in man: organization of callosal connections, related myelo- and cytoarchitecture, and putative boundaries of functional visual areas, *J Comp Neurol* 298:188, 1990.

14. Cowey A, Heywood CA: There's more to colour than meets the eye, *Behav Brain Res* 71:89, 1995.

15. Cowey A, Stoerig P: The neurobiology of blindsight, *Trends NeuroSci* 14:140, 1991.

16. Damasio AR, Damasio H, Van Hoesen GW: Prosopagnosia: anatomic basis and behavioral mechanisms, *Neurology* 32:331, 1982.

17. de Jong BM et al: The cerebral activity related to the visual perception of forward motion in depth, *Brain* 117:1039, 1994.

18. DeAngelis GC, Cumming BG, Newsome WT: Cortical area MT and the perception of stereoscopic depth, *Nature* 394:677, 1988.

19. DeAngelis GC, Newsome WT: Organization of disparity-selective neurons in macaque area MT, *J Neurosci* 19:1398, 1999.

20. Desimone R, Schein SJ: Visual properties of neurons in area V4 of the macaque: sensitivity to stimulus form, *J Neurophysiol* 57:835, 1987.

21. Desimone R et al: Contour, color and shape analysis beyond the striate cortex, *Vision Res* 25:441, 1985.

22. DeYoe EA, Van Essen DC: Segregation of efferent connections and receptive field properties in visual area V2 of the macaque, *Nature* 317:58, 1985.

23. DeYoe EA et al: Antibody labeling of functional subdivisions in visual cortex: Cat-301 immunoreactivity in striate and extrastriate cortex of the macaque monkey, *Visual Neurosci* 5:67, 1990.

24. DeYoe EA et al: Mapping striate and extrastriate visual areas in human cerebral cortex, *Proc Natl Acad Sci USA* 93:2382, 1996.

25. Distler C et al: Cortical connections of inferior temporal area TEO in macaque monkeys, *J Comp Neurol* 334:125, 1993.

26. Faugier-Grimaud S, Ventre J: Anatomic connections of inferior parietal cortex (area 7) with subcortical structures related to vestibulo-ocular function in a monkey *(Macaca fascicularis)*, *J Comp Neurol* 280:1, 1989.

27. Felleman DJ, Burkhalter A, Van Essen DC: Cortical connections of areas V3 and VP of macaque monkey extrastriate visual cortex, *J Comp Neurol* 379:21, 1997.

28. Felleman DJ, Van Essen DC: Distributed hierarchical processing in the primate cerebral cortex, *Cereb Cortex* 1:1, 1991.

29. Ferrera VP, Nealey TA, Maunsell JH: Responses in macaque visual area V4 following inactivation of the parvocellular and magnocellular LGN pathways, *J Neurosci* 14:2080, 1994.

30. Fujita I et al: Columns for visual features of objects in monkey inferotemporal cortex, *Nature* 360:343, 1992.

31. Gaska JP, Jacobson LD, Pollen DA: Spatial and temporal frequency selectivity of neurons in visual cortical area V3A of the macaque monkey, *Vision Res* 28:1179, 1988.

32. Gattass R, Sousa AP, Gross CG: Visuotopic organization and extent of V3 and V4 of the macaque, *J Neurosci* 8:1831, 1988.

33. Ghose GM, Ts'o DY: Form processing modules in primate area V4, *J Neurophysiol* 77:2191, 1997.

34. Girard P, Salin PA, Bullier J: Visual activity in areas V3a and V3 during reversible inactivation of area V1 in the macaque monkey, *J Neurophysiol* 66:1493, 1991.

35. Halgren E et al: Location of human face-selective cortex with respect to retinotopic areas, *Hum Brain Mapp* 7:29, 1999.

36. Heilman KM et al: Apraxia after a superior parietal lesion, *Cortex* 22:141, 1986.

37. Heywood CA, Gaffan D, Cowey A: Cerebral achromatopsia in monkeys, *Eur J Neurosci* 7:1064, 1995.

38. Hockfield S, Tootell RB, Zaremba S: Molecular differences among neurons reveal an organization of human visual cortex, *Proc Natl Acad Sci USA* 87:3027, 1990.

39. Horton JC, Hocking DR: Myelin patterns in V1 and V2 of normal and monocularly enucleated monkeys, *Cereb Cortex* 7:166, 1997.

40. Kaas JH: Human visual cortex: progress and puzzles, *Curr Biol* 5:1126, 1995.

41. Kaas JH: Theories of visual cortex organization in primates. In Rockland KS, Kaas JH, and Peters A (eds): Extrastriate cortex in primates, New York, 1997, Plenum Press.

42. Kobatake E, Tanaka K: Neuronal selectivities to complex object features in the ventral visual pathway of the macaque cerebral cortex, *J Neurophysiol* 71:856, 1994.

43. Lamotte RH, Acuna C: Defects in accuracy of reaching after removal of posterior parietal cortex in monkeys, *Brain Res* 139:309, 1978.

44. Law I et al: Parieto-occipital cortex activation during self-generated eye movements in the dark, *Brain* 121:2189, 1998.

45. Livingstone MS, Hubel DH: Specificity of cortico-cortical connections in monkey visual system, *Nature* 304:531, 1983.

46. Livingstone MS, Hubel DH: Connections between layer 4B of area 17 and the thick cytochrome oxidase stripes of area 18 in the squirrel monkey, *J Neurosci* 7:3371, 1987.

47. Lynch JC et al: Parietal lobe mechanisms for directed visual attention, *J Neurophysiol* 40:362, 1977.

48. Maunsell JH, Nealey TA, DePriest DD: Magnocellular and parvocellular contributions to responses in the middle temporal visual area (MT) of the macaque monkey, *J Neurosci* 10:3323, 1990.

49. Mishkin M, Ungerleider LG, Macko KA: Object vision and spatial vision: two cortical pathways, *Trends Neurosci* 6:414, 1983.

50. Movshon JA, Newsome WT: Visual response properties of striate cortical neurons projecting to area MT in macaque monkeys, *J Neurosci* 16:7733, 1996.

51. Munk MH et al: Visual latencies in cytochrome oxidase bands of macaque area V2, *Proc Natl Acad Sci USA* 92:988, 1995.

52. Nakamura H et al: The modular organization of projections from areas V1 and V2 to areas V4 and TEO in macaques, *J Neurosci* 13:3681, 1993.

53. Newsome WT, Pare EB: A selective impairment of motion perception following lesions of the middle temporal visual area (MT), *J Neurosci* 8:2201, 1988.

54. Newsome WT et al: Deficits in visual motion processing following ibotenic acid lesions of the middle temporal visual area of the macaque monkey, *J Neurosci* 5:825, 1985.

55. Olavarria JF, Van Essen DC: The global pattern of cytochrome oxidase stripes in visual area V2 of the macaque monkey, *Cereb Cortex* 7:395, 1997.

56. Roe AW, Ts'o DY: Visual topography in primate V2: multiple representations across functional stripes, *J Neurosci* 15:3689, 1995.

57. Rosa MGP: Visuotopic organization of primate extrastriate cortex. In Rockland KS, Kaas JH, and Peters A (eds): Cerebral cortex, New York, 1997, Plenum Press.

58. Sakata H et al: Parietal cortical neurons responding to rotary movement of visual stimulus in space, *Exp Brain Res* 61:658, 1986.

59. Salzman CD, Britten KH, Newsome WT: Cortical microstimulation influences perceptual judgements of motion direction, *Nature* 346:174, 1990.

60. Schein SJ, Desimone R: Spectral properties of V4 neurons in the macaque, *J Neurosci* 10:3369, 1990.

61. Selemon LD, Goldman-Rakic PS: Common cortical and subcortical targets of the dorsolateral prefrontal and posterior parietal cortices in the rhesus monkey: evidence for a distributed neural network subserving spatially guided behavior, *J Neurosci* 8:4049, 1988.

62. Seltzer B, Pandya DN: Afferent cortical connections and architectonics of the superior temporal sulcus and surrounding cortex in the rhesus monkey, *Brain Res* 149:1, 1978.

63. Sereno MI et al: Borders of multiple visual areas in humans revealed by functional magnetic resonance imaging, *Science* 268:889, 1995.

64. Shipp S, Zeki S: Segregation of pathways leading from area V2 to areas V4 and V5 of macaque monkey visual cortex, *Nature* 315:322, 1985.

65. Shiwa T: Corticocortical projections to the monkey temporal lobe with particular reference to the visual processing pathways, *Arch Ital Biol* 125:139, 1987.

66. Stepniewska I, Kaas JH: Topographic patterns of V2 cortical connections in macaque monkeys, *J Comp Neurol* 371:129, 1996.

67. Tanaka K et al: Coding visual images of objects in the inferotemporal cortex of the macaque monkey, *J Neurophysiol* 66:170, 1991.

68. Tootell RB, Hadjikhani N: Where is "dorsal v4" in human visual cortex? Retinotopic, topographic and functional evidence, *Cereb Cortex* 11:298, 2001.

69. Tootell RB, Hamilton SL, Silverman MS: Topography of cytochrome oxidase activity in owl monkey cortex, *J Neurosci* 5:2786, 1985.

70. Tootell RB, Taylor JB: Anatomical evidence for MT and additional cortical visual areas in humans, *Cereb Cortex* 5:39, 1995.

71. Tootell RB et al: Functional analysis of human MT and related visual cortical areas using magnetic resonance imaging, *J Neurosci* 15:3215, 1995.

72. Tootell RB et al: Functional analysis of V3A and related areas in human visual cortex, *J Neurosci* 17:7060, 1997.

73. Van Essen DC et al: The projections from striate cortex (V1) to areas V2 and V3 in the macaque monkey: asymmetries, areal boundaries, and patchy connections, *J Comp Neurol* 244:451, 1986.

74. Ventre J, Faugier-Grimaud S: Projections of the temporoparietal cortex on vestibular complex in the macaque monkey *(Macaca fascicularis)*, *Exp Brain Res* 72:653, 1988.

75. Wang G, Tanifuji M, Tanaka K: Functional architecture in monkey inferotemporal cortex revealed by in vivo optical imaging, *Neurosci Res* 32:33, 1998.

76. Watson JD et al: Area V5 of the human brain: evidence from a combined study using positron emission tomography and magnetic resonance imaging, *Cereb Cortex* 3:79, 1993.

77. Xiao Y, Zych A, Felleman DJ: Segregation and convergence of functionally defined V2 thin stripe and interstripe compartment projections to area V4 of macaques, *Cereb Cortex* 9:792, 1999.

78. Yeterian EH, Pandya DN: Corticostriatal connections of extrastriate visual areas in rhesus monkeys, *J Comp Neurol* 352:436, 1995.

79. Yoshida K, Benevento LA: The projection from the dorsal lateral geniculate nucleus of the thalamus to extrastriate visual association cortex in the macaque monkey, *Neurosci Lett* 22:103, 1981.

80. Yukie M, Iwai E: Direct projection from the dorsal lateral geniculate nucleus to the prestriate cortex in macaque monkeys, *J Comp Neurol* 201:81, 1981.

81. Yukie M, Iwai E: Laminar origin of direct projection from cortex area V1 to V4 in the rhesus monkey, *Brain Res* 346:383, 1985.

82. Zeki S: A century of cerebral achromatopsia, *Brain* 113:1721, 1990.

83. Zeki S: Cerebral akinetopsia (visual motion blindness), *Brain* 114:811, 1991.

84. Zeki S, Shipp S: Functional segregation within area V2 of macaque monkey visual cortex. In Kulikowski JJ, Dickinson CM, and Murray IJ (eds): *Seeing contour and colour: based on the proceedings of the Third International Symposium of the Northern Eye Institute, Manchester, England, August 9-13, 1987,* Oxford; New York, 1989, Pergammon Press.

85. Zeki S, Shipp S: Modular connections between areas V2 and V4 of macaque monkey visual cortex, *Eur J Neurosci* 1:494, 1989.

86. Zeki S et al: A direct demonstration of functional specialization in human visual cortex, *J Neurosci* 11:641, 1991.

87. Zeki SM: Representation of central visual fields in prestriate cortex of monkey, *Brain Res* 14:271, 1969.

88. Zeki SM: Cortical projections from two prestriate areas in the monkey, *Brain Res* 34:19, 1971.

89. Zeki SM: Colour coding in rhesus monkey prestriate cortex, *Brain Res* 53:422, 1973.

90. Zeki SM: The functional organization of projections from striate to prestriate visual cortex in the rhesus monkey, *Cold Spring Harb Symp Quant Biol* 40:591, 1975.

91. Zeki SM: Simultaneous anatomical demonstration of the representation of the vertical and horizontal meridians in areas V2 and V3 of rhesus monkey visual cortex, *Proc R Soc Lond B Biol Sci* 195:517, 1977.

92. Zeki SM: The third visual complex of rhesus monkey prestriate cortex, *J Physiol* 277:245, 1977.

93. Zeki SM: Uniformity and diversity of structure and function in rhesus monkey prestriate visual cortex, *J Physiol* 277:273, 1978.

94. Zihl J, von Cramon D, Mai N: Selective disturbance of movement vision after bilateral brain damage, *Brain* 106:313, 1983.

95. Zilles K, Clarke S: Architecture, connectivity, and transmitter receptors of human extrastriate visual cortex. In Rockland KS, Kaas JH, and Peters A (eds): Extrastriate cortex in primates, New York, 1997, Plenum Press.

CHAPTER 31

VISUAL DEPRIVATION

QIANG GU, JOANNE A. MATSUBARA, AND JAMIE D. BOYD

As shown in the previous chapters, much is known of the anatomic and functional organization of the lateral geniculate nucleus (LGN) and visual cortex. The central visual pathways are precisely wired to process features such as depth, motion, orientation, direction, color, contrast, and texture. The precise wiring is not fully formed at birth and is highly dependent on visual experience.

BINOCULAR RESPONSES IN VISUAL CORTEX

Hubel and Wiesel were the first to conduct animal experiments to demonstrate the role of visual experience on the development of the visual system.[66-68,126-128] Using young animals, Hubel and Wiesel deprived vision to one eye by suturing the eyelid shut. Several important findings on the role of monocular deprivation in the development of the visual system were made. First, although eyelid suture reduced retinal illumination by several log units and eliminated all patterned vision, it did not injure the eye in any way. The occluded eye usually developed axial myopia, but no other significant abnormality ensued. The researchers did not find any effects of monocular deprivation on the retina. Second, cells in the LGN layer connected to the deprived eye had smaller cell bodies than those cells receiving input from the normal eye. Although cells within deprived laminas were shrunken, they had normal center-surround receptive fields and responded briskly to visual stimulation. Third, cortical cells lost functional connections with the deprived eye, and most cortical cells encountered were activated only by the stimulation of the nondeprived eye. In normal animals without visual deprivation, most neurons in the visual cortex respond to visual input from either eye (binocular neurons). Only a few neurons can be activated exclusively by stimulation of either the left or the right eye (monocular neurons). Binocular neurons may respond equally well to both eyes or may show stronger response to one eye than to the other. According to their response preference to the left and right eye, cortical neurons were classified in seven ocular dominance classes by Hubel and Wiesel[66]; the distribution of cortical neurons in these ocular dominance classes can be displayed in an ocular dominance histogram (Figure 31-1, A).

Monocular eyelid suture caused many cortical neurons to stop responding to the deprived eye; therefore the ocular dominance histogram showed a shift of ocular dominance distribution of cortical neurons toward the nondeprived eye (Figure 31-1, B). The effect of eyelid suture on cortical neurons appears to be a result of competition between the two eyes' inputs because binocular eyelid suture, or rearing animals in the dark, could not induce the same cortical changes. In visual cortex of monocularly deprived animals, the strong input from the normal eye competes with the weak one from the deprived eye so that functional connections from the normal eye are retained and nonfunctional connections from the deprived eye are decayed. This kind of "winner-takes-all" phenomenon can be observed in many places in the developing visual system (see also Chapter 27) and follows the same rule as that for learning and memory postulated by the Canadian psychologist Donald Hebb.[52] Thus experience-dependent changes in ocular dominance are referred to as *ocular dominance plasticity*. Similar effects of monocular deprivation have been

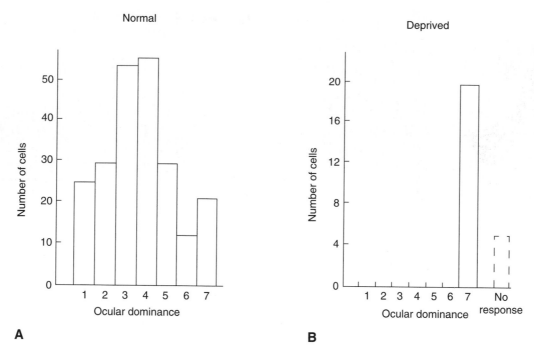

FIGURE 31-1   Ocular dominance histogram showing change of ocular preference of neurons in kitten visual cortex after monocular deprivation. Each cell was characterized according to whether it was driven solely by one eye (either left or right, group 1 or group 7), equally by both eyes (group 4), or somewhere in between (groups 2, 3, 5, and 6). **A,** Normal kitten. Most neurons responded to stimulation of either eye. **B,** Monocularly deprived kitten that had one eye (corresponding to group 1) sutured closed at about 10 days of age, and the duration of closure was 2.5 months. Neurons stopped responding to the deprived eye. (From Wiesel TN, Hubel DH: *J Neurophysiol* 26:1003, 1963.)

observed in other mammalian species such as the monkey, rat, mouse, and ferret.* The minimal amount of time needed to reliably produce a noticeable shift of ocular dominance is approximately 4 to 10 hours.[86,91,92,97,102]

Anatomic correlates of ocular dominance plasticity were demonstrated using transneuronal-tracing methods. When radioactively labeled proline is injected into one eye, it is taken up by retinal ganglion cells and transported through the LGN to the primary visual cortex. Therefore ocular dominance columns (introduced in Chapter 27) that represent the injected eye can be labeled. With normal visual experience, the dimensions of ocular dominance columns corresponding to either the left or the right eye are roughly equal. However, following monocular deprivation during development, ocular dominance columns devoted to the deprived eye can undergo a substantial shrinkage of territory in contrast to an expansion of the dimension of ocular dominance columns devoted to the nondeprived eye (Figure 31-2).

In line with these results, computer reconstructions of single geniculocortical axonal terminals revealed that the complexity of the terminal arborization was less for the deprived eye, while the afferents serving the nondeprived eye expanded[2] (Figure 31-3). Thus visual deprivation could cause both functional and structural changes of ocular dominance domains in the visual cortex.

ORIENTATION AND DIRECTION SELECTIVITY IN VISUAL CORTEX

Hubel and Wiesel found that monocular deprivation had a profound effect on neurons in immature visual cortex, whereas few effects were detected with monocular deprivation in adult animals. Immediately after birth, neurons in the visual cortex are immature. Their responses to visual stimulation are sluggish and lack any specificity. The latency and specificity of the responses can be improved with normal, or prevented with abnormal, visual experience during postnatal development.

Neurons in the visual cortex exhibit more complex response patterns than those of retinal gan-

*References 5, 25, 40, 44, 69, 70, 85.

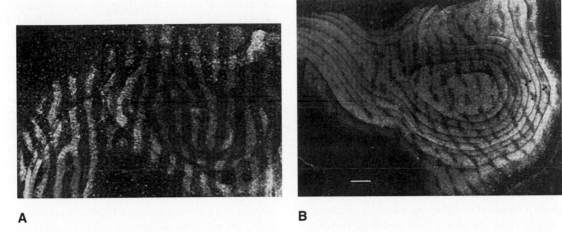

A   **B**

FIGURE 31-2 Change of ocular dominance columns in macaque monkey visual cortex after monocular deprivation. Radioactive proline was injected into the normal eye and transported to the visual cortex to reveal the projections of that eye. In these sections, cut parallel to the cortical surface, white areas show labeled terminals in layer 4. **A,** Normal monkey. The stripes representing the injected eye (bright) and noninjected eye (dark) have roughly equal spacing. **B,** Monocularly deprived monkey that had one eye sutured closed from birth for 18 months. The bright stripes, representing label in layer 4 from the open, injected eye are widened, the dark ones (closed eye) are greatly narrowed. (Scale bar = 1 mm.) (From Hubel DH, Wiesel TN, LeVay S: *Philos Trans R Soc Lond B Biol Sci* 278:377, 1977.)

glion cells and LGN relay cells. Although the latter respond to stimulation using spots of light, cortical neurons usually respond to stimulation of bars of light with a preferred orientation and direction of motion. It appears that these features are also susceptible to experience-dependent modifiability in the immature visual cortex. Early studies have shown that orientation selectivity requires visual experience to be maintained or developed fully.[127,128] When kittens were raised in environments in which visual experience was limited to contours of a single orientation, an alteration in the distribution of orientation preference in the cortex was observed, with more cells preferring orientations near the experienced orientation than other orientations.[15,60] Additional investigations made it clear that any bias in the distribution of orientation preferences is induced on the cortical level and not in the LGN.[32,109]

Direction selectivity, like orientation selectivity and binocularity, first appears at the level of the primary visual cortex. This property is present in attenuated form in cortical neurons recorded from young kittens lacking visual experience.[6,67] When kittens were raised in a controlled environment in which contours move in one direction only, the large majority of direction-selective cells in the cortex preferred movement in that direction.[29,36,119,122] Another way to modify direction selectivity of cortical neurons is to rear animals in stroboscopic illumination,

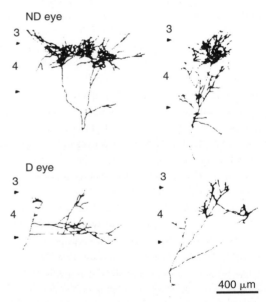

FIGURE 31-3 Change of lateral geniculate nucleus terminals in kitten visual cortex after monocular deprivation. Reconstructions of geniculocortical arbors revealed a dramatic reduction in complexity of the deprived eye (*D*) as compared with that of the nondeprived eye (*ND*). Two representative examples serving for each eye are shown. The duration of monocular deprivation was 33 days. The numbers *3* and *4* indicate cortical layers, and the *arrowheads* indicate the border of cortical layers. (From Antonini A, Stryker MP: *Science* 260:1819, 1993.)

in which there is ample experience of pattern without retinal image motion.[28,99] This environment of "directional deprivation" radically reduced the proportion of direction selective neurons in the visual cortex.[28,30,99]

Critical Period for Experience-Dependent Modifications

An important feature of these experience-dependent modifications is that changes of neuronal responses can be made only within a transient "critical period" during early postnatal development, but not thereafter in adult animals.* By applying visual deprivation in animals at different ages and by measuring physiologic changes after a fixed period of visual deprivation, one can determine quantitatively the magnitude of changes associated with the deprivation and can then define the critical period of visual cortex plasticity. Thus it can be determined at what ages (1) an effect can be found, (2) an effect is maximal, or (3) there is no effect. For ocular dominance plasticity in the cat, the critical period starts at 3 weeks of age, peaks at 4 to 6 weeks, declines from 6 weeks until around 5 months, then has a plateau of reduced plasticity until it finally ends between 9 months and 1 year of age.[37,68,72,98,127] The critical period of ocular dominance plasticity varies with the layer of cortex studied. There is evidence that the critical period in layer IV ends earlier than the critical period for cells in other layers.[37,83,94,113] A recent study suggests that even within the same cortical layer, plasticity may not be at the same level. Some neurons may have greater ability to change responses to stimulation than other neurons depending on the expression level of transmitter receptors that they possess.[81]

In addition to cats, the critical period for ocular dominance changes has been studied in a number of other mammalian species. The critical periods vary among different species. In mice and rats the critical period starts around postnatal day 17, peaks at postnatal day 28, and ends at postnatal day 35.[40,44,85] In ferrets the critical period starts around postnatal day 32, peaks around postnatal day 42, and ends around postnatal day 100.[70] In the macaque monkey the critical period is initiated soon after birth, peaks around 1 month of age, and ends before 2 years of age.[83] Clinical observations indicate that visual cortex plasticity in humans starts between birth and 6 months of age, peaks at 1 to 2 years of age, and declines between 2 and 8 years of age.[33] The critical period for

the induction of changes in orientation selectivity appears to be identical to that for the induction of the effects of monocular occlusion.[14] The critical period for alteration of direction selectivity seems to end earlier than the critical period for ocular dominance changes or orientation selectivity.[13,34-36]

Why is a critical period for activity-dependent modification in visual cortex necessary? It is well established that binocular vision is crucial for stereopsis, which requires precise corresponding inputs from both eyes. When the distance between the two eyes becomes larger during development, cortical neurons fine-tune their connections to both eyes. In the species mentioned previously, the critical periods coincide with the times of greatest growth of the head and eyes.

Mechanisms Underlying Plasticity

The mechanisms behind the cellular interactions at the heart of ocular dominance plasticity have been examined pharmacologically by, for example, intracortical infusion of chemicals that block or mimic activities of a particular molecule of interest. The ocular dominance shift that normally occurs in the visual cortex after monocular occlusion can be prevented if neurons are silenced by intracortical infusion of the Na^+ channel blocker tetrodotoxin (TTX), which blocks action potentials.[111] Because the LGN inputs are not affected by the TTX treatment, this experiment shows the dependence of plasticity on activity in the target cortical neurons. Ocular dominance shifts can also be prevented by artificially increasing cortical activity by infusion of glutamate, an excitatory amino acid neurotransmitter, or an antagonist of γ-aminobutyric acid (GABA), an inhibitory neuorotransmitter.[108,110,114] In both of these cases, normal activity of cortical neurons is disturbed. The extra cortical activity reduces the signal/noise ratio of cortical responses, again leading to the conclusion that normal activity in the postsynaptic cells is necessary for synaptic changes. One theory is that a postsynaptic cortical neuron compares the activity of terminals driven by the two eyes with its own activity and actively maintains connections with terminals that tend to be active at the same time the cortical cell is active itself (just how a cortical neuron might maintain its connections is discussed later). Altering normal cortical activity disrupts this comparison and prevents ocular dominance shifts. Among the excitatory and inhibitory receptors in the visual cortex, the *N*-methyl-D-aspartate (NMDA) receptor and $GABA_A$ receptor appear to be key receptors underlying visual cortex plasticity.[80,108,110]

---

*References 31, 37, 68, 72, 98, 113.

Cortical plasticity can be modified by far-reaching axons that arise from several subcortical centers and innervate all cortical areas and layers in a rather diffuse fashion. These subcortical centers in the basal forebrain, locus coeruleus, and raphe nucleus modulate the excitability of cortical neurons by releasing acetylcholine, noradrenaline, and serotonin, respectively.

Kasamatsu and Pettigrew showed that noradrenaline could affect ocular dominance plasticity.[76,103] Depletion of noradrenaline by 6-hydroxydopamine (6-OHDA), a neurotoxin that kills most noradrenergic terminals, prevented ocular dominance shifts in young animals, whereas infusion of noradrenaline in visual cortex enhanced plasticity in kittens and even restored it to some extent in adult animals.[53,76,103] Later studies demonstrate that blockade of noradrenergic β_1-receptor prevented ocular dominance plasticity.[77] Acetylcholine and serotonin have also been shown to be involved in ocular dominance plasticity.[8,47,48,124] Intracortical infusion of muscarinic M_1 cholinergic receptor antagonists suppressed ocular dominance changes, as did intracortical infusion of a serotonin $5-HT_{2c}$ receptor antagonist.[47,124]

The cellular mechanisms that link activation of receptors on cortical neurons to changes in plasticity appear to involve several intracellular second messenger systems such as the phosphatidylinositol and cyclic adenosine monophosphate (cAMP) cascades. It has been shown that both a high lithium level, which blocks phosphatidylinositol turnover, and pharmacologic inhibition of the cAMP-dependent protein kinase (PKA) reduce ocular dominance plasticity in kitten visual cortex.[9,75] The activation of second-messenger-dependent protein kinases and phosphatases likely triggers further downstream cascades, leading to gene expressions, which then result in activity-dependent synaptic changes.

Many different processes are likely involved in the maintenance of connections between cortical cells and LGN terminals. Lately, much attention has been focused on the neurotrophin family. Neurotrophins are structurally related proteins that support survival, growth, and differentiation of distinct populations of neurons and include nerve growth factor (NGF), brain-derived neurotrophic factor (BDNF), neurotrophin-3 (NT-3), and neurotrophin-4/5 (NT-4/5). Experimental manipulation of NGF, NT-4/5, and BDNF levels affects ocular dominance plasticity in the developing visual cortex and in adult visual cortex.* Manipulation of NT-4/5 or BDNF levels

*References 12, 20, 39, 42, 46, 49, 65, 84, 85, 104.

also perturbed the formation of ocular dominance columns in kitten visual cortex, and BDNF was found to have a hypertrophic action on geniculocortical terminals in developing, but not in adult, cat visual cortex.[18,19,50] Together, these data suggest that NGF, BDNF, and NT-4/5 are required for visual cortex development and plasticity.

CLINICAL IMPLICATIONS OF EXPERIENCE-DEPENDENT CHANGES
Changes during Development
Much of the work discussed thus far, which examined the basic mechanism of how experience changes the developing visual system, used severe forms of deprivation, such as complete monocular occlusion. However, there is accumulating evidence that moderate disruptions of visual experience caused by clinically relevant conditions, such as strabismus, anisometropia, and glaucoma, can also lead to changes in the central visual system. These changes have been observed both in humans and in nonhuman primate models.

Amblyopia. As discussed previously, the visual system is most susceptible to experience-dependent changes during development. If a young child experiences abnormal visual experience, there may be a loss of visual function that persists even after the optical or ocular problems are corrected. Amblyopia, or "lazy eye," often develops when unequal refractive power (anisometropia) or misalignment of the visual axis (strabismus) of the two eyes interferes with focused and balanced binocular vision early in development. This leads to a condition in which information from the affected eye is not processed properly because of binocular competition and visual acuity is reduced relative to the normal eye. Thus amblyopia is a disease of the development of the central visual system.

What are the changes that take place in the central visual pathways that lead to the loss of acuity seen in amblyopia? One might suppose that the deficit in amblyopia is similar to the deficit seen in monocular occlusion, namely, a shrinkage of cortical territory devoted to the deprived eye in the primary visual cortex. It appears, however, that although shrinkage of ocular dominance columns does occur in primates when one eye is completely deprived of form vision soon after birth, effects are not as clear in the visual cortex after less extreme forms of deprivation.[64,69,83] In an experimental primate model of anisometropia, retinal blur resulted when one eye underwent atropinization since birth, yet unlike the monocular deprivation experiments described previously, only a moderate amount of column shrinkage was reported.[54] In one naturally occurring case of anisometropic amblyopia in a monkey, ocular dominance column sizes were found to be normal.[63] However, despite minimal effects on the ocular dominance columns, functional deficits in the blurred eye were evident in both the atropinized and the naturally anisometropic eye, showing that shrinkage of ocular dominance columns alone cannot account for the functional deficits in amblyopia.

In parallel with the primate studies, Horton and Stryker[64] examined the width of ocular dominance columns in visual cortex of a human amblyope postmortem. They used staining for the metabolic enzyme cytochrome oxidase (CO), which is proportional to brain activity levels. Normal CO staining is continuous in layer 4C, the primary LGN input layers, because activity driven by the two eyes is about equal. If one eye is lost or damaged, the ocular dominance columns of the damaged eye become pale staining because they are less active without the driving input of the LGN. Horton and Stryker's patient was diagnosed as having anisometropia at age 5, developed amblyopia, and sustained damage to the optic nerve of his good eye several months before his death. The latter loss facilitated CO mapping of ocular dominance columns, which, as in the amblyopic monkey, were completely normal in width.

Although both eyes may drive roughly equal amounts of cortical territory, other changes in the visual cortex of persons with anisometropic amblyopia have been reported. In amblyopic monkeys, CO staining shows a pattern of dark bands that are centered on, but narrower than, the ocular dominance columns of both eyes. The dark bands are separated by narrow pale staining bands that straddle the borders between ocular dominance columns. These borders are zones of binocular processing in visual cortex, where information from the two eyes is combined. Reduced CO activity in these regions suggests that binocular activity is reduced, which may impair neuronal function in anisometropic amblyopia.[63]

Strabismus. Disruption of binocular interactions in visual cortex is also found, of course, in the amblyopia that develops following strabismus (i.e., the misalignment of the two eyes). This misalignment results in diplopia (double vision), which affected children may compensate for by fixating with one eye and suppressing vision from the other. Suppression of the deviated eye is most common, but in some cases suppression may alternate between normal and deviated eye. Both forms lead to amblyopia.

In experimental animals, strabismus can be induced by surgical manipulations of the extraocular muscles. Monkeys made strabismic as juveniles, like children, may develop amblyopia. The visual cortex of strabismic amblyopic monkeys shows structural changes somewhat different than those of anisometropic amblyopic monkeys.[41,62] In layer 4C, especially in the parvocellular recipient sublayer, alternating dark and light CO stripes are often seen, suggesting that suppression is causing the cortical territory of the deviated eye to be less active. The width of the dark and light columns are approximately equal, however, suggesting that cortical territory is not lost by the deviated eye. Approximately equally sized ocular dominance columns were also seen in a human with strabismic amblyopia, assessed with the CO method following loss of the fellow eye.[61] In this case anatomic markers of binocular deficits were seen, such as a reduced CO stain at the borders of ocular dominance columns. In strabismic monkeys, staining for the structural protein neurofilament and for myelin is also reduced at ocular dominance columns borders; curiously, Nissl staining for cell bodies is enhanced at the borders, although this appears to be the result of denser staining of individual cells and not of larger numbers of cells.[41]

Suppression after induction of strabismus is such a strong effect that it can be induced in adult animals, as well as in development.[62] In this study, adult monkeys were made strabismic, and the extent to which each animal fixated with either eye was noted. Animals that fixated with one eye exclusively, while suppressing the other, showed darker staining in the center of the ocular dominance columns of the fixating eye compared with the suppressed eye, both within layer 4 and in the superficial layers. The binocular border zones of both eyes' columns were pale, suggesting loss of binocular function. The ocular dominance columns as assessed by transport of anatomic tracers were of about equal width for the two eyes, as would be expected given the developmental studies and the fact that these animals were past the critical period for ocular dominance column modification. Animals that showed weak fixation preference, tending to alternate fixation between the deviated and nondeviated eye, did not show differential staining of ocular dominance columns for the

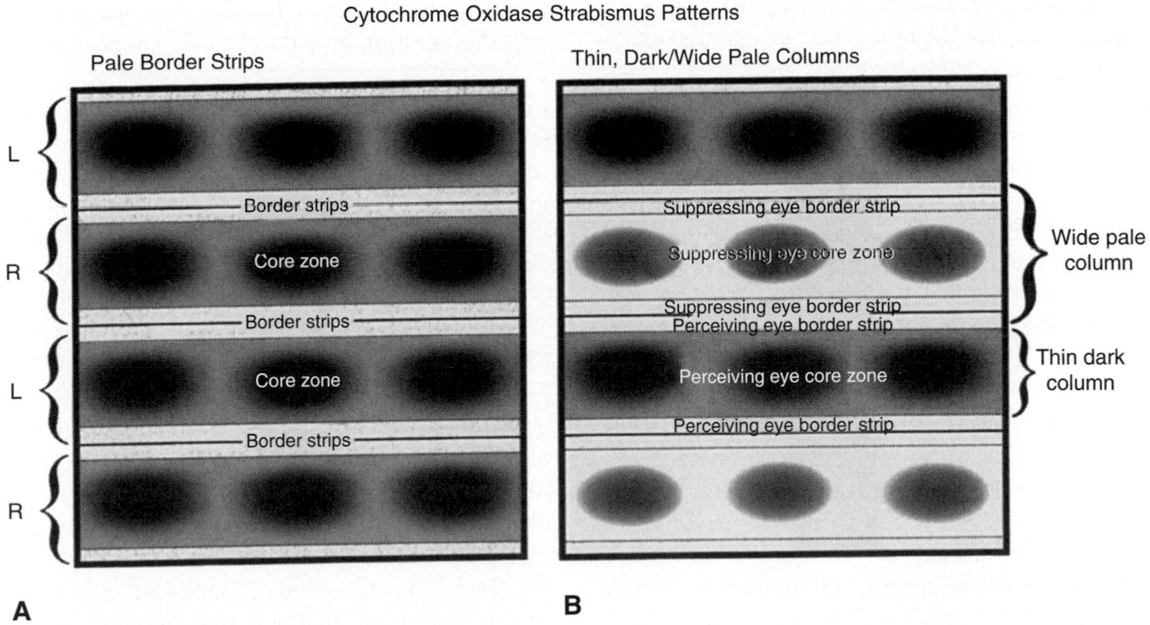

Cytochrome Oxidase Strabismus Patterns

FIGURE 31-4 Schematic diagrams showing the two patterns of cytochrome oxidase (CO) activity induced by experimental strabismus in monkeys. **A,** Pale border strips prevailed in regions of cortex where CO activity was lost in the binocular border strips, from disruption of ocular alignment, but metabolic activity remained strong in the monocular core zones serving each eye. This pattern is seen only in cortex representing the central 15 degrees and in monkeys with a weak fixation preference. **B,** Thin, dark alternating with wide pale columns were seen in cortex where CO activity was reduced in both eyes' binocular border strips and one eye's monocular core zones. Presumably, CO was lowered in the suppressed eye's core zones. This pattern was seen throughout the cortex in animals with a strong fixation preference but only in the peripheral cortex of those with a weak fixation preference. (From Horton JC, Hocking DR, Adams DL: *J Neurosci* 19:7111, 1999.)

two eyes in the representation of central vision, although they tended to suppress the temporal retina in the peripheral representation (Figure 31-4). Instead, pale borders, suggesting loss of binocular function, and dark monocular centers were seen for both sets of ocular dominance columns. Thus the CO staining patterns correlate with the monkeys' fixation patterns, suggesting that the reduced CO staining was truly a result of suppression.

The pattern of connectivity between cortical columns is also affected in strabismus. In visual cortex of normal monkeys, local, horizontal cortical connections link ocular dominance columns of both similar and opposite eye preference.[87] In animals made strabismic at birth, however, horizontal connections from one set of ocular dominance columns skip over columns from the other eye, preferentially targeting only columns of the same eye.[120]

Functional Deficits in Amblyopia and Strabismus.
In addition to the anatomic data on the visual cortex of persons with amblyopia, there is a wealth of information on the electrophysiologic changes that occur in amblyopia. The electrophysiologic changes often correlate with behavioral deficits in amblyopic patients and awake, behaving primates. Human psychophysics and primate electrophysiology reveal a deficit in spatial vision. Responses through the amblyopic eye have lower contrast sensitivity, lower spatial resolution, larger receptive fields, and lower optimal spatial frequency.[79,93] Animal studies suggest a correlation between the profundity of the amblyopia and electrophysiologic changes in neuronal responses recorded in area V1. However, not all of the loss of visual function can be explained by the electrophysiologic deficits in V1, suggesting that extrastriate visual areas are also affected in amblyopia.[78]

In anisometropic monkeys with severe amblyopia, it was reported that the amblyopic eye was able to drive fewer neurons than the nonamblyopic eye[93]; in persons with less severe anisometropia and in persons with strabismus, the number of cells driven by the two eyes was more nearly equal.[79] The physiologic results thus support the anatomic findings that ocular dominance columns of the amblyopic eye do not appreciably shrink, except in severe amblyopia.

In humans with amblyopia, stereopsis is often impaired, especially in persons with strabismus, but also in those with anisometropic amblyopia. Cortical binocularity is also greatly reduced in amblyopic monkeys. In normal monkeys, many cells outside of layer 4 can be driven by stimulating either eye, whereas in amblyopic monkeys, most neurons are excited by only one eye.[79,93] Interestingly, there is some evidence that inhibitory interactions may retain binocularity, so a cell excited by one eye can be inhibited by the other eye.[116] These types of interactions may be involved in generating the suppression seen in persons with strabismic amblyopia.

Abnormalities of neural activity have also been recorded in human visual cortex using evoked potentials and functional imaging techniques.[1,7] Reduced responses through the amblyopic eye were found in both primary visual cortex and in extrastriate cortex, including V2, V3, and V3A.[7] The difference in the magnitude of activation through the amblyopic eye compared with the normal eye did not correlate strongly with the behavioral deficit, which, as discussed previously, is greatest for high spatial frequencies and lower contrasts. Nevertheless, the greatest difference in responses between the two eyes was found at higher spatial frequencies, at least in some subjects.

Changes in Adulthood

During the critical period, monocular deprivation causes the ocular dominance columns devoted to the deprived eye to undergo substantial shrinkage (see Figure 31-2). This led to the notion that experience-dependent changes were possible only during the development of the visual system (i.e., before the closure of the critical period). However, whereas some effects, such as the expansion and shrinkage of ocular dominance columns, are possible only during the critical period, other effects of visual deprivation are evident in the mature visual cortex. Namely, if an adult primate is subjected to monocular deprivation or even more subtle forms of deprivation, such as in the example of suppression following strabismus given previously, the activity of neurons is dramatically reduced and a measurable loss of CO activity associated with the deprived eye is present in the LGN and V1.[55-59,62,71] Metabolic activity and synaptic connections play an important role in maintaining the structural and functional integrity of neurons within the adult central nervous system (CNS).[24] A loss of afferent connections is

known to cause target neurons to atrophy and undergo transneuronal degeneration.[51,73,101] In the clinical setting, retinal diseases in which photoreceptors or retinal ganglion cells are damaged may cause a reduction in visually evoked neuronal activity and may thus cause an associated loss of neurons in the target nuclei of the adult CNS. By the same logic, a surgical or laser procedure that affects the inner retina may also result in an associated loss or change in the adult CNS.

Glaucoma. Primary open-angle glaucoma is an example of retinal disease in which elevated intraocular pressure (IOP) causes degenerative effects on the optic nerve and retinal ganglion cells.[105-107] Although the site of primary damage is at the level of the retinal ganglion cell axon, transneuronal changes have been seen at the level of the LGN and V1. With use of a primate model of glaucoma, studies have shown that unilateral elevated IOP affects the size, density, and number of neurons in the LGN.[125] Both magnocellular and parvocellular layers are affected, but there appears to be a slightly greater loss in the magnocellular layers.[21,26,121,125] Transneuronal degenerative effects caused by elevated IOP also include a loss of immunoreactivity for parvalbumin, a calcium-binding protein of projection neurons in the LGN.[129] The most likely explanation for these degenerative effects is that elevated IOP causes a reduction of metabolic activity along the retinogeniculate pathway. In fact, decreased metabolic activity of LGN neurons after elevated IOP was observed with use of CO histochemistry, in which lighter CO staining in the LGN neurons correlates with a decrease in their metabolic activity.[26]

Loss of activity is also evident beyond the LGN, in the primary visual cortex, V1. The LGN projects to layer 4C and to the CO blobs in layers 2 and 3 of V1. After unilateral elevated IOP, layer 4C contains a series of dark- and light-staining CO bands, which represent the ocular dominance columns of the normal (dark CO) and elevated IOP (light CO) eye[27,82] (Figure 31-5, *D*, *F*, and *H*). The CO blobs overlying the ocular dominance columns of the glaucomatous eye also demonstrate a shrinkage and reduction in CO staining (Figure 31-5, *E* and *G*). A time-course study revealed that CO staining is affected in layer 4C first and later in the CO blobs of layers 2 and 3.[82]

Pan-Retinal Photocoagulation. Laser photocoagulation is used to treat several disorders of the retina,

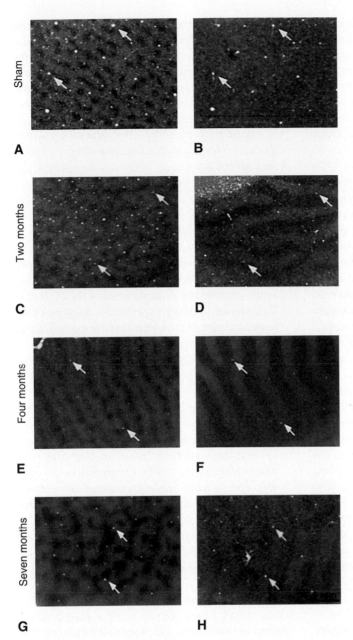

FIGURE 31-5   Cytochrome oxidase (CO)–stained tangential sections through layers 2 and 3 and 4C of primary visual cortex in sham operated (**A, B**), 2 months (**C, D**), 4 months (**E, F**) and 7 months (**G, H**) after elevated intraocular pressure (IOP). Alignment between pairs of tangential sections is shown by the *arrows,* which point to the cross sections of penetrating blood vessels. The CO blob pattern seen in the sham operated (**A**) and at 2 months after elevated IOP (**C**) differ from the pattern seen at 4 months (**E**) and 7 months after elevated IOP (**G**). At 4 and 7 months after elevated IOP, rows of pale shrunken CO blobs alternate with rows of robust CO blobs. In layer 4, alternating rows of light (elevated IOP) and dark (normal eye) CO bands are seen starting at 2 months after elevated IOP (**D**) to 7 months after elevated IOP (**F, H**). (From Lam D: Cortical consequences of elevated intraocular pressure in a primate model of glaucoma, master's thesis, British Columbia, 2001, University of British Columbia.)

including proliferative diabetic retinopathy. In a recent study, pan-retinal photocoagulation (PRP) treatment analogous to the Diabetic Retinopathy Study Research Group (DRS/ETDRS) protocol, was performed on one eye of normal monkeys.[38,89] Several hundred laser spots were placed in the mid-peripheral retina, extending from 20 to 50 degrees from the fovea. Animals were sacrificed at 20 hours, 12 days, 6 months, and 13 months after PRP. Retinal histology revealed that the predominant damage occurred in the outer nuclear layer, with loss of photoreceptors. Retinal ganglion cells appeared to

be spared. The visual cortex of these monkeys was assessed for reduction of metabolic activity with use of CO histochemistry and immunohistochemistry for Zif-268, an immediate early gene product shown to be expressed in neurons in an activity-dependent manner.[22] PRP resulted in a reduction of Zif-268 immunostaining (at 20 hours after PRP) and CO activity (at 12 days and 6 month after PRP) in the lasered eye's ocular dominance columns in approximately 50% of the peripheral visual field representation of area V1. Reduction of CO activity in the cortical representation of both the laser and interlaser sites was present and suggests that the extent of the visual field damage seen in the visual cortex is greater than the site occupied by the laser burn. Whether the increase in the extent of the visual field damage is caused by central, cortical mechanisms is unknown. However, another possible explanation is that PRP causes greater damage, as a result of indirect photochemical injury, than that represented by the visible retinal scars.[89,100]

Redistribution of Cortical Plasticity Markers. How does the adult brain respond to the reduction in neural activity associated with visual deprivation? What role does cortical plasticity, the ability of neurons to regain function after loss of sensory inputs, play in the mature cortex? Several studies have addressed these issues in both sensory and motor systems.[16,23,43] In the visual cortical studies after elevated IOP or PRP mentioned previously, CO staining was combined with an immunohistochemical survey of several neurochemicals.[82,89] Immunohistochemical levels of synaptophysin, a synaptic vesicle protein, and growth-associated protein (GAP-43), an axonal growth cone protein, were both found to be higher in V1 after elevated IOP or after PRP.* Because synaptophysin and GAP-43 are normally expressed at low levels in adult brain and have been implicated in neuronal remodeling, it is possible that their upregulation represents a mechanism by which the adult brain could respond to visual deprivation.[74,88,95,96,112] Combined with earlier studies, these results suggest that synaptic and axonal connections reorganize and rewire in the visual cortex of adult primates in response to reduced neural activity associated with visual deprivation.†

KEY POINTS

- Visual deprivation can have profound effects, both functionally and structurally, on visual cortical neurons.
- Experience-dependent modifications of cortical ocular dominance, orientation preference, and direction preference can be made within a so-called critical period during early postnatal development, but not thereafter in adult visual cortex.
- Ocular dominance plasticity, although caused by competition between LGN afferents, is dependent on normal activity of cortical neurons; cortical neurons actively choose to maintain termi-

nals driven through the open eye at the expense of terminals driven through the deprived eye.
- Ascending projections from subcortical centers can modulate synaptic plasticity in cortex by release of serotonin, acetylcholine, and noradrenaline. These act through various second-messenger systems in cortical neurons.
- Neurotrophins have also been shown to play important roles in visual cortex plasticity.
- Amblyopia is a disease of the development of the central visual system. It is caused by degraded vision (e.g., occlusion, anisometropia, strabismus) during a critical period and results in loss of visual acuity in adulthood.
- Ocular dominance column width in primary visual cortex is not usually altered in amblyopia. Instead, the borders of ocular dominance columns, normally zones of binocular processing, are affected.
- Functionally, the selectivity and sensitivity of responses through the amblyopic eye are degraded, and there are fewer binocular interactions.
- Even in adults, disruptions in retinal activity can lead to transneuronal changes in the LGN and in visual cortex.
- Increased IOP, as occurs in glaucoma, causes a reduction in metabolic activity in the LGN and a decrease in neuronal size and number in the denervated laminas. Both increased IOP and laser photocoagulation, which damages mostly photoreceptors while leaving ganglion cells intact, lead to reduced activity in the ocular dominance columns of the affected eye in V1.
- After visual deprivation, molecules associated with axonal growth and remodeling upregulate in V1 of adult animals.

ACKNOWLEDGMENTS

Qiang Gu is a joint scholar of British Columbia Health Research Foundation and Vancouver Hospital and Health Sciences Center.

REFERENCES

1. Anderson SJ, Holliday IE, Harding GF: Assessment of cortical dysfunction in human strabismic amblyopia using magnetoencephalography (MEG), *Vis Res* 39:1723, 1999.
2. Antonini A, Stryker MP: Rapid remodeling of axonal arbors in the visual cortex, *Science* 260:1819, 1993.
3. Baekleandt V et al: Alterations in GAP-43 and synapsin immunoreactivity provide evidence for synaptic reorganization in adult cat dorsal lateral geniculate nucleus following retinal lesions, *Eur J Neurosci* 6:754, 1994.
4. Baekleandt V et al: Long-term effects of retinal lesions on growth-associated protein 43 (GAP-43) expression in the visual system of adult cats, *J Neurosci Lett* 208:113, 1996.

---

*References 10, 11, 17, 45, 82, 89, 90, 115, 117, 123.
†References 3, 4, 23, 43, 56, 58, 118.

5. Baker F, Grigg P, Von Noorden G: Effects of visual deprivation and strabismus on the response of neurons in the visual cortex of the monkey, including studies on the striate and prestriate cortex in the normal animal, *Brain Res* 66:185, 1974.

6. Barlow HB, Pettigrew JD: Lack of specificity of neurones in the visual cortex of young kittens, *J Physiol* 218:98P, 1971.

7. Barnes GR et al: The cortical deficit in humans with strabismic amblyopia, *J Physiol* 533:281, 2001.

8. Bear MF, Singer W: Modulation of visual cortical plasticity by acetylcholine and noradrenaline, *Nature* 320:172, 1986.

9. Beaver CJ et al: Cyclic AMP-dependent protein kinase mediates ocular dominance shifts in cat visual cortex, *Nat Neurosci* 4:159, 2001.

10. Benowitz LI et al: Anatomical distribution of the growth-associated protein GAP-43/B-50 in the adult rat brain, *J Neurosci* 8:339, 1988.

11. Benowitz LI et al: Localization of the growth-associated phosphoprotein GAP-43 (B-50, F1) in the human cerebral cortex, *J Neurosci* 9:990, 1989.

12. Berardi N et al: Monocular deprivation effects in the rat visual cortex and lateral geniculate nucleus are prevented by nerve growth factor (NGF): I. Visual cortex, *Proc R Soc Lond B Biol Sci* 251:17, 1993.

13. Berman N, Daw NW: Comparison of the critical periods for monocular and directional deprivation in cats, *J Physiol* 265:249, 1977.

14. Blakemore C: Developmental factors in the formation of feature extracting neurons. In Worden F, Schmitt F (eds): *The neurosciences, third study program,* Cambridge, Mass, 1994, MIT Press.

15. Blakemore C, Cooper GF: Development of the brain depends on the visual environment, *Nature* 228:477, 1970.

16. Bloom F: CNS plasticity: a survey of opportunities. In Bignami A et al (eds): *Central nervous system plasticity and repair,* New York, 1985, Raven Press.

17. Buckley KM, Floor E, Kelly RB: Cloning and sequence analysis of cDNA encoding p38, a major synaptic vesicle protein, *J Cell Biol* 105:2447, 1987.

18. Cabelli RJ, Hohn A, Shatz CJ: Inhibition of ocular dominance column formation by infusion of NT-4/5 or BDNF, *Science* 267:1662, 1995.

19. Cabelli RJ et al: Blockade of endogenous ligands of trkB inhibits formation of ocular dominance columns, *Neuron* 19:63, 1997.

20. Carmignoto G et al: Effects of nerve growth factor on neuronal plasticity of the kitten visual cortex, *J Physiol* 464:343, 1993.

21. Chaturvedi N, Hedley-Whyte ET, Dreyer EB: Lateral geniculate nucleus in glaucoma, *Am J Ophthalmol* 116:182, 1993.

22. Chaudhuri A, Matsubara JA, Cynader MS: Neuronal activity in primate visual cortex assessed by immunostaining for the transcription factor Zif268, *Vis Neurosci* 12:35, 1995.

23. Chino YM: Adult plasticity in the visual system, *Can J Physiol Pharmacol* 73:1323, 1995.

24. Cowan W: Anterograde and retrograde transneuronal degeneration in the central and peripheral nervous system. In Ebbesson S, Nauta W (eds): *Contemporary research methods in neuroanatomy,* New York, 1970, Springer-Verlag.

25. Crawford ML et al: Physiological consequences of unilateral and bilateral eye closure in macaque monkeys: some further observations, *Brain Res* 84:150, 1975.

26. Crawford ML et al: Glaucoma in primates: cytochrome oxidase reactivity in parvo- and magnocellular pathways, *Invest Ophthalmol Vis Sci* 41:1791, 2000.

27. Crawford ML et al: Experimental glaucoma in primates: changes in cytochrome oxidase blobs in V1 cortex, *Invest Ophthalmol Vis Sci* 42:358, 2001.

28. Cynader M, Berman N, Hein A: Cats reared in stroboscopic illumination: effects on receptive fields in visual cortex, *Proc Natl Acad Sci USA* 70:1353, 1973.

29. Cynader M, Berman N, Hein A: Cats raised in a one-directional world: effects on receptive fields in visual cortex and superior colliculus, *Exp Brain Res* 22:267, 1975.

30. Cynader M, Chernenko G: Abolition of direction selectivity in the visual cortex of the cat, *Science* 193:504, 1976.

31. Cynader M, Timney BN, Mitchell DE: Period of susceptibility of kitten visual cortex to the effects of monocular deprivation extends beyond six months of age, *Brain Res* 191:545, 1980.

32. Daniels JD, Norman JL, Pettigrew JD: Biases for oriented moving bars in lateral geniculate nucleus neurons of normal and stripe-reared cats, *Exp Brain Res* 29:155, 1977.

33. Daw N: *Visual development,* New York, 1995, Plenum Press.

34. Daw NW, Ariel M: Properties of monocular and directional deprivation, *J Neurophysiol* 44:280, 1980.

35. Daw NW, Berman NE, Ariel M: Interaction of critical periods in the visual cortex of kittens, *Science* 199:565, 1978.

36. Daw NW, Wyatt HJ: Kittens reared in a unidirectional environment: evidence for a critical period, *J Physiol* 257:155, 1976.

37. Daw NW et al: Critical period for monocular deprivation in the cat visual cortex, *J Neurophysiol* 67:197, 1992.

38. Diabetic Retinopathy Study Research Group: Diabetic retinopathy study: report 6. Design, methods and baseline results, *Invest Ophthalmol Vis Sci* 21:149, 1981.

39. Domenici L et al: Antibodies to nerve growth factor (NGF) prolong the sensitive period for monocular deprivation in the rat, *Neuroreport* 5:2041, 1994.

40. Fagiolini M et al: Functional postnatal development of the rat primary visual cortex and the role of visual experience: dark rearing and monocular deprivation, *Vis Res* 34:709, 1994.

41. Fenstemaker SB, Kiorpes L, Movshon JA: Effects of experimental strabismus on the architecture of macaque monkey striate cortex, *J Comp Neurol* 438:300, 2001.

42. Galuske RA et al: Differential effects of neurotrophins on ocular dominance plasticity in developing and adult cat visual cortex, *Eur J Neurosci* 12:3315, 2000.

43. Gilbert CD: Adult cortical dynamics, *Physiol Rev* 78:467, 1998.

44. Gordon JA, Stryker MP: Experience-dependent plasticity of binocular responses in the primary visual cortex of the mouse, *J Neurosci* 16:3274, 1996.

45. Goslin K et al: Development of neuronal polarity: GAP-43 distinguishes axonal from dendritic growth cones, *Nature* 336:672, 1988.

46. Gu Q, Liu Y, Cynader MS: Nerve growth factor-induced ocular dominance plasticity in adult cat visual cortex, *Proc Natl Acad Sci USA* 91:8408, 1994.

47. Gu Q, Singer W: Effects of intracortical infusion of anticholinergic drugs on neuronal plasticity in kitten striate cortex, *Eur J Neurosci* 5:475, 1993.

48. Gu Q, Singer W: Involvement of serotonin in developmental plasticity of kitten visual cortex, *Eur J Neurosci* 7:1146, 1995.

49. Hanover JL et al: Brain-derived neurotrophic factor overexpression induces precocious critical period in mouse visual cortex, *J Neurosci* 19:RC40, 1999.

50. Hata Y et al: Brain-derived neurotrophic factor expands ocular dominance columns in visual cortex in monocularly deprived and nondeprived kittens but does not in adult cats, *J Neurosci* 20:RC57, 2000.

51. Headon MP, Sloper JJ, Powell TP: Initial hypertrophy of cells in undeprived laminae of the lateral geniculate nucleus of the monkey following early monocular visual deprivation, *Brain Res* 238:439, 1982.

52. Hebb D: *The organization of behaviour,* New York, 1949, Wiley.

53. Heggelund P, Imamura K, Kasamatsu T: Reduced binocularity in the noradrenaline-infused striate cortex of acutely anesthetized and paralyzed, otherwise normal cats, *Exp Brain Res* 68:593, 1987.

54. Hendrickson AE et al: Effects of early unilateral blur on the macaque's visual system. II. Anatomical observations, *J Neurosci* 7:1327, 1987.

55. Hendry SH: Delayed reduction in GABA and GAD immunoreactivity of neurons in the adult monkey dorsal lateral geniculate nucleus following monocular deprivation or enucleation, *Exp Brain Res* 86:47, 1991.

56. Hendry SH, Jones EG: Reduction in number of immunostained GABAergic neurones in deprived-eye dominance columns of monkey area 17, *Nature* 320:750, 1986.

57. Hendry SH, Jones EG: Activity-dependent regulation of GABA expression in the visual cortex of adult monkeys, *Neuron* 1:701, 1988.

58. Hendry SH, Kennedy MB: Immunoreactivity for a calmodulin-dependent protein kinase is selectively increased in macaque striate cortex after monocular deprivation, *Proc Natl Acad Sci USA* 83:1536, 1986.

59. Hendry SH et al: Distribution and plasticity of immunocytochemically localized GABAA receptors in adult monkey visual cortex, *J Neurosci* 10:2438, 1990.

60. Hirsch HV, Spinelli DN: Visual experience modifies distribution of horizontally and vertically oriented receptive fields in cats, *Science* 168:869, 1970.

61. Horton JC, Hocking DR: Pattern of ocular dominance columns in human striate cortex in strabismic amblyopia, *Vis Neurosci* 13:787, 1996.

62. Horton JC, Hocking DR, Adams DL: Metabolic mapping of suppression scotomas in striate cortex of macaques with experimental strabismus, *J Neurosci* 19:7111, 1999.

63. Horton JC, Hocking DR, Kiorpes L: Pattern of ocular dominance columns and cytochrome oxidase activity in a macaque monkey with naturally occurring anisometropic amblyopia, *Vis Neurosci* 14:681, 1997.

64. Horton JC, Stryker MP: Amblyopia induced by anisometropia without shrinkage of ocular dominance columns in human striate cortex, *Proc Natl Acad Sci USA* 90:5494, 1993.

65. Huang ZJ et al: BDNF regulates the maturation of inhibition and the critical period of plasticity in mouse visual cortex, *Cell* 98:739, 1999.

66. Hubel D, Wiesel T: Receptive fields, binocular interaction and functional architecture in cat's visual cortex, *J Physiol* 160:109, 1962.

67. Hubel D, Wiesel T: Receptive fields of cells in striate cortex of very young, visually inexperienced kittens, *J Neurophysiol* 26:994, 1963.

68. Hubel DH, Wiesel TN: The period of susceptibility to the physiological effects of unilateral eye closure in kittens, *J Physiol* 206:419, 1970.

69. Hubel DH, Wiesel TN, LeVay S: Plasticity of ocular dominance columns in monkey striate cortex, *Philos Trans R Soc Lond B Biol Sci* 278:377, 1977.

70. Issa NP et al: The critical period for ocular dominance plasticity in the Ferret's visual cortex, *J Neurosci* 19:6965, 1999.

71. Jones EG et al: Activity-dependent regulation of gene expression in adult monkey visual cortex, *Cold Spring Harb Symp Quant Biol* 55:481, 1990.

72. Jones KR, Spear PD, Tong L: Critical periods for effects of monocular deprivation: differences between striate and extrastriate cortex, *J Neurosci* 4:2543, 1984.

73. Kalil R, Fedynyshyn J: Axotomy induces two cytologically distinct types of cell death in the dorsal lateral geniculate nucleus (LGN) of the adult rat, *Soc Neurosci Abstr* 24:1303, 1998.

74. Kanus P, Betz H, Rehm H: Expression of synaptophysin during postnatal development of the mouse brain, *J Neurochem* 47:1302, 1986.

75. Kasamatsu T, Ohashi T, Imamura K: Lithium reduces ocular dominance plasticity in kitten visual cortex, *Brain Res* 558:157, 1991.

76. Kasamatsu T, Pettigrew JD: Depletion of brain catecholamines: failure of ocular dominance shift after monocular occlusion in kittens, *Science* 194:206, 1976.

77. Kasamatsu T, Shirokawa T: Involvement of beta-adrenoreceptors in the shift of ocular dominance after monocular deprivation, *Exp Brain Res* 59:507, 1985.

78. Kiorpes L, McKee SP: Neural mechanisms underlying amblyopia, *Curr Opin Neurobiol* 9:480, 1999.

79. Kiorpes L et al: Neuronal correlates of amblyopia in the visual cortex of macaque monkeys with experimental strabismus and anisometropia, *J Neurosci* 18:6411, 1998.

80. Kleinschmidt A, Bear MF, Singer W: Blockade of "NMDA" receptors disrupts experience-dependent plasticity of kitten striate cortex, *Science* 238:355, 1987.

81. Kojic L et al: Columnar distribution of serotonin-dependent plasticity within kitten striate cortex, *Proc Natl Acad Sci USA* 97:1841, 2000.

82. Lam D: Cortical consequences of elevated intraocular pressure in a primate model of glaucoma, master's thesis, British Columbia, 2001, University of British Columbia.

83. LeVay S, Wiesel TN, Hubel DH: The development of ocular dominance columns in normal and visually deprived monkeys, *J Comp Neurol* 191:1, 1980.

84. Lodovichi C et al: Effects of neurotrophins on cortical plasticity: same or different? *J Neurosci* 20:2155, 2000.

85. Maffei L et al: Nerve growth factor (NGF) prevents the shift in ocular dominance distribution of visual cortical neurons in monocularly deprived rats, *J Neurosci* 12:4651, 1992.

86. Malach R, Ebert R, Van Sluyters RC: Recovery from effects of brief monocular deprivation in the kitten, *J Neurophysiol* 51:538, 1984.

87. Malach R et al: Relationship between intrinsic connections and functional architecture revealed by optical imaging and in vivo targeted biocytin injections in primate striate cortex, *Proc Natl Acad Sci USA* 90:10469, 1993.

88. Masliah E et al: Reactive synaptogenesis assessed by synaptophysin immunoreactivity is associated with GAP-43 in the dentate gyrus of the adult rat, *Exp Neurobiol* 113:131, 1991.

89. Matsubara J et al: The effects of panretinal photocoagulation on the primary visual cortex of the adult monkey, *Trans Am Ophthal Soc* 99:71, 2001.

90. Meiri KF, Pfenninger KH, Willard MB: Growth-associated protein, GAP-43, a polypeptide that is induced when neurons extend axons, is a component of growth cones and corresponds to pp46, a major polypeptide of a subcellular fraction enriched in growth cones, *Proc Natl Acad Sci USA* 83:3537, 1986.

91. Mioche L, Singer W: Chronic recordings from single sites of kitten striate cortex during experience-dependent modifications of receptive-field properties, *J Neurophysiol* 62:185, 1989.

92. Movshon JA, Dursteler MR: Effects of brief periods of unilateral eye closure on the kitten's visual system, *J Neurophysiol* 40:1255, 1977.

93. Movshon JA et al: Effects of early unilateral blur on the macaque's visual system: III. Physiological observations, *J Neurosci* 7:1340, 1987.

94. Mower GD et al: Dark rearing prolongs physiological but not anatomical plasticity of the cat visual cortex, *J Comp Neurol* 235:448, 1985.

95. Nelson RB et al: Gradients of protein kinase C substrate phosphorylation in primate visual system peak in visual memory storage areas, *Brain Res* 416:387, 1987.

96. Neve RL et al: The neuronal growth-associated protein GAP-43 (B-50, F1): neuronal specificity, developmental regulation and regional distribution of the human and rat mRNAs, *Brain Res* 388:177, 1987.

97. Olson CR, Freeman RD: Progressive changes in kitten striate cortex during monocular vision, *J Neurophysiol* 38:26, 1975.

98. Olson CR, Freeman RD: Profile of the sensitive period for monocular deprivation in kittens, *Exp Brain Res* 39:17, 1980.

99. Olson CR, Pettigrew JD: Single units in visual cortex of kittens reared in stroboscopic illumination, *Brain Res* 70:189, 1974.

100. Parver LM: Photochemical injury to the foveomacula of the monkey eye following argon blue-green panretinal photocoagulation, *Trans Am Ophthalmol Soc* 98:365, 2000.

101. Pearson HE, Stoffler DJ: Retinal ganglion cell degeneration following loss of postsynaptic target neurons in the dorsal lateral geniculate nucleus of the adult cat, *Exp Neurol* 116:163, 1992.

102. Peck CK, Blakemore C: Modification of single neurons in the kitten's visual cortex after brief periods of monocular visual experience, *Exp Brain Res* 22:57, 1975.

103. Pettigrew JD, Kasamatsu T: Local perfusion of noradrenaline maintains visual cortical plasticity, *Nature* 271:761, 1978.

104. Pizzorusso T et al: TrkA activation in the rat visual cortex by antirat trkA IgG prevents the effect of monocular deprivation, *Eur J Neurosci* 11:204, 1999.

105. Quigley HA, Addicks EM: Chronic experimental glaucoma in primates: II. Effect of extended intraocular pressure elevation on optic nerve head and axonal transport, *Invest Ophthalmol Vis Sci* 19:137, 1980.

106. Quigley HA, Dunkelberger GR, Green WR: Retinal ganglion cell atrophy correlated with automated perimetry in human eyes with glaucoma, *Am J Ophthalmol* 107:453, 1989.

107. Quigley HA et al: Chronic glaucoma selectively damages large optic nerve fibers, *Invest Ophthalmol Vis Sci* 28:913, 1987.

108. Ramoa AS, Paradiso MA, Freeman RD: Blockade of intracortical inhibition in kitten striate cortex: effects on receptive field properties and associated loss of ocular dominance plasticity, *Exp Brain Res* 73:285, 1988.

109. Rauschecker JP: Neuronal mechanisms of developmental plasticity in the cat's visual system, *Hum Neurobiol* 3:109, 1984.

110. Reiter HO, Stryker MP: Neural plasticity without postsynaptic action potentials: less-active inputs become dominant when kitten visual cortical cells are pharmacologically inhibited, *Proc Natl Acad Sci USA* 85:3623, 1988.

111. Reiter HO, Waitzman DM, Stryker MP: Cortical activity blockade prevents ocular dominance plasticity in the kitten visual cortex, *Exp Brain Res* 65:182, 1986.

112. Schreyer DJ, Skene JH: Fate of GAP-43 in ascending spinal axons of DRG neurons after peripheral nerve injury: delayed accumulation and correlation with regenerative potential, *J Neurosci* 11:3738, 1991.

113. Shatz CJ, Stryker MP: Ocular dominance in layer IV of the cat's visual cortex and the effects of monocular deprivation, *J Physiol* 281:267, 1978.

114. Shaw C, Cynader M: Disruption of cortical activity prevents ocular dominance changes in monocularly deprived kittens, *Nature* 308:731, 1984.

115. Skene JH et al: A protein induced during nerve growth (GAP-43) is a major component of growth-cone membranes, *Science* 233:783, 1986.

116. Smith EL III et al: Residual binocular interactions in the striate cortex of monkeys reared with abnormal binocular vision, *J Neurophysiol* 78:1353, 1997.

117. Sudhof TC et al: A synaptic vesicle protein with a novel cytoplasmic domain and four transmembrane regions, *Science* 238:1142, 1987.

118. Tighilet B, Hashikawa T, Jones EG: Cell- and lamina-specific expression and activity-dependent regulation of type II calcium/calmodulin-dependent protein kinase isoforms in monkey visual cortex, *J Neurosci* 18:2129, 1998.

119. Tretter F, Cynader M, Singer W: Modification of direction selectivity of neurons in the visual cortex of kittens, *Brain Res* 84:143, 1975.

120. Tychsen L, Burkhalter A: Neuroanatomic abnormalities of primary visual cortex in macaque monkeys with infantile esotropia: preliminary results, *J Pediatr Ophthalmol Strabismus* 32:323, 1995.

121. Vickers JC et al: Magnocellular and parvocellular visual pathways are both affected in a macaque monkey model of glaucoma, *Aust NZ J Ophthalmol* 25:239, 1997.

122. Vital-Durand F, Jeannerod M: Role of visual experience in the development of optokinetic response in kittens, *Exp Brain Res* 20:297, 1974.

123. Voigt T, De Lima AD, Beckmann M: Synaptophysin immunohistochemistry reveals inside-out pattern of early synaptogenesis in ferret cerebral cortex, *J Comp Neurol* 330:48, 1993.

124. Wang Y, Gu Q, Cynader MS: Blockade of serotonin-2C receptors by mesulergine reduces ocular dominance plasticity in kitten visual cortex, *Exp Brain Res* 114:321, 1997.

125. Weber AJ et al: Experimental glaucoma and cell size, density, and number in the primate lateral geniculate nucleus, *Invest Ophthalmol Vis Sci* 41:1370, 2000.

126. Wiesel T, Hubel D: Effects of visual deprivation on morphology and physiology of cells in the cat's lateral geniculate body, *J Neurophysiol* 26:978, 1963.

127. Wiesel T, Hubel D: Single-cell responses in striate cortex of kittens deprived of vision in one eye, *J Neurophysiol* 26:1003, 1963.

128. Wiesel TN, Hubel DH: Comparison of the effects of unilateral and bilateral eye closure on cortical unit responses in kittens, *J Neurophysiol* 28:1029, 1965.

129. Yucel YH et al: Loss of neurons in magnocellular and parvocellular layers of the lateral geniculate nucleus in glaucoma, *Arch Ophthalmol* 118:378, 2000.

SECTION 12

PUPIL

RANDY KARDON

CHAPTER 32

THE PUPIL

RANDY KARDON

The pupillary opening appears to occupy a central location, but if carefully measured, it is actually situated slightly inferior and nasal to the center of the cornea. The major functions of the pupil are outlined in Figure 32-1 and are summarized as follows.

First, pupil movement in response to changing light intensity aids in optimizing retinal illumination to maximize visual perception. In dim light, dilation of the pupil provides an immediate means for maximizing the number of photons reaching the retina, which in turn supplements the slower dark adaptive mechanisms involving retinal gain control at the photoreceptor and bipolar cell level. With exposure to bright light, pupil constriction can reduce retinal illumination by up to 1.5 log units within 1 to 2 seconds. Although this reduction in retinal illumination is only a portion of the 12 log unit range of light sensitivity of the retina, it provides an important and immediate contribution to early light adaptation.[47] Patients with a fixed immobile pupil are usually symptomatic during an abrupt change in illumination; they may be photophobic when they are subjected to sudden increases in light, and they may not be able to discern objects in their environment when they first enter dim lighting conditions. These symptoms are described by patients with an immobile pupil because compensatory retinal adaptation is not fast enough. This emphasizes the important role of the pupil in optimizing visual perception in a timely fashion over a wide range of lighting conditions of the environment.

Second, the diameter of the pupil can also contribute to improving (up to a point) the image quality of the retina when the steady-state pupil diameter is small. A small pupil reduces the degree of chromatic and spherical aberration.[10,57] Part of the reason is that a smaller aperture size limits the light rays entering the optical system to the central cornea and lens, avoiding more peripheral portions of the cornea and lens, where aberrations are greater. In recent years, with the advent of refractive surgery of the cornea, the role of pupil diameter in controlling aberration in the optical system has become more clinically apparent. After refractive surgery, younger patients, who usually have larger pupils in dim light compared with older individuals, often experience bothersome symptoms of glare and image degradation, especially at night, as a result of optical aberrations. The area of the pupil is large enough in these patients to exceed the corneal optical zone of refractive surgery. Most refractive surgeons attempt to address this problem by carefully measuring the pupil diameter in dim lighting conditions preoperatively and then adjusting the optical zone of corneal refractive surgery according to pupil diameter. Despite these measurements, many patients still may experience glare and optical aberrations during dim lighting conditions. To this end, some refractive surgeons have found that topical drops that produce miosis may reduce pupil diameter enough in dim lighting conditions (without affecting accommodation) to alleviate the symptoms of aberration. There is a limit to the beneficial optical effects of a small pupil because constriction beyond a certain diameter results in image degradation as a result of increased diffraction and reduction of retinal illumination below an optimal level.[11] Therefore there exists an optimal range of pupil diameter for vision, and this size may vary somewhat, depending on the individual optical characteristics of a person's eye.

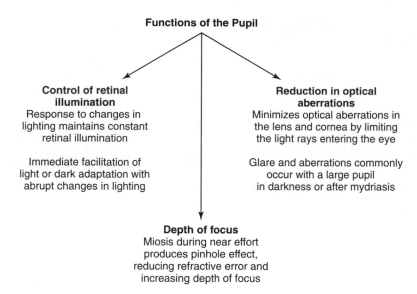

FIGURE 32-1   Functions of the pupil include control of retinal illumination, reduction in optical aberrations, and improved depth of focus.

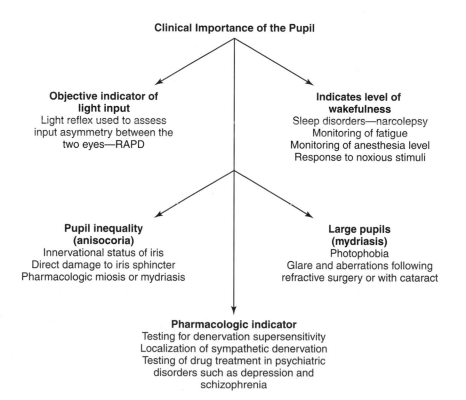

FIGURE 32-2   Clinical importance of the pupil. *RAPD,* Relative afferent pupillary defect.

Third, a small pupil increases the depth of focus of the eye's optical system, similar to the known pinhole effect of camera lenses used for photography.[9] When a subject views objects at near, not only the accommodation power of the eye changes but the near response of pupil contraction helps bring objects into better focus by increasing the depth of focus afforded by the smaller aperture size.

Besides the physiologic functions of the pupil explained earlier and outlined in Figure 32-1, the pupil diameter and its movement under different conditions also provide an important indicator used for clinical assessment of a patient. The clinical aspects of pupil function (Figure 32-2) consist of (1) pupil movement as an objective indicator of afferent input, (2) pupil diameter as an indicator of wakefulness, (3) pupil inequality as a reflection of autonomic nerve output to each iris, (4) the influence of pupil diameter on the optical properties of the eye, and (5) the pupil response to drugs as a means of monitoring pharmacologic effects.

The pupil acts as an objective indicator of the amount of light transduction by the visual system. In this sense the pupil can be used to monitor retinal light sensitivity. This is extremely useful in the clinical setting because the amount of transient pupil contraction to a light stimulus or the steady-state diameter of the pupil under constant illumination can reflect the health of the retina and optic nerve and may be used to detect disease. The most common clinical test for assessing input asymmetry between the two eyes is the alternating light test, commonly referred to as the *swinging flashlight test.* As a light is alternated back and forth between the right and left eyes, the clinician observes the pupil movements in response to the light. If the two eyes are matched with respect to retinal and optic nerve input, the pupil movements appear similar when either eye is stimulated. However, if one eye's input has been diminished because of disease affecting the retina or optic nerve, the pupil responses to light shown in that eye become noticeably less during the alternating light test. When this input asymmetry is observed during the alternating light test, it is called a *relative afferent pupillary defect* (RAPD): RAPDs are discussed in greater length in a subsequent portion of this chapter.

Pupil diameter can also be used to determine the extent of midbrain supranuclear inhibition, which is also related to an individual's state of wakefulness. An excited, aroused person will have larger-diameter pupils because of the increase in central inhibition of the parasympathetic nerves innervating the iris

sphincter, which originate in the midbrain, and the increase in sympathetic tone to the dilator muscle. Conversely, a sleepy individual, a fatigued individual, or one under the influence of general anesthesia or narcotics will have smaller pupils as a result of central disinhibition at the level of the midbrain. Careful monitoring of the diameter of the pupil in this setting may be clinically useful for ascertaining the presence of sleep disorders such as narcolepsy, the level of anesthesia, or the presence of narcotics. The extent of pupil dilation to sensory stimuli such as pain or sound may also serve as an objective indicator of how intact the sensory input is.

Inequality of the pupils, termed *anisocoria,* is another important clinical state of the pupils because it may represent autonomic nerve interruption to the iris from the sympathetic or parasympathetic nervous system, direct damage to the iris sphincter muscle, or pharmacologic exposure of the iris to mydriatic or miotic drugs. The clinical significance of anisocoria and the various causes of it are covered in more detail later in this chapter.

Large pupils may produce clinically significant visual symptoms in the form of aberrations in form and color of images, particularly at night or after dilating drops, when pupil diameter is largest. A large nonmobile pupil resulting from scarring, dilating drops, or damage to the iris sphincter muscle or its nerve supply may produce extreme sensitivity to light. This is because the normal function of the pupil in controlling retinal illumination is impaired.

The pupil may be used clinically as a pharmacologic indicator of peripheral or central drug effects. With topical delivery of drugs into each eye with eyedrops, the sensitivity of the iris sphincter or dilator muscle can be compared between the two eyes because, under normal conditions, the two eyes should be matched in their response. Dilute concentrations of cholinergic or adrenergic drops, which normally cause little, if any, pupil response, may produce asymmetric exaggerated mydriasis (adrenergic, sympathomimetic drugs) or constriction (cholinergic, parasympathetic drugs) if the iris has been deprived of its nerve innervation for as little as a few days. In cases of unilateral oculosympathetic nerve damage, topical drugs such as cocaine may be used to confirm the diagnosis. Once the diagnosis of an oculosympathetic lesion is confirmed, hydroxyamphetamine drops may be used a few days later to localize the lesion to the preganglionic or the postganglionic site along the sympathetic nervous system chain (covered in more detail later in this chapter). The pupil response to topical inhibitors of narcotics (naloxone) has also been used to study the effect of narcotic tolerance in addicted individuals. Pupillary responses to psychosensory stimuli may also be used in the near future to aid in the diagnosis and monitoring of treatment in psychiatric disorders such as depression and schizophrenia.

In this chapter the physiology of the normal pupil is discussed, and examples of abnormalities of pupil function are also shown to apply what is known about normal pupil physiology to understanding various pathologic states. The reader who is interested in pursuing these subjects in much greater detail is advised to consult the excellent book by Loewenfeld.[42]

The Neuronal Pathway of the Pupil Light Reflex and Near Pupil Response

To understand the major factors that can affect the diameter and movement of the pupil to various stimuli, it is important to know the basic neuronal pathway for the pupil light reflex and near response. This is schematically depicted in Figure 32-3. The pupil light reflex consists of three major divisions of neurons that integrate the light stimulus to produce a pupil contraction: (1) an afferent division, (2) an interneuron division, and (3) an efferent division.

The afferent division consists of retinal input from photoreceptors, bipolar neurons, and ganglion cells. Axons of retinal ganglion cells from each eye provide light input information that is conveyed by synapses to interneurons located in the pretectal olivary nucleus of the midbrain. In turn, these interneurons distribute pupil light input to neurons in the right and left Edinger-Westphal nuclei through crossed (decussating) and uncrossed (nondecussating) connections. From here, the neurons of the Edinger-Westphal nucleus send their preganglionic parasympathetic axons along the oculomotor nerve to synapse at the ciliary ganglion in each orbit. The neurons in the ciliary ganglion give rise to postganglionic parasympathetic axons that travel in the short ciliary nerves to the globe, where they synapse with the iris sphincter muscle.

The pupil constriction to a near stimulus involves activation of neurons in the rostral brainstem that relay their signal to the same Edinger-Westphal neurons that are activated in the light reflex. Therefore the efferent pathway for the near pupil constriction is the same as for the light reflex, but the input pathway to the Edinger-Westphal nucleus differs.

The integration of the pupil light reflex and pupil near response, including the anatomy of the involved neurons, their receptive field properties, and their response to various attributes of light stimuli, has been recently reviewed.[28] In the following sections, these neuronal pathways are summarized.

Afferent Arm of the Pupil Light Reflex

The neural integration of the pupil light reflex begins with the afferent pathway in the retina, consisting of the photoreceptors, bipolar cells, and ganglion cells. For many years, it was disputed whether it was the rods or cones that contribute to the pupil light reflex and whether these were the same photoreceptors as those contributing to visual perception. Extensive experimental and psychophysical work has shown that the neuronal pathways mediating the pupil light reflex and visual perception share the same photoreceptors. There are no separate photoreceptors for vision and different ones for the pupil light reflex. Because of this, almost all changes in stimulus condition that produce a difference in visual perception also produce a comparable change in pupil responsiveness. These include changes in retinal adaptation, wavelength of light, stimulus duration, and stimulus light intensity. In fact, in almost every way measured, the pupil responses to light parallel those of visual perception. For example, the wavelength-sensitivity profile of pupil threshold as the color of light is changed from blue to red exactly parallels the same wavelength-sensitivity profile of visual perception. The shift in sensitivity is also the same as the eye is changed from a condition of light adaptation to dark adaptation (Purkinje shift), providing further evidence that the same photoreceptors are used for both pupil and vision. Patients with various abnormalities of rods and cones can be shown to have the same deficits in color vision or lack of appropriate sensitivity change during dark adaptation when the results of visual threshold are compared with pupil threshold to light stimuli.[50] Both rods and cones contribute to the pupil light reflex, but to a different extent depending on the lighting conditions.

Under conditions of dark adaptation and in response to low-intensity lights, the pupil light reflex becomes a sensitive light meter and is mediated primarily by rods, giving rise to low-amplitude pupil contractions. However, with brighter light stimuli and under conditions of greater light adaptation, the cones dominate most of the pupil light reflex and give rise to larger pupil contractions, compared with rod input. Therefore the rods are primarily responsible

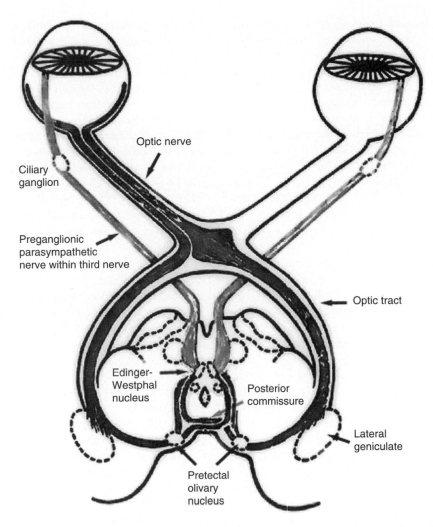

Optic nerve

Ciliary ganglion

Preganglionic parasympathetic nerve within third nerve

Optic tract

Edinger-Westphal nucleus

Posterior commissure

Lateral geniculate

Pretectal olivary nucleus

FIGURE 32-3   Diagram of the nerve pathways involved in the pupil light reflex. Afferent input from the nasal retina crosses to the contralateral side, and the pupil input from retinal ganglion cell axons exits the optic tract in the brachium of the superior colliculus to synapse at the pretectal olivary nucleus. The temporal retinal input from the same eye follows a similar course on the ipsilateral side. The neurons in the pretectal olivary nucleus send crossed and uncrossed fibers by way of the posterior commissure to the Edinger-Westphal nucleus on each side. From here, the preganglionic parasympathetic fibers travel with the oculomotor nerve and then synapse at the ciliary ganglion. The postganglionic parasympathetic neurons pass from the ciliary ganglion by way of the short ciliary nerves to the iris sphincter muscle.

for the pupil's ability to give rise to small contractions in response to low-intensity lights under conditions of dark adaptation—they provide a high sensitivity to the pupil light reflex at low light levels. The cones provide the input responsible for the larger pupil contractions that are easily observed under direct clinical observation, occurring at suprathreshold levels of light, mainly under photopic conditions. Loewenfeld[39] has summarized the extensive literature on this subject and should be consulted by the reader desiring a more complete discussion of this topic. It is also believed that the bipolar cells, which receive in-

put from the photoreceptors, are the same neurons providing input to the pupil light reflex as those mediating visual perception.

Although it appears that the pupil and visual systems share the same photoreceptor input (and presumably bipolar cell input), the story for ganglion cell input is far less clear. The ganglion cells are the first neurons in the afferent chain to give rise to action potentials (the photoreceptors and bipolar cells give rise to generator potentials). Over the years, many anatomic and physiologic studies have been carried out in an attempt to classify retinal ganglion cells on the basis of their cell body size, dendritic field, axonal diameter, and electric firing properties. This information has been collected in a number of species, most notably the cat and monkey. With use of histologic labeling techniques, the projections of the ganglion cell axons to the lateral geniculate body and midbrain have been studied. Loewenfeld[39] has summarized the properties of the major classes of ganglion cells in the retina and their projections. According to these studies, it appears that three main types of ganglion cells make up the primate retina: the α, β, and γ cells. In the cat these correspond to the Y, X, and W cells, respectively.

A separate class of ganglion cells (the primate γ cells and the cat W cells) appear to be primarily responsible for conveying the classic pupil light reflex input to the midbrain. These cells may also play a role in other visually evoked reflexes (e.g., eye position control), projecting to the superior colliculus and also to the accessory optic system. The γ cells have small cell bodies and thin, slowly conducting axons, with large-sized receptive fields. They respond primarily to incremental changes in light intensity and are relatively insensitive to movement. These cells project almost exclusively to the midbrain and not to the lateral geniculate nucleus. The ganglion cell type (γ cell) that mediates afferent pupil input is densest in the central retina. The ganglion cells in the central area also have more of a one-to-one relationship with photoreceptor and bipolar cells, in contrast to those in the peripheral retina, where many more photoreceptors and bipolar cells map to one ganglion cell (convergence). Therefore it is the central density of ganglion cells, their approximate one-to-one mapping with photoreceptors and bipolar cells, and their receptive field properties that account for the greater amplitude of pupil response to stimuli in the central visual field and the central field "weighting" of the pupil light reflex. It has been estimated that the number of ganglion cells conveying light input to the classic pupil light reflex pathway are far fewer than those primary conveying visual, perceptual input (approximately 1000 pupil ganglion cells compared with 1 million visual perception ganglion cells) (Paul Gamlin, personal communication, 1995).

As stated earlier, there appears to be a separate type of ganglion cell mediating the classic midbrain pupil light reflex. However, there is also evidence that ganglion cells conveying visual information to the occipital cortex may also play a role in modulation of pupil movement in response to different types of visual stimuli. For example, patients with isolated occipital infarcts have homonymous visual field defects that show corresponding pupil defects to small (2 degrees in diameter) focal lights presented to the same cortically blind visual field area. This phenomenon has been reported previously, but only recently has the correspondence between the shape characteristic of the homonymous pupil and visual field defect been fully appreciated.* This correspondence provides compelling evidence for a role of cortical mediation of the pupil light reflex when small, focal light stimuli are used. In addition, the pupil has also been shown to respond to changes in complex stimuli such as spatial frequency, motion, and contrast, providing additional evidence for a higher-level cortical process that is capable of mediating pupil contractions to visual stimuli.† Such evidence implies that other types of ganglion cells, in addition to the classic luminance responding cells that project to the midbrain, may also participate in the pupil reflex, perhaps the same ones that also mediate visual perception.

The Interneuron Arm of the Pupil Light Reflex

The ganglion cell axons conveying light input to the classic pupil light reflex pathway become separate from the rest of the ganglion cell axons at the distal portion of the optic tract before the lateral geniculate nucleus. As in the visual input pathway, the pupil ganglion cell axons from the nasal retina (temporal field) decussate at the chiasm to the opposite side, and the axons from the temporal retina (nasal field) stay on the same side. Therefore pupil ganglion cell axons from homonymous areas of the visual field (temporal field from the contralateral eye and nasal field from the ipsilateral eye) distribute within the optic tract. From there, they travel in the brachium of the superior colliculus and synapse in the midbrain with the next neurons in the light reflex located at the olivary pretectal nucleus. These neurons represent interneurons because they serve to integrate the afferent input coming from the retina with the efferent output of the pupil light reflex exiting the midbrain.

The receptive field properties of the pretectal neurons have recently been elucidated in the awake primate.[18,19] These interneurons are the "way-station" for the converging receptive field impulses of the retinal ganglion cells from the retina and are fewer in num-

---

*References 1, 3, 4, 12, 20-23, 26, 30, 44, 46.
†References 5, 6, 13, 49, 54, 58, 59.

ber, summating the ganglion cell input at this location. The receptive field of each pretectal neuron has been found to receive input from ganglion cells over a large area of retina (up to 20 degrees). Some of these neurons exhibit a "flat" response, firing equally well from input over its entire receptive field. However, another subset exhibits a "foveal-weighted" response, discharging at a higher frequency when a stimulus is placed near the center of the visual field (and receptive field of the neuron). This may partly explain why the pupil light reflex appears to be more sensitive to light coming from the center of the visual field.

Patients with damage to their central visual field have also been found to show an obvious decrease in the pupil light reflex in the affected eye compared with the fellow eye, which may relate to the receptive field properties of the pretectal interneurons. The pretectal neurons discharge at a frequency that is linear to the log of intensity of the light stimulus given. However, not all of these neurons respond in the same range; it appears that some are more sensitive in different ranges of intensities, so together, there is an interneuron response covering at least a 4 log unit range of input. Neurons in the pretectum send crossed and uncrossed fibers, through the posterior commissure, to the small population of neurons comprising the paired Edinger-Westphal nuclei. This allows afferent input from the pretectal nucleus on each side to be distributed almost equally to the pupil efferent pathway originating in the Edinger-Westphal nucleus. Damage to the posterior commissure from tumors compressing the dorsal midbrain from above (e.g., pinealomas) or from encephalitis (e.g., tertiary syphilis) may block the impulse pathway from the pretectal neurons to the Edinger-Westphal nucleus. This situation can result in a loss of the pupil light reflex but spares the near pupil response (which originates from a more rostral location in the midbrain, before synapsing with the Edinger-Westphal nucleus), causing a light-near dissociation of the pupil.

The uncrossed pathway appears to have evolved during development of binocularity and stereovision. Animals with eyes located more to the side of the head (e.g., birds, rabbits) have almost completely crossed pathways with no significant uncrossed component. That is why shining a light in one eye of these animals produces an almost totally crossed input to the pretectum, which then sends an almost completely crossed output to the Edinger-Westphal nucleus. The result is that only the pupil of the eye being stimulated will contract.

Cats are between birds and primates in this evolutionary respect, with approximately 70% of their pupil pathway crossed. Placing a pet cat so that one of its eyes points more toward a light produces a greater reaction of the pupil in the eye facing the light, causing an anisocoria. In humans, in whom the crossed and uncrossed pathways are almost equal, the direct and consensual pupil light reflex is equal. This is why illuminating one eye normally does not result in pupil inequality (anisocoria). Similarly, input deficits to one eye caused by damage to the retina or optic nerve should not normally produce an anisocoria in humans.

In some individuals the crossed pathway slightly exceeds the uncrossed pathway in both the retina and midbrain, leading to a slightly greater pupil response in the eye stimulated compared with the pupil contraction of the fellow eye, similar to cats, but not to the same extent. This consensual deficit, termed *contraction anisocoria*, is small and can usually be recognized only with the aid of pupillographic recordings.

The Efferent Arm of the Pupil Light Reflex

The efferent arm of the pupil light reflex is diagrammatically summarized in Figure 32-4, which also shows the site of common lesions along this pathway that may be encountered in clinical practice. The neurons in the Edinger-Westphal nucleus send preganglionic axons into the right and left fascicle of the oculomotor nerve (third nerve) to join the motor axons destined for the eye muscles, as well as the preganglionic accommodative fibers that originate in nearby nuclei. The right and left fascicles of the third nerve exit the midbrain through the subarachnoid space, where each continues as the third nerve toward the orbital apex. The pupillary preganglionic fibers are located on the superior aspect of the oculomotor nerve as it exits the midbrain, but soon come to lie on the medial aspect.[34] This is why aneurysms of the circle of Willis that lie in this area, such as aneurysms of the posterior communicating artery, often cause pupillary efferent deficits early on, because of the medial location of the artery with respect to the oculomotor nerve. After passing through the cavernous sinus to the orbital apex, the preganglionic pupillary fibers and accommodative fibers synapse in the ciliary ganglion (parasympathetic ganglion). A lesion at this site may produce an Adie's pupil. From here, the last neurons in the chain, the postganglionic neurons, pass into the eye by way of the short ciliary nerves, where they innervate the iris sphincter muscle. The

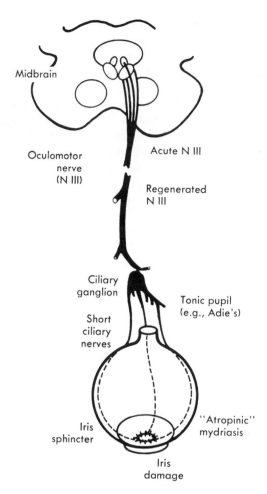

Midbrain

Oculomotor
nerve
(N III)

Acute N III

Regenerated
N III

Ciliary
ganglion

Short
ciliary
nerves

Tonic pupil
(e.g., Adie's)

Iris
sphincter

"Atropinic"
mydriasis

Iris
damage

FIGURE 32-4 Innervation of the iris sphincter, from the Edinger-Westphal nucleus by way of oculomotor nerve, ciliary ganglion, and short ciliary nerves, with some of the causes of a fixed dilated pupil.

strict. This triad of ocular vergence, accommodation, and pupil contraction is called the *near response*. Despite many contentions in the literature claiming that this pupil constriction is exclusively dependent on either convergence or accommodation, clinical and experimental data indicate that any one of the three functions can be selectively abolished or elicited without affecting the others. These experimental and clinical observations have resulted in general agreement that the impulses that cause accommodation, convergence, and pupil constriction must arise from different cell groups within the oculomotor nucleus and travel by way of separate fibers to their effector muscles. Accommodation, convergence, and pupillary constriction are associated movements and are not tied to one another in the manner usually referred to by the term *reflex*. They are controlled, synchronized, and associated by supranuclear connections, but they are not caused by one another. The components of the near pupil reflex were recently summarized.[28,34]

The miosis of the near response and the pupillary constriction to light have a single final common efferent pathway from the Edinger-Westphal nucleus to the iris sphincter by way of the ciliary ganglion. They primarily differ in the origin of the supranuclear pathways that are elicited by light and near that both converge on the Edinger-Westphal nucleus. With a near stimulus, such as accommodation, the pupil normally constricts even with no change in retinal luminance. It is important to realize that this near reflex of the pupil is mediated by the same efferent nerve pathway originating from the same neurons in the Edinger-Westphal nucleus that mediate the pupil light reflex. There does not appear to be a separate neuronal efferent pathway that mediates the near pupil constriction.

However, the supranuclear control over this response is different from the one mediating the light reflex. In the case of the light reflex, the supranuclear input comes from the pretectal nucleus, as described in the previous section. In the case of the near reflex involving accommodation, convergence, and miosis, the supranuclear input is thought to originate from cortical areas surrounding visual cortex and from cortical areas within the frontal eye fields. The cortical neurons providing input for the near reflex are thought to synapse at least once, before passing ventral toward the visceral neurons overlying the oculomotor complex in the midbrain. This is because a cortical lesion in this area does not produce atrophy within the oculomotor nuclear complex (it is at least one synapse removed). It is

postganglionic accommodative fibers, which outnumber the pupil fibers 30:1, supply the ciliary muscle within the ciliary body of the eye. The postganglionic pupillary neurons appear to innervate the iris sphincter muscle in a segmental distribution over approximately 20 clock-hour sections. This is why lesions of the ciliary ganglion, such as in Adie syndrome, usually cause sectors of the iris sphincter to become acutely denervated, with loss of the pupil contraction only in these segments.

The Pupil Near Reflex and Accommodation

When fixation of the eye is shifted from a far to a near object of interest, the eyes converge, the intraocular lenses accommodate, and both pupils con-

also important to realize that the near reflex consists of convergence of the eyes, accommodation, and pupil contraction, all of which should be thought of as comovements and, as stated earlier, are not strictly dependent on one another. Any one of the three comovements may occur in the absence of the others, as discussed by Loewenfeld.[37] Because the supranuclear pathway for the near reflex passes ventral in the midbrain and the supranuclear pathway for the light reflex passes dorsal in the midbrain, the two systems may be differentially affected by disease processes.

The supranuclear neuronal input from a near visual task stimulates the pupil constrictor neurons located in the visceral part of the Edinger-Westphal nuclei. The same supranuclear neuronal input also stimulates the more numerous accommodative neurons, located nearby in the remaining visceral portion of the Edinger-Westphal nucleus. These preganglionic neurons give rise to accommodative axons that travel together with the pupil preganglionic light reflex neurons within the oculomotor nerve to synapse at the ciliary ganglion in the orbit (see previous section). The postganglionic parasympathetic accommodative axons, which innervate the smooth muscle of the ciliary body, outnumber the postganglionic light reflex axons, which innervate the iris sphincter muscle in a ratio of 30:1. As mentioned previously, this ratio has some clinical relevance in the setting of damage to the postganglionic parasympathetic axons. Such denervation can occur as a result of an Adie's pupil or trauma or after orbital surgery. After acute injury, the surviving nerve cell bodies within the ciliary ganglion sprout axons and grow toward the ciliary body muscle and the iris sphincter after about 8 to 12 weeks. Because the accommodative cell bodies outnumber the pupil light reflex cell bodies, almost all of the axonal sprouts reaching the iris sphincter muscle originate from the accommodative cell bodies. This reinnervation of the iris sphincter is therefore aberrant because the pupil sectors that were denervated still do not respond to light, but they now contract in response to activation of the accommodative neurons, hence producing a light-near dissociation of the pupil reflex.

In summary, with a near stimulus, both the accommodative neurons (which mediate ciliary muscle contraction) and light reflex neurons (which mediate iris sphincter contraction) in the Edinger-Westphal visceral motor nuclei are stimulated from a supranuclear level. This gives rise to a separate neuronal output of accommodative and light reflex

preganglionic neurons by way of the oculomotor nerve to the ciliary ganglion, which in turn gives off separate postganglionic innervation to the ciliary body and iris sphincter muscles. The preganglionic and postganglionic light reflex pathway make use of the same neurons to mediate pupil contraction to either near or light stimuli.[26]

Pupil Reflex Dilation: Central and Peripheral Nervous System Integration

Normally, when the pupil dilates, two integrated processes take place: The iris sphincter relaxes, and the iris dilator contracts, helping actively pull the pupil open.[38,39] Because the iris sphincter is stronger than the dilator muscle, pupil dilation does not readily occur until the sphincter muscle relaxes. Relaxation of the iris sphincter is accomplished by supranuclear inhibition of the Edinger-Westphal nucleus at a central nervous system level, most notably from the reticular activating formation in the brainstem. It appears from animal studies that this neuronal inhibitory pathway involves the central nervous system's sympathetic class of neurons. These sympathetic neurons pass through the periaqueductal gray area and innervate the pupil efferent neurons at the Edinger-Westphal nucleus and at the synapse there is an α_2-adrenergic receptor activation.[35] When this central inhibition is active, the preganglionic parasympathetic output from the Edinger-Westphal nucleus is suppressed, resulting in a relative relaxation of the iris sphincter and pupil dilation. When this inhibition is inactive, such as during sleep, with anesthesia, or with narcotics, the preganglionic neurons fire at a high rate, causing miosis. The neurons of the Edinger-Westphal nucleus are unique in this respect because their baseline discharge frequency, without any input, is high. If all input to these neurons is disconnected, they fire at a high rate, which results in a sustained pupil contraction and miosis. This is why deep sleep or anesthesia, which reduces almost all inhibitory supranuclear input to the Edinger-Westphal nucleus, results in small pupils.

Alternatively, during a state of wakefulness, the supranuclear inhibition is active and the neurons of the Edinger-Westphal nucleus are suppressed, causing the pupils to become larger again. If a light stimulus is given at this point, a train of neuronal impulses from the retina and then the pretectal interneuron will arrive at the Edinger-Westphal nucleus, which momentarily overcomes this inhibition, causing the pupil to constrict. If the light is turned off or the retina begins to become light adapted, the supranuclear inhibition again dominates, causing a reflex dilation of the pupil.

Almost all of the conditions mentioned previously cause changes in pupil diameter resulting from the modulation of the neuronal output from the Edinger-Westphal nucleus. In addition, the same factors causing a reflex dilation of the pupil also result in an increase in output to the peripheral sympathetic nervous system innervating the iris dilator muscle. The sympathetic nerve activity can be thought of as a "turbocharge" for pupil dilation. Peripheral sympathetic nerve activation is not a requirement for pupil dilation to occur (parasympathetic inhibition alone can accomplish that to some extent), but it greatly enhances the dynamics of pupil dilation in terms of speed and maximal pupil diameter attained.

The sympathetic outflow to the iris dilator muscle can be thought of as a paired three-neuron chain (Figure 32-5) without decussations. The first neuron originates in the hypothalamus and descends through the brainstem on each side into the lateral column of the spinal cord, where it synapses at the cervicothoracic level of C7-T2. The second preganglionic neuron leaves this level of the spinal cord and travels over the apical pleura of the lung and into the spinal rami to synapse at the superior cervical ganglion at the level of the carotid artery bifurcation on the right and left side of the neck. The third neuron, the postganglionic neuron, follows a long course along the internal carotid artery into the head and orbit. As these neurons pass through the cavernous sinus, they are in brief association with the abducens and then the trigeminal

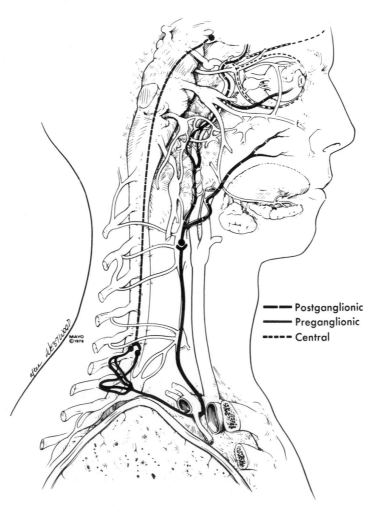

Postganglionic
Preganglionic
Central

Figure 32-5 Sympathetic innervation to the eye, showing the three-neuron chain of central, preganglionic, and postganglionic fibers. (From Maloney WF et al: *Am J Ophthalmol* 90:394, 1980.)

nerve before entering the orbit and distributing to the iris dilator muscle via the long ciliary nerves.[32]

In addition to the neuronal mechanisms involved in pupil dilation, humoral mechanisms also may contribute to pupil diameter. Circulating catecholamines in the blood (e.g., a bolus released from the adrenal glands) may act directly on the iris dilator muscle either through the bloodstream or, potentially, indirectly through the tears, resulting in mydriasis. Clinical conditions that influence the integration of the parasympathetic inhibition, sympathetic stimulation, and humoral release of neurotransmitters may take various forms and may affect the dynamics of reflex dilation in a characteristic manner that may be diagnostic of clinical conditions. This is revisited later in this chapter when pupil inequality and conditions that impede pupil dilation are discussed.

Other Neuronal Input to the Iris

In addition to the autonomic nerves supplying the iris, sensory innervation to the iris is provided by the ophthalmic division of the trigeminal nerve.[24,48] However, these sensory nerves may play an additional role in modulating pupil diameter. It is well known to cataract surgeons that mechanical and chemical irritation of the eye can cause a strong miotic response that is noncholinergic and fails to reverse with autonomically acting drugs. In rabbits and cats the response seems to be caused by the release of substance P or closely related peptides from the sensory nerve endings, but in monkeys and humans, substance P has little or no miotic effect. Almegard, Stjernschantz, and Bill[2] report that cholecystokinin (in nanomolar amounts) caused contraction of isolated iris sphincter from monkeys and humans. Intracameral injections in monkeys caused miosis that was not prevented by tetrodotoxin or indomethacin, indicating that the miosis was not caused by either stimulation of nerve endings or release of prostaglandins but by direct action on sphincter receptors. The cholecystokinin antagonist lorglumide caused competitive inhibition of the response.

STRUCTURE OF THE IRIS

Iris Sphincter, Iris Dilator, and Iris Color

It is important to understand the structure of the iris and its histology to understand how the iris tissue accommodates changes in pupil diameter during contraction and dilation and how disorders of the iris tissue affect pupil movement. The iris can be divided into two main layers: the posterior leaf and the anterior leaf (Figure 32-6). The posterior iris leaf contains the dilator muscle, the sphincter muscle, and the posterior pigmented epithelium. From a front view of the iris, the dilator muscle is located circumferentially, in the midperiphery of the iris.

The sphincter muscle is located just inside the pupillary border; its circumference is made up of

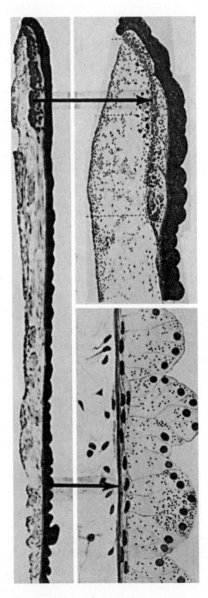

FIGURE 32-6 Histology of the iris in cross section. Upper arrow points to sphincter muscle drawn in higher magnification; lower arrow points to dilator muscle of bleached preparation drawn in higher magnification. (From Saltzmann M: *Anatomy and histology of the human eye-ball*, Chicago, 1912, University of Chicago Press.)

approximately 20 motor segments connected together but innervated individually by postganglionic branches of the ciliary nerve. In the normal iris these segments receive nerve excitation in a roughly simultaneous fashion, and the entire circumference contracts in concert. Both the dilator and sphincter muscles are derived embryologically from the anterior layer of the two layers of posterior pigmented epithelium.

The more superficial, anterior iris leaf consists of connective tissue stroma with cells, blood vessels, and nerves supplying the sphincter and dilator, but there is no epithelial layer in primate species. The different components of the posterior and anterior iris undergo structural alterations to accommodate changes in pupil diameter during contraction and dilation.[45]

During pupil contraction, the outer circumference of the iris, called the *outer ciliary ring* (which contains the dilator), enlarges in area as the pupil becomes smaller and the iris tissue spreads out to compensate for the reduction in pupil diameter. The area of the inner circumference of the iris, called the *inner ciliary ring* or *collarette* (which contains the sphincter), remains relatively constant as the pupil becomes smaller despite the increasing area taken up by iris tissue. Consequently, as the pupil becomes small, compaction of iris tissue in the inner collarette poses a mechanical limitation to iris movement. This results in a nonlinear "leveling off" of how much the pupil can contract in response to stronger light stimuli. These mechanical nonlinearities introduced by the rearrangement of iris tissue at the extremes of pupil dilation and contraction have been extensively studied by Loewenfeld.[40]

The mechanical nonlinearities are important because they impose limitations on the range of pupil diameter over which the extent of pupil movement can be used for assessing neuronal reflexes to light stimuli or near stimuli or for pharmacologic testing of the pupil. For example, a person with small, 3-mm diameter pupils in dim light would obviously not show as large a pupil contraction to a standard light stimulus compared with a person with 5-mm diameter pupils, but the retina and optic nerves of both persons may be completely normal. A similar situation would occur if one attempts to quantify the response to a topical miotic or mydriatic agent. Therefore the structure of the iris can pose physical constraints on pupil movement in response to sensory stimuli or pharmacologic agents, and this should be considered carefully when comparing the response in different eyes.

The color of the iris is determined by its mesodermal and ectodermal components. In Caucasians, the stroma is relatively free of pigment at birth. The stroma absorbs the long wavelengths of light, allowing the shorter (blue) wavelengths to pass through to the pigmented epithelium, where they are reflected back, causing the iris to appear blue. If pigmentation does not develop in the anterior stromal layers, the iris remains blue throughout life. If the stroma becomes denser and contains significant numbers of melanosomes, the blue color gives way to gray. The accumulation of pigment in the iris melanocytes of individuals destined to have nonblue irides occurs during the first year of life and is dependent on sympathetic innervation of the melanocytes (derived from neural crest cells). Interruption of the oculosympathetic nerve supply to one eye during this time period usually results in heterochromia, with the denervated iris remaining blue. In a heavily pigmented iris, the fine pattern of iris vessels is hidden by pigment and the surface of the iris looks brown and velvety.

PROPERTIES OF LIGHT AND THEIR EFFECT ON PUPIL MOVEMENT

Properties of light stimulating the retina that affect the pupil response include intensity, duration, temporal frequency, area, perimetric location, state of retinal adaptation, wavelength, and spatial frequency. There is a wealth of information on how these properties of light stimuli affect the pupillary response with regard to latency and amplitude of movement. Loewenfeld[41,42] has presented the most complete review of this topic in her book on the pupil, which should be consulted for a detailed literature review and for examples illustrating these different light effects. In general, the amplitude of pupil movement increases in proportion to the log light intensity of the stimulus, whereas the latency time of the pupil light reflex (time from stimulus onset to beginning of pupil contraction) becomes shorter (Figure 32-7). With increasing duration of light stimulus, the contraction amplitudes become greater and more prolonged. With long-duration light stimuli, after an initial contraction, the pupil may undergo oscillations (hippus) and undergo slow dilation, or "pupil escape," because of light adaptation (see Figure 32-7). Table 32-1 summarizes the different light effects.

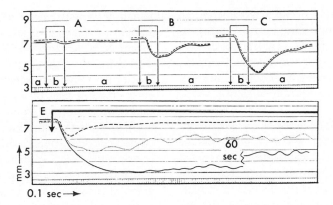

FIGURE 32-7 *A, B,* and *C,* Dark-adapted normal subject. Light flashes, *b,* of increasing intensity were given to the right eye to produce increasing pupillary constriction. Latent period decreases with intensity of flash. Both pupils were recorded simultaneously using an infrared pupillography device. The right pupil tracing (*solid line*) and the left pupil tracing (*broken line*) move in synchrony. *E,* Reactions of the pupil to prolonged light of different intensities. At the dimmest intensity there was a short pupil light constriction and the pupil dilated (escaped) during the light stimulus. At the brighter intensities, the contractions were larger and more sustained, also exhibiting oscillations (hippus). (From Lowenstein O, Loewenfeld IE: In Davso H [ed]: *The eye,* vol 3, New York, 1962, Academic Press.)

Most investigations of the pupillary light reflex have focused on the response of the pupil to changes in light level because the neuronal pathway for this reflex was thought to respond only to stepwise changes in light intensity. With the advent of computer graphics and sophisticated software programs, more complex stimuli can be presented to allow properties of spatial frequency, color, motion, and luminance to be controlled more carefully. A number of investigators have taken advantage of this technology to investigate whether the pupil is capable of responding to visual stimuli that change in color or spatial frequency when the average luminance does not change.[21-25,28,31]

The results of these studies provide evidence that the pupil contracts to either an onset or offset of spatial frequency or color exchanges. From a practical standpoint, these responses allow the pupil response to be used as an objective indicator of visual acuity and color discrimination. From a theoretical standpoint, the pupil response to isoluminant stimuli provides a means to explore how and where different signals are processed in the visual system. From these studies it is becoming more apparent that visual cortex plays a role in modulating the pupil response to these complex stimuli, providing evidence that small pupil reflexes elicited by properties of visual stimuli besides luminance involve more than just midbrain processing.

RELATIVE AFFERENT PUPILLARY DEFECTS

Clinical Observation of the Pupil Light Reflex

One of the most important clinical uses of the pupil has to do with its role in assessing afferent input from the retina, optic nerve, and anterior visual pathways (chiasm, optic tract, and midbrain pathways). The pupil light reflex sums the entire neuronal input from the photoreceptors, bipolar cells, ganglion cells, and axons of ganglion cells. Therefore damage at any one of these sites along the visual pathway will reduce the amplitude of pupil movement in response to a light stimulus.[42,43] The pupil light reflex can show considerable variation even among normal individuals as a result of supranuclear influences on the midbrain pupillomotor center that are not related to afferent input of the retina and optic nerve. However, the pupil light reflex is symmetric between the two eyes of a normal individual. The normal symmetry of input between the two eyes allows the clinician to pick up any asymmetric damage between the two eyes by simply comparing how well the pupil contracts to a standard light shined into one eye compared with alternating the light over to the other eye.[36] Observation of the pupil movement in response to alternating the light back and forth between the two eyes (Figures 32-8 and 32-9) is the basis for the alternating light test or swinging flashlight test for assessing the RAPD.[51,52] The RAPD, or input asymmetry, can be quantified in log units using neutral density filters of increasing strength placed in front of the better responding eye. A log density filter that neutralizes or balances the asymmetry of pupil movement between the two eyes, until they are matched, is chosen and is taken as the log unit RAPD.

Another important property of the pupil light reflex is that when a diffuse light stimulus enters the eye, the entire area of the visual field is summated into the pupil response, with some increased weight given to the central 10 degrees.[42] The area summating properties of the pupil light reflex make the am-plitude of its movement roughly proportional to the amount of working visual field. Therefore damage to peripheral portions of the retina and visual field defects outside of the central field reduce the amplitude of the pupil light reflex. This is in contrast to other objective tests of visual function such as the Ganzfeld electroretinogram (which measures diffuse damage to the retina and not local damage) and visual evoked potentials (which are center weighted and therefore affected mainly be central field loss). The pupil light reflex is one of the few objective reflexes that can be used as a clinical test for detecting and quantifying abnormalities in either the retina,

TABLE 32-1
EFFECT OF PROPERTIES OF LIGHT STIMULI ON THE PUPILLARY LIGHT REFLEX

STIMULUS PROPERTY	EFFECT ON PUPILLARY LIGHT REFLEX
Light intensity	Amplitude of contraction increases linearly over at least a 3 log unit range of stimulus intensity (stimulus under photopic conditions). The entire stimulus-response function resembles an S-shaped curve. Latency time, the time from stimulus onset to the start of pupil contraction (200-450 msec), becomes more prolonged with dimmer light stimuli (in the range of 20-40 msec further delay/log unit decrement of light intensity).
State of light adaptation	In the dark-adapted state, the threshold light intensity needed to produce a pupil contraction becomes less as rods are brought into play. However, rods in the dark-adapted state do not produce as much increase in pupil contraction in response to increases in stimulus intensity, compared with cones in the mesopic and photopic states.
Duration	When stimulus duration is shorter than 70 msec, there is a reciprocal relationship between the duration and intensity, which is required to produce a given pupil contraction amplitude. With longer-duration stimuli, the pupil contracts more, there is a shorter latency time (up to a point), and the pupillary contraction is more sustained; however, pupil escape (relative dilation) may occur as a result of light adaptation.
Area	The pupillary light reflex shows much greater area summation properties than visual perception (for visual threshold of perception, summation is minimal with stimuli greater than 1 degree). With full-field Ganzfeld stimuli, the pupil threshold can be equal to visual threshold (or even smaller); with stimuli smaller than 1-2 degrees, visual threshold is usually more sensitive (by 0.5-1.0 log units).
Perimetric location	Under dark adaptation, the fovea shows a decreased sensitivity compared with surrounding retinal areas because of the lack of rods here. In mesopic and photopic adaptation, the pupil responds greatest in the central field; the temporal field response is usually greater than the nasal field response.
Spectral sensitivity	The wavelength sensitivity of the pupillary light reflex follows that of visual perception with a blue shift under dark adaptation and a peak sensitivity at green under photopic conditions.
Temporal frequency	The normal pupil cannot move much faster than 4 Hz because of the relatively slow contraction of smooth muscle. Animals with striated iris muscle (pigeons) can easily follow a 10-Hz stimulus. At frequencies from 9-25 Hz, the steady-state pupil diameter increases, indicating loss of sensitivity in neuronal integration of light within this frequency range.
Spatial frequency	When the change in average luminance across a stimulus patch is kept constant, the pupil undergoes small contractions when a sinusoidal grating is presented or when the grating bars are alternated between dark and light. The mechanism is thought to be independent of a luminance response. The greater the spatial frequency, the less the pupil contracts to the stimulus and this has been correlated with visual acuity.
Motion	Recent evidence suggests that the pupil may respond to a motion stimulus even under isoluminant conditions.

optic nerve, optic chiasm, or optic tract, and it is also able to detect regional visual field damage in the center or periphery.

Because the amount of the RAPD is correlated to a large extent with the amount of asymmetry of visual field deficit between the two eyes, it can also be used to help substantiate abnormal results of visual field testing.[8,25,31,53] This can often help the clinician determine whether a patient's visual field defects are reliable and reflect the true pathologic state. This correlation between the visual field asymmetry and the RAPD is also useful in following the course of disease to determine whether there is a worsening or improvement in function over time. In this respect, it is important to emphasize that the RAPD is a *relative* measure of the input of one eye compared with the other. Bilateral symmetric damage should not produce an RAPD. The relative nature of this measurement should also be kept in mind when interpreting changes over repeated patient visits. For example, a patient who exhibited a definite RAPD in one eye on the first visit may show no RAPD at all on the follow-up visit. This may represent improvement in the previously damaged eye. However, it may also indicate that there is now damage in what was previously

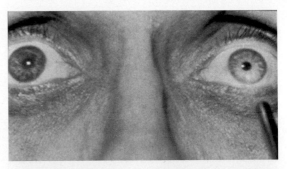
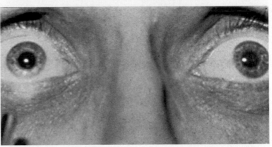

FIGURE 32-8 A patient is shown with a large relative afferent pupil defect of the right eye. In the top photograph a light is shined in the normal left eye and both pupils constrict to a small diameter. When the light is alternated to stimulate the right eye (*bottom photograph*), the pupils hardly constrict at all.

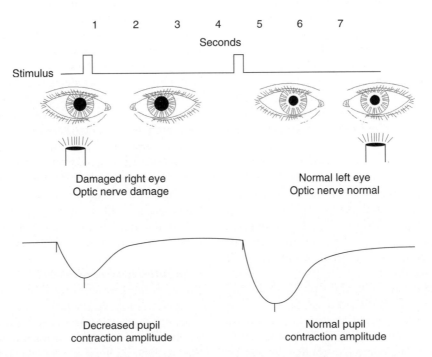

FIGURE 32-9 Pupillographic demonstration of a right relative afferent pupil defect. With short light pulses the pupil light reflex (*bottom tracings*) are of lesser amplitude when the stimulus was given to the right eye compared with stimulus to the left eye.

the better eye, matching the damage to the other eye, so that there are now symmetric visual field defects and no RAPD. Therefore it is always important to consider that the RAPD is a measurement of afferent input of one eye *relative* to the other eye.

Estimating the amount of the RAPD in log units is important to understand how much visual field damage (asymmetry between the two eyes) is present and whether it is consistent with the results of the visual field test. For example, a patient with a small amount of macular degeneration in one eye and not the other might be expected to have only a 0.3 log unit RAPD. However, if that patient had a 1.0 log unit RAPD, some other cause of visual loss, such as a previous branch retinal artery occlusion or optic neuropathy, would have to be considered. In addition, the area and extent of visual field loss would be expected to be more than that caused by a small amount of macular degeneration. The importance of quantifying the RAPD cannot be overemphasized. In general, in the case of unilateral visual damage, loss of the central 5 degrees of the visual field results in an RAPD of approximately 0.3 log units. Loss of the entire central area of field (10 degrees) causes about a 0.6 to 0.9 log unit RAPD. Each visual field quadrant outside of the macula is worth about 0.3 log units (Figure 32-10), but the temporal field loss seems to result in more loss of pupil input compared with the nasal field quadrants. Examples of the log unit magnitude of the RAPD expected for common clinical disorders is given in Table 32-2. The correlation between the relative afferent defect and the area and extent of visual field loss, however, is only approximate. Differences between the two may be important clues as to the cause and extent of damage to the anterior visual system.

Recent studies using computerized pupillography to more precisely quantify the log unit RAPD have also revealed that some normal subjects with normal visual fields and examination can have a small 0.3 log unit RAPD.[32,33,55] Therefore small RAPDs discovered incidentally in a patient without ocular complaints and a normal examination can probably be dismissed.

Estimating the amount of the pupillomotor input asymmetry (the RAPD) can also be done more subjectively, without using neutral density filters, by grading the asymmetry of pupil response as +1, +2, +3, or +4. This subjective grading can also be classified according to the amount of pupil escape or dilation of the pupils as the light is alternated to the other eye.[7] However, most subjective grading of

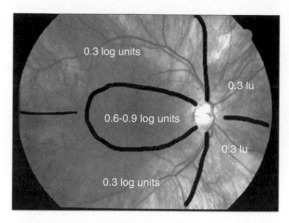

FIGURE 32-10 Approximate distribution of the amount of log unit relative afferent pupil defect expected for corresponding loss of input in the regions of the retina shown, assuming the other eye is normal.

the RAPD has serious limitations; it is subject to some large errors resulting from age variations in pupil diameter and pupil mobility. For example, a patient with small pupils and small pupil contractions to light may have a large RAPD that may appear deceptively small on the basis of the small differences in pupil excursion observed as the light is alternated between the two eyes. However, the amount of neutral density filter needed to dim the better eye until the small contractions are equal could easily approach 0.9 to 1.2 log units, representing substantial input damage. Estimating the size of an RAPD without using filters is much like estimating an ocular deviation "by Hirschberg" without doing a prism cover test. More accurate quantification of the RAPD is accomplished by determining the log unit difference needed to balance the pupil reaction between the two eyes using photographic neutral density filters, as described previously. If one pupil does not move well because of weakness of the sphincter or pharmacologic immobility, one can still check for a RAPD by observing the pupil that still works—and comparing its direct reaction with its consensual reaction.

Computerized Pupillometry

Various computerized, infrared-sensitive pupillometers are commercially available. Most of these elegant instruments can precisely record the dynamics of pupillary movement in the light or in the dark (Figure 32-11). Once recorded, the pupillary information can be analyzed by sophisticated software (see pupil tracings in the alternating light test, shown in Figure 32-9). This allows quantitative information

TABLE 32-2
COMMON DISEASES PRODUCING RELATIVE AFFERENT PUPILLARY DEFECTS (RAPD) AND EXPECTED MAGNITUDE OF DEFECT

CONDITION	SITE	LOG UNIT RAPD	INFLUENCING FACTORS
Intraocular hemorrhage	Anterior chamber or vitreous (dense)	0.6-1.2	Density of hemorrhage
Intraocular hemorrhage	Anterior chamber (diffuse)	0.0-0.3	Density of hemorrhage
Intraocular hemorrhage	Preretinal (central vein occlusion or diabetic)	0.0	Preretinal location does not significantly reduce light
Diffusing media opacity	Cataract or corneal scar	0.0-0.3 (in opposite eye)	Dispersion of light producing increase in light input
Unilateral functional visual field loss	None	0	
Central serous retinopathy (CSR) or cystoid macular edema (CME)	Retina (fovea)	0.3 log units	Area of retina involved
Central or branch retinal vein occlusion (CRVO, BRVO)	Inner retina	0.3-0.6 (nonischemic) 0.9 (ischemic)	Area of visual field defect and degree of ischemia
Central or branch retinal artery occlusion (CRAO, BRAO)	Inner retina	0.3-3.0	Area and location of retina involved
Retinal detachment	Outer retina	0.3-2.1	Area and location of detached retina (e.g., 0.6 log units for macula + 0.3 log units for each quadrant)
Anterior ischemic optic neuropathy	Optic nerve head	0.6-2.7	Extent and location of visual field defect
Optic neuritis (acute)	Optic nerve	0.6-3.0	Extent and location of visual field defect
Optic neuritis (recovered)	Optic nerve	0.0-0.6	No visual field defect, residual RAPD
Glaucoma	Optic nerve	Usually none, if symmetric damage to both eyes	Degree of visual field asymmetry between the two eyes correlates with the log unit RAPD
Compressive optic neuropathy	Optic nerve	0.3-3.0	Extent and location of visual field defect
Chiasmal compression	Optic chiasm	0.0-1.2	Asymmetry of visual field loss, unilateral central field involvement
Optic tract lesion	Optic tract	0.3-1.2 (in the eye with temporal field loss)	Incongruity of homonymous field defect, hemifield pupillomotor input asymmetry
Postgeniculate damage	Visual radiations Visual cortex	0.0	Stimulus light area (no RAPD but definite pupil perimetry defects)
Midbrain tectal damage	Olivary pretectal area of pupil light input region of midbrain	0.3-1.0	Similar to optic tract lesions, but no visual field defect

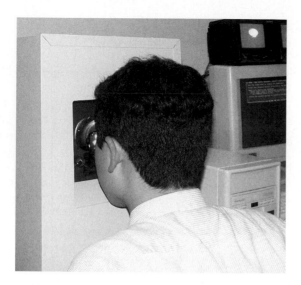

FIGURE 32-11 Computerized infrared pupillographic instrument, which records the bright image of both pupils simultaneously, is shown. This instrument can be used to give full-field light stimuli to either eye produced on a monochrome monitor inside of the box, or it may also be used to present focal light stimuli to provide a form of objective pupil perimetry.

about the pupillary light reflex to be assessed. In the near future, this may help automate the clinical determination of pupil input deficits caused by retinal and optic nerve diseases.[14,15,17,31-33] Such instrumentation is also useful for detecting and diagnosing causes of anisocoria (unequal pupils) when both pupils are recorded simultaneously (refer to the section on oculosympathetic defects).

Pupil Perimetry

The pupil light reflex may also be used to obtain objective information about the sensitivity of local areas of the visual field by recording small pupil contractions in response to focal light stimuli placed in different perimetric locations. An automated perimeter can be modified to record pupil responses to each focal light stimulus to produce a form of objective pupil perimetry.[26,30] A video camera is pointed at the pupil, and the amplitude of each light reaction is measured and stored in the computer. This has turned out to be helpful as an objective form of perimetry and as a way to localize lesions in the pupillary pathways (Figure 32-12). Pupil perimetry is also useful in cases of nonorganic, functional visual loss to show objectively that messages are indeed going normally into the brain from parts of the visual field in which the patient claims to see nothing.

EFFERENT PUPILLARY DEFECTS

Anisocoria

When a pupil inequality is seen, it usually means that damage has occurred to either the iris sphincter or dilator muscle, their innervation has been interrupted, or there are external pharmacologic factors influencing pupil movement (Figure 32-13). To sort out which muscle is not working right, it helps to know how the anisocoria is influenced by light. It is worth noting that an anisocoria always increases in the direction of action of the paretic iris muscle, just as an esotropia increases when gaze is in the direction of action of a weak lateral rectus muscle. If the iris sphincter is paretic, the lighting condition that normally brings into action that muscle accentuates the weakness; adding bright light tends to increase the anisocoria. Alternatively, if the iris dilator is paretic, the anisocoria is expected to increase as light is taken away because reflex dilation to darkness is impaired. Table 32-3 provides a summary of the common causes of anisocoria that are discussed in the following section.

Pupil Inequality That Increases in the Dark

In patients who have pupil inequality that increases in the dark, the problem is distinguishing Horner syndrome from a simple anisocoria (or physiologic anisocoria). In both of these conditions, the pupil inequality becomes greater in dim light but the dynamics of pupil dilation is impaired in oculosympathetic defects, but not in simple anisocoria. Other features also characterize simple anisocoria from Horner syndrome.

A simple anisocoria may vary from day to day, or even from hour to hour, and it is visible in about one fifth of the normal population. In some people it may be present most of the time, and the larger pupil may always be in the same eye. In other people it may come and go, and the larger pupil may often switch to the other eye. Physiologic anisocoria is not related to refractive error. The cause of physiologic anisocoria is not known with certainty, but current evidence favors a transient, asymmetric, supranuclear inhibition of the Edinger-Westphal nucleus. This would cause the pupil on the more inhibited side to be larger. If this mechanism is correct, it would also explain why any stimulus that transiently overcomes supranuclear inhibition, such as bright light, near stimulus, sleep, or anesthesia, causes the physiologic anisocoria to decrease. Simple anisocoria is considered benign.

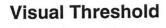

Visual Threshold

Visual testing time = 18 minutes

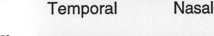

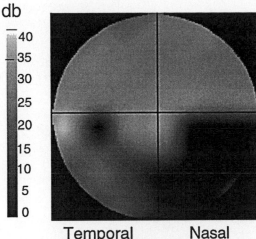

Pupil Contraction

Pupil testing time = 8 minutes

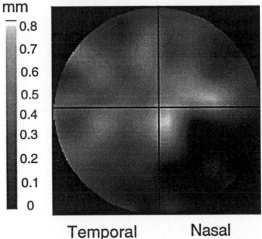

FIGURE 32-12   Example of a patient with anterior ischemic optic neuropathy showing the correspondence between the visual field and pupil field defect.

Clinically, Horner syndrome is recognized by looking for the associated signs, such as ptosis, "upside-down ptosis" of the lower lid, and in a fresh case, conjunctival injection, decreased sweating on the involved side, and in some cases, lowered intraocular pressure on the affected side. Pain on the side of the face with the smaller pupil (jaw, ear, and cheek pain) is often an important sign pointing to a carotid artery dissection as a cause of the Horner syndrome (Figure 32-14).

The characteristic dilation lag of the Horner's pupil can easily be seen in the office with a hand light shining from below. At the time the room lights are switched off, the reflex dilation of the two pupils should be simultaneously observed and the smaller pupil assessed to see whether it dilates slower than the other pupil does. Pupil dilation is normally a combination of sphincter relaxation and dilator contraction. This combination produces a prompt dilation in a normal pupil when the illumination is abruptly decreased. The patient with Horner syndrome has a weak dilator muscle in one iris, and as a result, that pupil dilates more slowly than the normal pupil (Figure 32-15). If the sympathetic lesion is complete, the affected pupil will dilate only by sphincter relaxation; this process takes longer than with an intact sympathetic innervation to the dilator muscle. This asymmetry of pupil dilation produces an anisocoria that becomes largest 4 to 5 seconds after the lights are turned out. Dilation of the eye with the oculosympathetic defect is a much slower process than most people imagine. After the lights have been out for 10 to 20 seconds, the anisocoria lessens as the sympathec-

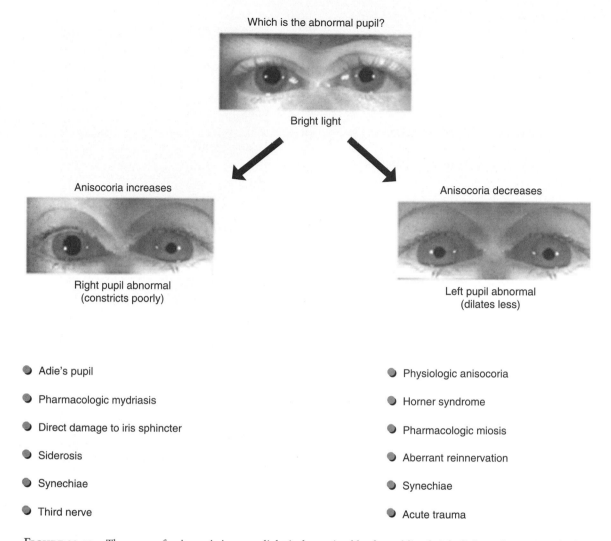

FIGURE 32-13 The cause of anisocoria in room light is determined by first adding bright light to determine whether the anisocoria increases (*left*) or decreases (*right*).

tomized pupil gradually catches up because of continual relaxation of the iris sphincter. The delayed dilation of the involved eye is a process referred to as *dilation lag* (see Figure 32-15). Often, the initial increase in anisocoria during the first few seconds of darkness can be accentuated by adding an auditory stimulus just after the lights are turned out. This causes the normal pupil to dilate forcefully in response to the extra sympathetic stimulation evoked by the loud noise, but in the eye with the oculosympathetic defect, there this maneuver has little effect. Comparison of the dynamics of dilation of the two pupils is a quick and simple way of distinguishing Horner syndrome from simple anisocoria, and it is a test that does not require pupillary drug testing. It works well most of the

time, especially in young people with mobile pupils, but if the dilation lag is inconclusive, cocaine eyedrops should be used to confirm the diagnosis of Horner syndrome.

Pharmacologic Diagnosis of Horner Syndrome with Cocaine

Cocaine's action is to block the reuptake of the norepinephrine that is normally released from the nerve endings. If, because of an interruption in the sympathetic pathway, norepinephrine is not being released, cocaine has no adrenergic effect. A Horner's pupil will dilate less to cocaine than the normal pupil, regardless of the location of the lesion. Forty-five minutes after cocaine drops have been placed in both eyes, the anisocoria should

TABLE 32-3
COMMON CAUSES OF ANISOCORIA AND ASSOCIATED FEATURES

CONDITION	CAUSE	ANISOCORIA	LIGHT RESPONSE	NEAR RESPONSE	SLIT LAMP	PHARMACOLOGIC TESTING
Acute Adie's pupil	Denervation of parasympathetic postganglionic nerves to pupillary sphincter (segmental)	Anisocoria increases in bright light	Segmental loss of light reaction in some sphincter areas around the circumference	Same areas where light response is lost also show loss of near constriction	Remaining innervated sphincter areas pucker with light and pull denervated segments	Supersensitivity to 0.1% pilocarpine Check response of both pupils in darkness after 30 minutes
Chronic Adie's pupil (greater than 8 wk after event)	Reinnervation of denervated sphincter segments by postganglionic accommodative nerves	May be no anisocoria in room light or affected pupil may be the smaller pupil	Poor response to light; poor dilation in darkness as a result of tonically contracted segments that have reinnervation	Light-near dissociation is present with good near effort from the patient	Similar appearance as in the acute state, reinnervated segments show diffuse contraction to near	As segments become reinnervated, cholinergic supersensitivity is lost Small, tonic pupil dilates normally to anticholinergics
Pharmacologic mydriasis (anticholinergic)	Scopolamine patch, eyedrops, plants (jimson weed)	Anisocoria increases in bright light	Loss of response to light; residual small reaction may occur with submaximal exposure or after sufficient time has elapsed	Same degree of loss of near response as loss of light response; near point of accommodation is more remote	Any residual light response of the sphincter is diffuse and not segmental	Subsensitivity to pilocarpine of all concentrations compared with the opposite unaffected eye (observed in dim light or darkness)
Pharmacologic mydriasis (adrenergic)	Low concentration of adrenergics found in over-the-counter eyedrops for red eyes, cocaine, Neo-Synephrine	Anisocoria increases in bright light, but not as much as in anticholinergic mydriasis	Diminished response to light, but dilator muscle can be overcome by strong sphincter constriction to bright light	Same diminished response as light reaction Near point of accommodation is unaffected and is normal	Besides diminished reaction, the pupil movement looks normal and is not segmental	Reversal of anisocoria with adrenergic blockade (dipyridamole or thymoxamine) May be overcome with pilocarpine
Damage to iris sphincter	Ischemia, angle-closure glaucoma, herpes zoster iritis, trauma, after anterior segment surgery	Anisocoria increases in bright light	Loss of response to light, some sphincter segments may be more affected than others	Usually affected to the same degree as the light reflex; may have normal accommodative amplitude	Transillumination defects may be present	Lack of response to 1% pilocarpine in damaged areas of the iris sphincter
Iron or copper mydriasis	Intraocular foreign body	Anisocoria increases in bright light	Loss of response to light, not usually segmental	Usually affected to the same degree as the light reflex	Usually heterochromia is present, with the iris being darker	May show cholinergic supersensitivity
Third nerve palsy	Trauma, compression, rarely ischemia	Anisocoria increases in bright light	Loss of response to light, not usually segmental unless aberrant regeneration is present	Usually affected to the same degree as the light reflex; accommodative amplitude is decreased	Usually symmetric weakness along the circumference of the sphincter to light reaction	May show cholinergic supersensitivity
Mechanically scarred iris	Trauma, iritis	Anisocoria increases in bright light	Loss of response to light when viewed without slit lamp	Usually affected to the same degree as the light reflex; accommodative amplitude is normal	Small movement of the scarred down iris can usually be observed; synechiae can often be seen after dilation	Lack of response to 1% pilocarpine
Physiologic anisocoria	Asymmetric inhibition at the Edinger-Westphal nucleus	Anisocoria decreases in bright light	Normal; normal dilation in response to darkness and auditory stimulation	Normal; anisocoria lessens with a good near response	Normal	Normal response to topical agents; cocaine lessens the anisocoria
Oculosympathetic defect (Horner syndrome)	Sympathetic nerve palsy; ptosis is usually present of the upper and lower lid; anhidrosis may be present	Anisocoria decreases in bright light	Normal; slow dilation in response to darkness and auditory stimulation	Normal; anisocoria lessens with a good near response	Normal; heterochromia is common if palsy occurred early in life	Cocaine increases the anisocoria; supersensitivity is usually demonstrated to adrenergic agents
Congenital pseudo-Horner syndrome	Unknown; anisocoria is often present in old photographs from infancy	Anisocoria decreases in bright light	Appears normal, but the smaller pupil does not dilate well to darkness or auditory stimulation	Normal; anisocoria lessens with a good near response	Normal	May give a false-positive cocaine test; when direct-acting agents or anticholinergic drops are used, the pupil still fails to dilate as well as the fellow eye

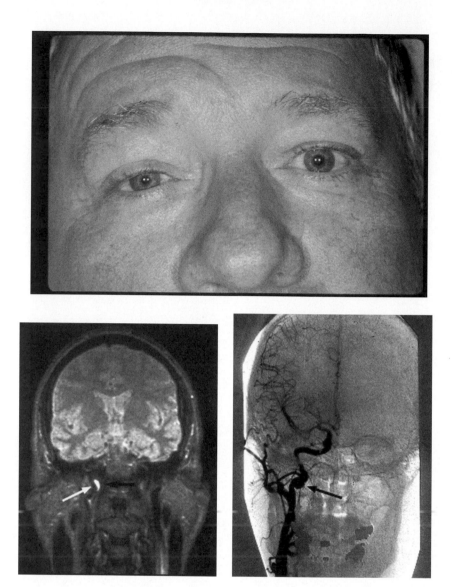

FIGURE 32-14   Example of a patient with acute Horner syndrome on the right with accompanying facial pain. Note the miosis and ptosis on the right eye. This patient had a dissection of the internal carotid artery demonstrated by the magnetic resonance imaging scan showing a bright signal in the wall of the carotid artery resulting from blood (white "comma" adjacent to carotid lumen in lower left; *arrow*). The dissection created a false lumen that appears as a focal enlargement of the lumen of the carotid artery demonstrated in the carotid angiogram on the right (*arrow*).

have clearly increased because the normal pupil has dilated more than the Horner's pupil.

A solution of 10% cocaine HCl drops in both eyes is recommended (never more than 2 drops) to be sure that the iris gets a full mydriatic dose; this high concentration of cocaine does not normally produce a corneal epithelial defect. It should be said that 2%, 4%, and 5% cocaine have also been used as a diagnostic test for Horner syndrome and work well. After 40 to 60 minutes have elapsed, the anisocoria is measured in room light. The patient should stay active during that time so that adequate sympathetic discharge is occurring (sleeping during this time might result in neither pupil dilating to cocaine). If there is little dilation of the eye with a suspected oculosympathetic defect and this pupil never dilated well in darkness before the drop was given, even after 30 seconds, a false-positive cocaine test

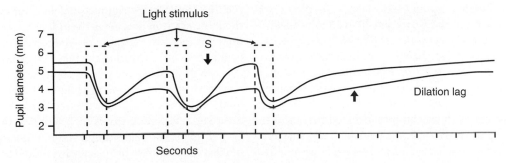

FIGURE 32-15 Example of a pupillographic demonstration of dilation lag of the pupil in the eye with Horner syndrome. The smaller pupil is slow to dilate, causing an increase in anisocoria during the early phase of dilation and accentuated by a loud sound (*S*). In the last part of the tracing, no further stimulus was given to allow the dilation lag to be observed in the tracing. The dilation lag is a delayed dilation of the smaller pupil; after 5 seconds in darkness, the smaller pupil slowly dilates as a result of inhibition of the sphincter muscle, despite loss of sympathetic nerve contribution to pupil dilation.

also must be considered. This can occur if the iris is in some way held in a miotic state by either scarring or aberrant reinnervation of the iris sphincter. In such cases, adding a direct-acting sympathomimetic agent to both eyes (i.e., 2.5% phenylephrine) at the conclusion of a positive cocaine test should easily dilate the iris of the suspected eye if there really is an oculosympathetic defect, and the cocaine-induced anisocoria should almost be eliminated. In some cases the 2.5% phenylephrine may even cause the eye with the oculosympathetic defect to have the larger pupil as a result of supersensitivity. Pseudo-Horner syndrome, caused by the reason's stated earlier, results in inadequate dilation to direct-acting sympathetic agents.

The likelihood of a diagnosis of Horner syndrome with cocaine testing increases in proportion to amount of anisocoria (measured 50 to 60 minutes after the instillation of cocaine). Unlike the hydroxyamphetamine test (used for localizing the lesion to either the preganglionic or postganglionic neuron), calculation of the change in the anisocoria from before to after cocaine application is unnecessary. It has been found that if there is at least 0.8 mm of pupillary inequality after cocaine, the presence of a Horner syndrome is highly likely.[29]

Pharmacologic Localization of the Denervation in Horner Syndrome

The site of the oculosympathetic lesion in Horner syndrome is a question of considerable clinical importance because many postganglionic defects are caused by benign vascular headache syndromes or more serious carotid dissections and a pregan-

glionic lesion is sometimes the result of the spread of a malignant neoplasm.

Hydroxyamphetamine eyedrops help localize the site of the lesion in Horner syndrome. The clinician would like to know where the lesion is because that knowledge directs the radiographic workup (e.g., to the internal carotid artery rather than to the pulmonary apex). Horner syndrome sometimes presents itself in such a characteristic setting that further efforts at localizing the lesion are not needed. This is true of patients with cluster headaches or after surgical procedures that interrupt the oculosympathetic chain in a known location.

Hydroxyamphetamine acts by releasing norepinephrine from storage in the sympathetic nerve endings. When the lesion is postganglionic, most, if not all, of the nerves are dead, and no norepinephrine stores are available for release. When the lesion is complete, a pupil like this will not dilate at all in response to hydroxyamphetamine. However, a period of almost 1 week from the onset of damage may be needed before the dying neurons and their stores of norepinephrine are gone. Therefore a hydroxyamphetamine test given within a week of a postganglionic lesion may give a false preganglionic localization if the norepinephrine stores have not yet disappeared. Horner's pupils resulting from preganglionic or central lesions dilate *at least* normally because the postganglionic neuron with its stores of norepinephrine, although disconnected, is still intact. In fact, when the lesion is in the preganglionic neuron, the Horner's pupil often becomes larger than the normal pupil—apparently resulting from "decentralization supersensitivity."

The hydroxyamphetamine test is simple: The pupils are measured *before* and 40 to 60 minutes *after* hydroxyamphetamine drops have been put in both eyes, and the change in anisocoria from the baseline predrop state to the postdrop state in room light is noted. If the Horner's pupil—the smaller one—dilates less than the normal pupil, the anisocoria increases and it can be concluded that the lesion is in the postganglionic neuron. If the smaller pupil dilates so well that it becomes the larger pupil, the lesion is preganglionic and the postganglionic neuron with its norepinephrine stores is still intact. The examiner should wait at least 2 to 3 days after using cocaine drops before using hydroxyamphetamine; cocaine seems to block hydroxyamphetamine's effectiveness because it blocks the uptake of hydroxyamphetamine into the postganglionic nerve terminal, thus inhibiting its action.

To understand how to better interpret the hydroxyamphetamine test, we studied hydroxyamphetamine mydriasis in patients with a known lesion location and in those in whom the location of the lesion is unknown. It appears that postganglionic lesions (along the carotid artery) can be separated from the nonpostganglionic lesions (in the brainstem, spinal cord, upper lung, and lower neck) with a degree of certainty that varies with the amount of change in anisocoria induced when the drops are put in both eyes.[16] An increase in the anisocoria of greater than 0.5 mm (change in anisocoria from prehydroxyamphetamine to posthydroxyamphetamine) makes a postganglionic lesion highly likely.

Congenital and Childhood Horner Syndrome

When a child has a unilateral ptosis and miosis, the first question is whether it is really Horner syndrome. The ptosis of Horner syndrome is moderate, never complete. Sometimes, the elevation of the lower lid (upside-down ptosis) is persuasive. A child with a congenital Horner syndrome and naturally curly hair has, on the affected side of the head, hair that seems limp and lank. The shape of the hair follicles apparently depends on intact sympathetic innervation, as does the iris pigment. A child with blond straight hair and pale blue eyes has no visible hair straightness or iris heterochromia. In children, iris color usually occurs after the first 9 to 12 months of life because of accumulation of melanosomes in iris melanocytes that are innervated by the sympathetic nerves. Therefore, if the iris in the eye with Horner syndrome does not develop pigmentation during this period (heterochromia occurs), it signifies that an oculosympathetic defect was present early in life; however, it does not indicate the cause or whether it was congenital or acquired during the first year of life.

Cocaine eyedrops may be of some help in diagnosing Horner syndrome in children. I have often used 10% drops with no ill effect, but I recommend a weaker solution (2 drops of 2% or 5% in each eye). If there is no significant dilation of the smaller pupil, a drop of 2.5% phenylephrine should then be administered to each eye to substantiate that the pupil can dilate to a direct-acting sympathomimetic agent and that this is not pseudo-Horner syndrome (see previous section on the cocaine test). Other signs may also be helpful for diagnosing Horner syndrome in children. The most telling sign is a hemifacial flush that can occur on the normally innervated side in contrast to the blanch that occurs on the side with the oculosympathetic defect when the infant is nursing or crying. In an air-conditioned office it may be hard to decide whether there is an asymmetry of sweating. A cycloplegic refraction can sometimes produce an atropinic flush everywhere except on the affected face and forehead and thus can unexpectedly solve the diagnostic problem.

In infants the hydroxyamphetamine drop test is not all that helpful in localizing the lesion because orthograde transsynaptic dysgenesis takes place at the superior cervical ganglion after an early interruption of the preganglionic oculosympathetic neuron. This results in fewer postganglionic neurons, even though there was no postganglionic injury, and this, in turn, produces weak mydriasis and ambiguous answers from the hydroxyamphetamine test in children.[56] Therefore, if it is used, the interpretation needs to take this into consideration. If, in response to hydroxyamphetamine, the affected eye with relative miosis dilates as well as or better than the fellow eye, it is probably a preganglionic lesion. However, any result showing less mydriasis in the affected eye compared with the fellow eye cannot be localized with certainty because of the reason listed earlier. Horner syndrome that has been clearly acquired in infancy should be evaluated for neuroblastoma—a treatable tumor—using a combination of imaging and of testing the urine for metabolites of adrenergic compounds secreted from the tumor.

Pupil Inequality That Is Increased in Bright Light

When the anisocoria increases with bright light, this implies that the larger pupil is abnormal and may not contract well to light because of direct damage to the iris sphincter muscle from trauma or surgery or because of ischemic atrophy, scarring (synechia) of the iris to the lens from previous inflammation, pharmacologic mydriasis, or denervation of the parasympathetic nerve supply to the iris sphincter (see Figure 32-4). The following sections outline the most important clinical observations and tests that may be needed to sort out the cause of the efferent pupil defect (see Table 32-2).

Examination of the Iris with High Magnification Using the Slit-Lamp Biomicroscope

Trauma to the globe usually results in a torn sphincter or an iris that shows transillumination defects at the slit lamp. The pupil is often not round, and there may be other evidence of ocular injury. Naturally, such a pupil does not constrict well to light. The residual reaction is often associated with the remaining normal sectors of the iris sphincter because the traumatic tears are usually segmental. An atrophic sphincter resulting from previous herpes zoster iritis may also reveal large geographic areas of transillumination defects seen with the slit lamp from previous ischemic vasculitic insults to the iris during the uveitis.

However, if the iris tissue looks normal, the examination is focused on whether any part of the iris sphincter is contracting with light. If some contraction occurs, it should be determined whether the residual contraction is diffuse over the whole circumference or segmental. If there is no segmental movement of the iris, the possibility of atropinic mydriasis should be considered.[27] However, a completely blocked light reaction can sometimes be seen when the sphincter is totally denervated by a preganglionic lesion (third nerve palsy) or a postganglionic lesion (fresh tonic pupil), in acute angle closure (iris ischemia), or in the presence of an intraocular iron foreign body (iron mydriasis). If the dilated pupil still has some response to light, the dilation could be caused by partial denervation of the sphincter or by incomplete atropinization or adrenergic mydriasis. When the light reaction is poor because the dilator muscle is in spasm (because of adrenergic mydriatics like phenylephrine), the pupil is large, the conjunctiva blanched, and the lid retracted. In such a case, the near point of accommodation is usually normal but may be slightly decreased as a result of spherical aberration and a shallow depth of field caused by the dilated pupil. However, in the case of adrenergic mydriasis, there usually is some light reaction to very bright lights

because the stronger iris sphincter can usually overcome pulling by the adrenergic effects on the dilator muscle.

If there is some residual light reaction, the next step is to look with the slit lamp for sector palsy of the iris sphincter. When the dilator is in a drug-induced adrenergic spasm or when the cholinergic receptors in the iris sphincter are blocked by an atropine-like drug, the entire sphincter muscle (all 360 degrees of it) is less effective. This is not the case when the postganglionic nerve fibers have been interrupted: Adie's pupils with a residual light reaction (about 90% of them) have segmental contractions of the remaining normal segments of the sphincter. Some preganglionic partial third nerve palsies also have regional sphincter palsies, but these can usually be attributed to an associated pre-existing diabetic autonomic neuropathy or aberrant regeneration. This means that when the examiner sees a pupil with a weak light reaction but no segmental palsy, he or she should consider a drug-induced mydriasis and then perhaps look again for lid and motility signs of a third nerve paresis.

Pharmacologic Response of the Iris Sphincter to Cholinergic Drugs

Cholinergic Supersensitivity. If weak pilocarpine (0.0625%, 0.1%, or 0.125%) is applied to both eyes and the affected (dilated) pupil constricts more than the normal pupil (actually becoming the smaller pupil in darkness), the iris sphincter has probably lost some of its innervation and has become supersensitive (Figure 32-16). Cholinergic supersensitivity can occur within 5 to 7 days. The conclusion that cholinergic supersensitivity exists assumes that corneal penetration of the drug is the same in each eye (i.e., both corneas are healthy and untouched, tear function is normal, and the eyelids are working properly in both eyes). It seems likely that with postganglionic denervation (damage at the ciliary ganglion or distal to it) the sphincter will show more supersensitivity than in the preganglionic case (third nerve palsy). However, it appears that the differences are not great. For all of these reasons, cholinergic supersensitivity of the iris sphincter is now considered only a confirmatory sign of Adie syndrome. In fact, the results of supersensitivity testing may be ambiguous in Adie syndrome, depending on the chronicity of the condition. As reinnervation takes place over time in Adie syndrome (with accommodative cholinergic nerves growing into the iris sphincter), the reinnervated sphincter segments may lose their cholinergic supersensitivity.[59] If a patient

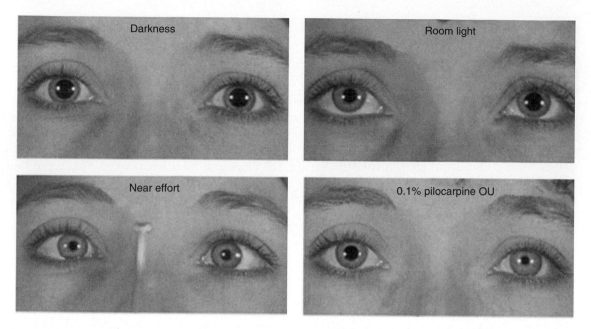

FIGURE 32-16 Example of Adie's pupil (*left*) showing little anisocoria in darkness (*upper left*) and an increasing anisocoria in room light (*upper right*). A light-near dissociation with a greater contraction of the left pupil to a near stimulus compared with light (*lower left*), indicating a chronic state resulting from reinnervation of the iris sphincter by accommodative neurons. The patient still exhibited signs of cholinergic supersensitivity (*lower right*), with the involved pupil contracting more to 0.1% pilocarpine than the fellow pupil.

shows the presence of cholinergic supersensitivity in one eye without any segmental palsies, other causes besides Adie's pupil should be reconsidered. Subtle signs of ptosis or diplopia should be looked for once more to leave no doubt that the oculomotor nerve is not affected. It is rare for an ambulatory patient to have an isolated sphincter palsy without other signs of oculomotor nerve palsy as a result of compressive damage to the intracranial third nerve caused by a tumor or aneurysm.

Testing of iris cholinergic sensitivity is best performed when comparing an affected eye with its fellow, normal eye. Testing for whether cholinergic supersensitivity is present in both eyes, without comparing the response with the normal fellow eye in the same subject, is problematic because there is considerable variation in the cholinergic response among different individuals. Even some normal eyes can respond to 0.05% pilocarpine, so for supersensitivity testing to be the most meaningful, the test is best used in the setting of unilateral causes.

Subsensitivity of the Iris Sphincter to Cholinergic Testing. If the normal pupil constricts only a small amount to dilute cholinergic agents and the dilated pupil not at all, the mydriasis may be caused by the presence of an anticholinergic drug like atropine,

which inhibits the receptors on the iris sphincter muscle. A stronger concentration of pilocarpine is then needed to settle this point. If, on application of 1% pilocarpine in each eye, the affected pupil does little or nothing and the unaffected pupil constricts normally, the pupil is not larger because of nerve denervation, but rather, because of a problem in the sphincter muscle itself. The following are different nonneuronal causes of mydriasis:

- Anticholinergic mydriasis (e.g., scopolamine, cyclopentolate, atropine)
- Traumatic iridoplegia (Look for sphincter tears, appearing as divots at the pupil border; pigment dispersion on the corneal endothelium of lens; and angle recession.)
- Angle-closure glaucoma (ischemia of the iris sphincter that occurs during the time when the intraocular pressure is high)
- Previous herpes zoster iritis causing direct damage to the iris sphincter
- Synechiae causing a bound-down iris that is mechanically immobile
- Fixed pupil following anterior segment surgery

The cause for a loss of function of the iris muscle following anterior segment surgery is unknown. In some cases with a postoperative rise in intraocular pressure, the cause may be an ischemic insult to

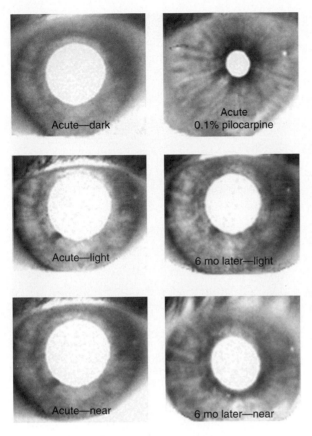

FIGURE 32-17 Infrared iris transillumination in Adie's pupil. The iris sphincter appears as a dark ring at the pupillary border when it contracts, as observed with infrared iris transillumination. In the patient shown, almost all of the iris sphincter was denervated, except for the segment at the 7 o'clock meridian, which darkened when made to contract with light or near (*left center,* and *left bottom panel*). With low-dose pilocarpine, the rest of the sphincter muscle that was denervated is the area where supersensitivity was present. Every area darkened after the pilocarpine, except the normal segment at the 7 o'clock position, which remains lighter (not contracted), as shown in the *upper right panel*. After 6 months, the pupil started to become smaller and contracted to near (*bottom right panel*), but it remained unresponsive to light, except for the 7 o'clock segment (*center right panel*).

the iris sphincter. An autoimmune process may be responsible, but it has not been proven. It may be related to the same process as Urrets-Zavalia syndrome, in which a dilated, fixed pupil may occur following penetrating keratoplasty.

Adie's Tonic Pupil: Postganglionic Parasympathetic Denervation

Young adults (more commonly women than men) may suddenly find that one pupil is large or that they cannot focus as well with one eye at near. Slit-lamp examination usually shows segmental denervation of the iris sphincter, with some remaining normal segments still reacting to light. Within the first week, supersensitivity of the iris and ciliary muscle to cholinergic substances can be demonstrated. After about 2 months, nerve regrowth is active and fibers originally bound for the ciliary muscle (they outnumber the sphincter fibers by 30:1) start arriving (aberrantly) at the iris sphincter and the ciliary muscle. The light reaction of the denervated segments does not return, but the reinnervated segments now show contraction to a near stimulus. This produces the characteristic "light-near dissociation" of Adie syndrome (Figure 32-16), as well as a return of some accommodative ampli-

tude. Therefore the presence of light-near dissociation in this setting is a sign of a chronic Adie's pupil with reinnervation and is not a sign of an acute Adie's pupil. The pupil contraction to a near stimulus is often tonic, being slow to dilate when gaze is shifted to a distant target. Although there is also some return of accommodative amplitude, the dynamics of focusing in the affected eye are also slowed and not normal. Patients often complain of difficulties when trying to refocus from near to far because the relaxation of accommodation is slower in the affected eye. Eventually, the affected pupil becomes the smaller of the two pupils, especially in dim light, as a result of the amount of reinnervation by cholinergic accommodative neurons, which keep the sphincter in a contracted state. It turns out that the segmental palsy of the iris sphincter in Adie syndrome and the individual sphincter segment responses to light, near and pilocarpine, can be seen especially well by infrared video recording of transillumination of the iris (Figure 32-17). Many of these patients also lack normal motor jerk reflexes and may also have decreased vibratory sensation, indicating a similar process occurring in the spinal cord neurons. However, Adie syndrome is not associated with any major neurologic disorder or significant dysfunction. The cause of Adie's pupil is not well understood, but it has been hypothesized that an immune reaction may mediate the damage to ciliary ganglion and spinal neurons. Younger children may get an Adie's pupil after having chickenpox. After about 10 years, almost 50% of patients with Adie's pupil show evidence of a similar process occurring in the other eye.

Pupil Involvement in Third Nerve Palsy

There is an old clinical rule of thumb stating that if the pupillary light reaction is spared in the setting of a third nerve palsy, the palsy is probably not caused by compression or injury, but more likely, it is caused by small vessel disease, such as might be seen in diabetes. It is still a fairly good rule, provided one bears in mind that a small but definite number of pupil-sparing third nerve palsies are caused by midbrain infarcts and should have neuroimaging studies. Because the preganglionic parasympathetic nerves for the pupil light reflex are located on the medial side of the intracranial portion of the third nerve as it exits the midbrain, compression of the third nerve in this location results in some element of iris sphincter palsy. The most common cause of this would be an aneurysm (i.e., of the posterior communicating artery) or pituitary apoplexy (sudden lateral expansion of a pituitary adenoma pressing on the medial aspect of the third nerve). Pupil involvement is often incomplete, so it is important to look for iris sphincter weakness by observing for anisocoria in bright light. In the absence of aberrant regeneration (from chronic compression), we have yet to observe a case of pupil involving third nerve palsy from an aneurysm that showed segmental palsies; all of the cases so far have shown symmetric involvement of the iris sphincter over its circumference. Some patients with ischemic third nerve palsy and diabetes have shown mild pupil involvement with elements of segmental palsies. It appears that these patients may have had preexisting pupil involvement from diabetic autonomic neuropathy.

Aberrant Regeneration in the Third Nerve

The third cranial nerve carries bundles of nerves supplying different extraocular muscles (medial rectus, inferior rectus, inferior oblique, superior rectus, and levator palpebrae muscles), as well as preganglionic parasympathetic nerves to the iris sphincter and ciliary body. Injury to the third nerve and glial scaffolding, through which individual nerve bundles pass, causes the nerve fibers to regrow, and they often end up in the wrong place. For

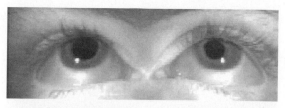
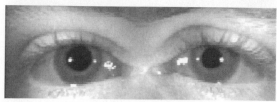
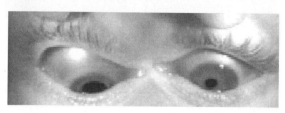

FIGURE 32-18 Primary aberrant regeneration of the left third nerve following chronic compression of the oculomotor nerve by a meningioma. In darkness (*top* and *center panels*) the left pupil is the smaller of the two pupils as a result of innervation by motor nerves. Nerves that normally would have supplied the inferior rectus muscle now are innervating the iris sphincter muscle, causing pupil contraction on downgaze (*lower panel*).

example, the eye may inappropriately turn in when the patient is trying to look down, or the pupil may inappropriately constrict with depression, adduction, or supraduction of the globe (Figure 32-18). With eyelid involvement, the lid fissure may widen with infraduction, adduction, or supraduction of the eye. Aberrant regeneration of the oculomotor nerve may be primary or secondary. In secondary aberrant regeneration, a third nerve palsy precedes the aberrant regeneration by at least 8 weeks. In primary aberrant regeneration, there is no preceding nerve palsy; the damage to the nerve slowly progresses simultaneous with the process of aberrant regeneration. Primary aberrant regeneration is clinically important to recognize because it is almost always caused by a slow compression of the intracranial third nerve by a tumor or aneurysm.

Light-Near Dissociation: Evaluation of the Near Response

The pupil response to a near effort should be observed as a standard part of the pupil evaluation. Any time the pupil light reaction seems weak, it is important to check to see whether the pupils constrict bet-

TABLE 32-4
CAUSES OF LIGHT-NEAR DISSOCIATION OF THE PUPIL

CAUSE	LOCATION	MECHANISM
Severe loss of afferent light input to both eyes	Anterior visual pathway (retina, optic nerves, chiasm)	Damage to the retina or optic nerve pathways
Loss of pretectal light input to Edinger-Westphal nucleus	Tectum of the midbrain	Infectious (Argyll Robertson pupils) or compression (pinealoma) or ischemia (stroke)
Adie syndrome	Iris sphincter	Aberrant reinnervation of sphincter by accommodative neurons
Third nerve aberrant reinnervation	Iris sphincter	Aberrant reinnervation of sphincter by accommodative neurons or medial rectus neurons

TABLE 32-5
CAUSES OF POOR PUPIL DILATION IN DARKNESS

CAUSE	LOCATION	MECHANISM
Past inflammation or surgical trauma	Posterior iris surface or sphincter	Scarring or synechiae of the iris resulting from past iritis
Acute trauma	Sphincter	Prostaglandin release causing sphincter spasm
Adie tonic pupil Third nerve aberrant reinnervation	Sphincter	Aberrant reinnervation of iris sphincter by accommodative or extraocular motor neurons that are not inhibited in darkness
Pharmacologic miosis	Iris sphincter	Cholinergic influence
Unilateral episodic spasm of miosis	Postganglionic parasympathetic neuron	Uninhibited episodic activation of postganglionic neurons
Congenital miosis (bilateral)	Sphincter	Developmental abnormality
Fatigue, sleepiness	Edinger-Westphal nucleus	Loss of inhibition at midbrain from reticular activating formation
Lymphoma, inflammation, infection	Periaqueductal gray matter	Interruption of inhibitory fibers to the Edinger-Westphal nucleus
Central acting drugs	Reticular activating formation, midbrain	Narcotics, general anesthetics
Old age (bilateral miosis)	Reticular activating formation, midbrain	Loss of inhibition at midbrain from reticular activating formation
Oculosympathetic defect	Sympathetic neuron interruption	Horner syndrome

ter to near than they do to light. If they do, this is called a *light-near dissociation.* Causes of light-near dissociation are summarized in Table 32-4. These are categorized by three major mechanisms:

1. Loss of light input resulting from severe damage to the afferent visual system (retina or optic nerve pathways)
2. Interruption of the light input pathways to the Edinger-Westphal nucleus from the pretectum (Argyll Robertson pupils, dorsal midbrain syndrome)
3. Aberrant regeneration of the pupillary sphincter from accommodative fibers (Adie

syndrome) or extraocular muscle neurons from the oculomotor nerve (medial rectus fibers or accommodative fibers from third nerve aberrant regeneration)

When the Pupil Fails to Dilate
When one or both pupils stay small and miotic, even in darkness, a number of reasons may be responsible (Table 32-5). To better understand the different possible mechanisms it is important to understand what normally happens in darkness to allow the pupil to dilate. When a light stimulus is terminated, two mechanisms cause the pupil to di-

late. The majority of pupil dilation comes about from inhibition to the Edinger-Westphal nucleus in the midbrain. This reduces the firing of the preganglionic parasympathetic neurons in the Edinger-Westphal nucleus, causing relaxation of the iris sphincter. Within a few seconds, sympathetic nerve firing increases, serving to augment the pupil dilation by active contraction of the dilator muscle. The combined inhibition of the iris sphincter and stimulation of the iris dilator is a carefully integrated neuronal reflex. The inability of the pupil to dilate in darkness may result from the following causes:

1. Mechanical limitations of the pupil (scarring)
2. Pharmacologic miosis
3. Aberrant reinnervation of cholinergic neurons to the iris sphincter that are not normally inhibited in darkness (accommodative or extraocular motor neurons)
4. Lack of inhibitory input signal getting to the Edinger-Westphal nucleus
5. Lack of sympathetic input to the dilator muscle

REFERENCES

1. Alexandridis E, Krastel H, Reuther R: Disturbances of the pupil reflex associated with lesions of the upper visual pathway, *Albrecht von Graefes Arch Klin Exp Ophthalmol* 209:199, 1979.
2. Almegrad B, Stjernschantz J, Bill A: Cholecystokinin contracts isolated human and monkey iris sphincters: a study with CCK receptor antagonists, *Eur J Pharmacol* 211:183, 1992.
3. Barbur JL, Forsyth PM: Can the pupil response be used as a measure of visual input associated with the geniculo-striate pathway? *Clin Vis Sci* 1:107, 1986.
4. Barbur JL, Harlow AJ, Sahraie A: Pupillary responses to stimulus structure, colour, and movement, *Ophthal Physiol Opt* 12:137, 1992.
5. Barbur JL, Keenleyside MS, Thomson WD: Investigation of central visual processing by means of pupillometry. In Kulikowski JJ, Dickinson CM, Murray IJ (eds): *Seeing colour and contour*, Oxford, 1989, Pergamon Press.
6. Barbur JL, Thomson WD: Pupil response as an objective measure of visual acuity, *Ophthal Physiol Opt* 7:425, 1987.
7. Bell RA et al: Clinical grading of relative afferent pupillary defects, *Arch Ophthalmol* 111:938, 1993.
8. Brown RH et al: The afferent pupillary defect in asymmetric glaucoma, *Arch Ophthalmol* 105:1540, 1987.
9. Campbell FW: The depth of field of the human eye, *Optica Acta* 4:157, 1957.
10. Campbell FW, Green DG: Optical and retinal factors affecting visual resolution, *J Physiol* 181:576, 1965.
11. Charman WN, Jenning JAM, Whitefoot H: The refraction of the eye in relation to spherical aberration and pupil diameter, *Vis Res* 17:737, 1978.
12. Cibis G, Campos E, Aulhorn E: Pupillary hemiakinesia in supragenicula lesions, *Arch Ophthalmol* 93:1322, 1975.
13. Cocker KD, Moseley MJ: Visual acuity and the pupil grating response, *Clin Vis Sci* 7:143, 1992.
14. Cox TA: Pupillography of a relative afferent pupillary defect, *Am J Ophthalmol* 101:320, 1986.
15. Cox TA: Pupillographic characteristics of simulated relative afferent pupillary defects, *Invest Ophthalmol Vis Sci* 30:1127, 1989.
16. Cremer SA et al: Hydroxyamphetamine mydriasis in Horner's syndrome, *Am J Ophthalmol* 110:71, 1990.
17. Fison PN, Garlick DJ, Smith SE: Assessment of unilateral afferent pupillary defects by pupillography, *Br J Ophthalmol* 63:195, 1979.
18. Gamlin PDR, Clarke RJ: The pupillary light reflex pathway of the primate, *J Am Optom Assoc* 66:415, 1995.
19. Gamlin PDR, Zhang H, Clarke RJ: Luminance neurons in the pretectal olivary nucleus mediate the pupillary light reflex in the rhesus monkey, *Exp Brain Res* 106:177, 1995.
20. Hamann K et al: Videopupillographic and VER investigations in patients with congenital and acquired lesions of the optic radiation, *Ophthalmologica* 178:348, 1979.
21. Harms H: Grundlagen, Methodik und Bedeutung der Pupillenperimetrie fur die Physiologie und Pathologie des Schorgans, *Albrecht von Graefes Arch Klin Exp Ophthalmol* 149:1, 1949.
22. Hellner KA, Jensen W, Muller A: Video processing pupillographic perimetry in hemianopsia, *Klin Mbl Augenheik* 172:731, 1978.
23. Hellner K, Jensen W, Muller-Jensen A: Video-processing pupillography as a method for objective perimetry in pupillary hemiakinesia. In Greve EL (ed): *The proceedings of the second international visual field symposium, Tubingen, 1976, Doc Ophthalmol Proc Series,* vol 14, The Hague, 1977, Dr W Junk Publishers.
24. Huhtala A: Origin of myelinated nerves in the rat iris, *Exp Eye Res* 22:259, 1976.
25. Johnson LN, Hill RA, Bartholomew MJ: Correlation of afferent pupillary defect with visual field loss on automated perimetry, *Ophthalmology* 95:1649, 1988.
26. Kardon RH: Pupil perimetry. In *Current opinion in ophthalmology*, vol 3, Philadelphia, 1992, Current Science.
27. Kardon RH: Anatomy and physiology of the pupil. Section III. The autonomic nervous system: pupillary function, accommodation, and lacrimation. In Miller NM, Newman NJ (eds): *Walsh and Hoyt's clinical neuro-ophthalmology*, vol 1, ed 5, Baltimore, 1998, Williams & Wilkins.
28. Kardon RH, Corbett JJ, Thompson HS; Segmental denervation and reinnervation of the iris sphincter as shown by infrared videographic transillumination, *Ophthalmology* 105:313, 1998.
29. Kardon RH, Haupert C, Thompson HS: The relationship between static perimetry and the relative afferent pupillary defect, *Am J Ophthalmol* 115:351, 1993.
30. Kardon RH, Kirkali PA, Thompson HS: Automated pupil perimetry, *Ophthalmology* 98:485, 1991.
31. Kardon RH et al: Critical evaluation of the cocaine test in the diagnosis of Horner's syndrome, *Arch Ophthalmol* 108:384, 1990.
32. Kawasaki A, Moore P, Kardon RH: Variability of the relative afferent pupillary defect, *Am J Ophthalmol* 120:622, 1995.
33. Kawasaki A, Moore P, Kardon RH: Long-term fluctuation of relative afferent pupillary defect in subjects with normal visual function, *Am J Ophthalmol* 122:875, 1996.
34. Kerr FWL, Hollowell OW: Location of pupillomotor and accommodation fibres in the oculomotor nerve: experimental observations on paralytic mydriasis, *J Neurol Neurosurg Psychiatr* 27:473, 1964.
35. Koss MC: Pupillary dilation as an index of central nervous system alpha2-adrenoceptor activation, *J Pharmacol Methods* 15:1, 1986.
36. Levatin P: Pupillary escape in disease of the retina or optic nerve, *Arch Ophthalmol* 62:768, 1959.

37. Loewenfeld IE: The light reflex. In *The pupil: anatomy, physiology and clinical applications,* vol 1, Ames, Iowa, and Detroit, Mich, 1993, Iowa State University Press and Wayne State University Press.

38. Loewenfeld IE: Methods of pupil testing. In *The pupil: anatomy, physiology and clinical applications,* vol 1, Ames, Iowa, and Detroit, Mich, 1993, Iowa State University Press and Wayne State University Press.

39. Loewenfeld IE: Reactions to darkness. In *The pupil: anatomy, physiology and clinical applications,* vol 1, Ames, Iowa, and Detroit, Mich, 1993, Iowa State University Press and Wayne State University Press.

40. Loewenfeld IE: The reaction to near vision. In *The pupil: anatomy, physiology and clinical applications,* vol 1, Ames, Iowa, and Detroit, Mich, 1993, Iowa State University Press and Wayne State University Press.

41. Loewenfeld IE: Reflex dilation. In *The pupil: anatomy, physiology and clinical applications,* vol 1, Ames, Iowa, and Detroit, Mich, 1993, Iowa State University Press and Wayne State University Press.

42. Loewenfeld IE, Newsome DA: Iris mechanics: I. Influence of pupil diameter on dynamics of pupillary movements, *Am J Ophthalmol* 71:347, 1971.

43. Lowenstein O, Kawabata H, Loewenfeld I: The pupil as indicator of retinal activity, *Am J Ophthalmol* 57:569, 1964.

44. Narasaki S et al: Videopupillographic perimetry and its clinical application, *Jpn J Ophthalmol* 18:253, 1974.

45. Newsome DA, Loewenfeld IE: Iris mechanics: II. Influence of pupil diameter on details of iris structure, *Am J Ophthal* 71:553, 1971.

46. Reuther R, Alexandridis E, Krastel H: Disturbances of the pupil reflex associated with cerebral infraction in the posterior cerebral artery territory, *Arch Psychiatr Nervenkr* 229:249, 1981.

47. Rushton WAW: Visual adaptation: the Ferrier lecture, *Proc R Soc Biol Lond* 162:20. 1965.

48. Saari M et al: Wallerian degeneration of the myelinated nerves of cat iris after denervation of the ophthalmic division of the trigeminal nerve: an electron microscopic study, *Exp Eye Res* 17:281, 1973.

49. Slooter, JH, van Noren D: Visual acuity measured with pupil responses to checkerboard stimuli, *Invest Ophthalmol Vis Sci* 19:105, 1980.

50. ten Doesschate J, Alpern M: Response of the pupil to steady state retinal illumination: contribution by cones, *Science* 149:989, 1965.

51. Thompson HS, Corbett JJ: Asymmetry of pupillomotor input, *Eye* 5:36, 1991.

52. Thompson HS, Corbett JJ, Cox TA: How to measure the relative afferent pupillary defect, *Surv Ophthalmol* 26:39, 1981.

53. Thompson HS et al: The relationship between visual acuity, pupillary defect, and visual field loss, *Am J Ophthalmol* 93:681, 1982.

54. Ukai K: Spatial pattern as a stimulus to the pupillary system, *J Opt Soc Am* 1094, 1985.

55. Volpe NJ et al: Portable pupillography of the swinging flashlight test to detect afferent pupillary defects, *Ophthalmology* 107:1913, 2000.

56. Weinstein JM, Zweifel TJ, Thompson HS: Congenital Horner's syndrome, *Arch Ophthalmol* 98:1074, 1980.

57. Westheimer G: pupil diameter and visual resolution, *Vis Res* 4:39, 1964.

58. Young RSL, Han B, Wu P: Transient and sustained components of the pupillary responses evoked by luminance and color, *Vis Res* 33:437, 1993.

59. Young RSL, Kennish J: Transient and sustained components of the pupil response evoked by achromatic spatial patterns, *Vis Res* 33:2239, 1993.

SECTION 13

CIRCULATION

ALBERT ALM

CHAPTER 33

OCULAR CIRCULATION

GEORGE A. CIOFFI, ELISABET GRANSTAM, AND ALBERT ALM

Over the past several decades, extensive investigations have examined the vascular anatomy, both gross and ultrastructural, of the eye. Particular attention has been given to the vascular supply of the posterior pole and optic nerve. In addition, research into the role of the vascular endothelium in regulation of vascular tone has increased our understanding of the blood flow regulation in both the healthy and the diseased eye.

Evidence that vascular factors contribute to the pathogenesis and development of various ocular diseases continues to accumulate. New sophisticated, in vivo analysis techniques, such as ultrasound color Doppler imaging and laser Doppler flowmetry, allow better assessment of the hemodynamic status of the eye. In response to the recognition that different analysis techniques have led to conflicting observations, experimental models have been developed to provide an additional tool with which to interpret the effects of blood flow alterations on the eye. A comprehensive understanding of the normal vascular anatomy and physiology of the eye is essential to understand the potential contributions of the vascular system to disease.

ANATOMY

Two separate vascular systems are involved in the nutrition of the eye: the retinal vessels and the uveal, or ciliary, vessels. The uveal blood vessels include the vascular beds of the iris, the ciliary body, and the choroid. The main function of the choroid is to serve the outer retina. In some lower mammals, such as rabbits and guinea pigs, the retinal tissues are almost completely dependent on the choroid because retinal vessels are found only within a small area of the retina or are totally lacking. In many higher mammals, including humans and other primates, the retina depends on both the retinal vessels and the choroid.

In humans the ocular vessels are derived from the ophthalmic artery, which is a branch of the internal carotid.[175] The ophthalmic artery branches into the central retinal artery, the posterior ciliary arteries, and several anterior ciliary arteries.[136] Figure 33-1 shows schematically the blood vessels of the human eye. The central retinal artery enters the optic nerve approximately 10 mm behind the eyeball and appears within the eye at the optic disc, where it branches into four major vessels each supplying one quadrant of the retina. Small arterioles and veins interdigitate in a characteristic way within the retina (Figure 33-2). A capillary-free zone surrounds the arterioles, probably because of high local oxygen tension, which causes vascular remodeling during maturation.[145,195]

In humans the orbital contents receive their vascular supply from several arteries, including the ophthalmic artery, the meningolacrimal artery (a branch from the middle meningeal artery), and the palpebral arteries, which branch from the facial artery.[224] The middle meningeal artery and the facial artery belong to the external carotid arterial system. The ophthalmic artery provides most of the blood supply to the eye and is the first branch of the internal carotid artery, arising as the internal carotid artery turns to pierce the dura and emerge from the cavernous sinus. The vascular supply to the intraorbital optic nerve, retina, and choroid arises predominantly from the ophthalmic arterial circulation by way of the posterior ciliary arteries, the central retinal artery, and the pial vascular network along the optic nerve.[225,227] The ophthalmic artery exits the intracranial cavity through the optic

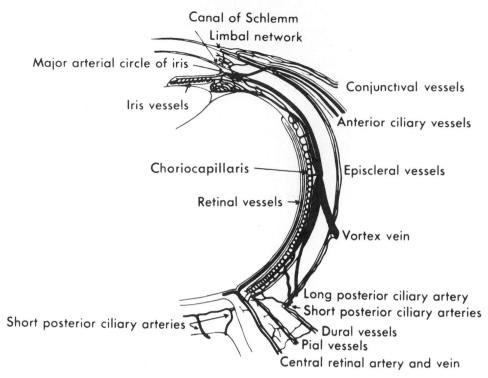

FIGURE 33-1 Blood vessels of the human eye. (Modified from Leber T: Circulations and Ernährungsverhältnisse des Auges. In Graefe A, Saemisch T [eds]: *Handbuch der gesamten Augenheilkunde,* Leipzig, Germany, 1903, Springer-Verlag.)

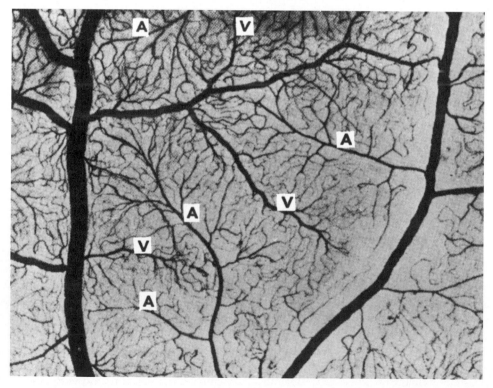

FIGURE 33-2 Field from equatorial zone in retina. *Left,* vein; *right,* artery. Note interdigitation of venae efferentes (*V*) with arteriae afferentes (*A*). Note also capillary-free zone around artery (From Michaelson J, Campbell ACP: *Trans Ophthalmol Soc UK* 60:71, 1940).

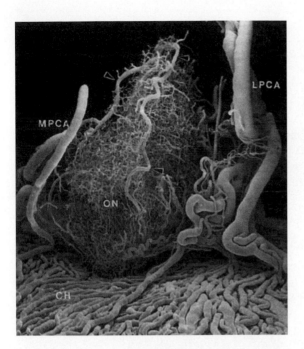

FIGURE 33-3 Posterior view of a vascular corrosion casting of a primate eye. The optic nerve enters the posterior aspect of the globe, with adjacent groups of posterior ciliary arteries. Pial arteries (*arrowheads*) course along the optic nerve. *CH*, Choroid; *LPCA*, lateral posterior ciliary arteries; *MPCA*, medial posterior ciliary arteries; *ON*, optic nerve. (From Cioffi GA: Vasculature of the anterior optic nerve and peripapillary choroid. In Ritch R, Shields MB, Krupin T [eds]: *The glaucomas*, St Louis, 1996, Mosby.)

canal and, in most individuals, lies inferolateral to the optic nerve. The ophthalmic artery has several intraorbital collateral vessels with the external carotid artery system. The most significant collaterals are the lacrimal and the ethmoidal anastomoses. The ocular branches of the ophthalmic artery are the central retinal artery and one to five posterior ciliary arterial trunks. These trunks branch into the main posterior ciliary arteries (Figure 33-3). Most individuals have two to three posterior ciliary trunks, which supply the medial and lateral posterior ciliary arteries. Each main posterior ciliary artery further divides into several short posterior ciliary arteries, just before or after entering the sclera. In addition, medial and lateral long posterior ciliary arteries arise from the ciliary trunks, travel anterior along the outside of the globe, before penetrating the sclera at the horizontal meridian of the globe. The long posterior ciliary arteries supply the iris, ciliary body, and the anterior region of the choroid.

The short posterior ciliary arteries course anterior after branching from the main posterior ciliary arteries and pierce the sclera immediately adjacent to the optic nerve, predominantly in the nasal and temporal region (Figure 33-4). Occasionally, short posterior ciliary arteries may have extrascleral anastomosis. The short posterior ciliary arteries supply the posterior choroid and most of the anterior optic nerve. The size and shape of the area of the choroid and optic nerve supplied by each short posterior ciliary artery is variable among subjects and even between the eyes of a single individual. Some short posterior ciliary arteries course, without branching, through the sclera directly into the choroid, whereas others divide within the sclera to provide branches to both the choroid and the anterior optic nerve. Often, the medial and lateral short posterior ciliary arteries anastomose and form an elliptic circle around the optic nerve, the arterial circle of Zinn and Haller. Branches derived from the circle of Zinn and Haller include recurrent pial branches, choroidal branches, and branches penetrating the optic nerve. This arterial circle is usually intrascleral, but occasionally, an incomplete extrascleral arterial network is present. Human intravascular corrosion castings have demonstrated that the anastomoses between the lateral and medial short posterior ciliary arteries form a complete elliptic circle around the optic nerve in 77% of the eyes but that 43% of these eyes have narrowed segments along the interarterial anastomoses.[224]

The venous drainage of the orbit generally does not follow the arterial supply. The orbital veins, in common with those of the head and neck, contain no valves. The largest of the orbital veins is the superior ophthalmic vein, which accommodates most of the orbital venous effluent. The venous drainage of the retina and the anterior optic nerve is almost exclusively through the central retinal vein and its tributaries, which subsequently empties into the superior ophthalmic vein. Most of the choroid is drained through the vortex venous system that empties into the superior and inferior ophthalmic veins. It is often difficult to identify an inferior ophthalmic vein independent from the superior ophthalmic vein; numerous anastomoses are generally present between them. Both vessels drain into the cavernous sinus. However, the inferior ophthalmic vein occasionally drains into the pterygoid plexus through the inferior orbital tissue.

The retinal vessels are distributed within the inner two thirds of the retina, whereas the outer layers, including the photoreceptors, are avascular and

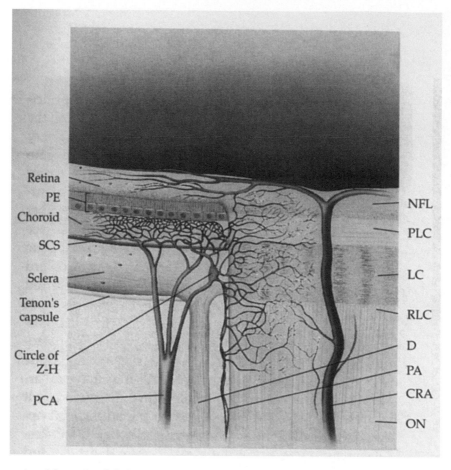

Figure 33-4   Arterial supply of the anterior optic nerve (*ON*) showing the contribution from the circle of Zinn-Haller (*Z-H*), the pial arteries (*PA*), and the central retinal artery (*CRA*). *D*, Dura mater; *LC*, laminar region; *NFL*, nerve fiber layer; *PCA*, posterior ciliary artery; *PLC*, prelaminar region; *RLC*, retrolaminar region. (From Cioffi GA: Vasculature of the anterior optic nerve and peripapillary choroid. In Ritch R, Shields MB, Krupin T [eds]: *The glaucomas*, St Louis, 1996, Mosby.)

---

nourished from the choroid (Figure 33-5). An avascular zone, which enables light to reach the central photoreceptors without encountering a single blood vessel, is seen centrally in the fovea (Figure 33-6; see also Color Plate 22). Arteries and veins are located within the nerve fiber layer (Figure 33-7). The capillaries are arranged in a laminated fashion with two layers of flat capillary networks in a large part of the retina.[195,319] In the central part of the retina, these capillary networks are dense and may become three or four layered, whereas in the periphery the networks are less dense and reduced to a single layer. The extreme peripheral inner retina is avascular. A separate superficial layer of capillaries, the radial peripapillary capillaries, extends from the optic disc, with its main extensions in the upper and lower temporal directions. A cil-

ioretinal artery is sometimes seen. It is a direct branch from the ciliary arteries, emerging from the rim of the optic cup and supplying a small area of the retina.

The retrobulbar part of the optic nerve is supplied by branches from the central retinal artery and from pial vessels, whereas the intraocular part of the nerve receives no branches from the central retinal artery, with the exception of the most superficial layers of the optic disc. The remaining part of the anterior optic nerve and the lamina cribrosa receive their main supply through direct branches from choroidal arteries and short posterior ciliary arteries.[139] The peripapillary choriocapillaris does not contribute to the vascular supply of the optic nerve. The posterior ciliary arteries branch behind the globe into 10 to 20 short poste-

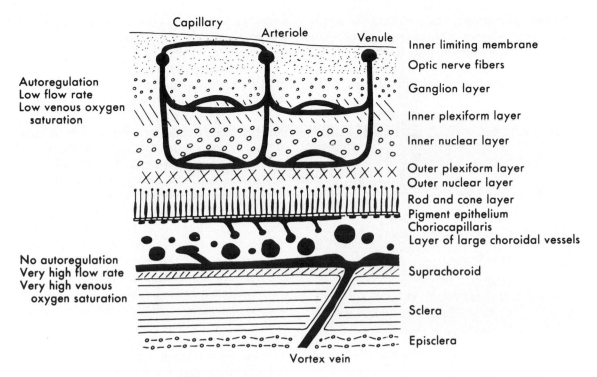

FIGURE 33-5 Retinal capillaries are distributed within inner layers of retina. The outer layer, 130 μm thick, has no blood vessels. It is nourished mainly from choroidal capillaries.

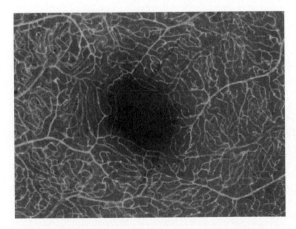

FIGURE 33-6 Foveal avascular zone. Immunohistochemical stain of the vascular endothelium in the retina. Note the central foveal avascular zone is devoid of both larger vessels and capillaries.

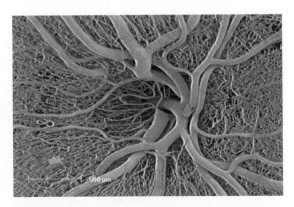

FIGURE 33-7 Anterior (retinal) view of vascular corrosion casting from a human eye. The depth of the normal optic nerve cup is outlined by the optic nerve vasculature. The central retinal artery and central retinal vein can be identified from the central/nasal portion of the optic nerve.

rior ciliary arteries and, as a rule, two long posterior ciliary arteries. The short posterior ciliary arteries pierce the sclera at the posterior pole and form the choriocapillaris, a dense, one-layered network adjacent to Bruch's membrane and the reti-

nal pigment epithelium. In the posterior pole the choriocapillaris is arranged in a lobular fashion with alternating feeding arterioles and draining venules and the transition from arteriole to choriocapillaris is unusually abrupt[137,336] (Figure 33-8). In the equatorial area and at the periphery, the lobular arrangement becomes gradually replaced by more spindle- or ladder-shaped patterns.[336] Interarterial and intervenous shunts between medium-sized vessels have been observed in the human choroid.[336] The

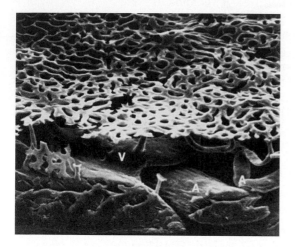

FIGURE 33-8   Scanning electron micrograph of cast of cat choroid. Choroidal arteries (*A*) and veins (*V*) are seen beneath choriocapillaris. Note abrupt transition from arterioles to choriocapillaris. (From Risco JM, Nopanitaya W: *Invest Ophthalmol Vis Sci* 19:5, 1980.)

long posterior ciliary arteries furnish a sector each in the nasal and temporal periphery of the choroid, respectively.[137]

The anterior ciliary arteries are the major source of blood supply to the anterior uvea.[327] They travel with the rectus muscles, pierce the sclera anteriorly to form an intramuscular circle, and with the long posterior ciliary arteries, form the major iridial circle of the iris, which is the main supply of the iris and the ciliary body (Figure 33-9). They also send some recurrent branches to the peripheral choroid.[101]

The vascular supply of the ciliary processes is complex, and large species variations have been observed.[206] In the human eye, the vascular anatomy of the ciliary processes has been described and divided into three regions[101] (Figures 33-9 and 33-10). The first region consists of anterior arterioles with a capillary network situated mainly at the broadened base of the anterior edge of the major ciliary processes. The capillaries drain into venules located deep in the ciliary processes with little connection to the other vascular territories or to the marginal ciliary vein. These vessels form a transition zone between the fenestrated capillaries of the ciliary processes and the nonfenestrated capillaries of the iris. The second region is also derived from the an-

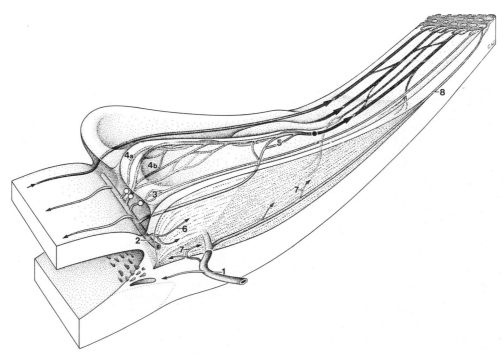

FIGURE 33-9   Schematic drawing of the vascular architecture in the human ciliary body, sagittal section. *1*, Perforating branches of the anterior ciliary arteries. *2*, Major arterial circle of iris. *3*, First vascular territory. *4*, Second vascular territory. *4a*, Marginal route. *4b*, Capillary network in the center of this territory. *5*, Third vascular territory. *6* and *7*, Arterioles to the ciliary muscle. *8*, Recurrent choroidal arteries. *Light circles,* Terminal arterioles. *Dark circle,* Efferent venous segment. (Modified from Funk R, Rohen JW: *Exp Eye Res* 51:651, 1990.)

terior portion of the major ciliary processes, but these vessels drain into a broad marginal vein at the inner edge of the ciliary processes. The third and final region provides blood to the posterior portion of the major ciliary processes and the minor ciliary processes. If exposed to epinephrine, the terminal arterioles of the two first vascular territories show marked focal constrictions.[101] This may be to protect the blood-aqueous barrier; a sympathetic tone prevents breakdown of the blood-aqueous barrier when arterial blood pressure is suddenly raised.[38]

Retinal venous blood is drained by a central retinal vein that leaves the eye through the optic nerve and drains into the cavernous sinus. Choroidal blood leaves the eye by way of the vortex veins, as a rule, one vein in each quadrant of the posterior pole of the eye. Blood from the anterior uvea is drained mainly through the vortex veins, although there are minor anastomotic communications with anterior episcleral vessels. Aqueous humor is drained into these episcleral vessels from collector channels leaving the canal of Schlemm. These episcleral veins, containing aqueous humor, were described by Ascher.[19]

Experimental occlusion of the retinal arteries in pigs has demonstrated that these vessels are end arteries without any anastomoses.[76] Occlusion of retinal vessels therefore destroys the inner retinal layers.[280] Irreparable damage occurs if ocular ischemia exceeds 1 hour.[100] Occlusion of choroidal arterioles

destroys the outer layers of the retina.[66] Interarterial shunts between medium-sized choroidal arteries may reduce the damage caused by occlusion of a single large or medium-sized choroidal artery, but the anatomic continuity of the choriocapillaris does not prevent choroidal ischemia.[336] Occlusion of a terminal choroidal arteriole likely cannot be compensated by flow through adjacent venules because an adequate pressure gradient promoting blood flow is not maintained. The situation is different in the anterior segment of the eye, where the anastomotic circles supplied by the anterior and long posterior ciliary arteries permit rather extensive muscle surgery without anterior segment ischemia.

FINE STRUCTURE AND BLOOD-OCULAR BARRIERS

The fine structure of the various vascular beds of the eye differs significantly with corresponding differences in permeability. All vascular beds are highly permeable to lipid-soluble substances, such as oxygen and carbon dioxide, which pass readily through the endothelial cells. Water also diffuses rapidly through the vessel wall, most likely both between and through the endothelial cells. For water-soluble substances, the permeability of the vessel wall is determined by the structure of the capillary endothelium. Capillaries may be classified as continuous, fenestrated, or discontinuous. Continuous capillaries are

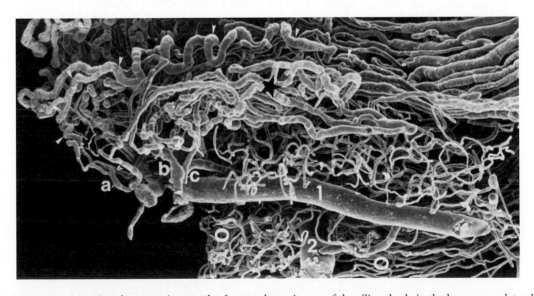

FIGURE 33-10   Scanning electron micrograph of a vascular resin cast of the ciliary body in the human eye; lateral aspect. *1,* Branch of the long posterior ciliary artery bending into the major arterial circle of the iris. *2,* Further branch of the major arterial circle of the iris. *a,* Anterior arterioles of the major processes (*arrows*). *b,* Arteriole for the central portion of the major process. *c,* Arteriole for the minor processes (*asterisk*). *Circles,* Ciliary muscle capillaries. Note the marginal venule (*arrowheads*). (From Funk R, Rohen JW: *Exp Eye Res* 51:651, 1990.)

the most impermeable type, and they can be found, for example, in mesentery, skeletal muscle, and brain. Adjacent endothelial cells are connected by more or less continuous networks of tight junctions (zonula occludentes). The wall of fenestrated capillaries is thin, with fenestrations covered by a thin, porous membrane. They are generally found in tissues where there are large fluid movements between the intravascular and extravascular compartments, such as the kidney, the intestinal mucosa, exocrine and endocrine glands.[182] Liver, spleen, and bone marrow contain discontinuous capillaries that permit blood cells to pass easily through the capillary walls. Continuous and fenestrated capillaries are represented in the eye, but no discontinuous capillaries are found.

Functional studies have demonstrated that even the continuous capillaries behave as porous membranes and that there are two populations of pores. The smaller pores, with a diameter of approximately 9 nm, are practically impermeable to albumin and large proteins.[231] They correspond to small interruptions in the junctional bindings between the

cells.[52] Large pores are much less frequent and have an estimated diameter of 24 to 70 nm.[115] They may be caused by occasional wide slits between endothelial cells.

Continuous capillaries in various tissues show a wide range of permeability because of a difference in continuity and complexity of the junctions corresponding to a difference in number and size of small pores. Thus the small pores of cerebral vessels have been estimated to have a diameter as small as 0.8 nm, and the endothelial permeability of the brain is less than 1% of that in skeletal muscle and less than 0.1% of that in the mesentery.[67,86] The tight junctions between the endothelial cells in the cerebral capillaries are the anatomic counterpart of the blood-brain barrier. The retina, being part of the brain, has a similar arrangement, the blood-retinal barrier, with tight junctions between the endothelial cells or the retinal capillaries (Figure 33-11) and between the cells of the retinal pigment epithelium.[68,153] A defect in the blood-retinal barrier exists at the level of the optic disc, where water-soluble

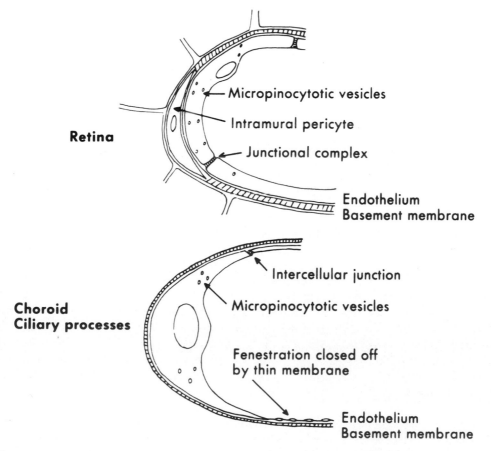

FIGURE 33-11   Schematic representation of capillary wall in retina and in ciliary process and choroid.

substances may enter the anterior optic nerve by diffusion from the extravascular space of the choroid.[114] The junctions of the capillaries of the prelaminar optic nerve may be less tight than those of the retina, as indicated by the relative presence of the endothelium-specific antigen PAL-E in the two vascular beds. The absence of PAL-E is used as a marker of the blood-brain barrier. PAL-E is expressed in most capillaries and veins but is generally absent from microvessels involved in the blood-brain and blood-ocular barriers. It was recently demonstrated that the capillaries of the prelaminar part of the optic nerve, unlike those of the retina, stained markedly for PAL-E.[270]

In the anterior segment of the eye, there is a corresponding blood-aqueous barrier that has tight junctions between the endothelial cells of the iris capillaries and between the nonpigmented cells of the ciliary epithelium.[279,281,323] Within the eye, variation in the degree of "leakiness" of tight junctions is considerable. Thus the permeability of the retinal capillaries is similar to that of cerebral vessels with no, or only minimal, leakage to fluorescein, or even sodium ions, whereas the junctional complexes of the primate iris vessels have a complexity intermediate between cerebral vessels and those of striated muscle.[96,114,318] Species differences exist; the iris vessels of the cat seem to be more permeable than those of primates.[22]

Because the blood-ocular barriers are largely impermeable even to small water-soluble substances, such as glucose and amino acids, vital metabolic substrates have to be transported through these barriers by means of carrier-mediated transport systems. Such transport systems can be found both in the blood-aqueous and the blood-retinal barriers.[13,200,247,317]

Rapid, modest, and reversible increments in permeability can occur even in cerebral vessels through a variety of stimuli, including drugs such as histamine, serotonin, and bradykinin.[67] This is assumed to take place through contractions of the endothelial cells in the cerebral venules causing widening of intracellular clefts. A receptor-mediated increase in vascular permeability has been observed in the rat iris, where isoproterenol increases permeability to carbon particles through development of clefts between the endothelial cells of the venules.[303,304] Thus it may be expected that some variation in the permeability of the blood-aqueous and blood-retinal barriers is normal.

Several ocular diseases and surgical trauma alter the permeability of the blood-ocular barriers. Thus the integrity of these barriers is of primary concern for the clinician. Ocular fluorophotometry permits clinical assessment of the permeability of the blood-retinal and blood-aqueous barriers, and this technique has been used to demonstrate increased permeability of the blood-retinal barrier in diabetes and arterial hypertension and of the blood-aqueous barrier after surgery.[170,171,268]

The retinal capillaries have a diameter of 5 to 6 μm.[175] The continuous layer of endothelial cells is surrounded by a thick basement membrane, within which is a discontinuous layer of intramural pericytes. There is a gradual transition between pericytes and smooth muscle cells in both terminal arterioles and venules. Pericytes are pluripotent cells that have been suggested to be involved in regulation of the microcirculation; in the permeability of the capillary wall; in modulation of endothelial cell growth and angiogenesis; in the immune system of the central nervous system; and as a progenitor for several cell types, including vascular smooth muscle cells, bone-producing cells, and phagocytes.[73-75,149,178,311] They are small cells with long processes that run parallel with the long axis of the microvessels and give off shorter processes that encircle the capillary walls. In the retina, pericyte processes cover a larger part of the circumference of the capillary endothelial tubes than in the brain.[94] They are located within basal lamina and are in intimate contact with the endothelial cells by peg and socket contacts, adhesion plaques, and gap junctions.[56,74,149] They express protein typical of contractile cells (i.e., actin and myosin).[74,149,178,311] Thus the pericytes contain the morphologic basis for contraction and deformation of the walls of the microvessels, although there seems to be heterogeneity of the contractile properties of the pericytes along the vascular bed. Nehls and Drenckhahn[208] report that pericytes of the true capillaries have little or no actin, but there is no doubt that precapillary and postcapillary pericytes do contract in vitro. Norepinephrine and histamine, but not endothelin, vasopressin, or acetylcholine, induced action potentials in cultured bovine retinal capillary pericytes.[144] Pericytes contract in the presence of angiotensin II, bradykinin, or serotonin and relax in the presence of adrenergic β_2-receptor agonists, nitric oxide, carbon dioxide, forskolin, or adenosine.* On the basis of these findings, it has been suggested that retinal pericytes may have an important role in regulation of the microcirculation.[17,149] Because of the pluripotent capacity of the pericytes, other roles must also be considered. Although vasoactive agents have been

---

*References 18, 127, 129, 188, 290, 339.

shown to change the caliber of capillaries in isolated whole mounted retina, Butryn et al.[53] found caliber changes only in larger vessels and not in capillaries in vivo after an intravitreal injection of vasoactive agents in rats.[276]

Thus much remains to be done to determine the main function of the retinal pericytes. It seems obvious that they play an important role in supporting the fragile capillary walls. Systemic hypertension in rats produces changes in retinal pericytes, and one could speculate that the early loss of pericytes in diabetes contributes to the formation of microaneurysms.[71,324] Their contacts with the endothelial cells indicate close collaboration in regulating the function of the capillaries. The capillaries are mainly exchange vessels and the contractile properties of the pericytes may be useful in this respect. Contraction may be tangential as well as circumferential.[207] In vascular beds without tight barriers, tangential contraction may deform endothelial cells and widen the interendothelial junctions.[178] Also, pericytes are more numerous and tend to have longer processes on the venous side of the capillaries and postcapillary venules.[149] Thus contraction of pericytes could have a more pronounced effect on fluid movement across the capillary wall than on vascular resistance because the ratio of precapillary to postcapillary resistance determines the hydrostatic pressure in the capillaries rather than flow resistance.[91] In the retina the exchange of fluid between blood and tissue is small, and at present there is no direct evidence that this is an important role for the retinal pericytes. One may speculate on their ability to convert to active macrophages. If this occurs in the retina, pericytes may be useful in clearing debris (e.g., disc hemorrhages), and they may also play a role in the immune response of the retina, as has been suggested for the brain.[311]

In the ciliary processes and the choroid, the capillaries are different from those of the retina and the iris (see Figure 33-11) in that these tissues contain fenestrated capillaries.[25,150] In the choriocapillaris the fenestrations are more numerous and larger in the submacular area compared with the periphery.[299] Such fenestrae result in high permeability to low-molecular-weight substances, and in both the ciliary processes and the choroid, the permeability even to substances as large as myoglobin (molecular weight 17,000) is high. Still larger albumin and gamma globulin molecules (molecular weight 67,900 and 156,000, respectively) also pass at high rates when compared with the conditions in many other tissues.[34] For the choriocapillaris, this high

permeability is probably necessary to maintain a high concentration of glucose at the retinal pigment epithelium and to permit passage of proteins involved in the supply of vitamin A to the retina.[43]

The uveal capillaries are wider than those of the retina, and the branches of the choriocapillaris are considered unusually wide. It was surprising, therefore, that only approximately 5% of intraarterially injected microspheres with a diameter of 8 to 10 m could pass through the rabbit choroid, whereas approximately 50% of these spheres passed through the vascular beds of the anterior uvea.[14] Casts from the rabbit choroid indicate that the spheres are caught in narrow or flat segments of the capillaries.[41]

TECHNIQUES FOR MEASURING OCULAR BLOOD FLOW

With increasing evidence that alterations in ocular blood flow are involved in the pathogenesis or contribute to the development of various ocular diseases, including diabetic retinopathy, glaucoma, and macular degeneration, a plethora of techniques for evaluating and monitoring the vascular status of the eye has evolved. These techniques have been used in both experimental animal models and human clinical investigations. Although each technique may provide valuable information about the status of a particular vascular bed within the eye, each one has limitations that must be taken into account while interpreting their measurements. The techniques that are clinically available measure either velocity of cells or fluorescein in the vascular bed or transit times for intravascular substances. None of these measurements can be translated into blood flow unless the precise diameter of the vessels at the site of measurement or information on the volume of the total retinal vascular bed is known. Still, when results obtained with available clinical techniques are cautiously interpreted in the light of what we know about the physiology and pharmacology of blood flow, valuable information can be gained. Much of our most accurate information regarding blood flow in the healthy eye has been derived from techniques that can be used only in animal experiments. Species differences do exist, but in most cases, results obtained in nonhuman primates are likely to be relevant for the human eye. For studies on the effect of various diseases on retinal blood flow or on the role of primary changes in ocular blood flow as part of the cause of disease, the lack of suitable animal models is a problem. A few techniques that have proved particularly useful are presented here along with some recent clinical techniques.

Techniques Used in Animal Experiments

Invasive, quantitative investigations of ocular blood flow have been performed in animals with a variety of techniques, including intravascular microspheres injections, iodoantipyrine autoradiography, hydrogen clearance, krypton washout, labile liposomes, oxygen tension assessment, and glucose consumption. For animal experiments, four basic techniques have proved valuable. With direct cannulation of the uveal veins, the blood flow within the uveal tract has been measured in both rabbits and cats.[30,31] In cats a large intrascleral venous plexus permits sampling of venous blood from either the anterior uvea or the posterior choroid. This plexus has been used to determine arteriovenous differences of oxygen and glucose.[7,315] A similar plexus exists in the retrobular space of the rabbit eye. Retinal arteriovenous differences can be studied in a variety of animals, including the pig, in which the retinal veins form a ring-shaped plexus around the optic nerve within the retrobulbar space.[318]

Intravascular injections of radioactively labeled and nonlabeled colored microspheres permit determination of blood flow to the different tissue beds within the eye.[9,221,229] Regional blood flow can be assessed by analyzing the distribution of particles (microspheres) injected into the systemic blood stream. Ideally, the relative quantity of particles recovered in each organ, compared with the total number of injected particles, equals the fraction of the cardiac output to the organ. The precision of the various microsphere techniques depends on several factors, including the number of microspheres trapped in the tissue sample. The accuracy of blood flow measurements within small tissue samples, such as the retina, the iris, or the optic nerve, can be improved if the number of samples is increased.[148] Precision of microsphere blood flow measurements can be further improved by the use of colored microsphere injections and microscopic counting of the imbedded microspheres.[106,229]

Continuous recording of the oxygen tension in the vitreous body close to the retina can give information on changes in retinal blood flow.[8] Studies of the oxygen profile within the retina with microelectrodes have the advantage of supplying information on the relative importance of the choroidal and retinal circulation in providing oxygen to the retina.[3] Glucose consumption in vivo can be studied by determining the tissue uptake of labeled 2-deoxy-D-glucose. Although it is not a direct measure of blood flow, this technique gives an estimate of alterations in metabolic demands and has proved useful for studying the effects of increased intraocular pressure (IOP) on the retina and the optic nerve.[40,289]

Clinical Methods

With the increasing clinical evidence that vascular abnormalities may be involved in the development of glaucomatous optic neuropathy at least in some eyes, many of the clinical techniques developed to assess ocular blood flow have focused on the optic nerve.[140] Conventional ocular hemodynamic measurements (including fluorescein fundus angiography, ocular thermocoupling and pulsatile ocular blood flow calculations) have been supplemented by these newer techniques (including color Doppler imaging, blue-field entoptic phenomenon, laser Doppler velocimetry and flowmetry, transcranial Doppler, and magnetic resonance imaging), and the combination has increased our understanding of the hemodynamic status of the eye in health and disease. Many of these techniques have been adapted to investigate hemodynamic alterations, not only in glaucoma but also in diverse disorders such as diabetic retinopathy, macular degeneration, retinal dystrophies, and nonglaucomatous optic neuropathies. However, each of these techniques has limitations, and not a single method provides comprehensive measurements for all the ocular tissues.[62,140] In addition, many of these techniques have lacked validation (assessment of reproducibility and accuracy) before implementation. Understanding the limitations and the theoretic assumptions of each of these techniques allows more prudent application in the clinical arena.

Fluorescein angiography is the basic technique for studies on retinal blood flow in clinical practice. Conventionally, fluorescein angiograms have been used to gather qualitative information about the vascular anatomy, patency, and integrity within the eye, but more recent attempts have been made to obtain quantitative or semiquantitative information. Quantitative angiogram techniques are based on the assumption that there is a constant relationship between fluorescence and fluorescein concentration.[248] Thus densitometric measurements of film can be used to calculate the mean transit time of the retinal circulation from fluorescein angiograms.[146] The mean transit time (MTT) is the ratio of blood volume to blood flow. The calculation is based on mathematics derived for a bolus injection, and it requires that the complete concentration-time curve can be reconstructed.[248] A major limitation is that the dye bolus reaching the eye after an injection into the antecubital vein is highly variable and confounded by a variety of factors. Together with the rapid recirculation of dye, this makes extrapolation of the downslope of the venous curve difficult. Analysis based on impulse-response relations improve reliability of MTT determinations from curves with a badly defined bolus compared with conventional analysis based on semilogarithmic extrapolation.[288] This makes it possible to construct time curves for the fluorescein concentrations in retinal arteries and veins. If the complete dye curves can be reconstructed, the MTT can be determined. The MTT (expressed in seconds) can be calculated as follows: vascular volume/flow through the vascular bed. MTT is the average time that a fluorescein molecule spends in the vascular bed, and it corresponds to the time necessary to renew all blood within the vascular bed.

The problems with recirculation have made it attractive to choose other parameters with which to analyze fluorescein angiograms. From the initial part of the curves, it is possible to measure the arteriovenous passage time (AVP), that is, the time it takes from the first appearance of the dye in an artery close to the disc until it appears in the nearby vein.[331] As long as the vascular volume is unknown, these techniques cannot be used to directly measure blood flow, but they may still provide valuable information on the effect of ocular disease on the retinal vascular bed.[314]

An interesting approach to obtaining a perfect bolus is the introduction of fluorescein into liposomes that can be released by laser in the retinal arteries[159,205,338] (Figure 33-12). The lack of choroidal background gives a beautiful demonstration of single retinal capillaries even outside the macula, and combined with high-speed angiography and image analysis, this technique should provide new opportunities for measuring various aspects of local retinal blood flow.

When choroidal circulation is being studied, indocyanine green (ICG) is a more suitable dye.[45] ICG has two significant advantages over fluorescein angiography for choroidal angiography. The fluo-

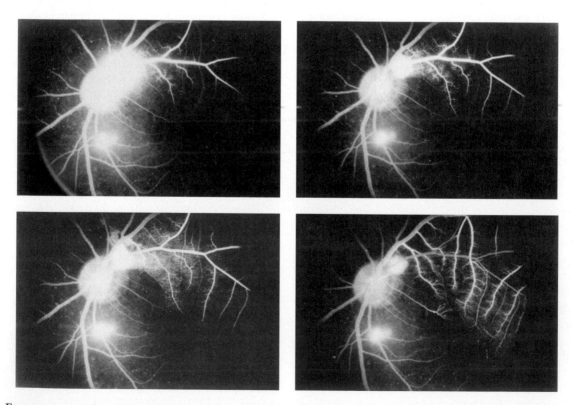

FIGURE 33-12   Fluorescein angiogram with targeted dye delivery in a monkey retina. Fluorescein is incapsulated in lipid vesicles and injected intravenously. Fluorescein is then released in the retinal artery by heating the artery with an argon laser. (Courtesy R. Zeimer, PhD.)

rescence of ICG is not blocked by the pigment epithelium as it fluoresces at near infrared, and ICG is almost completely bound to proteins, which means that it does not easily pass the walls of the choriocapillaris. Single choroidal vessels can be observed even late in the angiogram (Figure 33-13). Despite these obvious advantages, the technique has not become a routine clinical tool. The need for a special camera and frequent difficulty in interpretation of ICG angiograms have somewhat limited widespread acceptance. An obvious use for ICG is to examine subretinal neovascular membranes, where it is a valuable complement to, but not a substitute for, fluorescein angiography[134] (see Figure 33-13). Image analysis techniques have demonstrated that the choroidal filling pattern is fairly constant for the same individual (Figure 33-14), and interpretation of ICG-angiograms based on image analysis may be a viable approach to clinical studies on choroidal blood flow.[90,162]

The principle of frequency shift of a signal induced by moving objects, the Doppler shift has been widely used for estimation of ocular blood flow. The signal can be either optical (laser Doppler velocimetry) or auditory (ultrasound color Doppler imaging). The first measurement of blood flow velocity in any tissue was made in the rabbit retina, and the first measurement in the human eye was presented only 2 years later.[254,309] Currently available instruments permit absolute measurements of flow velocity in large retinal vessels by bidirectional laser Doppler flowmetry.[256] The laser Doppler signal can also be used to estimate blood volume, which enables semiquantitative measurements of blood flow.[258] Microvascular laser Doppler flowmetry is primarily sensitive to blood flow changes in the superficial layers of the anterior optic nerve and retina, with a theoretic depth of tissue penetration of 1000 μm.[163,236] Recently, laser Doppler flowmetry has been combined with a scanning laser system to visualize the perfusion of selected areas of the retina and anterior optic nerve.[196,198] With a confocal scanning device, one can investigate various depths of tissue.[61,237] The results of the measurements are highly dependent on the selection of measurement area.[46] The brightness of the illuminated fundus and ocular pulsatility related to the cardiac pulse also influence the measurements.[300,321]

In color Doppler velocimetry, ultrasound is the signal used for detection of the Doppler shift induced by moving red blood cells.[1] With this technique, Doppler shift information is superimposed in color on a conventional gray-scale two-dimensional B-scan structure image.[329] The ophthalmic and central retinal vessels are particularly suitable for measurements with color Doppler imaging, and the resistance index (RI) is the most reproducible measurement parameter.[132,264] RI is calculated from the peak systolic (PSV) and end-diastolic velocity (EDV) as follows: (PSV − EDV)/PSV. The correlation between RI and vascular resistance in vivo is unclear. No study has evaluated the technique in

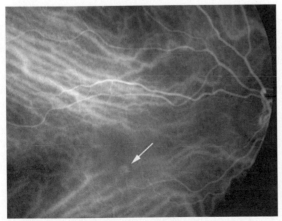

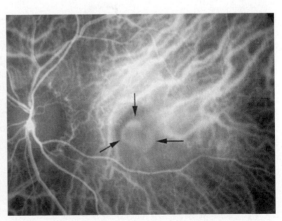

A

B

FIGURE 33-13 Indocyanin green choroidal angiograms. **A,** White arrow shows a "hot spot" in an eye where fluorescein angiography identified an occult subretinal neovascular membrane. **B,** Black arrows outline a neovascular membrane in an eye where fluorescein angiography identified a classical subretinal neovascular membrane. (Courtesy Urban Eriksson, MD.)

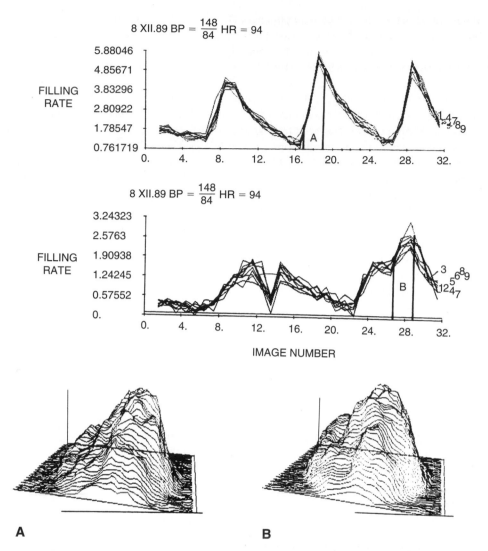

FIGURE 33-14 Computer-based reconstruction of choroidal filling in the healthy human eye with indocyanine green (ICG). The angiogram is recorded with a CCD camera and images are stored at a rate of 15 frames per second. The frames are aligned and divided into a grid pattern with 150 sectors, each sector corresponding to a fundus area of about 0.25 mm² (roughly corresponding to the size of a choroidal lobule). The change in average gray level for each area is recorded as a function of time, and the first derivate of that function is the instantaneous filling rate of that particular sector of the choroid. The two top curves represent the filling rates of nine clustered choroidal sectors on two different occasions in the same individual. Cyclic variation in filling rates corresponds to heart rate. The two three-dimensional surfaces at the bottom of the graph represent the filling rates during systole (**A** and **B**) in all 150 choroidal sectors included in the angiogram, where the x- and y-axes correspond to fundus location and the z-axis to filling rate. Note the similarity of the two filling patterns despite marked difference in heart rate (*HR*). For details see Klein et al.[162] *BP*, Blood pressure. (Courtesy R.W. Flower.)

---

the eye, and studies on cerebral vessels have not confirmed a useful correlation between RI and cerebrovascular resistance.[310] Vessels as small as the short posterior ciliary arteries may be imaged with color Doppler techniques, although the reproducibility and accuracy of these measurements are suspect.

Another quantitative index of tissue blood velocity can be obtained by use of the laser speckle phenomenon.[301,302] The method is currently under development, and most of the published data have been obtained in animals.[308] However, some promising measurements in humans have also been performed.[302]

When the retina is illuminated with blue light at a wavelength of 430 nm, the retinal shadow produced by circulating leukocytes flowing through the macular capillaries can be observed and is called the *blue-field entoptic phenomenon.*[285] Leukocyte velocity is estimated by the test subject matching the speed of the perceived leukocytes to the speed of computer-simulated particles on a video screen.[252] The method is subjective and is based on the assumption that the macular capillaries have a fixed diameter and that the number of capillaries open to flow is constant. If these requirements are met, leukocyte velocity is proportional to blood flow through the macular area. The subject is also asked to estimate the number of moving leukocytes. The value of this information is less clear because factors besides blood flow may affect the number of leukocytes perceived by the subject. Thus, unlike velocity, it depends on the amount of retinal irradiance, and it cannot be excluded that changes in the retinal environment, such as pH, PO_2 or PCO_2 also has an affect on the number of leukocytes perceived.[235]

Pneumatonometric measurement of ocular pulse amplitude has been developed for estimation of the pulsatile component of ocular blood flow.[168,282] It is believed that pulsatile ocular blood flow techniques primarily measure the pulsatile component of the choroidal blood flow. Laser interferometric measurement of fundus pulsations adds another aspect of pulsatility of the eye.[274,275] Ocular pulsatility is influenced by axial length and refractive error of the eye, as well as blood pressure changes and posture.[246,320] Because the ratio of pulsatile to nonpulsatile ocular blood flow cannot be assumed to be constant, especially in the event of changes in systemic blood pressure, pulsatile blood flow is likely a poor estimate of total ocular blood flow.[274]

RATE OF BLOOD FLOW AND OXYGEN SUPPLY

With use of many of the previously described techniques, the following information regarding the normal ocular blood flow has been obtained. Blood flow within the undisturbed eye of anesthetized nonhuman primates is presented in Figure 33-15, along with other nonocular tissues for comparison. Blood flow values reported for the human retina, 35 and 80 l/min, are similar to the flow values obtained in nonhuman primates.[85,257] The mean retinal circulation time in humans has been reported to be approximately 3 to 5 seconds.[78,146,288]

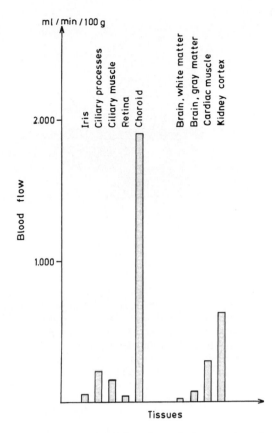

FIGURE 33-15 Blood flow through tissues of monkey eye. Flow through other tissues is included for comparison. (Values for blood flow through ocular tissues from Alm, Bill, and Young, 1973.[12] Values for extraocular tissues are taken from Folkow and Neil, 1971.[91])

In nonhuman primates, regional differences in blood flow through the retina and choroid are significant: Blood flow near the fovea and around the optic nerve is much higher than blood flow in the peripheral retina[11] (Figure 33-16). As shown in Figure 33-15, blood flow through the choroid is extremely high, and if the combined retinal and choroidal blood flow per 100 g retina is calculated, the resulting figure is about 10 times that of gray matter of the brain. Interestingly, a corresponding difference in metabolic requirements does not exist. Consequently, oxygen extraction from each milliliter of uveal blood is low. For example, the arteriovenous difference for choroidal blood oxygenation in cats is approximately 3%, and the difference for mixed blood from the choroid and anterior uvea is 4% to 5%.[7] Similar figures have been obtained for mixed uveal blood in other species, such as dogs and pigs.[65,316] In contrast, the oxygen content of retinal

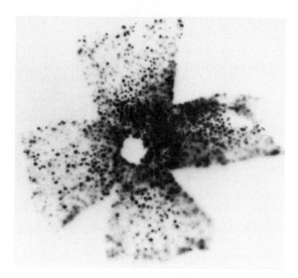

Figure 33-16 Autoradiograph of flat mount of monkey choroid after injection of labeled microspheres into left heart ventricle. Flow is proportional to number of microspheres per unit area. High flow in central choroid corresponds to the fovea and the region around the optic nerve. Four incisions were made from periphery into choroid. Optic nerve gave central hole. (Technique reported in Alm and Bill.[9]) (From Alm A: Microcirculation of the eye. In Mortillaro NA [ed]: *The physiology and pharmacology of the microcirculation,* vol 1, New York, 1983, Academic Press.)

venous blood in humans is approximately 38% lower than that in arterial blood.[147] A similar figure was obtained in a study with direct measurements of the oxygen content of venous blood from pigs.[316]

Despite the low oxygen extraction from choroidal blood, the choroid is of great importance for the supply of nutrients to the outer layers of the retina. This is evident not only for primates in which the avascular fovea is nourished by the choroid but also in lower mammals, in which a major part of the nutrients consumed by the retina is derived from the choroidal blood vessels. Thus in anesthetized cats approximately 80% of the oxygen consumed by the retina is delivered by the choroid.[9] The corresponding figure for the primates is 65%.[11] In pigs, the total consumption in vivo of oxygen and glucose is 330 and 150 nmol/min, respectively.[316] Approximately 60% of the oxygen and 75% of the glucose are delivered by the choroidal vessels. The dependence of the retina on both retinal and choroidal blood flow is illustrated by the retinal tissue oxygen tension profile[3] (Figure 33-17).

Undoubtedly, the high rate of blood flow through the uvea is important. In addition to providing the uvea with a high oxygen tension, thereby enhancing the diffusion of oxygen into the retina, the uvea's high blood flow rate is believed to protect

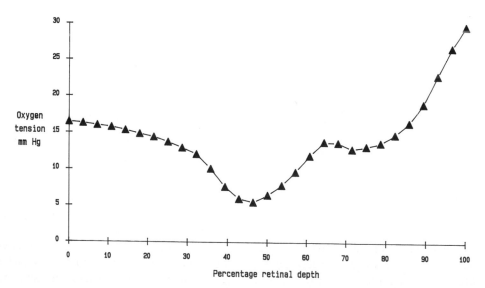

Figure 33-17 Oxygen tension profile through the cat retina. Oxygen tension was determined with a microelectrode. In this example, oxygen tension at the internal limiting membrane (*left on the graph*) is 33 mm Hg, stays at that level for the first 20% of retinal depth and then falls to a minimum of approximately 5 mm Hg at a depth most likely corresponding to the inner nuclear layer. It then increases toward the choroid with a maximum of almost 85 mm Hg close to the choriocapillaris, clearly demonstrating the dual supply of oxygen to the retina. (Courtesy V.A. Alder, S. Cringle, and D-Y. Yu.)

the eye from thermal damage even under extreme conditions (e.g., an Arctic snowstorm, a Finnish sauna bath, or observation of bright objects). A high rate of choroidal blood flow may also prevent damage from elevation in tissue temperature when light is focused on the fovea.[41,232]

In many tissues the entire capillary bed is not open or perfused at a given time. The number of open capillaries likely depends on the metabolic needs of the tissue. The precapillary sphincter or arteriolar smooth muscle regulates opening and closing of the capillary beds. Thus only part of the capillaries are open in skeletal muscles during rest, while maximal exercise may increase blood flow tenfold to twentyfold.[91] The opening and closing of capillaries in response to the tissue need is termed *vasomotion*, although this term is sometimes also used for rhythmic changes in flow through a tissue. Such rhythmic changes in overall flow can probably be expected to occur in any tissue with a stable metabolism in which blood flow is affected by the metabolic by-products. Continuous measurements of the oxygen tension in the vascularized part of the retina of the anesthetized cat and monkey show fluctuations of a low frequency, which indicates that the metabolic milieu fluctuates within a narrow range; in turn, this might be expected to lead to similar fluctuations in flow.[49] Studies with laser Doppler flowmetry have demonstrated such rhythmic changes in both vascular volume and red cell velocity in the superficial optic nerve, retina, and choroid, with the most pronounced but slow changes in the optic nerve.[258] These fluctuations were out of phase by almost 180 degrees, resulting in much smaller fluctuations in flow. Whether these fluctuations are caused by variation in the number of open capillaries or changes in volume of the small venules is unclear. In a study with direct observation of the retinal and choroidal vasculature, no precapillary sphincters were found; the blood flow appeared to be uninterrupted in all capillaries observed.[97,98] In the retina of young cats, some spontaneous contractions and dilations occur in the small arterioles and precapillary sphincters, but there is much less vasomotion in the retinal vessels of adult cats.[176] Also, results obtained with the blue-field simulation technique support the assumption that all retinal capillaries are open. Thus, when the intraocular pressure is artificially increased, leukocyte velocity is initially reduced, but within a minute or two velocity is restored. If some capillaries were closed, one would expect them to open as

a result of the reduced perfusion pressure and the autoregulatory response would then be perceived as an increased density of leukocytes with lower velocities rather than velocity returning to baseline.[255]

CONTROL OF CIRCULATION
The Vascular Endothelium

The vascular endothelium is a confluent monolayer of flattened, rhomboid-shaped cells that line the intimal surface of all blood vessels. The layer, previously thought to be a passive barrier, is now believed to be an active participant in vasomotor regulation. Over the past several decades, the endothelium has been shown to play a role in vasomotor tone, coagulation, vascular structure, and immune responses.[227] The endothelial-derived factors work in concert with vasoactive nerves, exogenous and endogenous vasoactive substances, and metabolic activities to influence blood flow. It is involved in regulation of vascular tone, platelet activity, and vascular permeability.[154,204] The importance of the vascular endothelium as a selective barrier for exchange between blood and tissue has long been recognized. Both in the brain and retina, the endothelium provides a barrier function. The blood-brain and blood-retinal barriers prevent circulating non–lipid-soluble vasoactive substances from reaching the vascular smooth muscles. The vascular endothelial cells also inactivate vasoactive substances such as norepinephrine, serotonin, bradykinin, and adenosine, in addition to converting the inactive precursor angiotensin I to angiotensin II. As a consequence, many drugs that act directly on vascular smooth muscles have an effect on the retinal vessels, only if they are injected into the vitreous body instead of intravascularly. In addition, systemically administered drugs may have an effect in diseased vessels with a damaged endothelium but not in normal vessels.

The vascular endothelium regulates the vascular tone by releasing potent vasoactive agents. Endothelial cells synthesize prostacyclin (PGI_2) from arachidonic acid. PGI_2 is a vasodilator and a potent inhibitor of platelet aggregation.[204] Nitric oxide synthase (NOS), the enzyme involved in the synthesis of nitric oxide (NO) from L-arginine, is present in vascular endothelial cells in the retina and in the vascular endothelium of the uvea.[58,194,332] Stimulation of endothelial muscarinic receptors induces the release of NO, which stimulates the guanylate cyclase in vascular smooth muscle, causing an increase in cyclic guanine monophosphate (cGMP) and relaxation.[102,203] The vasodilatory effect of acetylcholine depends on an intact vascular endothelium.[103]

In addition, the vascular endothelium has the capacity to synthesize vasoactive peptides, the endothelins (ETs), a family of 21–amino acid peptides, of which ET-1 and ET-3 are associated with blood vessels in the eye.[57,334] After their release from the vascular endothelial cells, ETs interact with ETA and ETB receptors, both of which have been detected in the vascular smooth muscle of choroidal and retinal blood vessels and in cultured retinal pericytes.[189,292] Stimulation of ETA and ETB receptors located on vascular smooth muscle results in vasoconstriction, whereas activation of ETB receptors located on the vascular endothelium elicits vascular relaxation by means of inducing formation of NO and prostacyclin.[135,160,187]

Endothelium-derived NO is released under both resting and bradykinin- or acetylcholine-stimulated conditions in vitro.[128,335] In vivo studies in experimental animals and humans using L-arginine analogs as competitive inhibitors of NOS have demonstrated the presence of a vasodilating NO-tone in the uvea, retina, and optic nerve head. NO possibly plays a role in the vasodilatory response to flickering light.* The role for PGI$_2$ and ETs in the regulation of normal blood flow is less clear. It seems that ETs might be involved in hyperoxia-induced vasoconstriction through activation of ETA receptors.[69,306] ET does not pass through the blood-retinal barrier and has no direct effect on retinal blood flow when injected into the bloodstream, but it does cause significant vasoconstriction if injected into the vitreous body of cats.[112,218] An indirect effect of intravascular ET-1 may occur through release of NO from the vascular endothelium as has been observed for blood flow through the optic nerve in cats.[218]

Complex interactions between endothelium-derived agents, vascular endothelium, and contractile vascular smooth muscle cells or pericytes most likely occur under normal conditions.[186] A disturbed endothelial cell function can be demonstrated in systemic disease, such as hypertension and diabetes mellitus, and may be involved in ocular disorders as well.[59,113,272] These findings have lead to the many recent investigations of vasoactive agents, aimed at selectively increasing perfusion pressure to various vascular beds in the eye, in an attempt to preserve visual function by preventing ischemic insults.[172]

*References 51, 72, 110, 164, 165, 179, 185, 271.

Perfusion Pressure

The perfusion pressure, the pressure promoting blood flow through a tissue, is the difference between the pressure in the arteries entering the tissue (*Pa*) and the veins leaving it (*Pv*). The relationship between blood flow (*BF*), perfusion pressure, and vascular resistance (*R*) is expressed by the following equation:

$$BF = \frac{Pa - Pv}{R}$$

The pressure within the retrobulbar arteries that supply the ocular tissues (*Pa*) cannot be determined accurately with available clinical methods. Ophthalmodynamometry is based on the appearance of pulsations and cessation of blood flow through the central retinal artery at increased IOP. Elevated IOP is used to reduce blood flow through the ophthalmic artery, which results in a corresponding reduction in the pressure fall between the internal carotid and the peripheral ocular arteries. Consequently, the pressure readings measured are closer to those existing in the internal carotid artery than to those in the arteries of the undisturbed eye. However, a reasonable estimation for the normal pressure in the ocular arteries, the mean arterial pressure, can be calculated. The mean arterial pressure is an arithmetically derived approximation and is equal to the diastolic pressure plus one third of the pulse pressure. For example, if the blood pressure measured in the brachial artery is 140/80 mm Hg, the mean arterial blood pressure at the level of the heart is 100 mm Hg. Sitting or standing, with the eyes positioned at 25 cm above the heart, the pressure in the internal carotid at the level of the ophthalmic artery is approximately 80 mm Hg. The difference corresponds to a blood column with a height of 25 cm. A further reduction in blood pressure takes place along the ophthalmic artery. In rabbits this pressure drop has been estimated to be 14 mm Hg.[32] In nonhuman primates the difference between mean arterial blood pressure and the mean pressure in the anterior ciliary arteries, at the point where they enter the eye, is 20 to 25 mm Hg.[180] Thus a reasonable estimate of the pressure in the arteries entering the eye is 60 to 70 mm Hg in the upright position. A change to a supine position increases this pressure.

A good estimate of the pressure in the veins leaving the eye (Pv) can be made by measuring the IOP because these two pressures are almost equal at both normal and elevated IOP.[33,180] Thus, with an IOP of 15 mm Hg, the normal perfusion pressure for ocular blood flow is approximately 50 mm Hg, and it may be considerably lower in healthy individuals without any obvious disturbance of normal eye function.

Spontaneous pulsations, which can be visualized in the central retinal vein at the optic disc, are a consequence of the pressure within the vein being nearly equal to the IOP, while at peak pulse pressure the vein and other parts of the ocular vascular bed expand slightly. This leads to small changes in blood volume within the eye, and as a consequence the IOP also varies with the pulse. The variation in IOP is 1 to 2 mm Hg.

Outside the eye, the pressure in the ocular veins is lower than the IOP because tissue pressure surrounding these vessels is lower. In the typical human eye the mean pressure in the episcleral veins is 7 to 8 mm Hg.[337] In anesthetized monkeys the episcleral venous pressure at a spontaneous IOP of 14 mm Hg was 10 to 11 mm Hg, whereas increasing IOP above 35 mm Hg had little effect on the pressure in the episcleral veins.[181] The pressure in the vortex veins just outside the globe may be expected to be similar to that in the episcleral veins. This means that there may be a pressure drop of 5 to 10 mm Hg in the ocular veins as they pass through the sclera, resulting in partial collapse of the veins.[28] Small elevations in the extraocular venous pressure tend to reverse this collapse and reduce the pressure drop without affecting the intraocular venous pressure. At larger elevations of the pressure in the extraocular veins, part of the pressure is transmitted into the intraocular veins, causing venous congestion (Figure 33-18). Congested ocular veins with capillary leakage and hemorrhages are seen when the intracranial pressure or the pressure within the sheath of the optic nerve is increased.[138] Another example may be the engorgement of retinal veins seen in early diabetic retinopathy, which indicates that the transmural pressure in the capillaries is increased.

As explained previously, the transmural pressure (the pressure inside the vessel minus the pressure outside the vessel) in the intraocular veins and the venous side of the capillaries is small. In a study in rabbits, the pressure in the choroidal veins was approximately 2 mm Hg above the IOP.[180] Thus even a small increase in intravascular pressure may raise the transmural pressure to several times its normal value. This raises the possibility that the development of microaneurysms in diabetic retinopathy may in part be caused by venous stasis. Clinical reports have suggested that in patients with impaired blood flow to one eye, diabetic retinopathy in that

eye is less pronounced than in the other eye.[105] In this situation it seems likely that a reduction of the transmural pressure in the veins and capillaries contributes to protection of the walls of the vessels.

The ocular perfusion pressure (Pa − Pv) can be reduced by either a reduction in arterial pressure or an increase in IOP. From the earlier equation, it follows that a reduction in perfusion pressure does re-

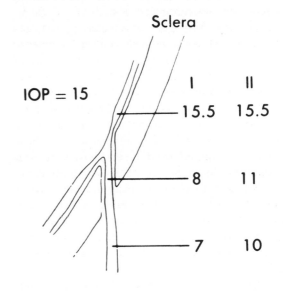

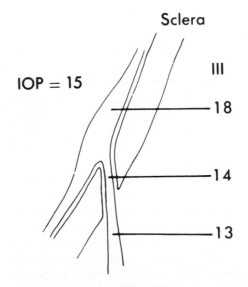

FIGURE 33-18 At an intraocular pressure (*IOP*) of 15 mm Hg, the vortex vein is partially collapsed where it enters the sclera. Venous pressure at this point is practically equal to IOP, I. A small rise in extraocular venous pressure does not change uveal venous pressure unless there is a change in IOP, II. A large rise in pressure in the extraocular part of the vortex vein raises pressure in the choroid and produces intraocular venous congestion, III.

sult in a reduction in ocular blood flow (BF) unless the vascular resistance (R) is reduced to the same extent as the perfusion pressure. In most tissues, such as the brain and the kidney, a reduction in vascular resistance occurs when the perfusion pressure is reduced. This autoregulation of blood flow tends to ensure constant levels of flow despite moderate variations in perfusion pressure. However, the presence or absence of autoregulation varies among species and even among tissue beds of a single organ of a specific species. Autoregulation has been demonstrated in the vascular beds of the anterior uvea in cats and monkeys and in the retina in rabbits, cats, pigs, and monkeys.[8,9,11,36,89] However, blood flow through the anterior uvea of rabbits is not autoregulated.[36] In most studies examining autoregulation, the ocular perfusion pressure is reduced by elevating the IOP; however, as expected, at least in cats, reductions in blood pressure have the same effect on retinal oxygen tension as elevations in IOP.[8] The mechanisms behind autoregulation are believed to be twofold: myogenic and metabolic.[91] Each of these components, as a rule, operate in concert. The stimuli for the myogenic mechanism are variations in the transmural pressure difference. When this pressure difference is decreased, as with increased IOP, the activity of pacemaker cells in the arteriolar wall is reduced, resulting in reduced arteriolar tone and consequently lowered vascular resistance.

In the typical human eye, information regarding the effect of increased IOP on uveal blood flow is minimal, but blood flow through the retina and optic nerve is autoregulated.[249,255,261] In these studies the upper limit for autoregulation of retinal blood flow is consistently low, approximately 30 mm Hg. Autoregulation also means that blood flow should remain normal if blood pressure is increased. However, a sufficiently large elevation in blood pressure overwhelms autoregulation, resulting in an increase in blood flow. Such a mechanism has been observed in the human eye, where an increase in blood pressure of 40% increases retinal blood flow.[262] In the latter study, and several other studies, arterial blood pressure was increased by exercise, which can be expected to produce a mixed response to a change in sympathetic tone and true autoregulatory capacity of the vascular bed.

Considering the deleterious effect of glaucoma on the optic nerve, the effect of increased IOP on blood flow through the anterior optic nerve is of special interest. However, the anterior optic nerve, at least within the superficial nerve fiber layer and the prelaminar region, does not seem to differ from the retina with respect to blood flow, perfusion pressure, and autoregulation. At least in healthy eyes, blood flow through the prelaminar region of the optic nerve is autoregulated both in monkey and human eyes.[73,250,289] The situation may be different in older adults or in disease states. In a study on aged monkeys that had been on an atherogenic diet for several years, increased glucose metabolism, suggesting reduced blood flow, was seen in the retina and in the optic nerve at an IOP that was within the autoregulatory range for healthy, young monkeys.[141] The autoregulation of blood flow through the anterior optic nerve is also of interest because small vessels originate from branches of choroidal and ciliary arteries that apparently do not alter resistance in response to increased IOP. It is possible that changes in optic nerve vascular resistance are mediated by the vascular endothelium that can induce vasodilation in response to changes in blood flow.[223,244] For the choroid, the situation is different. Moderate elevations in IOP result in concomitant reductions in choroidal blood flow in both cats and monkeys.[9,11] Figure 33-19 summarizes the effects of reductions in ocular perfusion pressure on blood flow through the various vascular beds of the primate eye.

The lack of autoregulation of choroidal blood flow is of interest because most ocular vascular beds are autoregulated. The lack of response of choroidal blood vessels to elevations in IOP suggests that pacemaker cells do not operate in the choroidal arterioles. In extreme circumstances when mean arterial pressure is modified by partial occlusion of the thoracic vena cava, a modest response has been elicited in the rabbit choroid, either as a result of a true myogenic response or induced by changes in vasomotor nerve tone.[161] The stimulus for the metabolic mechanism is believed to be local accumulation of vasodilatory metabolites, such as carbon dioxide and hypoxia. The choroidal vessels respond to carbon dioxide and thus could be expected to show some "metabolic autoregulation." However, the choroidal arteriovenous difference for carbon dioxide is normally small.[7] Even significant reductions in choroidal blood flow cause only a minor increase in tissue carbon dioxide tension and, consequently, no measurable effect on choroidal vascular resistance. At low levels of choroidal blood flow, further reductions may be expected to cause a significant accumulation of vasodilatory metabolites and thus some autoregulatory response.

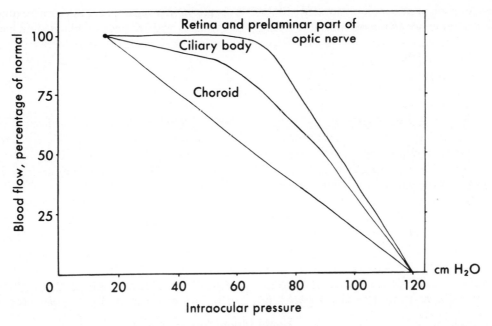

FIGURE 33-19 When intraocular pressure (IOP) is increased, there is no decrease in retinal blood flow and optic nerve head blood flow up to a certain level. Change in flow in ciliary body is also small. In the choroid, even moderate increments in eye pressure reduce blood flow. At high IOP, further increments in pressure reduce flow in all intraocular tissues.

As a result of the autoregulation of retinal blood flow, the oxygen tension in the inner parts of the retina is maintained at a constant level even during large variations in IOP or blood pressure.[8] The reduction in choroidal blood flow, which follows moderate increments in IOP, does not seem to reduce the supply of nutrients to the retina because the extraction of oxygen and glucose from each milliliter of blood is increased. Thus the net extraction is maintained at the same level despite large variations in blood flow[7,316] (Figure 33-20).

NERVOUS CONTROL OF BLOOD FLOW

Histologic studies and stimulation experiments have revealed a rich and powerful supply of vasoactive autonomic nerves to the various vascular beds of the uvea, but not in the retina (Figure 33-21). Sympathetic nerves, derived from the superior cervical sympathetic ganglion, innervate the central retinal artery up to the lamina cribrosa, but not beyond, and sympathectomy has no effect on retinal blood flow in the primate eye, whereas all uveal vascular beds are innervated.[79,174,191] Many sympathetic nerves contain neuropeptide Y (NPY). In several species, including primates, NPY immunoreactive nerves have been observed close to uveal blood vessels. Their distribution resembles that of the adrenergic innervation.[295] Ocular parasympathetic nerves with effects on ocular blood flow include the oculomotor and the facial nerves. The facial nerve innervates mainly choroidal vessels.[267] The transmitter is probably vasoactive intestinal peptide (VIP), and vascular nerves with VIP-like immunoreactivity have also been found in the human eye.[297] Sensory nerves of trigeminal origin containing the peptides substance P (SP) and calcitonin gene-related peptide (CGRP) are also associated with uveal blood vessels, mainly in the ciliary body and, to some extent, in the choroid.[294,296] Several neuropeptides have been shown to have an effect on ocular vessels. Thus NPY has a direct contractile effect on bovine retinal vessels in vitro and enhances the effect of noradrenaline in the proximal part or these vessels.[242] CGRP relaxes precontracted bovine retinal arteries and increases blood flow through the ciliary body in monkeys when administered intracamerally.[15,243] Intravenously administered pituitary adenylate cyclase activating polypeptide (PACAP) increases choroidal blood flow in rabbits.[214]

Sympathetic stimulation reduces blood flow through all parts of the uvea in rabbits, cats, and

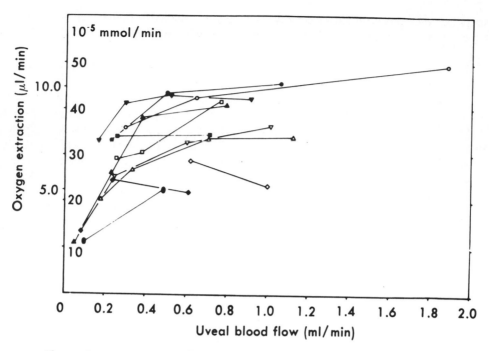

FIGURE 33-20   Changes in oxygen extraction from blood passing through the uvea when blood flow is reduced by increase in intraocular pressure. (From Alm A, Bill A: *Acta Physiol Scand* 80:19, 1970.)

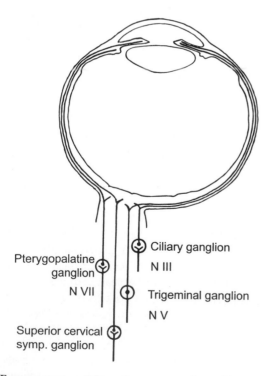

FIGURE 33-21   Schematic representation of innervation of ocular blood vessels.

monkeys, whereas retinal blood flow is unaffected.[5,10,29] In most species, only α-receptors seem to be present in the uvea.[10,22] In the anterior uvea of cats and rats, neurogenic vasoconstriction is mediated by adrenergic α_1-receptors.[157,166] In some species, stimulation of the cervical sympathetic chain may induce vasodilation that is revealed only after effective blockade of the adrenergic α-receptors. In the rat, but not in the pig, this vasodilation is mediated by adrenergic β_1-receptors.[158,298] Also, at least in rabbits, the entire vasoconstrictive response is not adrenergic because it is only partially eliminated after α-adrenergic blockade. It is reasonable to assume that the nonadrenergic component is caused by NPY, as is the case in other vascular beds.[111] One important physiologic role of the sympathetic nerves in ocular blood flow control is to help maintain the blood flow at a suitable level during sudden elevations in blood pressure.[38] Such elevations, occurring in everyday life in acute stress situations and during work, are the result of a general increase in sympathetic activity. Left unchecked, these responses would cause overperfusion of the eye, resulting in breakdown of the blood-aqueous and blood-retinal barriers. However, with simultaneous activity in the sympathetic nerves to the eye, these effects are prevented. Thus sympathetic activity assists autoregulatory mechanisms in maintaining the intraocular blood flow and volume constant.

The role of the parasympathetic nerves in the eye is much less clear than that of the sympathetic nerves. Oculomotor nerve stimulation has significant, complex effects on blood flow through the anterior uvea, but it has no obvious effect on choroidal or retinal blood flow.[42,293] Thus blood flow through the iris is reduced in rabbits, cats, and monkeys, whereas blood flow through the ciliary body is reduced in rabbits but increased in cats and monkeys. The latter effect may be caused by vasodilatory metabolites accumulated during contraction of the ciliary muscle. The vasoconstriction in the iris is a combined aminergic and cholinergic effect. The nature of the aminergic transmitter and its physiologic role are unknown. The cholinergic component is muscarinic, and it results in a cholinergic vasoconstrictor effect in conscious rabbits. It is interesting to note that this tone is almost eliminated by pentobarbital anesthesia. As previously stated, the vasodilating effect of acetylcholine is caused by a receptor-mediated release of NO. Vasoactive cholinergic nerves in lower species are mainly vasoconstrictive, but in mammals most vascular beds lack cholinergic vasoactive innervation. The coronary vessels form an exception with dual cholinergic regulation of vascular tone: vasoconstrictive cholinergic nerves and vasodilatory endothelial receptors. The iridial vessels are another example. A cholinergic vasoconstrictor tone is present also in primates, but topical application of neostigmine causes a substantial vasodilation in the anterior uvea of monkeys.[12,293] This discrepancy may be accounted for by the different vasoactive effects of acetylcholine when acting directly on vascular smooth muscle and when acting on vascular endothelial cells. The normal cholinergic tone in the anterior uvea releases acetylcholine that acts mainly on the vascular smooth muscles, causing them to contract. Neostigmine treatment, on the other hand, probably results in large amounts of acetylcholine and a direct cholinergic effect on the vascular endothelium. The endothelial cells then respond by releasing NO.

Intracranial stimulation of the facial nerve in rabbits, cats, and monkeys causes a moderate vasodilation in the anterior uvea and a significant vasodilation in the choroid.[217] The effect cannot be blocked by atropine and can be simulated by vasoactive intestinal peptide.[216] In cats the effect on choroidal blood flow of facial nerve stimulation at 5 Hz is mediated by NO, whereas higher stimulation frequencies induce an additional vasodilation that seems to be independent of NO.[215] The physiologic role of these potent, vasodilatory, "peptidergic" nerves may be the reflexive increase in choroidal blood flow induced by light.[233]

A peculiar type of neural influence on the blood vessels is seen in rabbits. Localized stroking of the iris in this animal gives rise to a local dilation of the arteriole that spreads over the iris. The vascular permeability is increased, miosis is prolonged, and IOP is raised.[277] A substance with vasodilating and smooth muscle–contracting properties is released when stroking the iris.[16] This substance, irin, seems to be a single prostaglandin or a mixture of several.[51] It is interesting to note that aspirin, which inhibits the synthesis of prostaglandins, modifies the effects of paracentesis in the rabbit eye.[210] Mechanical or electrical stimulation of the sensory nerve to the eye produces a reaction similar to that of stroking the iris, but surprisingly, nerve stimulation seems to cause little release of prostaglandins.[77] The effect of sensory nerve stimulation seems to be mediated by SP and CGRP.[44,222] Prostaglandins and SP have similar effects on the anterior segment of the rabbit eye, and there seems to be some interaction between them. Thus the miosis caused by prostaglandin application depends on an intact trigeminal innervation. Indomethacin pretreatment, which inhibits prostaglandin synthesis, reduces the effects of intracamerally injected SP.[184]

Although vascular nerves with SP and CGRP immunoreactivity have been observed in the human eye, mainly in the ciliary body, their effect on blood flow is unknown. There are large species differences in the ocular effects of these transmitters.[294,296] In rabbits, but not in cats, intracameral injections of SP cause substantial vasodilation in the ciliary body, whereas in cats a similar effect can be achieved with CGRP.[183,222] In rabbits, SP causes an accumulation of inositol-triphosphate (IP_3) and contraction of the iris sphincter, but the human iris sphincter does not contract as a response to SP and there is an accumulation of cyclic adenosine monophosphate instead of IP_3.[305]

EFFECT OF DRUGS ON THE BLOOD FLOW THROUGH THE EYE

Intravenous and close-arterial injections of vasoactive drugs often have different effects on choroidal blood flow.[60] Intravenous injections have an effect on most vascular beds of the body, which influences the arterial blood pressure and thus the ocular perfusion pressure. As discussed previously, choroidal blood flow lacks autoregulation; thus effects of systemically administered vasoactive drugs on choroidal blood flow are most likely secondary to changes in the systemic cardiovascular status (i.e., systemic blood pressure and pulse rate). Although the other vascular beds of the eye are autoregulated, the ability of vascular beds within the diseased eye may be altered or even absent. Thus systemic administration of vasodilators can be expected to have little or no effect on ocular blood flow. They might even reduce ocular blood flow, if given in sufficient doses to cause systemic vasodilation and reduce blood pressure. Therefore, in general, no therapeutic benefit is to be expected from systemic administration of vasodilators. Topical application with eye drops may circumvent this problem. In phakic eyes therapeutic concentrations can be expected to be present only in the anterior segment and anterior uvea. In the phakic eye, there is no evidence that topically applied medications reach the posterior segment of the eye (retina, optic nerve, and posterior uvea) in concentrations sufficient to have therapeutic effects. A study in monkeys with color Doppler imaging demonstrated that retrobulbar injections of epinephrine decrease velocities in the retrobulbar vessels, whereas topical application of eye drops had no significant effect.[209] Retrobulbar or close-arterial injections may give therapeutic concentrations in the posterior pole of the eye without systemic effects. However, they may still have a limited effect on retinal blood flow because the blood-retinal barrier prevents most drugs from reaching the smooth muscles of the retinal vessels. The effect of adenosine on retinal blood flow is a good example. Adenosine is an endogenously released substance involved in hypoxic vasodilation.[107,266,322] An intravenous injection has no effect on blood flow through the retina in cats.[240] Papaverine, on the other hand, which is a lipid-soluble adenosine uptake inhibitor that can pass through the blood-retinal barrier, causes a significant increase in oxygen tension in the vitreous close to the retina in cats when administered systemically.[4] Also, intravitreal injections of adenosine dilate retinal vessels.[55,108]

The state of the vascular endothelium may decide the effect of some vasoactive drugs, either because of a breakdown of the barrier or because of loss of responsiveness of a diseased endothelium. Hayreh et al.[142] showed that an intravenous infusion of serotonin had no effect on retinal vessels in healthy monkeys but caused a transient occlusion

or delayed filling on fluorescein angiograms in monkeys that had been on a diet intended to promote atherosclerosis. Discontinuation of the atherogenic diet for 5 to 12 months abolished vasoconstrictor effect, suggesting a repair of a damaged endothelium.

At present, there seems to be no indication for the use of vasodilators in ocular therapy; however, there are other reasons to investigate the pharmacology of ocular blood vessels. Some drugs that are used for other purposes, such as the treatment of glaucoma, have known effects on vascular smooth muscles in other tissues. They can be expected to have a direct effect on blood flow in the anterior segment of the eye through direct penetration. As they reduce the IOP, they can also have a modest indirect effect on ocular blood flow by increasing ocular perfusion pressure. In particular, blood flow through the choroid is affected, but blood flow in the retina and the optic nerve is also affected, especially if the autoregulatory response is deficient.

Vasoconstrictors

Topical administration of epinephrine reduces blood flow through the anterior uvea in monkeys, and vasoconstriction in the uvea is provoked by arterial injections of dihydroergotamine.[6,27] α_2-Adrenoceptor agonists induce vasoconstriction in the anterior segment of the cat eye.[167] Studies of the effects of various drugs on the oxygen tension of the vitreous body close to the retina indicate that none of the vasoconstricting drugs—norepinephrine, angiotensin, or dihydroergotamine—have any effect on retinal vascular resistance.[4] In the case of epinephrine, the blood-retinal barrier may be decisive for the lack of effect. Norepinephrine applied outside the blood-retinal barrier in vitro constricts retinal arteries, and retinal vessels bind adrenergic agonists, indicating the presence of both α_1- and α_2-receptors.[93,152] Angiotensin does not contract retinal vessels in vitro, but it may effect other ocular vessels.[219] It contracts isolated human posterior ciliary arteries, and receptors for angiotensin II have been identified in bovine retinal pericytes, which contract in vitro when exposed to angiotensin II.[24,188]

Vasodilators

Acetylcholine, papaverine, aminophylline, theophylline, and amyl nitrite, but not nicotinic acid, dilate uveal blood vessels, and topical administration of pilocarpine or neostigmine increases blood flow through the anterior uvea in monkeys.[12,27,29,213] The oxygen tension in the vitreous body close to the retina in cats is unaffected by arterial administrations of the vasodilators isoproterenol, histamine, nicotinic acid, and xanthinol nicotinate, but it is significantly increased by papaverine, most likely because of its ability to pass the blood-retinal barrier (see previous discussion).[4]

The retinal vessels lack sympathetic innervation, and the blood-retinal barrier protects the vascular smooth muscles from circulating catecholamines. Thus there is no reason to expect a sympathetic tone of the retinal vessels. Still, binding sites for adrenergic β-receptor agonists have been found in retinal vessels, but they do not seem to be involved in regulation of flow.[87] Adrenergic β-receptor agonists do not contract retinal vessels either in vitro or after an intraarterial injection.[4,152]

Cholinergic receptors and the ability to synthesize acetylcholine have been demonstrated in retinal vessel preparations.[88] The presence of an endothelium-dependent relaxation of retinal arteries in vitro suggests an endothelial origin for these receptors.[23] Endothelial receptors may also explain the binding sites for β_1- and β_2-agonists in retinal vessels because β-adrenergic agonists have no effect on retinal vessels either in vitro or after intravitreal or intraarterial injections.[4,55,87,152]

Oral administration of the methylxanthine derivative pentoxifylline increases leukocyte velocity in the macular capillaries studied with the blue-field simulation technique both in healthy individuals and in patients with diabetes.[286,287] Calcium channel blockers, administered systemically, increase blood flow through the anterior optic nerve in cats but have little effect on retinal blood flow in cats, in healthy human eyes, or in eyes with open-angle or normal tension glaucoma.[130,133,283,330]

Metabolic Control of Ocular Blood Flow

In the brain and the retina, high tissue concentrations of oxygen produce vasoconstriction and low concentrations produce vasodilation. These effects seem to be at least partly mediated by ETs and adenosine, respectively.[107,266,306,322] High concentrations of carbon dioxide lead to vasodilation, and low concentrations lead to vasoconstriction. Similar effects are seen in the optic nerve of rabbits under conditions of hypercapnia and hyperoxia.[228] In the uvea of adult cats and rabbits, the effect of moderate oxygen excess or lack seems to be too small to be detected.[30] However, the effect of alterations in the systemic oxygenation status on some of the vascular beds of the uvea may be masked by the larger effects on total uveal blood flow. Photographic studies of

the iris vessels of the albino rabbit indicate that they respond with contraction and dilation at increased and reduced levels of oxygen tension, respectively.[291] Excessive carbon dioxide causes marked vasodilation in all parts of the uvea.[9]

Arterial oxygen tension has a significant effect on retinal vascular tone and blood flow in the human eye. Breathing pure oxygen constricts retinal vessels and reduces blood flow 60%, with little if any effect on choroidal blood flow.[95,251,260] The vasoconstriction is not sufficient to prevent a rise in retinal oxygen tension.[2,8] Hyperoxia reduces and hypoxia increases leukocyte velocity in the macular capillaries.[82]

In immature eyes a high oxygen concentration in the inhaled gas has dramatic effects on both humans and experimental animals: vasoconstriction, inhibition of vascular development, and eventually, obliteration of the vessels[20] (Figure 33-22). After withdrawal of the excess oxygen, vasoproliferation, retinal edema, and hemorrhage may result. These changes produce retinopathy of prematurity that may lead to traction detachment of the retina and blindness.

Inhalation of 7% carbon dioxide in 21% oxygen results in moderate dilation of visible retinal vessels.[95] However, significant dilation of the small resistance vessels occurs, and at an arterial carbon dioxide tension of 80 mm Hg, retinal blood flow is increased by 300% to 400% in cats.[9] With combinations of carbon dioxide and oxygen, the oxygen tension in the inner parts of the retina can be increased by more than 300%.[8] Increased carbon dioxide tension increases leukocyte velocity in the macular capillaries and choroidal blood flow in the human eye.[131,260] It also reduces the vasoconstriction induced by high oxygen tension.[230]

Breathing pure oxygen increases the oxygen tension of choroidal venous blood and, consequently, the amount of oxygen delivered by the choroid to the retina. However, this is not enough to supply the entire thickness of the retina in case of a retinal arterial occlusion.[241] Adding 4% to 6% carbon dioxide to the oxygen increases choroidal blood flow and oxygen supply to the retina and may help relieve vascular spasm. The clinical value of inhaling such a mixture of oxygen and carbon dioxide is doubtful. It had no effect in fully developed retinal venous occlusions, whereas some improvement was reported for selected cases of preocclusion of retinal veins.[278] Thus clinical data are currently insufficient to support the value of oxygen, with or without added carbon dioxide, in the treatment of retinal vascular occlusions.

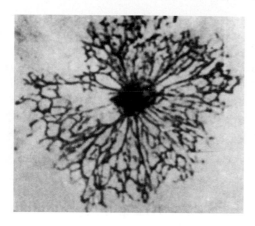

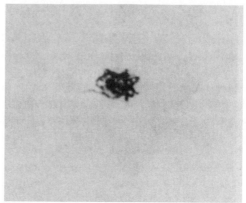

A   **B**

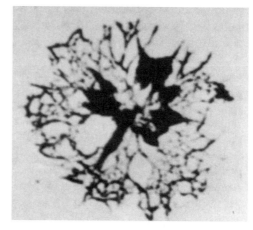

C

Figure 33-22 **A,** Healthy mouse retina at 1 day old. **B,** Total vasoobliteration after 5 days in 98% to 100% oxygen. **C,** Five days after return to air. New vessels have grown into retina and into vitreous (dense central vessel). (India ink injection.) (From Ashton N: *Br J Ophthalmol* 52:505, 1968.)

Illumination of the retina influences retinal metabolism and blood flow. The photoreceptors consume more oxygen in the dark and preretinal oxygen tension is 26% lower in dark-adapted rabbits compared with that of light-adapted animals.[177,313,340] The rabbit retina is avascular, and increased oxygen consumption in the photoreceptor layer affects the oxygen tension in the inner layers of the retina. However, the situation is different in a vascularized retina. Studies of glucose consumption in the nonhuman primate retina during different lighting conditions show that glucose uptake in the photoreceptor layer is higher in darkness than during constant daylight illumination but that the difference in glucose uptake in the inner retinal layers is not significant[40] (Figure 33-23, *bottom*). Flickering light at 4 to 8 Hz, on the other hand, increased glucose uptake in the ganglion cell layer (Figure 33-23, *top*). Also in the vascularized retina of pigs and cats, oxygen and glu-

cose consumption are independent of the level of constant light in the inner retina, but they are greatly reduced in the outer retina (photoreceptors) when the dark-adapted retina is exposed to light.[48,325,326] During diffuse luminance flicker, a modest increase in retinal blood flow occurs (39%) and a significant increase (256%) in blood flow through the optic nerve occurs in cats.[50,164,259] The effect is mediated by NO, and a corresponding increase in preretinal K^+ concentration occurs, indicating a close coupling between retinal neuronal activity and optic nerve head blood flow.[50,51,164] Flickering light also has an effect on retinal blood flow in the human eye. A brief increase in retinal blood flow velocity occurs when light is turned on after a period of darkness, and during flicker a modest (3% to 4%) increase in retinal arterial and venous diameters occurs, as does an increase in leukocyte velocity in the macular capillaries.[92,253,269]

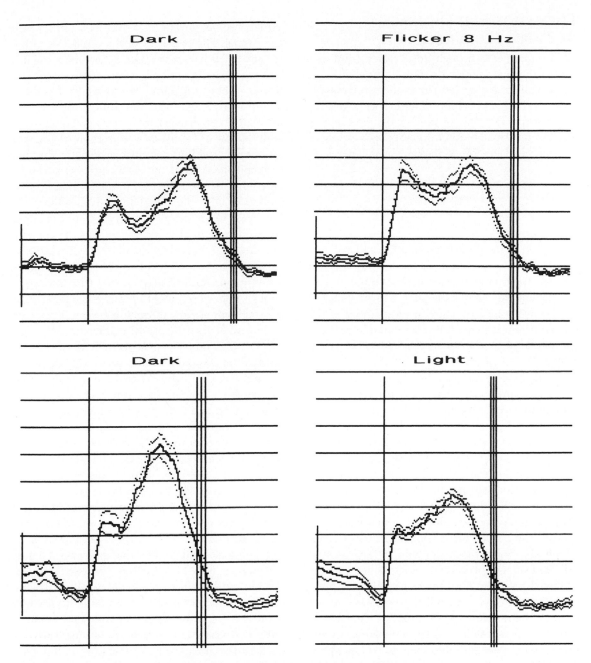

FIGURE 33-23 Optical density profiles from autoradiograms of the central retina at a position 1 to 4 mm temporal to the optic disc at different lighting conditions after an intravenous injection of labeled 2-deoxy-D-glucose. High density indicates high glucose uptake. Vitreous to the left, triple vertical lines indicate position of retinal pigment epithelium. *Top*, Flickering light increases glucose uptake in ganglion cell layer compared with glucose uptake in the dark. *Bottom*, The glucose uptake in the photoreceptor layer is lower during constant illumination than in darkness. (Technique reported in Bill and Sperber.[40]) (Courtesy A. Bill and G. Sperber.)

FORMATION AND DRAINAGE OF TISSUE FLUID IN THE EYE

Fluid movement through small pores from one compartment to another depends on the hydrostatic and colloid osmotic pressures in the two compartments and the permeability of the barrier or wall between them. The flow of fluid across the capillary wall through small ion-permeable pores is expressed by a modified concept of Starling's hypothesis:

$$F = C \times [(P_{hc} - P_{ht}) + (P_{collt} - P_{collc})]$$

where
  C = Constant
  P_{hc} = Mean hydrostatic pressure in capillary
  P_{collc} = Mean colloid osmotic pressure in capillary
  P_{ht} = Hydrostatic pressure in tissue fluid
  P_{collt} = Colloid osmotic pressure in tissue fluid

The hydrostatic pressure in most tissues of the eye corresponds to the IOP. However, in the suprachoroidal space, it is believed to be less by several millimeters of mercury.[80] Outside the eye, in the orbit, the hydrostatic pressure is close to zero. The blood-aqueous and blood-retinal barriers prevent passage of large molecules, such as proteins, into the aqueous humor, vitreous body, and extracellular spaces of the iris and the retina. This results in a colloid osmotic pressure in these compartments that is close to zero. In the extracellular spaces of the ciliary processes and the choroid, the situation is different. The capillary beds in these two regions are permeable even to proteins, which leads to a protein content in these compartments between 60% and 70% of that in plasma.[34,35] The normal colloid osmotic pressure in plasma is approximately 25 mm Hg. Thus the colloid osmotic pressure in the stroma of the ciliary processes and the choroid is approximately 16 mm Hg. This means that there is a colloid osmotic pressure gradient, tending to absorb fluid into the vessels, which corresponds to approximately 25 mm Hg across the capillary walls of the iris and the retina and 9 mm Hg across the capillary walls of the ciliary processes and the choroid. The hydrostatic pressure in the capillaries is obviously higher than that in the veins and higher than the IOP. This results in a hydrostatic pressure gradient over the capillary walls in the eye, tending to move fluid into the extravascular compartments by ultrafiltration. In the choriocapillaris of the rabbit, the average pressure has been determined to be approximately 10 mm Hg above the IOP.[180] Thus in the choroid the colloid osmotic and the average hydrostatic pressure gradients are

similar and net flow of fluid over the capillary wall is minimal. The pressures in the capillaries of the iris and retina have never been determined, and it is unknown whether there is a net inflow or outflow through these capillaries. However, it has been demonstrated that the net inflow or outflow through the iris capillaries is negligible compared with the rate of formation and outflow of aqueous humor.[37] Ultrafiltration must take place through the capillary walls of the ciliary processes to provide fluid for the aqueous humor formation. It is unclear whether the rate of aqueous formation adjusts itself to the net ultrafiltration from the blood vessels or whether the latter is adjusted to the rate of secretion. A hybrid model in which the extravascular albumin concentration plays a central role is a likely possibility.[34] The pores that are large enough to be permeable to proteins are fewer than the small pores. Flow through large pores depends mainly on hydrostatic pressure differences.[34]

The high protein concentration of the tissue fluid in the choroid and the absence of protein in the tissue fluid in the retina have an interesting consequence. The colloid osmotic pressure of the choroidal tissue fluid tends to cause water movement through the pigment epithelium from the retina into the choroid. This may be one of several important mechanisms for the attachment of the rest of the retina to the pigment epithelium.

Lymph vessel–like structures have been observed in the choroid of nonhuman primates, but they are probably not necessary for the removal of extravascular proteins.[169] The sclera is permeable even to large molecules and proteins that have passed out of the vascular beds of the ciliary processes, and the choroid can leave the eye mainly by direct flow or diffusion through the sclera.[34] Because the sclera is permeable even to proteins, the colloid osmotic pressure has no effect on transscleral flow. The adequate hydrostatic pressure gradient promoting flow through the sclera is inadequate. This pressure gradient is of the same order as the IOP because the pressure in the orbit is about zero and the pressure in the suprachoroidal space is almost as high as the IOP. There is a pressure gradient, albeit small, between the anterior chamber and the suprachoroidal space. Part of the aqueous humor is drained by this pressure gradient into the suprachoroidal space through the tissue spaces of the ciliary muscle. In monkeys, such flow is pronounced; in adult humans, it seems to be less than 15% of the total drainage although the low level may be caused by age rather than a true species difference.[37,39]

OCULAR BLOOD FLOW
IN OCULAR DISEASE

To date, most clinical studies have addressed the correlation between blood flow and other signs of ocular disease. Long-term studies are needed to determine to what extent disturbed hemodynamics may be causative or simply a consequence of disease. In addition, longitudinal studies are necessary to determine how medical or surgical therapy may modify ocular blood flow to provide beneficial effects to the eye. Correlation between disease and hemodynamics has been examined for many common ocular disorders.

Diabetes Mellitus

In diabetes mellitus a number of factors may influence blood flow regulation in the eye. Acutely elevated blood glucose levels affect vascular endothelial cell function and contractility of retinal pericytes.[190,328] In cultured bovine retinal vascular endothelial cells, increased environmental glucose levels attenuate expression of NOS and synthesis of NO is reduced.[59] On the other hand, in the early streptozotocin-diabetic (STZ) rat model, a normal action of NO has been found in the ocular and peripheral vascular beds.[47,110] Other experimental studies in this diabetes model have revealed increased expression of messenger ribonucleic acid (mRNA) for endothelins and increased leukocyte entrapment in retinal blood vessels despite normal leukocyte flow velocity.[70,203]

In the human eye, there are many indications that retinal vessels are affected by diabetes. Reduced retinal vasoconstriction in response to inspired oxygen is an early sign in diabetes, and the normal reduction of retinal blood flow observed during hyperoxia is progressively impaired in diabetic patients with retinopathy.[93,118] Arterial flow pulsatility is reduced in mild retinopathy but increases with progression and becomes above normal in severe retinopathy.[84] The autoregulatory response of retinal blood flow to an increased IOP is also progressively impaired in persons with diabetes.[284] Studies on retinal blood flow with laser Doppler flowmetry have demonstrated an increase in retinal blood flow that is related to the duration of the disease and metabolic control, with the exception of eyes with marked capillary nonperfusion where retinal blood flow is reduced.[116,122,123] Even in these eyes there may in fact be a relative increase in flow because panretinal photocoagulation therapy of proliferative diabetic retinopathy reduces arterial pulsatility and venous diameters, improves the response to hyperoxia, and reduces retinal blood flow.[83,121,192,234]

The situation may be different in the choroid. In early STZ-induced diabetes in rats, choroidal blood flow is normal; however, studies in human eyes with color Doppler imaging, as well as studies on choroidal pulsatility, indicate reduced choroidal blood flow in eyes of patients with diabetes.[110,173,272,307]

Divergent results obtained from clinical studies would be expected if metabolic control, blood glucose levels, duration of the disease, and stage of the retinopathy all affect retinal blood flow. In chronic disease the level of glycosylated hemoglobin (HbA$_{1c}$) is an indicator of long-term metabolic control. Duration of disease has been found to be of importance for the development of impaired endothelial function.[239] Acetylcholine-induced vasodilation has been reported to be more attenuated in rats with poor metabolic control, measured as a high level of HbA$_{1c}$, than in animals with more moderately elevated HbA$_{1c}$ levels.[263] In humans with type 1 diabetes mellitus of long duration, a reduced response to NO-inhibition with N^G-monomethyl-L-arginine (L-NMMA) has been observed in the uveal vessels.[273] In addition, acute changes in blood glucose levels may affect retinal blood flow. Atherton et al.[21] found that intravenous glucose infusions increased retinal blood flow in the anesthetized cat by 33% based on flow calculations from high-speed fluorescein angiograms. An increase in preretinal oxygen tension after glucose administration has also been reported in healthy and in diabetic dogs.[81] In human eyes, Grunwald et al.[120] reported that normoglycemia achieved with an insulin injection reduced retinal blood flow and that the effect was largest in those patients with a short disease duration.

In summary, the bulk of the studies done on human eyes indicate that there is little effect on retinal blood flow in early diabetic patients whose disease is well controlled, although some effect on the reactivity of the retinal vessels can be observed even at this stage. As the retinopathy progresses, a gradual increase in retinal blood flow occurs until capillary nonperfusion becomes prominent. Panretinal photocoagulation is followed by an immediate reduction of retinal blood flow, presumably as a consequence of improved metabolic conditions in the remaining retina.

Glaucoma

A noticeable rise in eye pressure, as often seen in angle-closure glaucoma, may be expected to cause ischemia within the anterior optic nerve and retina and may damage both of these tissues. The situation in chronic open-angle glaucoma is different. Both experimental and clinical studies support the assumption that optic nerve blood flow is as efficiently autoregulated as retinal blood flow. However, these studies have been performed on healthy eyes and most likely under constant illumination. The metabolic demands on the retina under anesthesia and constant illumination are rather low, whereas under other conditions, the eye may be more vulnerable to an increased IOP.[39] Age and atherosclerosis also likely affect autoregulation of blood flow. Thus Hayreh et al.[141] reported that increased IOP caused a higher level of anaerobic glycolysis in the retina and anterior optic nerve of aged monkeys kept on an atherogenic diet compared with young monkeys, suggesting a deficient autoregulation of blood flow. It seems reasonable that the autoregulation is deficient in some elderly glaucoma patients. In one group of patients with glaucoma who were studied with the blue-field entoptoscope, the average upper limit for normal leukocyte velocity was an IOP of approximately 25 mm Hg, compared with approximately 30 mm Hg in healthy eyes.[119] Obviously, if autoregulation is deficient, reducing IOP and thus increasing ocular perfusion should be a rational therapeutic approach.

Other abnormalities of the circulation of blood to the anterior optic nerve have been proposed as potential causative factors in the development of glaucomatous optic neuropathy. Population surveys have demonstrated a relationship between open-angle glaucoma and systemic hypertension and between open-angle glaucoma and diabetes.[201,312] Patients with progressive visual field loss are more likely to have nocturnal arterial hypotension.[109,143,193] Disorders associated with vasospasm, such as migraine headaches or cold hands and feet, are more commonly seen in patients with glaucoma, both with and without elevated IOP.[104,226,238] Furthermore, elevated levels of prothrombin fragments have been reported in untreated patients with open-angle glaucoma, possibly contributing to the increased prevalence of retinal venous thrombosis in glaucoma.[220]

Additional studies have suggested that the blood flow in the peripapillary region and the retrobulbar space is significantly reduced in eyes exhibiting glaucomatous optic nerve damage.* In the optic nerve, evidence of decreased blood flow accompanied with visual field damage has been reported in patients with glaucoma.[126,199,211] Many of these studies remain controversial because the validity of the various hemodynamic measurement techniques remains under investigation. The hypothesis that circulatory abnormalities are related to the development of glaucomatous optic neuropathy is well supported by these clinical associations. As reasonable as this hypothesis may be, ischemia has never actually been demonstrated to cause, or even contribute to, glaucomatous optic neuropathy. The direct evidence that ischemia is related to glaucoma, as a causative factor, is lacking. Vascular disease may merely be an associated finding.[63]

Aging and Macular Degeneration

Many common ocular diseases are associated with aging. In macular degeneration, hemodynamic abnormalities have been sited as both potential causative agents and as part of the pathologic process. Retinal capillaries are known to show substantial changes, including localized narrowing, constriction, caliber irregularity, and occlusion in aged rats.[26] Blue-field entoptic investigations have suggested that, in healthy human subjects, retinal macular blood flow decreases with age. The 20% decrease in average velocity with age is similar to the age-related decrease in number of cells observed in the human foveal ganglion cell layer.[123] With use of laser Doppler flowmetry, choroidal blood flow has been shown to decrease with age. This change is probably related to the decrease in density and diameter of the choriocapillaries that occurs with increasing age.[117] In addition, average choroidal blood flow measured with the same technique is lower in the nonexudative stages of macular degeneration than that of age-matched controls, and the effect is caused mainly by a decrease in blood flow volume.[125] Hemodynamic abnormalities in the retrobulbar circulation have been found to occur in greater frequency in macular degeneration and may play a role in the pathogenesis.[64,99,151] Further longitudinal studies are needed to determine whether these alterations in the choroidal blood flow play a role in the development of choroidal neovascularization and whether blood flow measurements may help identify subjects with macular degeneration at risk for developing choroidal neovascularization.

---

*References 54, 155, 197, 212, 245, 265, 333.

References

1. Aburn NS, Sergott RC: Orbital colour Doppler imaging, *Eye* 7:39, 1993.
2. Alder VA, Cringle SJ: The effect of the retinal circulation on vitreal oxygen tension, *Curr Eye Res* 4:121,1985.

3. Alder VA, Cringle SJ, Constable IJ: The retinal oxygen profile in cats, *Invest Ophthalmol Vis Sci* 24:30, 1983.

4. Alm A: Effects of norepinephrine, angiotensin, dihydroergotamine, papaverine, isoproterenol, nicotinic acid and xanthinol nicotinate on retinal oxygen tension in cats, *Acta Ophthalmol* 50:707, 1972.

5. Alm A: The effect of sympathetic stimulation on blood flow through the uvea, retina, and optic nerve in monkeys, *Exp Eye Res* 25:19, 1977.

6. Alm A: The effect of topical l-epinephrine on regional ocular blood flow in monkeys, *Invest Ophthalmol Vis Sci* 19:487, 1980.

7. Alm A, Bill A: Blood flow and oxygen extraction in the cat uvea at normal and high intraocular pressures, *Acta Physiol Scand* 80:19, 1970.

8. Alm A, Bill A: The oxygen supply to the retina: I. Effects of changes in intraocular and arterial blood pressures and in arterial PO_2 and PCO_2 on the oxygen tension in the vitreous body of the cat, *Acta Physiol Scand* 84:261, 1972.

9. Alm A, Bill A: The oxygen supply to the retina: II. Effects of high intraocular pressure and of increased arterial carbon dioxide tension on uveal and retinal blood flow in cats: a study with labelled microspheres including flow determinations in brain and some other tissues, *Acta Physiol Scand* 84:306, 1972.

10. Alm A, Bill A: The effect of stimulation of the sympathetic chain on retinal oxygen tension and uveal, retinal and cerebral blood flow in cats, *Acta Physiol Scand* 88:84, 1973.

11. Alm A, Bill A: Ocular and optic nerve blood flow at normal and increased intraocular pressures in monkeys *(Macaca irus)*: a study with radioactively labelled microspheres including flow determinations in brain and some other tissues, *Exp Eye Res* 15:15, 1973.

12. Alm A, Bill A, Young FA: The effects of pilocarpine and neostigmine on the blood flow through the anterior uvea in monkeys: a study with radioactively labelled microspheres, *Exp Eye Res* 15:31, 1973.

13. Alm A, Törnquist P, Mäepea O: The uptake index method applied to studies on the blood-retinal barrier: II. Transport of several hexoses by a common carrier, *Acta Physiol Scand* 113:81, 1981.

14. Alm A, Törnquist P, Stjernschantz J: Radioactively labeled microspheres in regional ocular blood flow determinations, *Bibl Anat* 16:24, 1977.

15. Almegård B, Andersson SE: Vascular effects of calcitonin gene-related peptide (CGRP) and cholecystokinin (CCK) in the monkey eye, *J Ocular Pharmacol* 9:77, 1993.

16. Ambache N, Kavanagh L, Whiting J: Effect of mechanical stimulation on rabbit eyes: release of active substance in anterior chamber perfusate, *J Physiol* 176:378, 1965.

17. Anderson DR: Glaucoma, capillaries and pericytes: 1. Blood flow regulation, *Ophthalmologica* 210:257, 1996.

18. Anderson DR, Davis EB: Glaucoma, capillaries and pericytes: 5. Preliminary evidence that carbon dioxide relaxes pericyte contractile tone, *Ophthalmologica* 210:280, 1996.

19. Ascher KW: *The aqueous veins,* Springfield, Ill, 1961, Charles C Thomas.

20. Ashton N: *Lecture,* William Mackenie centenary symposium, Glasgow, Scotland, 1968.

21. Atherton A et al: The effect of acute hyperglycaemia on the retinal circulation on the normal cat, *Diabetologia* 18:233, 1980.

22. Bellhorn RW: Permeability of blood-ocular barriers of neonatal and adult cats to fluorescein-labeled dextrans of selected molecular sizes, *Invest Ophthalmol Vis Sci* 21:282, 1981.

23. Benedito S et al: Role of the endothelium in acetylcholine-induced relaxation and spontaneous tone of bovine isolated retinal small arteries, *Exp Eye Res* 52:575, 1991.

24. Berg-Nyborg NC, Nielsen PJ: Angiotensin-II contracts isolated human posterior ciliary arteries, *Invest Ophthalmol Vis Sci* 31:2471, 1990.

25. Bernstein MH, Hollenberg MJ: Fine structure of the choriocapillaris and retinal capillaries, *Invest Ophthalmol* 4:1016, 1965.

26. Bhutto IA, Amemiya T: Retinal vascular changes during aging in Wistar Kyoto rats: application of corrosion cast and scanning electron microscopy, *Ophthalmic Res* 27:249, 1995.

27. Bill A: Aspects of physiological and pharmacological regulation of uveal blood flow, *Acta Soc Med Ups* 67:122, 1962.

28. Bill A: Aspects of regulation of the uveal venous pressure in rabbits, *Exp Eye Res* 1:193, 1962.

29. Bill A: Autonomic nervous control of uveal blood flow, *Acta Physiol Scand* 56:70, 1962.

30. Bill A: A method for quantitative determination of blood flow through the cat uvea, *Arch Ophthalmol* 67:156, 1962.

31. Bill A: Quantitative determination of uveal blood flow in rabbits, *Acta Physiol Scand* 55:101, 1962.

32. Bill A: Blood pressure in the ciliary arteries of rabbits, *Exp Eye Res* 2:20, 1963.

33. Bill A: The uveal venous pressure, *Arch Ophthalmol* 69:780, 1963.

34. Bill A: Capillary permeability to and extravascular dynamics of myoglobin, albumin and gammaglobulin in the uvea, *Acta Physiol Scand* 73:204, 1968.

35. Bill A: A method to determine osmotically effective albumin and gammaglobulin concentrations in tissue fluids, its application to the uvea and a note on the effects of capillary "leaks" on tissue fluid dynamics, *Acta Physiol Scand* 73:511, 1968.

36. Bill A: Effects of acetazolamide and carotid occlusion on the ocular blood flow in unanesthetized rabbits, *Invest Ophthalmol* 13:954, 1974.

37. Bill A: Blood circulation and fluid dynamics in the eye, *Physiol Rev* 55:383, 1975.

38. Bill A, Linder M, Linder J: The protective role of ocular sympathetic vasomotor nerves in acute arterial hypertension. In Proceedings of the Ninth European Conference on Microcirculation, Antwerp, Belgium, 1976, *Bibl Anat* 16:30, 1977.

39. Bill A, Phillips CI: Uvoscleral drainage of aqueous humor in human eyes, *Exp Eye Res* 12:275, 1971.

40. Bill A, Sperber G: Aspects of oxygen and glucose consumption in the retina: effects of high intraocular pressure and light, *Graefes Arch Clin Exp Ophthalmol* 228:124, 1990.

41. Bill A, Sperber G, Ujiie K: Physiology of the choroidal vascular bed, *Int Ophthalmol* 6:101, 1983.

42. Bill A, Stjernschantz J, Alm A: Effects of hexamethonium, biperiden and phentolamine on the vasoconstrictive effects of oculomotor nerve stimulation in rabbits, *Exp Eye Res* 23:614, 1976.

43. Bill A, Törnquist P, Alm A: The permeability of the intraocular blood vessels, *Trans Ophthalmol Soc UK* 100:332, 1980.

44. Bill A et al: Substance P-release on trigeminal nerve stimulation: effects on pupil, eye pressure and capillary permeability, *Acta Physiol Scand* 106:371, 1979.

45. Bishoff PM, Flower RW: Ten years experience with choroidal angiography using indocyanine green dye: a new routine examination or an epilogue? *Doc Ophthalmol* 60:235, 1985.

46. Bohdanecka Z et al: Influence of acquisition parameters on hemodynamic measurements with the Heidelberg retina flowmeter at the optic disc, *J Glaucoma* 7:151, 1998.

47. Brands MW, Fitzgerald SM: Acute endothelium-mediated vasodilation is not impaired at the onset of diabetes, *Hypertension* 32:541, 1998.

48. Braun RD, Linsenmeier RA, Goldstick TK: Oxygen consumption in the inner and outer retina of the cat, *Invest Ophthalmol Vis Sci* 36:542, 1995.

49. Braun RD, Linsenmeier RA, Yancey CM: Spontaneous fluctuations in oxygen tension in the cat retina, *Microvasc Res* 44:73, 1992.

50. Buerk DG, Riva CE, Cranstoun SD: Frequency and luminance-dependent blood flow and K(+) ion changes during flicker stimuli in cat optic nerve head, *Invest Ophthalmol Vis Sci* 36:2216, 1995.

51. Buerk DG, Riva CE, Cranstoun SD: Nitric oxide has a vasodilatory role in cat optic nerve head during flicker stimuli, *Microvasc Res* 52:13, 1996.

52. Bundgaard M: The three-dimensional organization of tight junctions in a capillary endothelium revealed by serial-section electron microscopy, *J Ultrastruct Res* 88:1, 1984.

53. Butryn RK et al: Vasoactive agonists do not change the caliber of retinal capillaries of the rat, *Microvasc Res* 50:80, 1995.

54. Butt Z et al: Measurement of ocular blood flow velocity using colour Doppler imaging in low tension glaucoma, *Eye* 9:29, 1995.

55. Campochiaro PA, Sen A: Adenosine and its agonists cause retinal vasodilation and hemorrhage: implications for ischemic retinopathies, *Arch Ophthalmol* 107:412, 1989.

56. Carlson ES: Fenestrated subendothelial basement membranes in human retinal capillaries, *Invest Ophthalmol Vis Sci* 30:1923, 1989.

57. Chakravarthy U et al: Immunoreactive endothelin distribution in ocular tissues, *Invest Ophthalmol Vis Sci* 35:2448, 1994.

58. Chakravarthy U et al: Nitric oxide synthase activity and expression in retinal capillary endothelial cells and pericytes, *Curr Eye Res* 14:285, 1995.

59. Chakravarthy U et al: Constitutive nitric oxide synthase expression in retinal vascular endothelial cells is suppressed by high glucose and advanced glycation end products, *Diabetes* 47:945, 1998.

60. Chandra SR, Friedman E: Choroidal blood flow: II. The effects of autonomic agents, *Arch Ophthalmol* 87:67, 1972.

61. Chauhan BC, Smith FM: Confocal scanning laser Doppler flowmetry: experiments in a model flow system, *J Glaucoma* 6:237, 1997.

62. Cioffi GA: Three assumptions: ocular blood flow and glaucoma, *J Glaucoma* 7:6, 1998.

63. Cioffi GA, Wang L: Optic nerve blood flow in glaucoma, *Semin Ophthalmol* 14:2000, 1999.

64. Ciulla TA et al: Color Doppler imaging discloses reduced ocular blood flow velocities in nonexudative age-related macular degeneration, *Am J Ophthalmol* 128:75, 1999.

65. Cohan BE, Cohan S: Flow and oxygen saturation in the anterior ciliary vein of the dog eye, *Am J Physiol* 205:60, 1963.

66. Collier RH: Experimental embolic ischemia of the choroids, *Arch Ophthalmol* 77:683, 1967.

67. Crone C: The Malpighi lecture: from "Porositates carnis" to cellular microcirculation, *Int J Microcirc Clin Exp* 6:101, 1987.

68. Cunha-Vaz JG, Shakib M, Ashton N: Studies on the permeability of the blood-retinal barrier, *Br J Ophthalmol* 50:441, 1966.

69. Dallinger S et al: Endothelin-1 contributes to hyperoxia-induced vasoconstriction in the human retina, *Invest Ophthalmol Vis Sci* 41:864, 2000.

70. Deng D et al: Diabetes-induced vascular dysfunction in the retina: role of endothelins, *Diabetologia* 42:1228, 1999.

71. de Oliveira F: Pericytes in diabetic retinopathy, *Br J Ophthalmol* 50:134, 1966.

72. Deussen A, Sonntag M, Vogel R: L-arginine-derived nitric oxide: a major determinant of uveal blood flow, *Exp Eye Res* 57:129, 1993.

73. Diaz-Flores L, Gutierrez R, Varela H: Angiogenesis: an update, *Histol Histopathol* 9:807, 1994.

74. Diaz-Flores L et al: Microvascular pericytes: a review of their morphological and functional characteristics, *Histol Histopathol* 6:269, 1991.

75. Diaz-Flores L et al: Pericytes as a supplementary source of osteoblasts in periosteal osteogenesis, *Clin Orthop* 275:280, 1992.

76. Dollery CT et al: Focal retinal ischaemia: I. Ophthalmoscopic and circulatory changes in focal retinal ischaemia, *Br J Ophthalmol* 50:283, 1966.

77. Eakins KE: Prostaglandin and nonprostaglandin mediated breakdown of the blood-aqueous barrier, *Exp Eye Res* 25(suppl):483, 1977.

78. Eberli B, Riva CE, Feke GT: Mean circulation time of fluorescein in retinal vascular segments, *Arch Ophthalmol* 97:145, 1979.

79. Ehinger B: Adrenergic nerves to the eye and to related structures in man and the cynomolgus monkey, *Invest Ophthalmol* 5:42, 1966.

80. Emi K, Pederson JE, Toris CB: Hydrostatic pressure of the suprachoroidal space, *Invest Ophthalmol Vis Sci* 30:233, 1989.

81. Ernest JT, Goldstick TK, Engerman RL: Hyperglycemia impairs retinal oxygen autoregulation in normal and diabetic dogs, *Invest Ophthalmol Vis Sci* 24:985, 1983.

82. Fallon TJ, Maxwell CD, Kohner EM: Retinal vascular autoregulation in conditions of hyperoxia and hypoxia using the blue field entoptic phenomenon, *Ophthalmology* 92:701, 1985.

83. Feke GT et al: Laser Doppler measurements of the effect of panretinal photocoagulation on retinal blood flow, *Ophthalmology* 89:757, 1982.

84. Feke GT et al: Retinal circulatory changes related to retinopathy progression in insulin-dependent diabetes mellitus, *Ophthalmology* 92:1517, 1985.

85. Feke GT et al: Blood flow in the normal human retina, *Invest Ophthalmol Vis Sci* 30:58, 1989.

86. Fenstermacher JD, Johnson JA: Filtration and reflection coefficients of the rabbit blood-brain barrier, *Am J Physiol* 211:341, 1966.

87. Ferrari-Dileo G: Beta$_1$ and beta$_2$ adrenergic binding sites in bovine retina and retinal blood vessels, *Invest Ophthalmol Vis Sci* 29:695, 1988.

88. Ferrari-Dileo G, Davis EB, Anderson DR: Biochemical evidence for cholinergic activity in retinal blood vessels, *Invest Ophthalmol Vis Sci* 30:473, 1989.

89. Ffytche TJ et al: Effects of changes in intraocular pressure on the retinal micro-vasculature, *Br J Ophthalmol* 58:514, 1974.

90. Flower RW, Fryczkowski AW, McLeod DS: Variability in choriocapillaris blood flow distribution, *Invest Ophthalmol Vis Sci* 36:1247, 1995.

91. Folkow B, Neil E: *In circulation*, New York, 1971, Oxford University Press.

92. Formaz E, Riva CE, Geiser M: Diffuse luminance flicker increases retinal vessel diameter in humans, *Curr Eye Res* 16:1252, 1997.

93. Forster BA, Ferrari-Dileo G, Anderson DR: Adrenergic alpha$_1$ and alpha$_2$ binding sites are present in bovine retinal blood vessels, *Invest Ophthalmol Vis Sci* 28:1741, 1987.

94. Frank RN, Turczyn TJ, Das A: Pericyte coverage of retinal and cerebral capillaries, *Invest Ophthalmol Vis Sci* 31:999, 1990.

95. Frayser R, Hickam JB: Retinal vascular response to breathing increased carbon dioxide and oxygen concentrations, *Invest Ophthalmol* 3:427, 1964.

96. Freddo TF, Raviola G: Freeze-fracture analysis of the interendothelial junctions in the blood vessels of the iris in *Macaca mulatta, Invest Ophthalmol Vis Sci* 23:154, 1982.

97. Friedman E, Oak SM: Choroidal microcirculation in vivo, *Bibl Anat* 7:129, 1965.

98. Friedman E, Smith TR, Kuwabara T: Retinal microcirculation in vivo, *Invest Ophthalmol* 3:217, 1964.

99. Friedman E et al: Ocular blood flow velocity in age-related macular degeneration, *Ophthalmology* 102:640, 1995.

100. Fujino T, Hamasaki DI: Effect of intraocular pressure on the electroretinogram, *Arch Ophthalmol* 78:757, 1967.

101. Funk R, Rohen JW: Scanning electron microscopic study on the vasculature of the human anterior eye segment, especially with respect to the ciliary processes, *Exp Eye Res* 51:651, 1990.

102. Furchgott RF: Role of endothelium in responses of vascular smooth muscle, *Circ Res* 53:557, 1983.

103. Furchgott RF, Zawadzki JV: The obligatory role of the endothelium in the relaxation of arterial smooth muscle by acetylcholine, *Nature* 398:373, 1980.

104. Gasser P, Flammer J: Blood-cell velocity in the nailfold capillaries of patients with normal-tension and high-tension glaucoma, *Am J Ophthalmol* 111:585, 1991.

105. Gay AJ, Rosenbaum AL: Retinal artery pressure in asymmetric diabetic retinopathy, *Arch Ophthalmol* 75:758, 1966.

106. Geijer C, Bill A: Effects of raised intraocular pressure on retinal, prelaminar and retrolaminar optic nerve blood flow in monkeys, *Invest Ophthalmol Vis Sci* 18:1030, 1979.

107. Gidday JM, Park TS: Adenosine-mediated autoregulation of retinal arteriolar tone in the piglet, *Invest Ophthalmol Vis Sci* 34:2713, 1993.

108. Gidday JM, Park TS: Microcirculatory responses to adenosine in the newborn pig retina, *Pediatr Res* 33:620, 1993.

109. Graham SL et al: Ambulatory blood pressure monitoring in glaucoma: the nocturnal dip, *Ophthalmology* 102:61, 1995.

110. Granstam E, Granstam S-O: Regulation of uveal and retinal blood flow in STZ-diabetic and non-diabetic rats: involvement of nitric oxide, *Curr Eye Res* 19:330, 1999.

111. Granstam E, Nilsson SFE: Non-adrenergic sympathetic vasoconstriction in the eye and some other facial tissues in the rabbit, *Eur J Pharmacol* 175:175, 1990.

112. Granstam E, Wang L, Bill A: Ocular effects of endothelin-1 in the cat, *Curr Eye Res* 11:325, 1992.

113. Granstam E et al: Endothelium-dependent vasodilation in the uvea of hypertensive and normotensive rats, *Curr Eye Res* 17:189, 1998.

114. Grayson MC, Laties AM: Ocular localization of sodium fluorescein, *Arch Ophthalmol* 85:600, 1971.

115. Grotte G: Passage of dextran molecules across the blood-lymph barrier, *Acta Chir Scand (Suppl)* 211:1, 1965.

116. Grunwald JE, DuPont J, Riva CE: Retinal haemodynamics in patients with early diabetes mellitus, *Br J Ophthalmol* 80:327, 1996.

117. Grunwald JE, Hariprasad SM, DuPont J: Effect of aging on foveolar choroidal circulation, *Arch Ophthalmol* 116:150, 1998.

118. Grunwald JE et al: Altered retinal vascular response to 100% oxygen breathing in diabetes mellitus, *Ophthalmology* 91:1447, 1984.

119. Grunwald JE et al: Retinal autoregulation in open-angle glaucoma, *Ophthalmology* 91:1690, 1984.

120. Grunwald JE et al: Effect of an insulin-induced decrease in blood glucose on the human diabetic retinal circulation, *Ophthalmology* 94:1614, 1987.

121. Grunwald JE et al: Diabetic glycemic control and retinal blood flow, *Diabetes* 39:602, 1990.

122. Grunwald JE et al: Total retinal volumetric rate in diabetic patients with poor glycemic control, *Invest Ophthalmol Vis Sci* 33:356, 1992.

123. Grunwald JE et al: Effect of aging on retinal macular microcirculation: a blue field simulation study, *Invest Ophthalmol Vis Sci* 34:3609, 1993.

124. Grunwald JE et al: Retinal hemodynamics in proliferative diabetic retinopathy: a laser Doppler velocimetry study, *Invest Ophthalmol Vis Sci* 34:66, 1993.

125. Grunwald JE et al: Foveolar choroidal blood flow in age-related macular degeneration, *Invest Ophthalmol Vis Sci* 39:385, 1998.

126. Grunwald JE et al: Optic nerve and choroidal circulation in glaucoma, *Invest Ophthalmol Vis Sci* 39:2329, 1998.

127. Haefliger IO, Chen Q, Anderson DR: Effect of oxygen on relaxation of retinal pericytes by sodium nitroprusside, *Graefes Arch Clin Exp Ophthalmol* 235:388, 1997.

128. Haefliger IO, Flammer J, Lüscher TF: Nitric oxide and endothelin-1 are important regulators of human ophthalmic artery, *Invest Ophthalmol Vis Sci* 33:2340, 1992.

129. Haefliger FO, Zschauer A, Anderson DR: Relaxation of retinal pericyte contractile tone through the nitric oxide-cyclic guanosine monophosphate pathway, *Invest Ophthalmol Vis Sci* 35:991, 1994.

130. Harino S, Riva CE, Petrig BL: Intravenous nicardipine in cats increases optic nerve head but not retinal blood flow, *Invest Ophthalmol Vis Sci* 33:2885, 1992.

131. Harino S et al: Rebreathing into a bag increases human retinal macular blood velocity, *Br J Ophthalmol* 79:380, 1995.

132. Harris A et al: Test/retest reproducibility of color Doppler imaging assessment of blood flow velocity in orbital vessels, *J Glaucoma* 4:281, 1995.

133. Harris A et al: Hemodynamic and visual function effects of oral nifedipine in patients with normal-tension glaucoma, *Am J Ophthalmol* 124:296, 1997.

134. Hasegawa Y et al: Klinische anwendung von indozyaningrün-angiographie zur diagnose choroidaler neovaskulärer erkrankungen, *Fortsch Ophthalmol* 85:410, 1988.

135. Haynes WG, Webb DJ: Endothelin as a regulator of cardiovascular function in health and disease, *J Hypertens* 16:1081, 1998.

136. Hayreh SS: The ophthalmic artery: III. Branches, *Br J Ophthalmol* 46:212, 1962.

137. Hayreh SS: Segmental nature of the choroidal vasculature, *Br J Ophthalmol* 59:631, 1975.

138. Hayreh SS: Optic disc edema in raised intracranial pressure: V. Pathogenesis, *Arch Ophthalmol* 95:1553, 1977.

139. Hayreh SS: Pathogenesis of optic nerve damage and visual field defects. In Heilman LK, Richardson KT (eds): *Glaucoma,* Stuttgart, Germany, 1978, Georg Thieme Verlag KG.

140. Hayreh SS: Evaluation of optic nerve head circulation: review of the methods used, *J Glaucoma* 6:319, 1997.

141. Hayreh SS, Bill A, Sperber GO: Effects of high intraocular pressure on the glucose metabolism in the retina and optic nerve in old atherosclerotic monkeys, *Graefes Arch Clin Exp Ophthalmol* 232:745, 1994.

142. Hayreh SS, Piegors DJ, Heistad DD: Serotonin-induced constriction of ocular arteries in atherosclerotic monkeys: implications for ischemic disorders of the retina and optic nerve head, *Arch Ophthalmol* 115:220, 1997.

143. Hayreh SS et al: Nocturnal arterial hypotension and its role in optic nerve head and ocular ischemic disorders, *Am J Ophthalmol* 117:603, 1994.

144. Helbig H et al: Membrane potentials in retinal capillary pericytes: excitability and effect of vasoactive substances, *Invest Ophthalmol Vis Sci* 33:2105, 1992.

145. Henkind P, de Oliveira F: Development of the retinal vessels in the rat, *Invest Ophthalmol* 6:520, 1967.

146. Hickam JB, Frayser R: A photographic method for measuring the mean retinal circulation time using fluorescein, *Invest Ophthalmol* 4:876, 1965.

147. Hickam JB, Frayser R, Ross J: A study of retinal venous blood oxygen saturation in human subjects by photographic means, *Circulation* 27:375, 1963.

148. Hillerdal M, Sperber GO, Bill A: The microsphere method for measuring low blood flows: theory and computer simulations applied to findings in the rat cochlea, *Acta Physiol Scand* 130:229, 1987.

149. Hirschi KK, D'Amore PA: Pericytes in the microvasculature, *Cardiovasc Res* 32:687, 1996.

150. Holmberg Å: The ultrastructure of the capillaries in the ciliary body, *Arch Ophthalmol* 62:949, 1979.

151. Hosal BM et al: Color Doppler imaging of the retrobulbar circulation in age-related macular degeneration, *Eur J Ophthalmol* 8:234, 1998.

152. Hoste AM et al: Effect of alpha-1 and beta agonists on contraction of bovine retinal resistance arteries in vitro, *Invest Ophthalmol Vis Sci* 30:44, 1989.

153. Hudspeth AJ, Yee AG: The intercellular junctional complexes of retinal pigment epithelia, *Invest Ophthalmol* 12:354, 1973.

154. Huxley VH: Physiological regulation of capillary permeability, *J Reconstr Microsurg* 4:34, 1988.

155. Kaiser HJ et al: Blood-flow velocities of the extraocular vessels in patients with high-tension and normal-tension primary open-angle glaucoma, *Am J Ophthalmol* 123:320, 1979.

156. Kalsner S: Cholinergic constriction in the general circulation and its role in coronary artery spasm, *Circ Res* 65:237, 1989.

157. Kawarai M, Koss MC: Sympathetic vasoconstriction in the rat anterior choroid is mediated by alpha-1-adrenoceptors, *Eur J Pharmacol* 363:35, 1998.

158. Kawarai M, Koss MC: Sympathetic vasodilation in the rat anterior choroid mediated by beta-1-adrenoceptors, *Eur J Pharmacol* 368:227, 1999.

159. Khoobehi B et al: Measurement of retinal blood velocity and flow rate in primates using a liposome-dye system, *Ophthalmology* 96:905, 1989.

160. Kiel JW: Endothelin modulation of choroidal blood flow in the rabbit, *Exp Eye Res* 71:543, 2000.

161. Kiel JW, Shepherd AP: Autoregulation of choroidal blood flow in the rabbit, *Invest Ophthalmol Vis Sci* 33:2399, 1992.

162. Klein GJ, Baumgartner RH, Flower RW: An image processing approach to characterizing choroidal blood flow, *Invest Ophthalmol Vis Sci* 31:629, 1990.

163. Koelle JS et al: Depth of tissue sampling in the optic nerve head using laser Doppler flowmetry, *Lasers Med Sci* 8:49, 1993.

164. Kondo M, Wang L, Bill A: The role of nitric oxide in hyperaemic response to flicker in the retina and optic nerve in cats, *Acta Ophthalmol Scand* 75:232, 1997.

165. Koss MC: Role of nitric oxide in maintenance of basal anterior choroidal blood flow in rats, *Invest Ophthalmol Vis Sci* 39:559, 1998.

166. Koss MC, Gherezghiher T: Adrenoceptor subtypes involved in neurally evoked sympathetic vasoconstriction in the anterior choroid of cats, *Exp Eye Res* 57:441, 1993.

167. Koss MC, Gherezghiher T: Ocular effects of alpha-2-adrenoceptor activation in anesthetized cats, *J Ocul Pharmacol* 10:149, 1994.

168. Krakau CET: Calculation of the pulsatile ocular blood flow, *Invest Ophthalmol Vis Sci* 33:2754, 1992.

169. Krebs W, Krebs IP: Ultrastructural evidence for lymphatic capillaries in the primate choroids, *Arch Ophthalmol* 106:1615, 1988.

170. Krogsaa B et al: The blood-retinal barrier permeability in essential hypertension, *Acta Ophthalmol* 61:541, 1983.

171. Krogsaa B et al: Blood-retinal barrier permeability versus diabetes duration and retinal morphology in insulin dependent diabetic patients, *Acta Ophthalmol* 65:686, 1987.

172. Kwon YH, Mansberger SL, Cioffi GA: Ganglion cell death in glaucoma: mechanisms and neuroprotective strategies, *Ophthalmol Clin North Am* 13:465, 2000.

173. Langham ME et al: Choroidal blood flow in diabetic retinopathy, *Exp Eye Res* 52:167, 1991.

174. Laties AM: Central retinal artery innervation, *Arch Ophthalmol* 77:405, 1967.

175. Leber T: Circulations and ernährungsverhältnisse des auges. In Graefe A, Saemisch T (eds): *Handbuch der gesamten augenheilkunde,* Leipzig, Germany, 1903, Springer-Verlag.

176. Lemmingson W: Über das vorkommen von vasomotion im retinalkreislauf, *Graefes Arch Clin Exp Ophthalmol* 176:368, 1968.

177. Linsenmeier RA: Effects of light and darkness on oxygen distribution and consumption in cat retina, *J Genet Physiol* 88:521, 1986.

178. Lonigro AJ et al: Hypotheses regarding the role of pericytes in regulating movement of fluid, nutrients, and hormones across the microcirculatory barrier, *Diabetes* 45(suppl 1): S38, 1996.

179. Luksch A et al: Effects of systemic NO synthase inhibition on choroidal and optic nerve head blood flow in healthy subjects, *Invest Ophthalmol Vis Sci* 41:3080, 2000.

180. Mäepea O: Pressure in the anterior ciliary artery, choroidal veins and choriocapillaris, *Exp Eye Res* 54:731, 1992.

181. Mäepea O, Bill A: The pressure in the episcleral veins, Schlemm's canal and the trabecular meshwork in monkeys: effects of changes in intraocular pressure, *Exp Eye Res* 49:645, 1989.

182. Majno G: Ultrastructure of the vascular membrane. In *Handbook of physiology,* vol 3, Baltimore, 1965, Williams & Wilkins.

183. Mandahl A: Effects of substance P on regional ocular blood flow, intraocular pressure and blood-aqueous barrier in rabbits, *Acta Ophthalmol* 67:378, 1989.

184. Mandahl A, Bill A: Ocular responses to antidromic trigeminal stimulation, intracameral prostaglandin E1 and E2, capsaicin and substance P, *Acta Physiol Scand* 112:331, 1981.

185. Mann RM et al: Nitric oxide and choroidal blood flow regulation, *Invest Ophthalmol Vis Sci* 36:925, 1995.

186. Martin AR et al: Retinal pericytes control expression of nitric oxide synthase and endothelin-1 in microvascular endothelial cells, *Microvasc Res* 59:131, 2000.

187. Masaki T et al: Molecular and cellular mechanism of endothelin regulation: implications for vascular function, *Circulation* 84:1457, 1991.

188. Matsugi T, Chen Q, Anderson DR: Contractile responses of cultured bovine retinal pericytes to angiotensin II, *Arch Ophthalmol* 115:1281, 1997.

189. McDonald DM et al: Characterization of endothelin A (ET$_A$) and endothelin B (ET$_B$) receptors in cultured bovine retinal pericytes, *Invest Ophthalmol Vis Sci* 36:1088, 1995.

190. McGinty A et al: Effect of glucose on endothelin-1-induced calcium transients in cultured bovine retinal pericytes, *J Biol Chem* 274:25250, 1999.

191. Menage MJ et al: Retinal blood flow after superior cervical ganglionectomy: a laser Doppler study in the cynomolgus monkey, *Br J Ophthalmol* 78:49, 1994.

192. Mendivil A, Cuartero V: Ocular blood flow velocities in patients with proliferative diabetic retinopathy after scatter photocoagulation: two years of follow-up, *Retina* 16:222, 1996.

193. Meyer JH, Brandi-Dohrn J, Funk J: Twenty-four hour blood pressure monitoring in normal tension glaucoma, *Br J Ophthalmol* 80:864, 1996.

194. Meyer P et al: Localization of nitric oxide synthase isoforms in porcine ocular tissues, *Curr Eye Res* 18:375, 1999.

195. Michaelson IC: *Retinal circulation in man and animals*, Springfield, Ill, 1954, Charles C Thomas.

196. Michelson G, Schmauss B: Two dimensional mapping of the perfusion of the retina and optic nerve head, *Br J Ophthalmol* 79:1126, 1995.

197. Michelson G, Groh MJ, Langhans M: Perfusion of the juxtapapillary retina and optic nerve head in acute ocular hypertension, *Ger J Ophthalmol* 5:315, 1996.

198. Michelson G et al: Principle, validity, and reliability of scanning laser Doppler flowmetry, *J Glaucoma* 5:99, 1996.

199. Michelson G et al: Visual field defect and perfusion of the juxtapapillary retina and the neuroretinal rim area in primary open-angle glaucoma, *Graefes Arch Clin Exp Ophthalmol* 236:80, 1998.

200. Miller S, Steinberg RH: Transport of taurine, L-methionine and 3-0-methyl-D-glucose across frog retinal pigment epithelium, *Exp Eye Res* 23:177, 1976.

201. Mitchell P et al: Open-angle glaucoma and diabetes: the Blue Mountains Eye Study, Australia, *Ophthalmology* 104:712, 1997.

202. Reference deleted in proofs.

203. Moncada S, Radomski MW, Palmer RMJ: Endothelium-derived relaxing factor: identification as nitric oxide and role in the control of vascular tone and platelet function, *Biochem Pharmacol* 37:2495, 1988.

204. Moncada S, Vane JR: Pharmacology and endogenous roles of prostaglandins endoperoxides, thromboxane A$_2$ and prostacyclin, *Pharmacol Rev* 30:293, 1979.

205. Mordon S et al: Laser-induced release of liposome-encapsulated dye: a new diagnostic tool, *Lasers Med Sci* 13:181, 1998.

206. Morrison JC, DeFrank MP, Van Buskirk EM: Comparative microvascular anatomy of mammalian ciliary processes, *Invest Ophthalmol Vis Sci* 28:1325, 1987.

207. Murphy DD, Wagner RC: Differential contractile response of cultured microvascular pericytes to vasoactive agents, *Microcirculation* 1:121, 1994.

208. Nehls V, Drenckhahn D: Heterogeneity of microvascular pericytes for smooth muscle type alpha-actin, *J Cell Biol* 113:147, 1991.

209. Netland PA, Siegner SW, Harris A: Color Doppler ultrasound measurements after topical and retrobulbar epinephrine in primate eyes, *Invest Ophthalmol Vis Sci* 38:2655, 1997.

210. Neufeld AH, Jampol LM, Sears ML: Aspirin prevents the disruption of the blood-aqueous barrier in the rabbit eye, *Nature* 238:58, 1972.

211. Nicolela MT, Hnik P, Drance SM: Scanning laser Doppler flowmeter study of retinal and optic disk blood flow in glaucomatous patients, *Am J Ophthalmol* 122:775, 1996.

212. Nicolela MT et al: Ocular hypertension and primary open-angle glaucoma: a comparative study of their retrobulbar blood flow velocity, *J Glaucoma* 5:308, 1996.

213. Niesel P: *Messungen von experimentell erzeugten aenderungen der aderhautdurchblutung be kaninchen*, Basel, Switzerland, 1962, S Karger AG.

214. Nilsson SFE: PACAP-27 and PACAP-38: vascular effects in the eye and some other tissues in the rabbit, *Eur J Pharmacol* 253:17, 1994.

215. Nilsson SFE: The significance of nitric oxide for parasympathetic vasodilation in the eye and other orbital tissues in the cat, *Exp Eye Res* 70:61, 2000.

216. Nilsson SFE, Bill A: Vasoactive intestinal peptide (VIP): effects on the eye and on regional blood flow, *Acta Physiol Scand* 121:385, 1984.

217. Nilsson SFE, Linder J, Bill A: Characteristics of uveal vasodilation produced by facial nerve stimulation in monkeys, cats and rabbits, *Exp Eye Res* 40:841, 1985.

218. Nishimura K et al: Effects of endothelin-1 on optic nerve head blood flow in cats, *J Ocular Pharmacol Ther* 12:75, 1996.

219. Nyborg NCB et al: Angiotensin II does not contract bovine retinal resistance arteries in vitro, *Exp Eye Res* 50:469, 1990.

220. O'Brien C et al: Activation of the coagulation cascade in untreated primary open-angle glaucoma, *Ophthalmology* 104:725, 1997.

221. O'Day DM et al: Ocular blood flow measurements by nuclide labelled microspheres, *Arch Ophthalmol* 86:205, 1971.

222. Oksala O: Effects of calcitonin gene-related peptide and substance P on regional blood flow in the cat eye, *Exp Eye Res* 47:283, 1988.

223. Olesen S-P, Clapham DE, Davies PF: Haemodynamic shear stress activates a K$^+$ current in vascular endothelial cells, *Nature* 331:168, 1988.

224. Olver JM, Spalton DJ, McCartney ACE: Microvasculature study of the retrolaminar optic nerve in man: the possible significance in anterior ischaemic optic neuropathy, *Eye* 4:7, 1990.

225. Onda E et al: Microvasculature of the human optic nerve, *Am J Ophthalmol* 120:92, 1995.

226. Orgül S, Flammer J: Headache in normal-tension glaucoma patients, *J Glaucoma* 3:292, 1994.

227. Orgül S, Meyer P, Cioffi GA: Physiology of blood flow regulation and mechanisms involved in optic nerve perfusion, *J Glaucoma* 4:427, 1995.

228. Orgül S et al: Optic nerve vasomotor effects of arterial blood gases, *J Glaucoma* 4:317, 1995.

229. Orgül S et al: Measurement of optic nerve blood flow with nonradioactive colored microspheres in rabbits, *Microvascular Res* 51:175, 1996.

230. Pakola SJ, Grunwald JE: Effects of oxygen and carbon dioxide on human retinal circulation, *Invest Ophthalmol Vis Sci* 34:2866, 1993.

231. Pappenheimer JR: Passage of molecules through capillary walls, *Physiol Rev* 33:387, 1953.

232. Parver LM, Auker C, Carpenter DO: Choroidal blood flow as a heat dissipating mechanism in the macula, *Am J Ophthalmol* 89:641, 1980.

233. Parver LM, Auker CR, Carpenter DO: Choroidal blood flow: III. Reflexive control in human eyes, *Arch Ophthalmol* 101:1604, 1983.

234. Patel V et al: Retinal blood flow in diabetic retinopathy, *Br Med J* 305:678, 1992.

235. Petrig BL, Riva CE: Optimal strategy in using the blue field simulation technique for the measurement of macular blood flow. In: Noninvasive assessment of the visual system, *Technical Digest Series* 3:76, 1990.

236. Petrig BL, Riva CE, Hayreh SS: Laser Doppler flowmetry and optic nerve head blood flow, *Am J Ophthalmol* 127:413, 1999.

237. Petrig BL et al: Confocal laser Doppler system for measurements of blood velocity in retinal vessels and flow in the optic nerve through the undilated pupil, *Lasers Light Ophthalmol* 8:137, 1998.

238. Phelps CD, Corbett J: Migraine and low-tension glaucoma: a case-control study, *Invest Ophthalmol Vis Sci* 26:1105, 1985.

239. Pieper GM: Enhanced, unaltered and impaired nitric oxide-mediated endothelium-dependent relaxation in experimental diabetes mellitus: importance of disease duration, *Diabetologia* 42:204, 1999.

240. Portellos M et al: Effects of adenosine on ocular blood flow, *Invest Ophthalmol Vis Sci* 36:1904, 1995.

241. Pournaras CJ et al: Diffusion of O_2 in the retina of anesthetized miniature pigs in normoxia and hyperoxia, *Exp Eye Res* 49:347, 1989.

242. Prieto D, Simonsen U, Nyborg KCB: Regional involvement of an endothelium-derived contractile factor in the vasoactive actions of neuropeptide Y in bovine isolated retinal arteries, *Br J Pharmacol* 116:2729, 1995.

243. Prieto D et al: Calcitonin gene-related peptide is a potent vasodilator of bovine retinal arteries in vitro, *Exp Eye Res* 53:399, 1991.

244. Ralevic V et al: Substance P is released from the endothelium of normal and capsaicin-treated rat hind-limb vasculature, in vivo, by increased flow, *Circ Res* 66:1178, 1990.

245. Rankin SJ et al: Color Doppler imaging and spectral analysis of the optic nerve vasculature in glaucoma, *Am J Ophthalmol* 199:685, 1995.

246. Ravalico G et al: Pulsatile ocular blood flow variations with axial length and refractive error, *Ophthalmologica* 211:271, 1997.

247. Reddy VN: Dynamics of transport systems in the eye: Friedenwald lecture, *Invest Ophthalmol Vis Sci* 18:1000, 1979.

248. Riva CE, Feke GT, Ben-Sira I: Fluorescein dye-dilution technique and retinal circulation, *Am J Physiol* 234:H315, 1978.

249. Riva CE, Grunwald JE, Petrig BL: Autoregulation of human retinal blood flow: an investigation with laser Doppler velocimetry, *Invest Ophthalmol Vis Sci* 27:1706, 1986.

250. Riva CE, Grunwald JE, Sinclair SH: Laser Doppler measurement of relative blood velocity in the human optic nerve head, *Invest Ophthalmol Vis Sci* 22:241, 1982.

251. Riva CE, Grunwald JE, Sinclair SH: Laser Doppler velocimetry study of the effect of pure oxygen breathing on retinal blood flow, *Invest Ophthalmol Vis Sci* 24:47, 1983.

252. Riva CE, Petrig B: Blue field entoptic phenomenon and blood velocity in the retinal capillaries, *J Opt Soc Am* 70:1234, 1980.

253. Riva CE, Petrig BL, Grunwald JE: Near infrared retinal laser Doppler velocimetry, *Lasers Ophthalmol* 1:211, 1987.

254. Riva C, Ross B, Benedek GB: Laser Doppler measurements of blood flow in capillary tubes and retinal arteries, *Invest Ophthalmol Vis Sci* 11:936, 1972.

255. Riva CE, Sinclair SH, Grunwald, JE: Autoregulation of retinal circulation in response to decrease of perfusion pressure, *Invest Ophthalmol Vis Sci* 21:34, 1981.

256. Riva CE et al: Bidirectional LDV system for absolute measurements of retinal blood speed, *Appl Opt* 18:2302, 1979.

257. Riva CE et al: Blood velocity and volumetric flow rate in human retinal vessels, *Invest Ophthalmol Vis Sci* 26:1124, 1985.

258. Riva CE et al: Rhythmic changes in velocity, volume, and flow of blood in the optic nerve head tissue, *Microvasc Res* 40:361, 1990.

259. Riva CE et al: Flicker evoked increase in optic nerve head blood flow in anesthetized cats, *Neurosci Lett* 128:291, 1991.

260. Riva CE et al: Choroidal blood flow in the foveal region of the human ocular fundus, *Invest Ophthalmol Vis Sci* 35:4273, 1994.

261. Riva CE et al: Autoregulation of human optic nerve head blood flow in response to acute changes in ocular perfusion pressure, *Graefes Arch Clin Exp Ophthalmol* 235:618, 1997.

262. Robinson F et al: Retinal blood flow autoregulation in response to an acute increase in blood pressure, *Invest Ophthalmol Vis Sci* 27:722, 1986.

263. Rodriguez-Manas L et al: Endothelial dysfunction and metabolic control in streptozotocin-induced diabetic rats, *Br J Ophthalmol* 123:1495, 1998.

264. Rojanapongpun P, Drance SM: Velocity of ophthalmic arterial flow recorded by Doppler ultrasound in normal subjects, *Am J Ophthalmol* 115:174, 1993.

265. Rojanapongpun P, Drance SM, Morrison BJ: Ophthalmic artery flow velocity in glaucomatous and normal subjects, *Br J Ophthalmol* 77:25, 1993.

266. Roth S et al: Concentrations of adenosine and its metabolites in the rat retinal/choroid during reperfusion after ischemia, *Curr Eye Res* 16:875, 1997.

267. Ruskell GL: Facial parasympathetic innervation of the choroidal blood vessels in monkeys, *Exp Eye Res* 12:166, 1971.

268. Sanders DR et al: Quantitative assessment of postsurgical breakdown of the blood-aqueous barrier, *Arch Ophthalmol* 101:131, 1983.

269. Scheiner AJ et al: Effect of flicker on macular blood flow assessed by the blue field simulation technique, *Invest Ophthalmol Vis Sci* 35:3436, 1994.

270. Schlingemann RO et al: Vascular expression of endothelial antigen PAL-E indicates absence of blood-ocular barriers in the normal eye, *Ophthalmic Res* 29:130, 1997.

271. Schmetterer L et al: The effect of systemic nitric oxide-synthase inhibition on ocular fundus pulsations in man, *Exp Eye Res* 64:305, 1997.

272. Schmetterer L et al: Fundus pulsation measurements in diabetic retinopathy, *Graefes Arch Clin Exp Ophthalmol* 235:283, 1997.

273. Schmetterer L et al: Nitric oxide and ocular blood flow in patients with IDDM, *Diabetes* 46:653, 1997.

274. Schmetterer L et al: Noninvasive investigations of the normal ocular circulation in humans, *Invest Ophthalmol Vis Sci* 39:1210, 1998.

275. Schmetterer L et al: A comparison between laser interferometric measurement of fundus pulsation and pneumotonometric measurement of pulsatile ocular blood flow: 1. Baseline considerations, *Eye* 14:39, 2000.

276. Schonfelder U et al: In situ observation of living pericytes in rat retinal capillaries, *Microvasc Res* 56:22, 1998.

277. Sears M: Miosis and intraocular pressure changes during manometry, *Arch Ophthalmol* 63:707, 1960.

278. Sedney SC: *Photocoagulation in retinal vein occlusion,* The Hague, 1976, Junk.

279. Shabo AL, Maxell DS: The blood-aqueous barrier to tracer protein: a light and electron microscopic study of the primate ciliary process, *Microvasc Res* 4:142, 1972.

280. Shakib M, Ashton N: Ultrastructural changes in focal retinal ischemia, *Br J Ophthalmol* 50:325, 1966.

281. Shiose Y: Electron microscopic studies on blood-retinal and blood-aqueous barrier, *Jpn J Ophthalmol* 14:73, 1971.

282. Silver DM et al: Estimation of pulsatile ocular blood flow from intraocular pressure, *Acta Ophthalmol* 191(suppl):25, 1989.

283. Sinclair AM, Hughes AD, Sever PS: Effect of nifedipine and glyceryl trinitrate on retinal blood flow in normal subjects, *J Hum Hypertens* 7:399, 1993.

284. Sinclair SH et al: Retinal vascular autoregulation in diabetes mellitus, *Ophthalmology* 89:748, 1982.

285. Sinclair SH et al: Investigation of the source of the blue field entoptic phenomenon, *Invest Ophthalmol Vis Sci* 30:668, 1989.

286. Sonkin PL, Sinclair SH, Hatchell DL: The effect of pentoxifylline on retinal capillary blood flow velocity and whole blood viscosity, *Am J Ophthalmol* 115:775, 1993.

287. Sonkin PL et al: Pentoxifylline increases retinal capillary blood flow velocity in patients with diabetes, *Arch Ophthalmol* 111:1647, 1993.

288. Sperber GO, Alm A: Retinal mean transit time determined with an impulse-response analysis from video fluorescein angiograms, *Acta Ophthalmol Scand* 75:532, 1997.

289. Sperber GO, Bill A: Blood flow and glucose consumption in the optic nerve, retina and brain: effects of high intraocular pressure, *Exp Eye Res* 41:639, 1985.

290. Speyer CL, Steffes CP, Ram JL: Effects of vasoactive mediators on the rat lung pericyte: quantitative analysis of contraction on collagen lattice matrices, *Microvasc Res* 57:134, 1999.

291. Stefansson E et al: Iris arteriolar diameters in hypoxia and hyperoxia: a photographic study in albino guinea pigs, *Invest Ophthalmol Vis Sci* 24:741, 1983.

292. Stitt AW et al: Endothelin-like immunoreactivity and receptor binding in the choroid and retina, *Curr Eye Res* 15:111, 1995.

293. Stjernschantz J, Bill A: Effect of intracranial stimulation of the oculomotor nerve on ocular blood flow in the monkey, cat and rabbit, *Invest Ophthalmol Vis Sci* 18:90, 1979.

294. Stone RA, Kuwayama Y: Substance P-like immunoreactive nerves in the human eye, *Arch Ophthalmol* 103:1207, 1985.

295. Stone RA, Laties AM, Emson PC: Neuropeptide Y and the ocular innervation of rat, guinea pig, cat and monkey, *Neuroscience* 17:1207, 1986.

296. Stone RA, McGlinn AM: Calcitonin gene-related peptide immunoreactive nerves in human and rhesus monkey eyes, *Invest Ophthalmol Vis Sci* 29:305, 1988.

297. Stone RA et al: Vasoactive intestinal polypeptide-like immunoreactive nerves to the human eye, *Acta Ophthalmol* 64:12, 1986.

298. Su E-N et al: Adrenergic and nitrergic neurotransmitters are released by the autonomic system of the pig long posterior ciliary artery, *Curr Eye Res* 13:907, 1994.

299. Sugita S, Hamasaki M, Higashi R: Regional difference in fenestration of choroidal capillaries in Japanese monkey eye, *Jpn J Ophthalmol* 26:47, 1982.

300. Sullivan P et al: The influence of ocular pulsatility on scanning laser Doppler flowmetry, *Am J Ophthalmol* 128:81, 1999.

301. Suzuki Y: Laser speckle velocimetry of retinal blood flow with simultaneous measurement of retinal vessel diameter, *J Jpn Ophthalmol Soc* 98:393, 1994.

302. Suzuki Y et al: Measurement of blood flow velocity in retinal vessels utilizing laser speckle phenomenon, *Jpn J Ophthalmol* 35:4, 1991.

303. Szalay J: Effect of beta adrenergic agents on blood vessels of the rat iris: II. Morphological modifications of the vessel wall, *Exp Eye Res* 31:299, 1980.

304. Szalay J et al: Effect of beta adrenergic agents on blood vessels of the rat iris: I. Permeability to carbon particles, *Exp Eye Res* 31:289, 1980.

305. Tachado SD et al: Species differences in the effects of substance P on inositol triphosphate accumulation and cyclic AMP formation, and on contraction in isolated iris sphincter of the mammalian eye: differences in receptor density, *Exp Eye Res* 53:729, 1991.

306. Takagi C et al: Endothelin-1 action via endothelin receptors is a primary mechanism modulating retinal circulatory response to hyperoxia, *Invest Ophthalmol Vis Sci* 37:2099, 1996.

307. Tamaki Y et al: Blood velocity in the ophthalmic artery determined by color Doppler imaging in normal subjects and diabetics, *Jpn J Ophthalmol* 37:385, 1993.

308. Tamaki Y et al: Noncontact, two-dimensional measurement of retinal microcirculation using laser speckle phenomenon, *Invest Ophthalmol Vis Sci* 35:3825, 1994.

309. Tanaka T, Riva C, Ben-Sira I: Blood velocity measurements in human retinal vessels, *Science* 186:830, 1974.

310. Taylor GA et al: Intracranial blood flow: quantification with duplex Doppler and color Doppler flow US, *Radiology* 176:231, 1990.

311. Thomas WE: Brain macrophages: on the role of pericytes and perivascular cells, *Brain Res* 31:42, 1999.

312. Tielsch JM et al: Hypertension, perfusion pressure, and primary open-angle glaucoma: a population-based assessment, *Arch Ophthalmol* 113:216, 1995.

313. Tillis TN et al: Preretinal oxygen changes in the rabbit under conditions of light and darkness, *Invest Ophthalmol Vis Sci* 29:988, 1988.

314. Tomic L et al: Comparison of retinal transit times and retinal blood flow: a study in monkeys, *Invest Ophthalmol Vis Sci* 42:752, 2001.

315. Törnquist P: Capillary permeability in cat choroid studied with the single injection technique, *Acta Physiol Scand* 106:425, 1979.

316. Törnquist P, Alm A: Retinal and choroidal contribution to retinal metabolism in vivo: a study in pigs, *Acta Physiol Scand* 106:351, 1979.

317. Törnquist P, Alm A: Carrier-mediated transport of amino acids through the blood-retinal and blood-brain barriers: a study with the uptake index method, *Graefes Arch Clin Exp Ophthalmol* 224:21, 1986.

318. Törnquist P, Alm A, Bill A: Studies on ocular blood flow and retinal capillary permeability to sodium in pigs, *Acta Physiol Scand* 106:343, 1979.

319. Toussaint D, Kuwabara T, Cogan DG: Retinal vascular patterns, *Arch Ophthalmol* 65:575, 1961.

320. Trew DR, Smith SE: Postural studies in pulsatile ocular blood flow: I. Ocular hypertension and normotension, *Br J Ophthalmol* 75:66, 1991.

321. Tsang AC et al: Brightness alters Heidelberg retinal flowmeter measurements in an in vitro model, *Invest Ophthalmol Vis Sci* 40:795, 1999.

322. Van Wylen DGL et al: Increases in cerebral interstitial fluid adenosine concentration during hypoxia, local potassium infusion, and ischemia, *J Cereb Blood Flow Metab* 6:522, 1986.

323. Vegge T: A study of the ultrastructure of the small iris, *Z Zellforsch Mikosk Anat* 123:195, 1972.

324. Wallow IHL et al: Systemic hypertension produces pericyte changes in retinal capillaries, *Invest Ophthalmol Vis Sci* 34:420, 1993.

325. Wang L, Kondo M, Bill A: Glucose metabolism in cat outer retina: effects of light and hyperoxia, *Invest Ophthalmol Vis Sci* 38:48, 1997.

326. Wang L, Törnquist P, Bill A: Glucose metabolism of the inner retina in pigs in darkness and light, *Acta Physiol Scand* 160:71, 1997.

327. Wilcox LM et al: The contribution of blood flow by the anterior ciliary arteries to the anterior segment of the primate eye, *Exp Eye Res* 30:167, 1980.

328. Williams SB et al: Acute hyperglycemia attenuates endothelium-dependent vasodilation in humans in vivo, *Circulation* 97:1695, 1998.

329. Williamson TH, Baxter GM, Dutton GN: Colour Doppler velocimetry of the arterial vasculature of the optic nerve head and orbit, *Eye* 7:74, 1993.

330. Wilson RP et al: A color Doppler analysis of nifedipine-induced posterior ocular blood flow changes in open-angle glaucoma, *J Glaucoma* 6:231, 1997.

331. Wolf S et al: Video fluorescein angiography: method and clinical application, *Graefes Arch Clin Exp Ophthalmol* 227:145, 1989.

332. Yamamoto R et al: The localization of nitric oxide synthase in the rat eye and related cranial ganglia, *Neuroscience* 54:189, 1993.

333. Yamazaki Y, Drance SM: The relationship between progression of visual field defects and retrobulbar circulation in patients with glaucoma, *Am J Ophthalmol* 124:287, 1997.

334. Yanagisawa Y et al: A novel vasoconstrictor peptide produced by vascular endothelial cells, *Nature* 332:311, 1988.

335. Yao K et al: Endothelium-dependent regulation of vascular tone of the porcine ophthalmic artery, *Invest Ophthalmol Vis Sci* 32:1791, 1991.

336. Yoneya S, Tso MOM: Angioarchitecture of the human choroids, *Arch Ophthalmol* 105:681, 1987.

337. Zeimer RC et al: A practical venomanometer: measurement of episcleral venous pressure and assessment of the normal range, *Arch Ophthalmol* 101:1447, 1983.

338. Zeimer RC et al: A potential method for local drug and dye delivery in the ocular vasculature, *Invest Ophthalmol Vis Sci* 29:1179, 1988.

339. Zschauer AOA, Davis EB, Anderson DR: Glaucoma, capillaries and pericytes: 4—beta-adrenergic activation of cultured retinal pericytes, *Ophthalmologica* 210:276, 1996.

340. Zuckerman R, Weiter JJ: Oxygen transport in the bullfrog retina, *Exp Eye Res* 30:117, 1980.

SECTION 14

EXTRAOCULAR MUSCLES/ EYE MOVEMENTS

LANCE M. OPTICAN

THE EXTRAOCULAR MUSCLES

JOHN D. PORTER, FRANCISCO H. ANDRADE, AND ROBERT S. BAKER

A thorough understanding of the gross and microscopic anatomy of the orbit and the extraocular muscles is a prerequisite to understanding the physiology of ocular motility. The requirements of vision place special demands on the muscles of rotation of the globe, and these muscles are understandably unique in embryologic origin, microscopic structure, and contractile characteristics. This chapter reviews the well-recognized issues of gross anatomy in light of the needs of the clinician, highlights the unique features of extraocular biology, and reviews new work in orbital anatomy regarding pulley systems and their impact on our understanding of ocular motor control. Consideration is given to advances in the cell and molecular biology of the eye muscles because rapid advances support improvements in management of eye alignment and movement disorders. Finally, attention is given to the interactions of the novel properties of the extraocular muscles with pharmaceuticals and disease processes.

ANATOMY OF THE BONY ORBIT

The bony orbit is roughly conical with the apex dorsal and medial. All of the nerves to the structures of the orbit, including the optic nerve, enter at this apex. Most of the extraocular muscles have their origin around a circular rim of connective tissue surrounding the orbital apex. The orbital walls are all roughly triangular, expanding in area from posterior to anterior. All of the bones to the orbit are thin, with the exception of the lateral wall, which is strong. The orbital rim forms the transition of the orbit to the bones of the face and is characterized by thickened bone able to withstand impact and protect the globe. The medial orbital walls

are roughly parallel to each other, and the roof and floor of the orbits are also on the same plane in healthy individuals. The lateral orbital walls form an angle of approximately 90 degrees with each other, and thus 45 degrees with the medial orbital wall (Figure 34-1). As noted previously, the extraocular muscles usually have their origin at the apex and proceed anteriorly to attach onto the globe. The exception to this is the inferior oblique muscle, which has its origin on the medial orbital wall, wrapping around the eye inferiorly, and the superior oblique muscle, with a physiologic origin at the superior portion of the medial orbital wall, where it goes through the trochlea.

THE GLOBE AND ORBITAL FAT AND FASCIA

The eye is suspended in the orbit by the extraocular muscles, orbital fat, and orbital connective tissue. The eye rotates within this suspending apparatus and often is likened to a ball-and-socket joint. This is an appealing analogy because the orbit is prone to be affected by many of the same diseases as joints, such as rheumatoid arthritis, myositis, tendinitis, and trauma. However, the orbit is not a true ball-and-socket joint. The eye does not rotate on a fluid-filled capsule, as do the bones of a joint. Nevertheless, a low-friction rotational surface is created by the complex arrangement of fat and fibrous tissue filling the orbit around the globe and extraocular muscle. All elements of the soft tissue of the orbit are connected to other elements and to the bony orbit by an elaborate network of fibrous septa (Figure 34-2). A particularly dense condensation of this septal network envelops the distal portion of the extraocular muscles and connects the distal muscle

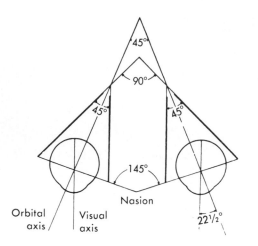

FIGURE 34-1 Angles formed by the walls of the orbit. (From Duke-Elder S, Wybar KC: The anatomy of the visual system. In Duke-Elder S [ed]: *System of ophthalmology,* vol 2, St Louis, 1961, Mosby.)

segments to each other. This portion of fibrous tissue is called *Tenon's capsule.* In the past the distinctness of this capsule has perhaps been overstated. The work of Koornneef[49-51] has illustrated the extensive fibrous connections throughout the orbit and has shown the difficulty in defining a separate and distinct anteriorly placed Tenon's capsule. The extent of the interconnectedness of this fibrous network is clearly, if unfortunately, illustrated by the far-reaching consequences of orbital trauma or hemorrhage. The medial wall, roof, and floor of the orbit are prone to fracture from nondirect blunt impact to the globe or the orbital rim. When a fracture occurs, the adjacent nasal sinuses are often disrupted with herniation and entrapment of the fat, fascia, and sometimes, muscle of the orbit.

An orbital floor fracture entrapping the inferior rectus muscle causes a limitation in upgaze, as would be expected. Less expected is the severe limitation in upward movement of the globe that may accompany fracture-entrapment of inferior fat and fibrous tissue only. This consequence, now frequently documented by sophisticated imaging, occurs because the fat and fascia of the orbital floor are strongly connected to the inferior rectus and inferior oblique muscles. These connections explain a motility abnormality greater than would be expected if the extent of these connections were not known. Similarly, a hemorrhage in the inferior orbit created by extraocular muscle surgery or by orbital surgery can result in a limitation in upgaze and downgaze by causing fibrosis in the normally

delicate fibrous septa surrounding the inferior rectus and inferior oblique muscles. The recently elucidated fibrous pulley system may contribute to the extent of motility abnormality created by trauma to pertinent segments of the orbit.

EXTRAOCULAR MUSCLE GROSS ANATOMY

Five of the six extraocular muscles (excluding the inferior oblique) have their origin at the orbital apex, around the annulus of Zinn. The annulus of Zinn surrounds the entry of the optic nerve into the orbit and is placed at the most posterior medial aspect of the orbit. The inferior oblique muscle has its origin on the nasal bony orbit and mirrors the position of the superior oblique muscle as it passes through the trochlea.

The rectus muscles are all close to 40 mm in length, the lateral being slightly longer than the medial because of its trajectory from the medial orbit around the globe to a temporal insertion. Each muscle receives its innervation at the junction of the posterior and middle third. Helveston et al.[38] have created a table of measurements for the extraocular muscles. Medial and lateral rectus muscles follow the medial and lateral walls of the orbit, respectively, until they pass through their pulleys just posterior to the equator of the globe. At this point, they begin to follow the curve of the globe and insert into the sclera by a tendinous attachment (Figure 34-3). The superior and inferior rectus muscles follow the roof and floor of the orbit, respectively, with the superior rectus being separated from the roof of the orbit by the levator palpebrae superioris muscle. These muscles also pass through pulleys positioned just posterior to the equator of the globe. They then follow the curve of the globe and insert by a tendon into the sclera. The position of the tendinous insertion of each muscle in relation to the corneal limbus is referred to as the *spiral of Tillaux* (Figure 34-4).

Apt[2] analyzed the rectus muscle insertions and established a set of normal values for distances from the anterior and posterior limbus to the insertion of the muscles. He also established the width of insertion and distances between insertions. The medial rectus muscle attaches closest to the corneal-scleral junction, followed by the inferior rectus, the lateral rectus, and finally, the superior rectus, attaching most posterior on the globe.

The distance from the insertion to the limbus has been considered by some clinicians to be relevant to

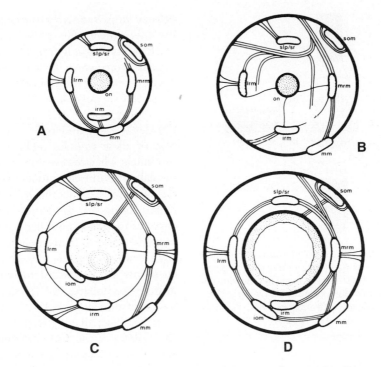

FIGURE 34-2 Four highly schematic drawings illustrating the directions of connective tissue septa of different eye muscles in the orbit. **A,** Areas near the orbital apex. **B,** Areas posterior from, but close to, the hind surface of the eye. **C,** Area lying a little anterior from hind surface of the eye. **D,** Area close to the equator of the eye. *iom,* Inferior oblique muscle; *irm,* inferior rectus muscle; *lrm,* lateral rectus muscle; *mm,* Müller's muscle; *mrm,* medial rectus muscle; *on,* optic nerve; *slp/sr,* superior levator palpebrae/superior rectus muscle complex; *som,* superior oblique muscle. (From Koornneef L: *Spatial aspects of orbital musculo-fibrous tissue in man: a new anatomical and histological approach,* Amsterdam, 1976, Swets and Zeitliinger.)

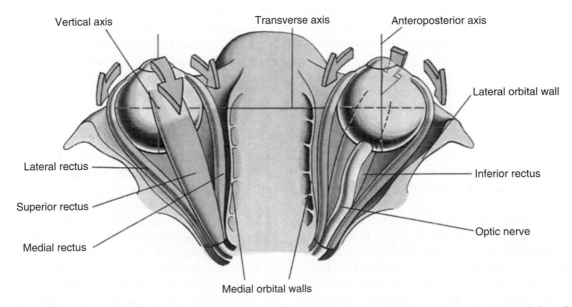

FIGURE 34-3 The orbits from above showing the medial and lateral recti and the superior rectus (*left*) and the inferior rectus (*right*), indicating the vectors of force of contraction of each muscle around a point of central rotation. (From Gray H, Williams PL, Bannister LH: *Gray's anatomy: the anatomical basis of medicine and surgery,* ed 38, New York, 1995, Churchill Livingstone.)

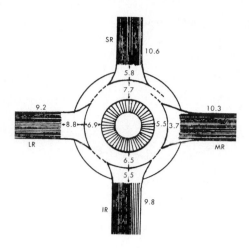

Figure 34-4   Diagramatic view of front of the right eye, drawn to scale, showing insertions of rectus muscles. All figures are in millimeters. Spiral made by insertions of oculorotatory muscle tendons is indicated by *dotted line,* called the *spiral of Tillaux.* (From Scobee RG: *The oculorotatory muscles,* St Louis, 1952, Mosby.)

choosing the amount of recession surgery to be performed for strabismus. Helveston et al.[38] recommend making recession measurements from the limbus instead of from the muscle insertion because of the variability of the insertion location. For example, they found the medial rectus insertion to occur anywhere from 3 to 6 mm from the limbus. Kushner, Lucchese, and Morton[52] systematically studied the effect of measuring from the limbus in recession surgery and found that the correlation with good outcome was all accounted for by the amount of recession from the insertion. Furthermore, Kushner et al.[54] have shown that the prediction of response to strabismus surgery is not significantly improved by inclusion of axial length or refractive error. It appears then that variability in insertion location and axial length need not influence recession amount from the insertion as determined by standard tables of preoperative deviation.

The superior oblique muscle arises from the frontal suture, superomedial to the annulus of Zinn and the medial rectus muscle origin. It travels superomedially in the orbit until it reaches the trochlea on the superomedial orbital wall, where it is redirected posteriorly, inferiorly, and toward the globe, where it travels over the circumference of the globe, finally inserting in a superior posterolateral position on the globe. The tendon makes an angle of approximately 55 degrees, with the visual axis of the globe in the primary position. The inferior

oblique muscle mirrors the path of the superior oblique muscle after it has passed through the trochlea. Its origin is from the orbital plate of the maxilla, from which it wraps around the inferior circumference of the globe to attach in an inferior posterolateral position on the globe (Figure 34-5).

The function of the medial and lateral rectus muscles is easily understood because the contraction of these muscles makes a relatively simple movement when the eye is in primary position. The medial rectus muscles adduct the eye and the lateral rectus muscles abduct the eye. However, it is worth remembering that most eye movements are more complex than this simplified schematic, and all eye muscles receive a change in innervation with virtually every eye movement. A number of fundamental points are important for conceptualizing the primary, secondary, and tertiary functions of extraocular muscles:

1. The eye rotates about a central point. The center of rotation of the eye is, for all intent and purpose, the geometric center of the eye. Translational movements of the globe are small and can be disregarded for the purposes of schematic understanding. This central rotation point means that when the front of the eye moves up, the back of the eye moves down; when the front of the eye moves right, the back of the eye moves left, and vice versa and so forth.

2. In primary position, the visual axis of the eye is aligned with the medial wall of the orbit and forms a 45-degree angle with the lateral wall. This means that the insertion of the superior and inferior rectus muscles forms an angle of approximately 23 degrees with the visual axis of the eye, and the angle of insertion of the superior and inferior oblique muscles forms an angle of 55 degrees with the visual axis (see Figure 34-5).

3. The extraocular muscles, with the exception of the inferior oblique muscle, originate from the posterior medial orbit at the annulus of Zinn. As each muscle contracts, its insertion moves toward the origin.

With these principles in mind, each fundamental movement of the eye initiated by individual extraocular muscles can be discerned. For example, in movements from primary position, the medial and lateral rectus muscles purely adduct and abduct the eye, respectively. However, in primary position, the superior and inferior rectus muscles have more complex actions, and to simplify and isolate the ac-

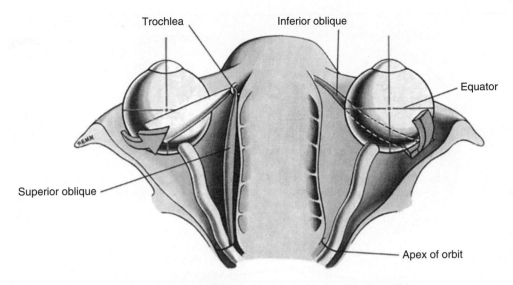

Trochlea   Inferior oblique

Equator

Superior oblique

Apex of orbit

FIGURE 34-5   Superior (*left*) and inferior (*right*) oblique muscles showing rotational directions (*arrows*) around the point of central rotation in relationship to the medial and lateral orbital walls. (From Gray H, Williams PL, Bannister LH: *Gray's anatomy: the anatomical basis of medicine and surgery,* ed 38, New York, 1995, Churchill Livingstone.)

tions of these muscles, it is best to have the patient looking 23 degrees in abduction. In this position the superior rectus is primarily an elevator and the inferior rectus muscle is primarily a depressor. The oblique muscles are somewhat more complex but still understandable on the basis of the aforementioned fundamental points. In adduction the superior oblique muscle has a strong depressor action and the inferior oblique muscle has a strong elevator action because these muscles insert behind the center of rotation of the globe. Thus, when the superior oblique muscle contracts, the back of the eye moves upward and the front of the eye moves downward; the opposite occurs for the inferior oblique muscle. In abduction the torsional aspects of these muscles become more prominent, with the superior oblique muscle being an incyclotorter (inward rotation) and the inferior oblique muscle an excyclotorter (outward rotation). The secondary and tertiary actions of the muscles are more or less prominent, depending on the position of gaze. The secondary action of the superior and inferior rectus muscles is adduction. The tertiary action of the superior rectus muscle is incyclotorsion, and that of the inferior rectus muscle is excyclotorsion. The primary action of the oblique muscles depends on the position of gaze, as noted previously. The tertiary action of the superior oblique muscle is abduction, especially in downgaze; the tertiary action of the inferior oblique muscle is abduction, espe-

cially in upgaze. All of these actions can be deduced by imagining the eye in the gaze position in question, then conceptualizing movement of the insertion toward the origin as contraction takes place with the central point of rotation of the eye remaining relatively fixed.

PULLEY SYSTEMS

Although not as distinct an anatomic structure as the trochlea of the superior oblique muscle, there are pulley systems for each of the four rectus muscles; it is somewhat surprising that details of their structure have come to light only relatively recently. The presence of muscle pulleys improves our understanding of clinical and theoretical ocular motility. Figure 34-6 demonstrates the anatomic position of muscle pulleys schematically, and a thorough discussion on the contribution of muscle pulleys to oculomotor physiology is given in Chapter 35.

The first evidence for extraocular muscle pulleys fixed to the orbital walls came when high-quality magnetic resonance imaging (MRI) showed the paths of rectus muscle bellies remaining relatively fixed in the orbit during large ocular rotations after surgical transposition of their insertions.[62] This led to more thorough MRI and anatomic investigations of the pulleys, including their identification for all rectus muscles and structural characterization as

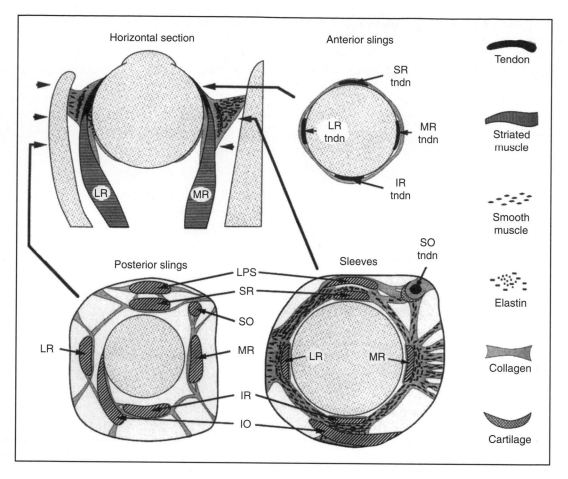

FIGURE 34-6   Diagramatic representation of the structure of the orbital connective tissues, including the rectus muscle pulleys. The three coronal views are represented at the levels indicated by *arrows* in horizontal section. *IO,* Inferior oblique; *IR,* inferior rectus; *LPS,* levator palpebral superioris; *LR,* lateral rectus; *MR,* medial rectus; *SO,* superior oblique; *SR,* superior rectus; *tndn,* tendon. (From Demer JL, Miller JM, Poukens V: *J Pediatr Ophthalmol Strabismus* 33:208, 1996.)

fibroelastic sleeves, consisting of dense bands of collagen and elastin suspended from the orbit and adjacent extraocular muscle sleeves by bands of similar composition.[16] The muscle pulleys contain smooth muscle, giving them the capacity to relax and contract.[75] They also have the orbital layer of extraocular muscle inserting into them, allowing further manipulation of their position in the orbit. These capabilities provide adjustment of the vector forces of the extraocular muscles on the globe in different gaze positions and during different movements, substantially simplifying the central innervation changes necessary to effect eccentric positions of gaze (see Chapters 35 and 36).

From a clinical standpoint, it has been demonstrated that the location of the pulleys may influence the effect of Faden procedures and the cause of incomitant strabismus.[17] The innervation of the smooth muscle suspension component of the muscle pulleys has a variety of neurotransmitters associated with them, suggesting the existence of excitatory and inhibitory control of the pulley suspension mechanism.

SKELETAL MUSCLE PROTOTYPE: STRUCTURE-FUNCTION OF A TYPICAL SKELETAL MUSCLE FIBER

The muscle fiber is the fundamental structural and functional unit of skeletal muscle. Individual muscle fibers are multinucleate syncytia surrounded by a cell membrane, the *sarcolemma.* The nuclei are elliptical in shape, exhibit a prominent nucleolus, and primarily lie just beneath the sarcolemma.

Rather than the usual circumstance of one nucleus being the controller for an entire cell, skeletal muscle adapts to its multinucleate state by having each nucleus exert influence over a longitudinal region of the muscle fiber, known as a *nuclear domain.* An organized array of contractile filaments provides the means by which muscle fibers perform their key role—shortening. Muscle fibers variably use both aerobic and anaerobic metabolism to provide the energy for the contractile process, so there are fiber type–specific differences in mitochondrial content. For readers interested in more details, Engel and Franzini-Armstrong[24] have published a thorough treatise on muscle biology.

The process of muscle development, or myogenesis, has been well documented.[31] Muscle fibers are formed in two waves of myogenesis: primary and secondary. In each wave the individually nucleated muscle precursor cells, termed *myoblasts,* fuse with one another to form multinucleate myotubes with centrally placed nuclei and little surrounding cytoplasm. As the myotube matures, its diameter increases as it accrues contractile elements and mitochondria, and the nuclei move to their definitive location at the periphery of the fiber. Adult skeletal muscles retain a quiescent stem cell population that allows regeneration. After muscle damage has occurred, the regenerative process recapitulates development as the precursor cells in the adult, now known as *satellite cells,* proliferate to produce myoblasts, which fuse to form new muscle fibers.

Muscle Fiber Structure-Function Correlations

Muscle is an ideal structure-function model because cellular properties directly determine the two key traits of muscle function: contraction speed and fatigue resistance. Contraction speed, in turn, is a function of two factors: (1) the types of contractile proteins expressed in a given muscle fiber and (2) the apparatus that links activation of the muscle fiber from a motor nerve to the production of a muscle contraction, excitation-contraction coupling. Fatigue resistance is a direct consequence of cellular metabolism, with more fatigable muscle fibers utilizing glycolysis, whereas fatigue-resistant muscle fibers depend on oxidative mechanisms for energy production. A basic understanding of the structural and functional elements of a skeletal muscle fiber and how they determine the fiber's contraction speed and fatigue properties follows.

The central contractile unit of a skeletal muscle fiber is the sarcomere (Figure 34-7). Each sarcomere is approximately 2 to 3 μm long. End-to-end arrangement of sarcomeres produces the characteristic longitudinal banding pattern of striated muscle. Sarcomeres are formed by the ordered arrangement of thick and thin filaments. Thin filaments are polymers of α-actin, whereas thick filaments consist of aggregates of myosin light and heavy chains. Two proteins that modulate the contractile process, troponin and tropomyosin, attach to the α-actin backbone. A muscle contraction, or twitch, consists of the sliding of actin and myosin filaments relative to one another, while the length of the filaments remains constant.

Skeletal muscles generally have only one type of α-actin. By contrast, there is considerable heterogeneity in myosin expression, with as many as 10 different myosin heavy-chain genes expressed in skeletal muscle (each myosin type or isoform is the product of a different gene).[100] Each myosin is energetically suited to a particular speed of contraction and rate of use and thus is one determinant of contraction speed.

The regular arrangement of actin and myosin filaments within each sarcomere gives rise to the characteristic striated pattern of skeletal muscle sarcomere (see Figure 34-7). Each sarcomere is composed of a dark, anisotropic band (A band) flanked on either side by a light, isotropic band (I band). I bands contain actin filaments exclusively, whereas the dark A bands are composed of both actin and myosin filaments. The A band exhibits a lighter H zone at its center because of the presence of only myosin filaments. An M line, containing proteins that interconnect and stabilize adjacent myosin filaments, bisects the H zone. The filaments of the I band are attached to the narrow, dense Z line, which marks the longitudinal boundary of each sarcomere. Contraction of the muscle fiber occurs by shortening of the sarcomere and is accomplished by the actin filaments sliding along the myosin filaments toward the center of the A band (Figure 34-8). This process shortens the I band and H zone, while the length of the actin and myosin filaments themselves, and of the A band, remains constant. Troponin and tropomyosin facilitate the process by alternatively blocking or allowing the interaction of actin and myosin filaments in response to calcium signals.

Individual sarcomeres are linked together longitudinally so that the small length changes that occur at each sarcomere are additive and can then produce large changes in overall muscle fiber length. Each end-to-end string of sarcomeres is known as a

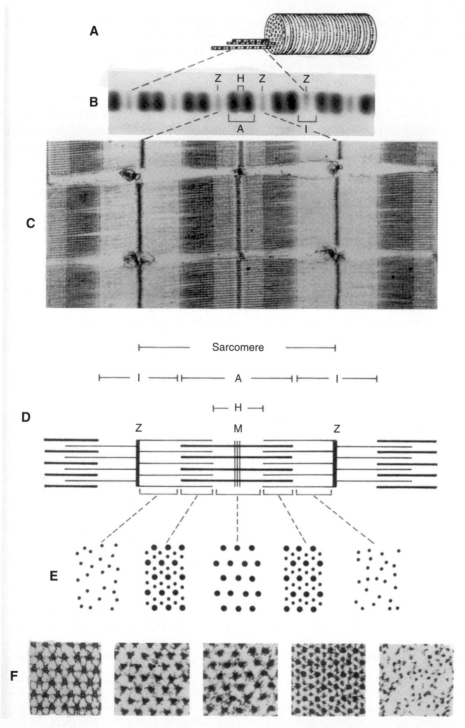

Figure 34-7   Organization of contractile filaments into a sarcomere. **A,** Schematic showing how a single muscle fiber (*large cylinder*) is composed of myofibrils (*small cylinders*). **B,** Banding pattern seen for a single myofibril with the light microscope. **C,** Electron micrograph illustrating arrangement of banding pattern in the sarcomere. **D,** Schematic of pattern of myofilaments depicted in (**C**). **E** and **F,** Cross sections of sarcomere at different sites in the sarcomere, schematically and with electron photomicrographs. Figures illustrate patterned arrangement of actin and myosin filaments. (From Engel AG, Franzini-Armstrong C: *Myology,* vol 1, New York, 1994, McGraw-Hill.)

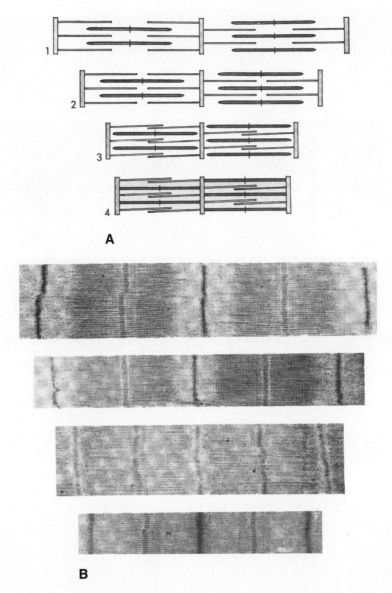

FIGURE 34-8 Illustration of skeletal muscle contractile process. **A,** Change in sarcomere length during a muscle contraction. Schematic shows a sarcomere at different muscle lengths. At rest (*1*), actin (*thin filaments*) and myosin (*thick filaments*) overlap is limited but allows the two to interact as a contraction is initiated. As actin filaments slide relative to one another in muscle shortening (*2*), the width of both the H zone and the I band decrease. As filaments begin to overlap (*3* and *4*), the I band is reduced or absent, whereas the A band does not change in width. Note that during muscle contraction, the length of the myosin and actin filaments themselves does not change. **B,** Electron micrographs corresponding to the four diagrams in (**A**). There is a clinically and scientifically important issue regarding sarcomere length. If sarcomeres are too long (e.g., in a stretched muscle), contractions are weakened because there is little side-to-side contact surface for actin and myosin filaments to interact. Alternatively, if sarcomeres are too short (e.g., in an overcontracted muscle), the total excursion possible by filaments sliding relative to one another is severely limited. (From Huxley HE: *Sci Am* 213:18, 1965.)

myofibril (Figure 34-9, *A*). Myofibrils are separated from one another by a membranous calcium storage system, the sarcoplasmic reticulum. Tubular invaginations of the sarcolemma, the T-tubule system, bring the sarcolemma into direct contact with elements of the sarcoplasmic reticulum.

Muscle Mode of Contraction

Mammalian skeletal muscles consist almost exclusively of fibers that undergo all-or-none action potentials; these fibers are called *twitch fibers*. The process of excitation-contraction coupling links acetylcholine release by a motor nerve terminal at

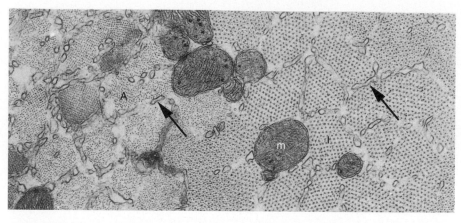

A

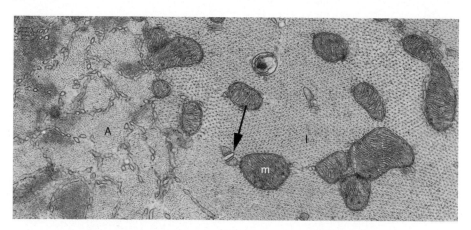

B

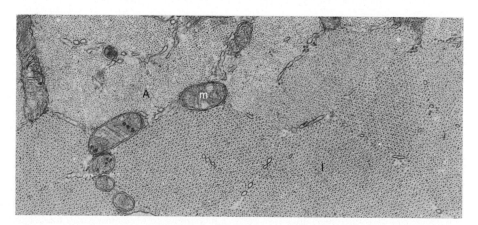

C

FIGURE 34-9   Electron photomicrograph illustrating extraocular twitch and tonic muscle fibers in cross section. Mitochondrial (*m*) and A and I bands are indicated in each panel. **A,** Appearance of a fast-twitch muscle fiber, with small myofibrils that are well defined by sarcoplasmic reticulum (*arrows*). This is a global intermediate singly innervated fiber from extraocular muscle, but arrangement of myofibrils resembles a typical fast-twitch skeletal muscle fiber. **B,** The myofibrils in this fiber are less well defined than those in (**A**), particularly in the I band regions. *Arrow* points to a triad, with the central T tubule and two surrounding elements of sarcoplasmic reticulum. This fiber is an extraocular orbital multiply innervated type that is not typically found in skeletal muscle. It exhibits both twitch and tonic contractions. **C,** This muscle fiber is a global layer multiply innervated fiber type. Traits are typical of tonic, nontwitch, muscle fibers normally found in amphibians. The fiber has little sarcoplasmic reticulum and large ill-defined myofibrils in both A and I bands. This arrangement contributes to a slow excitation-contraction coupling process and its slow contractions.

TABLE 34-1
SKELETAL MUSCLE FIBER CLASSIFICATION SCHEMES

Classification				
Brooke and Kaiser[8]	I	IIA	IIB	IIC
Burke et al.[11]	S	FR	FF	F (int.)
Gauthier and Lowey[34]	Red (slow) oxidative	Red (fast) oxidative	White glycolytic	—
Peter et al.[68]	Slow-twitch oxidative	Fast-twitch oxidative/ glycolytic	Fast-twitch glycolytic	—
Physiology[12,18]				
Twitch contraction time	Slow	Intermediate	Fast	Fast
Twitch tension	Very low	Low	High	Intermediate
Fatigue resistance	Resistant (high)	Resistant (moderate)	Sensitive	Intermediate

Modified from Spencer RF, Porter JD: *Rev Oculomot Res* 2:33, 1988.

the neuromuscular junction to a muscle contraction. Interaction of acetylcholine with muscle cell surface receptors located adjacent to the nerve terminal results in depolarization of the sarcolemma and a propagated action potential along the fiber surface. This action potential is conveyed to the interior of the muscle fiber by the T tubules. T-tubule depolarization subsequently opens sarcoplasmic reticulum calcium release channels, and there is a rapid elevation in intracellular free calcium levels. Calcium, in turn, acts on the troponin-tropomyosin complex to allow direct interaction of adjacent actin and myosin filaments. Finally, the sliding of actin and myosin filaments relative to one another produces muscle fiber shortening. The contraction is rapidly terminated because calcium pumps in the sarcoplasmic reticulum efficiently resequester free calcium. In this scheme, fast-twitch fibers have well-developed T tubule and sarcoplasmic reticulum systems, so the contractile process is rapid, whereas slow-twitch fibers exhibit the opposite properties. The energy requirement for muscle contraction is provided by adenosine triphosphate (ATP) cleavage via a myofibrillar ATPase. Both anaerobic (glycolytic) or aerobic (mitochondrial oxidative) mechanisms participate in muscle fiber energetics.

In contrast to this typical excitation-contraction coupling scheme for twitch fiber contraction, some adult vertebrate skeletal muscle fiber types are multiply innervated (i.e., multiple nerve contacts along their length) and do not propagate action potentials. Instead, these fibers undergo slow, graded contractions in the regions immediately adjacent to each neuromuscular junction. In these fibers the neuromuscular junctions are small, the myofibrils

are large, and the T-tubule and sarcoplasmic reticulum systems are sparse (see Figure 34-9, *C*). These nontwitch fibers are rare in mammalian skeletal muscle.

TRADITIONAL SKELETAL MUSCLE FIBER TYPES

The structural characteristics that determine contractile properties are not independently regulated; however, a muscle fiber, for example, may exhibit interrelated properties that maximize contraction speed but minimize fatigue resistance. Muscle fibers are organized in this way to allow them to specialize for specific functional roles while maximizing peak energy efficiency. The presence of clear patterns in the covariation of skeletal muscle fiber traits has been used to develop muscle fiber–type classification schemes. These classification schemes are a convenient means of understanding muscle function and also are of considerable diagnostic value because several neuromuscular and autoimmune diseases preferentially involve specific muscle fiber types. The major muscle classifications agree on three to four fiber types in typical skeletal muscle: (1) slow twitch, fatigue resistant (red or type I); (2) fast twitch, fatigue resistant (intermediate or type IIA); (3) fast twitch, fatigable (white or type IIB); and (4) fast twitch, intermediate (type IIC or IIX/D)[8,11,34,68] (Table 34-1). These traditional morphologic muscle fiber types have distinct functional identities and are found in virtually every mammalian skeletal muscle.[12,18] Individual muscle or muscle group role specializations then are achieved by regulation of the relative content of these four muscle fiber types.

STRUCTURAL ORGANIZATION OF EXTRAOCULAR MUSCLES

Extraocular Muscle Overview

Although the extraocular muscles clearly are striated muscles, they are highly specialized to the extent that the "rules" that govern traditional skeletal muscle do not always apply to this muscle group. The extraocular muscles have a diverse functional repertoire. The ability to maintain fixation on visual targets is essential for clear vision and must be accomplished within very fine tolerances, or diplopia results. Extraocular muscle also must precisely respond to polymodal sensory signals in production of smooth changes in eye position in vestibuloocular, optokinetic, vergence, and pursuit movements that track or stabilize visual targets. In addition to the slow reflexive and voluntary eye movements, the eye muscles execute reorienting saccadic eye movements that may exceed speeds of 600 degrees per second. In all, extraocular muscle contraction speeds must execute eye movement types that vary in velocity by 10,000-fold; such a wide dynamic range of tasks is not assigned to other skeletal muscles. Because of these diverse functional requirements, the extraocular muscles exhibit what is arguably the greatest diversity of any mammalian skeletal muscle. As we have seen, patterned variations in the characteristics responsible for muscle fiber contraction, speed, and fatigue resistance form the basis for skeletal muscle fiber–type classification schemes. Given the diverse requirements placed on extraocular muscle, it should be no surprise that the traditional classification schemes cannot be applied to extraocular muscle.

Layered Organization and Blood Supply

Extraocular muscles exhibit a distinctive layered organization (Figure 34-10). In a cross section through the midbelly of a rectus muscle, two distinct regions are observed, each with different fiber-type content: (1) an outer orbital layer adjacent to the periorbital and orbital bone and (2) an inner global layer adjacent to the optic nerve and eye. The orbital layer consists of smaller-diameter fibers and typically is C-shaped, encompassing the global layer except for a gap left adjacent to the optic nerve or globe. Although the global layer extends the full muscle length, inserting through a well-defined tendon, the orbital layer ends before the muscle becomes tendinous. Unlike the rectus muscle organization, the orbital layer of the oblique muscles sometimes completely encircles the global layer. The levator palpebrae superioris muscle does not exhibit the layered organization, instead appearing to have only a

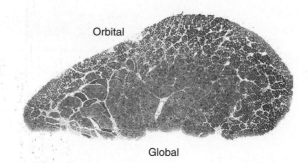

FIGURE 34-10   Light microscope view showing the layers of the lateral rectus muscle from monkey. The orbital layer is the small fiber layer that forms a "c," with the open part of the c downward in this illustration. Fiber diameter is notably larger in the global layer. Distinct orbital and global layers are present in all rectus and oblique muscles.

global layer. The organization of the extraocular muscles is readily accessible to both basic research and morphopathologic evaluation because the two muscle layers and the fiber types in these layers can be recognized by most routine histologic stains.

Recent findings suggest a novel division of labor among the extraocular muscle layers. The orbital layer apparently acts only on the extraocular muscle pulleys, positioning them for optimal kinematics, whereas the global layer inserts directly on the sclera to move the globe.[21]

Muscular branches from the ophthalmic artery supply the extraocular muscles. A lateral muscular branch supplies the superior rectus muscle and a portion of the lateral rectus muscle. The lacrimal artery supplies the rest of the lateral rectus muscle. A medial muscular branch supplies the inferior and medial rectus muscles and a portion of the inferior oblique muscle. The infraorbital artery supplies the rest of the inferior oblique muscle. Finally, the superior muscular branch of the ophthalmic artery supplies the superior oblique muscle. In comparison with other skeletal muscles, the extraocular muscles possess a highly extensive network of vessels[103] (Figure 34-11). The blood supply to the orbital layer is much more extensive than that of the global layer. This highly developed blood supply and correspondingly high blood flow rate is not surprising in view of the continuous activity of the extraocular muscles.[104]

Extraocular Muscle Fiber Types

Six distinct muscle fiber types are present in the extraocular muscles (Figures 34-12 and 34-13).

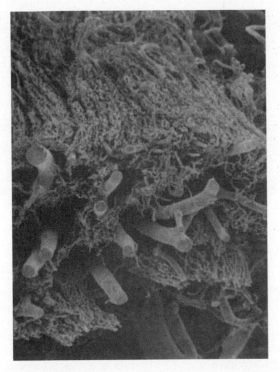

A

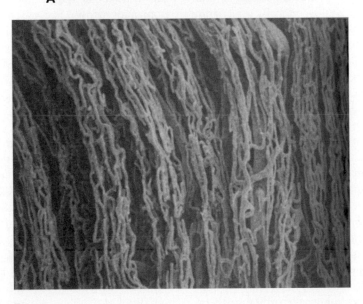

B

FIGURE 34-11 Illustration of the extensive blood supply to the extraocular muscles in humans. These scanning electron photomicrographs were obtained by perfusing the vasculature with plastic, digesting away the tissues, and then coating the plastic casts of the blood vessels with gold so that they could be imaged with the scanning electron microscope. **A,** Cut edge of a rectus muscle, showing the large arteries and veins. **B,** Micrograph of capillary bundles running in the same direction as rectus muscle fibers. (From Porter JD, Baker RS: Anatomy and embryology of the ocular motor system. In Miller NR, Newman NJ [eds]: *Walsh and Hoyt's clinical neuro-ophthalmology,* vol 1, ed 5, Baltimore, 1998, Williams & Wilkins.)

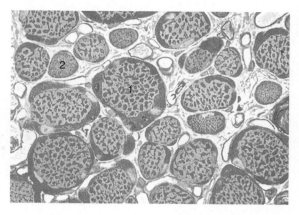

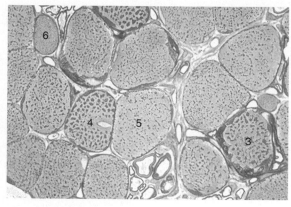

A   **B**

FIGURE 34-12   Light photomicrographs of the two layers of a monkey rectus muscle, showing the six fiber types present in monkey extraocular muscles. **A,** Orbital layer. *1,* Orbital singly innervated fiber type. *2,* Orbital multiply innervated fiber type. **B,** Global layer. *3,* Global red singly innervated fiber type. *4,* Global intermediate singly innervated fiber type. *5,* Global white singly innervated fiber type. *6,* Global multiply innervated fiber type.

Although these fiber types are best documented in monkeys, humans exhibit similar fiber types.[92,93] The fiber types are designated according to their layer distribution (orbital or global), innervation type (singly or multiply), and mitochondrial content (red, intermediate, or white). Fiber-type traits are summarized in Table 34-2, and there are several extensive reviews of the extraocular muscle fiber classification scheme.[71,74,93] An identifying trait of extraocular muscle is the presence of an extraocular muscle-specific myosin that is not expressed in any other skeletal muscles except for the larynx. This myosin is found, at the least, in the orbital singly innervated fiber type and may be in other global layer fiber types.[9,83,99-101]

Orbital Singly Innervated Fiber (see Figure 34-13, *A*). Orbital singly innervated fibers represent the predominant fiber type (80%) in the orbital layer of rectus and oblique muscles. A single neuromuscular junction is present at approximately the middle of each fiber. Morphologically, orbital singly innervated fibers contain small myofibrils, allowing rapid access of calcium in the sarcoplasmic reticulum to the contractile filaments, and high mitochondrial content. At midbelly, fiber diameter is largest and these fibers taper proximally and distally. Mitochondria form characteristically large clusters, particularly at midbelly. Histochemical staining profile shows this fiber to be fast twitch and fatigue resistant, arguably the most fatigue resistant of mammalian skeletal muscle fiber types.

Myosin expression is heterogeneous, with expression of a unique myosin gene that is expressed in only extraocular and laryngeal muscles and a developmental myosin isoform not typically seen in adult skeletal muscle. Consistent with the high mitochondrial and oxidative enzyme content, individual orbital singly innervated muscle fibers are ringed by capillaries. The overall profile is consistent with rapid, highly fatigue-resistant muscle contractions.

Orbital Multiply Innervated Fiber (see Figures 34-9, *B*, and 34-13, *B*). The orbital multiply innervated fiber accounts for the remainder of fibers (20%) in the orbital layer. Unlike other adult skeletal muscle fibers, small, multiple nerve terminals are distributed along the length of individual muscle fibers. The orbital multiply innervated fiber exhibits considerable structural variation along its length. In its center this type has traits consistent with fast-twitch contraction. By contrast, proximal and distal to the fiber center this fiber type exhibits slow myofibrillar ATPase and the fine structural characteristics of slowly contracting fibers. Myosin heavy-chain expression is consistent with this profile in that midfiber regions stain for a fast isoform and proximal/distal regions stain for developmental myosin isoform and the slow myosin isoform. Physiologic studies suggest that orbital multiply innervated fibers exhibit twitch capability in midbelly and nontwitch contractions in proximal and distal fiber segments.[41] Collectively, the features of this

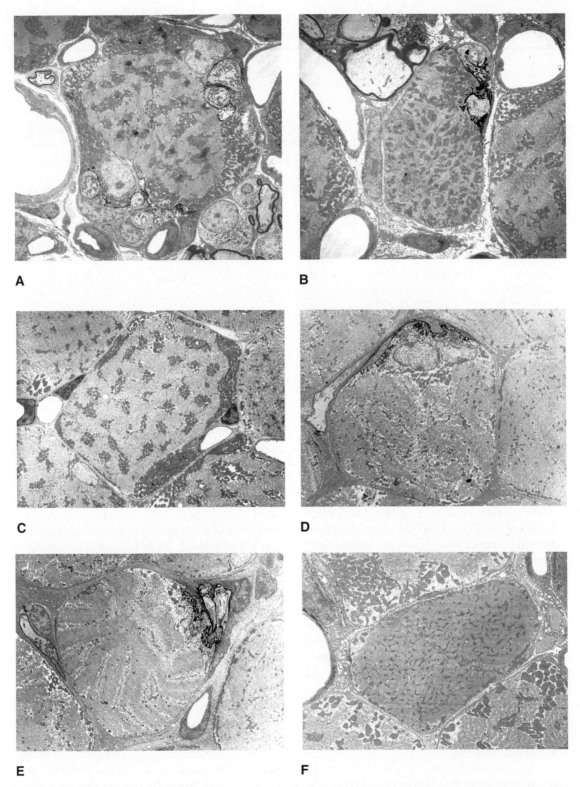

FIGURE 34-13 Electron photomicrographs of the six fiber types present in monkey extraocular muscles. **A,** Orbital singly innervated fiber type. **B,** Orbital multiply innervated fiber type. **C,** Global red singly innervated fiber type. **D,** Global intermediate singly innervated fiber type. **E,** Global white singly innervated fiber type. **F,** Global multiply innervated fiber type.

Table 34-2
EXTRAOCULAR MUSCLE FIBER TYPES

Fiber Types	Orbital SIF	Orbital MIF	Global red SIF	Global int. SIF	Global white SIF	Global MIF
Classification number	1	2	3	4	5	6
Myofibril size	Small	Large	Small	Small	Small	Large
Sarcoplasmic reticulum development	Moderate	Low	Moderate	High	High	Poor
Mitochondria (number, size)	Many, large	Few to many, small	Many, large	Many, moderate	Few, small	Few, small
Energy metabolism	Oxidative/glycolytic	Oxidative	Oxidative/modestly glycolytic	Moderately oxidative/moderately glycolytic	Glycolytic	Weakly oxidative/weakly glycolytic
Presumed contraction mode/speed*	Fast twitch	Mixed (twitch/tonic)	Fast twitch	Fast twitch	Fast twitch	Slow tonic
Presumed fatigue resistance*	High	Moderate	High	Intermediate	Slow	Poor

Modified from Spencer RF, Porter JD: *Rev Oculomot Res* 2:33, 1988.
*Properties are inferred from structural appearance, histochemical enzyme–staining patterns, and myosin immunocytochemistry.

fiber type are unlike any that previously have been described in skeletal muscle, and it is difficult to draw conclusions regarding its function.

Global Red Singly Innervated Fiber (Fig. 34-13, C). Approximately one third of the muscle fibers in the global layer are global red singly innervated fibers. The histochemical, ultrastructural, and myosin heavy-chain expression profile of this fiber type closely resembles that of the orbital singly innervated fiber. However, the global type does not exhibit the longitudinal variations in ultrastructure and does not coexpress the developmental myosin isoforms. Moreover, these fibers express the IIA myosin isoform throughout their length. Together, these observations suggest similarities with the skeletal IIA fiber type, but the high mitochondrial content is greatly different from typical IIA fibers. Functionally, the fiber profile suggests that global red singly innervated fibers are fast twitch and highly fatigue resistant.

Global Intermediate Singly Innervated Fiber (see Figures 34-9, A, and 34-13, D). The global intermediate singly innervated fiber type constitutes approximately one fourth of the fibers in the global layer. Myofibrillar ATPase and ultrastructural char-

acteristics indicate that this is a fast-twitch fiber type, with myosin isoform immunoreactivity characteristic of type II fibers, probably type IIB. Moderate levels of oxidative enzymes and anaerobic enzymes are apparent. Numerous medium-sized mitochondria are distributed singly or in small clusters. Myofibrillar size and sarcoplasmic reticulum content are intermediate between the other two types of global singly innervated fibers. Overall, this profile fits that of a fast-twitch fiber with an intermediate level of fatigue resistance, probably lying between skeletal types IIA and IIB in fatigability.

Global White Singly Innervated Fiber (see Figure 34-13, E). The last global singly innervated fiber type makes up approximately one third of the global layer. The fibers are most analogous to skeletal type IIB fibers with respect to the modest levels of oxidative enzymes, high anaerobic metabolic capacity, and fast-type ATPase profile. The myosin heavy-chain profile is most likely of the IIB type. Few small mitochondria are singly arranged between the myofibrils. The overall fiber profile is consistent with a fast-twitch type that is used only sporadically because of low fatigue resistance.

Global Multiply Innervated Fiber (see Figures 34-9, C, and 34-13, F). Global multiply innervated fibers constitute the remaining tenth of the global layer. Numerous small superficial grapelike endings are distributed along the longitudinal extent of individual fibers of this type. A novel type of sensory nerve terminal, known as the *myotendinous cylinder* or *palisade ending,* is associated with the myotendinous junction of this fiber type. These fibers contain few small mitochondria that are arranged singly between the myofibrils. The myofibrils are large, and sarcoplasmic reticulum development is so poor that myofibril separation is often indistinct. The large myofibrils mean that the calcium source, the sarcoplasmic reticulum, and the contractile filaments are spatially far apart, resulting in slow contractions. The ultrastructural profile of this fiber resembles that of slow, tonic muscle fibers in amphibians. The myosin expression profile includes slow-twitch (type I), slow tonic, and α-cardiac myosin heavy-chain isoforms. Like amphibian muscles, the global multiply innervated fiber type exhibits a slow, graded, nonpropagated response after either neural or pharmacologic activation.[13] This fiber type has no counterpart in other human skeletal muscle. The finding of a phylogenetically primitive muscle fiber type in one of the fastest skeletal muscles is difficult to reconcile, unless one considers a potential role in either fine foveating movements of the eye or as part of a specialized proprioceptive apparatus.

Division of Labor in Extraocular Muscle

The goal of correlative anatomic and physiologic studies of extraocular muscle has been to uncover any association of specific muscle fiber types with defined eye movement functions. The segregation of function among different motor unit types has been a long debated issue in the field of oculomotor system research. An early concept of extraocular muscle suggested that the separate extraocular muscle fiber types subserved distinct classes of eye movement. However, intraoperative electromyographic studies performed by Scott and Collins[85] demonstrated that all of the extraocular muscle fiber types participate in all classes of eye movement. Different fiber types were recruited at specific eye positions, regardless of what type of eye movement was used. Robinson's model[80] has muscle fiber types activated at particular eye positions for movement and maintenance of gaze position. In this scheme the orbital singly innervated and global red singly innervated fiber types become active well in the off-direction of a muscle's plane of action, with recruitment of first the global intermediate and then the global white singly innervated fiber types. This model is consistent with the fatigue resistance of the various singly innervated fiber types. Robinson[80] also suggests that the two multiply innervated fiber types become active around primary position, aiding in small adjustments of eye position.

A recent view of extraocular muscle function requires some reexamination of the functional roles of the six distinct muscle fiber types. The active pulley hypothesis states that the global layer is responsible for eye movements, whereas the orbital layer functions in coordinated movement of the extraocular muscle pulleys.[21] Consistent with this view, the less-well-developed orbital layer in rodent extraocular muscles correlates with the presence of muscle pulleys that are simpler than those in primates.[46] Taken together, the orbital fiber types then may be recruited in a position-dependent fashion, as proposed by Scott and Collins,[85] but for the purpose of coordinating pulley movement with eye movement.

EXTRAOCULAR MUSCLE DEVELOPMENT

The extraocular muscles are set apart from other skeletal muscles as early as the time of their embryonic origin. In contrast to the somatic origin of most skeletal muscles, they are derived from two sources of cephalic mesodermal cells: the prechordal plate and cranial paraxial mesoderm.[69,88,97,98] A prior notion that the extraocular muscles originate from the neural crest is only partially correct. Studies have established that the myoblasts that form the extraocular muscles arise from cranial mesoderm, whereas the orbital connective tissues originate from neural crest.

Embryonic Origin of Extraocular Muscle

Two theories exist regarding the early events in the ontogenesis of the extraocular muscles. One holds that each muscle condenses from one of three distinct precursors, separately and at distinct times.[35,36] The alternative theory is that the extraocular muscles develop concurrently from a single mesenchymal condensation that subsequently divides into separate superior and inferior mesodermal complexes.[86,87] Individual extraocular muscles may receive contributions from both mesodermal complexes (medial and lateral recti) or may arise from only one or the other complex (remainder of the oculorotatory muscles plus the levator palpebrae superioris). During organogenesis, the developing brainstem also is segmented into regions known as *rhombomeres;* these regions give rise to the cranial nerves.[57] Each of the oculomotor nerves arises from particular rhombomeres, consistent with the segmental nature of the cranial nerves. Studies suggest that aggregates of myoblasts may be contacted by oculomotor nerves before migration and carry their innervation with them into the developing orbit.[98] Whether innervation first occurs in the orbit or while myoblasts are still adjacent to the neural tube, the close proximity of the extraocular muscles' primordia may actually facilitate development of anomalous innervation of eye muscles. The classic clinical example of this relationship is Duane retraction syndrome, wherein the congenital absence of the abducens nerve results in the "inappropriate" innervation of the lateral rectus by the oculomotor nerve.

Extraocular Myogenesis

After originating from prechordal and paraxial mesoderm, extraocular muscle precursor cells migrate to the orbit and form condensations around the developing eye. These myoblasts then proceed through the same general scheme of myogenesis that has been described for other skeletal muscles.[9,69] In macaque monkeys, myoblasts fuse to form primary myotubes before embryonic day 62, whereas secondary myotubes appear between embryonic days 62 and 92 (term in the monkey is 165 days) (Figure 34-14). Early neuromuscular contacts are observed at least as early as embryonic day 62.[69] Within a month thereafter, the characteristic cytologic features of singly innervated and multiply innervated fiber types are apparent and all primary and secondary generation fibers are generated and maturing. The phylogenetically "old" global multiply innervated fibers are the first to form, and fibers in the orbital layer mature last. Development recapitulates phylogeny because the primitive multiply innervated fiber type that is common in amphibians matures before phylogenetically "newer" twitch-fiber types. Although the early events in myogenesis are virtually identical to the well-studied pattern in other skeletal muscles, during later stages of muscle fiber differentiation of eye, muscle diverges from the typical skeletal muscle pattern. Final maturation of extraocular muscle fiber types occurs postnatally.[69]

Critical Period in Extraocular Muscle Development

The visual and oculomotor systems develop in parallel over the first few years of life. Hubel and Wiesel[39,40] pioneered the critical period concept in the visual system. The visual cortex of mammals is anatomically and physiologically immature at birth, with key properties such as binocularity and depth perception developing during a species-specific postnatal window. Inappropriate visual experience (by experimental design or as a result of strabismus) disrupts the formation of ocular dominance columns in the visual cortex, resulting in the loss of stereopsis and often severe reductions in visual acuity (amblyopia). Recent evidence suggests that the extraocular muscles may exhibit a critical period in parallel with that of the visual system.

Unlike some skeletal muscles essential for life, the extraocular muscles are immature at birth. Neonatal eye movements are poorly coordinated and inaccurate during at least part of the first year. Thus substantial postnatal differentiation of extraocular muscle fiber types is observed at molecular, cellular, structural, and functional levels. The definitive adult properties of the extraocular muscles are shaped by the activation patterns that they experience in the postnatal period. Experimental manipulations of visuomotor development (monocular deprivation, dark rearing) produce severe deficiencies in visuomotor coordination, extraocular muscle motor units, and the molecular and contractile properties of the extraocular muscles.[10,55,82,89] In rats expression of the extraocular muscle-specific myosin is suppressed by alterations in visual experience during the first 45 days of life.[10] Moreover, a strain of monkeys that is prone to congenital esotropia exhibits maldevelopment of the extraocular muscles.[70] Considered together, these findings support the notion that alterations in extrinsic sensory cues have profound consequences for the development of the extraocular muscles. The concept of an eye muscle critical period then must be considered in assessing the consequences of, and designing treatments for, strabismus.

EXTRAOCULAR MUSCLE GENETICS

Gene Expression Profiling

Completion of the human genome project is providing researchers with new tools to develop molecular definitions for cell and tissue types that thus far have been defined on the basis of structural parameters. This is a major advance

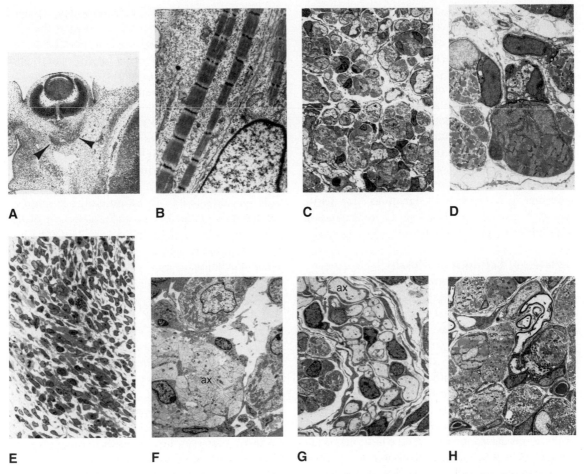

FIGURE 34-14   Light and electron photomicrographs of developing rat extraocular muscle. **A** and **B,** Light photomicrographs of rat orbital at embryonic day 14. Eye development is still at the eye cup stage, with prominent lens. *Arrowheads* indicate developing extraocular muscle behind the eye. **B,** Higher magnification shows condensation of primary myotubes. **C,** Electron photomicrograph of developing primary myotube at embryonic day 14. Note the developing myofibrils, only two of which are evident in this myotube. **D,** Electron photomicrograph of intramuscular axons (*ax*) at embryonic day 18, with absence of any separation between adjacent axons. **E,** Electron photomicrograph of developing extraocular muscle at postnatal day 7, with both primary and secondary myotubes present. Secondary myotubes initially develop immediately adjacent to primary myotubes and separate later. **F,** At postnatal day 7, intramuscular ocular motor nerve axons (*ax*) are now separated by one another by Schwann cell processes, but are not yet myelinated. **G,** A simple nerve terminal is present on a multiply innervated fiber at postnatal day 7. This fiber type is the first of the six extraocular muscle fiber types to reach mature state. **H,** Intramuscular nerves are myelinated and muscle fiber type differentiation is evident by postnatal day 14. Note a myelinated axon cut longitudinally loses its myelin and forms a primitive nerve terminal, capping what is a singly innervated fiber type.

because differences between, for example, a retinal photoreceptor and an extraocular muscle fiber, ultimately are a function of the differential pattern of gene expression in the two cell types. That a photoreceptor expresses rhodopsin, whereas a muscle fiber does not, would be widely assumed and thus not viewed as a particularly useful piece of information. However, knowledge of the overall patterns in gene expression that collectively give the photoreceptor and the muscle fiber their distinct identities has been unapproachable by routine molecular biology methods. In the last few years differential display polymerase chain reaction (PCR), deoxyribonucleic acid (DNA) microarray, and serial analysis of gene expression techniques have allowed researchers to move beyond analysis of only a few genes at a time to create tissue-specific gene expression profiles by *simultaneously* evaluating the expression of thousands of genes.

Although, as noted in this chapter, considerable structural and functional differences exist between extraocular and other skeletal muscles, little is known of the underlying mechanistic differences in gene expression. The extraocular muscle-specific myosin stood alone as a molecular signature of this muscle group. Studies using gene profiling techniques have identified both additional genes novel to extraocular muscle and hundreds of genes with expression patterns that uniquely specify extraocular muscle over other craniofacial and limb muscles.[67,78] In the next few years, the approach of discovering such "molecular signatures" for tissue types will give rise to a new level of understanding of cellular structure and function.

Genetics of Extraocular Muscle and Correlates for Strabismus

Although the molecular genetics of skeletal muscle development has received considerable attention, little is known about developmental mechanisms operating at the gene expression level in extraocular muscle. Given the broadly based differences between extraocular and other skeletal muscles, it is logical to expect that there are eye muscle–specific transcription factors and signal transduction mechanisms to direct myoblasts toward formation of these specialized muscles. A clue to understanding specific mechanisms in extraocular myogenesis has come from studies of the Rieger syndrome gene, paired homeodomain-like protein 2, or *Pitx2*. Humans with mutations in one *Pitx2* allele exhibit malformations of the anterior segment of the eyes, the teeth, and the umbilicus. An embryo-lethal null mutation of *Pitx2* in mice also produces dysgenesis of the extraocular muscles.[48] These data suggest that *Pitx2* lies early in the cascade responsible for morphogenesis of eye muscle. Mutations in as yet unidentified genes downstream from *Pitx2* may play a mechanistic role in extraocular muscle development and thereby may be causative factors in congenital strabismus.

Although the last 10 years have been a period of considerable progress in identification of the genetic basis for many neurologic diseases, little attention has been directed toward the inheritance of ocular motility disorders.[26] Studies by Engle et al.[25,27-30] have established genetic linkage for four types of congenital fibrosis of extraocular muscle (CFEOM) and congenital ptosis. Patients with CFEOM1 exhibit ptosis and downward and outward deviation of the eyes (Figure 34-15). These studies assist in the identification of candidate disease genes and ultimately may allow development of new treatment regimens. Data suggest that, instead of being a primary muscle disease, CFEOM1 involves neuron pool–specific loss of oculomotor motor neurons in the same ways that congenital absence of abducens motor neurons is linked to Duane syndrome and oculomotor/trochlear motor neuron absence leads to extraocular muscle developmental abnormalities in a knockout mouse model.[30,63,72] Collectively, these data suggest that genes playing key roles in either extraocular muscle or oculomotor motor neuron development may be vulnerable to mutation and therefore potential etiologic factors in uncharacterized disorders of eye alignment or movement. Engle[26] has reviewed possible genetic involvement in other ocular deviations.

EXTRAOCULAR MUSCLE PHYSIOLOGY

The extraocular muscles exhibit the greatest structural diversity amongst mammalian skeletal muscles. Whether the number of morphologically different fiber types is in response to functional requirements or a developmental consequence of the anatomic location of the extraocular muscles is unclear.[71] However, because muscle properties are often a function of usage patterns, the fiber type heterogeneity of these muscles is clearly suggestive of functional versatility.

Physiologically, the extraocular muscles have been characterized as being weak, fast, and fatigue resistant. Under isometric conditions, extraocular muscles have short contraction (time required to reach peak twitch force) and half-relaxation (time from peak to half-peak twitch force) times compared with prototypical fast muscles. Forces measured during maximal tetanic contractions of extraocular muscles are just fractions of those obtained from limb muscles, even when normalized to muscle cross-sectional area[19,32,56] (Figures 34-16 and 34-17). Moreover, their twitches are unusually shallow and the twitch/tetanus ratio is lower than in most muscles. This characteristic is particularly evident when the force responses to increasing stimulation frequency are plotted, and a shift down and to the right in the force-frequency relationship becomes obvious (see Figure 34-17, *B*). All of these properties of extraocular muscles may reflect a combination of factors: (1) faster than normal calcium transients during contraction, accomplished by the abundant sarcoplasmic reticulum;

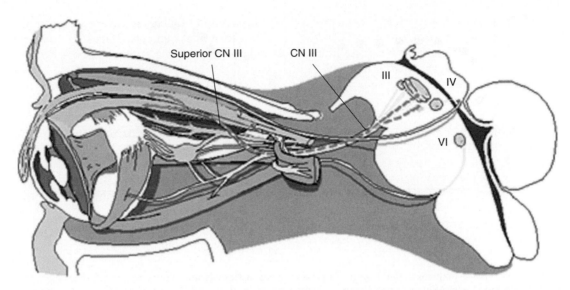

FIGURE 34-15 Schematic showing lateral view of the brainstem and orbit with proposed mechanism for congenital fibrosis of extraocular muscle type 1 (*CFEOM1*). *Dotted subnuclei of the oculomotor nucleus* and *dotted superior division of the oculomotor nerve* indicate that these structures representing the superior rectus and levator palpebrae superioris muscles are abnormal or absent in CFEOM1 patients. *CN,* Cranial nerve. (From Engle EC: The genetics of strabismus: Duane, Moebius, and fibrosis syndromes. In Traboulsi EI [ed]: *Genetic diseases of the eye: a textbook and atlas,* New York, 1998, Oxford University Press.)

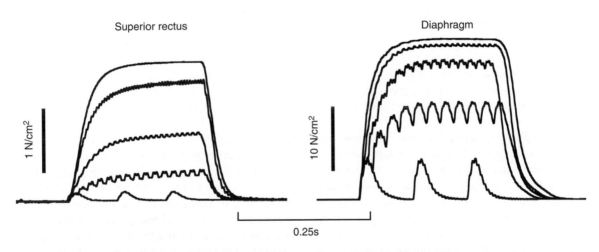

FIGURE 34-16 Muscle force production in extraocular muscle versus the diaphragm. Force tracings for rat superior rectus muscle in response to increasing stimulation frequencies (increasing from bottom, 10 to 300 Hz). By comparison, the diaphragm summates individual stimulations into maximum tetanic force more rapidly (stimulation frequency increasing from bottom, 10 to 200 Hz) and has higher total force production. Forces generated by extraocular muscle are an order of magnitude smaller than those in diaphragm. Note difference in force scales.

(2) displacement of contractile material by other intracellular and extracellular structures; (3) the presence of less–readily excitable nontwitch fibers; and (4) differences in the kinetics of actomyosin, a possibility at least in those fibers that express extraocular muscle-specific myosin.[3]

The estimation of shortening velocity by isotonic contractions (force-velocity relationship) of whole muscles composed of a heterogeneous fiber population is a complex "average" of the speed of all of the muscle fibers.[15] Few studies have attempted to determine the force-velocity relationship of extraocular

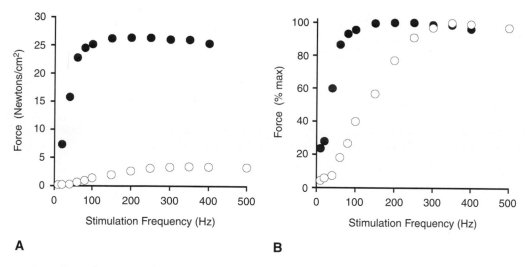

Figure 34-17   Force-frequency relationship comparison of rat superior rectus (*open circles*) with diaphragm (*filled circles*). **A,** Absolute force-frequency relationship, with force normalized to muscle cross-sectional area. This illustrates the significantly higher force produced in diaphragm versus extraocular muscle, even when corrected to the smaller fiber diameter in extraocular muscle. **B,** Relative force-frequency relationship, expressed as percentage of maximum force. Note that higher stimulation frequencies are required for the superior rectus to reach maximum force.

muscles. By this technique, the extraocular muscles appear to be at least as fast as the prototypical fast muscle, extensor digitorum longus. This finding is somewhat surprising because the extensor digitorum longus muscle is a homogeneous fast muscle, whereas the extraocular muscles are integrated by mixed populations of fiber types, although most extraocular muscle fibers express type II (fast) myosin isoforms.

The passive mechanical load that the extraocular muscles work against is relatively small (eyeball itself, suspensory connective tissue). This has been postulated as one reason for the substantial fatigue resistance of the extraocular muscles.[33] This argument neglects the extra load produced by the coactivation of antagonist muscles during eye movements. Moreover, because the absolute force that the extraocular muscles can generate is also small (see Figures 34-16 and 34-17, *A*), it is more relevant to present the passive mechanical load as a fraction of maximal force produced by the muscles. Most skeletal muscles work approximately 25% to 40% of their maximal force (or velocity), maximizing power and efficiency. Possibly, the overall design of the eye and its motor system is such that the extraocular muscles work within this optimal range. Because the load is largely unchangeable and the extraocular muscles normally have high activity rates, fatigue may not be a concern. Other muscles have similar profiles: The diaphragm muscle is constantly active and does not fatigue under most, if not all, physiologic conditions. It is only when the load is altered, such as placing an inspiratory resistor, or the muscle itself is damaged that fatigue ensues. In this context, studies using artificially induced fatigue of the extraocular muscles might be a tool to understand the physiology of the muscles, even without a clear biologic correlate in the intact system.

Extraocular Motor Units
Skeletal muscles and their motor neurons are organized into motor units—one motor neuron plus the muscle fibers that it innervates. The size of a motor unit is the number of muscle fibers that are innervated by a single motor neuron. The ability of a skeletal muscle to increment force therefore depends on the range of available motor unit sizes—if the average motor unit is large, force can be increased or decreased only in large increments, and the opposite for small motor units. The small motor unit size seen in extraocular muscle (10 muscle fibers per motor neuron) is consistent with the precise incrementation of force that is required in fixation and eye movements. The globe represents a small, fixed, and typically unchanging load for the extraocular muscles, although disease, trauma, or surgical intervention can alter resistance. The small motor unit size of extraocular muscle then allows precise targeting of eye movements and fine adjustments to prevent diplopia.

Goldberg and Shall[37] have compared and contrasted extraocular motor unit types with the better studied spinal cord units, noting the presence of slow, fatigable, and nontwitch types not found at the level of the spinal cord. Physiologic studies have not yet identified six distinct motor unit types corresponding to all six extraocular muscle fiber types, perhaps reflecting subtle differences in fatigue among the three global singly innervated fiber types. Goldberg and Shall[37] also reported that several of the tenets of spinal motor units might not apply to extraocular units, including different criteria for fatigue, the possibility of individual motor units containing more than one muscle fiber type, and the lack of linear force summation during motor unit recruitment.

Extraocular Muscle Proprioception

A typical skeletal muscle relies on specialized stretch receptors, neuromuscular spindles, and Golgi tendon organs to provide monosynaptic feedback of muscle length and tension information for precise regulation of motoneuron discharge rate. Because the globe is small and represents a fixed load, compensatory stretch reflexes may not be necessary and have not been found in oculomotor motor neurons.[45] Neuromuscular spindles and Golgi tendon organs have been identified in the extraocular muscles of some species, including humans. Although these spindles are smaller and more delicate than those in other striated muscles, their structure is similar, consisting of groups of fine, cross-striated muscle fibers with a rich nerve supply enclosed in a thin, oval capsule of fibrous tissue. The unique morphology and species differences in the presence or absence of neuromuscular spindles may relate to the notion that the extraocular muscles have no requirements to adjust for a changing external load. It then appears that neuromuscular spindles and Golgi tendon organs do not seem to be major sensory receptors in extraocular muscle.

A sensory receptor unique to extraocular muscle, the myotendinous cylinder or palisade ending, appears to be the predominant sensory end organ in extraocular muscle[79] (Figure 34-18). Palisades are specifically associated with a particular extrafusal muscle fiber type, the global multiply innervated fiber. Steinbach and Smith[95] suggest that these sensory endings may provide important afferent information regarding spatial localization of the extraocular muscles. The association of palisade endings with the global multiply innervated fiber type (a nontwitch muscle fiber) suggests that the information that arises from this receptor does not mediate rapid adjustments in muscle force, but rather that eye muscle proprioception may contribute to long-term recalibration of the motor system. Donaldson[23] suggests that abnormalities of extraocular muscle proprioception may be etiologic in some types of human squint strabismus. For a thorough treatment of the proprioceptive apparatus in extraocular muscle, see Donaldson's review.[23]

PHARMACOLOGY: CLINICAL APPLICATIONS, INCLUDING STRABISMUS

Because extraocular muscle is remarkably different from other skeletal muscles, the response of this muscle group to therapeutic and toxic agents is not predictable from what is known about other skeletal muscles. The following sections discuss agents with clinical applications for which extraocular muscle exhibits a differential response.

Botulinum Toxin

Botulinum toxin type A has come into use for a variety of movement disorders, including ophthalmic applications in blepharospasm and strabismus. The primary action of botulinum toxin is blockade of the calcium-dependent release of acetylcholine at the neuromuscular junction. Focal injection of botulinum toxin produces denervation atrophy of all skeletal muscle fiber types. Fiber size and fiber type–specific characteristics are restored after motor neuron sprouting reestablishes innervation.

As in other skeletal muscles, botulinum toxin causes reversible denervation of the orbicularis oculi muscle, providing only temporary relief of blepharospasm. Sprouting restores innervation within a couple of months and the patient experiences return of eyelid spasms. However, botulinum toxin has different consequences when used as an alternative to traditional strabismus surgery.[83,91]

Unlike its use in other neuromuscular disorders, single injections of botulinum toxin can be highly effective in permanent correction of strabismus[59-61,83,94] (Figure 34-19). This result likely is caused, at least in part, by the fact that botulinum toxin produces specific, long-term changes in extraocular muscle.[91] Specifically, permanent alterations occur in orbital singly innervated fibers. Considered together, there is significant potential in taking advantage of the novel interactions of therapeutic agents with extraocular muscle fiber types for management of ocular alignment and motility disorders.

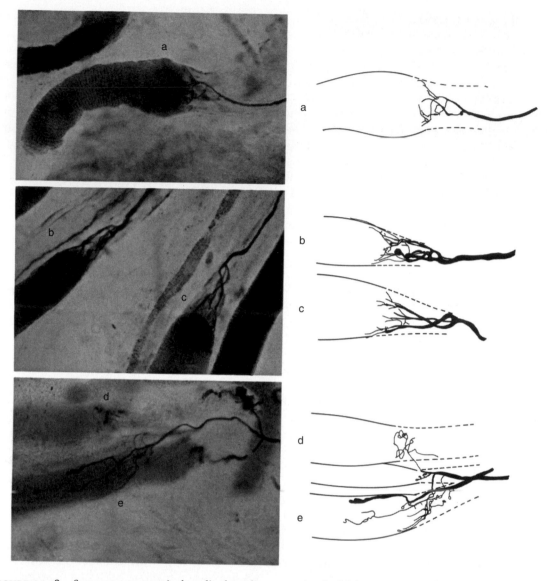

FIGURE 34-18   Sensory nerve terminals, palisade endings, associated with human extraocular muscle. Endings (*a* to *e*) in photomicrographs at *left* are shown schematically in drawings at *right*. Note location of palisade endings at myotendinous junction of muscle fibers. (From Richmond FJR et al: *Invest Ophthalmol Vis Sci* 25:471, 1984.)

Channel Blocking Agents

Succinylcholine is a depolarizing blocker of neuro-muscular transmission in typical mammalian skeletal muscle fiber types. By contrast, in extraoc-ular muscle, succinylcholine selectively activates the multiply innervated fibers. (Although the global type clearly is involved, the degree of activa-tion of orbital multiply innervated fibers is un-clear.) Succinylcholine has value in strabismus surgery because it induces graded contractions that produce ocular alignment under general anes-thesia approximating that seen in the awake pa-

tient[64] (Figure 34-20). On one hand, these data highlight functional differences in extraocular muscles, and on the other, they have been inter-preted to indicate that the multiply innervated fiber types play a role in the establishment of pri-mary ocular alignment.

Calcium channel blockers, such as diltiazem and verapamil, interfere with excitation-contracting coupling in cardiac and vascular smooth muscle by blocking entry of extracellular calcium. The poor development of the sarcoplasmic reticulum in ex-traocular muscle multiply innervated fibers suggests

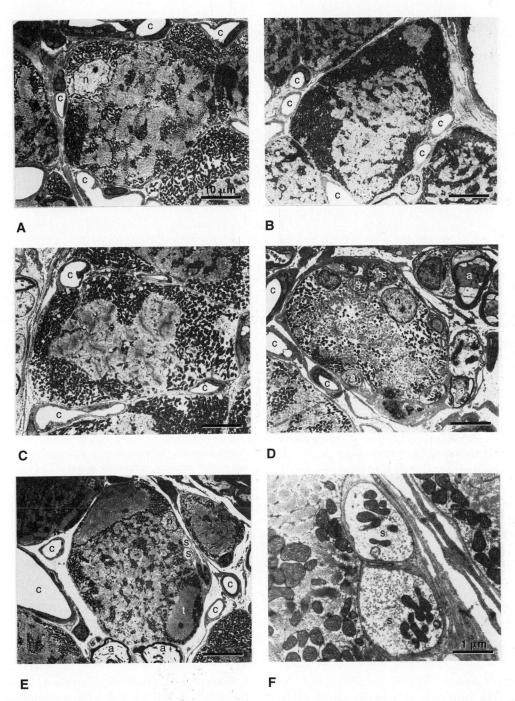

FIGURE 34-19 Electron photomicrographs of orbital singly innervated muscle fibers after injection of botulinum toxin type A. **A,** Normal orbital singly innervated muscle fiber from untreated monkey. Note the extensive capillary network (*c*) that surrounds the fiber. **B** and **C,** Formation of tubular aggregates (overproliferation of sarcoplasmic reticulum) in orbital singly innervated fibers within 7 to 14 days of botulinum toxin injection. Aggregates are particularly apparent among the mitochondrial clusters around the periphery of fibers. Note migration of mitochondria from the center to the periphery of the muscle fibers. **D,** By 28 days after toxin injection, some fibers have regressed to an undifferentiated state, although neuromuscular junctions (*s*) are still present. *a,* Axon. **E** and **F,** At 35 days after injection, tubular aggregates (*t*) persist, but there is some hypertrophy of preterminal axons (*a*) and axon terminals (*s*), indicative of sprouting to form new neuromuscular junctions following botulinum paralysis. (**A-E,** bars = 5 μm; **F,** bar = 0.5 μm.) (Adapted from Spencer RF, McNeer KW: *Arch Ophthalmol* 105:1703, 1987.)

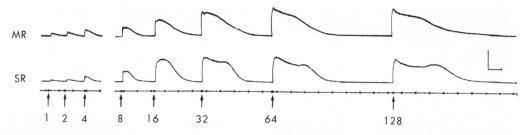

FIGURE 34-20   Effect of increasing dosage (in μg/kg, given intravenously) of succinylcholine on tension of cat medial rectus muscle. Successively larger doses increase baseline muscle force via the multiply innervated fiber system. *MR*, Medial rectus; *SR*, superior rectus. (Calibrations = 10 g tension, 1 minute.) (From Eakins KE, Katz RL: *Br J Pharmacol* 26:205, 1966.)

that the contractile process in these fibers is dependent on extracellular calcium, rather than intracellular stores, and thus might be antagonized by cardioactive and vasoactive calcium blockers. Jacoby et al.[42] demonstrated that reduction in extracellular calcium concentration greatly reduces the tension development in extraocular muscle global multiply innervated fibers and tested the hypothesis that diltiazem then would alter resting eye position. Diltiazem produces a severe reduction in tension development in isolated multiply innervated fibers and causes short-term alterations in eye position when injected into single extraocular muscles. The identification of specific means to block tension development in the global multiply innervated fiber type should facilitate studies of the functional role of this fiber type in fixation and eye movements and has potential for treatment of strabismus.

Local Anesthetic Toxicity

The aminoacyl class of local anesthetics widely used in ophthalmology is highly myotoxic. However, patients rarely experience ptosis and diplopia when these agents are used in ophthalmic procedures. This observation is consistent with experimental findings that retrobulbar bupivacaine causes only mild pathologic conditions in monkeys[73] (Figure 34-21). Specifically, global white singly innervated fibers exhibited pathologic changes after bupivacaine injections. Extraocular muscle sparing then may relate to the high mitochondrial content of many of the extraocular muscle fiber types, which potentially allows management of the intracellular calcium overload produced by local anesthetics. The intramuscular consequences associated with direct injection of anesthetic into muscles may, in a dose-dependent fashion, overload the extraocular muscle calcium scavenging capacity and thus be more severe.

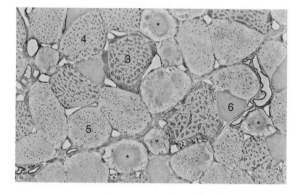

FIGURE 34-21   Effect of retrobulbar injection of bupivacaine on monkey extraocular muscle. Light photomicrograph of global layer of monkey rectus muscle 14 days after anesthetic injection. Scattered fibers, typically global white singly innervated fibers, exhibit peripheral damage to contractile filaments (*asterisks*). *3*, Global red singly innervated fiber type. *4*, Global intermediate singly innervated fiber type. *5*, Global white singly innervated fiber type. *6*, Global multiply innervated fiber type.

DISEASE RESPONSIVENESS OF EXTRAOCULAR MUSCLE

An important consequence of the unusual properties of extraocular muscle is their differential involvement in a variety of neuromuscular and autoimmune disorders. It appears that novel constitutive or adaptive traits of the eye muscles cause them to be preferentially involved or spared by disease.[71] In essence, constitutive properties of the extraocular muscles necessary for their day-to-day function may fortuitously be responsible for their sparing in muscular dystrophy or selective targeting in ocular myasthenia gravis. Understanding the relationship between eye muscle properties and pathogenic mechanisms will not only aid knowledge of extraocular muscle biology but may yield insight into devastating disorders.

Strabismus

The extent to which alterations in extraocular muscle are a cause or a consequence of strabismus is unknown. A major difficulty in assessing muscle pathologic conditions associated with strabismus has been an inability to obtain representative samples of fibers in both orbital and global layers from routine strabismus surgery. Because the orbital layer ends before the tendon of insertion into the sclera, resections normally do not yield an adequate sample for pathologic analysis. The few reports of extraocular muscle alterations in strabismus have not yielded a consistent pattern in muscle pathology.[5,58] An exception to this is the "overacting" muscles from overacting inferior oblique of congenital fibrosis of extraocular muscle, in which prominent central aggregates of mitochondria have been observed in global intermediate singly innervated fibers of the overcontracted muscle.[30,90] There also are reports of structural alterations in the specialized extraocular muscle proprioceptors, the palisade endings, in strabismus.[20,22] These are amenable to study in resected material because palisade endings are located at the distal myotendinous junction.

Various structural and functional alterations of extraocular muscle as a consequence of muscle resection have been reported.[14,53,81] Adaptive changes at the level of the sarcomere would be anticipated both in strabismus and after surgical correction of strabismus, but have been difficult to address (see Figure 34-8). The hypothetical basis for adjustment of sarcomere number is valid: Chronic changes in the length of a muscle alter the degree of overlap of actin and myosin filaments. If there is too much or too little overlap, contraction is, at best, highly inefficient or, at worst, severely restricted. One report suggests that extraocular muscle gains or loses sarcomeres to maintain optimal length of the remaining sarcomeres.[84] A better understanding of the manner in which sarcomere length and number is regulated in extraocular muscle might prove of significant value for improvements in the treatment of strabismus.

Myasthenia Gravis

The extraocular muscles are the earliest detected and often the sole target in some patients with myasthenia gravis. This clinical finding might result from either the low tolerance of ocular alignment systems for errors that produce diplopia or a reduced safety factor at oculomotor neuromuscular junctions. Recent efforts have focused on the potential role of muscle group–specific differences in acetylcholine receptors (AChR) in the cause of ocu-lar myasthenia. Kaminski et al.[43,44] suggest that the retention of fetal AChR subunit in adult extraocular muscle may provide a target for this autoimmune disease. However, the hypothesis linking AChR isoform to ocular susceptibility to myasthenia does have two caveats: (1) Although ptosis is a common symptom, the fetal AChR is not found in the levator palpebrae superioris; and (2) there are conflicting reports regarding muscle group–specific distribution of fetal AChR subunit when studied at the messenger ribonucleic acid level. The notion that properties of extraocular muscles or oculomotor neurons may result in a lowered safety factor for neuromuscular transmission remains a compelling potential cause of ocular myasthenia gravis.

Graves Ophthalmopathy

The involvement of extraocular muscle, and sparing of other skeletal muscles, in Graves ophthalmopathy does not appear to be a muscle issue per se, but rather can largely be ascribed to a disease process that specifically targets orbital fibroblasts. The extraocular muscles enlarge as a result of an abnormal accumulation of glycosaminoglycans in the connective tissues, thereby compressing all orbital tissues. The pathogenic mechanism underlying Graves ophthalmopathy most likely involves circulating T cells, directed against an antigen on thyroid follicular cells, recognizing this same antigen on orbital fibroblasts. Interferon-γ, interleukin-1alpha, and tumor necrosis factor are present in the orbital connective tissue of patients with ophthalmopathy and act preferentially on orbital fibroblasts to stimulate their proliferation, as well as glycosaminoglycan production.[4] The preferential involvement of orbital fibroblasts in Graves ophthalmopathy may be a consequence of their unusual neural crest origin. Observations that the sarcomeric organization of the muscle fibers remains intact are consistent with the hypothesis that this disease principally targets fibroblasts. However, other reports suggest that extraocular muscle fibers proper may be targeted by cell-mediated cytotoxicity.[6]

Muscular Dystrophy

The extraocular muscles exhibit a novel response to muscular dystrophy because they are spared in otherwise devastating Duchenne muscular dystrophy and are involved in oculopharyngeal muscular dystrophy. Sparing of extraocular muscle in Duchenne muscular dystrophy is mechanistically interesting because knowledge of muscle protective strategies not only advances our understanding of the basic biology of these muscles but may yield treatment options for the patient with Duchenne muscular dystrophy. This is an active area of investigation and is discussed subsequently. The targeting of oculopharyngeal muscular dystrophy is much less well understood, but it has been linked to expansion of a GCG repeat in the poly(A) binding protein 2 gene (*PABP2*). The hallmark pathologic signs in pharyngeal and extraocular muscle (nuclear filament accumulation) presumably result from a gain in function of the *PABP2* gene.[7]

Duchenne muscular dystrophy is an X-linked recessive disease that is characterized by degeneration in most types of skeletal muscle. Mutations are particularly common in the dystrophin gene because it is among the largest known genes and therefore is more susceptible to sporadic mutations. The most widely held theory of pathogenesis is that the absence of the protein dystrophin (i.e., dystrophinopathy) leads to sarcolemmal destabilization, thereby disrupting myofiber calcium homeostasis and triggering calcium-activated protease activity. An alternative theory is that muscle degeneration is a result of elevated free radical production.

Interestingly, extraocular muscle is structurally and functionally spared in Duchenne muscular dystrophy and in animal models of dystrophinopathy and sarcoglycanopathy (limb girdle muscular dystrophy).[47,76,77] These disorders involve components of a transmembrane dystrophin-glycoprotein complex thought to play both mechanical stabilization and cell signaling roles. Extraocular muscle normally has all the known members of the dystrophin-glycoprotein complex[1] (Figure 34-22). These muscles normally exhibit high calcium flux and reactive oxygen species production as a result of the high contractile rates and respiratory activity. The mechanisms for calcium and reactive oxygen species homeostasis then are enhanced in extraocular muscle to survive normal metabolic stresses. Extraocular muscle can adapt in ways that preclude elevated calcium and/or free radicals—a viable mechanism for their sparing in the muscular dystrophies. Alternatively, there may be adaptations at the level of the dystrophin-glycoprotein complex that lead to extraocular muscle survival.[76]

Mitochondrial Myopathies

Mitochondrial myopathies represent functionally significant, developmental, or age-linked skeletal muscle disorders. Ocular signs are the most characteristic clinical feature in chronic progressive external ophthalmopathy, Kearns-Sayre syndrome, and a variety of mitochondrial encephalomyopathies.

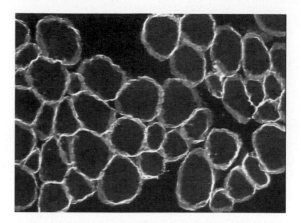

FIGURE 34-22 Fluorescence micrograph of mouse extraocular muscle stained with an antibody for dystrophin. Dystrophin is part of a multiprotein complex, the dystrophin-glycoprotein complex, that connects the muscle fiber internal skeleton to the surrounding connective tissue, thereby stabilizing the sarcolemma during muscle contraction. Dystrophin is associated with the muscle fiber sarcolemma; thus staining rings each muscle fiber. In Duchenne muscular dystrophy and its animal models, dystrophin is lost from the extraocular sarcolemma but muscle fibers are spared the pathologic conditions that are seen in other skeletal muscles.

However, analyses of extraocular muscle in the mitochondrial myopathies are relatively rare, often reporting nonspecific alterations, and are difficult to interpret because of past failures to understand how normal extraocular muscle differs from skeletal muscle.[96] Extraocular muscle dependence on oxidative energy metabolism is a result of their high metabolic rate and may be what targets this muscle group in the mitochondrially inherited diseases. During normal mitochondrial respiration, a small percentage of the oxygen used is incompletely reduced. The resulting reactive oxygen species are thought to act locally in mitochondria to alter membrane properties, disrupt protein functions, and mutate mitochondrial DNA (mtDNA). Over the course of a lifetime, the functionally compromised mitochondria accumulate within cells and, in theory, are ultimately responsible for the "ragged red" muscle fibers that characterize the mitochondrial myopathies. Compelling evidence in support of this view includes the finding that (1) the identical mtDNA base substitutions that characterize the acquired mitochondrial myopathies are observed in all extraocular muscles of elderly control human subjects[65] and (2) mitochondrial cytochrome c oxidase exhibits an aging-dependent defect density five to six times higher in eye muscle than in limb muscle, diaphragm, or even heart.[66] Taken together, there is a compelling argument that extraocular muscle targeting in mitochondrial myopathy directly relates to the high degree of oxidative stress in this unique muscle group.

CONCLUSION

Like skeletal muscle, extraocular muscle indeed is voluntary, striated muscle. However, the biology of the extraocular muscles is best understood if one is not biased by the vast literature on skeletal muscle. Instead, it must be recognized that the molecular, cellular, biochemical, structural, and functional properties of this muscle group are often at variance with the more traditional skeletal muscles. Developmental processes that, at least in part, are unique to eye muscle act to shape the properties of this novel muscle group. The diverse tasks demanded of extraocular muscle by an array of eye movement control systems, from the phylogenetically primitive vestibulo-ocular reflex to highly evolved vergence eye movements, help shape the muscle phenotype. The novel properties of the eye muscles, in turn, lead to differential responses to pharmaceuticals and disease processes that must be taken into account by both scientists and clinicians.

REFERENCES

1. Andrade FH, Porter JD, Kaminski HJ: Eye muscle sparing by the muscular dystrophies: lessons to be learned? *Microsc Res Tech* 48:192, 2000.
2. Apt L: An anatomical reevaluation of rectus muscle insertions, *Trans Am Ophthalmol Soc* 78:365, 1980.
3. Asmussen G, Gaunitz U: Mechanical properties of the isolated inferior oblique muscle of the rabbit, *Pflugers Arch* 392:183, 1981.
4. Bahn RS: The fibroblast is the target cell in the connective tissue manifestations of Graves' disease, *Int Arch Allergy Immunol* 106:213, 1995.
5. Berard-Badier M et al: Ultrastructural studies of extraocular muscles in ocular motility disorders: II. Morphological analysis of 38 biopsies, *Graefes Arch Clin Exp Ophthalmol* 208:193, 1978.
6. Blau HM et al: Thyroglobulin-independent, cell-mediated cytotoxicity of human eye muscle cells in tissue culture by lymphocytes of a patient with Graves' ophthalmopathy, *Life Sci* 32:45, 1983.
7. Brais B et al: Short GCG expansions in the PABP2 gene cause oculopharyngeal muscular dystrophy, *Nat Genet* 18:164, 1998.
8. Brooke MH, Kaiser KK: Muscle fiber types: how many and what kind? *Arch Neurol* 23:369, 1970.
9. Brueckner JK, Itkis O, Porter JD: Spatial and temporal patterns of myosin heavy chain expression in developing rat extraocular muscle, *J Muscle Res Cell Motil* 17:297, 1996.
10. Brueckner JK, Porter JD: Visual system maldevelopment disrupts extraocular muscle-specific myosin expression, *J Appl Physiol* 85:584, 1998.
11. Burke RE et al: Physiological types and histochemical profiles in motor units of the cat gastrocnemius, *J Physiol* 234:723, 1973.
12. Burke RE et al: Motor units in cat soleus muscle: physiological, histochemical and morphological characteristics, *J Physiol* 238:503, 1974.
13. Chiarandini DJ, Stefani E: Electrophysiological identification of two types of fibres in rat extraocular muscles, *J Physiol* 290:453, 1979.
14. Christiansen S et al: Fiber hypertrophy in rat extraocular muscle following lateral rectus resection, *J Pediatr Ophthalmol Strabismus* 25:167, 1988.
15. Claflin DR, Faulkner JA: Shortening velocity extrapolated to zero load and unloaded shortening velocity of whole rat skeletal muscle, *J Physiol* 359:357, 1985.
16. Clark RA, Miller JM, Demer JL: Location and stability of rectus muscle pulleys: muscle paths as a function of gaze, *Invest Ophthalmol Vis Sci* 38:227, 1997.
17. Clark RA et al: Posterior fixation sutures: a revised mechanical explanation for the fadenoperation based on rectus extraocular muscle pulleys, *Am J Ophthalmol* 128:702, 1999.
18. Close RI: Dynamic properties of mammalian skeletal muscles, *Physiol Rev* 52:129, 1972.
19. Close RI, Luff AR: Dynamic properties of inferior rectus muscle of the rat, *J Physiol (Lond)* 236:259, 1974.
20. Corsi M et al: Morphological study of extraocular muscle proprioceptor alterations in congenital strabismus, *Ophthalmologica* 200:154, 1990.
21. Demer JL, Oh SY, Poukens V: Evidence for active control of rectus extraocular muscle pulleys, *Invest Ophthalmol Vis Sci* 41:1280, 2000.
22. Domenici-Lombardo L et al: Extraocular muscles in congenital strabismus: muscle fiber and nerve ending ultrastructure according to different regions, *Ophthalmologica* 205:29, 1992.
23. Donaldson IM: The functions of the proprioceptors of the eye muscles, *Philos Trans R Soc Lond B Biol Sci* 355:1685, 2000.
24. Engel AG, Franzini-Armstrong C: *Myology,* New York, 1994, McGraw-Hill.
25. Engle E: A genetic approach to congenital extraocular muscle disorders, *J Child Neurol* 14:34, 1999.
26. Engle EC: The genetics of strabismus: Duane, Mobius and fibrosis syndromes. In Traboulsi EI (ed): *Genetic diseases of the eye: a textbook and atlas,* New York, 1998, Oxford University Press.
27. Engle EC et al: Mapping a gene for congenital fibrosis of the extraocular muscles to the centromeric region of chromosome 12, *Nat Genet* 7:69, 1994.
28. Engle EC et al: Congenital fibrosis of the extraocular muscles (autosomal dominant congenital external ophthalmoplegia): genetic homogeneity, linkage refinement, and physical mapping on chromosome 12, *Am J Hum Genet* 57:1086, 1995. (Published erratum appears in *Am J Hum Genet* 58:252, 1996.)
29. Engle EC et al: A gene for isolated congenital ptosis maps to a 3-cM region within 1p32-p34.1, *Am J Hum Genet* 60:1150, 1997.
30. Engle EC et al: Oculomotor nerve and muscle abnormalities in congenital fibrosis of the extraocular muscles, *Ann Neurol* 41:314, 1997.
31. Franzini-Armstrong C, Fischman DA: Morphogenesis of skeletal muscle fibers. In Engel AG, Franzini-Armstrong C (eds): *Myology,* New York, 1994, McGraw-Hill.

32. Frueh BR et al: Contractile properties and temperature sensitivity of the extraocular muscles, the levator and superior rectus of the rabbit, *J Physiol* 475:327, 1994.

33. Fuchs AF, Binder MD: Fatigue resistance of human extraocular muscles, *J Neurophysiol* 49:28, 1983.

34. Gauthier GF, Lowey S: Distribution of myosin isoenzymes among skeletal muscle fiber types, *J Cell Biol* 81:10, 1979.

35. Gilbert P: The origin and development of the extrinsic ocular muscles in the domestic cat, *J Morphol* 81:151, 1947.

36. Gilbert PW: The origin and development of the human extrinsic ocular muscles, *Contrib Embryol* 36:61, 1957.

37. Goldberg SJ, Shall MS: Motor units of extraocular muscles: recent findings, *Prog Brain Res* 123:221, 1999.

38. Helveston EM et al: Surgical treatment of congenital esotropia, *Am J Ophthalmol* 96:218, 1983.

39. Hubel DH, Wiesel TN: Binocular interaction in striate cortex of kittens reared with artificial squint, *J Neurophysiol* 28:1041, 1965.

40. Hubel DH, Wiesel TN: The period of susceptibility to the physiological effects of unilateral eye closure in kittens, *J Physiol* 206:419, 1970.

41. Jacoby J, Chiarandini DJ, Stefani E: Electrical properties and innervation of fibers in the orbital layer of rat extraocular muscles, *J Neurophysiol* 61:116, 1989.

42. Jacoby J et al: Diltiazem reduces the contractility of extraocular muscles in vitro and in vivo, *Invest Ophthalmol Vis Sci* 31:569, 1990.

43. Kaminski HJ, Kusner LL, Block CH: Expression of acetylcholine receptor isoforms at extraocular muscle endplates, *Invest Ophthalmol Vis Sci* 37:345, 1996. (Published erratum appears in *Invest Ophthalmol Vis Sci* 37:6A, 1996).

44. Kaminski HJ, Ruff RL: Ocular muscle involvement by myasthenia gravis, *Ann Neurol* 41:419, 1997.

45. Keller EL, Robinson DA: Absence of a stretch reflex in extraocular muscles of the monkey, *J Neurophysiol* 34:908, 1971.

46. Khanna S, Porter JD: Evidence for rectus extraocular muscle pulleys in rodents, *Invest Ophthalmol Vis Sci* 42:1986, 2001.

47. Khurana TS et al: Absence of extraocular muscle pathology in Duchenne's muscular dystrophy: role for calcium homeostasis in extraocular muscle sparing, *J Exp Med* 182:467, 1995.

48. Kitamura K et al: Mouse Pitx2 deficiency leads to anomalies of the ventral body wall, heart, extra- and periocular mesoderm and right pulmonary isomerism, *Development* 126:5749, 1999.

49. Koornneef L: The architecture of the musculo-fibrous apparatus in the human orbit, *Acta Morphol Neerl Scand* 15:35, 1977.

50. Koornneef L: Details of the orbital connective tissue system in the adult, *Acta Morphol Neerl Scand* 15:1, 1977.

51. Koornneef L: New insights in the human orbital connective tissue: result of a new anatomical approach, *Arch Ophthalmol* 95:1269, 1977.

52. Kushner BJ, Lucchese NJ, Morton GV: Should recessions of the medial recti be graded from the limbus or the insertion? *Arch Ophthalmol* 107:1755, 1989.

53. Kushner BJ, Vrabec M: Theoretical effects of surgery on length tension relationships in extraocular muscles, *J Pediatr Ophthalmol Strabismus* 24:126, 1987.

54. Kushner BJ et al: Factors influencing response to strabismus surgery, *Arch Ophthalmol* 111:75, 1993.

55. Lennerstrand G, Hanson J: Contractile properties of extraocular muscle in cats reared with monocular lid closure and artificial squint, *Acta Ophthalmol* 57:591, 1979.

56. Luff AR: Dynamic properties of the inferior rectus, extensor digitorum longus, diaphragm and soleus muscles of the mouse, *J Physiol* 313:161, 1981.

57. Lumsden A, Keynes R: Segmental patterns of neuronal development in the chick hindbrain, *Nature* 337:424, 1989.

58. Martinez AJ, Biglan AW, Hiles DA: Structural features of extraocular muscles of children with strabismus, *Arch Ophthalmol* 98:533, 1980.

59. McNeer KW, Tucker MG, Spencer RF: Botulinum toxin management of essential infantile esotropia in children, *Arch Ophthalmol* 115:1411, 1997.

60. McNeer KW, Tucker MG, Spencer RF: Botulinum toxin therapy for essential infantile esotropia in children, *Arch Ophthalmol* 116:701, 1998.

61. McNeer KW, Tucker MG, Spencer RF: Management of essential infantile esotropia with botulinum toxin A: review and recommendations, *J Pediatr Ophthalmol Strabismus* 37:63, 2000.

62. Miller JM, Demer JL, Rosenbaum AL: Effect of transposition surgery on rectus muscle paths by magnetic resonance imaging, *Ophthalmology* 100:475, 1993.

63. Miller NR et al: Unilateral Duane's retraction syndrome (type 1), *Arch Ophthalmol* 100:1468, 1982.

64. Mindel JS et al: Succinyldicholine and the basic ocular deviation, *Am J Ophthalmol* 95:315, 1983.

65. Muller-Hocker J et al: Different in situ hybridization patterns of mitochondrial DNA in cytochrome C oxidase-deficient extraocular muscle fibres in the elderly, *Virchows Arch* 422:7, 1993.

66. Muller-Hocker J et al: Defects of the respiratory chain in various tissues of old monkeys: a cytochemical-immunocytochemical study, *Mech Ageing Dev* 86:197, 1996.

67. Niemann CU, Krag TO, Khurana TS: Identification of genes that are differentially expressed in extraocular and limb muscle, *J Neurol Sci* 179:76, 2000.

68. Peter JB et al: Metabolic profiles of three fiber types of skeletal muscle in guinea pigs and rabbits, *Biochemistry* 11:2627, 1972.

69. Porter JD, Baker RS: Prenatal morphogenesis of primate extraocular muscle: neuromuscular junction formation and fiber type differentiation, *Invest Ophthalmol Vis Sci* 33:657, 1992.

70. Porter JD, Baker RF: Developmental adaptations in the extraocular muscles of *Macaca nemestrina* may reflect a predisposition to strabismus, *Strabismus* 1:173, 1993.

71. Porter JD, Baker RS: Muscles of a different 'color': the unusual properties of the extraocular muscles may predispose or protect them in neurogenic and myogenic disease, *Neurology* 46:30, 1996.

72. Porter JD, Baker RS: Absence of oculomotor and trochlear motoneurons leads to altered extraocular muscle development in the Wnt-1 null mutant mouse, *Brain Res Dev Brain Res* 100:121, 1997.

73. Porter JD et al: Extraocular myotoxicity of the retrobulbar anesthetic bupivacaine hydrochloride, *Invest Ophthalmol Vis Sci* 29:163, 1988.

74. Porter JD et al: Extraocular muscles: basic and clinical aspects of structure and function, *Surv Ophthalmol* 39:451, 1995.

75. Porter JD et al: Structure-function correlations in the human medial rectus extraocular muscle pulleys, *Invest Ophthalmol Vis Sci* 37:468, 1996.

76. Porter JD et al: The sparing of extraocular muscle in dystrophinopathy is lost in mice lacking utrophin and dystrophin, *J Cell Sci* 111:1801, 1998.

77. Porter JD et al: Extraocular muscle is spared despite the absence of an intact sarcoglycan complex in gamma- or delta-sarcoglycan-deficient mice, *Neuromuscul Disord* 11:197, 2001.

78. Porter JD et al: Extraocular muscle is defined by a fundamentally distinct gene expression profile, *Proc Nat Acad Sci* 98:12062, 2001.

79. Richmond FJ et al: Palisade endings in human extraocular muscles, *Invest Ophthalmol Vis Sci* 25:471, 1984.

80. Robinson DA: The functional behavior of the peripheral ocular motor apparatus: a review. In Kommerell G (ed): *Disorders of ocular motility,* Munich, 1978, Bergman.

81. Rosenbaum AL et al: Length-tension properties of extraocular muscles in patients with esotropia and intermittent exotropia, *Am J Ophthalmol* 117:791, 1994.

82. Rothblat LA, Schwartz ML, Kasdan PM: Monocular deprivation in the rat: evidence for an age-related defect in visual behavior, *Brain Res* 158:456, 1978.

83. Scott AB: Botulinum toxin injection into extraocular muscles as an alternative to strabismus surgery, *Ophthalmology* 87:1044, 1980.

84. Scott AB: Change of eye muscle sarcomeres according to eye position, *J Pediatr Ophthalmol Strabismus* 31:85, 1994.

85. Scott AB, Collins CC: Division of labor in human extraocular muscle, *Arch Ophthalmol* 90:319, 1973.

86. Sevel D: A reappraisal of the origin of human extraocular muscles, *Ophthalmology* 88:1330, 1981.

87. Sevel D: The origins and insertions of the extraocular muscles: development, histologic features, and clinical significance, *Trans Am Ophthalmol Soc* 84:488, 1986.

88. Sohal GS, Ali AA, Ali MM: Ventral neural tube cells differentiate into craniofacial skeletal muscles, *Biochem Biophys Res Commun* 252:675, 1998.

89. Sparks DL et al: Long- and short-term monocular deprivation in the rhesus monkey: effects on visual fields and optokinetic nystagmus, *J Neurosci* 6:1771, 1986.

90. Spencer RF, McNeer KW: Structural alterations in overacting inferior oblique muscles, *Arch Ophthalmol* 98:128, 1980.

91. Spencer RF, McNeer KW: Botulinum toxin paralysis of adult monkey extraocular muscle: structural alterations in orbital, singly innervated muscle fibers, *Arch Ophthalmol* 105:1703, 1987.

92. Spencer RF, Porter JD: Innervation and structure of extraocular muscles in the monkey in comparison to those of the cat, *J Comp Neurol* 198:649, 1981.

93. Spencer RF, Porter JD: Structural organization of the extraocular muscles, *Rev Oculomot Res* 2:33, 1988.

94. Spencer RF et al: Botulinum toxin management of childhood intermittent exotropia, *Ophthalmology* 104:1762, 1997.

95. Steinbach MJ, Smith DR: Spatial localization after strabismus surgery: evidence for inflow, *Science* 213:1407, 1981.

96. Suomalainen A et al: Autosomal dominant progressive external ophthalmoplegia with multiple deletions of mtDNA: clinical, biochemical, and molecular genetic features of the 10q-linked disease, *Neurology* 48:1244, 1997.

97. Wachtler F et al: The extrinsic ocular muscles in birds are derived from the prechordal plate, *Naturwissenschaften* 71:379, 1984.

98. Wahl CM, Noden DM, Baker R: Developmental relations between sixth nerve motor neurons and their targets in the chick embryo, *Dev Dyn* 201:191, 1994.

99. Wasicky R et al: Muscle fiber types of human extraocular muscles: a histochemical and immunohistochemical study, *Invest Ophthalmol Vis Sci* 41:980, 2000.

100. Weiss A, Leinwand LA: The mammalian myosin heavy chain gene family, *Annu Rev Cell Dev Biol* 12:417, 1996.

101. Wieczorek DF et al: Co-expression of multiple myosin heavy chain genes, in addition to a tissue-specific one, in extraocular musculature, *J Cell Biol* 101:618, 1985.

102. Winters LM, Briggs MM, Schachat F: The human extraocular muscle myosin heavy chain gene (MYH13) maps to the cluster of fast and developmental myosin genes on chromosome 17, *Genomics* 54:188, 1998.

103. Woodlief NF: Initial observations on the ocular microcirculation in man: I. The anterior segment and extraocular muscles, *Arch Ophthalmol* 98:1268, 1980.

104. Wooten GF, Reis DJ: Blood flow in extraocular muscle of cat, *Arch Neurol* 26:350, 1972.

CHAPTER 35

THREE-DIMENSIONAL ROTATIONS OF THE EYE

CHRISTIAN QUAIA AND LANCE M. OPTICAN

MOVEMENTS OF THE EYE

Each eye is controlled by six extraocular muscles and has six degrees of freedom: three for rotation and three for translation. However, the amount of translation possible is limited, approximately 2 mm along the anteroposterior axis and 0.5 mm in the frontal plane.[1] Thus the globe can be well approximated as a spherical joint with its center fixed in the head. With this approximation, we need to consider only rotations around three orthogonal axes passing through the center of the eye. These three axes define a system of coordinates for describing ocular rotations. Unfortunately, the mathematical description of rotations of solid objects is much more complicated than that for translations. The final position reached after translations along the three space axes is independent of their order (e.g., x-axis followed by y-axis movement yields the same position as y followed by x. In contrast, the final orientation reached after a sequence of rotations around different axes depends on their order. For example, in the two panels of Figure 35-1, a camera, starting from the same initial orientation (left column), is rotated around the same pair of axes (arrows in the figure), but in different order. Clearly, the final orientations (right column) are different for the two sequences of rotations. This would not be the case for translations. Thus rotations are said to be *noncommutative*. The dependence of the final orientation on the sequence of rotations makes the study of eye movements less intuitive than one might hope. However, careful attention to the definitions of eye orientation and rotation, and to the choice of mathematical tools used to quantify them, can greatly facilitate our thinking about eye rotations.

This latter element is particularly important. In fact, translations and the resulting positions can be described by simply specifying the three Cartesian coordinates of the center of the eye. This more familiar, Euclidean space of translations is flat, and moving in only one direction never results in getting back to the initial position. In contrast, rotations and the resulting orientations cannot be described by any simple (i.e., intuitive) set of three coordinates. One of the fundamental reasons for this complexity is that the space of all rotations is curved. This can be easily noted by considering that if one keeps rotating an object around the same axis, eventually (after 360 degrees) it will get back to its initial orientation. To address the inherent complexity of rotations, several mathematical tools have been developed over the last 150 years. These tools include quaternions, sequences of rotations, rotation matrices, and rotation vectors. Although all of these methods are equivalent (they all describe the same rotations), each method has both advantages and disadvantages in different applications.[21]

QUANTIFYING EYE ROTATIONS

The first issue that must be addressed when describing rotations or orientations of the eye is whether to consider the three orthogonal axes of rotation as fixed in space, fixed in the head, or moving with the eye. Of course, keeping the axes fixed in space would be of little help because the eye muscles move the eye relative to the head. The

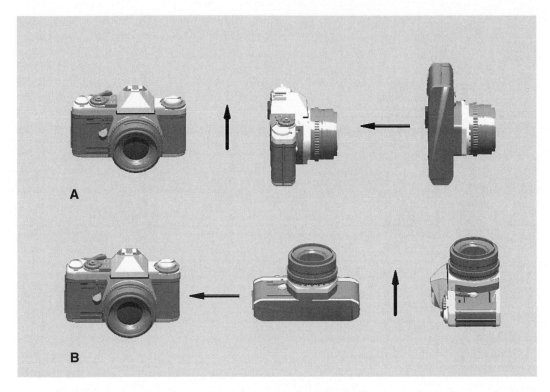

FIGURE 35-1 Noncommutativity of rotations. The image on the *right of each arrow* is obtained by rotating the image on its left around an axis collinear with the arrow. **A,** The camera first rotates 90 degrees around a vertical axis and then 90 degrees around a horizontal axis. **B,** The order of rotations is reversed. The final orientation of the camera is clearly different in the two cases. (From Quaia C, Optican LM: *J Neurophysiol* 79:3197, 1998.)

other two solutions have both advantages and disadvantages; the decision of which one to use depends on the specific oculomotor task under study.

Eye-Fixed Coordinates

Eye-fixed reference frames are based on consideration of a mechanical mounting system for rotations, such as for a camera. The simplest way to make a camera mount is to have one axis for panning the camera left or right (yaw or vertical axis), one for tilting it up or down (pitch or horizontal axis), and one for twisting it clockwise or counterclockwise about the lens' axis (roll or torsion axis). These axes are nested, one within the other, in a system or gimbals. (*Note:* The way the gimbals are nested specifies the mathematical order of the rotations; thus the order in which the gimbals are moved is irrelevant.) Eye-fixed systems are defined by the order of their rotations.[10] There are three rotation axes, so six sequences of rotations are possible. These eye-fixed coordinate systems are not useful for the general treatment of rotations because they favor one axis over the others (the first, which

is independent of the other two). Nonetheless, two eye-fixed systems were commonly used in the past and are therefore briefly mentioned here. The Fick system starts with a horizontal rotation around the vertical axis, followed by a vertical rotation around the new horizontal axis, and finally a torsional rotation about the new line of sight. The Helmholtz system starts with a vertical rotation around the horizontal axis, followed by a horizontal rotation around the new vertical axis, and finally a torsional rotation about the new line of sight. The left column of Figure 35-2 shows a Fick gimbal, and the right column shows a Helmholtz gimbal (torsional axes not shown). The movements in the eye-fixed axis cases have been decomposed into two rotations. The first position (top row) shows the eye looking straight ahead, in *primary* position. When the eye rotates from primary position around the head-fixed horizontal or vertical axis, it is said to move into a *secondary* position. This is shown in the middle row for Fick and Helmholtz gimbals. Note that the first Fick rotation turns the eye to the left, whereas the first Helmholtz rotation turns the

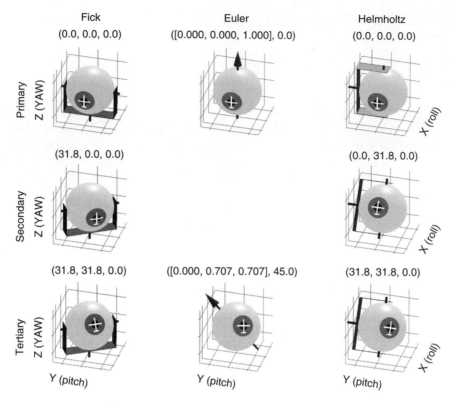

Figure 35-2   Demonstration of head-fixed and eye-fixed coordinate systems. *Left column* shows positions reached by rotations around one of the six systems of eye-fixed axes (Fick). Because these axes move with the eye (torsion axis not shown), they can be represented by a gimbal system. In the Fick system the order of rotations is horizontal, vertical, torsional. *Middle column* shows a rotation around a head-fixed axis (Euler). With Euler axis, there is only one rotation, about an axis that is tilted appropriately. *Right column* shows another eye-fixed system of axes (Helmholtz). In the Helmholtz system the order of rotations is vertical, horizontal, torsional. Gaze angles are referred to as *primary (top row,* looking straight ahead), *secondary (middle row,* on the horizontal or vertical meridian), or *tertiary (bottom row,* off both the horizontal and vertical meridians). As can be seen from the middle row, a rotation around one eye-fixed axis moves the eye into a secondary position. *Note:* All of these tertiary orientations correspond to a 45-degree rotation up and to the left. In Fick coordinates that corresponds to (31.8, 31.8, 0), in Helmholtz coordinates to (31.8, 31.8, 0), and in head-fixed coordinates to ($[0, 1, 1]/\sqrt{2}$, 45).

eye upward. The bottom row shows the eye rotated away from the horizontal or vertical meridian, into what is called a *tertiary* position.

Head-Fixed Coordinates

When using head-fixed axes, the description of rotations that we prefer (because it seems to be the most intuitive) is the so-called axis-angle form (see Figure 35-2, middle column), which follows from Euler's theorem. This theorem states that *any orientation of a rigid body with one point fixed can be achieved, starting from a reference orientation, by a single rotation around an axis (through the fixed point) along a unit-length vector, n̂, by an angle, φ.*[9] Euler's theorem highlights an aspect common to all of the methods that can be used to represent rotary

motion: the need to define a *reference orientation.* Although its choice is totally arbitrary, the one most commonly adopted in eye movement research is the orientation with the head upright and the eye looking straight ahead. The three main axes of rotation then point straight ahead (x-axis, roll or torsion rotations), straight to the left (y-axis, pitch or vertical rotations), and straight up (z-axis, yaw or horizontal rotations). The x-, y-, and z-axes define a right-handed system of head-fixed coordinates *(x, y, z)* that describe, for each eye orientation, Euler's axis of rotation, n̂. (*Note:* In a right-handed coordinate system, the direction that the eye turns for a positive angle is the direction that the fingers of the right hand curl when the thumb points along the axis n̂.) With this convention, for example, if

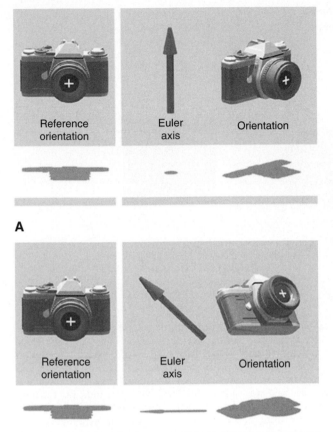

FIGURE 35-3 Representation of eye orientation using the axis-angle form. For each panel the reference orientation is shown on the left. **A,** The camera is rotated 45 degrees to the left, and the corresponding Euler axis points straight up, (0, 0, 1), in the *xyz* coordinate system (see text). **B,** The camera is rotated 45 degrees up and to the left around the axis, $(0, 1, 1)/\sqrt{2}$. Note that the central cross on the camera's lens appears twisted with respect to the vertical axis, even though Euler axis has no torsional component. (Reprinted from Quaia C, Optican LM: *J Neurophysiol* 79:3197, 1998.)

the eye is rotated 45 degrees to the left, its orientation is described by ([0, 0, 1], 45), as that orientation is achieved by rotating the eye, starting from the reference orientation, by 45 degrees around the vertical axis (0, 0, 1) (see Figure 35-2, middle column, top row and Figure 35-3, *A*; note that we are looking at the camera from the front, so the *x*-, *y*-, and *z*-axes point out of the page, to the right, and up, respectively). Similarly, if the eye is rotated 45 degrees up and to the left, its orientation is ([0, 1, 1] $\sqrt{2}$, 45) (see Figure 35-2 middle column, bottom row and Figure 35-3, *B*). (*Note:* When eye orientations are discussed in the context of Listing's law, a slightly different reference orientation is chosen for convenience. See subsequent discussion.)

False Torsion

The examples of rotations about different axes shown in Figure 35-2 demonstrate an interesting effect of the noncommutativity of rotations. Note that all three rotations were designed to point the eye 45 degrees up and 45 degrees to the left. In the

Euler axis case (middle column), this entails a single rotation of amplitude 45 degrees around an axis tipped 45 degrees from the vertical, $(0, 1, 1)/\sqrt{2}$. In the eye-fixed axes cases, this entails two rotations of magnitude 45 degrees/$\sqrt{2}$ (approximately 31.8 degrees) around the first two gimbal axes. If rotations were commutative, like translations, the final eye orientation in each case would be the same. However, it is clear from the bottom row that the final orientations are not the same (i.e., rotations are not commutative).

Figure 35-4 shows the three tertiary orientations from Figure 35-2 plotted together. The graph has been rotated so that you are looking directly down the line of sight of the Fick coordinate system (white cross). Note that the Fick cross is upright (i.e., rotations in the Fick coordinate system preserve the gravitational vertical on the retina, as is obvious from the gimbals in Figure 35-2). The eyeball itself is drawn rotated around an Euler axis (light gray cross). In this case we see that both the eccentricity of the eye and its torsion are slightly different from the

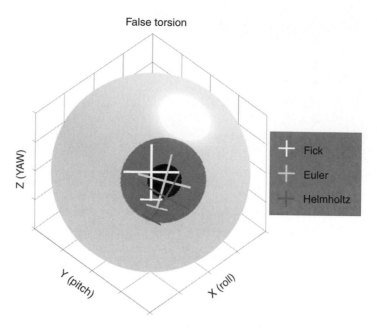

FIGURE 35-4 Noncommutativity of rotations and false torsion resulting from equivalent rotations around eye-fixed and head-fixed axes. Eye orientation is indicated by the *crosses* (Fick, *white;* Euler, *light gray;* Helmholtz, *dark gray*). In this figure the eye has been rotated 45 degrees around an axis tilted 45 degrees ([0, 1, 1]/√2, 45) *middle column, bottom row of Figure 35-3*). The view of the graph has been rotated around to Fick coordinates (31.8, 31.8, 0). Thus the Fick axis appears centered and upright, which follows because Fick rotations preserve the gravitational vertical on the retina. The Euler and Helmholtz crosses are progressively displaced and twisted from the Fick cross. This indicates the noncommutativity of rotations. Under normal circumstances, the eye assumes the orientation given by the Euler rotation (Listing's law). The Fick cross is rotated clockwise from there (from the eye's point of view), and the Helmholtz cross is rotated counterclockwise. In all cases this orientation was achieved without any rotations about the torsional axes. Thus the twists of the local reference frame are referred to as *false torsions.*

Fick case. A voluntary eye movement to this location would have this orientation (Listing's laws, see following discussion). Finally, the dark gray cross shows the final orientation reached by rotations around the Helmholtz axes. Its cross is even further eccentric and twisted than the Euler cross. (*Note:* The distance between the crosses is a function of the size of the eye rotation; as the eye rotation shrinks in size, so does the difference between the eccentricity and twist of the crosses.) These twists are called *false torsions* because they do not arise from rotations about a torsional axis. Obviously, the difference in eccentricity of these three crosses can be eliminated by adjusting the size of the horizontal and vertical rotations for the Fick and Helmholtz systems. However, the difference in the twists persists unless a nonzero torsional rotation is introduced.

The difference between true torsion and false torsion is one of the most confusing aspects of the study of eye rotations. It arises because we think about the eye in two different ways. As a globe, we need a way to describe all of its rotations in a con-

sistent system linked to the head. As an eye, we think of how the gravitational vertical in the visual world will be projected on the retina. When the eye rotates about an Euler axis (fixed in the head) with zero torsional component, the local vertical (which is fixed to the eye) is carried around to a new orientation. Although the twist of the local vertical is real (i.e., it does not line up with the gravitational vertical in the new orientation), it did not arise from a twist around the Euler torsional axis (x-axis). It arose because the eye-fixed axes were carried around by a rotation in a curved space, and hence the eye-fixed axes themselves changed. It was not a true torsion (i.e., a rotation around the head-fixed, torsional axis). The existence of false torsion shows that pointing the eye involves both directing the line of gaze and choosing a final torsion (three degrees of freedom). However, the brain chooses the final orientation as a function of the horizontal and vertical rotations in a simple but nonintuitive way, thus reducing the number of degrees of freedom of the eye from three to two.

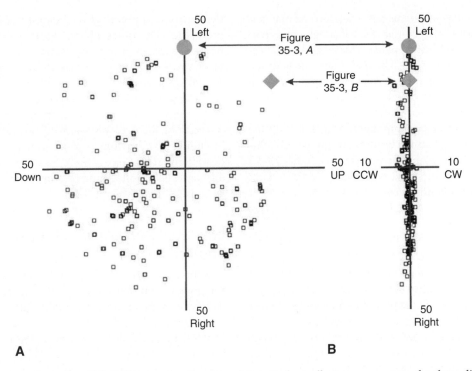

A   **B**

FIGURE 35-5 Example of Listing's plane in a human subject. Each small square represents the three-dimensional components of the tip of the Euler axis from one eye orientation. **A,** Front view, vertical and horizontal components. **B,** Side view, vertical and torsional components. The large gray circles represent the orientation shown in Figure 35-3, *A,* whereas the *large gray diamonds* represent the orientation shown in Figure 35-3, *B.* Note that the horizontal component is reversed because in Figure 35-3 we were looking at the vectors from the front, whereas here they are plotted from the camera's point of view. (Adapted from Crawford JD: Listing's law: what's all the hubbub? In Harris LR, Jenkin M [eds]: *Vision and action,* Cambridge, 1998, Cambridge University.)

LISTING'S LAW

Each eye has three rotational degrees of freedom, but the direction of gaze has only two degrees of freedom because the eye can rotate about the line of sight without changing the direction of gaze. This situation is called *kinematic redundancy* and implies that each direction of gaze corresponds to an infinite number of different eye orientations.[3] Despite this potential redundancy, observation of actual eye orientations reveals that the brain constrains the torsion to be a function of the horizontal and vertical orientation. This reduces the number of degrees of freedom to two. Each gaze direction (achieved with saccadic or smooth pursuit movements) corresponds to a unique eye orientation, regardless of previous movements and orientations. This observation, known as *Donder's law,* holds when the head is kept fixed; it was further extended by Listing to actually specify the space of possible orientations.[11] This is *Listing's law,* which states that if the vectors describing the eye orientations attained by a subject having his or her head fixed in space are plotted, they lie in or near a plane (the so-called Listing's plane).[11] Figure 35-5 shows an example of orientation measurements made from a human subject, where each point indicates the orientation of the eye during a period of fixation.[2] Figure 35-5, *A,* shows the vertical and horizontal components of the Euler axis (from the subject's point of view), whereas Figure 35-5, *B,* shows their vertical and torsional components. As an example, on top of the human data we have added two symbols indicating where the Euler axis for the camera orientations shown in Figure 35-3, *A* (large circles) and *B* (large diamonds), would be in this graph (note that the horizontal component is reversed because in Figure 35-3 we were looking at the vectors from the front and not from the camera's point of view). It is clear that the points in Figure 35-5 form a thin, pancakelike cloud (i.e., they lie near Listing's plane).

With the head upright, Listing's plane is normally tilted backward (approximately 20 degrees); that is, it is not aligned with the vertical plane.[24]

However, the data are usually transformed to a new coordinate system so that the torsional axis is perpendicular to Listing's plane. This was done, for example, in Figure 35-5. The major advantage of using this information is that Listing's law then simply states that only eye orientations with zero torsion are allowed. (*Note:* This refers to an axis with no torsional component, which is not the same as saying that the brain sends no torsional innervation to the oblique muscles; see Table 35-1.) This lack of a torsional component of the axis of rotation should not be confused with the alignment of the retina with the local gravitational vertical, as noted previously.

It must be stressed that Listing's law is enforced only when the head is fixed; it breaks down when the head is moving. When the head turns, the vestibuloocular reflex (VOR) counterrotates the eye, so the visual world is kept (approximately) stable on the retina. When this involves head motions with the eyes in an elevated or depressed position, accumulated VOR slow phases can carry the eye out of Listing's plane by as much as 30 degrees; the saccade generator compensates for this by adding a predic-

TABLE 35-1
Muscle Actions with the Eye in Primary Position

Muscle	Primary	Secondary	Tertiary
Lateral rectus	Abduction	None	None
Medial rectus	Adduction	None	None
Superior rectus	Elevation	Intorsion	Adduction
Inferior oblique	Extorsion	Elevation	Abduction
Inferior rectus	Depression	Extorsion	Adduction
Superior oblique	Intorsion	Depression	Abduction

The axis of action is perpendicular to the plane formed by the center of the eye and the (functional) origin and insertion of the muscle. Each axis has some orientation, which can be described with head-fixed coordinates. The head-fixed axis where most of the force is generated by the muscle gives rise to its primary action. The axis with the next most force gives rise to the secondary action, and the axis with the least force projection gives rise to the tertiary action. Note that muscles work in pairs. From primary position, the lateral and medial recti muscles move the eye horizontally, the superior rectus muscle and the inferior oblique muscle elevate the eye, the inferior rectus muscle and the superior oblique muscle depress the eye, and the superior oblique muscle and the inferior oblique muscle twist the eye. This classification is difficult to maintain once the eye moves away from primary position because the functional origin of the muscles is changed by the pulleys.

tive torsional component to the innervation of the preceding VOR quick phase.[4] Furthermore, when binocular orientations are considered, Listing's plane varies as a function of the depth of the target, so Listing's plane for each eye rotates outward as the eyes rotate inward during vergence.[15] This implies that Listing's law cannot arise from a mechanical property of the oculomotor plant but rather must be enforced by providing it with the appropriate innervation signals (here *plant* refers to the system being controlled by the brain; i.e., the globe, extraocular muscles, and orbital tissues).

Neural Control of Ocular Orientation

The most important issue in the study of the eye rotations is to understand how the brain generates three-dimensional neural signals that can accurately control the orientation of the eyes, suppress ocular drift, and (when necessary) enforce Listing's law. To address this question, we have to start by identifying the innervation signals that need to be supplied to the extraocular muscles to produce realistic eye movements.

With use of the biomechanical model of the eye plant developed by Robinson, it is possible to show that, because of the viscoelastic properties of the orbital tissues, the torque applied to the eyeball to generate an eye movement can always be interpreted as the sum of three components: a *step* (i.e., a signal proportional to the current eye eccentricity), a *slide* (i.e., a low-pass filtered version of the velocity profile), and a *pulse* (i.e., a signal proportional to the velocity of the eyes).[14, 18] The step compensates for the elastic forces that tend to drag the eyeball toward its resting position, whereas the slide and the pulse compensate for the viscosity of the muscles and orbital tissues (Figure 35-6, *A*). If the pulse, slide, and step are not matched to the dynamics of the oculomotor plant, a postsaccadic ocular drift ensues (Figure 35-6, *B*).

The brain controls the generation of this torque through innervation signals (Figure 35-7, *B*), but the torques are delivered to the eyeball by the extraocular muscles. Unfortunately, the muscles are not good actuators, especially at high speeds of shortening or lengthening; consequently, the innervation signal must take the characteristics of the muscles, as well as of the globe and orbital tissues, into account. More precisely, an analysis of Robinson's model of the plant reveals that, in the process of transferring the force to the tendons, each muscle absorbs both a *step* and a *pulse* of force. The former is proportional to the length of the muscle, whereas the latter is proportional to its speed of shortening (or lengthening). The muscles behave so poorly that approximately 90% of the energy produced during a saccadic eye movement (Figure 35-7, *A*) is dissipated by the muscles, and only the remaining 10% is actually used to rotate the eyeball (Figure 35-7, *C* and *D*, pulse). Even during periods of fixation, only 23% of the innervation force is transferred to the tendons, and the remaining 77% is used to maintain the length of the muscles (see Figure 35-7, *C* and *D*, step). In other words, to deliver the appropriate torque to the eyeball (see Figure 35-7, *D*; note tenfold gain increase for this graph), an extra, and much larger, innervation force (see Figure 35-7, *B*) must be supplied to account for the loss in the extraocular muscles (see Figure 35-7, *C*).

The decomposition of the innervation signal into the force absorbed by the muscles and the force delivered to the tendons, as well as the decomposition of these forces into their basic components, follows from the properties of the eye plant and thus holds for any movement, regardless of its dynamics or of the innervation pattern. It cannot be stressed enough that the only signal that must exist in the brain is the overall innervation command, which is carried by the motoneurons. In contrast, the various signals described previously (pulse, slide, and step for the orbital tissues, and pulse and step for the muscles) are the result of an objective, but artificial, decomposition that we have applied to the overall command; these components do not need to exist as separate signals in the brain. However, because each of these signals compensates for different forces, their adaptation requirements are different. Accordingly, the only reason-

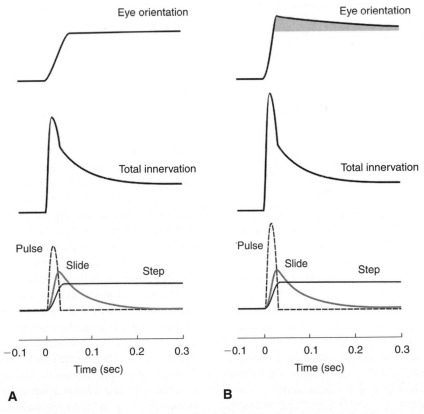

FIGURE 35-6 Components of the innervation signal. The innervation signal is the sum of three components: a pulse, a slide, and a step. **A,** When the three signals are appropriately matched, the eyes move quickly to the target and stop abruptly. In this case the eye orientation follows the step of innervation. **B,** If the components are mismatched (in this case the pulse is too large), the eyes drift uncontrollably toward the target. The step is no longer a faithful representation of eye orientation.

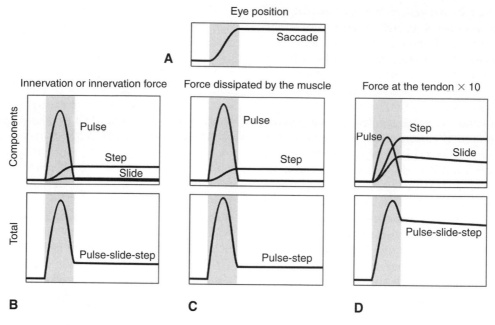

FIGURE 35-7   Distribution of forces between extraocular muscles and orbital tissues. **A,** Schematic saccadic eye movement. **B,** The saccadic innervation consists of a pulse, slide, and step, which generate corresponding forces in the muscles. **C,** Most of the pulse and the step are used to change muscle length. Thus the muscle itself "eats up" most of the force. **D,** The remaining force delivered to the tendon consists of a small piece of the pulse, the slide, and part of the step. (*Note:* The forces in **D** are magnified approximately 10 times.) The ratio of the pulse dissipated by the muscle and the pulse delivered to the tendon is about 20. The ratio of the step dissipated to that delivered is approximately 3.3. (*Second row* shows components of innervation and force; *third row* shows total innervation and force; the *gray area* indicates saccade duration.)

able way to guarantee that they are always appropriate is to compute them separately and then to sum them together, with adaptable weights, at the level of the motoneurons.

However, this does not imply that these signals have to be computed independently from each other. In fact, because they are associated with physical signals that are related to each other (e.g., eye velocity and orientation are related because the latter is a function of the history of the former), these neural signals must also be related to each other (i.e., they must be *matched*). This matching is important because the purpose of eye movements is to serve vision and any mismatch in these signals causes the eyes to drift uncontrollably (see Figure 35-6, *B*), degrading vision.[25] The simplest way to guarantee accurate control is to generate one of the three signals and then compute the other two from that signal.

Robinson[19] recognized this matching problem almost 30 years ago and proposed a solution for the one-dimensional case (i.e., for rotations around a single axis). In this simplified case there is a direct

proportionality between muscle length and eye orientation and between eye velocity and rate of change of muscle length. This implies that the step component relative to the eye muscles is always directly proportional to the step component relative to the orbital tissues, and they can be lumped together into a single step. The same holds true for the pulse components, so the overall innervation force can then be seen simply as the sum of a pulse, a slide, and a step. Robinson[19] proposed that in this case, the step of innervation can be computed by simply integrating (in the mathematical sense) the pulse. Similarly, the slide can be computed by low-pass filtering of the pulse. This works well because, for rotations around one axis, the orientation (associated with the step component when matching is perfect) is equal to the integral of angular velocity (also associated with the pulse component under matching conditions).

Unfortunately, when rotations around arbitrary axes in three dimensions must be considered, things get far more complicated. First, in the general case there is no direct proportionality between muscle length and eye orientation; accordingly, the step signals relative to the orbital tissues (step$_{OT}$) and to the muscles (step$_M$) cannot be lumped together. On the other hand, the two pulse signals are both still proportional to the rate of change of muscle length and may still be lumped together. Thus the overall innervation command can now be seen as a three-dimensional composite of four signals: pulse-slide-step$_{OT}$-step$_M$. Second, and more important, *in three dimensions the derivative of eye orientation is not equal to eye angular velocity.*[9] This inequality, which is true for any rigid body rotating around a point fixed in space, is a result of the noncommutativity of rotations (see Figure 35-1).

The noncommutativity of rotations has several consequences, but one of the most important (and least intuitive) for oculomotor control is that, to keep the vectors describing the instantaneous orientation of the eye in a plane (e.g., Listing's plane) as it moves, the angular velocity vector about which the eye is spinning must tilt *out* of that plane.[22] This applies to all rotations where the gaze does not go through a great circle on the eye centered on primary position (e.g., no tilt of the angular velocity axis for a rotation from up and left 45 degrees to down and right 45 degrees, which goes through primary position, but a tilt is needed for a rotation from up and left 45 degrees to down and left 45 degrees). This tilt of the angular velocity axis is given by the so-called half-angle rule; that is, if the eyes are elevated 45 degrees up and one wants to rotate the eyes from, say, left 10 degrees to right 10 degrees, the axis of angular velocity must be tipped back from the vertical by 22.5 degrees for the orientation axis to stay in Listing's plane[23] (Figure 35-8, *B*, dashed line). In other words, to ensure that the orientation vector (and its derivative) has no torsional component during the movement, the angular velocity vector must have a torsional component whose amplitude is a function of the orientation of the eyes.

How does all of this influence the task of generating the innervation command appropriate to rotate the eyes in three dimensions? If the pulse of innervation has to encode the angular velocity of the eyes, the implications are straightforward: First, the brain has to generate a pulse encoding the appropriate angular velocity signal, tipped out of Listing's plane if orientation has to be confined to that plane. Second, and more important, the step component relative to the orbital tissues (step$_{OT}$) must be computed by passing the pulse through some rotational operator; simply integrating it does not produce the desired signal because angular velocity

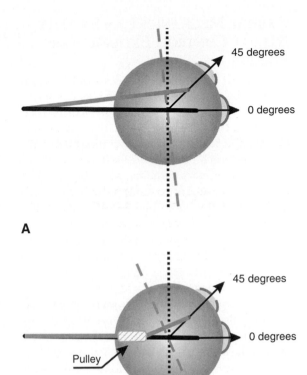

A

B

FIGURE 35-8   Axis of action of the horizontal recti for two different models of orbital mechanics. The schematics are a scaled version of an actual human orbit. **A,** If the muscles can move freely in the orbit, the muscular path does not change much whether the eye is in primary position *(black solid line)* or elevated by 45 degrees *(gray solid line)*. Correspondingly, the axis of action *(black dotted and gray dashed lines)* is approximately fixed in the orbit. **B,** If the path of the muscles through the orbit is constrained by pulleys *(hatched oval)*, the muscular path from the origin to the pulleys is essentially constant in the orbit, regardless of the orientation in the eye. However, the axis of action of the muscles changes dramatically with orientation; the magnitude of this change is clearly a function of the position of the pulleys. (*Note:* The axis of action is collinear with the angular velocity vector about which the eye would spin if moved by that pair of muscles.) (Modified from Quaia C, Optican LM: *J Neurophysiol* 79:3197, 1998.)

is not the derivative of orientation.[22] In contrast, the slide and the muscle's step component (step$_M$) can still be computed as in the one-dimensional case. Finally, the four components must be summed together in the correct proportions at the level of the motoneurons.

Orbital Mechanics Can Simplify Neural Control: Extraocular Pulleys

The abstract discussions of muscles and rotations can now be linked by considering how the orbital geometry of muscles determines the axis of rotation of the eye. Classically, the muscle actions were described in terms of how much they rotated the eye around each of the head-fixed axes when the eye was in primary position (see Table 35-1). A more accurate analysis considers that each muscle tends to turn the eye around a specific axis, called the *axis of action* of the muscle. By definition, the axis of action is the unit-length vector that is perpendicular to the plane determined by the three points: center of the eye, origin of the muscle, and insertion of the muscle.

The solution we outlined previously for generating the pulse, slide, and step is based on the assumption that the axes of action of the muscles are fixed in the orbit (i.e., the axes do not change when the eye moves). In this case there is a one-to-one correspondence between shortening velocity of the muscle and angular velocity of the eye. However, it has been demonstrated that the axes of action of the extraocular muscle are not fixed in the orbit.[12] Instead, they vary as a function of the orientation of the eye. The reason for this dependency is that the muscle's path, which determines its axis of action, is constrained so that the belly of the muscle moves only slightly during eye rotations.[12,13,20] Anatomic studies have shed light on the underlying mechanism, showing that each rectus muscle passes through a ring or sleeve near the equator of the globe.[7,8] The ring is made of collagen and is linked to Tenon's fascia, adjacent muscles, and the wall of the orbit by bands consisting of collagen, elastin, and smooth muscle.[16] This anatomic structure forms a functional pulley.[5]

How does the presence of these pulleys affect oculomotor control? The mechanical effect of the pulleys is to make the axes of action of the extraocular muscles vary dramatically as a function of the orientation of the eye. Before the pulleys were discovered, it was assumed that the axis of action of each rectus muscle was perpendicular to the plane formed by its origin on the annulus of Zinn, its insertion, and the center of the globe. Under these conditions (see Figure 35-8, *A*), changing the orientation of the eye (e.g., from straight ahead to 45 degrees up) only minimally affected the axis of action of the other muscles (in this case the horizontal recti muscles). However, with orbital pulleys (see Figure 35-8, *B*), the axis of action of each mus-

cle is now perpendicular to the plane formed by the location of its pulley, its insertion on the globe, and the center of the globe. In other words, the pulley acts as the functional point of origin of the muscle. If we now consider what happens when the eye is elevated, we see that the axes of action of the muscles change considerably (see Figure 35-8, *B*).

Quantitatively, it can be shown that if the orbital pulleys are properly located, the velocity of contraction of the muscles (which, as pointed out previously, is associated with the viscous force that must be compensated by the pulse of innervation) closely approximates the derivative of eye orientation, and not eye angular velocity.[17] The derivative of the eye orientation signal, unlike angular velocity, is confined to Listing's plane whenever the orientation is. Accordingly, it becomes much easier to implement Listing's law: All that is needed to keep the orientation of the eye in Listing's plane is to generate the pulse of innervation in that plane. Furthermore, if both step components of innervation are computed by integrating the pulse, the resulting movement has only small postsaccadic drifts, certainly small enough not to impede vision.

Thanks to the presence of the pulleys, it becomes much easier to compute all of the components of the innervation signal. However, this simplification must not be confused with a mechanical implementation of Listing's law. If the brain sends a pulse of innervation that has a nonzero torsional component (i.e., an Euler axis that is not in Listing's plane), the eye rotates out of Listing's plane. Indeed, during head-free gaze shifts, the VOR rotates the eyes opposite of any head rotation. If the head rotates out of Listing's plane, the VOR is constantly violating Listing's law and the saccade generator must compute torsional components to compensate for this.[4] Thus Listing's law must be implemented in the brain, although the pulleys make the required computations much simpler than they would be if the muscle axes were fixed in the orbit.

This neural simplification requires more than just a proper placement of the pulleys (they have to be located between the equator and the posterior pole of the globe, in the position that causes the angular velocity vector to tilt half as much as the change in elevation; that is, to generate the half-angle rule). As the eye turns, the pulleys must also move. More precisely, as a muscle contracts, its pulley must be pulled backward so that the distance between the location of the pulley and the insertion point of the muscle on the globe is approximately constant. This behavior was indeed found by Demer, Oh, and Poukens[6] with high-resolution magnetic resonance imaging studies of the human orbit.

The mechanism proposed to achieve such a dynamic relocation of the pulleys turns out to be simple, albeit surprising. It has been known for a long time that the fibers that make up each extraocular muscle can be histologically differentiated into two groups: the global fibers and the orbital fibers.[11] It turns out that whereas the global fibers of the rectus muscles go through the pulley and insert anterior to the globe's equator, the orbital fibers insert directly on the pulley.[6] Thus, when the whole muscle contracts, part of its tension is delivered to the globe and part is delivered to the pulley itself, moving it as required.

SUMMARY

The brain faces a difficult problem when controlling rotations of the eye because ocular drift suppresses vision; gaze direction has only two degrees of freedom, whereas the eye has three; and angular velocity is not the derivative of orientation (i.e., rotations are noncommutative). The extraocular muscles and the orbital pulleys form a mechanism for rotating the eye in three dimensions. The advantage of this configuration is that if the pulleys are in the right place, generating the innervation signals appropriate to control ocular rotations without ocular drift and to enforce Listing's Law becomes easier.[17] This neural simplification requires a more complex orbital mechanism: The pulleys must change the axes of action of the extraocular muscles as a function of eye orientation. However, it appears to be simpler, and perhaps more reliable, to control the location of the pulleys rather than to implement neural circuitry to perform noncommutative operations. The overall complexity of the system is thereby reduced.

ACKNOWLEDGMENTS

We are grateful to Drs. C.M. Schor, J.D. Crawford, and D. Tweed for comments and suggestions.

REFERENCES

1. Carpenter RHS: *Movements of the eyes,* London, 1977, Psion.

2. Crawford JD: Listing's law: what's all the hubbub? In Harris LR, Jenkin M (eds): *Vision and action,* Cambridge, 1998, Cambridge University.

3. Crawford JD, Vilis T: How do motor systems deal with the problems of controlling three-dimensional rotations? *J Motor Behav* 27:89, 1995.

4. Crawford JD et al: Three-dimensional eye-head coordination during gaze saccades in the primate, *J Neurophysiol* 81:1760, 1999.

5. Demer JL, Miller JM, Poukens V: Surgical implications of the rectus extraocular muscle pulleys, *J Pediatr Ophthalmol Strabismus* 33:208, 1996.

6. Demer JL, Oh SY, Poukens V: Evidence for active control of rectus extraocular muscle pulleys, *Invest Ophthalmol Vis Sci* 41:1280, 2000.

7. Demer JL et al: Evidence for fibromuscular pulleys of the recti extraocular muscles, *Invest Ophthalmol Vis Sci* 36:1125, 1995.

8. Demer JL et al: Innervation of extraocular pulley smooth muscle in monkeys and humans, *Invest Ophthalmol Vis Sci* 38:1774, 1997.

9. Goldstein H: *Classical mechanics,* ed 2, Reading, Mass, 1980, Addison-Wesley.

10. Haslwanter T: Mathematics of three-dimensional eye rotations, *Vision Res* 35:1727, 1995.

11. Leigh RJ, Zee DS: *The neurology of eye movements,* ed 3, New York, 1999, Oxford University Press.

12. Miller JM: Functional anatomy of normal human rectus muscles, *Vision Res* 29:223, 1989.

13. Miller JM, Robins D: Extraocular muscle side slip and orbital geometry in monkeys, *Vision Res* 27:381, 1987.

14. Miller JM, Robinson DA: A model of the mechanics of binocular alignment, *Comput Biomed Res* 17:436, 1984.

15. Mok D et al: Rotation of Listing's plane during vergence, *Vision Res* 32:2055, 1992.

16. Porter JD et al: Structure-function correlations in the human medial rectus extraocular muscle pulleys, *Invest Ophthalmol Vis Sci* 37:468, 1996.

17. Quaia C, Optican LM: Commutative saccadic generator is sufficient to control a 3-D ocular plant with pulleys, *J Neurophysiol* 79:3197, 1998.

18. Robinson DA: The mechanics of human saccadic eye movement, *J Physiol (Lond)* 174:245, 1964.

19. Robinson DA: Models of the saccadic eye movement control system, *Kybernetik* 14:71, 1973.

20. Simonsz HJ et al: Sideways displacement and curved path of recti eye muscles, *Arch Ophthalmol* 103:124, 1985.

21. Tweed D: Kinematic principles of three-dimensional gaze control. In Fetter M, et al: *Three-dimensional kinematics of eye, head and limb movements,* Amsterdam 1997, Harwood.

22. Tweed D, Vilis T: Implications of rotational kinematics for the oculomotor system in three dimensions, *J Neurophysiol* 58:823, 1987.

23. Tweed D, Vilis T: Geometric relations of eye position and velocity vectors during saccades, *Vision Res* 30:111, 1990.

24. Tweed D, Cadera W, Vilis T: Computing three-dimensional eye position quaternions and eye velocity from search coil signals, *Vision Res* 30:97, 1990.

25. Westheimer G, McKee SP: Visual acuity in the presence of retinal-image motion, *J Opt Soc Am* 65:847, 1975.

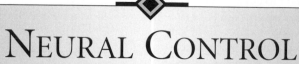

NEURAL CONTROL OF EYE MOVEMENTS

CLIFTON M. SCHOR

OCULOMOTOR CONTROL

Three Fundamental Visual Sensory-Motor Tasks

The neural control of eye movements is organized to optimize performance of three general perceptual tasks. One task is to resolve the visual field while we move, either by translation or rotation through space (self-motion). Our body motion causes the image of the visual field to flow across the retina, and reflexive eye movements reduce or stabilize this image motion to improve visual performance. The second task is to resolve objects whose position or motion is independent of the background field (object motion). Eye movements improve visual resolution of individual objects by maintaining alignment of the two foveas with both stationary and moving targets over a broad range of directions and distances of gaze. The third task is to explore space and shift attention from one target location to another. Rapid eye movements place corresponding images on the two foveas as we shift gaze between targets lying in different directions and distances of gaze.

Three Components of Eye Rotation

All three perceptual tasks require three-dimensional control of eye position. These dimensions are controlled by separate neural systems. As described in Chapter 35, three pairs of extraocular muscles provide control of horizontal, vertical, and torsional position of each eye. Eye movements are described as combined rotations about three principal axes as illustrated in Figure 36-1. Horizontal rotation occurs about the vertical z-axis, vertical rotation

about the horizontal x-axis, and torsion about the line of sight or y-axis. As described in Chapter 35, the amount of rotation about each of the three principal axes that is needed to describe a certain direction of gaze and torsional orientation of the eye depends on the order of sequential rotations (e.g., horizontal, followed by vertical and then torsional).[117] Some oculomotor tasks, such as retinal image stabilization, use all three degrees of freedom, whereas other tasks, such as voluntary gaze shifts, require only two degrees of freedom (i.e., gaze direction and eccentricity from primary position). As described by Donders' law, torsional orientation of the eye is determined by horizontal and vertical components of eye position. Ocular torsion is independent of the path taken by the eye to reach a given eye position and is constrained by the gaze direction. Listing's law quantifies the amount of ocular torsion at any given eye position, relative to the torsion of the eye in primary position of gaze.

Binocular Constraints on Eye Position Control

Binocular alignment of retinal images with corresponding retinal points places additional constraints on the oculomotor system. Because the two eyes view the world from slightly different vantage points, the retinal image locations of points subtended by near objects differ slightly in the two eyes. This disparity can be described with three degrees of freedom (horizontal, vertical, and torsional components) that are analogous to the angular rotations of the eye shown in Figure 36-1. The main task of binocular eye alignment is to minimize horizontal and vertical dispari-

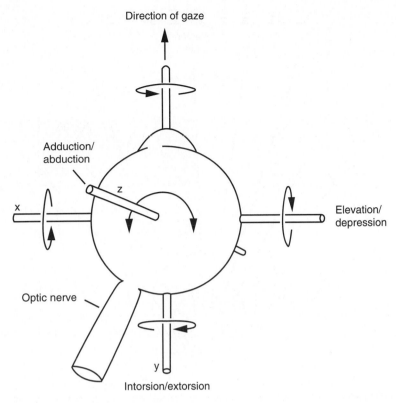

FIGURE 36-1 The three principal axes of eye rotation. Horizontal rotation occurs about the vertical axis (z), vertical rotation about the transverse axis (x), and torsion about the anteroposterior axis (y). (From Goldberg ME, Eggers HM, Gouras D: The ocular motor system. In Kandel ER, Schwartz JH, Jessell TM [eds]: *Principles of neural science,* ed 3, Norwalk, Conn, 1991, Appleton and Lange.)

ties and cyclodisparities subtended by near targets on the two foveas. This requires a conjugate system that rotates the two eyes in the same direction and amount and a disconjugate system that rotates the visual axes in opposite directions. As described by Hering,[41] a common gaze direction for the two eyes is achieved by a combination of conjugate and disconjugate movements that are controlled by separate systems. The *version* system controls conjugate movements and the *vergence* system controls disconjugate movements. Pure version and vergence movements are described, respectively, by the isovergence and isoversion contours shown in Figure 36-2. The isovergence circle describes the locus of points that stimulate the same vergence angle in all directions of gaze.[80] A different isovergence circle exists at each viewing distance. The isoversion lines describe the locus of points that stimulate the same version angle over a range of viewing distances in a common direction of gaze relative to the head. Pure vergence movements occur along any of the isoversion lines and not just along the central or midsagittal plane. Fixation

changes along any other contour result from a combination of version and vergence movements. Both version and vergence movements are described as combinations of horizontal, vertical, and torsional rotations. For example, there can be horizontal and vertical version and vergence movements. Torsional rotations are usually called *cyclorotations* (e.g., cycloversion or cyclovergence). Hering's law implies that there is equal innervation of yoked muscle pairs: "one and the same impulse of will directs both eyes simultaneously as one can direct a pair of horses with single reins."[41] The law should not be taken literally because common gaze commands from higher levels are eventually parceled into separate innervation sources in the brainstem that control individual muscles in the two eyes.

Feedback and Feed-Forward Control Systems

The oculomotor system requires feedback to optimize sensory stimuli for vision with a sufficiently high degree of precision. Feedback provides information

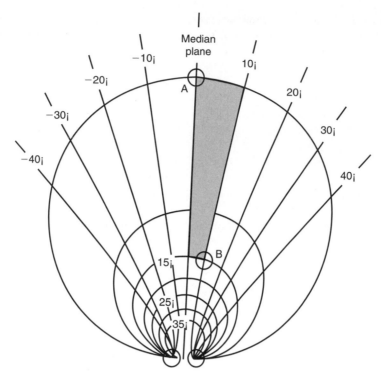

FIGURE 36-2   Geometric representation of the two components of eye movements by locations of the intersections of the two visual axes. The value in degrees marked along each isovergence circle denotes the convergence angle, and the value in degrees marked on the hyperbola isoversion lines denotes the visual direction when a line is not close to the eyes.

about motor response errors on the basis of their sensory consequences, such as unwanted retinal image motion or displacement. This visual error information usually arrives too late to affect the current movement because the time delays in the visual system are approximately 50 to 100 milliseconds. Instead, it is used to adaptively adjust motor responses to minimize subsequent errors. Oculomotor systems use sensory information to guide eye movements in two different ways: Motor responses can be guided in a closed-loop mode with an ongoing feedback signal that indicates the difference between the desired and actual motor response, or they can operate without concurrent feedback in an open-loop mode. The closed-loop feedback mode is used to reduce internal system errors or external perturbations. A physical example of a closed-loop system is the thermostatic regulation of room temperature; if the outside temperature drops, the furnace will turn on so that the room temperature stays constant. Motor responses also can be controlled in an open-loop mode, without a concurrent feedback signal. A physical example of an open-loop system is a water faucet; if the pressure drops, the flow of water will also drop

because the valve does not compensate for the pressure drop.

The mode of the response depends on the latency of the response, its duration, and its velocity. In most examples, visual feedback in a closed-loop system is used to maintain or regulate a fixed position or to slow movements of the eyes when there is adequate time to process the error signal. Errors in eye posture or movement are sensed from displacement of the object of regard from the fovea or slippage of the retinal image, and negative feedback control mechanisms attempt to reduce the errors to zero during the response.

Feed-forward control systems do not use concurrent visual feedback and are described as open-loop systems. These systems can respond to nonvisual (extraretinal) stimuli, or they respond to advanced visual information with short latencies and brief durations. For example, brief rapid head movements stimulate vestibular signals that evoke compensatory eye movements to stabilize the retinal image. These head movements can produce retinal image velocities of 300 to 400 degrees per second, yet the eyes respond with a counterrotation within 14 milliseconds of the movement.[55] The oculomotor response to head motion must rely on vestibular signals because retinal image velocities produced by head rotation exceed the upper velocity limit for sensing motion by the human eye. Retinal image velocities that exceed this upper limit appear as blurred streaks rather than as moving images. Visual feedback is not available when the response to head rotation begins because the latency is too short to use concurrent visual feedback. A minimum of 50 milliseconds is needed to activate cortical areas that initiate ocular following, such that any motor response with a shorter latency must occur without concurrent visual feedback.[72] Some open-loop systems, such as brief rapid gaze shifts (*saccades*), respond to visual information sensed before the movement rather than during the movement. Their response is too brief to be guided by negative visual feedback. Accuracy of a feed-forward system is evaluated after the response is completed. Visually sensed posttask errors are used by feed-forward systems to improve the accuracy of subsequent open-loop responses in an adaptive process that calibrates motor responses. Calibration minimizes motor errors in systems that do not use visual feedback during their response. All feed-forward oculomotor systems are calibrated by adaptation, and this plasticity persists throughout life.

Hierarchy of Oculomotor Control

The following sections present a functional classification of eye position and movement control systems used to facilitate three general perceptual tasks, as well as a hierarchical description of their neuroanatomic organization. A hierarchy of neural control exists within each of the functional categories of eye movements that plans, coordinates, and executes motor activity. Three pairs of extraocular muscles that rotate each eye about its center of rotation are at the bottom of this hierarchy. The forces applied by these muscle pairs to the eye are controlled at the level above by the motor nuclei of cranial nerves III, IV, and VI. Motor neurons in these nuclei make up the final common pathway for all classes of eye movements. Axon projections from these neurons convey information to the extraocular muscles for executing both slow and fast eye movements. Above this level, premotor nuclei in the brainstem coordinate the combined actions of several muscles to execute horizontal, vertical, and torsional eye rotations. These gaze centers orchestrate the direction, amplitude, velocity, and duration of eye movements. Interneurons from the premotor nuclei all converge on motor nuclei in the

final common pathway. Premotor neurons receive instructions from supranuclear regions, including the superior colliculus (SC); the substantia nigra; the cerebellum; frontal cortical regions, including the frontal eye fields (FEF) and supplementary eye fields (SEF); and extrastriate regions, including the medial temporal visual area (MT), the medial superior temporal visual area (MST), the lateral intraparietal area, and the posterior parietal area (PP). These higher centers plan the desired direction and distance of binocular gaze in three-dimensional space. They transform sensory visual stimuli into motor commands. They determine when and how fast to move the eyes to fixate selected targets in a natural complex scene or to return them to a remembered gaze location. The following sections discuss the hierarchical control for each of three functional classes of eye movements. The next section describes the final common pathway that conveys innervation for all classes of eye movements.

Final Common Pathway

Cranial Nerves III, IV, and VI and Motor Nuclei. Cranial nerves III, IV, and VI represent the final common pathway as defined by Sherrington[108] for all classes of eye movements. All axon projections from these cranial nuclei carry information for voluntary and reflex fast and slow categories of eye movements.[53] The oculomotor (III), trochlear (IV), and abducens (VI) nuclei innervate the six extraocular muscles, iris, and ciliary body. The abducens nucleus innervates the ipsilateral lateral rectus muscle. Premotor interneurons also project from VI to the contralateral oculomotor nucleus (III) for control of the contralateral medial rectus muscle to produce yoked movements on lateral gaze that are consistent with Hering's law. The trochlear nucleus innervates the contralateral superior oblique muscle. The oculomotor nucleus innervates the ipsilateral medial rectus, inferior rectus, inferior oblique, and contralateral superior rectus muscles. The anterior portion of the oculomotor nucleus also contains motor neurons that control pupil size and accommodation in a specialized region called the *Edinger-Westphal nucleus.*[36] Afferents from this nucleus synapse in the ciliary ganglion before innervating their target muscles.[121] The regions of the oculomotor nucleus that control various eye muscles are illustrated in Figure 36-3.

Motor Neuron Response. The motor neurons control both the position and velocity of the eye. They receive inputs from burst and tonic cells in

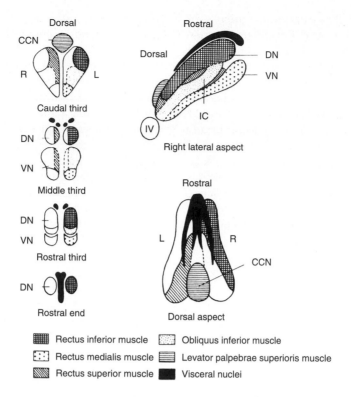

FIGURE 36-3   Representation of motor neurons for right extraocular muscles in the oculomotor nucleus of monkey. Transverse sections at levels as indicated in the complex. Lateral and dorsal views are shown to the right. *CCN*, Caudal central nucleus; *DN*, dorsal nucleus; *IC*, intermediate column; *IV*, trochlear nucleus; *VN*, ventral nucleus. (From Warwick R: *J Comp Neurol* 98:449, 1953.)

premotor nuclei. The tonic inputs are responsible for holding the eyes steady, and the more phasic, or burstlike, inputs are responsible for initiating all eye movements to overcome orbital viscosity and for controlling eye movements. As illustrated in Figure 36-4,[93] all motoneurons have the following characteristics:

1. They have on-off directions (they increase their firing rate in the direction of agonist activity).
2. All cells participate in all classes of eye movements, including steady fixation.
3. Each cell (especially tonic) has an eye position threshold at which it begins to fire. Motoneurons have thresholds that range from low to high. Cells with low thresholds begin firing when the eye is in the off field of the muscle that it innervates. Cells with higher thresholds can begin to fire after the eye has moved past the primary position by as much as 10 degrees into the on field of the muscle. The graded thresholds of motoneurons are responsible for the recruitment of active cells as the eyes move into the field of action for the muscle.

4. Contractile force is increased by increasing the frequency of spike potentials for a given neuron. Once their threshold is exceeded, all cells increase their firing rate as the eye moves further along in the on direction of the muscle until they saturate. Cells increase their firing rate linearly as the eye moves into their on field.

FUNCTIONAL CLASSIFICATION INTO THREE GENERAL CATEGORIES
Stabilization of Gaze Relative to the External World

Movements of the head during locomotion tasks such as walking are described by a combination of angular rotations and linear translations. The oculomotor system keeps gaze fixed in space during these head movements by using extraretinal and retinal velocity information about head motion.

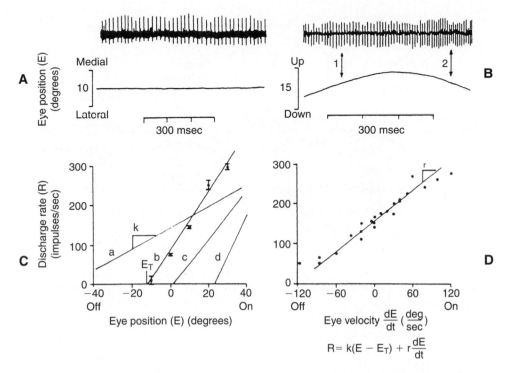

FIGURE 36-4 Discharge rate of oculomotor neurons in relation to eye movement. **A,** The steady firing rate is shown when the eye is stationary. **B,** The rate-position curve illustrates an increase of firing rate with eye position for four neurons. **C,** The firing rate is shown during a slow voluntary eye movement. The arrows indicate points where the eye passes through the same position with velocity of opposite signs, and the associated firing rate is different. **D,** Firing rate is plotted for a single unit and a particular deviation of the eye as a function of eye velocity. (From Robinson DA, Keller EL: *Bibl Ophthalmol* 82:7, 1972).

The primary extraretinal signal comes from accelerometers in the vestibular apparatus.

Extraretinal Signals. The vestibular system contains two types of organs that transduce angular and linear acceleration of the head into velocity signals[69,109] (Figure 36-5). Three semicircular canals lie on each side of the head in three orthogonal planes that are approximately parallel to a mirror-image set of planes on the contralateral side of the head. These canals are stimulated by brief angular rotations of the head and the resulting reflexive ocular rotation is referred to as the *vestibuloocular reflex* (angular VOR). In addition, two otoliths (the utricle and sacculus) transduce linear acceleration caused by head translation, as well as head pitch (tilt about the interaural axis) and roll (tilt about the nasooccipital axis), into translation velocity and head orientation signals (linear VOR). These signals stimulate eye rotations that are approximately equal and opposite to

the motion of the head. This stabilization reflex has a short 7- to 15-millisecond latency because it is mediated by only three synapses and is accurate for head turns at velocities in excess of 300 degrees per second.[48,55] Hair cells in the canals can be stimulated by irrigating one ear with cold water. This produces a caloric-vestibular nystagmus that causes the eyes to rotate slowly to the side of the irrigated ear.[17] These slow-phase movements are interrupted by fast saccadic eye movements that reset eye position in the reverse direction (fast phase). A sequence of slow and fast phases is referred to as *jerk nystagmus* (Figure 36-6). Head rotations about horizontal, vertical, and nasooccipital axes produce VOR responses with horizontal, vertical, and torsional counterrotations of the slow phase of the nystagmus.[106]

To be effective, these reflex eye rotations must stabilize the retinal image. If the axis of angular head rotation coincided with the center of eye rotation, perfect compensation would occur if angular eye

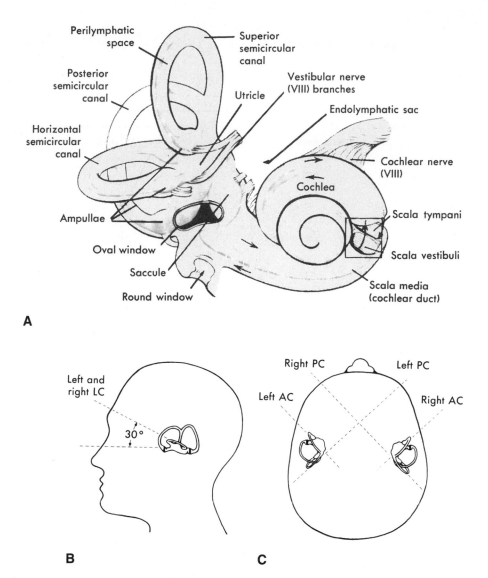

Figure 36-5   Vestibular end organs in the human temporal bone. Three canals transduce angular head acceleration and two otoliths, the sacculus and utricle, transduce linear acceleration and head orientation. Right labyrinth is viewed from horizontal aspect (**A**). The canals are in three orthogonal planes that are approximately parallel to a mirror image set of planes on the contralateral side of the head that lie roughly in the pulling direction of the three muscle planes. **B,** Lateral canals. **C,** Anterior and posterior vertical canals. *AC,* Anterior vertical canal; *LC,* lateral canal; *PC,* posterior vertical canal. (**A,** Drawings by Ernest W. Beck; courtesy Beltone Electronics Corp, Chicago, Ill; **B** and **C,** From Barber HO, Stickwell CW: *Manual of electronystagmography,* St Louis, 1976, Mosby.)

velocity equaled angular head velocity. However, the axis of head rotation is the neck and not the center of eye rotation, such that when the head rotates, the eyes both rotate and translate with respect to the visual field. This is exacerbated during near viewing conditions. The eye must rotate more than the head to stabilize the retinal image motion of a nearby target caused by angular head movements. Indeed, the gain of the VOR increases with convergence.[110] Mismatches between eye and head velocity also oc-

cur with prescription spectacles that magnify or minify retinal image motion. Because the VOR responds directly to vestibular and not visual stimuli, its response is classified as open loop. The VOR compensates for visual errors by adapting its gain in response to retinal image slip to produce a stabilized retinal image.[69] Perfect compensation would occur if angular eye velocity were equal and opposite to angular head velocity while viewing a distant scene. However, empirical measures show that at high os-

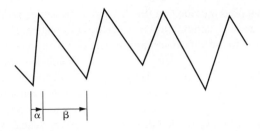

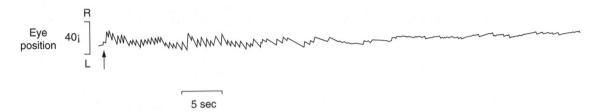

Eye position 40₁

5 sec

FIGURE 36-6 Optokinetic nystagmus and vestibuloocular reflex are composed of a slow phase (β) that rotates the eye in a direction that stabilizes the retinal image and a fast phase (α) that resets the eye's position. This figure illustrates the vestibuloocular response to sustained rotation. The slow phase is in the direction opposite to head rotation. Horizontal position is plotted against time. The reflex gradually habituates and disappears by approximately 30 seconds. (From Miller, Neil R [eds]: *Walsh and Hoyt's clinical neuro-ophthalmology*, ed 4, Baltimore, 1982, Williams & Wilkins.)

cillation frequencies (2 Hz), compensation by the VOR is far from perfect, and yet the world appears stable and single during rapid head shaking without any perceptual instability or oscillopsis.[23] Thus perception of a stable world requires that the visual system be aware of both the amount of head rotation and the inaccuracy of compensatory eye movements so that it can anticipate any residual retinal image motion during the head rotation.

Retinal Signals. Head motion also produces whole-field retinal image motion of the visual field (optic flow).[20] These retinal signals stimulate reflexive compensatory eye rotations that stabilize the retinal image during slow or long-lasting head movements. The eyes follow the moving field with a slow phase that is interrupted by resetting saccades (fast phase) one to three times per second.[15] This jerk nystagmus is called *optokinetic nystagmus* (OKN), and it complements the VOR by responding to low-velocity sustained head movements such as those that occur during walking and posture instability. Like the VOR, OKN also responds with horizontal, vertical, and cyclic eye rotations to optic flow about vertical, horizontal, and nasooccipital axes.[16]

The optokinetic response to large fields has two components, including an early and a delayed segment (OKNe and OKNd, respectively). OKNe is a

short-latency ocular following response (less than 50 milliseconds) that constitutes the rapid component of OKN, and OKNd builds up slowly after 7 seconds of stimulation.[72,86] OKNe is likely to be mediated by the pursuit pathway.[70] The delayed component is revealed by the continuation of OKNd in darkness (optokinetic after nystagmus, OKAN). OKNd results from a velocity memory or storage mechanism.[19,86] The time constant of the development of the OKAN matches the time constant of decay of the cupula in the semicircular canals.[92] Thus OKAN builds up so that vision can compensate for loss of the vestibular inputs during prolonged angular rotation that might occur in a circular flight path. OKN can be used clinically to evaluate visual acuity objectively by measuring the smallest texture size and separation in a moving field that elicits the reflex.

Neurocontrol of Stabilization Reflexes

Vestibuloocular Reflex. The transducer that converts head rotation into a neural code for driving the VOR consists of a set of three semicircular canals paired on each side of the head.[69] The horizontal canals are paired, and the anterior canal on one side is paired with the posterior canal on the contralateral side (see Figure 36-5). Opponent pairs also exist; therefore, when one canal is stimulated by a given head rotation, its paired member on the contralateral side is inhibited. For example, downward and forward head motion to the left causes increased firing of the vestibular nerve for the left anterior canal and decreased firing of the vestibular nerve projections from the right posterior canal. The three canals lie roughly in the pulling directions of the three muscle planes.[69] Thus the left anterior canal and right posterior canal are parallel to the muscle planes of the left eye vertical recti and the right eye obliques. Pathways for the horizontal VOR are illustrated in Figure 36-7 for a leftward head rotation.[53] Excitatory innervation projects from the left medial vestibular nucleus to the right abducens nucleus to activate the right lateral rectus muscle, and an interneuron from the right abducens nucleus projects to the left oculomotor nucleus to activate the left medial rectus muscle. The

abducens serves as a premotor nucleus to coordinate conjugate horizontal movements to the ipsilateral side in accordance with Hering's law.

The cerebellar flocculus is essential for adaptation of the VOR to optical distortions such as magnification. The flocculus receives excitatory inputs from retinal image motion (retinal slip) and head velocity information (canal signals) and inhibitory inputs from neural correlates of eye movements that provide a negative feedback signal.[56] Adaptation occurs only if retinal image motion and head turns occur together.[45] The gain of the VOR is adapted to decrease whenever retinal slip and head turns are in the same direction and increase whenever they are in opposite directions. Following adaptation, an error correction signal is projected from the flocculus by Purkinje cells to floccular target neurons in the vestibular nucleus to make appropriate changes in VOR gain.[56]

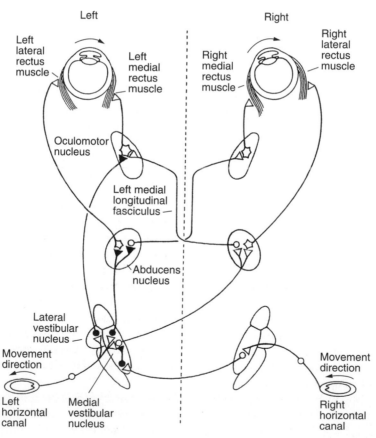

FIGURE 36-7   Pathways of the horizontal vestibuloocular reflex in the brainstem for leftward head rotation. Inhibitory connections are shown as filled neurons, excitatory connections as unfilled neurons. Leftward head rotation stimulates the left horizontal canal and inhibits the right horizontal canal. This results in an increased discharge rate in the right lateral and left medial rectus and decreased discharge rate in the left lateral and right medial rectus. (From Goldberg ME, Eggers HM, Gouras P: The ocular motor system. In Kandel ER, Schwartz JH, Jessell TM [eds]: *Principles of neural science,* ed 3, Norwalk, Conn, 1991, Appleton and Lange.)

Optokinetic Nystagmus. The visual stimulus for OKN is derived from optic flow of the retinal image.[3,33,120] The retina contains ganglion cells that respond exclusively to motion in certain directions or orientations. This information passes along the optic nerve, decussates at the chiasm, and projects to the cortex via the geniculate body or to the midbrain by way of the accessory optic tract[42] (Figure 36-8). This tract has several nuclei in the pretectal area. One pair of these nuclei, the nucleus of the optic tract (NOT), is tuned to horizontal target motion to the ipsilateral side (i.e., nasal-to-temporal motion). The lateral and medial terminal nuclei are tuned for vertical target motion.[83] Neurons in these nuclei receive subcortical inputs only from the contralateral eye. They have large receptive fields and respond to large textured stimuli moving in specific directions. Stimulation of the right NOT with rightward motion causes following movements of both eyes to the right or ipsilateral side, and similarly, stimulation of the left NOT with leftward motion causes leftward conjugate following

movements. Each NOT projects signals through the inferior olive to the vestibular nuclei and possibly to the flocculus by way of the climbing fibers of the cerebellum.[33] The NOT provides a visual signal to the vestibular nucleus, and the motor response is the same as that for velocity signals originating from the semicircular canals.

The cortical region that organizes motion signals is the MST. This region is important for generating motion signals for both pursuit and OKN.[3] Binocular cortical cells receive projections from both eyes and code ipsilateral motion from the contralateral visual field at higher velocities than the subcortical system.[120] The cortical cells project to the ipsilateral NOT.

Until the age of 3 to 4 months, the monocular subcortical projections predominate because the cortical projection has not yet developed.[96] As a result, OKN in infancy is driven mainly by the crossed subcortical input. The consequence is that monocular stimulation evokes OKN only with temporal-to-nasal motion but not with nasal-to-temporal motion. After 3 to 4 months of development, the infant's cortical projections predominate and horizontal OKN responds to both monocular temporalward and nasalward image motion. The cortical projections to the NOT fail to develop in infantile esotropia, and as adults, these patients exhibit the same asymmetric OKN pattern as that observed in immature infants.[104] This anomalous projection is responsible for a disorder known as *latent nystagmus,* in which a jerk nystagmus occurs when one eye is occluded with the slow phase directed toward the side of the covered eye. During monocular fixation, the stimulated retina increases the activity of neurons in the contralateral NOT through subcortical crossed projections, but it is unable to innervate the ipsilateral NOT through the ineffective cortical-tectal projection. The result is that both eyes' positions are drawn to the side of the stimulated NOT (i.e., the side of the covered eye). The fixation error is corrected with a saccade, and a repeated sequence is described as latent or occlusion nystagmus (LN).[25]

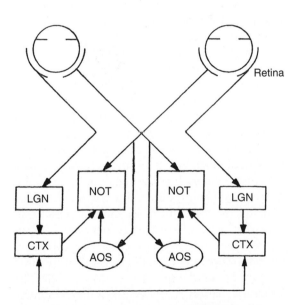

FIGURE 36-8 Simplified schematic illustrating the inputs to the nucleus of the optic tract (*NOT*) from subcortical crossed retinal projections and cortical-tectal projections. Each NOT gets direct retinal input from the contralateral nasal retina, which is excited by temporal-to-nasal motion. It also receives indirect cortical input (*CTX*) from the temporal retina of the ipsilateral eye, which tends to be excited more by nasal-to-temporal motion, as well as input via the accessory optic system (*AOS*) and input from the contralateral visual cortex via the corpus callosum. *LGN,* Lateral geniculate nucleus. (Adapted from Hoffmann KP, Distler C, Ilg U: *J Comp Neurol* 321:150, 1992.)

Foveal Gaze Lock (Maintenance of Foveal Alignment with Stationary and Slowly Moving Targets)

Static Control of Eye Alignment (Fixation). The oculomotor system enhances visual resolution by maintaining alignment of the fovea with attended stationary and moving targets.[50,122] During fixation of stationary targets, the eyes sustain foveal alignment over a wide range of target locations in the visual field. Gaze direction is controlled by a combination of eye position in the orbit and head position.[52] Gaze mainly is controlled by eye position for targets lying at eccentricities of less than 15 degrees from primary position.[7] Steady fixation at larger gaze eccentricities is accomplished with a combination of head and eye position. Holding eye fixation at large eccentricities (more than 30 degrees) without head movements is difficult to sustain, and the eye drifts intermittently toward primary position in gaze-evoked nystagmus.[1] This drift is exacerbated by alcohol.[9] Even within the 15-degree range, the fixating eye is not completely stationary. It exhibits physiologic nystagmus that is composed of slow horizontal, vertical, and torsional drifts (0.1 degree per second); microsaccades (less than 0.25 degree); and a small-amplitude (less than 0.01 degree) high-frequency tremor (40 to 80 Hz).[14] Some of the drifts and saccades are error producing, whereas others are error correcting when they serve to continually minimize motion and adjust the alignment of the target of regard with the fovea.[50,119] The high-frequency tremor reflects the noise possibly originating from asynchronous firing of individual motoneurons that is filtered by the mechanical properties of the eye.

Stereoscopic depth perception is enhanced by accurate binocular fixation.[95,97] Precise bifoveal alignment requires that the eyes maintain accurate convergence at the distance of the attended target. Small constant errors of convergence during attempted binocular fixation (less than 15 arcmin) are referred to as *fixation disparity,* and these can impair stereo performance.[6,77] Fixation disparity is a closed-loop error because it occurs in the presence of retinal image feedback from binocular disparity. Fixation disparity results from incomplete nullification of an open-loop error of convergence known as *heterophoria.* Heterophoria equals the difference between the convergence stimulus and the convergence response measured under open-loop conditions (e.g., monocular occlusion). The magnitude of fixation disparity increases monotonically with the disparity stimulus to convergence when it is varied with horizontal prisms.[77] The slope of this function is called the *forced-duction fixation disparity curve.*[77] Shallow slopes of these curves indicate that the heterophoria is reduced by adaptation during binocular or closed-loop conditions.[95] Vergence adaptation is rapid; for example, when convergence is stimulated for only 1 minute with a convergent disparity and one eye is then occluded, the convergence response persists in the open-loop state.[95] Typically, the convergent disparity is produced by prisms that deflect the perceived direction of both eyes' images inward, or in the nasalward direction (i.e., the base of the prism before each eye is temporalward or "base-out"). This adapted change in heterophoria is constant in all directions of gaze and is termed *concomitant adaptation.* Prism adaptation is in response to efforts by closed-loop disparity vergence to nullify the open-loop vergence error (heterophoria). Prism adaptation improves the accuracy of binocular alignment and stereodepth performance.

Horizontal vergence equals the horizontal component of the angle formed by the intersection of the two visual axes, and it is described with three different units of measurement or scales that include the degree, prism diopter (PD), and meter angle (MA). *Prism diopters* equal 100 times the tangent of the angle. *Meter angles* equal the reciprocal of the viewing distance (specified in meters) at which the visual axes intersect as measured from the center of eye rotation. A target at 1 meter stimulates 1 MA of convergence (approximately 3.4 degrees) and 1 diopter of accommodation. PD can be computed from MA by the product of MA and the interpupillary distance (IPD), measured in centimeters. For example, convergence at a viewing distance of 50 cm by two eyes with a 6-cm IPD equals either 2 MA or 12 PD. The advantage to units in MA is that the magnitude of the stimulus to accommodation in diopters is approximately equal to the magnitude of the stimulus to convergence, assuming that both are measured from a common point such as the center of eye rotation. This assumption produces large errors for viewing distances less than 20 cm because accommodation is usually measured in reference to the corneal apex that is 13 mm anterior to the center of eye rotation. The advantage to units in PD is that they are easily computed from the product of MA and IPD. The advantage to units in degrees is that they accurately quantify asymmetric convergence where targets lie at different distances from the two eyes.

The Maddox classification[58] describes open- and closed-loop components that make up the horizontal vergence response. The classification includes three open-loop components that influence heterophoria. These include an adaptable intrinsic bias (tonic vergence), a horizontal vergence response to monocular depth cues (proximal vergence), and a horizontal vergence response that is coupled with accommodation by a neurologic cross-link known as *accommodative-convergence.* Tonic vergence has an innate divergence posture (5 degrees) known as the *anatomic position of rest*.[91] Tonic vergence adapts rapidly to compensate for vergence errors during the first 6 weeks of life. At birth the eyes diverge during sleep, but after 6 weeks the visual axes are nearly parallel during sleep.[89] The adapted vergence, measured in an alert state, in the absence of binocular stimulation and accommodative effort, is called the *physiologic position of rest.* The physiologic position of rest equals the sum of tonic vergence and the anatomic position of rest. Tonic vergence adaptation ability continues throughout life to compensate for trauma, disease, and optical distortions from spectacles and aging factors.

Proximal vergence describes the open-loop vergence response to distance percepts stimulated by monocular depth cues such as size, overlap, linear perspective, texture gradients, and motion parallax.[68,123] This proximal response accounts for a large portion of the convergence response to changing distance.[46,102] The open-loop convergence response is also increased by efforts of accommodation.[5,73] The eyes maintain approximately two thirds of an MA of convergence (4 PD) for every diopter of accommodation.[77] A target at 1 meter stimulates 1 MA of convergence (approximately 3.4 degrees) and 1 diopter of accommodation. Therefore, when the eyes accommodate 1 diopter, the accommodative-convergence response increases by approximately 2.3 degrees or 4 PD, which is only 68% of the convergence stimulus. The sum of the three open-loop components of convergence typically lag behind the convergence stimulus and produce an open-loop divergence error (exophoria) that is usually less than 2 degrees under far viewing conditions and 4 degrees at near viewing distances.[11] *Esophoria* describes open-loop vergence errors caused by excessive convergence that lead the stimulus. The distribution of heterophoria in the general population is not gaussian or normally distributed. It is narrowly peaked at approximately a mean close to zero, indicating that binocular errors of eye alignment are minimized by an adaptive calibration process.[114] During closed-loop stimulation, vergence error is reduced to less than one tenth of a degree by the component of the Maddox classification controlled by visual feedback, disparity vergence, which is stimulated by retinal image disparity. Variation in any of the three open-loop components of convergence influences the magnitude of heterophoria and the resulting closed-loop fixation disparity. Fixation disparity acts as a stimulus to maintain activity of disparity vergence so

that it continues to sustain its nulling response of the underlying heterophoria during attempted steady binocular fixation.[95] Other dimensions of vergence also adapt to disparity stimuli. Vertical vergence adapts to vertical prism before one eye and cyclovergence adapts to optically produced cyclodisparity stimuli.[62,100,103,115]

Dynamic Control of Eye Alignment (Smooth Tracking Responses to Open- and Closed-Loop Stimuli)

Conjugate Smooth Pursuit Tracking. Smooth following pursuit movements allow the eyes to maintain foveal alignment with a moving target that is voluntarily selected.[51,85] *Pursuit* is the conjugate component of smooth following eye movement responses to target motion. As described subsequently, disconjugate following responses to changes in target distance are called *smooth vergence*. Conjugate pursuit differs from the delay portion of OKN, which is a reflex response to optic flow of the entire visual field. A conflict occurs between the pursuit and optokinetic systems when the eyes pursue an object that is moving across a stationary background. Pursuit stabilizes the moving target on or near the fovea, but it causes optic flow or retinal slip of the stationary background scene. Conflicts can also occur between pursuit and the VOR if gaze is controlled with head tracking movements. Stabilizing the retinal image of a moving object with head movements produces a vestibular signal from the canals. Consequently, pursuit of a small moving target against a stationary background with eye or head movements requires that OKN and the VOR be ignored or suppressed. This is accomplished most effectively when the background lies at a different distance than the pursuit target.[44]

Pursuit responds to target velocities ranging from several minutes of arcsec to more than 175 degrees per second.[85] The gain or accuracy of pursuit is reduced as target velocity increases higher than 100 degrees per second.[74] The VOR has a much higher velocity range than pursuit. This can be demonstrated by comparing two views of one's index finger. One can either keep the finger stationary while shaking the head rapidly from side to side at 2 to 3 Hz or shake the finger at the same frequency without moving the head. The eye cannot follow the moving finger, but it can follow the stationary finger while shaking the head even though the head-relative motion is identical in these two examples. The pursuit response is more accurate when the target motion is predictable, such as with pendular motion.[113] Pursuit errors are reduced by modifying pursuit velocity and with small catch-up saccades. The combination of pursuit and catch-up saccades that appear at low stimulus velocities in patients with pursuit deficits is termed *cogwheel pursuit.* The ratio of eye velocity over target velocity (gain) or accuracy of pursuit is normally affected by target visibility (contrast), as well as drugs and fatigue.[79,87]

The pursuit response to sudden changes in target velocity has a short latency (80 to 130 milliseconds) and is composed of two general phases: *open loop* and *closed loop*[57] (Figure 36-9). Pursuit is initiated during the open-loop phase and is maintained during the closed-loop phase. The open-loop response is divided into an early and late component. The early component is a feed-forward phase that lasts for only 20 milliseconds. During this early phase, there is a rapid acceleration of the eye (40 to 100 degrees per second) that is in the correct direction but is independent of the stimulus velocity and initial retinal image position.[57] During the late open-loop component, which lasts 80 milliseconds, the initiation of pursuit depends strongly on target velocity and retinal image position.[13] Eye accelera-

tion is highest in response to targets imaged near the fovea and decreases sharply with increasing eccentricity up to 21 degrees. These open-loop components are calibrated by adaptation.[13]

Pursuit is maintained during the closed-loop phase, in response to negative feedback from retinal image velocity (retinal slip) and position, as well as an internal estimate of target velocity relative to the head. If the eye lags behind the stimulus, the retinal image velocity is not nulled, leaving a residual retinal image slip and position error away from the fovea. The pursuit system accelerates to correct both retinal position and velocity errors.[87] When pursuit is accurate and there is no retinal error, the eye continues to pursue the target without the eye-referenced signals. Pursuit is maintained by an internal estimate of target velocity or a head-referenced motion signal that is computed from a combination of retinal slip and an internal representation of eye velocity.[85] This can be demonstrated by attempting to fixate an ocular floater or a retinal afterimage that is located near the fovea. Attempts to foveate the stabilized retinal image lead to smooth following eye movements even though the retinal image is always motionless. The eye is tracking an internal correlate of its own motion that causes the target to appear to move with respect to the head.

Disconjugate Smooth Vergence Tracking. Foveal alignment of targets that move slowly in depth is maintained by smooth vergence following eye movements.[21,46] In addition to improving stereoscopic depth perception, smooth vergence provides information about changing target distance that affects size and depth perception.[12,31,43] Slow changes in smooth vergence respond to body sway and posture instability. Although smooth vergence responses can be inaccurate during natural rapid head movements, when the head is stationary, these response are accurate at temporal frequencies up to 1 Hz.[88] At higher frequencies, accuracy is reduced but can improve with small disparity stimuli.[21] It is likely that accuracy of smooth vergence is task dependent. Smooth vergence accuracy is more demanding for spatial localization tasks that lack depth cues other than for disparity compared with tasks that have ample monocular cues for direction and distance. The accuracy of smooth vergence responses to changing disparity improves with predictable target motion.[88] Stimuli for smooth vergence tracking include magnitude and velocity of retinal image disparity and perceptual cues to motion in depth,

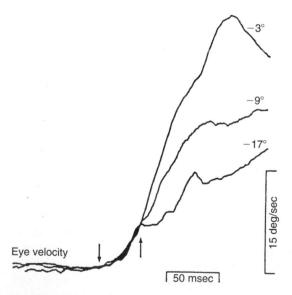

FIGURE 36-9 Eye velocity during the onset of pursuit to a 15-degree per second ramp target motion, the ramp of motion beginning at different eccentricities as indicated at the right portion of each trace. The velocity of the early component (indicated by *arrows*) was the same for all starting positions, but the velocity of the late component varied. (From Lisberger SG, Westbrook LE: *J Neurosci* 5:1662, 1985.)

including size looming.[21,68,88] Smooth vergence tracking is susceptible to fatigue and central nervous system suppressants.[88]

Adaptable Interactions between Smooth Pursuit and Smooth Vergence. In natural scenes, motion of a target in the frontoparallel plane is tracked binocularly with conjugate smooth pursuit. However, in conditions of anisometropia corrected with spectacle lenses, the image motion of the two eyes is magnified unequally, producing variations of binocular disparity that increase with target eccentricity from the optical centers of the lenses. Tracking motion of targets in the frontoparallel plane then requires both smooth pursuit and smooth vergence eye movements such that one eye moves more than the other does. The oculomotor system can adapt to the binocular disparity that changes predictably with eye position. Adaptation produces open-loop nonconjugate variations of heterophoria that compensate for the horizontal and vertical disparities produced by the unequal magnifiers during smooth vergence tracking responses.[98] After only 1 hour of pursuit tracking experience with anisometropic spectacles, one eye can be occluded and the two eyes continue to move unequally during monocular tracking.[99] The adapted heterophoria is coupled to vary with both eye position and direction of eye movement.[37]

Neurocontrol of Smooth Foveal Tracking

Smooth Pursuit Tracking System. Smooth following eye movements result from cortical motion signals in extrastriate cortex in areas MT and MST that lie in the superior temporal sulcus.[2,49] Area MT encodes speed and direction of visual stimuli in three dimensions relative to the eye. MT receives inputs from the primary visual cortex and projects visual inputs to area MST and the FEF. Cells in MST fire in concert with head-centric target movement (i.e., they combine retinal and efference copy signals).[75] Each hemisphere of the MST codes motion to the ipsilateral side. Cells have two types of visual motion sensitivity; they respond to motion of large-field patterns and small spots, but the direction preferences for the two stimulus types are opposite. The antidirectional large-field responses could facilitate pursuit of small targets moving against a far stationary field and motion parallax stimuli. Efference from MST and FEF projects ipsilaterally to the NOT to generate OKN and to the dorsal lateral pontine premotor nuclei (DLPN) for pursuit tracking.[33] Velocity signals are projected from DLPN to the floccular region and to the vermis lobules VI

and VII of the cerebellum.[33] The flocculus is thought to maintain pursuit eye movements during steady constant tracking, whereas the vermis is important when the target velocity changes or when pursuit is initiated. The role of the cerebellum is to sort out eye and head rotations in the tracking process and to sort out the ocular pursuit signal from visual and eye-head motor inputs.[76] From here, activity passes through parts of the vestibular nuclei, which perform the necessary neural integration of the velocity signal to a position signal that is sent to the eye muscle motor neurons.

Smooth Vergence Tracking System. Vergence results from the combined activity of intrinsic tonic activity, accommodative vergence, and responses to binocular disparity and perceived distance.[53] The sensory afferent signals for vergence (binocular disparity and blur) are coded in the primary visual cortex (area V1).[84] Some cells in V1 incorporate vergence to code egocentric (head-referenced) distance.[116] Cells in area MT and MST respond to retinal disparity and changing size.[24,59,94] Cells in the parietal cortex respond to motion in depth.[18] Efferent commands for vergence appear in cells in the FEF.[35] In the midbrain the premotor nucleus reticularis tegmenti pontis (NRTP), located just ventral to the rostral portion of the paramedian pontine reticular formation (PPRF), receives projections from the FEF and the SC.[34] The NRTP projects to the cerebellum and appears to be associated with vergence and accommodation.[78] The posterior interposed nucleus of the cerebellum projects to supraoculomotor regions that contain near response cells in the mesencephalic reticular formation.[63,128] The supraoculomotor nucleus contains both burst and tonic neurons.[66] The burst cells code velocity signals for smooth vergence, and the tonic neurons code position signals to maintain static vergence angle. Excitatory connections of the supraoculomotor nucleus project to the oculomotor nucleus, driving the medial recti.[47,129] Inhibitory connections project to the abducens nucleus to inhibit the lateral rectus muscle.[66] The supraoculomotor nucleus relays control of both accommodative and disparity vergence.[47]

Foveal Gaze Shifts: Target Selection and Foveal Acquisition

Rapid Conjugate Shifts of Gaze Direction (Saccadic Eye Movements). Saccades are fast, yoked eye movements that have a variety of functions.[10,118] They produce the quick phase of the VOR and OKN to prevent turning the eyes to their mechanical limits. They reflexively shift gaze in response to novel stimuli that appear unexpectedly away from the point of fixation. Saccades shift gaze during reading from one group of words to another. Saccades search novel scenes to assist in acquiring information. They also return gaze to remembered spatial locations. Two primary functions in all of these tasks are to move the eye rapidly from one position to another and then to maintain the new eye position. The rapid movement is controlled by a pulse-and-slide innervation pattern, and the position is maintained by a step innervation.

The separate components of innervation for the saccade match the characteristics of the plant (i.e., globe, muscles, fat, and suspensory tissues). The rapid changes in orbital position are made by the saccade at a cost of considerable energy. Saccade velocities can approach 1000 degrees per second.[10] Achieving these high velocities requires a phasic level of torque to overcome the viscosity of orbital tissues, most of which is in the muscles.[91] The phasic-torque is generated by a large brief force resulting from a pulse or burst of innervation. The torque is dissipated or absorbed by the muscles, so the force developed by the pulse of innervation does not reach the tendon (see Chapter 35). At the end of the saccade, a lower constant force resulting from a step innervation generates a tonic level of torque that is needed to hold the eye still against the elastic restoring forces of the orbital tissues.[118] The eye positions resulting from the pulse and step forces must be equal to produce rapid gaze shifts. Pulse-step mismatches result

in rapid and slow components of gaze shifts. For example, if the pulse is too small, the saccade slides (postsaccadic drift, called a *glissade*) to the new eye position at the end of the rapid phase of the saccade. The slide component is adaptable, as has been shown by long-term exposure to artificially imposed retinal image slip immediately after each saccade.[82] The adapted postsaccadic drift cannot be explained by an adjustment of the pulse/step ratio, suggesting that the slide innervation is an independent third component of saccadic control (pulse-slide-step). Slide innervation produces a phasic-torque in addition to the pulse component that adjusts the duration and velocity of the saccade so that its amplitude matches the position maintained by the step component.[82] The pulse, slide, and step are all under independent, cerebellar control, with the primary goal of protecting vision by preventing retinal slip and a secondary goal of making accurate saccades.

The amplitude of the saccade determines its dynamic properties (e.g., peak velocity, duration). The main sequence diagram plots these two dynamic parameters as a function of amplitude[8] (Figure 36-10). As saccade amplitude increases from 0.1 to 10 degrees, duration increases from 20 to 40 milliseconds and peak velocity increases from 10 to 400 degrees per second. Peak velocity saturates for saccades larger than 20 degrees, such that the amplitude of larger saccades increases primarily with duration. Abnormal saccade amplitudes (dysmetria) can be either too small (hypometric) or too large (hypermetric). Large gaze shifts are normally

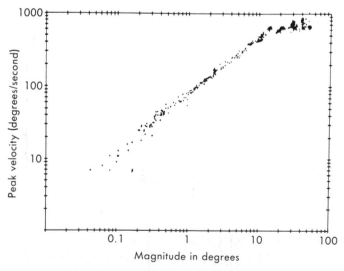

FIGURE 36-10   Main sequence diagram. Peak velocity is plotted against magnitude of human saccadic eye movements. (From Bahill AT, Clark MR, Stark L: *Math Biosci* 24:191, 1975.)

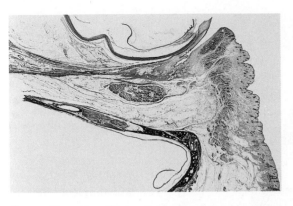

COLOR PLATE 1 Photomicrograph of the lower eyelid and inferior fornix at the level of the inferior rectus and inferior oblique muscles. The capsulopalpebral head of the inferior rectus muscle surrounds the inferior fornix as a portion of the suspensory apparatus of the inferior fornix. The palpebral conjunctiva adheres firmly to the underlying connective tissue, whereas the bulbar conjunctiva is less fixed.

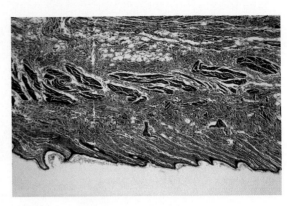

COLOR PLATE 2 Superficial musculoaponeurotic system investing orbicularis oculi muscle.

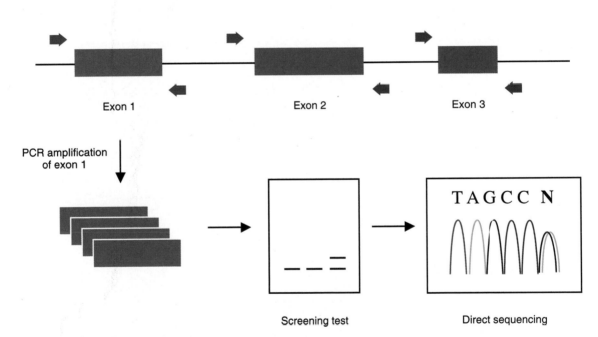

COLOR PLATE 3 Candidate gene screening. DNA comprising the three exons of a gene is amplified by the polymerase chain reaction. Each exon is then screened for mutations, and when a variant is detected, this is directly sequenced to identify the specific mutation.

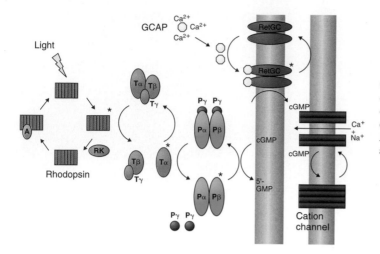

COLOR PLATE 4 Phototransduction cascade. *A,* Arrestin; *GCAP,* guanylate cyclase activating protein; *P,* phosphodiesterase; *RetGC,* retinal guanylate cyclase; *RK,* rhodopsin kinase; *T,* transducin; *,* activated.

COLOR PLATE 5 Rhodopsin mutations. Schematic diagram of the rhodopsin molecule indicating the location of mutations referred to in the text. The intradiscal domain is the site of the disulfide bond between cysteines 110 and 187, and retinal is linked to lysine 296 within the seventh transmembrane helix. The carboxy-terminus lies within the cytoplasm.

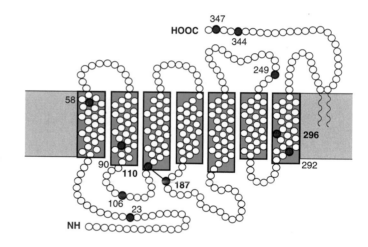

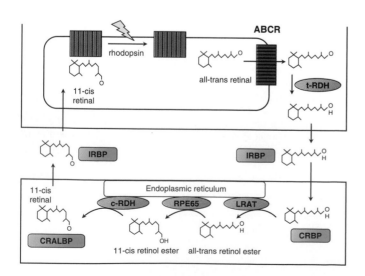

COLOR PLATE 6 Retinal (vitamin A) cycle. Recycling of retinal occurs via a complex cycle involving the photoreceptor outer segment (*top*) and the retinal pigment epithelial cell (*bottom*). Retinoid-binding proteins are shown in green and enzymes in lilac.

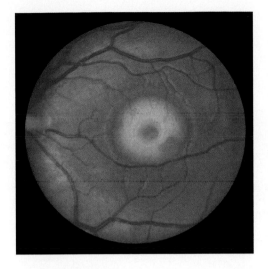

COLOR PLATE 7 Fundus photograph from a patient with Best vitelliform macular dystrophy (family SL76) and mutation Y85H (T357C) in the bestrophin gene. Arden index 1.3. (From Ponjavic V et al: *Ophthalmol Genetic* 20:251, 1999.)

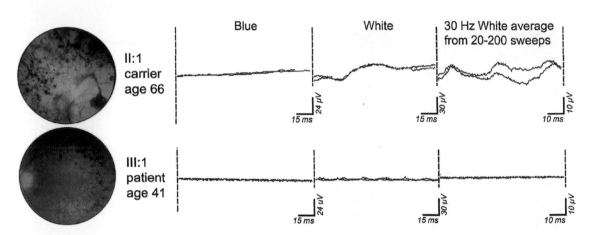

COLOR PLATE 8 Fundus appearance and full-field electroretinogram recordings from three patients with the exon 1 deletion in the *XLRS1* gene. (From Eksandh L: *Arch Ophthalmol* 118:1098, 2000.)

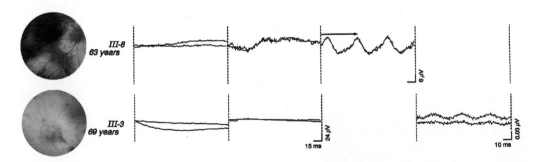

COLOR PLATE 9 Fundus photographs and full-field electroretinograms from a mother and a son in a family with X-linked retinitis pigmentosa with a microdeletion in the *RPGR* gene. *Right column:* (*Top*) Carrier shows attenuated vessels, spicular pigment, and atrophy of the central fundus. (*Bottom*) Patient shows typical bone-spicular pigmentary retinal degeneration. *Left column:* Shown are rod response to dim blue light, mixed cone-rod responses to white flashes, and isolated cone responses to a 30-Hz flickering light. (From Andréasson S et al: *Am J Ophthalmol* 124:95, 1997.)

Fundus appearance

Full-field ERG

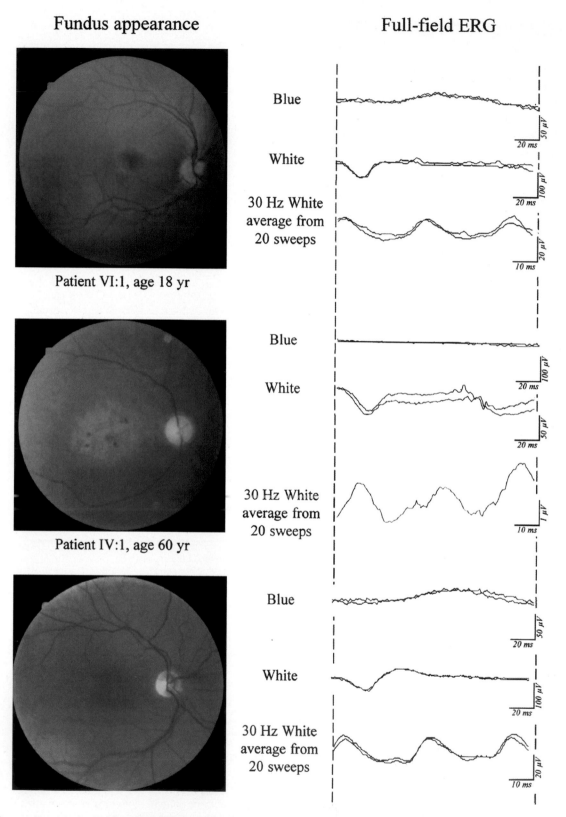

Patient VI:1, age 18 yr

Patient IV:1, age 60 yr

COLOR PLATE 10 Fundus photographs and full-field electroretinograms from two patients in a family with choroideremia and deletion of the entire *CHM* gene. (From Ponjavic V et al: *Ophthalmic Genetics* 16:143, 1995.)

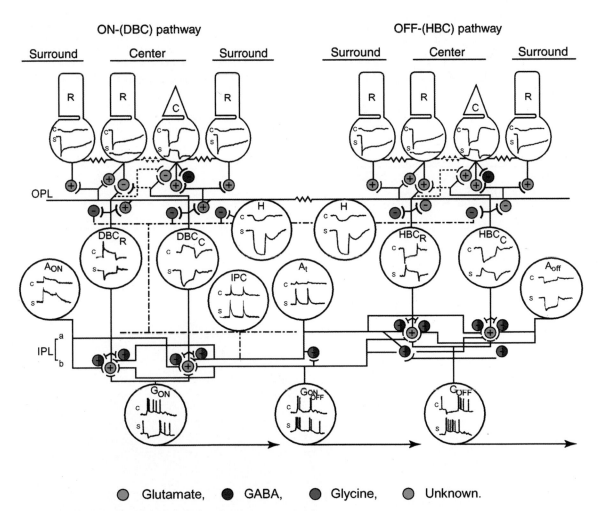

COLOR PLATE 11 Summary schematic diagram of major synapses that mediate CSARF of bipolar cells and ganglion cells in the retina. The left portion shows the ON or depolarizing bipolar cell (DBC) pathway and the right portion shows the OFF or hyperpolarizing bipolar cell (HBC) pathway. The upper trace in each cell is the voltage response to center illumination and the lower trace is the response to surround illumination. +, Sign-preserving chemical synapses; −, sign-inverting chemical synapses; and ⌇, electric synapses. Neurotransmitter color code: *blue*, glutamatergic; *red*, GABA-ergic; *green*, glycinergic; *yellow*, unknown. A_{OFF}, Sustained OFF amacrine cell; A_{ON}, sustained ON amacrine cell; A_{ON-OFF}, transient ON-OFF amacrine cell; C, cone; G_{OFF}, sustained OFF ganglion cell; G_{ON}, sustained ON ganglion cell; G_{ON-OFF}, ON-OFF ganglion cell; H, horizontal cell; HBC_R, HBC_C, DBC_R, *and* DBC_C, rod- and cone-dominated bipolar cells; IPC, interplexiform cell; IPL, inner plexiform layer; OPL, outer plexiform layer; R, rod.

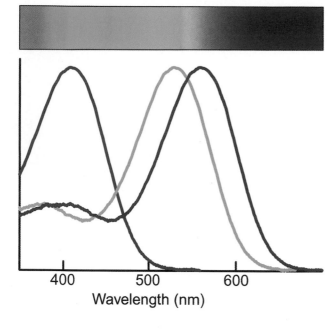

Color Plate 12 An example of absorption spectra of the three cone pigments plotted on a single axis. The l_{max} values of the S-, M-, and L-wavelength sensitive pigments are 414, 535, and 560 nm, respectively. The spectra are presented only in the so-called visible range of 400 to 700 nm. The absorption peaks are normalized to a common value. These spectra are measured from photoreceptor pigment molecules in solution. When measured in vivo, the spectra, and consequently the l_{max} values, are shifted to somewhat longer wavelengths as a result of the optical properties of various parts of the eye. Typically, cone spectral sensitivities are represented as the log of quantal sensitivity as a function of the wavelength of the light stimulus.

Color Plate 13 PA schematic representation of the boundaries of retinal color sensitivity in the retina of the right eye. The zones of color sensitivity for green, red, blue, and white are shown as nested overlapping shapes. It is generally assumed that relative cone sensitivities depend on the relative numbers of cells of a cone type in the retina, estimated to be 7% S-, 37% M-, and 56% L-wavelength sensing cones. The cone cells form a fixed mosaic pattern that influences the ability to discriminate color depending on location within the visual field.

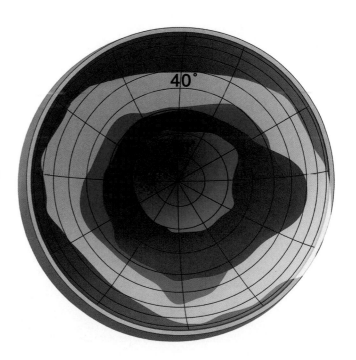

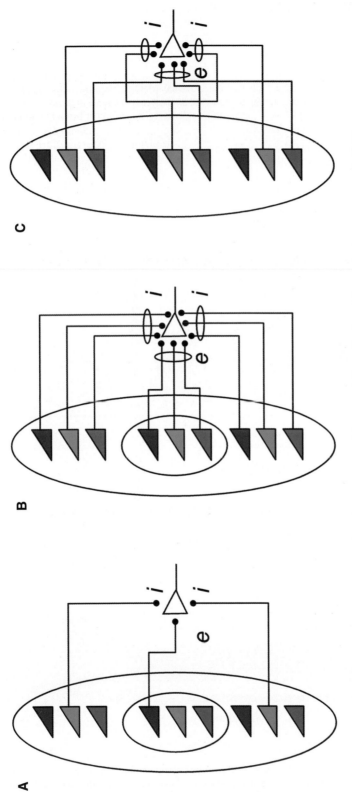

COLOR PLATE 14 A schematic representation of the potential contribution of three cone systems to receptive field neurons that display opponent mechanisms. **A,** The neuron (*open triangle*) receives excitatory inputs (*e*) from L-wavelength sensing cones (red) at its center and inhibitory inputs (*i*) from M-wavelength sensing cones (green) in the surround region. The type of receptive field neuron is terms a *red ON-center, green OFF-surround neuron.* **B,** The neuron receives L-, M-, and S-wavelength sensing (blue) cone excitatory inputs from the center portion and inhibitory inputs from the surround potion of its receptive field. This neuron represents a simple ON-center receptive field neuron and it responds primarily to spatial, not chromatic, attributes. **C,** The neuron receives S-wavelength sensing excitatory inputs and M-wavelength sensing inhibitory inputs from its entire receptive field. This neuron represents a blue ON-center, green OFF-surround receptive field neuron and responds only to color, not to spatial attributes.

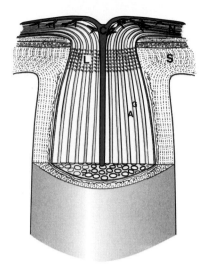

COLOR PLATE 15 Cross-sectional view of the optic nerve head. For simplification, only the central retinal artery (*C*) is shown. Retinal ganglion cell axons arising in the nerve fiber layer (*N*) course in bundles (*A*) within the optic nerve, separated by glia (*G*). The lamina cribrosa (*L*) is contiguous to the sclera (*S*).

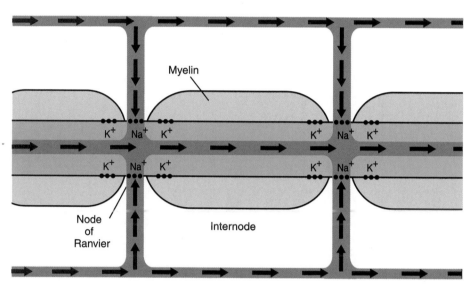

COLOR PLATE 16 Schematic of flow of positive ions (sodium) during the depolarization of a myelinated axon within the optic nerve. Sodium ions flow in through voltage-gated sodium channels at the nodes of Ranvier. Repolarization occurs through the efflux of potassium at voltage-gated potassium channels in the perinodal area.

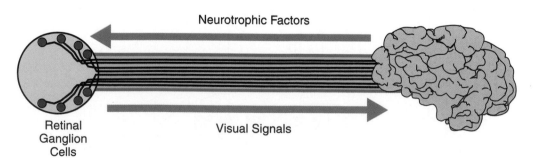

COLOR PLATE 17 Schematic of flow of visual information from the eye to the brain and of neurotrophic factors from the brain to the eye. Both occur by means of the axons of retinal ganglion cells, the former through electrical conduction, the latter through retrograde axonal transport.

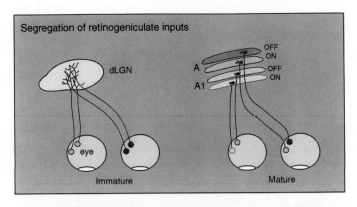

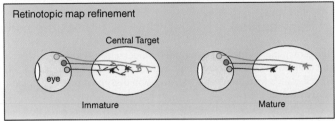

COLOR PLATE 18 The projection of retinal ganglion cells are organized into at least three distinct patterns. In the adult, projections from the two eyes to the dorsal lateral geniculate nucleus (dLGN) are segregated into eye-specific layers; in some animals, each eye layer is divided into ON and OFF sublaminas. The number of eye-specific layers varies from species to species; shown here are two eye layers in the ferret: layer A, which receives contralateral eye input, and layer A1, which is innervated by the ipsilateral eye. Furthermore, neighboring retinal ganglion cells project topographically to their targets, the superior colliculus, and the dLGN. During development, these projections patterns are not well defined and undergo a period of refinement before achieving the precision seen in the adult.

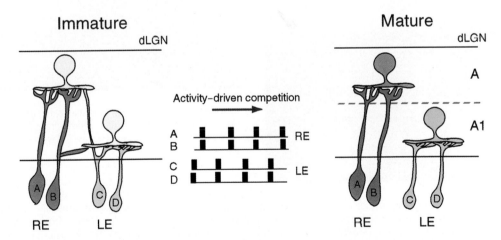

COLOR PLATE 19 An example of how synchronous versus asynchronous activity could lead to the segregation of retinal inputs to the dorsal lateral geniculate nucleus (dLGN). Initially, individual dLGN neurons (shown here for the dLGN in the left hemisphere) are innervated by ganglion cells from the two eyes. *A* and *B*, Right eye (*RE*). *C* and *D*, Left eye (*LE*). Although the spontaneous activity of cells *A* and *B* are synchronized, their activity is not correlated with the activity of cells *C* and *D*. Based on Hebbian mechanisms, the correlated firing of cells *A* and *B* will lead to the strengthening of their inputs and the weakening of the spurious input from *C*. Similarly, connections from *C* and *D* are costrengthened at the expense of cell *B*. By maturity, the projections of cells from the two eyes are segregated into eye-specific layers A and A1.

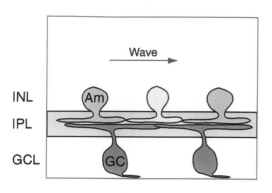
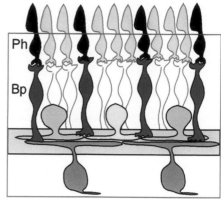

Early network   Mature network

COLOR PLATE 20 Retinogeniculate connections remodel concurrently with the assembly of the retinal circuitry. Retinal waves appear when connections between amacrine cells (*Am*) and ganglion cells (*GC*) form in the inner plexiform layer (*IPL*). As bipolar cell inputs form, waves persist, but soon disappear on photoreceptor (*Ph*) maturation. *GCL,* Ganglion cell layer; *INL,* inner nuclear layer.

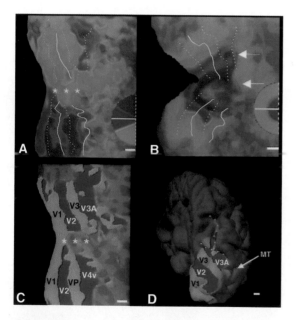

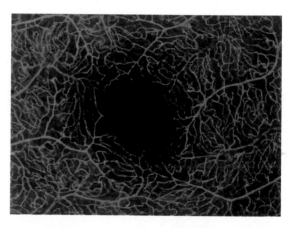

COLOR PLATE 22 Foveal avascular zone. Immunohistochemical stain of the vascular endothelium in the retina. Note the central foveal avascular zone is devoid of both larger vessels and capillaries.

COLOR PLATE 21 Maps of human visual areas, generated by functional imaging using retinotopically varying stimuli. The maps in **A** to **C** are flattened views of a right hemisphere, as if the cortex had been removed from the brainstem and flattened. Dorsal is to the top of each map, and ventral is to the bottom. In making the reconstructions, a cut (visible to the left of each figure) was made along the horizontal meridian representation of V1 to relieve the curvature of the cortical mantle and reduce distortion. **A,** A map of cortical response plotted as a function of the polar angle of an annular stimulus (see Chapter 30). **B,** A map of cortical response as a function of eccentricity of the annulus. In each case, *dashed* and *solid lines* show the boundaries of cortical areas, and the *asterisks* mark the location of the foveal representation. **C,** A map of local visual field sign, where yellow is a mirror-image representation, like V1, and blue is a non–mirror-image representation, like V2. Borders of V1, V2, V3/VP, and V3A can be identified in this fashion. **D,** The borders of the cortical areas determined from receptive field sign projected onto the three-dimensional reconstruction of the brain, showing the relationship of the cortical areas to the sulci and gyri. (Bars = 1 mm.) (From Tootell RB et al: *J Neurosci* 17:7060, 1997.)

accomplished with a sequence of hypometric saccades that are composed of a series of short-latency corrective saccades in the same direction.[10] The normal latency of a saccade to an unpredictable stimulus is 180 to 200 milliseconds.[14] However, corrective saccades occur with shorter latencies (100 to 150 milliseconds). Saccade latency can be reduced by a blank or gap interval before the saccade, resulting in an express saccade with latencies less than 100 milliseconds.[30] Saccade latencies to predictable target changes, such as occur in a tennis match, can be reduced to zero.[113]

Although saccades are too brief to use visual feedback during their response, they do use fast internal feedback based on an internal representation of eye position (efference copy signal) that helps control the position of the eye on a moment-to-moment basis.[90] Thus saccadic eye movements are not ballistic in that they are guided by extraretinal information during their flight. The goal of the saccade is to reach a specified direction in head-centric space. Normally, the perceived head-centric direction of a target does not change when the eye changes position. However, spectacle refractive corrections that magnify or minify the retinal image produce changes in perceived direction with eye position. Because the entrance pupil of the eye translates when the eye rotates, the eye views a nonfoveal eccentric target through a different part of the lens before the saccade than after the saccade, when the target is viewed directly along the line of sight. The prismatic power of the lens increases with distance from the optical center of the lens such that when viewing a target through a magnifier, the saccade amplitude needed to fixate an eccentric target is larger than the gaze eccentricity sensed before the saccade. Saccades are controlled by a feed-forward system that does not use visual feedback during the motor response. Consequently, initial saccadic responses to visual distortion produced by the magnifier are hypometric. However, using position errors after the saccade, the system adapts rapidly (within 70 trials) to minimize its errors.[26] In cases of anisometropia in which the retinal images are magnified unequally by the spectacle refractive correction, the saccadic system adapts to produce unequal or disconjugate saccades that align both visual axes with common fixation targets.[27,54,81] The same adaptive process is likely to calibrate the conjugate saccades and maintain that calibration throughout life in spite of developmental growth factors and injury.

Disconjugate Shifts of Gaze Distance (Near Response in Symmetric Convergence). Large abrupt shifts in viewing distance stimulate adjustments of several motor systems, including accommodation, convergence, and pupil constriction.[46] Separate control systems initiate and complete these responses.[107] Initially, the abrupt adjustments are controlled by feed-forward systems that do not use visual feedback until the responses are nearly completed. However, they are guided by fast feedback from efference copy signals to monitor both the starting point of the near response and the accuracy of its end point.[102,127] Visual feedback is unavailable during the response because the blur and disparity cues are too large at the beginning of the gaze shift to be sensed accurately. The motor responses are initiated by high-level cues for perceived distance and by voluntary shifts of attention. Retinal cues from blur and disparity are used as feedback only to refine the responses once the stimuli are reduced to amplitudes that lie within the range of visual sensitivity (i.e., as the eyes approach alignment at their new destination). The three motor systems are synchronized or coordinated with one another by cross-links. When they approach their new target destination, accommodation and convergence use visual feedback to refine their response.

The cross-couplings are demonstrated by opening the feedback loop for one motor system while stimulating a coupled motor system that is under closed-loop control. For example, accommodative convergence, measured during monocular occlusion, increases linearly with changes in accommodation stimulated by blur.[5,73] Similarly, convergence accommodation, measured during binocular viewing through pinhole pupils, increases linearly with changes in convergence stimulated by disparity.[29] The pupil constricts with changes in either accommodation or convergence to improve the clarity of near objects.[124] These interactions are greater during the dynamic changes in the near response than during the static end point of the response.[99]

The cross-couplings between accommodation and convergence are illustrated with a heuristic model[99] (Figure 36-11). Three of the Maddox components are represented in the model by an adaptable slow tonic component: the cross-links between accommodation and convergence, disparity-driven vergence, and blur-driven accommodation (fast phasic components).[58] The enhanced gain of the cross-link interactions associated with dynamic stimulation of vergence and accommodation results from the stimulation of the cross-links by the

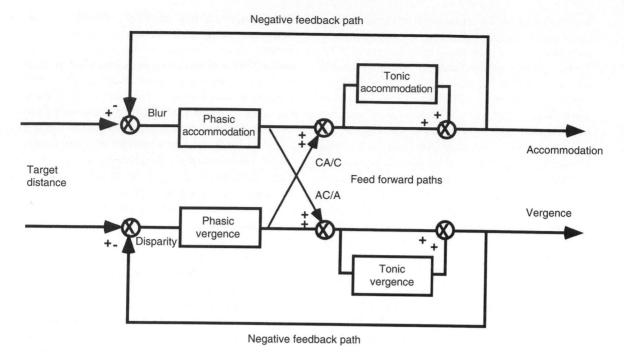

FIGURE 36-11 Model of cross-link interactions between vergence and accommodation. A fast phasic system drives the cross-links from accommodation to convergence (*AC/A*) and from convergence to accommodation (*CA/C*). The slow tonic system adapts to the faster phasic system and gradually replaces it. Cross-link innervation is reduced when the tonic system reduces the load on the fast phasic system. (From Kotulak J, Schor CM: *Invest Ophthal Vis Sci* 27:544, 1986.)

phasic, but not the tonic, components. When accommodation or convergence is stimulated, the faster transient-phasic system responds first, but it does not sustain its response. The slower and more sustained adaptable tonic system gradually takes over the load of keeping the eyes aligned and focused by resetting the level of tonic activity. Because the cross-links are mainly stimulated by the phasic component, accommodative vergence and vergence accommodation are stimulated more during the dynamic response than during steady fixation when the tonic components control eye alignment and focus.

Traditionally, only the horizontal component of vergence has been considered as part of the near response. However, vertical vergence and cyclovergence must also be adjusted during the near response to optimize the sensory stimulus for binocular vision.[4,101,117,119,125] The primary goal of the near response is to minimize large changes in horizontal and vertical disparities and cyclodisparities at the fovea that normally accompany large shifts in viewing distance. Horizontal disparities arise from targets that are nearer or farther than the convergence distance, assuming that the horopter equals the Vieth-Muller circle. The isovergence circle describes the locus of points that stimulates a constant vergence angle in all directions of gaze, and it is equivalent to the Vieth-Muller circle that was described in Chapter 19 (see Figures 19-4 and 36-2).[80] Convergence and divergence stimuli lie closer or farther, respectively, from the isovergence circle. Vertical disparities arise from targets in tertiary gaze directions at finite viewing distances because these targets lie closer to one eye than the other and their retinal images have unequal size and vertical eccentricity (vertical disparity) (Figure 36-12). Torsional disparities arise from elevated targets at finite viewing distances, because during convergence, Listing's law predicts that the horizontal meridians of the two eyes will be extorted in upward gaze and intorted in downward gaze.[117] These torsional eye postures produce incyclodisparity in upward gaze and excyclodisparity in downward gaze. With large shifts of viewing distance, horizontal and vertical disparities and cyclodisparities can exceed the stimulus operating range for continuous feedback control of disparity

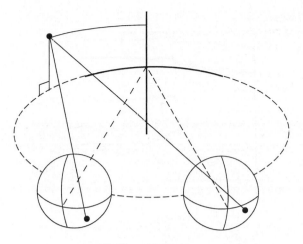

FIGURE 36-12 For convergence at a finite viewing distance, points in tertiary directions subtend unequal vertical visual angles at the two eyes, which produce vertical disparities.

---

vergence. Initially, the near response is stimulated by perceived distance, and voluntary changes in horizontal vergence respond without disparity feedback in feed-forward control. Unlike horizontal vergence, neither vertical vergence nor cyclovergence is normally under voluntary control. They participate in the near response through cross-couplings with motor responses that are under voluntary control. This allows potential vertical and torsional eye alignment errors to be reduced during the near response without feedback from retinal image disparity.

Empirical measures demonstrate that the gains for the three coupling relationships for horizontal and vertical vergence and cyclovergence are optimal for reducing disparity at the fovea to zero during the open-loop phase of the near response.[99,101,111,125] The tuned coupling gains for all three vergence components of the near response are the product of neural plasticity that adapts each of these cross-couplings to optimize binocular sensory functions.[67,71,100] Plasticity also exists for other couplings. For example, vertical vergence and cyclovergence can both be adapted to vary with head roll.[61,62] The coupling of pupil constriction with accommodation and convergence may also be under adaptive control. The pupil constriction component of the near response does not appear until the end of the second decade of life, suggesting that it responds to accommodative errors resulting from the aging loss of accommodative amplitude.[124] The pupil constriction component of the near response is an attempt to restore clarity of the near retinal image.

Interactions between Conjugate and Disconjugate Eye Movements (Asymmetric Vergence). In natural viewing conditions, it is rare for the eyes to converge symmetrically from one distance to another. Gaze usually is shifted between targets located at different directions and distances from the head. Rapid gaze shifts to these targets require a combination of conjugate saccades and disjunctive vergence. In asymmetric convergence the velocity of disparity vergence, accommodative vergence, and accommodation are enhanced when accompanied by gaze shifting saccades.[22,28,105] Without the saccade, symmetric vergence responses are sluggish, reaching velocities of only 10 degrees per second.[88] Symmetric vergence has a latency of 160 milliseconds and a response time of approximately 1 second. Similarly, accommodation that is not accompanied by a saccade has a peak velocity of only 4 degrees per second, a latency of approximately 300 to 400 milliseconds, and a response time of approximately 1 second. However, when accompanied by a saccade, vergence velocity approaches 50 degrees per second and accommodation velocity approaches 8 to 9 degrees per second.[22,105] Latency of accommodation accompanied by saccades is also reduced by 50%, so the accommodative response is triggered in synchrony with the saccade that has a latency of only 200 milliseconds. As shown in Figure 36-13, response times for both accommodation and accommodative vergence are reduced dramatically when accompanied by saccades. Figure 36-14 compares symmetric and asymmetric disparity vergence. The high-velocity asymmetric vergence appears to result in part from yoked saccades of unequal amplitude. These unequal saccades result from an asynchronous onset of binocular saccades. The abducting saccade begins before the adducting saccade, causing a brief divergence.[60,126] Additional accelerated vergence and accommodation responses appear to be triggered with the saccade.[64,65,126] Both the vergence and accommodation responses continue after the completion of the saccade, but overall the responses are completed in less time than when not accompanied by a saccade.

Neurocontrol of Foveal Gaze Shifts

Saccadic Gaze Shifting System. The FEF mediate voluntary control of contralateral saccades. The FEF is active whether or not saccades occur.[39] The

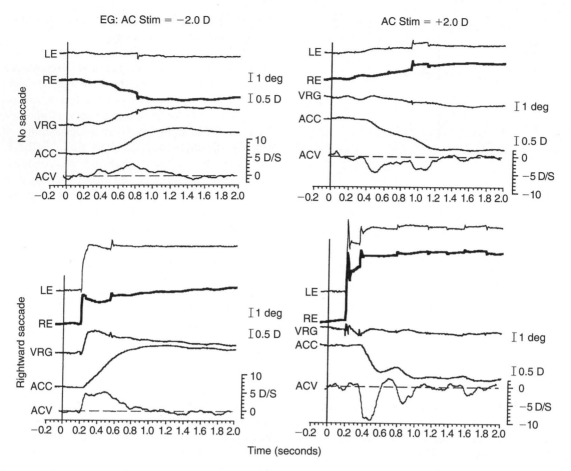

Figure 36-13 Examples of eye movement and accommodation traces during 6-degree rightward saccade (*bottom panels*) and no saccade (*top panels*) conditions. (*Left panel,* trials requiring *increased* accommodation; *right panel,* trials requiring *decreased* accommodation.) Time 0 corresponds to accommodation stimulation (*AC Stim*) onset. The following conventions apply: *ACC,* Accommodation (degrees); *ACV,* accommodation velocity (degrees/sec), derivative of ACC; *LE,* left (viewing) eye position; *RE,* right (nonviewing) eye position; *VRG,* vergence position (LE-RE). (Modified from Schor CM et al: *Vision Res* 39:3769, 1999.)

activity is related to visual attention, and when saccades occur, the related activity in the FEF precedes them by 50 milliseconds. The surface of the FEF has a coarse retinotopic organization. Stimulation of a particular area causes a saccade to change eye position in a specific direction and amplitude. These cells are active before saccades to certain regions of visual space. These regions are called the *movement field* of the cell, and they are analogous to the receptive fields of sensory neurons in the visual cortex. Stimulation of FEF cells in one hemisphere causes conjugate saccades to the contralateral side. Vertical saccades require stimulation of both hemispheres of the FEF. Modalities that can stimulate movement fields include vision, audition, and touch. The FEF project two main efferent pathways

for the control of saccades. One projection is to the SC. The other projection is to the midbrain, to the PPRF and the rostral interstitial medial longitudinal fasciculus (riMLF) for the control of horizontal and vertical saccades, respectively.[40,112] The fibers from the FEF descend to the ipsilateral SC and cross the midline to the contralateral PPRF. Neither the SC nor FEF are required exclusively to generate saccades. Either one of them can be ablated without abolishing saccades; however, if both are ablated, saccades are no longer possible. The function of the SC is to represent intended gaze direction resulting from combinations of head and eye position. Stimulation of a specific region in the intermediate layers of the colliculus can result in several combinations of head and eye position that achieve the

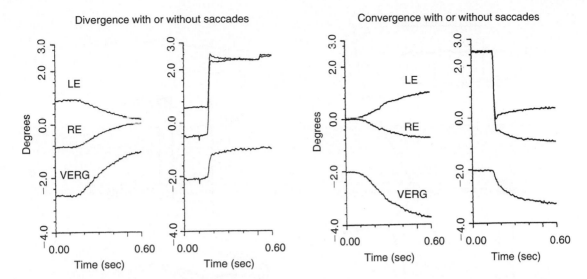

FIGURE 36-14 Vergence changes with or without an accompanying saccade, shown for a rhesus monkey. Vergence traces (right-left eye position) are offset for clarity. Convergence is negative. Note the increase in vergence velocity when a saccade is conjoined with vergence. The facilitation is greater for divergence because of the inherent divergence associated with horizontal saccades. *LE,* Left eye; *RE,* right eye; *VERG,* vergence change. (From Leigh JR, Zee DS: *The neurology of eye movements,* ed 3, Oxford, 1999, Oxford University Press.)

same gaze direction relative to the body.[32] Cells in the SC respond to all sensory modalities, including vision, audition, and touch. The spatial locations of all of these sensory stimuli are mapped in the colliculus relative to the fovea. As with the FEF, stimulation of one SC causes a conjugate saccade to the contralateral side; stimulation of both sides is necessary to evoke purely vertical saccades.

The output of the SC and FEF project to two premotor nuclei, the PPRF and the riMLF, which shape the velocity and amplitude of horizontal and vertical components of saccades, respectively.[40,49] The PPRF projects to the ipsilateral abducens nucleus, which contains motoneurons that innervate the ipsilateral lateral rectus muscle and interneurons that project to the contralateral oculomotor nucleus to innervate the medial rectus muscle. The PPRF also projects inhibitory connections to the contralateral PPRF and vestibular nucleus to reduce innervation of the antagonist during a saccade. The riMLF projects to the ipsilateral trochlear nucleus (IV) and to both oculomotor nuclei (III). Four types of neurons, including burst cells, tonic cells, burst-tonic cells, and pause cells, control saccades in several premotor sites. The pulse component of the saccade is controlled by medium-lead burst neurons (MLB). Long-lead burst neurons discharge up to 200 milliseconds before the saccade and receive input from the SC and FEF. They drive

MLB that begin discharging at a high frequency (300 to 400 spikes per second) immediately at the beginning of the saccade and throughout its duration. Duration of MLB activity ranges from 10 to 80 milliseconds. They project to the motor nuclei and control pulse duration and firing frequency, which determine saccade duration and velocity. Inhibitory burst neurons inhibit antagonist muscles by suppressing neurons in the contralateral abducens nucleus.

Initiation of the pulse is gated by the omnipause neuron (OPN), which is located in the nucleus of the dorsal raphe, below the abducens nucleus (Figure 36-15). Normally, the OPNs prevent saccades by constantly inhibiting burst cells. The OPN discharges continuously except immediately before and during saccades, when they pause. OPNs engage the saccade by releasing their inhibition of the burst cells. The same OPNs inhibit saccades in all directions.

On completion of the saccade, the new eye position is held by the discharge step of the tonic cell. Integrating the pulse derives the discharge rate of the premotor-tonic cell. At least two sites are known to integrate horizontal pulses: the medial vestibular nuclei and the nucleus prepositus hypoglossi. Pulses for vertical saccades are integrated in the interstitial nucleus of Cajal (INC). The flocculus of the cerebellum is also involved in integrating the velocity

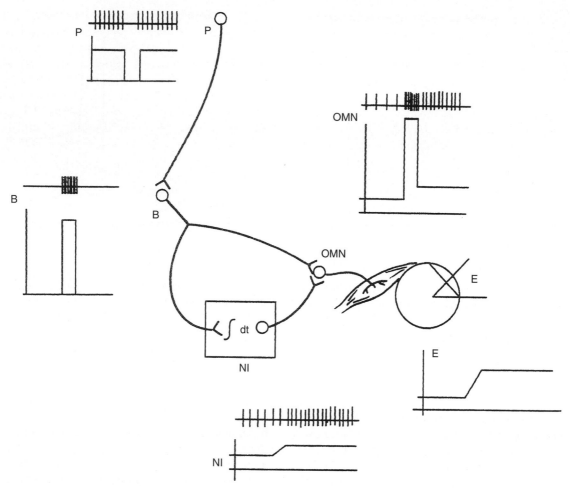

FIGURE 36-15 The relationship among omnipause cells (*P*), burst cells (*B*), and cells of the neural integrator (*NI*) in the generation of the saccadic pulse and step. Omnipause cells cease discharging just before each saccade, allowing the burst cells to generate the pulse. The pulse is integrated by the neural integrator to produce the step. The pulse and step combine to produce the innervational change on the ocular motoneurons (*OMN*) that produces the saccadic eye movement (*E*). Vertical lines represent individual discharges of neurons. Underneath the schematized neural (spike) discharge is a plot of discharge rate versus time. (From Leigh JR, Zee DS: *The neurology of eye movements*, ed 3, Oxford, 1999, Oxford University Press.)

signals to position signals controlling eye movements. Some anomalies that occur appear to result from lesions of the integrator. In these cases the eyes make a saccade and then drift back to primary position. Affected patients are unable to hold fixation away from primary position, and a jerk gaze nystagmus develops in which the slow-phase drift of the eyes is toward primary position and the fast-phase saccade is toward the desired eccentric gaze direction. Combined eye position and velocity signals are carried by burst-tonic neurons, which are active during ipsilateral saccades and inhibited during contralateral saccades.

Vergence Gaze Shifting System: The Near Triad and Interactions with Saccades. The supraoculomotor nucleus in the mesencephalic reticular formation contains near response cells. This is a heterogeneous population made up of cells that respond to accommodative stimuli or vergence stimuli or a combination of accommodation and vergence stimuli.[47,65,129] This nucleus contains burst, tonic, and burst-tonic cells that are characteristic of premotor nuclei for saccades. Velocity signals related to disparity stimuli activate burst cells, and a position signal from tonic innervation is derived by integration of the burst cell activity. These cells are believed to provide velocity and position signals to the medial rectus motoneurons in the control of vergence, as well as commands to the Edinger-Westphal nucleus to stimulate accommodation.[36] The Edinger-Westphal nucleus, located at the rostral portion of the midbrain at the oculomotor nucleus, contains parasympathetic motor neurons that project to the ciliary muscle and drive accommodation.[36] Each hemisphere of the Edinger-Westphal nucleus projects to its ipsilateral eye. Parasympathetic outflow of the Edinger-Westphal nucleus also results in miosis (pupillary contraction). Inhibition of the Edinger-Westphal nucleus causes pupil dilation.

Saccades enhance the velocity of both vergence and accommodation. Current models of saccade-vergence interactions suggest that OPNs in the midbrain gate the activity of both saccade bursters and vergence bursters.[126] Accelerated vergence caused by saccadic facilitation results from a release from inhibition of vergence bursters by reduced firing of the OPNs, which share their inhibition with saccadic and near response bursters. This facilitation is correlated with an augmentation of firing rate of a subset of convergence burst neurons of the near response cells.[64,65] This model has been developed further to include the potential for saccadic facilitation of accommodation.[64,65] Because near response cells provide innervation for both accommodation and vergence, release of inhibition from OPNs augments activity of both accommodation and vergence when associated with saccades.[105] This augmentation would not only enhance velocity of the near response but would also gate or synchronize innervation for vergence and accommodation with saccades.

NEUROLOGIC DISORDERS OF THE OCULOMOTOR SYSTEM

Neurologic disorders have greater variability across individuals than is found for the typical oculomotor system. The sources of variability come from the location and extent of lesions, associated anomalies or syndromes, different sources or causes of the problem, history of prior treatment interventions, and adaptive responses that attempt to compensate for the disorder. A multiperspective classification can reflect this individual variation. It views the anomaly in different ways and highlights different types of information about the condition. Its versatility describes the range of anomalous behaviors that may develop as a function of various combinations of causal factors. The pattern of associated conditions or syndromes facilitates estimating the prognosis for cosmetic and functional correction. Oculomotor disorders are classified in terms of behavioral descriptions, etiology, and neuroanatomic sites of involvement. Behavioral categories can be descriptive, such as the magnitude and direction of a strabismus (an eye turn), gaze restrictions, saccadic disorders, and nystagmus. They can also be described by an associated cluster of anomalies that collectively characterize a disease (syndrome). Categories of etiology include congenital, developmental, and acquired. Congenital disorders appear in early infancy (younger than 18 months). Developmental anomalies can result from interference of normal sensory-motor interactions during the first 6 years of life that constitute the critical period for visual development. Both congenital and developmental disorders are associated with anomalies throughout the oculomotor pathways, including sensory or afferent components of the visual system, and they are classified in terms of syndromes. Acquired disorders can result from trauma or disease and they are classified in terms of specific anatomic sites of involvement and by syndromes.[53]

Strabismus

Nonparalytic strabismus falls into both congenital and developmental categories. A strabismus or tropia describes a misalignment of the two eyes that is not corrected by disparity vergence during binocular fixation. In congenital and developmental forms of strabismus, the eye turn is usually concomitant, meaning that its amplitude does not vary with direction of gaze with either eye fixating. Nonparalytic strabismus usually is a horizontal deviation, where convergent and divergent eye turns are referred to as *esotropia* and *exotropia*, respectively. Esotropia is more common than exotropia in childhood. Infantile or early-onset esotropia appears within the first 18 months of life and is associated with two forms of nystagmus that include LN and asymmetric OKN, as well as cog-wheel temporalward pursuits (asymmetric pursuit), which were described earlier in this chapter. Esotropia is also associated with a vertical misalignment of the eyes when one eye is occluded, which is referred to as *dissociated vertical deviation* (DVD). When either the right or left eye is occluded, the covered eye rotates upward. This distinguishes DVD from a vertical strabismus in which one of the two eyes remains elevated with respect to the position of the other eye, independent of which eye is fixating. The combination of LN, asymmetric OKN, asymmetric pursuit, and DVD is termed *infantile strabismus syndrome*.[104] The presence of this syndrome in an adult is a retrospective indicator of an early age of onset for a strabismus. The early onset of eye misalignment prevents sensory fusion and causes one eye to be suppressed. This disrupts the development of both monocular and binocular sensory functions and can lead to the development of amblyopia, anomalous correspondence, and stereoblindness (see Chapter 19). Accommodative esotropia is a developmental form of nonparalytic strabismus that results from either large, uncorrected hyperopic refractive errors or abnormally large interactions between the cross-coupling of accommodation and convergence. Uncorrected hyperopia produces a mismatch between the stimulus between accommodation and convergence. Excessive convergence is caused by accommodative attempts to clear the retinal image and the cross-coupling between accommodation and convergence. The disparity-divergence system is unable to align the eyes and compensate for the accommodative esotropia.

Acquired strabismus usually results from lesions in the brainstem produced by trauma or disease that affect the integrity of the cranial nerves of the final common pathway. The lesions result in muscle palsies that cause deviations between the two visual axes that increase as gaze is directed into the field of action of the affected muscle (paralytic strabismus). The deviation of the paretic eye when the normal eye fixates (primary deviation) usually is smaller than the deviation of the normal eye when the paretic eye fixates (secondary deviation). This nonconcomitant variation of eye turn is a diagnostic feature of paralytic strabismus. Lesions of the third, fourth, and sixth nerves are called *complete ophthalmoplegia, trochlear palsy,* and *abducens palsy,* respectively. Ophthalmoplegia describes an immobilized eye resulting from paresis of several muscles innervated by the oculomotor nucleus, including the medial rectus, vertical recti, and inferior oblique muscles, as well as the levator of the lid. It is characterized by a fixed-dilated pupil and ptosis, with the eye remaining in a downward and abducted position. Abducens palsy is characterized by an esotropia that increases during abduction of the affected eye. Trochlear palsy is characterized by a hyperdeviation of the affected eye that increases during adduction and depression of the affected eye and head tilt to the side of the affected eye.

Gaze Restrictions

Lesions in premotor nuclei, supranuclear, and cortical sites restrict movements of both eyes. The MLF is the fiber bundle that interconnects premotor regions with the III, IV, and VI cranial nuclei. Any lesion that disconnects these fibers from the premotor to the motor nuclei is called *ophthalmoplegia* (Figure 36-16). Lesions caudal to the oculomotor nucleus cause exotropia and failure of adduction; however, convergence of the two eyes is spared. *Internuclear ophthalmoplegia* (INO) refers to an adduction failure caused by disruption of interneuron projections from the abducens nucleus to the contralateral oculomotor nerve nucleus. The affected eye is unable to adduct to the contralateral side, and the eye drifts in the temporalward direction. Sparing of convergence distinguishes this lesion from complete ophthalmoplegia. Patients with INO can develop a convergence nystagmus in an attempt to bring the exotropic eye into primary gaze. INO is classified as *anterior* if only adduction of one eye is affected and as *posterior* if both adduction of one eye and abduction of the other eye are affected. *One-and-a-half syndrome* is a combination of horizontal gaze palsy and INO that is caused by a lesion of the abducens (affecting the ipsilateral lateral rectus) and interneurons projecting from both abducens nuclei (affecting the ipsilateral and contralateral medial recti).

Foville syndrome is a unilateral lesion at or near the abducens nucleus that causes conjugate gaze palsy, contralateral limb paralysis, and ipsilateral facial paralysis. Lesions of the abducens nucleus block horizontal movement of both eyes to the side of the lesion because interneurons that project from the abducens nucleus to the contralateral oculomotor nucleus are also affected. Because the abducens is the final common pathway for all lateral conjugate eye movements, lesions there affect saccades, pursuit, and VOR. Lesions in the PPRF limit only horizontal saccades of both eyes to the ipsilateral side and cause drift of the eyes to the contralateral side. Lesions of the DLPN affect only horizontal pursuit toward the side of the lesion.

Lesions rostral to the oculomotor nucleus cause paralysis of vertical gaze (Parinaud syndrome) and failure of convergence but retention of normal horizontal gaze ability. Parinaud syndrome occurs with lesions in the vicinity of the riMLF and INC and affects all vertical eye movements, including saccades. It often results from tumors of the pineal gland that compress the SC and pretectal structures. Unilateral lesions in this area may also cause skew deviations in

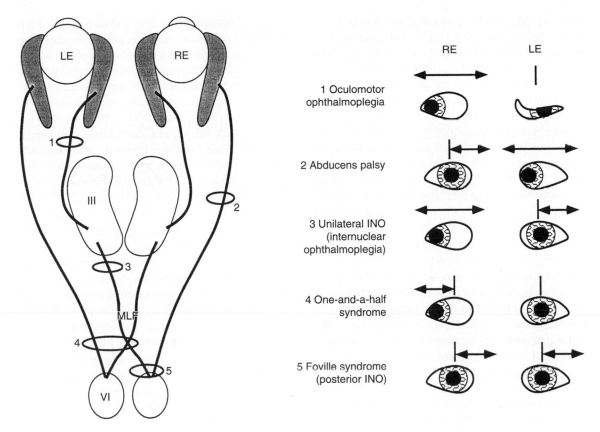

FIGURE 36-16 Subcortical disorders: gaze palsies. Eye positions shown reflect attempted right gaze in each case, but the arrows show the full range of horizontal gaze for each eye. *LE,* Left eye; *MLF,* medial longitudinal fasciculus; *RE,* right eye; *III,* oculomotor; *VI,* abducens. (Drawing by Scott B. Stevenson; courtesy University of Houston.)

which there is a vertical deviation of one eye. Unilateral lesions can also cause unilateral nystagmus, in which the affected eye has a slow upward drift and fast downward saccade (downbeat nystagmus).

Cortical lesions produce gaze restrictions of both saccades and pursuits. Lesions of the primary visual cortex produce blindness in the corresponding parts of the visual field contralateral to the lesion (scotoma). Pursuit and saccade targets presented in the scotoma are invisible to the patient. If the entire visual cortex in one hemisphere is destroyed, the vision near the fovea may be intact (macular sparing), allowing the patient to track targets over the full range of eye movements. As in the primary visual cortex, lesions in MT produce contralateral scotomas of the visual field. Saccades to fixed targets may be accurate, but pursuit responses to moving targets presented in the affected field will be absent or deficient. Lesions in MST produce visual effects similar to MT, but they also produce a unidirectional pursuit deficit for targets in both vi-

sual hemifields moving toward the side of the lesion. Lesions in the PP cortex produce attentional deficits, which make pursuit and saccades to small targets more difficult than larger ones. Lesions of the FEF produce a deficit for horizontal pursuit and OKN toward the side of the lesion and saccades to the contralateral side. Lesions to the SEF impair memory-guided saccades.

Saccade Disorders

Saccade disorders consist of abnormal metrics (velocity and amplitude) and inappropriate, spontaneous saccades that take the eye away from the target during attempted fixation. Saccades are classified as too fast or slow if their velocity does not fall within the main sequence plot of velocity versus amplitude (see Figure 36-10). However, saccade velocity may be normal while its amplitude is in error. If saccades are too small, the eye could start to make a large saccade and would accelerate to an appropriate high velocity but then be stopped short of the goal by a physical restriction or by rapid fatigue, such as in myasthenia gravis. Saccades can also be interrupted by other saccades in the opposite direction (back-to-back saccades) such as those observed in voluntary nystagmus. (These are truncated saccades.) Slow saccades can result from muscle palsies and a variety of anomalies in premotor neurons.[53]

Cerebellar disorders can cause saccade *dysmetria* (inaccuracy). Saccades can be too large (hypermetric) or too small (hypometric) relative to the target displacement. Inaccuracy can lead to macrosaccadic oscillations when the eye repeatedly attempts to correct its fixation errors with inaccurate saccades. Either the pulse or the step component of the saccade can be inaccurate (Figure 36-17). If the pulse is too small, the saccade is slow; if the step is not constant but decays, eye position drifts toward primary position. Repeated attempts to fixate eccentrically result in gaze-evoked nystagmus. If the pulse and step are mismatched, there is postsaccadic drift or glissade to the final eye position.

Cerebellar disorders and progressive supranuclear palsy can cause saccadic intrusions. These are conditions in which spontaneous saccades occur at the wrong time and move the eye away from the target during attempted fixation. Ocular flutter is characterized by rapid back-and-forth horizontal saccades without normal saccade latency or intersaccadic interval. Opsoclonus is ocular flutter in all directions. There are also square wave jerks that move the eye away from a point of fixation and then back again. These movements have a normal intersaccadic interval.

Nystagmus

Nystagmus is a regular pattern of to-and-fro movements of the eyes, usually with alternating slow and fast phases (see Figure 36-6). The direction of the nystagmus is specified according to the direction of the fast phase (e.g., "jerk right") because the fast phase is more visible than the slow phase. When the velocity of the eye oscillations is equal in both directions, the waveform is classified as pendular.

Congenital nystagmus (CN) appears early in life and often is associated with albinism, aniridia, and congenital achromatopsia. CN is a jerk waveform of nystagmus that has a null point or gaze direction where the amplitude is minimized. The differentiating characteristic of CN is that the speed of the slow phase increases exponentially, until a resetting quick phase occurs. In all other forms of nystagmus, the speed of the slow phase is constant or decreases before the quick phase. Persons with CN

can adopt a head turn to allow their gaze direction to coincide with the null point. Convergence also dampens CN, and some individuals adopt an esotropia in an attempt to block the nystagmus at the expense of binocularity (nystagmus blocking syndrome). Latent nystagmus, described earlier in this chapter, is a developmental form of nystagmus associated with early-onset esotropia or abnormal binocular vision, and it is thought to be related to asymmetric OKN that is also associated with disrupted development of binocular vision.[96]

Vestibular nystagmus can result from central and peripheral anomalies of the vestibular gaze stabilization system. The vestibular system is organized in a push-pull fashion in which the inputs from each side of the head are normally balanced when the head is stationary. When an imbalance exists, the eyes behave as if the head were constantly rotating. The amplitude of the nystagmus is highest when gaze deviates in the direction of the fast phase (Alexander's law). In some cases of vestibular nystagmus, the direction of the nystagmus reverses every 2 minutes (periodic alternating nystagmus). The reversal reflects the action of the normal cerebellar adaptive control mechanism to correct an imbalance in the vestibular system. Rebound nystagmus is a related condition associated with gaze-evoked nystagmus that was described earlier in this chapter. In gaze-evoked nystagmus, when fixation is held eccentrically, the slow phase is toward primary position. In rebound nystagmus the amplitude of the nystagmus is reduced after 35 seconds of sustained fixation. However, when the eyes return to primary position, the nystagmus reverses direction (rebound nystagmus). The attenuation and reversal of slow-phase direction demonstrates an attempt by the cerebellum to reduce the slow drifts during attempted steady fixation caused by a leaky tonic innervation for eye position.

Nystagmus can also have vertical and torsional components. For example, see-saw nystagmus is an acquired pendular form of nystagmus in which there is a combination of vertical and torsional oscillation of eye orientation. The eyes bob up and down by several degrees in opposite directions (skew movements). As one eye elevates and intorts, the other eye depresses and extorts. The exact cause is unknown, but see-saw nystagmus is associated with visual loss in bitemporal hemianopia and optic chiasm disorders. The nystagmus is thought to result from an inappropriate ocular tilt response (ocular counterroll during head tilt) orchestrated by the cerebellum in association with the otoliths.

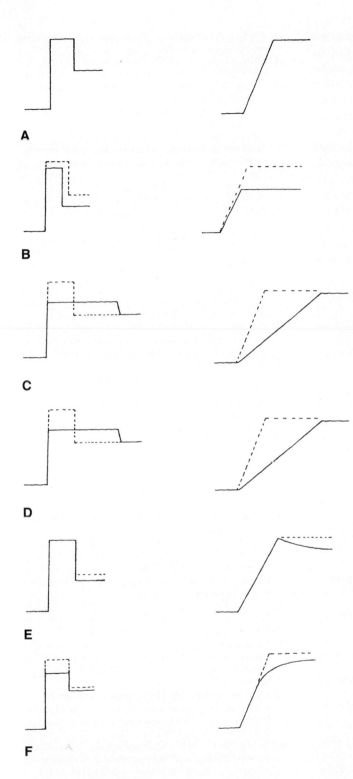

FIGURE 36-17   Disorders of the saccadic pulse and step. Innervation patterns are shown on the left, and eye movements on the right. Dashed lines indicate the normal response. **A,** Normal saccade. **B,** Hypometric saccade: pulse amplitude (width × height) is too small but pulse and step are matched appropriately. **C,** Slow saccade: decreased pulse height with normal pulse amplitude and normal pulse-step match. **D,** Gaze-evoked nystagmus: normal pulse, poorly sustained step. **E,** Pulse-step mismatch (glissade); step is relatively smaller than pulse. **F,** Pulse-step mismatch caused by internuclear ophthalmoplegia (INO). The step is larger than the pulse, therefore the eye drifts onward after the initial rapid movements. (From Leigh JR, Zee DS: *The neurology of eye movements,* ed 3, Oxford, 1999, Oxford University Press.)

All of the oculomotor anomalies described previously show some evidence of attempts by the oculomotor system to correct them using the same adaptive mechanisms that normally calibrate the various classes of eye movement systems. However, the anomalies are beyond the corrective range of

the adaptive processes. If it were not for these adaptive processes, these anomalies would be far more prevalent and the oculomotor system would be extremely susceptible to permanent injury resulting from disease and trauma. The consequences would be dramatic. For example, approximately 50 years ago a physician named John Crawford lost function of his vestibular apparatus as a result of an overdose of streptomycin used to treat tuberculosis located in his knee. He reported that every movement of his head caused vertigo and nausea, even when his eyes were open. If his eyes were shut, the symptoms intensified. He attempted to steady his head by lying on his back and gripping the bars at the head of the bed. However, even in this position the pulse beat in his head became a perceptible motion, disturbing his equilibrium. It is difficult to imagine how we would survive without the adaptive processes that continually calibrate our oculomotor system and allow us to distinguish between motion of our head and eyes from motion of objects in the world.

ACKNOWLEDGMENTS

Comments by James Maxwell and Lance Optican are appreciated.

REFERENCES

1. Able LA et al: Endpoint nystagmus, *Invest Ophthalmol Vis Sci* 17:539, 1977.
2. Albright TD: Centrifugal directional bias in the middle temporal visual area (MT) of the macaque, *Vis Neurosci* 2:177, 1989.
3. Albright TD: Cortical processing of visual motion. In Miles FA, Wallman J (eds): *Visual motion and its role in the stabilization of gaze*, New York, 1993, Elsevier.
4. Allen MJ, Carter JH: The torsion component of the near reflex, *Am J Optom* 44:343, 1967.
5. Alpern M, Ellen P: A quantitative analysis of the horizontal movements of the eyes in the experiments of Johannes Muller: I. Methods and results, *Am J Ophthalmol* 42:289, 1956.
6. Badcock DR, Schor CM: Depth-increment detection function for individual spatial channels, *J Opt Soc Am A* 2:1211, 1985.
7. Bahill AT, Adler D, Stark L: Most naturally occurring human saccades have magnitudes of 15 degrees or less, *Invest Ophthalmol* 14:468, 1975.
8. Bahill AT, Clark MR, Stark L: The main sequence: a tool for studying human eye movements, *Math Biosci* 24:191, 1975.
9. Baloh RW et al: Effect of alcohol and marijuana on eye movements, *Aviat Space Environ Med* 50:18, 1979.
10. Becker W: Metrics. In Wurtz RH, Goldberg ME (eds): *The neurobiology of saccadic eye movements*, New York, 1989, Elsevier.
11. Borish IM: *Clinical refraction*, ed 3, Chicago, 1970, Professional Press.
12. Bradshaw MF, Glennerster A, Rogers BJ: The effect of display size on disparity scaling from differential perspective and vergence cues, *Vision Res* 36:1255, 1996.
13. Carl JR, Gellman RS: Adaptive responses in human smooth pursuit. In Keller EL, Zee DS (eds): *Adaptive processes in visual and oculomotor systems: advances in the biosciences*, vol 57, Oxford, 1986, Pergamon Press.
14. Carpenter RHS: *Movements of the eyes*, ed 2, London, 1988, Pion.
15. Cheng M, Outerbridge JS: Optokinetic nystagmus during selective retinal stimulation, *Exp Brain Res* 23:129, 1975.
16. Cheung BSK, Howard IP: Optokinetic torsion: dynamics and relation to circular vection, *Vision Res* 31:1327, 1991.
17. Cogan DG: *Neurology of the ocular muscles*, ed 2, Springfield, Ill, 1956, Charles C Thomas.
18. Colby CL, Duhamel JR, Goldberg ME: Ventral intraparietal area of the macaque: anatomic location and visual response properties, *J Neurophysiol* 69:902, 1993.
19. Collewijn H: Integration of adaptive changes of the optokinetic reflex, pursuit and the vestibulo-ocular reflex. In Berthoz A, Melvill Jones G (eds): *Adaptive mechanisms in gaze control*, New York, 1985, Elsevier.
20. Collewijn H: The optokinetic contribution. In Carpenter RHS (ed): *Vision and visual dysfunction*, vol 8, *Eye movements*, Boca Raton, Fla, 1991, CRC Press.
21. Collewijn H, Erkelens CJ: Binocular eye movements and the perception of depth. In Kowler E (ed): *Eye movements and their role in visual and cognitive processes*, New York, 1990, Elsevier.
22. Collewijn H, Erkelens CJ, Steinman RM: Trajectories of the human binocular fixation point during conjugate and non-conjugate gaze-shifts, *Vision Res* 37:1049, 1997.
23. Collewijn H, Steinman RM, Erkelens CJ: Binocular fusion, stereopsis and stereoacuity with a moving head. In Regan D (ed): *Binocular vision*, London, 1991, Macmillan.
24. DeAngelis GC, Newsome WT: Organization of disparity-selective neurons in macaque area MT, *J Neurosci* 19:1398, 1999.
25. Dell'Osso LF, Schmidt D, Daroff RB: Latent, manifest latent and congenital nystagmus, *Arch Ophthalmol* 97:1877, 1979.
26. Deuble H: Separate adaptive mechanism for the control of reactive and volitional saccadic eye movements, *Vision Res* 35:3520, 1995.
27. Erkelens CJ, Collewijn H, Steinman RM: Asymmetrical adaptation of human saccades to anisometropia spectacles, *Invest Ophthalmol Vis Sci* 30:1132, 1989.
28. Enright JT: Changes in vergence mediated by saccades, *J Physiol (Lond)* 350:9, 1984.
29. Fincham EF, Walton J: The reciprocal actions of accommodation and convergence, *J Physiol (Lond)* 137:488, 1957.
30. Fischer B, Ramsperger E: Human express saccades: extremely short reaction times of goal directed eye movements, *Exp Brain Res* 57:191, 1984.
31. Foley JM: Primary distance perception. In Held R, Leibowitz HW, Teuber H-L (eds): *Handbook of sensory physiology*, vol VIII, *Perception*, Berlin, 1978, Springer Verlag.
32. Freedman EG, Sparks DL: Activity of cells in the deeper layers of the superior colliculus of the rhesus monkey: evidence for a gaze displacement command, *J Neurophysiol* 78:1669, 1997.
33. Fuchs AF, Mustari MJ: The optokinetic response in primates and its possible neuronal substrate. In Miles FA, Wallman J (eds): *Visual motion and its role in the stabilization of gaze*, New York, 1993, Elsevier.
34. Gamlin PD, Clarke RJ: Single-unit activity in the primate nucleus reticularis tegmenti pontis related to vergence and ocular accommodation, *J Neurophysiol* 73:2115, 1995.
35. Gamlin PD, Yoon K: An area for vergence eye movement in primate frontal cortex, *Nature* 407:1003, 2000.
36. Gamlin PD et al: Behavior of identified Edinger-Westphal neurons during ocular accommodation, *J Neurophysiol* 72:2368, 1994.
37. Gleason G et al: Directionally selective short-term non-conjugate adaptation of vertical pursuits, *Vision Res* 33:65, 1993.

38. Goldberg ME, Eggers HM, Gouras P: The ocular motor system. In Kandel ER, Schwartz JH, Jessell TM (eds): *Principles of neural science,* ed 3, Norwalk, Conn, 1991, Appleton and Lange.

39. Goldberg ME, Segraves MA: The visual and frontal cortices. In Wurtz RH, Goldberg ME (eds): *The neurobiology of saccadic eye movements,* New York, 1989, Elsevier.

40. Hepp K et al: Brainstem regions related to saccade generation. In Wurtz RH, Goldberg ME (eds): *The neurobiology of saccadic eye movements,* New York, 1989, Elsevier.

41. Hering E, Bridgeman B, Stark L: *The theory of binocular vision,* New York, 1977, Plenum Press.

42. Hoffmann KP, Distler C, Ilg U: Colossal and superior temporal sulcus contributions to receptive field properties in the macaque monkey's nucleus of the optic tract and dorsal terminal nucleus of the accessory optic tract, *J Comp Neurol* 321:150, 1992.

43. Hollins M, Bunn KW: The relation between convergence micropsia and retinal eccentricity, *Vision Res* 17:403, 1997.

44. Howard IP, Marton C: Visual pursuit over textured backgrounds in different depth planes, *Exp Brain Res* 90:625, 1997.

45. Ito M: Synaptic plasticity in the cerebellar cortex that may underlie the vestibulo-ocular adaptation. In Berthoz A, Melvill Jones G (eds): *Adaptive mechanisms in gaze control,* New York, 1985, Elsevier.

46. Judge SJ: Vergence. In Carpenter RHS (ed): *Vision and visual dysfunction,* vol 8, *Eye movements,* Boca Raton, Fla, 1991, CRC Press.

47. Judge SJ, Cumming BG: Neurons in the monkey midbrain with activity related to vergence eye movements and accommodation, *J Neurophysiol* 55:915, 1986.

48. Keller EL: Gain of the vestibulo-ocular reflex in monkey at high rotational frequencies, *Vision Res* 20:535, 1978.

49. Keller EL: The brainstem. In Carpenter RHS (ed): *Vision and visual dysfunction,* vol 8, *Eye movements,* Boca Raton, Fla, 1991, CRC Press.

50. Kowler E: The stability of gaze and its implications for vision. In Carpenter RHS (ed): *Vision and visual dysfunction,* vol 8, *Eye movements,* Boca Raton, Fla, 1991, CRC Press.

51. Kowler E et al: Voluntary selection of the target for smooth eye movement in the presence of superimposed, full-field stationary and moving stimuli, *Vision Res* 12:1789, 1984.

52. Land MF: Predictable eye-head coordination during driving, *Nature* 359:318, 1992.

53. Leigh JR, Zee DS: *The neurology of eye movements,* ed 3, Oxford, 1999, Oxford University Press.

54. Lemij HG, Collewijn H: Nonconjugate adaptation of human saccades to anisometropic spectacles: meridian-specificity, *Vision Res* 32:453, 1992.

55. Lisberger SG: The latency of pathways containing the site of motor learning in the monkey vestibulo-ocular reflex, *Science* 225:74, 1984.

56. Lisberger SG: The neural basis for learning of simple motor skills, *Science* 242:728, 1988.

57. Lisberger SG, Westbrook LE: Properties of visual inputs that initiate horizontal smooth pursuit eye movements in monkeys, *J Neurosci* 5:1662, 1985.

58. Maddox EC: *The clinical use of prism,* ed 2, Bristol, England, 1893, John Wright & Sons.

59. Maunsell JHR, Van Essen DC: Functional properties of neurons in middle temporal visual area of the macaque monkey: II. Binocular interactions and sensitivity to binocular disparity, *J Neurophysiol* 49:1148, 1983.

60. Maxwell JS, King WM: Dynamics and efficacy of saccade-facilitated vergence eye movements in monkeys, *J Neurophysiol* 68:1248, 1992.

61. Maxwell JS, Schor CM: Head-position-dependent adaptation of nonconcomitant vertical skew, *Vision Res* 37:441, 1997.

62. Maxwell JS, Schor CM: Adaptation of torsional eye alignment in relation to head roll, *Vision Res* 39:4192, 1999.

63. May PJ, Porter JD, Gamlin PD: Interconnections between the primate cerebellum and midbrain near-response regions, *J Comp Neurol* 315:98, 1992.

64. Mays LE, Gamlin PD: A neural mechanism subserving saccade-vergence interactions. In Findlay JM, Walker R, Kentridge RW (eds): *Eye movement research: mechanisms, processes and applications,* New York, 1995, Elsevier.

65. Mays LE, Gamlin PD: Neuronal circuitry controlling the near response, *Curr Opin Neurobiol* 5:763, 1995.

66. Mays LE, Porter JD: Neural control of vergence eye movements: activity of abducens and oculomotoneurons, *J Neurophysiol* 52:743, 1984.

67. McCandless JW, Schor CM: An association matrix model of context-specific vertical vergence adaptation, *Network Comput Neural Syst* 8:239, 1997.

68. McLin L, Schor CM, Kruger P: Changing size (looming) as a stimulus to accommodation and vergence, *Vision Res* 28:883, 1988.

69. Melvill Jones G: The vestibular contribution. In Carpenter RHS (ed): *Vision and visual dysfunction,* vol 8, *Eye movements,* Boca Raton, Fla, 1991, CRC Press.

70. Miles FA: The sensing of rotational and translational optic flow by the primate optokinetic system. In Miles FA, Wallman J (eds): *Visual motion and its role in the stabilization of gaze,* New York, 1993, Elsevier.

71. Miles FA, Judge SJ, Optican LM: Optically induced changes in the couplings between vergence and accommodation, *J Neurosci* 7:2576, 1987.

72. Miles FA, Kawano K, Optican LM: Short-latency ocular following responses of monkey: I—dependence on temporospatial properties of visual input, *J Neurophysiol* 56:1321, 1986.

73. Müller J: *Elements of physiology,* vol 2, London, 1843, Taylor and Walton (Translated by W Baly).

74. Myer CH, Lasker AG, Robinson DA: The upper limit for smooth pursuit velocity, *Vision Res* 25:561, 1985.

75. Newsome WT, Wurtz RH, Komatsu H: Relation of cortical areas MT and MST to pursuit eye movements: II. Differentiation of retinal from extraretinal inputs, *J Neurophysiol* 60:604, 1988.

76. Noda H, Warabi T: Responses of Purkinje cells and mossy fibers in the flocculus of the monkey during sinusoidal movements of a moving pattern, *J Physiol (Lond)* 387:611, 1987.

77. Ogle KN, Martens TG, Dyer JA: Oculomotor imbalance in binocular vision and fixation disparity, Philadelphia, 1967, Lea and Febiger.

78. Ohtsuka K, Maekawa H, Sawa W: Convergence paralysis after lesions of the cerebellar peduncles, *Ophthalmologica* 206:143, 1993.

79. O'Mullane G, Knox PC: Modification of smooth pursuit initiation by target contrast, *Vision Res* 39:3459, 1999.

80. Ono H: The combination of version and vergence. In Schor CM, Ciuffreda K (eds): *Vergence eye movements: basic and clinical aspects,* Boston, 1983, Butterworth-Heinemann.

81. Oohira A, Zee DS, Guyton DL: Disconjugate adaptation to long-standing, large-amplitude, spectacle-corrected anisometropia, *Invest Ophthalmol Vis Sci* 32:1693, 1991.

82. Optican LM, Miles FA: Visually induced adaptive changes in primate saccadic oculomotor control signals, *J Neurophysiol* 54:940, 1985.

83. Pasik T, Pasik P: Optokinetic nystagmus: an unlearned response altered by section of chiasma and corpus callosum in monkeys, *Nature* 203:609, 1964.

84. Poggio G: Mechanisms of stereopsis in monkey visual cortex, *Cereb Cortex* 3:195, 1995.

85. Pola J, Wyatt HJ: Smooth pursuit response characteristics, stimuli and mechanisms. In Carpenter RHS (ed): *Vision and visual dysfunction,* vol 8, *Eye movements,* Boca Raton, Fla, 1991, CRC Press.

86. Raphan T, Cohen B: Velocity storage and the ocular response to multidimensional vestibular stimuli. In Berthoz A, Melvill Jones G (eds): *Adaptive mechanisms in gaze control,* New York, 1985, Elsevier.

87. Rashbass C: The relationship between saccadic and smooth tracking eye movements, *J Physiol (Lond)* 159:326, 1961.

88. Rashbass C, Westheimer G: Disjunctive eye movements, *J Physiol (Lond)* 159:339, 1961.

89. Rethy I: Development of the simultaneous fixation from the divergent anatomic eye-position of the neonate, *J Ped Ophthalmol* 6:92, 1969.

90. Robinson DA: Oculomotor control signals. In Lennerstrand G, Bach-Y-Rita P (eds): *Basic mechanisms of ocular motility and their clinical implications,* Oxford, 1975, Pergamon Press.

91. Robinson DA: A quantitative analysis of extraocular muscle cooperation and squint, *Invest Ophthalmol* 14:801, 1975.

92. Robinson DA: Control of eye movements. In Brooks V (ed): Handbook *of physiology: section I—the nervous system,* Bethesda, Md, 1981, William & Wilkins.

93. Robinson DA, Keller EL: The behavior of eye movement motoneurons in the alert monkey, *Bibl Ophthalmol* 82:7, 1972.

94. Roy JP, Komatsu H, Wurtz RH: Disparity sensitivity of neurons in monkey extrastriate area MST, *J Neurosci* 12:2478, 1992.

95. Schor CM: Fixation disparity and vergence adaptation. In Schor CM, Ciuffreda K (eds): *Vergence eye movements: basic and clinical aspects,* Boston, 1983, Butterworth-Heinemann.

96. Schor CM: Development of OKN. In Miles FA, Wallman J (eds): *Visual motion and its role in the stabilization of gaze,* New York, 1993, Elsevier.

97. Schor CM: Binocular vision. In De Valois K (ed): *Seeing,* 2000, Academic Press.

98. Schor CM, Gleason J, Horner D: Selective nonconjugate binocular adaptation of vertical saccades and pursuits, *Vision Res* 30:1827, 1990.

99. Schor CM, Kotulak J: Dynamic interactions between accommodation and convergence are velocity sensitive, *Vision Res* 26:927, 1986.

100. Schor CM, Maxwell JS, Graf E: Plasticity of convergence-dependent variations of cyclovergence with vertical gaze, *Vision Res* 41:3353, 2001.

101. Schor CM, Maxwell JS, Stevenson SB: Isovergence surfaces: the conjugacy of vertical eye movements in tertiary positions of gaze, *Ophthalmic Physiol Opt* 14:279, 1994.

102. Schor CM et al: Negative feedback control model of proximal convergence and accommodation, *Ophthalmic Physiol Opt* 12:307, 1992.

103. Schor CM et al: Spatial aspects of vertical phoria adaptation, *Vision Res* 33:73, 1993.

104. Schor CM et al: Prediction of early onset esotropia from the components of the infantile squint syndrome, *Invest Ophthalmol Vis Sci* 38:719, 1997.

105. Schor CM et al: Saccades reduce latency and increase velocity of ocular accommodation, *Vision Res* 39:3769, 1999.

106. Seidman SH, Leigh RJ: The human torsional vestibulo-ocular reflex during rotation about an earth-vertical axis, *Brain Res* 504:264, 1989.

107. Semmlow JL et al: Disparity vergence eye movements exhibit preprogrammed motor control, *Vision Res* 34:335, 1994.

108. Sherrington C: *The integrative action of the nervous system,* ed 2, New Haven, Conn, 1947, Yale University Press.

109. Simpson JI, Graf W: The selection of reference frames by nature and its investigators. In Berthoz A, Melvill Jones G (eds): *Adaptive mechanisms in gaze control,* New York, 1985, Elsevier.

110. Snyder LH, King WM: Effect of viewing distance and the location of the axis of rotation on the monkey's vestibulo-ocular reflex (VOR): I. Eye movement responses, *J Neurophysiol* 67:861, 1992.

111. Somani RAB et al: Visual test of listing's law during vergence, *Vision Res* 38:911, 1998.

112. Sparks DL, Hartwich-Young R: The deep layers of the superior colliculus. In Wurtz RH, Goldberg ME (eds): *The neurobiology of saccadic eye movements,* New York, 1989, Elsevier.

113. Stark L, Vossius G, Young LR: Predictive control of eye tracking movements, *IRE Trans Hum Factors Electron* 3:52, 1962.

114. Tait EF: A report on the results of the experimental variation of the stimulus conditions in the responses of the accommodative convergence reflex, *Am J Optom* 10:428, 1933.

115. Taylor MJ, Roberts DC, Zee DS: Effect of sustained cyclovergence on eye alignment: rapid torsional phoria adaptation, *Invest Ophthalmol Vis Sci* 41:1076, 2000.

116. Trotter Y et al: Neural processing of stereopsis as a function of viewing distance in primate visual cortical area V1, *J Neurophysiol* 76:2872, 1996.

117. Tweed D: Visual-motor optimization in binocular control, *Vision Res* 37:1939, 1997.

118. Van Gisbergen JAM, Van Opstal AJ: Models. In Wurtz RH, Goldberg M (eds): *The neurobiology of saccadic eye movements,* New York, 1989, Elsevier.

119. Van Rijn LJ, Van der Steen J, Collewijn H: Instability of ocular torsion during fixation: cyclovergence is more stable than cycloversion, *Vision Res* 34:1077, 1994.

120. Wallman J: Subcortical optokinetic mechanisms. In Miles FA, Wallman J (eds): *Visual motion and its role in the stabilization of gaze,* New York, 1993, Elsevier.

121. Westheimer G, Blair S: The parasympathetic pathways to internal eye muscles, *Invest Ophthalmol* 12:193, 1973.

122. Westheimer G, McKee SP: Visual acuity in the presence of retinal image motion, *J Opt Soc Am* 65:47, 1975

123. Wick B, Bedell HE: Magnitude and velocity of proximal vergence, *Invest Ophthalmol Vis Sci* 30:755, 1989.

124. Wilhelm H, Schaeffel F, Wilhelm B: Age relation of the pupillary near reflex, *Klin Monatsbl Augenheilkd* 203:110, 1993.

125. Ygge J, Zee DS: Control of vertical eye alignment in three-dimensional space, *Vision Res* 35:3169, 1995.

126. Zee DS, FitzGibbon EJ, Optican LM: Saccade-vergence interactions in humans, *J Neurophysiol* 68:1624, 1992.

127. Zee DS, Levi L: Neurological aspects of vergence eye movements, *Rev Neurol (Paris)* 145:613, 1989.

128. Zhang H, Gamlin PD: Neurons in the posterior interposed nucleus of the cerebellum related to vergence and accommodation: I. Steady-state characteristics, *J Neurophysiol* 79:1255, 1998.

129. Zhang Y, Mays LE, Gamlin PD: Characteristics of near response cells projecting to the oculomotor nucleus, *J Neurophysiol* 67:944, 1992.

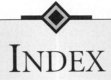

INDEX

Page numbers followed by f indicate figures; t, tables; b, boxes.

A

ABCR gene
  inherited retinal dystrophies, 363, 367t,
    373-375
  retinal pigment epithelium, 350
  visual adaptation, 597
ABCR protein, 417
Abducens palsy, 852
Aberrant regeneration in the third nerve, 740
Aberrations
  contrast sensitivity, 180-186
  glare sensitivity, 180-186
  visual acuity, 455
Abetalipoproteinemia, 360t
Abnormal adaptation in retinal disease,
  596-598
Abnormal retinal correspondence, 489-491
Absolute disparity, 492
Absorption, 455
Accessory lacrimal gland secretion, 36-37
Accessory optic system, 642f, 643
Accommodation, 197-199
  accommodative triad, 212
  adult eye optics and refraction, 169
  anatomy of accommodative apparatus,
    201-208
  anterior chamber, 202f
  anterior zonule, 209
  choroid, 202f
  ciliary body, 201-202
  ciliary muscle, 202-203, 204f
  composition of the eye, 200
  cornea, 202f
  crystalline lens, 207-208, 209f
  cycloplegia, 213
  defined, 200
  depth of field, 200-201
  depth of focus, 200-201
  fovea, 202f
  iris, 202f
  lens, 202f
  main zonular fibers, 205
  measurement of, 213-214
  mechanism of, 209-212
  near reflex, 212
  negative vergence, 200
  optical requirements for, 200-201
  optics of the eye, 199-200
  ora serrata, 202f
  pars plana, 201, 206f
  pharmacology of, 212-213
  positive vergence, 200
  presbyopia, 223-226
  pupil, 720-721
  retina, 202f
  sclera, 202f
  scleral spur, 202f
  spanning zonular fiber system, 205
  stimulus to, 212
  supraciliaris, 201-202
  tension zonular fiber system, 205
  tonic accommodation, 212

Accommodation—cont'd
  visual acuity, 201
  young eye optics and refraction, 162
  zonular fork, 205, 206f
  zonules, 202f, 203-207, 208f, 209-212
Accommodative-convergence neurologic
  cross-link, 840
Action potentials, 613-615
Active secretion in aqueous humor
  hydrodynamics, 238-240
Active transport in aqueous humor
  hydrodynamics, 243-244
Activity and retinogeniculate projection
  activity-dependent development,
    648-652
Acuity. *See* Visual acuity.
Adaptable interactions between smooth
  pursuit and smooth vergence, 843
Adaptation. *See* Visual adaptation.
Additive primary colors, 578
Adenosine A₁ agonists, 267
Adenosine triphosphate (ATP), 131-132
Adhesion
  cell adhesion molecules in retina, 321
  corneal epithelium, 51-53, 54f, 55f
  lens fiber cell differentiation, 128
Adie's pupil, 719-720, 733t, 737-738,
  739-740
Adrenergic mechanisms in aqueous humor
  hydrodynamics, 245-246, 259-261
Adult eyes, 167
  accommodation, 169
  aqueous humor, 169
  chart luminance, 171-172
  contrast, 173
  contrast sensitivity, 173
  contrast sensitivity recording, 174-175
  contrast sensitivity testing, 172-173
  cornea's role, 168, 169f
  crystalline lens' role, 168-169
  crystallins, 169
  definition and units, 173
  drifts, 171
  Foucalt gratings, 173-174
  Fourier transformation, 173-174
  glycosaminoglycan, 168
  halftones, 173
  Holobacterium halobium, 170
  lens, 117-118, 119f
  microsaccades, 171
  receptor size and spacing, 170-171
  resonance, 168
  retinal image, 167
  retina's role, 169-171
  rhodopsin, 170
  sine waves, 173-174
  square waves, 173-174
  targets, 173
  tremors, 171
  visible light waves, 167-173
  visual acuity as log MAR, 172
  visual acuity chart contrast, 172

Adult eyes—cont'd
  visual acuity testing, 171
  visual deprivations, 704-706
Advanced Glaucoma Intervention Study
  (AGIS), 564
Afferent arm of the pupil light reflex,
  716-718
Afferent axons, 658, 659f, 660f
After cataracts, 137, 142
Aging eyes, 186
  ametropia, 191-192
  aqueous humor hydrodynamics, 247t,
    248
  astigmatism, 190
  cataracts. *See* Cataracts.
  "completing the picture" illusion, 186-187
  contrast enhancement, 187-188
  Craik-Cornsweet-O'Brien illusion, 188
  edge sharpening, 188
  emmetropization, 192
  evolution of ocular components, 186
  "filling in information," 186-187
  gap figures, 187
  gene sharing, 186
  lens, 133-134
  myopia, 189-190
  nonoptical brain mechanisms that
    enhance retinal image, 186-189
  ocular circulation, 776
  pathologic myopia, 189-190
  physiologic myopia, 190
  presbyopia. *See* Presbyopia.
  prevalence, 189
  refractive errors, 189-191
  removing distractions, 189
  retina, 343
  school myopia, 190
  Vernier acuity, 188-189
  visual acuity, 464-465
  vitreous, 302-306
AGIS. *See* Advanced Glaucoma
  Intervention Study (AGIS).
AII amacrine cell type, 340-341
Airy disc, 455
Akinetopsia, 694
Aldose reductase, 145
Amacrine cells, 323f, 333-336
  AII amacrine cell type, 340-341
  displaced amacrine cells, 333, 335, 338
  light responses, 432
  synapses, 432
Amblyopia
  visual acuity, 467-468
  visual deprivations, 701-702, 703-704
Ametropia, 191-192
Anchoring fibrils, 51
Anchoring plaques, 51
ANF. *See* Atrial natriuretic factor (ANF).
Angioblastic meningiomas, 611
Angioscotometry, 447
Angle of anomaly, 490
Angular artery, 10f

Aniseikonia, 500-503
Anisocoria, 715, 719, 730-732, 733t, 736-737
Annulus of Zinn, 788-790
Anomaloscope, 584
Anterior ciliary vessels, 748f
Anterior cortex, 118f
Anterior ethmoidal artery, 10f
Anterior hyaloid, 294
Anterior internuclear ophthalmoplegia, 852
Anterior optic nerve, 749, 750f
Anterior polar cataracts, 142-143
Anterior pupillary membrane, 129
Anterior segment organizer, 129
Anterior suture, 118f
Anterior zonule, 209
Anteroposterior axis, 789f
Aphakia, 122
Apoptosis
    inherited retinal dystrophies, 377
    optic nerve, 620-621
    retina, 322
Apoptosome, 621
Apparent motion, 523
Aqueous humor, 237-238
    active secretion, 238-240
    active transport, 243-244
    adenosine A$_1$ agonists, 267
    adrenergic mechanisms, 245-246, 259-261
    adult eye optics and refraction, 169
    age, 247t, 248
    atrial natriuretic factor, 246, 247t
    biochemistry of aqueous humor
        formation, 241-242
    blood-aqueous barrier, 242-243, 244
    cell junctional mechanisms, 267-269
    cholinergic mechanisms, 244-245, 253-258
    cholinergic sensitivity of the outflow
        mechanism, alterations in, 258-261
    complex electron-dense substance in the
        JXT, 266-267
    composition of aqueous humor, 242, 244
    compounds that disrupt or remodel the
        structure of the meshwork and canal
        IW, 267
    conventional outflow, 253-258, 259-261
    corneal endothelium, 89
    corticosteroid mechanisms, 262-264,
        265f, 266f
    cytoskeletal and cell junctional
        mechanisms, 267-269
    diffusion, 238
    drainage, 248-249
    erythrocytes, 269
    exercise, 247t, 248
    facility of inflow, 240
    flare, 242
    fluid mechanics, 248-249
    formation of aqueous humor, 238-242,
        244
    glaucoma, 253, 258, 270
    Goldmann equation, 248
    guanylate cyclase activators, 246
    hyaluronidase and protease-induced
        facility increases, 267
    intraocular pressure. *See* Intraocular
        pressure (IOP).
    ketanserin, 246-248
    macromolecule-induced facility
        decreases, 270
    microtubules, 269
    myocilin, 263-264, 265f
    nitrovasodilators, 246, 247t
    outflow apparatus cholinergic sensitivity
        alterations, 258-261
    outflow biomechanics, 270-271
    particulate-induced facility decreases,
        269-270
    pharmacology, 244, 249-258
    physiology of aqueous humor
        formation, 238-240

Aqueous humor—cont'd
    pilocarpine, 244-245, 255-259, 260, 261
    plasma membrane proteins, 264-266
    prostaglandin mechanisms, 261-262,
        263t
    protease-induced facility increases, 267
    protein, 270
    protein kinase inhibitors, 256
    Schlemm's canal, 237, 250-253
    steady-state IOP, 248
    surgery, 247t, 248
    TIGR, 263-264, 265f
    trabecular meshwork. *See* Trabecular
        meshwork (TM).
    turnover constant, 240
    ultrafiltration, 238
    unconventional outflow, 258, 259f, 261,
        262t
    uveoscleral outflow, 258, 259f, 261, 262t
Arachnoid meninges, 610-611
Arcuate density, 330
Arden index, 415
Area 7a, 691
Area 17 of Brodmann. *See* Primary visual
    cortex.
Area V1. *See* Primary visual cortex.
Arginine, 399-400
Ascorbic acid, 131
Aspheric surfaces, 185
Asteroid hyalosis, 445
Astigmatism
    aging eye optics and refraction, 190
    young eye optics and refraction, 165
Astrocytes
    optic nerve, 608-610
    retina, 337
Asymmetric vergence, 847, 848f, 849f
ATP. *See* Adenosine triphosphate (ATP).
Atrial natriuretic factor (ANF), 246, 247t
Attenuation characteristics of a linear filter,
    517
Autosomal dominant retinitis pigmentosa,
    365
Autosomal recessive retinitis pigmentosa,
    365, 377
    inherited retinal dystrophies, 369-370
Axis of action, 828
Axons, 603-604, 606, 612-613
    conduction, 613-616
    counts and dimensions, 605-606
    injury, 619-626
    lateral geniculate nucleus, 658-659, 660f
    regeneration, 626
    transport, 616-617

B

BAB. *See* Blood-aqueous barrier (BAB).
Ball-and-socket joints, 125, 126f
Basal junctions, 331
Base, vitreous, 294f
Batten syndrome, 360t
Bcl-2 gene overexpression, 627
Beaded filaments, 125, 134
Beat frequency, 544
Berger's space, 294f
Best vitelliform macular dystrophy, 376
Bestrophin
    electroretinograms, 417
    inherited retinal dystrophies, 367t, 376
Binocular vision, 484, 506-507
    abnormal retinal correspondence,
        489-491
    absolute disparity, 492
    advantages to, 484
    angle of anomaly, 490
    binocular disparity, 488, 491-493
    binocular rivalry suppression, 505-506
    corresponding retinal points/areas, 487
    cover points, 488
    "crossed" diplopia, 486
    crossed disparity, 491

Binocular vision—cont'd
    diplopia, 486-487, 489
    disparity of the retinal images, 488,
        491-493
    distal disparity, 491
    egocenter, 485
    egocentric direction, 485-486
    fixation disparities, 492
    horizontal disparity angles, 488
    horopter, 488-489
    infant vision development, 543-547
    interocular blur suppression, 504-505
    local sign, 485
    longitudinal visual angles, 488
    neural control of eye movements, 830-
        831, 832f
    normal retinal correspondence, 487-489
    oculocentric direction, 485
    Panum's fusional area, 489, 492
    permanent-occlusion suppression, 506
    physiologic diplopia, 486-487
    proximal disparity, 491
    reconciliation of differences in
        oculocentric visual directions, 486
    relative disparity, 492
    retinal disparity, 488, 491-493
    retinal rivalry suppression, 505-506
    spatial form processing, 470, 480-481
    stereopsis. *See* Stereopsis.
    subjective angle, 490
    suppression, 489, 504-506
    suppression scotoma, 489
    suspension, 505
    uncrossed disparity, 491
    version and vergence ocular movement
        combinations, 485-486
    visual deprivations, 697-698, 699f
    visual direction, 485-487
    window experiment of Hering, 487
Biochemistry
    aqueous humor hydrodynamics, 241-242
    color vision, 579-583
    retina. *See* Retinal biochemistry.
    vitreous, 295-297
Biophysical aspects of vitreous, 297-301,
    305-306
Bipolar cells, 323f, 324f, 332-333, 429,
    430-432
Bitemporal hemianopsia, 644
Blepharospasm, 22-23
Blinking, 22
Bloch's law, 511, 512f
Blood supply
    extraocular muscles, 798, 799f
    optic nerve, 617-619
Blood-aqueous barrier (BAB)
    aqueous humor hydrodynamics, 242-
        243, 244
    trabecular meshwork, 242
Blood-ocular barrier, 753-756
Blood-retinal barrier, 297-301, 312-313
Blue arcs of the retina, 447-448
Blue-field entoptic phenomenon, 761
Botulinum toxin, 809, 811f
Bow region, lens, 118f
Bowman's layer, 49-51
Broad band cells, 664
Bruch's membrane, 326-327, 348, 349f
Brücke brightness enhancement effect, 522
Brunescent cataracts, 133
BSS PLUS solution, 89t, 91
BZIP transcription factors, 121

C

C wave in electroretinograms, 410
Calcium homeostasis
    cataracts, 140-141
    phototransduction, 391
    retinal biochemistry, 393
Callosal degeneration, 693
Calyces, 329

Camouflage breaking, 470
CAMs. *See* Cell adhesion molecules
  (CAMs) in retina.
Canal of Schlemm
  aqueous humor hydrodynamics, 237,
    250-253
  ocular circulation, 748f
Capillaries
  choriocapillaries, 348, 349, 349f
  discontinuous capillaries, 753-754
  fenestrated capillaries, 753-754
  lens, 129
  ocular circulation, 753-756, 774
Capsule, 117, 118f, 135-136
  presbyopia, 220-221
Cardinal points, 162-163
Cataracts, 117, 137
  after cataracts, 137, 142
  age-related cortical cataracts, 140-146,
    146-147, 148
  age-related nuclear cataracts, 137-140,
    146-147, 148
  aldose reductase, 145
  anterior polar cataracts, 142-143
  brunescent cataracts, 133
  calcium homeostasis, 140-141
  congenital cataracts, 142
  contrast sensitivity, 178-179
  cortical cataracts, 140-146, 146-147
  developing countries, 148
  diabetes, 145-146
  Elschnig's pearls, 142
  epidemiology, 146-147, 148
  extracapsular cataract extraction, 142
  formation, 117
  future advances, 147-149
  galactosemia and galactokinase
    deficiency, 143
  genetic advancements, 147-148
  glare sensitivity, 178-179
  globular degeneration, 141
  hereditary cataracts, 142
  hyperbaric oxygen treatments, 138
  infectious agent causes, 142
  infrared light exposure, 145
  intracapsular cataract extraction, 142
  microwave exposure, 145
  mixed cataracts, 141
  nigrescent cataracts, 133
  nuclear cataracts, 137-140, 146-147
  nuclear sclerotic cataracts, 138
  nutrition and formation, 148
  oxidative stress and, 138, 139, 146-147
  posterior capsular opacification, 137
  posterior subcapsular cataracts, 141
  radiation exposure, 143-144
  rubella cataracts, 142
  second sight, 138
  secondary cataracts, 137, 141-142,
    148-149
  sex and influence on, 146
  Soemmering's ring, 142
  steroid exposure, 145
  technologies and, 149
  UV light, 144
CD/DS proteoglycans. *See* Chondroitin
  sulfate/dermatan sulfate (CD/DS)
  proteoglycans.
Cell adhesion in corneal epithelium, 51-53,
  54f, 55f
Cell adhesion molecules (CAMs) in retina,
  321
Cell classes/types
  lateral geniculate nucleus, 657-658
  primary visual cortex, 674-678, 678-680
Cell death mechanisms in retinitis
  pigmentosa, 366
Cell distribution in retina, 321
Cell junctional mechanisms, 267-269
Cellular considerations of vitreous
  embryology, 293-294

Cellular retinaldehyde-binding protein, 374
Center-surround antagonistic receptive
  field organization (CSARFs), 430
Center-surround pattern, 582
Central inherited retinal dystrophies, 359
Central nervous system axonal
  regeneration, 626
Central nervous system integration with
  pupil, 721-723
Central retinal artery and vein, 748f
Central visual pathways, 641-643
  accessory optic system, 642f, 643
  bitemporal hemianopsia, 644
  Edinger-Westphal nucleus, 642
  extrastriate visual cortex. *See* Extrastriate
    visual cortex.
  homonymous hemianopsia, 645
  lateral geniculate nucleus. *See* Lateral
    geniculate nucleus (LGN).
  nasal hemianopsia, 645
  oculomotor nucleus, 642f
  optic chiasm, 642f, 644f
  optic nerve, 642f, 644f
  optic radiation, 642f, 644f
  optic tract, 642f, 644f
  pretectum, 642, 644f
  primary visual cortex. *See* Primary visual
    cortex.
  pulvinar, 642f, 643
  red nucleus, 642f
  retinogeniculate projection activity-
    dependent development. *See*
    Retinogeniculate projection activity-
    dependent development.
  substantia nigra, 642f
  superior colliculus, 641-642, 644f
  targets of retinal projections, 641-643
  visual deprivation. *See* Visual
    deprivations.
  visual field lesions, 644-645
CFEOM. *See* Congenital fibrosis of
  extraocular muscle (CFEOM).
CFF. *See* Critical flicker fusion (CFF).
C-fos gene, 76
cGMP-dependent channel regulation in
  phototransduction, 388-391
cGMP-gated cation channel in cone
  photoreceptors, 419
cGMP-gated cation channel proteins in
  inherited retinal dystrophies, 370
Channel blocking agents in extraocular
  muscles, 810-812
Chart luminance, 171-172
Chief ray in visual acuity, 454
Chief retractor of the upper eyelid, 20
Chievitz transient fiber, 320, 321
Childhood Horner Syndrome, 736
Children
  electroretinograms, 413-414
  infant vision development. *See* Infant
    vision development.
  young eye optics and refraction. *See*
    Young eye optics and refraction.
Cholesterol, 126
Cholinergic mechanisms in aqueous
  humor hydrodynamics, 244-245, 253-
  258
Cholinergic sensitivity of the outflow
  mechanism, alterations in, 258-261
Cholinergic supersensitivity in the pupil,
  737-738
Chondroitin sulfate/dermatan sulfate
  (CD/DS) proteoglycans, 56
Choriocapillaries, 348, 349, 349f
Choriocapillaris, 748f, 751, 752f, 756
Choroid
  accommodation, 202f
  ocular circulation, 754f, 756, 774
Choroideremia, 420
Chromatic aberrations, 184
Chromaticity stimulus, 514, 515f

Chromatopsia, 584
Chromophore cycle in phototransduction,
  385-387
Chromophores, lens, 133
CIGTS. *See* Collaborative Initial Glaucoma
  Treatment Study (CIGTS).
Ciliary body, 201-202
Ciliary muscle
  accommodation, 202-203, 204f
  presbyopia, 215-216, 217f, 218f, 219f,
    227-228
Ciliary processes, 754f, 756
Circulation, ocular. *See* Ocular circulation.
C-jun gene, 76
Classical crystallins, 124-125
Clinical aspects and implications
  corneal epithelium, 53-56
  inherited retinal dystrophies, 358-360,
    360-361
  motion processing, 526-527
  ocular circulation, 757-761
  optic nerve, 619
  perimetry and visual field testing, 562
  pupil, 714f, 715-716
  retinitis pigmentosa, 363-366
  temporal properties of vision, 522-523
  visual deprivations, 701-706
Cloquet's canal, 293, 294f
Closed loop, 842
Closure of eyelids, 22
CLUE (contact lens-use endotheliopathy)
  syndrome, 66
C-maf gene, 122
CO blobs, 673
Cocaine's action on pupil, 732-735, 736
Cogwheel pursuit, 842
Collaborative Initial Glaucoma Treatment
  Study (CIGTS), 564
Collagen
  corneal stroma, 81-84
  vitreous, 293, 295-297
Collarette, 724
Color vision, 578
  additive primary colors, 578
  anomaloscope, 584
  biochemistry of, 579-583
  center-surround pattern, 582
  chromatopsia, 584
  color blindness, 579
  complementary colors, 578
  convergence, 581
  daltonism, 579
  defects, 583-584
  deuteranomaly, 584
  deuteranopia, 583, 584
  dichromats, 583
  divergence, 581
  dyschromatopsia, 584
  G protein-coupled receptors, 579
  heterotrimeric G proteins, 579
  light and color, 578-579
  Maxwell's disc, 583
  molecular genetics of, 583
  monochromatic light, 578
  negative afterimage, 583
  OFF-response, 582
  ON-response, 582
  opponent processes, 582
  opsin-shift, 579
  optical physics, 578
  photoreceptor cells, 580-581
  prism, 578
  protanomaly, 583
  protanopia, 583, 584
  retina, signal processing in, 581-583
  signal processing in the retina, 581-583
  spatial form processing, 470
  testing, 583-584
  transducins, 579
  trichromacy, 580-581
  Young-Helmholtz hypothesis, 579, 582

Columns in primary visual cortex, 681-683
Complete ophthalmoplegia, 852
"Completing the picture" illusion, 186-187
Complex cells in primary visual cortex, 676
Complex electron-dense substance in the JXT, 266-267
Compression, 624-625
Compressive optic neuropathy, 605
Computerized pupillometry, 728-730
Concomitant adaptation, 840
Cone pedicles, 330-331
Cone photoreceptor cells, 323f, 328f
Cone photoreceptor pathways, 341-342
Cone rod homeobox (CRX), 375
Cone synaptic pathways, 429-430, 431f
Cone visual pigments, 387-388
Cone voltage responses, 426, 427f
Congenital cataracts, 142
Congenital fibrosis of extraocular muscle (CFEOM), 806, 807f
Congenital Horner Syndrome, 736
Congenital stationary night blindness (CSNB), 367t, 369, 370-371
Conjugate smooth pursuit tracking, 841-842
Conjunctiva
    dynamics of during ocular movements, 24-25
    embryology, 16, 17f
    eyelids, 19f, 20f
    morphology, 23-24
    stem cells of the ocular surface, 24
Conjunctival epithelial cells, 34f, 37f, 38, 39f
Conjunctival goblet cells, 38-39
Conjunctival vessels, 748f
Connective tissue, orbit, 7-9, 17f
Connexins, 126-127
Connexons, 332
Contact lenses
    contact lens-use endotheliopathy syndrome, 66
    contrast sensitivity, 178
    cornea, 94, 95f
    glare sensitivity, 178
Continuos capillaries, 753-754
Contraction, extraocular muscles, 795-797
Contraction anisocoria, 719
Contrast detection threshold, 476
Contrast sensitivity, 175-177, 186
    aberrations, 180-186
    adult eye optics and refraction, 172-173, 174-175
    aging eye optics and refraction, 187-188
    aspheric surfaces, 185
    cataracts, 178-179
    chromatic aberrations, 184
    contact lens wear, 178
    contrast luminance, 175
    corneal conditions, 178
    corneal edema, 176f, 177, 178
    defenses against light scattering, 184
    depth of field, 179
    depth of focus, 179-180, 181f, 182f, 183f
    destructive interference, 184
    intensity discrimination, 175
    keratoconus, 178
    light absorption, 186
    light scatterer vs. transmitter, 175
    light scattering, 183-184
    modulation transfer function, 179
    nephrotic cystinosis, 178
    opacified posterior capsules, 178-179
    opaqueness, 175
    penetrating keratoplasty, 178
    refractive surgery, 178
    spherical aberrations, 184-186
    stereopsis, 500
    visual acuity, 463
Contrast sensitivity function (CSF), 474-476
Conventional outflow in aqueous humor hydrodynamics, 253-258, 259-261

Convergence, 581
Cornea, 47
    accommodation, 202f
    adult eye optics and refraction, 168, 169f
    contact lenses, 94, 95f
    contrast sensitivity, 176f, 177, 178
    developmental abnormalities, 69-70
    drug penetration factors, 95-97
    edema, 176f, 177, 178
    embryology, 69-70
    endothelium. See Corneal endothelium.
    epithelium. See Corneal epithelium.
    glare sensitivity, 176f, 177, 178
    metabolism, 92-94
    nerves, 66-68
    neurotrophic ulcers, 68
    nutrition, 92-95
    optic vesicle, 69
    oxygen requirements, 93-94
    pharmacology, 95-97
    preservative use in ophthalmic preparations, 96-97
    retina and, 322f
    stroma. See Corneal stroma.
    vitamin A, 94-95
    xerophthalmia, 95
Corneal endothelium
    anatomy, 59, 60f, 61f
    aqueous humor solution, 89
    BSS PLUS solution, 89t, 91
    contact lens-use endotheliopathy syndrome, 66
    Descemet's membrane, 64, 65f, 66, 70
    fluid pump, 86
    glutathione-bicarbonate ringer's solution, 89
    guttata, 66, 68f
    ion transport, 87-88
    irrigating solutions, 88-91
    metabolic pump, 86
    morphometry, 59-66
    physiology, 86-87
    pleomorphism, 63, 67f
    polymegathism, 59, 63, 67f, 94, 95f
    temperature reversal, 86, 87f
    wound healing, 91-92
Corneal epithelium
    anatomy, 47-49, 50f, 51f, 52f
    anchoring fibrils, 51
    anchoring plaques, 51
    basement membrane, 49-51
    Bowman's layer, 49-51
    cell adhesion, 51-53, 54f, 55f
    c-fos gene, 76
    c-jun gene, 76
    clinical manifestations of abnormalities in, 53-56
    electrophysiology and ion transport, 77-80
    exfoliation holes, 48
    ion transport, 77-80
    lacrimal system, 37-38, 39f
    maintenance of and response to wounding, 70-77
    nonkeratinized epithelium, 48
    tear film, 37-38, 39f
    wound healing, 70-77
    zonula occludens, 53
Corneal stroma, 56-59, 80-81
    chondroitin sulfate/dermatan sulfate proteoglycans, 56
    collagen interactions, 81-84
    ground substance, 56
    hydration, 84-85
    keratin sulfate proteoglycans, 56
    keratocan, 56, 58
    keratocytes, 56, 58
    lumican, 56, 58
    mimecan, 56, 58
    proteoglycans, 56, 81-85
    stromal fibroblasts, 58
    wound healing, 85-86

Correlational models of motion perception, 525
Corresponding retinal points/areas in binocular vision, 487
Cortex
    extrastriate visual cortex. See Extrastriate visual cortex.
    primary visual. See Primary visual cortex.
    vitreous, 294, 294f, 296f
Cortical cataracts, 140-146, 146-147
Cortical plasticity marker redistribution, 706
Corticosteroid mechanisms in aqueous humor hydrodynamics, 262-264, 265f, 266f
Cover points in binocular vision, 488
Craik-Cornsweet-O'Brien illusion, 188
Cranial nerves III, IV, VI, 833, 834f
Critical flicker fusion (CFF), 513
    Brücke brightness enhancement effect, 522
    chromaticity stimulus, 514, 515f
    eccentricity, 514, 515f
    Ferry-Porter law, 513, 514, 518
    Granit-Harper law, 514-516
    luminance stimulus, 513-514
    perception and, 522
    perimetry and visual field testing, 570-571
    size of stimulus, 514-516
    Talbot-Plateau law, 517, 522
Critical periods/durations
    extraocular muscle development, 804
    temporal properties of vision, 511-513
    visual deprivations, 700
Crossed diplopia, 486
Crossed disparity, 491
CRX. See Cone rod homeobox (CRX).
Crystalline lens
    accommodation, 207-208, 209f
    adult eye optics and refraction, 168-169
    presbyopia, 220f, 221-223, 224f
Crystallins
    adult eye optics and refraction, 169
    lens fiber cell differentiation, 122, 124-125, 134
CSARFs. See Center-surround antagonistic receptive field organization (CSARFs).
CSF. See Contrast sensitivity function (CSF).
CSNB. See Congenital stationary night blindness (CSNB).
Curvature establishment and maintenance, lens, 133
Cyclic guanine monophosphate, 370, 388-391, 419
Cyclins in lens fiber cell differentiation, 122
Cyclopean, 481
Cycloplegia, 213
Cyclorotations, 831
Cytoskeletal and cell junctional mechanisms in aqueous humor hydrodynamics, 267-269
Cytoskeleton and lens fiber cell differentiation, 125, 134

D

Daltonism, 579
Dark light, 450
Dark trough in electroretinograms, 415
Dark-field microscopy, 303
Deep petrosal nerve, 31f
Defenses against light scattering, 184
Deformation phosphene, 449
DEM. See Direction of eye movement (DEM).
Demographic data in perimetry and visual field testing, 557-560
Denervation in Horner Syndrome, 735-736
Depolarized optic nerves, 614
Deprivations. See Visual deprivations.

Depth of field
  accommodation, 200-201
  contrast sensitivity, 179
  glare sensitivity, 179
Depth of focus
  accommodation, 200-201
  contrast sensitivity, 179-180, 181f, 182f, 183f
  glare sensitivity, 179-180, 181f, 182f, 183f
  pupil, 714f, 715
  young eye optics and refraction, 162
Descemet's membrane, 64, 65f, 66, 70
Destructive interference, 184
Deuteranomaly, 584
Deuteranopia, 583, 584
Developing countries and cataracts, 148
Development. See also Embryology.
  corneal abnormalities, 69-70
  extraocular muscles, 803-804
  infant vision. See Infant vision development.
  lens, 119-122
  sclera, 99-100
  visual acuity, 464
  visual deprivations, 701-704
Deviation values in perimetry and visual field testing, 560
Diabetes
  cataracts, 145-146
  ocular circulation, 775
Dichromats, 583
Diffraction in visual acuity, 454
Diffuse bipolar cells, 333
Diffusion
  aqueous humor hydrodynamics, 238
  vitreous, 305-306, 309, 310f, 311f
Digenic retinitis pigmentosa, 366
Dilation lag, pupil, 732, 735f
Dilation of pupil, 721-723, 741-742
Diplopia, 486-487, 489
Direction of eye movement (DEM), 532
Direction selectivity in visual cortex, 698-701
Disaccommodation theory of presbyopia, 229
Disconjugate shifts of gaze distance, 845-847
Disconjugate smooth vergence tracking, 842-843
Discontinuous capillaries, 753-754
Disparity of the retinal images, 488, 491-493
Disparity-defined form in spatial form processing, 470, 480-481
Displaced amacrine cells, 333, 335, 338
Displacement perimetry, 567-570
Dissociated vertical deviation (DVD), 851
Distal disparity in binocular vision, 491
Distal stimulus in visual acuity, 453
Distichiasis, 19
Divergence in color vision, 581
Donders' law
  neural control of eye movements, 830
  three-dimensional rotations of the eye, 823
Dopaminergic retinal neurons, 341
Doppler techniques in ocular circulation, 759-760, 770, 775
Dorsal lateral geniculate nucleus (dLGN).
  See Retinogeniculate projection activity-dependent development.
Dorsal streams
  extrastriate visual cortex, 689-691
  primary visual cortex, 683
Dorsal V3, 691
Dowling-Rushton relationship, 594
Doyne honeycomb retinal dystrophy, 376
Drainage in aqueous humor hydrodynamics, 248-249
Drifts, 171
Drugs. See Pharmacology.

Duchenne muscular dystrophy, 813-814
Dura meninges in optic nerves, 610-611
Dural vessels in ocular circulation, 748f
DVD. See Dissociated vertical deviation (DVD).
Dyads, 332, 337, 338f
Dynamic control of eye alignment, 841-843
Dyschromatopsia, 584
Dysgenetic lens, 122
Dysmetria, 854

E
Early development, lens, 119-122
Early Manifest Glaucoma Trial (EMGT), 562-564
Early visual processing, 532, 533f
Eccentricity in critical flicker fusion, 514, 515f
Edge sharpening, 188
Edinger-Westphal nucleus
  central visual pathways, 642
  neural control of eye movements, 833, 851
  pupil, 716, 719, 720-721, 721-722, 730
EFEMP1 gene, 367t, 376
Efferent arm of the pupil light reflex, 719-720
Efferent axons, 658-659, 661f
Egocenter, 485
Egocentric direction, 485-486
Electrolyte balance, lens, 132-133
Electrolyte secretion in lacrimal system, 33-38
Electrooculography, 415-416
Electrophysiology
  corneal epithelium, 77-80
  inherited retinal dystrophies, 360-361
  optic nerve, 613-616
Electroretinograms (ERG), 409-410, 411f, 412f
  ABCR protein, 417
  Arden index, 415
  bestrophin protein, 417
  c wave, 410
  children and, 413-414
  choroideremia, 420
  cyclic guanine monophosphate-gated cation channel in cone photoreceptors, 419
  dark trough, 415
  defect differences in retinal proteins, 417-420
  electrooculography, 415-416
  focal electroretinogram examination, 416-417
  general anesthesia, 413-414
  isolated rod and cone responses, 414-415
  light peak, 415, 416f
  measurement methods, 411-417
  multifocal electroretinogram examination, 416-417, 418f
  origin of retinal responses, 410-411, 412f
  peripherin/RDS protein, 419
  photopic responses, 415
  rhodopsin, 419
  rhodopsin kinase, 420
  RS protein, 417
  scotopic responses, 415
  temporal aspects of, 415
Ellipsoids, 329
Elschnig's pearls, 142
Embryology. See also Development.
  conjunctiva, 16, 17f
  cornea, 69-70
  extraocular muscles, 803-804
  eyelids, 16-17
  lacrimal system, 30, 40
  orbit, 3, 17f
  retina, 319-322
  sclera, 99-100
  vitreous, 293-294

EMGT. See Early Manifest Glaucoma Trial (EMGT).
Emmetropization
  aging eye optics and refraction, 192
  young eye optics and refraction, 163-164
Endochondral bones, 3
Endothelium, cornea. See Corneal endothelium.
End-stopped cells, 676
Energy
  lens, 131-132
  retinal biochemistry, 400-403
Entoptic phenomena, 441
  angioscotometry, 447
  asteroid hyalosis, 445
  blue arcs of the retina, 447-448
  dark light, 450
  deformation phosphene, 449
  flick phosphene, 445-446
  fundus reflex, 441, 442f
  Haidinger's brushes, 449
  halos, 443-444
  intrinsic gray of the retina, 450
  Maxwellian view, 448
  Maxwell's spot, 448-449
  Moore's lightning streaks, 445
  muscae volitantes, 444
  ocular media imperfections, 441-443
  outer plexiform layer, images arising from, 449
  pathologic halos, 443-444
  perimetry, 452
  phosphenes, 445-446, 449-450
  physiologic halos, 443-444
  pinhole method, 442, 444
  pressure phosphene, 449
  Purkinje figures, 446-447
  quick eye movement, 445-446
  retinal nerve fiber distribution, images influenced by, 447-448
  retinal photoreceptor properties, phenomena caused by, 450-452
  retinal vasculature, 446-447
  Stiles-Crawford effect, 450, 451f, 452f
  vitreoretinal sources of entoptic images, 445
  vitreous produced images, 444-445
Episcleral vessels, 748f
Epithelial cells
  conjunctival, 34f, 37f, 38, 39f
  lacrimal system, 37-38, 39f
  lens, 128
Epithelium
  cornea. See Corneal epithelium.
  lens, 117, 118f
  retinal pigment epithelium. See Retinal pigment epithelium (RPE).
ERG. See Electroretinograms (ERG).
Erythrocytes, 269
Esophoria, 841
Esotropia, 851
Evolution of ocular components, 186
Excitotoxicity, 613
Excretory system of lacrimal system, 40-42
Exercise and aqueous humor hydrodynamics, 247t, 248
Exfoliation holes, 48
Exophthalmos, 7
Exotropia, 851
Exposure duration in visual acuity, 463
External carotid arterial supply, 12-13
Extracapsular cataract extraction, 142
Extraocular muscles, 787, 815
  annulus of Zinn, 788-790
  anteroposterior axis, 789f
  blood supply, 798, 799f
  bony orbit anatomy, 787, 788f
  botulinum toxin, 809, 811f
  channel blocking agents, 810-812
  congenital fibrosis of extraocular muscle, 806, 807f

Extraocular muscles—cont'd
contraction, 795-797
critical period in extraocular muscle development, 804
development, 803-804
disease responsiveness of, 812-815
division of labor in, 803
Duchenne muscular dystrophy, 813-814
embryonic origin, 803-804
fascia, 787-788, 789f
fiber structure-function, 792-797
fiber types, 797, 798-803
gene expression profiling, 804-806
genetics, 804-806, 807f
global intermediate singly innervated fiber, 801f, 802
global multiply innervated fiber, 801f, 803
global red singly innervated fiber, 801f, 802
global white singly innervated fiber, 801f, 802
globe, 787-788, 789f
graves ophthalmopathy, 813
gross anatomy, 788-791
inferior rectus, 789f
lateral orbit wall, 789f
lateral rectus, 789f, 790
layered organization, 798
local anesthetic toxicity, 812
medial orbital walls, 789f
medial rectus, 789f, 790
mitochondrial myopathies, 814-815
motor units, 808-809
muscular dystrophy, 813-814
myasthenia gravis, 813
myoblasts, 793
myofibrils, 795, 796f
myogenesis, 804, 805f
myotendinous cylinder, 803
nuclear domain, 793
optic nerve, 789f
orbital fat, 787-788, 789f
orbital multiply innervated fiber, 800-802
orbital singly innervated fiber, 800, 801f
PABP2 gene, 814
palisade ending, 803
pharmacology, 809-812
physiology, 806-809
Pitx2 gene, 806
proprioception, 809, 810f
pulley systems, 791-792
rhombomeres, 804
sarcolemma, 792
sarcomeres, 793-795
satellite cells, 793
skeletal muscle fiber types, 797
spiral of Tillaux, 788, 790f
strabismus, 806, 809-812, 813
structural organization, 798-803
superior rectus, 789f
Tenon's capsule, 788
transverse axis, 789f
twitch fibers, 795
vertical axis, 789f
Extraocular pulleys, 828-829
Extraorbital branches of the ophthalmic artery, 12
Extraretinal signals in neural control of eye movements, 835-837
Extrastriate visual cortex
akinetopsia, 694
area 7a, 691
callosal degeneration, 693
connection patterns, 687
defining visual areas, 686-687
dorsal stream areas, 689-691
dorsal V3, 691
evidence for in humans, 692-693
functional imaging, 693

Extrastriate visual cortex—cont'd
functional specificity, 687, 688f, 694
histology, 686, 693-694
inferotemporal cortex, 692
lateral geniculate nucleus, 687
lateral intraparietal area, 691
MT, 689-690
parietal lobe areas, 691
processing streams in, 687-694
retinotopographic mapping, 686
retinotopy, 693
V1 compared, 687-694
V2, 687-689
V3, 691
V3A, 691
V3 proper, 691
V4, 691-692
V5, 689-690
ventral posterior area, 691
ventral stream areas, 691-692
Eye movements of others, monitoring, 166-167
Eyebrows, 17-18
Eye-fixed coordinates, 819-820
Eyelids, 18-20
blepharospasm, 22-23
blinking, 22
chief retractor of the upper eyelid, 20
closure, 22
conjunctiva, 19f, 20f
distichiasis, 19
embryology, 16-17
frontonasal process, 16
hair follicles, 20f
hemifacial spasm, 23
Hering's law, 21
inferior orbicularis, 19f
inferior septum, 19f
inferior tarsus, 19f
levator, 19f
levator aponeurosis, 19f
Lockwood's ligament, 19f
maxillary process, 16
meibomian glands, 20f
Meige syndrome, 23
movement of, 20-22
mucocutaneous junction, 20f
Müller's muscle, 21-22
muscles of Riolan, 18, 20f
opening of, 20-22
orbital fat, 19f
pathway for eyelid movement, 22
spasm, 22-23
superior septum, 19f
superior tarsus, 19f
sweat gland, 20f
Tenson's capsule, 19f
Whitnall's ligament, 19f
winking, 22

F
Face, 16, 25-27
conjunctiva. See Conjunctiva.
extraocular muscles, 787-788, 789f
eyebrows. See Eyebrows.
eyelids. See Eyelids.
forehead. See Forehead.
recognition in young eye optics and refraction, 164-166
superficial musculoaponeurotic system, 25-27
tissue, 7-9
Facial nerve VII, 31f
False torsion, 821-822
Fat, orbit, 7-9
FDT perimetry. See Frequency doubling technology (FDT) perimetry.
Feedback
lateral geniculate nucleus, 662, 663f
neural control of eye movements, 831-833

Feed-forward pathways/systems
lateral geniculate nucleus, 662, 663f
neural control of eye movements, 831-833
Fenestrated capillaries, 753-754
Ferry-Porter law, 513, 514, 518
Fetal vasculature, 129
FGF. See Fibroblast growth factors (FGF).
Fiber baskets, 329
Fiber cell differentiation, lens. See Lens fiber cell differentiation.
Fiber structure-function in extraocular muscles, 792-797
Fiber types in extraocular muscles, 797, 798-803
Fibroblast growth factors (FGF), 123-124
"Filling in information," 186-187
Final common pathway, 833-834
Fine structures in ocular circulation, 753-756
First-order motion, 523-525
Fixation, 839-841
Fixation disparities
binocular vision, 492
neural control of eye movements, 840
Flare in aqueous humor hydrodynamics, 242
Flick phosphene, 445-446
Flicker perimetry, 570-571
Fluid circulation, lens, 132-133
Fluid mechanics in aqueous humor hydrodynamics, 248-249
Fluid pump in corneal endothelium, 86
Fluorescein absorption in retinal pigment epithelium (RPE), 352-353
Fluorescein angiography in ocular circulation, 757-759
Fluorescein concentration and profiles in the vitreous, 297-301, 305-306, 312-313
Focal electroretinogram examination, 416-417
Focus factors in visual acuity, 455
Forced-choice preferential looking (FPL), 531
Forced-duction fixation disparity curve, 840
Forehead, 17-18
Foucalt gratings, 173-174
Fourier transformation, 173-174
Fovea
accommodation, 202f
centralis, 342
trochlearis, 5
vitreous, 294f
Foveal gaze lock, 839-843
Foveal gaze shifts, 843-851
Foveal vision, 343
Foville syndrome, 852
FoxE3, 122
FPL. See Forced-choice preferential looking (FPL).
Free calcium, lens, 132-133
Frequency doubling effect in perimetry and visual field testing, 567
Frequency doubling technology (FDT) perimetry, 565-567, 568f
Friedreich ataxia, 360t
Frontonasal process, eyelids, 16
Functional imaging in extrastriate visual cortex, 693
Functional integrity and temporal properties of vision, 522
Functional specificity in extrastriate visual cortex, 687, 688f, 694
Fundamental waveform and temporal properties of vision, 516
Fundus flavimaculatus, 367t, 373-375
Fundus imaging, 361
Fundus reflex, 441, 442f
Fusion in infant vision development, 543-545

Future advances/prospects
 inherited retinal dystrophies, 377
 lens, 147-149

G

G protein-coupled receptors in color
 vision, 579
GABA synaptic release, 397-398
GABA-ergic amacrine cells, 333
Galactosemia and galactokinase deficiency,
 143
Ganglion cells
 postnatal retinal ganglion cell, 627
 pupil, 717-718
 retina, 322f, 323f, 324f, 325f, 338-339,
  339
 retinal intercellular light responses and
  synaptic organization, 433-434
Gap figures, 187
Gap junctions, 126-127
Gaze restrictions, 852-853
Gaze tracking, 561
GBR solution. *See* Glutathione-bicarbonate
 ringer's (GBR) solution.
General anesthesia and electroretinograms,
 413-414
Genes and genetics
 ABCR gene, 350, 363, 367t, 373-375, 597
 augmentation in recessive and X-linked
  diseases, 377
 bcl-2 gene overexpression, 627
 candidate gene analysis, 363
 cataracts, 147-148
 c-fos gene, 76
 c-jun gene, 76
 c-maf gene, 122
 color vision, 583
 EFEMP1 gene, 367t, 376
 expression profiling, 804-806
 extraocular muscles, 804-806, 807f
 inherited retinal dystrophies, 362-363,
  366-376
 IRBP gene, 351
 linkage mapping, 362-363
 L-maf, 121-122
 NR2E3 gene, 375-376
 PABP2 gene, 814
 peripherin/RDS gene, 361, 366, 367t,
  368, 371-372
 Pitx2 gene, 806
 RDH5 gene, 597
 retinal dystrophies. *See* Inherited retinal
  dystrophies.
 retinitis pigmentosa, 364t
 RPE65 gene, 367t, 374, 597
 sharing, 186
 therapy strategies, 377
 vitreous, 293-294
Geometric theory of presbyopia, 229
Germinative zone, 117
Glabella, 3
Glands and ocular surface epithelia that
 secrete tears, 32
Glare sensitivity, 175-177, 186
 aberrations, 180-186
 aspheric surfaces, 185
 cataracts, 178-179
 chromatic aberrations, 184
 contact lens wear, 178
 contrast luminance, 175
 corneal conditions, 178
 corneal edema, 176f, 177, 178
 defenses against light scattering, 184
 depth of field, 179
 depth of focus, 179-180, 181f, 182f, 183f
 destructive interference, 184
 intensity discrimination, 175
 keratoconus, 178
 light absorption, 186
 light scatterer vs. transmitter, 175
 light scattering, 183-184

Glare sensitivity—cont'd
 Miller-Nadler glare tester, 177
 modulation transfer function, 179
 nephrotic cystinosis, 178
 opacified posterior capsules, 178-179
 opaqueness, 175
 penetrating keratoplasty, 178
 refractive surgery, 178
 spatial form processing, 473-474
 spherical aberrations, 184-186
Glaucoma
 Advanced Glaucoma Intervention Study,
  564
 aqueous humor hydrodynamics, 253,
  258, 270
 Early Manifest Glaucoma Trial, 562-564
 Normal Tension Glaucoma Study, 562
 ocular circulation, 775-776
 optic nerve, 625
 visual deprivations, 704
Glia, 615
Glial cells, 336-337
Glial mantle of Fuchs, 608
Gliosis, 623
Glissade, 844
Global intermediate singly innervated fiber,
 801f, 802
Global multiply innervated fiber, 801f, 803
Global red singly innervated fiber, 801f,
 802
Global white singly innervated fiber, 801f,
 802
Globe
 extraocular muscles, 787-788, 789f
 orbit, 6-7
Globular degeneration, 141
Glucose and retinal biochemistry, 400
Glucose concentration, vitreous, 299f
Glutamate homeostasis, 394-396
Glutamate receptors, 396-397
Glutamate transporters, 393-394
Glutamatergic synapses between
 photoreceptors and second-order
 retinal neurons, 426-428
Glutamatergic transmission, 391-397
Glutathione, 130-131
Glutathione-bicarbonate ringer's (GBR)
 solution, 89
Glycine homeostasis, 398
Glycinergic amacrine cells, 333
Glycosaminoglycan, 168
Goldmann equation, 248
Graded potentials, optic nerve, 613
Gradient models of motion perception, 525
Granit-Harper law, 514-516
Grating acuity
 infant vision development, 535-536, 537f
 spatial form processing, 476
Graves ophthalmopathy, 813
Gray scale in perimetry and visual field
 testing, 560
Greater superior petrosal nerve, 31f
Ground substance in corneal stroma, 56
Growth, lens, 128, 147
Growth factor therapy in inherited retinal
 dystrophies, 377
Growth factors in lens fiber cell
 differentiation, 123-124, 128
Guanylate cyclase activating proteins, 370
Guanylate cyclase activators, 246
Guttata, 66, 68f

H

Haidinger's brushes, 449
Hair follicles, eyelids, 20f
Halftones, 173
Halos, 443-444
Harmonics, 516
Head-fixed coordinates, 820-821
Hemifacial spasm, 23
Henle fiber layer, 327

Hereditary cataracts, 142
Hering's law, 21
Heterophoria, 840
Heterotrimeric G proteins, 579
Hierarchy of oculomotor control, 833
Hierarchy of visual processing, 532-534
High-contrast acuity, 470-473
High-pass resolution perimetry, 571, 573f
Hill of vision, 552
Holobacterium halobium, 170
Holocrine secretion, 33
Homonymous hemianopsia, 645
Horizontal cell responses in retinal
 intercellular light responses and
 synaptic organization, 428
Horizontal cell synapses in retinal
 intercellular light responses and
 synaptic organization, 428-429
Horizontal cells, retina, 323f, 331-332
Horizontal disparity angles in binocular
 vision, 488
Horner syndrome, 730-731, 732-736
Horopter, 488-489
Hyaluronic acid in vitreous, 293, 295-297
Hyaluronidase and protease-induced
 facility increases in aqueous humor
 hydrodynamics, 267
Hydration
 corneal stroma, 84-85
 sclera, 100-101, 102
Hydrogen peroxide, lens, 130, 131
Hydroxyamphetamine test, 735-736
Hyperacuities
 infant vision development, 545
 spatial form processing, 477
 visual acuity, 457t, 458-459, 464
Hyperbaric oxygen treatments, 138
Hypercolumns in primary visual cortex, 681
Hypothalamus, 613

I

IGF. *See* Insulin-like growth factor (IGF).
Image segmentation, 522
Immune activation, optic nerve, 622-623
Incremental threshold in perimetry and
 visual field testing, 552, 553f
Indoleamine accumulating amacrine cell
 type (A17), 341
Induced effects, stereopsis, 501
Inequality that increases in bright light,
 pupil, 736-737
Inequality that increases in the dark, pupil,
 730-732, 734f, 735f
Infant vision development, 531, 547-548
 assessment methodologies, 531-532
 beat frequency, 544
 binocular vision, 543-547
 direction of eye movement, 532
 early visual processing, 532, 533f
 forced-choice preferential looking, 531
 fusion, 543-545
 grating acuity, 535-536, 537f
 hierarchy of visual processing, 532-534
 hyperacuities, 545
 late visual processing, 532, 533f
 middle visual processing, 532, 533f
 motion, 539-540, 541f, 542f
 ocular-following movements, 532
 optokinetic nystagmus, 532
 preferential looking, 531
 processing hierarchy, 532-534
 response waveform development,
  537-539, 540f
 spatiotemporal vision, 534-535, 536f
 stereopsis, 545-547, 548f
 stereothreshold, 545-547, 548f
 temporal resolution, 536-537, 538f
 TNO test, 546
 transient VEPs, 531
 Vernier acuity, 541-543, 544f
 visual evoked potentials, 531-532

Infantile strabismus syndrome, 852
Infectious agent causes of cataracts, 142
Inferior marginal arcade, 10f
Inferior orbicularis, 19f
Inferior orbital fissure, 31f
Inferior rectus, 789f
Inferior septum, 19f
Inferior tarsus, 19f
Inferotemporal cortex, 692
Inflammation, optic nerve, 624
Information processing and retinal
  biochemistry, 391-400
Infraorbital artery, 10f
Infraorbital groove, 31f
Infraorbital nerve, 31f
Infrared light exposure and cataracts, 145
Inherited retinal dystrophies, 358
  ABCR gene, 363, 367t, 373-375
  abetalipoproteinemia, 360t
  all-*trans*-retinyl ester isomerohydrolase,
    373, 374
  apoptosis, 377
  autosomal recessive retinitis pigmentosa,
    369-370
  Batten syndrome, 360t
  best vitelliform macular dystrophy, 376
  bestrophin, 367t, 376
  candidate gene analysis, 363
  cellular retinaldehyde-binding protein,
    374
  central dystrophies, 359
  cGMP-gated cation channel proteins,
    370
  11-*cis*-retinol dehydrogenase, 375
  class I mutants, 369
  class II mutants, 369
  class III mutants, 369
  clinical classification, 358-360
  clinical examination and investigations,
    360-361
  cone rod homeobox, 375
  congenital stationary night blindness,
    367t, 369, 370-371
  current management, 376-377
  Doyne honeycomb retinal dystrophy,
    376
  EFEMP1 gene, 367t, 376
  electrophysiology, 360-361
  Friedreich ataxia, 360t
  functional characteristics of rhodopsin,
    368-369
  fundus imaging, 361
  future prospects, 377
  gene augmentation in recessive and
    X-linked diseases, 377
  gene therapy strategies, 377
  genetic linkage mapping, 362-363
  growth factor therapy, 377
  guanylate cyclase activating proteins, 370
  inheritance pattern, 361-362
  Kearns-Sayre syndrome, 360t, 361
  Laurence-Moon/Bardet-Biedl syndrome,
    360t
  macular dystrophies, 359, 376
  Malattia Leventinese retinal dystrophy,
    367t, 376
  molecular genetic techniques, 362-363
  molecular genetics, 366-376
  mutations, 369
  neural retina leucine zipper, 375
  NR2E3 gene, 375-376
  PDE enzyme, 370
  peripheral dystrophies, 359
  peripherin/RDS gene, 361, 366, 367t,
    368, 371-372
  photoreceptor apoptosis manipulation,
    377
  photoreceptor structural proteins, 371-373
  photoreceptor transplantation, 377
  photoreceptor-specific-nuclear receptor,
    375-376

Inherited retinal dystrophies—cont'd
  phototransduction cascade proteins,
    366-371
  protein, cellular retinaldehyde-binding,
    374
  protein, photoreceptor structural,
    371-373
  protein, rim, 367t, 373-375
  protein, ROM-1, 371-372
  protein, serum retinal-binding, 375
  proteins, phototransduction cascade,
    366-371
  proteins of undermined function, 376
  psychophysics, 361
  Refsum syndrome, 360t
  retinal guanylate cyclases, 367t, 370
  retinal pigment epithelium
    transplantation, 377
  retinitis pigmentosa. *See* Retinitis
    pigmentosa.
  retinol metabolism, 373-375
  rhodopsin, 366-369
  ribozyme treatment in dominant
    disorders, 377
  rim protein, 367t, 373-375
  rod cGMP phosphodiesterase, 370
  ROM-1 protein, 361, 366, 371-372
  RPE65 gene, 367t, 374
  serum retinal-binding protein, 375
  Stargardt disease/fundus flavimaculatus,
    367t, 373-375
  structural characteristics of rhodopsin,
    368-369
  syndromic dystrophies, 359-360
  therapy, 376-377
  transcription factors, 375-376
  transplantation of photoreceptors and
    retinal pigment epithelium, 377
  Usher syndromes, 360t, 372
  vitamin A metabolism, 373-375
  X-linked retinoschisis, 372-373
Inhibitory transmission in retinal
  biochemistry, 397-399
Injury signal, optic nerve, 622
Inner ciliary ring, 724
Inner neuroblastic layers, 320
Inner nuclear layer, 323f, 325f, 331-336
Inner plexiform layer, 323f, 325f, 337, 338f
Inner psychophysics, 453
Inner segments of the photoreceptors, 348,
  349f
Innervation, 101
INO. *See* Internuclear ophthalmoplegia
  (INO).
Inputs in primary visual cortex, 672-674,
  683-684
Insulin-like growth factor (IGF), 123-124
Intensity discrimination, 175
Interaction effects in visual acuity, 463-464
Interactions between conjugate and
  disconjugate eye movements, 847,
  848f, 849f
Intercellular junction, 754f
Internal carotid artery, 9-12, 10f
Interneuron arm of pupil light reflex,
  718-719
Interneuron cells in lateral geniculate
  nucleus, 657
Internuclear ophthalmoplegia (INO), 852
Interocular blur suppression, 504-505
Interplexiform cells, 323f, 336, 432-433
Interpretation of visual field information,
  557-564
Interstitial amacrine cells, 333
Interstitial cells, 337
Intracapsular cataract extraction, 142
Intracranial optic nerve, 605, 618
Intramural pericyte, 754f
Intraocular pressure (IOP), 237, 246-248,
  266-267
  adrenergic mechanisms, 245-246

Intraocular pressure (IOP)—cont'd
  corticosteroid mechanisms, 262-264
  cytoskeletal and cell junctional
    mechanisms, 269
  fluid mechanics, 248-249
  macromolecule-induced facility
    decreases, 270
  outflow apparatus sensitivity, 259, 261
  outflow biomechanics, 270
  particulate-induced facility decreases,
    269-270
Intraorbital optic nerve, 604-605, 618
Intrinsic gray of the retina, 450
Ion transport
  corneal endothelium, 87-88
  corneal epithelium, 77-80
IOP. *See* Intraocular pressure (IOP).
IRBP gene, 351
Iris
  accommodation, 202f
  ocular circulation, 748f
  pupil, 723-724, 733t, 737-739
Irrigating solutions, corneal endothelium,
  88-91
Ischemia, 623-624
Isolated rod and cone responses in
  electroretinograms (ERG), 414-415

J

Jerk nystagmus, 835
Junctional complex, ocular circulation, 754f

K

K cell physiology, 656-659, 664-665
Kearns-Sayre syndrome, 360t, 361
Keratin sulfate (KS) proteoglycans, 56
Keratocan, 56, 58
Keratoconus, 178
Keratocytes, 56, 58
Keratoplasty, penetrating, 178
Ketanserin, 246-248
KIF3A protein, 392-393
Kinematic redundancy, 823
Kinetic perimetry, 554, 555f
KS proteoglycans. *See* Keratin sulfate (KS)
  proteoglycans.

L

Lacrimal artery, 10f
Lacrimal gland, 30-32
  accessory lacrimal gland secretion, 36-37
  deep petrosal nerve, 31f
  electrolyte secretion, 33-37
  embryology, 30
  facial nerve VII, 31f
  greater superior petrosal nerve, 31f
  inferior orbital fissure, 31f
  infraorbital groove, 31f
  infraorbital nerve, 31f
  lacrimal nerve, 31f
  main lacrimal gland secretion, 33-36,
    37f, 38f
  maxillary nerve, 31f
  merocrine secretion, 34
  protein secretion, 33-37
  signal transduction pathway, 35, 37f
  sphenopalatine ganglion, 31f
  sphenopalatine nerves, 31f
  trigeminal nerve V, 31f
  vidian nerve, 31f
  water secretion, 33-37
  zygomatic nerve, 31f
Lacrimal gland fossa, 5
Lacrimal system
  conjunctival epithelial cells, 34f, 37f,
    38, 39f
  conjunctival goblet cells, 38-39
  corneal epithelial cells, 37-38, 39f
  electrolyte secretion, 33-38
  embryology of lacrimal excretory
    system, 40

Lacrimal system—cont'd
  excretory system, 40-42
  holocrine secretion, 33
  lacrimal gland. *See* Lacrimal gland.
  lacrimal pump theory, 41
  lipids, 32-33
  meibomian gland secretion of lipids,
    32-33
  mucins, 38-39
  nasolacrimal groove, 40
  punctum, 40
  tear film. *See* Tear film.
  water secretion, 33-38
Lactate accumulation, lens, 129
Lactate concentration, vitreous, 299f
Lactate metabolism and retinal
    biochemistry, 400-401
Landolt's Cs, 457, 459, 460, 463
Late visual processing, 532, 533f
Latent nystagmus, 839
Lateral geniculate nucleus (LGN), 641,
    642f, 644f, 656f
  afferent axons, 658, 659f, 660f
  anatomical organization, 655-659
  axons, 658-659
  broad band cells, 664
  cell classes, 657-658
  circuit neurochemistry, 662-664
  efferent axons, 658-659, 661f
  extrastriate visual cortex, 687
  feedback, 662, 663f
  feed-forward pathways, 662, 663f
  interneuron cells, 657
  K cell physiology, 656-659, 664-665
  layers and maps, 656-657
  M cell physiology, 656-659, 664-665
  M lesions, 665-667
  optic chiasm, 656f
  optic nerve, 605, 612, 656f
  optic radiations, 656f
  P cell physiology, 656-659, 664-665
  P lesions, 665-667
  parallel processing, 664-667
  primary visual cortex, 670f, 673-678
  ratios, 661-662
  receptive field properties, 661-662
  relay cells, 657
  retina, 656f
  striate cortex, 656f
  structural organization, 655-659
  transfer ratios, 662
  triad, 662
  visual signal regulation, 659-664
  visual signals to cortex, 655
Lateral intraparietal area (LIP) of
    extrastriate visual cortex, 691
Lateral orbit wall, extraocular muscles, 789f
Lateral palpebral artery, 10f
Lateral rectus, extraocular muscles, 789f,
    790
Laurence-Moon/Bardet-Biedl syndrome,
    360t
Layer IVB of Brodmann, 674
Layered organization of extraocular
    muscles, 798
Layers and connections of primary visual
    cortex, 672-674, 675f, 676f
Layers and maps of lateral geniculate
    nucleus, 656-657
Lazy eye. *See* Amblyopia.
Lens, 117
  accommodation, 202f
  adult lens anatomy, 117-118, 119f
  aging, changes with, 133-134
  anterior cortex, 118f
  anterior pupillary membrane, 129
  anterior segment organizer, 129
  anterior suture, 118f
  aphakia, 122
  ascorbic acid, 131
  ATP, 131-132

Lens—cont'd
  bow region, 118f
  bZIP transcription factors, 121
  capillary network, 129
  capsule, 117, 118f, 135-136
  cataracts. *See* Cataracts.
  cell metabolism problems, 129-131
  chromophores, 133
  c-maf, 122
  crystalline lens. *See* Crystalline lens.
  curvature establishment and
    maintenance, 133
  dysgenetic lens, 122
  early development, 119-122
  electrolyte balance, 132-133
  energy production, 131-132
  epithelial cell communication, 128
  epithelium, 117, 118f
  fetal vasculature, 129
  fiber cell differentiation. *See* Lens fiber
    cell differentiation.
  fluid circulation, 132-133
  FoxE3, 122
  free calcium, 132-133
  future advances, 147-149
  germinative zone, 117
  glutathione, 130-131
  growth, 128, 147
  hydrogen peroxide, 130, 131
  lactate accumulation, 129
  L-maf, 121-122
  maf family of transcription factors,
    121-122
  nuclear region, 118f
  oxidants within and around lens, 130
  oxidative damage protection, 130-131
  oxidative stress, 129-131
  Pax-6, 119-121
  Pitx3, 122
  posterior cortex, 118f
  presbyopia, 222, 226-227, 229
  primary vitreous body, 121
  protein stability, 129
  proteins and aging, 134
  prox1, 122
  refraction, 118-119, 133
  retina, 322f
  sox1, 122
  suspensory ligaments, 118f
  sutures, 117, 118f, 134-135
  transcription factors, 119-122
  transparency, 118-119, 133
  tunica vasculosa lentis, 129
  umbilical suture, 134
  vascular support during development,
    129
  water balance, 132-133
  zonules, 118, 119f, 136-137
Lens fiber cell differentiation, 122-124
  adhesion, 128
  anterior segment organizer, 129
  ball-and-socket joints, 125, 126f
  beaded filaments, 125, 134
  cholesterol, 126
  classical crystallins, 124-125
  connexins, 126-127
  crystallins, 122, 124-125, 134
  cyclins, 122
  cytoskeleton, 125, 134
  epithelial cell communication, 128
  fibroblast growth factors, 123-124
  gap junctions, 126-127
  growth factors, 123-124, 128
  insulin-like growth factor, 123-124
  lipids, 125-126
  major intrinsic polypeptide, 126
  microtubules, 125
  MP20, 127-128
  N-cadherin, 128
  organelle degradation, 128
  proteins, 126-128

Lens fiber cell differentiation—cont'd
  taxon specific crystallins, 124-125
  vascular support during development, 129
  vimentin, 125, 134
Lenticular sclerosis, 227, 228-229
Leptomeninges, 610
Levator, eyelids, 19f
Levator aponeurosis, 19f
LGN. *See* Lateral geniculate nucleus (LGN).
Light
  absorption, 186
  color and, 578-579
  induced responses, 354-355
  path, 311
  peak and electroretinograms, 415, 416f
  pupil and, 716-720, 724-725, 725-728,
    726t, 740-741
  Retinal intercellular light responses and
    synaptic organization. *See* Retinal
    intercellular light responses and
    synaptic organization.
  scatterer vs. transmitter, 175
  scattering, 183-184
  sensitivity factors in perimetry and
    visual field testing, 552-553
Limbal network, 748f
Line orientation receptors, 166
Linear filters, 517
Linear systems, 516
Linkage mapping, 362f
LIP of extrastriate visual cortex. *See* Lateral
    intraparietal area (LIP) of extrastriate
    visual cortex.
Lipids
  lacrimal system, 32-33
  lens fiber cell differentiation, 125-126
  tear film, 32-33
Listing's law, 823-824
L-maf, 121-122
Local anesthetic toxicity and extraocular
    muscles, 812
Local image features, 669
Local sign in binocular vision, 485
Lockwood's ligament, 19f
Long posterior ciliary artery, 748f, 751
Longitudinal visual angles in binocular
    vision, 488
Long-range motion mechanism, 524
Low-contrast letter acuity, 470-473
Lumican, 56, 58
Luminance
  critical flicker fusion frequency, 513-514
  spatial form processing, 470-478
  temporal properties of vision, 520
  visual acuity, 462-463
Lymphatic drainage, 14
Lyonization, 366

M

M cell physiology, 656-659, 664-665
M lesions, 665-667
Macromolecule-induced facility decreases,
    270
Macula lutea, 342
Macular degeneration, 776
Macular dystrophies, 359, 376
Macular edema, 309, 310f, 310t
Maculopapillary bundle, 339
Maf family of transcription factors,
    121-122
Magnocellular pathways, 522
Main lacrimal gland secretion, 33-36, 37f,
    38f
Main zonular fibers, 205
Maintenance of foveal alignment with
    stationary and slowly moving targets,
    839-843
Major arterial circle of iris, 748f
Major intrinsic polypeptide (MIP), 126
Malattia Leventinese retinal dystrophy,
    367t, 376

MAR. *See* Minimum angle of resolution (MAR).
Marcus Gunn pupil, 612
Mast cells, 611
Mature vitreous body anatomy, 294-295
Maxillary artery, 10f
Maxillary bone, 3
Maxillary nerve, 31f
Maxillary process, eyelids, 16
Maxwellian view, 448
Maxwell's disc, 583
Maxwell's spot, 448-449
Mean-modulated flicker, 520
Measurement methods
  accommodation, 213-214
  electroretinograms, 411-417
  ocular circulation, 756-761
Medial orbital walls of extraocular muscles, 789f
Medial rectus of extraocular muscles, 789f, 790
Medial strut, 4
Medium-contrast acuity, 470-473
Meibomian glands
  eyelids, 20f
  lacrimal system, 32-33
Meige syndrome, 23
Membranous bones, orbit, 3
Meninges, optic nerve, 610-611
Meningothelial cells, 611
Meridional variations in acuity, 463
Merocrine secretion, 34
Metabolic buffer function, vitreous, 309-311
Metabolic control of blood flow, 771-773
Metabolic pump, corneal endothelium, 86
Meter angles, 840
Mexican hat sensitivity profile, 477
Michelson contrast, 466, 467f
Microcircuitry, primary visual cortex, 678-681
Microglia, 610
Microglial cells, 337
Micropinocytotic vesicles, 754f
Microsaccades, 171
Microtubules
  aqueous humor hydrodynamics, 269
  lens fiber cell differentiation, 125
Microwave exposure and cataracts, 145
Middle meningeal artery, 10f
Middle visual processing, 532, 533f
Midget bipolar cells, 333
Midget cell system, 342
Miller-Nadler glare tester, 177
Mimecan, 56, 58
Minimum angle of resolution (MAR), 458
Minimum discriminable and visual acuity, 457t, 458-459
Minimum resolvable and visual acuity, 457-458, 459-461
Minimum visible and visual acuity, 456-457
MIP. *See* Major intrinsic polypeptide (MIP).
Mitochondrial myopathies, 814-815
Mixed cataracts, 141
Modulation transfer function (MTF), 179
Modules, primary visual cortex, 681-683
Molecular genetics
  color vision, 583
  inherited retinal dystrophies, 362-363, 366-376
  vitreous, 293-294
Molecular mechanisms of aging, vitreous, 302-303
Monads, 337
Monitoring other's eye movements, 166-167
Monochromatic light, 578
Monovision, 499
Moore's lightning streaks, 445

Morphology, conjunctiva, 23-24
Morphometry, corneal endothelium, 59-66
Motion processing, 523
  apparent motion, 523
  clinical applications of motion processing, 526-527
  correlational models of motion perception, 525
  first-order motion, 523-525
  gradient models of motion perception, 525
  infant vision development, 539-540, 541f, 542f
  long-range motion mechanism, 524
  motion adaptation, 523
  motion aftereffect, 523
  motion perception models, 524-525
  neural encoding of motion, 525-526
  perceptual evidence for unique motion processing, 523-525
  perimetry and visual field testing, 567-570
  psychophysical evidence for unique motion processing, 523-525
  second-order motion, 523-525
  spatial form processing, 470, 478-479
Motion-in-depth, 503-504
Motor neuron responses, 833-834, 835f
Motor units, extraocular muscles, 808-809
Movement, recognizing, 167
Movement field of cells, 848
Movement of eyelids, 20-22
Movements of the eye
  neural control. *See* Neural control of eye movements.
  three-dimensional rotations. *See* Three-dimensional rotations of the eye.
MP20, 127-128
MTF. *See* Modulation transfer function (MTF).
Mucins, 38-39
Mucocutaneous junction, eyelids, 20f
Müller cells
  retina, 322, 323f, 327, 329, 336-337
  retinal pigment epithelium, 348, 349f
Müller's muscle, 21-22
Multifactorial theory of presbyopia, 230
Multifocal electroretinogram examination, 416-417, 418f
Multiple visual field assessments to determine progression, 561-562
Muscae volitantes, 444
Muscles of Riolan, 18, 20f
Muscular branch, orbit, 10f
Muscular dystrophy, 813-814
Mutations, inherited retinal dystrophies, 369
Myasthenia gravis, 813
Myelin, optic nerve, 606-608, 615-616
Myoblasts, 793
Myocilin, 263-264, 265f
Myofibrils, extraocular muscles, 795, 796f
Myogenesis, extraocular muscles, 804, 805f
Myoids, 329
Myopia, 189-190
Myotendinous cylinder, extraocular muscles, 803

N

Nasal hemianopsia, 645
Nasofrontal artery, 10f
Nasolacrimal groove, 40
N-cadherin, 128
Near reflex, 212
Near response
  neural control of eye movements, 845-847
  pupil, 720-721, 740-741
Near triad and interactions with saccades, 850-851
Necrosis, 620

Negative afterimage, 583
Negative vergence, 200
Nephrotic cystinosis, 178
Nerve fiber bundle defects, 604
Nerve fiber layer
  optic nerve, 603-604
  retina, 325f, 339
Nerve pathways, pupil, 716-723
Nerves
  cornea, 66-68
  cranial nerves III, IV, VI, 833, 834f
  deep petrosal nerve, 31f
  facial nerve VII, 31f
  greater superior petrosal nerve, 31f
  infraorbital nerve, 31f
  lacrimal nerve, 31f
  maxillary nerve, 31f
  ophthalmic division of the trigeminal nerve, 723
  optic nerve. *See* Optic nerve.
  sphenopalatine nerves, 31f
  trigeminal nerve V, 31f
  vidian nerve, 31f
  zygomatic nerve, 31f
Nervous control of blood flow, 767-769
Neural control of eye movements
  abducens palsy, 852
  accommodative-convergence, 840
  adaptable interactions between smooth pursuit and smooth vergence, 843
  anatomic position of rest, 841
  anterior internuclear ophthalmoplegia, 852
  asymmetric vergence, 847, 848f, 849f
  binocular constraints on eye position control, 830-831, 832f
  closed loop, 842
  cogwheel pursuit, 842
  complete ophthalmoplegia, 852
  components of eye rotation, 830, 831f
  concomitant adaptation, 840
  conjugate smooth pursuit tracking, 841-842
  cranial nerves III, IV, VI and motor nuclei, 833, 834f
  cyclorotations, 831
  disconjugate shifts of gaze distance, 845-847
  disconjugate smooth vergence tracking, 842-843
  disorders, 851-856
  dissociated vertical deviation, 851
  Donders' law, 830
  dynamic control of eye alignment, 841-843
  dysmetria, 854
  Edinger-Westphal nucleus, 833, 851
  esophoria, 841
  esotropia, 851
  exotropia, 851
  extraretinal signals, 835-837
  feedback systems, 831-833
  feed-forward systems, 831-833
  final common pathway, 833-834
  fixation, 839-841
  fixation disparity, 840
  forced-duction fixation disparity curve, 840
  foveal gaze lock, 839-843
  foveal gaze shifts, 843-851
  Foville syndrome, 852
  gaze restrictions, 852-853
  glissade, 844
  heterophoria, 840
  hierarchy of oculomotor control, 833
  infantile strabismus syndrome, 852
  interactions between conjugate and disconjugate eye movements, 847, 848f, 849f
  internuclear ophthalmoplegia, 852
  jerk nystagmus, 835

Neural control of eye movements—cont'd
latent nystagmus, 839
maintenance of foveal alignment with
stationary and slowly moving targets,
839-843
meter angles, 840
motor neuron response, 833-834, 835f
movement field of cells, 848
near response in symmetric
convergence, 845-847
near triad and interactions with
saccades, 850-851
neurocontrol of foveal gaze shifts,
847-851
neurocontrol of smooth foveal tracking,
843
neurocontrol of stabilization reflexes,
837-839
nystagmus, 854-856
ocular orientation, 824-829
one-and-a-half-syndrome, 852
open loop, 842
ophthalmoplegia, 852, 853f
optokinetic nystagmus, 837, 839
physiologic position of rest, 841
posterior internuclear ophthalmoplegia,
852
prism diopters, 840
pursuit component of smooth following
eye, 841
rapid conjugate shifts of gaze direction,
843-845
retinal signals, 837
saccade disorders, 853-854, 855f
saccades, 833, 850-851
saccadic eye movements, 843-845
saccadic gaze shifting system, 847-850
smooth pursuit tracking system, 843
smooth tracking responses to open- and
closed-loop stimuli, 841-843
smooth vergence, 841
smooth vergence tracking system, 843
stabilization of gaze relative to the
external world, 834-839
static control of eye alignment, 839-841
strabismus, 851-852
target selection and foveal acquisition,
843-851
trochlear palsy, 852
vergence gaze shifting system, 850-851
vergence systems, 831
version systems, 831
vestibuloocular reflex, 835-838
visual sensory-motor tasks, 830
Neural control of ocular orientation,
824-829
Neural encoding of motion, 525-526
Neural processing in young eyes, 164, 165f
Neural retina leucine zipper, 375
Neurite extension inhibition, 626-627
Neurite extension substrates, 627
Neurochemistry, 391-400
Neurocontrol of foveal gaze shifts, 847-851
Neurocontrol of smooth foveal tracking,
843
Neurocontrol of stabilization reflexes,
837-839
Neurotrophic ulcers, 68
Neurulation, retina, 319
Nigrescent cataracts, 133
Nitric oxide synthesis (NOS), 399-400
Nitrovasodilators, 246, 247t
Nodes of Ranvier, 615
Noncommutative rotations, 818
Nonkeratinized corneal epithelium, 48
Nonoptical brain mechanisms that
enhance retinal image, 186-189
Normal retinal correspondence in
binocular vision, 487-489
Normal Tension Glaucoma Study, 562
Normal visual acuity, 461

NOS. *See* Nitric oxide synthesis (NOS).
NR2E3 gene, 375-376
Nuclear cataracts, 137-140, 146-147
Nuclear domain, extraocular muscles, 793
Nuclear region, lens, 118f
Nuclear sclerotic cataracts, 138
Numeric values in perimetry and visual
field testing, 560
Nutrition
cataracts and, 148
cornea and, 92-95
Nystagmus, 839, 854-856

O

OCT. *See* Optical coherence tomography
(OCT).
Ocular circulation, 747
aging, 776
anatomy, 747-753
animal experiments to measure ocular
blood flow, 757
anterior ciliary vessels, 748f
anterior optic nerve, 749, 750f
blood-ocular barriers, 753-756
blue-field entoptic phenomenon, 761
canal of Schlemm, 748f
capillaries, 753-756, 774
central retinal artery and vein, 748f
choriocapillaris, 748f, 751, 752f, 756
choroid, 754f, 756, 774
ciliary processes, 754f, 756
clinical methods to measure ocular
blood flow, 757-761
conjunctival vessels, 748f
continuos capillaries, 753-754
diabetes mellitus, 775
discontinuous capillaries, 753-754
Doppler techniques, 759-760, 770, 775
drugs, effect on blood flow, 769-773
dural vessels, 748f
endothelium basement membrane, 754f
episcleral vessels, 748f
fenestrated capillaries, 753-754
fine structures, 753-756
fluorescein angiography, 757-759
glaucoma, 775-776
intercellular junction, 754f
intramural pericyte, 754f
iris vessels, 748f
junctional complex, 754f
limbal network, 748f
long posterior ciliary artery, 748f, 751
macular degeneration, 776
major arterial circle of iris, 748f
measurement of ocular blood flow,
756-761
metabolic control of blood flow, 771-773
micropinocytotic vesicles, 754f
nervous control of blood flow, 767-769
oxygen supply, 761-763, 771-772
perfusion pressure, 764-767, 768f
pial vessels, 748f
rate of blood flow, 761-763
retina, 754f
retinal vessels, 748f
short posterior ciliary arteries, 748f, 749,
750-751
tissue fluid formation and drainage, 774
vascular endothelium, 763-764, 770
vasoconstrictors, 770
vasodilators, 770-771
vasomotion, 763
vortex vein, 748f
Ocular dominance, 673
Ocular dominance plasticity, 697-698,
700-701
Ocular media imperfections, 441-443
Ocular orientation, 824-829
Ocular surface
conjunctiva. *See* Conjunctiva.
eyebrows. *See* Eyebrows.

Ocular surface—cont'd
eyelids. *See* Eyelids.
face. *See* Face.
forehead. *See* Forehead.
lacrimal system. *See* Lacrimal system.
orbit. *See* Orbit.
Ocular-following movements in infants,
532
Oculocentric direction in binocular vision,
485
Oculomotor nucleus in central visual
pathways, 642f
OFF channels, 323-324, 325t
OFF-response, 582
OKN. *See* Optokinetic nystagmus (OKN).
Oligodendrocytes, 606-608
OLM. *See* Outer limiting membrane
(OLM).
ON-channels, 323-324, 325f
One-and-a-half-syndrome, 852
ON-OFF-cells, 433-434
ON-response, color vision, 582
Opacified posterior capsules, 178-179
Opaqueness, 175
Open loop, 842
Opening of eyelids, 20-22
Ophthalmic artery, 10-13
Ophthalmic division of the trigeminal
nerve, 723
Ophthalmic facial anatomy and physiology,
16
conjunctiva. *See* Conjunctiva.
eyebrows. *See* Eyebrows.
eyelids. *See* Eyelids.
face. *See* Face.
forehead. *See* Forehead.
Ophthalmoplegia, 852, 853f
Opponent processes in color vision, 582
Opsin protein, 424
Opsin-shift, 579
Optic nerve, 603
action potentials, 613-615
angioblastic meningiomas, 611
apoptosis, 620-621
apoptosome, 621
arachnoid meninges, 610-611
astrocytes, 608-610
axon counts and dimensions, 605-606
axonal conduction, 613-616
axonal injury, 619-626
axonal regeneration, 626
axonal transport, 616-617
axons, 603-604, 606, 612-613
bcl-2 gene overexpression, 627
blood supply, 617-619
central nervous system axonal
regeneration, 626
central visual pathways, 642f, 644f
chiasm, 605, 618
clinical implications of axonal injury,
619
compression, 624-625
compressive optic neuropathy, 605
depolarized, 614
dura meninges, 610-611
electrophysiology, 613-616
excitotoxicity, 613
extraocular muscles, 789f
glaucoma, 625
glia, 615
glial mantle of Fuchs, 608
gliosis, 623
graded potentials, 613
hypothalamus, 613
immune activation, 622-623
inflammation, 624
injury signal, 622
intracranial optic nerve, 605, 618
intraorbital optic nerve, 604-605, 618
ischemia, 623-624
lateral geniculate nucleus, 605, 612, 656f

Optic nerve—cont'd
 leptomeninges, 610
 Marcus Gunn pupil, 612
 mast cells, 611
 meninges, 610-611
 meningothelial cells, 611
 microglia, 610
 microscopic anatomy and cytology,
  606-612
 myelin, 606-608, 615-616
 necrosis, 620
 nerve fiber bundle defects, 604
 nerve fiber layer, 603-604
 neurite extension inhibition, 626-627
 neurite extension substrates, 627
 nodes of Ranvier, 615
 oligodendrocytes, 606-608
 optic canal, 605, 618
 optic nerve head, 617-618
 optic tract, 605, 618
 pachymeninges, 610
 papilledema, 625-626
 phagocytosis, 622-623
 pia meninges, 610-611
 postnatal retinal ganglion cell, 627
 pretectal nuclei, 612
 primary visual cortex, 670f
 regeneration, 626-627
 resting potential, 614
 retina, 322f, 339
 retinal blood supply, 617
 retinal ganglion cell axons, 603-604,
  612-613, 619-622
 retinal ganglion cell electrophysiology,
  613
 retinopetal projections, 613
 retinotopy, 604-605
 saltatory conduction, 615
 signaling of axonal injury, 621-622
 superior colliculus, 612-613
 swinging flashlight test, 612
 synaptic transmissions, 613
 therapies of axonal injury, 622
 topographic anatomy, 603-605
 transection, 623
 Uhthoff's phenomenon, 616
 vascular biology, 618-619
Optic radiations
 central visual pathways, 642f, 644f
 lateral geniculate nucleus, 656f
 primary visual cortex, 670f
Optic strut, 5
Optic tracts
 central visual pathways, 642f, 644f
 optic nerve, 605, 618
 primary visual cortex, 670f
Optic vesicle, cornea, 69
Optical aberration reduction, 713, 714f
Optical coherence tomography (OCT),
  303-305, 307
Optics and refraction
 adult eyes. See Adult eyes.
 aging eyes. See Aging eyes.
 contrast sensitivity. See Contrast
  sensitivity.
 glare sensitivity. See Glare sensitivity.
 tissue light scattering, 175-177
 young eyes. See Young eye optics and
  refraction.
Optokinetic nystagmus (OKN)
 infant vision development, 532
 neural control of eye movements, 837,
  839
Ora serrata, 202f
Orbit
 angular artery, 10f
 anterior ethmoidal artery, 10f
 arteries, 9-13
 bones of, 3-6
 branching order of ophthalmic artery, 11
 connective tissue, 7-9, 17f

Orbit—cont'd
 embryology, 3, 17f
 endochondral bones, 3
 exophthalmos, 7
 external carotid arterial supply, 12-13
 extraocular muscles, 787, 788f
 extraorbital branches of the ophthalmic
  artery, 12
 fascial tissue, 7-9
 fat, 7-9, 19f, 787-788, 789f
 fovea trochlearis, 5
 glabella, 3
 globe, 6-7
 inferior marginal arcade, 10f
 infraorbital artery, 10f
 internal carotid arterial supply, 9-12
 internal carotid artery, 10f
 lacrimal artery, 10f
 lacrimal gland fossa, 5
 lateral palpebral artery, 10f
 lymphatic drainage, 14
 maxillary artery, 10f
 maxillary bone, 3
 medial strut, 4
 membranous bones, 3
 middle meningeal artery, 10f
 muscular branch, 10f
 nasofrontal artery, 10f
 ocular branches of the ophthalmic
  artery, 12
 ophthalmic artery, 10-13
 optic strut, 5
 orbital branches of the ophthalmic
  artery, 12
 osteology/fractures, 3-6
 posterior ciliary artery, 10f
 proptosis, 7
 recurrent meningeal artery, 10f
 sphenoid bone, 3
 superior alveolar artery, 10f
 superior marginal arcade, 10f
 supraorbital artery, 10f
 supraorbital ridges, 3
 supratrochlear artery, 10f
 thyroid eye disease, 7
 vasculature, 9-14
 venous drainage, 13-14
 zygomaticofacial artery, 10f
 zygomaticotemporal artery, 10f
Orbital multiply innervated fiber, 800-802
Orbital singly innervated fiber, 800, 801f
Ordinary visual acuity, 457-458, 459-461
Organelle degradation in lens fiber cell
  differentiation, 128
Orientation selectivity in visual cortex,
  698-701
Origin of retinal responses in
  electroretinograms, 410-411, 412f
Outer ciliary ring, pupil, 724
Outer limiting membrane (OLM), 336,
  348, 349f
Outer neuroblastic layers, retina, 320
Outer nuclear layer, retina, 323f, 325f, 327-330
Outer plexiform layer
 images arising from, 449
 retina, 325f, 330-331
Outer psychophysics, 453
Outer segments of the photoreceptors, 348,
  349f
Outflow apparatus cholinergic sensitivity
  alterations, 258-261
Outflow apparatus sensitivity, 259, 261
Outflow biomechanics, 270-271
Output of retina, 586
Outputs, primary visual cortex, 674, 675f,
  676f, 683-684
Oxidants within and around lens, 130
Oxidative damage protection, lens, 130-131
Oxidative stress, lens, 129-131
Oxidative stress and cataracts, 138, 139,
  146-147

Oxygen concentration, vitreous, 300f
Oxygen requirements of cornea, 93-94
Oxygen supply and consumption, 402-403,
  761-763, 771-772

P

P cells
 lateral geniculate nucleus, 656-659,
  664-665
 retina, 339
P lesions, 665-667
PABP2 gene, 814
Pachymeninges, 610
Palisade ending in extraocular muscles, 803
Pan-retinal photocoagulation (PRP),
  704-706
Panum's fusional area (PFA), 489, 492
Papilledema, 625-626
Parallel inputs and outputs in primary
  visual cortex, 683-684
Parallel processing in lateral geniculate
  nucleus, 664-667
Parasol ganglion cells, 339
Parietal lobe areas in extrastriate visual
  cortex, 691
Pars plana, 201, 206f
Particulate-induced facility decreases,
  269-270
Parvocellular pathways, 522
Pathologic halos, 443-444
Pathologic myopia, 189-190
Pathway for eyelid movement, 22
Pattern deviation probability plots in
  perimetry and visual field testing,
  560-561
Pax-6, 119-121
PCO. *See* Posterior capsular opacification
  (PCO).
PDE enzyme, 370
Penetrating keratoplasty, 178
Perception
 acuity. *See* Visual acuity.
 adaptation. *See* Visual adaptation.
 binocular vision. *See* Binocular vision.
 color vision. *See* Color vision.
 critical flicker fusion frequency, 522
 entoptic phenomena. *See* Entoptic
  phenomena.
 infants. *See* Infant vision development.
 motion processing, 523-525
 perimetry and visual field testing. *See*
  Perimetry and visual field testing.
 spatial form processing. *See* Spatial form
  processing.
 temporal properties. *See* Temporal
  properties of vision.
Perfusion pressure, 764-767, 768f
Perimetry and visual field testing, 572-573
 Advanced Glaucoma Intervention Study,
  564
 clinical trials and progression, 562
 Collaborative Initial Glaucoma
  Treatment Study, 564
 critical flicker fusion, 570-571
 demographic data, 557-560
 deviation values, 560
 displacement perimetry, 567-570
 Early Manifest Glaucoma Trial, 562-564
 entoptic phenomena, 452
 flicker perimetry, 570-571
 frequency doubling effect, 567
 frequency doubling technology
  perimetry, 565-567, 568f
 gaze tracking, 561
 gray scale, 560
 high-pass resolution perimetry, 571, 573f
 hill of vision, 552
 incremental threshold, 552, 553f
 interpretation of visual field
  information, 557-564
 kinetic perimetry, 554, 555f

Perimetry and visual field testing—cont'd
  light sensitivity factors, 552-553
  methods of conducting perimetry,
    553-557
  motion-automated perimetry, 567-570
  multiple visual field assessments to
    determine progression, 561-562
  new perimetric test procedures, 564-572
  Normal Tension Glaucoma Study, 562
  numeric values, 560
  pattern deviation probability plots,
    560-561
  progression identification approaches,
    562-564
  psychophysical basis for perimetry,
    552-553
  pupil, 730, 731f
  reliability indices, 557-560
  "repeatable," 562
  short-wavelength automated perimetry,
    565, 566f
  single visual field analysis, 557-561
  standard automated perimetry, 554-556
  suprathreshold screening procedures,
    553-554
  Swedish Interactive Threshold
    Algorithm, 554, 556-557, 558f, 560
  temporal modulation perimetry,
    570-571, 572f
  test information, 557-560
  threshold estimation procedures,
    554-557
  total deviation probability plots,
    560-561
  true progression, 562
  visual field indices, 560, 561f
  visual field progression, 561-564
  Weber fraction, 552, 553f
  "worsening of sensitivity," 562
Peripheral dystrophies, 359
Peripheral nervous system integration and
    pupil, 721-723
Peripherin/RDS gene, 361, 366, 367t, 368,
    371-372
Peripherin/RDS protein, 419
Permanent occlusion suppression in
    binocular vision, 506
PFA. See Panum's fusional area (PFA).
pH regulation, 403
Phagocytosis
  optic nerve, 622-623
  retinal pigment epithelium, 349
Pharmacology
  accommodation, 212-213
  aqueous humor hydrodynamics, 244,
    249-258
  cornea, 95-97
  extraocular muscles, 809-812
  ocular circulation, 769-773
  pupil, 732-736, 737-739
Phase offsets in stereopsis, 500
Phase segmentation in temporal properties
    of vision, 522
Phase shifts in temporal properties of
    vision, 516
Phosphenes, 445-446, 449-450
Phosphodiesterase activation, 388, 389f
Photopic responses in electroretinograms,
    415
Photoreceptors
  color vision, 580-581
  cone pedicles, 330-331
  cone photoreceptor cells, 323f, 328f
  cone photoreceptor pathways, 341-342
  cone rod homeobox, 375
  cone synaptic pathways, 429-430, 431f
  cone visual pigments, 387-388
  cone voltage responses, 426, 427f
  inherited retinal dystrophies, 371-373,
    375-376, 377
  retina, 322f, 323f, 325f, 327-330

Photoreceptors—cont'd
  retinal intercellular light responses and
    synaptic organization, 424-426
  retinal pigment epithelium, 349-350
  rod cGMP phosphodiesterase, 370
  rod photoreceptor cells, 323f, 328f
  rod photoreceptor pathways, 323, 324f,
    339-341
  rod spherules, 330, 331f
  rod synaptic pathways, 429-430, 431f
  rod voltage responses, 426, 427f
  visual adaptation, 588-595
Photostasis, 587-588
Phototransduction, 382
  calcium homeostasis, 391
  cGMP-dependent channel regulation,
    388-391
  chromophore cycle, 385-387
  cone visual pigments, 387-388
  inherited retinal dystrophies, 366-371
  KIF3A protein, 392-393
  phosphodiesterase activation, 388, 389f
  retina, 327
  retinal intercellular light responses and
    synaptic organization, 424
  rhodopsin activation, 382-385
  rhodopsin inactivation, 385
  rim protein, 385
  S-modulin, 385
  transducin, 388, 389f
  vitamin A, 387
Physical basis in visual acuity, 453-455
Physiologic diplopia, 486-487
Physiologic factors in visual acuity, 456
Physiologic halos, 443-444
Physiologic myopia, 190
Physiologic position of rest, 841
Physiology
  aqueous humor hydrodynamics, 238-240
  corneal endothelium, 86-87
  extraocular muscles, 806-809
  vitreous, 306-311
  young eye optics and refraction, 164-167
Pia meninges, 610-611
Pial vessels in ocular circulation, 748f
Pilocarpine (PILO), 244-245, 255-259, 260,
    261
Pinhole method in entoptic phenomena,
    442, 444
Pitx3, 122
Pitx2 gene, 806
Plasma membrane proteins, 264-266
Pleomorphism, 63, 67f
Polymegathism, 59, 63, 67f, 94, 95f
Positional offsets in stereopsis, 500
Positive vergence, 200
Posterior capsular opacification (PCO),
    137
Posterior ciliary artery, 10f
Posterior cortex, lens, 118f
Posterior hyaloid, 294
Posterior internuclear ophthalmoplegia,
    852
Posterior precortical vitreous pocket
    (PPVP), 303
Posterior subcapsular cataracts, 141
Posterior vitreous detachment (PVD),
    306-309
Postganglionic parasympathetic
    denervation, pupil, 739-740
Postnatal retinal ganglion cell, 627
Postreceptoral mechanisms in visual
    adaptation, 595-596
Postsynaptic receptors, 398-399
PPVP. See Posterior precortical vitreous
    pocket (PPVP).
Preferential looking in infant vision
    development, 531
Presbyopia, 197-199, 214-215
  accommodative performance loss,
    223-226

Presbyopia—cont'd
  age changes in capsules, 220-221
  age changes in human ciliary muscle,
    215-216, 219f, 227-228
  age changes in rhesus ciliary muscle,
    215, 216f, 217f, 218f, 219f, 227-228
  age changes in zonules, 216-220
  aging eye optics and refraction, 190-191
  capsule changes, 220-221
  ciliary muscle age changes, 215-216,
    217f, 218f, 219f, 227-228
  correcting, 230-231
  crystalline lens growth, 220f, 221-223,
    224f
  disaccommodation theory of, 229
  geometric theory of, 229
  human ciliary muscle changes, 215-216
  lens hardness, increases in, 226-227
  lens paradox, 222, 229
  lenticular sclerosis, 227, 228-229
  multifactorial theory of, 230
  optical compensation for, 230
  rhesus ciliary muscle changes, 215
  Schacher's theory of, 229-230
  Scheimpflug slit-lamp measurements,
    221
  surgical compensation for, 230-231
  theories of, 228-230
  zonule changes, 216-220
Pressure phosphene, 449
Pretectal nuclei, 612
Pretectum, 642, 644f
Prevalence in aging eye optics and
    refraction, 189
Primary eye position, 819, 820f, 824
Primary visual cortex, 642f, 644f, 669, 684
  area 17 of Brodmann, 669-670
  area V1, 669-670
  cell classes, 678-680
  cell types, 674-678
  CO blobs, 673
  columns, 681-683
  complex cells, 676
  connections within, 680
  dorsal streams, 683
  end-stopped cells, 676
  extrastriate visual cortex compared,
    687-694
  functional architecture, 681-683
  hypercolumns, 681
  inputs, 672-674, 683-684
  lateral geniculate nucleus, 656f
  lateral geniculate nucleus differences,
    670f, 674-678
  lateral geniculate nucleus inputs, 670f,
    673-674
  layer IVB of Brodmann, 674
  layers and connections, 672-674, 675f,
    676f
  local image features, 669
  microcircuitry, 678-681
  modules, 681-683
  ocular dominance, 673
  optic chiasma, 670f
  optic nerve, 670f
  optic radiations, 670f
  optic tracts, 670f
  outputs, 674, 675f, 676f, 683-684
  parallel inputs and relationship to
    parallel outputs, 683-684
  processing dynamics, 680-681
  receptive field properties, 674-678
  road map or organization, 669-672
  simple cells, 676
  stria of Gennari, 669, 674
  striate cortex, 669
  superior colliculus, 670f
  ventral streams, 683
Primary vitreous, 293
  lens, 121
Prism, 578

Prism diopters, 840
Probability summation over time, 513
Processing hierarchy in infant vision development, 532-534
Processing streams in extrastriate visual cortex, 687-694
Programmed cell death, 322
Progression identification approaches in perimetry and visual field testing, 562-564
Proliferation factor controls, retina, 321
Proliferative vitreoretinopathy (PVR), 355
Proprioception and extraocular muscles, 809, 810f
Proptosis, 7
Prostaglandin mechanisms in aqueous humor hydrodynamics, 261-262, 263t
Protanomaly, 583
Protanopia, 583, 584
Protease-induced facility increases in aqueous humor hydrodynamics, 267
Proteins
    aqueous humor hydrodynamics, 256, 270
    inherited retinal dystrophies, 361, 366-371, 371-376
    lacrimal gland, 33-37
    lens, 126-128, 129, 134
    phototransduction, 385
    retinal pigment epithelium, 351, 352f
    ROM-1 protein, 361, 366, 371-372
    RS protein, 417
Proteoglycans
    corneal stroma, 56, 81-85
    sclera, 100-101
Prox1, 122
Proximal disparity in binocular vision, 491
Proximal stimulus in visual acuity, 453
PRP. See Pan-retinal photocoagulation (PRP).
Psychophysical basis for perimetry, 552-553
Psychophysical evidence for unique motion processing, 523-525
Psychophysical techniques in visual adaptation, 588
Psychophysics, 361
Pulleys, 791-792, 828-829
Pulse force, 825, 826f
Pulse signal, 824, 825f
Pulvinar, 642f, 643
Punctum, 40
Pupil, 713-716
    aberrant regeneration in the third nerve, 740
    accommodation, 720-721
    Adie's pupil, 719-720, 733t, 737-738, 739-740
    afferent arm of the pupil light reflex, 716-718
    anisocoria, 715, 719, 730-732, 733t, 736-737
    central nervous system integration, 721-723
    childhood Horner Syndrome, 736
    cholinergic supersensitivity, 737-738
    clinical importance, 714f, 715-716
    cocaine's action on, 732-735, 736
    collarette, 724
    computerized pupillometry, 728-730
    congenital Horner Syndrome, 736
    contraction anisocoria, 719
    denervation in Horner Syndrome, 735-736
    depth of focus, 714f, 715
    dilation, 721-723, 741-742
    dilation lag, 732, 735f
    Edinger-Westphal nucleus, 716, 719, 720-721, 721-722, 730
    efferent arm of the pupil light reflex, 719-720
    functions, 713-715

Pupil—cont'd
    ganglion cells, 717-718
    Horner syndrome, 730-731, 732-736
    hydroxyamphetamine test, 735-736
    inequality that increases in bright light, 736-737
    inequality that increases in the dark, 730-732, 734f, 735f
    inner ciliary ring, 724
    interneuron arm of pupil light reflex, 718-719
    iris, 723-724, 733t, 737-739
    light properties and effect on pupil movement, 724-725, 726t
    light reflex, 716-720, 725-728
    light-near dissociation, 740-741
    Marcus Gunn pupil, 612
    near response, 720-721, 740-741
    nerve pathways, 716-723
    ophthalmic division of the trigeminal nerve, 723
    optical aberration reduction, 713, 714f
    outer ciliary ring, 724
    perimetry, 730, 731f
    peripheral nervous system integration, 721-723
    pharmacology, 732-736, 737-739
    postganglionic parasympathetic denervation, 739-740
    Purkinje shift, 716
    reflex, 720
    relative afferent pupillary defect, 715, 726-728, 729t
    retinal illumination control, 713, 714f
    size and visual acuity, 463
    slit-lamp biomicroscope, 737
    swinging flashlight test, 715
    third nerve palsy, 733t, 740
Purkinje figures, 446-447
Purkinje shift, 716
Pursuit component of smooth following eye, 841
PVD. See Posterior vitreous detachment (PVD).
PVR. See Proliferative vitreoretinopathy (PVR).

Q
Qualitative stereopsis, 494-496
Quantifying eye rotations, 818-822
Quantitative stereopsis, 494-496
Quick eye movement, 445-446

R
Radiation exposure and cataracts, 143-144
RAPD. See Relative afferent pupillary defect (RAPD).
Rapid conjugate shifts of gaze direction, 843-845
Rate of blood flow, 761-763
Ratios in lateral geniculate nucleus, 661-662
RDH5 gene, 597
Receptive field
    lateral geniculate nucleus, 661-662
    primary visual cortex, 674-678
    visual adaptation, 595-596
Receptor size and spacing, 170-171
Receptoral mechanisms in visual adaptation, 588-595
Recognizing faces, 164-166
Recognizing movements, 167
Reconciliation of differences in oculocentric visual directions, 486
Recurrent meningeal artery, 10f
Red nucleus, 642f
Redistribution of cortical plasticity markers, 706
Reference orientation, 820
Reflex, pupil, 720

Refraction, lens, 118-119, 133
Refractive defocus, stereoacuity with, 498-500
Refractive errors
    aging eye optics and refraction, 189-191
    visual acuity, 461-462
Refractive surgery, 178
Refsum syndrome, 360t
Regeneration, optic nerve, 626-627
Relative afferent pupillary defect (RAPD), 715, 726-728, 729t
Relative disparity in binocular vision, 492
Relay cells, 657
Reliability indices in perimetry and visual field testing, 557-560
Removing distractions in the aging, 189
"Repeatable" in perimetry and visual field testing, 562
Resonance, 168
Response waveform development, 537-539, 540f
Resting potential, optic nerve, 614
Retina, 319, 322-323
    abnormal adaptation in retinal disease, 596-598
    abnormal retinal correspondence, 489-491
    accommodation, 202f
    adult eye optics and refraction, 167, 169-171
    aging changes, 343
    AII amacrine cell type, 340-341
    amacrine cells, 323f, 333-336
    apoptosis, 322
    arcuate density, 330
    astrocytes, 337
    basal junctions, 331
    binocular vision, 488, 491-493, 505-506
    biochemistry. See Retinal biochemistry.
    bipolar cells, 323f, 324f, 332-333
    blood supply, 617
    blood-retinal barrier, 297-301, 312-313
    blue arcs of the retina, 447-448
    Bruch's membrane, 326-327
    calyces, 329
    cell adhesion molecules, 321
    cell distribution, 321
    central retinal artery and vein, 748f
    Chievitz transient fiber, 320, 321
    color vision, 581-583
    cone pedicles, 330-331
    cone photoreceptor cells, 323f, 328f
    cone photoreceptor pathways, 341-342
    connexons, 332
    cornea, 322f
    diffuse bipolar cells, 333
    displaced amacrine cells, 333, 335, 338
    dopaminergic retinal neurons, 341
    dyads, 332, 337, 338f
    electrophysiology and function. See Electroretinograms (ERG).
    ellipsoids, 329
    embryology, 319-322
    entoptic phenomena, 446-447, 447-448, 450-452
    fiber baskets, 329
    fovea centralis, 342
    foveal vision, 343
    functional organization, 323-324
    GABA-ergic amacrine cells, 333
    ganglion cell layer, 323f, 325f, 338-339
    ganglion cells, 322f, 323f, 324f, 339
    glial cells, 336-337
    glycinergic amacrine cells, 333
    Henle fiber layer, 327
    histologic organization, 324-339, 342-343
    horizontal cells, 323f, 331-332
    illumination control, 713, 714f
    indoleamine accumulating amacrine cell type, 341

Retina—cont'd
inherited retinal dystrophies. *See*
Inherited retinal dystrophies.
inner neuroblastic layers, 320
inner nuclear layer, 323f, 325f, 331-336
inner plexiform layer, 323f, 325f, 337,
338f
intercellular light responses and synaptic
organization. *See* Retinal intercellular
light responses and synaptic
organization.
interplexiform cells, 323f, 336
interstitial amacrine cells, 333
interstitial cells, 337
intrinsic gray of the retina, 450
lateral geniculate nucleus, 656f
lens, 322f
macula lutea, 342
maculopapillary bundle, 339
microglial cells, 337
midget bipolar cells, 333
midget cell system, 342
monads, 337
Müller cells, 322, 323f, 327, 329, 336-337
myoids, 329
nerve fiber layer, 325f, 339
neural control of eye movements, 837
neurulation, 319
ocular circulation, 748f, 754f
OFF channels, 323-324, 325f
ON-channels, 323-324, 325f
optic nerve, 322f, 339, 603-604, 612-613,
619-622
outer limiting membrane, 336
outer neuroblastic layers, 320
outer nuclear layer, 323f, 325f, 327-330
outer plexiform layer, 325f, 330-331
P cells, 339
parasol ganglion cells, 339
photoreceptor cells, 322f, 323f, 325f,
327-330
phototransduction, 327
pigment epithelium. *See* Retinal pigment
epithelium (RPE).
programmed cell death, 322
proliferation factor controls, 321
rod photoreceptor cells, 323f, 328f
rod photoreceptor pathways, 323, 324f,
339-341
rod spherules, 330, 331f
sclera, 322f
second-order cells, 322f
triads, 330, 331
visual acuity, 455-456, 462
visual adaptation, 586-587, 596-598
vitreoretinal interface, 295, 296f
vitreoretinal interface imaging, 303-305
vitreoretinal sources of entoptic images,
445
vitreous, 306-309
young eye optics and refraction, 164
Retinal biochemistry, 382, 403
arginine, 399-400
calcium homeostasis at synaptic
terminals, 393
energy consumption in rod outer
segment, 401-402
energy metabolism, 400-403
energy supply, 400-401
GABA synaptic release, 397-398
glucose metabolism, 400
glucose supply, 400
glutamate homeostasis, 394-396
glutamate receptors, 396-397
glutamate transporters, 393-394
glutamatergic transmission, 391-397
glycine homeostasis, 398
information processing, 391-400
inhibitory transmission, 397-399
lactate metabolism, 400-401
neurochemistry, 391-400

Retinal biochemistry—cont'd
nitric oxide synthesis, 399-400
oxygen supply and consumption,
402-403
pH regulation, 403
phototransduction. *See*
Phototransduction.
postsynaptic receptors, 398-399
ribbon synapses, 392-393
synaptic release at ribbon synapses,
392-393
taurine, 399
Retinal intercellular light responses and
synaptic organization
amacrine cell light responses, 432
amacrine cell synapses, 432
bipolar cell output synapses, 430-432
bipolar cell responses, 429
center-surround antagonistic receptive
field organization, 430
cone synaptic pathways, 429-430, 431f
cone voltage responses, 426, 427f
ganglion cell responses, 433-434
glutamatergic synapses between
photoreceptors and second-order
retinal neurons, 426-428
horizontal cell responses, 428
horizontal cell synapses, 428-429
interplexiform cell responses and
synapses, 432-433
neuron organization and light responses,
422-424
ON-OFF-cells, 433-434
opsin protein, 424
photoreceptor coupling, 424-426
photoreceptor responses and synapses,
424-426
phototransduction, 424
rod synaptic pathways, 429-430, 431f
rod voltage responses, 426, 427f
Schiff-base linkage, 424
spontaneous excitatory postsynaptic
currents, 428
S-potentials, 428
Retinal pigment epithelium (RPE), 323f,
325-327, 325f, 348-349
ABCR gene, 350
all-*trans*-retinal, 350, 351, 352f
Bruch's membrane, 348, 349f
choriocapillaries, 348, 349, 349f
fluorescein absorption, 352-353
function, 349-355
inner segments of the photoreceptors,
348, 349f
IRBP gene, 351
light-induced responses, 354-355
Müller cells, 348, 349f
outer limiting membrane, 348, 349f
outer segments of the photoreceptors,
348, 349f
phagocytosis, 349
photoreceptor outer segment turnover,
349-350
proliferative vitreoretinopathy, 355
proteins, 351, 352f
retinoid metabolism, 350-351, 352f
retinol, 350-351, 352f
retinol-binding protein, 351
transplantation and inherited retinal
dystrophies, 377
transport, 351-353
transthyretin, 351
visual cycle, 350-351, 352f
water transport, 353
Retinitis pigmentosa, 363
autosomal dominant retinitis
pigmentosa, 365
autosomal recessive retinitis pigmentosa,
365, 377
cell death mechanisms, 366
clinical features, 363-366

Retinitis pigmentosa—cont'd
digenic retinitis pigmentosa, 366
genes and loci for, 364t
linkage mapping, 362f
lyonization, 366
rhodopsin, 369-370
X-linked retinitis pigmentosa, 365-366,
377
Retinogeniculate projection activity-
dependent development, 646, 652
activity alone is insufficient, 651-652
activity before vision is spatially and
temporally patterned, 649-650
activity's role, 648-649
cell networks, 650-651
refinement during development,
646-648
refinement through activity, 648-649
Retinol metabolism in inherited retinal
dystrophies, 373-375
Retinopetal projections in optic nerve,
613
Retinotopographic mapping in extrastriate
visual cortex, 686
Retinotopy
extrastriate visual cortex, 693
optic nerve, 604-605
Reverse contrast, 463
Rhesus ciliary muscle changes, 215
Rhodopsin
adult eye optics and refraction, 170
electroretinograms, 419, 420
inherited retinal dystrophies, 366-369
phototransduction, 382-385
retinitis pigmentosa, 369-370
visual adaptation, 591-594, 594-595,
596-597
Rhombomeres, 804
Ribbon synapses in retinal biochemistry,
392-393
Ribozyme treatment in dominant
disorders, 377
Rim protein
inherited retinal dystrophies, 367t,
373-375
phototransduction, 385
Rod cGMP phosphodiesterase, 370
Rod photoreceptor cells, 323f, 328f
Rod photoreceptor pathways, 323, 324f,
339-341
Rod spherules, 330, 331f
Rod synaptic pathways, 429-430, 431f
Rod voltage responses, 426, 427f
ROM-1 protein, 361, 366, 371-372
RPE. *See* Retinal pigment epithelium
(RPE).
RPE65 gene
inherited retinal dystrophies, 367t, 374
visual adaptation, 597
RS protein, 417
Rubella cataracts, 142
Rushton's paradox, 594

S
Saccade disorders, 853-854, 855f
Saccades, 833, 850-851
Saccadic eye movements, 843-845
Saccadic gaze shifting system, 847-850
Saltatory conduction, optic nerve, 615
Sarcolemma, 792
Sarcomeres, 793-795
Satellite cells, 793
Scatter, 455
Schacher's theory of presbyopia, 229-230
Scheimpflug slit-lamp measurements, 221
Schiff-base linkage, 424
Schlemm's canal (SC)
aqueous humor hydrodynamics, 237,
250-253
ocular circulation, 748f
School myopia, 190

Sclera
    accommodation, 202f
    anatomy, 97-99
    embryology and development, 99-100
    hydration, 100-101, 102
    innervation, 101
    permeability, 101-103
    proteoglycans, 100-101
    retina, 322f
    wound healing, 101
Scleral spur, 202f
Scotopic responses in electroretinograms (ERG), 415
Second sight, 138
Secondary cataracts, 137, 141-142, 148-149
Secondary eye position, 819, 820f, 824
Secondary vitreous, 293
Second-order cells, retina, 322f
Second-order motion, 523-525
Selective adaptation, 521
Sensor for physiology of surrounding structures, 311-313
Serum retinal-binding protein, 375
Sex and influence on cataracts, 146
Short posterior ciliary arteries, 748f, 749, 750-751
Short-wavelength automated perimetry (SWAP), 565, 566f
Signal processing in the retina, 581-583
Signal transduction pathway, 35, 37f
Signaling of axonal injury, 621-622
Simple cells in primary visual cortex, 676
Sine waves, 173-174
Single visual field analysis, 557-561
Sinusoidal grating targets, 465-467
SITA. See Swedish Interactive Threshold Algorithm (SITA).
Skeletal muscle fiber types, 797
Slide component of three-dimensional rotations of the eye, 824, 825f
Slit-lamp biomicroscope, 737
SMAS. See Superficial musculoaponeurotic system (SMAS).
S-modulin, 385
Smooth pursuit tracking system, 843
Smooth tracking responses to open- and closed-loop stimuli, 841-843
Smooth vergence, 841
Smooth vergence tracking system, 843
Snellen charts, 470, 471f-472f
Snellen's letters, 457-458, 459f, 460, 461, 462f, 464f
Social seeing, 167
Soemmering's ring, 142
Sox1, 122
Spanning zonular fiber system, 205
Spasm, eyelids, 22-23
Spatial distortions, 500-503
Spatial effects, 518
Spatial form processing, 481
    binocular disparity-defined form, 470, 480-481
    camouflage breaking, 470
    color, 470
    contrast detection threshold, 476
    contrast sensitivity function, 474-476
    cyclopean, 481
    disparity-defined form, 470, 480-481
    glare susceptibility, 473-474
    grating acuity, 476
    high-contrast acuity, 470-473
    hyperacuities, 477
    low-contrast letter acuity, 470-473
    luminance-define objects, 470-478
    medium-contrast acuity, 470-473
    Mexican hat sensitivity profile, 477
    motion-defined objects, 470, 478-479
    Snellen charts, 470, 471f-472f
    spatial contrast, 474
    spatial filters, 476-477
    spatial Fourier analysis, 476-477

Spatial form processing—cont'd
    spatial frequency, 474, 500
    spatial frequency discrimination threshold, 476
    texture-defined form, 470, 479-480
    two-dimensional images, 477-478
Spatiotemporal contrast sensitivity function, 518, 519f
Spatiotemporal vision in infant vision development, 534-535, 536f
Specification of the stimulus in visual acuity, 453-455
Speed of retinal adjustments, 586-587
Sphenoid bone, 3
Sphenopalatine ganglion, 31f
Sphenopalatine nerves, 31f
Spherical aberrations, 184-186
Spiral of Tillaux, 788, 790f
Spontaneous excitatory postsynaptic currents, 428
S-potentials in retinal intercellular light responses and synaptic organization, 428
Square waves, 173-174
Stabilization of gaze relative to the external world, 834-839
Standard automated perimetry, 554-556
Stargardt disease/fundus flavimaculatus, 367t, 373-375
Static control of eye alignment, 839-841
Steady-state IOP, 248
Stem cells of the ocular surface, 24
Step force in three-dimensional rotations of the eye, 825, 826f
Step signal in three-dimensional rotations of the eye, 824, 825f
Stereopsis, 493-494
    aniseikonia, 500-503
    contrast effects and, 500
    induced effects, 501
    infant vision development, 545-547, 548f
    monovision, 499
    motion-in-depth, 503-504
    phase offsets, 500
    positional offsets, 500
    qualitative stereopsis, 494-496
    quantitative stereopsis, 494-496
    refractive defocus, stereoacuity with, 498-500
    spatial distortions, 500-503
    spatial frequency and, 500
    stereoacuity, 496-500
    stereothreshold, 496-500
Stereothreshold
    infant vision development, 545-547, 548f
    stereopsis, 496-500
Steroid exposure and cataracts, 145
Stiles-Crawford effect, 450, 451f, 452f
Strabismus
    extraocular muscles, 806, 809-812, 813
    neural control of eye movements, 851-852
    visual deprivations, 702-704
Stria of Gennari, 669, 674
Striate cortex. See Primary visual cortex.
Stroma, corneal. See Corneal stroma.
Subjective angle in binocular vision, 490
Substantia nigra, 642f
Superficial musculoaponeurotic system (SMAS), 25-27
Superior alveolar artery, 10f
Superior colliculus (SC)
    central visual pathways, 641-642, 644f
    optic nerve, 612-613
    primary visual cortex, 670f
Superior marginal arcade, 10f
Superior rectus, extraocular muscles, 789f
Superior septum, 19f
Superior tarsus, 19f
Suppression in binocular vision, 489, 504-506

Suppression scotoma in binocular vision, 489
Supraciliaris, 201-202
Supraorbital artery, 10f
Supraorbital ridges, 3
Suprathreshold screening procedures in perimetry and visual field testing, 553-554
Supratrochlear artery, 10f
Surface, ocular
    conjunctiva. See Conjunctiva.
    eyebrows. See Eyebrows.
    eyelids. See Eyelids.
    face. See Face.
    forehead. See Forehead.
    lacrimal system. See Lacrimal system.
    orbit. See Orbit.
Surgery
    aqueous humor hydrodynamics, 247t, 248
    presbyopia, 230-231
Surround effects and temporal properties of vision, 518-520
Suspension in binocular vision, 505
Suspensory ligaments, lens, 118f
Sutures, lens, 117, 118f, 134-135
SWAP. See Short-wavelength automated perimetry (SWAP).
Sweat gland, 20f
Swedish Interactive Threshold Algorithm (SITA), 554, 556-557, 558f, 560
Swinging flashlight test
    optic nerve, 612
    pupil, 715
Synaptic release at ribbon synapses in retinal biochemistry, 392-393
Synaptic transmissions, optic nerve, 613
Syndromic dystrophies, 359-360

T
Talbot-Plateau law, 517, 522
Targets
    adult eye optics and refraction, 173
    central visual pathways, 641-643
    neural control of eye movements, 843-851
    visual acuity, 463
Taurine, 399
Taxon specific crystallins in lens fiber cell differentiation, 124-125
Tear film, 32
    conjunctival epithelial cells, 34f, 37f, 38, 39f
    conjunctival goblet cells, 38-39
    corneal epithelial cells, 37-38, 39f
    electrolyte secretion, 33-38
    glands and ocular surface epithelia that secrete tears, 32
    holocrine secretion, 33
    lacrimal gland. See Lacrimal gland.
    lipids, 32-33
    meibomian gland secretion of lipids, 32-33
    mucins, 38-39
    water secretion, 33-38
Technologies and cataracts, 149
Temperature reversal in corneal endothelium, 86, 87f
Temporal aspects of electroretinograms (ERG), 415
Temporal modulation perimetry, 570-571, 572f
Temporal properties of vision, 511
    attenuation characteristics of a linear filter, 517
    Bloch's law, 511, 512f
    Brücke brightness enhancement effect, 522
    clinical applications of measurements, 522-523
    critical duration, 511-513

Temporal properties of vision—cont'd
critical flicker fusion frequency. *See* Critical flicker fusion (CFF).
functional integrity, 522
fundamental waveform, 516
harmonics, 516
image segmentation, 522
linear filters, 517
linear systems, 516
luminance-pedestal flicker, 520
magnocellular pathways, 522
mean-modulated flicker, 520
mechanisms underlying, 521-522
parvocellular pathways, 522
perception, 522
phase segmentation, 522
phase shifts, 516
probability summation over time, 513
selective adaptation, 521
spatial effects, 518
spatiotemporal contrast sensitivity function, 518, 519f
surround effects, 518-520
Talbot-Plateau law, 517, 522
temporal contrast sensitivity, 516-518
temporal summation, 511-513
Temporal resolution in infant vision development, 536-537, 538f
Tenon's capsule, extraocular muscles, 788
Tension zonular fiber system, 205
Tenson's capsule, 19f
Tertiary eye position, 820, 824
Tertiary vitreous, 293
Test information in perimetry and visual field testing, 557-560
Testing color vision, 583-584
Texture-defined form, 470, 479-480
Therapy
axonal injury, 622
inherited retinal dystrophies, 376-377
Third nerve palsy, 733t, 740
Three-dimensional rotations of the eye, 818, 819f, 829
axis of action, 828
Donders' law, 823
extraocular pulleys, 828-829
eye-fixed coordinates, 819-820
false torsion, 821-822
head-fixed coordinates, 820-821
kinematic redundancy, 823
Listing's law, 823-824
neural control of ocular orientation, 824-829
noncommutative rotations, 818
primary eye position, 819, 820f, 824
pulse force, 825, 826f
pulse signal, 824, 825f
quantifying eye rotations, 818-822
reference orientation, 820
secondary eye position, 819, 820f, 824
slide component of, 824, 825f
step force, 825, 826f
step signal, 824, 825f
tertiary eye position, 820, 824
Threshold estimation procedures in perimetry and visual field testing, 554-557
Thyroid eye disease, 7
Tissue fluid formation and drainage in ocular circulation, 774
Tissue light scattering, 175-177
TM. *See* Trabecular meshwork (TM).
TNO test, 546
Tonic accommodation, 212
Torsion, 821-822
Total deviation probability plots in perimetry and visual field testing, 560-561
Trabecular meshwork (TM), 237, 249-250, 266-267
adrenergic mechanisms, 259-261

Trabecular meshwork (TM)—cont'd
blood-aqueous barrier, 242
cholinergic mechanisms, 253-258
cytoskeletal and cell junctional mechanisms, 268-269
hyaluronidase and protease-induced facility increases, 267
macromolecule-induced facility decreases, 270
outflow biomechanics, 270
particulate-induced facility decreases, 269-270
Transcription factors
inherited retinal dystrophies, 375-376
lens, 119-122
Transducins
color vision, 579
phototransduction, 388, 389f
Transfer ratios in lateral geniculate nucleus, 662
Transient VEPs, 531
Transparency, lens, 118-119, 133
Transplantation of photoreceptors and retinal pigment epithelium, 377
Transthyretin, 351
Transverse axis, extraocular muscles, 789f
Tremors in adult eye optics and refraction, 171
Triads
accommodative triad, 212
lateral geniculate nucleus, 662
near triad and interactions with saccades, 850-851
retina, 330, 331
Trichromacy, 580-581
Trigeminal nerve V, 31f
Trochlear palsy, 852
True progression in perimetry and visual field testing, 562
Tunica vasculosa lentis, 129
Turnover constant in aqueous humor hydrodynamics, 240
Twitch fibers, 795
Two-dimensional images, 477-478

U
Uhthoff's phenomenon, 616
Ultrafiltration in aqueous humor hydrodynamics, 238
Ultrastructural aspects of vitreous, 295-297, 298f
Ultraviolet light and cataracts, 144
Umbilical suture, lens, 134
Unconventional outflow in aqueous humor hydrodynamics, 258, 259f, 261, 262t
Uncrossed disparity in binocular vision, 491
Usher syndromes, 360t, 372
Uveoscleral outflow in aqueous humor hydrodynamics, 258, 259f, 261, 262t

V
V1, 669-670. *See also* Primary visual cortex.
V2, 687-689
V3, 691
V3A, 691
V4, 691-692
V5, 689-690
Vasoconstrictors, 770
Vasodilators, 770-771
Vasomotion, 763
Ventral posterior area of extrastriate visual cortex, 691
Ventral streams
extrastriate visual cortex, 691-692
primary visual cortex, 683
VEPs. *See* Visual evoked potentials (VEPs).
Vergence gaze shifting system, 850-851
Vergence systems and neural control of eye movements, 831

Vernier acuity
aging eye optics and refraction, 188-189
infant vision development, 541-543, 544f
Version and vergence ocular movement combinations, 485-486
Version systems and neural control of eye movements, 831
Vertical axis, extraocular muscles, 789f
Vestibuloocular reflex (VOR), 835-838
Vidian nerve, 31f
Vimentin, 125, 134
Visible light waves in adult eye optics and refraction, 167-173
Visual acuity, 453
aberrations, 455
absorption, 455
accommodation, 201
adult eye optics and refraction, 171, 172
aging, 464-465
Airy disc, 455
amblyopia, 467-468
chief ray, 454
contrast, 463
criteria for, 456-459
developmental aspects, 464
diffraction, 454
distal stimulus, 453
exposure duration, 463
factors influencing, 461-465
focus factors, 455
hyperacuity, 457t, 458-459, 464
inner psychophysics, 453
interaction effects, 463-464
Landolt's Cs, 457, 459, 460, 463
luminance, 462-463
meridional variations in acuity, 463
Michelson contrast, 466, 467f
minimum angle of resolution, 458
minimum discriminable, 457t, 458-459
minimum resolvable, 457-458, 459-461
minimum visible, 456-457
normal visual acuity, 461
ordinary visual acuity, 457-458, 459-461
outer psychophysics, 453
physical basis, 453-455
physiologic factors, 456
proximal stimulus, 453
pupil size, 463
refractive error, 461-462
retinal anatomy, 455-456
retinal eccentricity, 462
reverse contrast, 463
scatter, 455
sinusoidal grating targets, 465-467
Snellen's letters, 457-458, 459f, 460, 461, 462f, 464f
specification of the stimulus, 453-455
target and eye movements, 463
Visual adaptation, 586-587
ABCR gene, 597
abnormal adaptation in retinal disease, 596-598
Dowling-Rushton relationship, 594
output of retina, 586
photoreceptor activation and inactivation, 588-595
photostasis, 587-588
postreceptoral mechanisms, 595-596
psychophysical techniques, 588
RDH5 gene, 597
receptive field, 595-596
receptoral mechanisms, 588-595
retinal disease, 596-598
rhodopsin bleaching, 591-594
rhodopsin mutations, 596-597
rhodopsin visual cycle, 594-595
RPE65 gene, 597
Rushton's paradox, 594
speed of retinal adjustments, 586-587
structural mechanisms, 587-588
visual cycle, 594-595

Visual cycle
  retinal pigment epithelium, 350-351, 352f
  visual adaptation, 594-595
Visual deprivations, 697, 706
  adulthood, changes in, 704-706
  amblyopia, 701-702, 703-704
  binocular responses in visual cortex,
    697-698, 699f
  clinical implications, 701-706
  cortical plasticity marker redistribution,
    706
  critical periods, 700
  development, changes during, 701-704
  direction selectivity in visual cortex,
    698-701
  glaucoma, 704
  ocular dominance plasticity, 697-698,
    700-701
  orientation selectivity in visual cortex,
    698-701
  pan-retinal photocoagulation, 704-706
  redistribution of cortical plasticity
    markers, 706
  strabismus, 702-704
Visual direction in binocular vision,
  485-487
Visual evoked potentials (VEPs), 531-532
Visual field lesions, 644-645
Visual field testing. *See* Perimetry and
  visual field testing.
Visual perception
  acuity. *See* Visual acuity.
  adaptation. *See* Visual adaptation.
  binocular vision. *See* Binocular vision.
  color vision. *See* Color vision.
  entoptic phenomena. *See* Entoptic
    phenomena.
  infants. *See* Infant vision development.
  perimetry and visual field testing. *See*
    Perimetry and visual field testing.
  spatial form processing. *See* Spatial form
    processing.
  temporal properties. *See* Temporal
    properties of vision.
Visual sensory-motor tasks, 830
Visual signal regulation, 659-664
Visual signals to cortex, 655
Vitamin A
  cornea, 94-95
  inherited retinal dystrophies, 373-375
  phototransduction, 387
Vitreoretinal interface, 295, 296f
Vitreoretinal interface imaging, 303-305
Vitreoretinal sources of entoptic images,
  445
Vitreous, 293, 294f, 313
  aging of, 302-306
  anatomy, 293-295
  anterior hyaloid, 294
  base, 294f
  Berger's space, 294f
  biochemical aspects, 295-297

Vitreous—cont'd
  biophysical aspects, 297-301, 305-306
  blood-retinal barrier permeability,
    297-301, 312-313
  body cavity filling-up function, 306-309
  cellular considerations of embryology,
    293-294
  Cloquet's canal, 293, 294f
  collagen, 293, 295-297
  cortex, 294, 294f, 296f
  dark-field microscopy, 303
  diffusion barrier between anterior and
    posterior segment of the eye, 309,
    310f, 311f
  diffusion kinetics, 305-306
  embryology, 293-294
  entoptic phenomena, 444-445
  fluorescein concentration and profiles,
    297-301, 305-306, 312-313
  fovea, 294f
  glucose concentration, 299f
  hyaluronic acid, 293, 295-297
  lactate concentration, 299f
  light path, 311
  macular edema, 309, 310f, 310t
  mature vitreous body anatomy, 294-295
  metabolic buffer function, 309-311
  molecular considerations of embryology,
    293-294
  molecular mechanisms of aging, 302-303
  optical coherence tomography, 303-305,
    307
  oxygen concentration, 300f
  physiology, 306-311
  posterior hyaloid, 294
  posterior precortical vitreous pocket,
    303
  posterior vitreous detachment, 306-309
  primary vitreous, 293
  retina's support function, 306-309
  secondary vitreous, 293
  sensor for physiology of surrounding
    structures, 311-313
  structural changes in aging, 303, 304f, 305f
  structural considerations of embryology,
    293
  tertiary vitreous, 293
  ultrastructural aspects, 295-297, 298f
  vitreoretinal interface, 295, 296f
  vitreoretinal interface imaging, 303-305
  Weiger's ligament, 294f
  Worst's interpretation, 303, 305f
VOR. *See* Vestibuloocular reflex (VOR).
Vortex vein, 748f

W

Water balance, lens, 132-133
Water secretion
  lacrimal gland, 33-37
  lacrimal system, 33-38
  tear film, 33-38

Water transport in retinal pigment
  epithelium, 353
Weber fraction, 552, 553f
Weiger's ligament, 294f
Whitnall's ligament, 19f
Window experiment of Hering, 487
Winking, 22
"Worsening of sensitivity" in perimetry
  and visual field testing, 562
Worst's interpretation, 303, 305f
Wound healing
  corneal endothelium, 91-92
  corneal epithelium, 70-77
  corneal stroma, 85-86
  sclera, 101

X

Xerophthalmia, 95
X-linked retinitis pigmentosa, 365-366,
  377
X-linked retinoschisis, 372-373

Y

Young eye optics and refraction, 161, 167.
  See also Infant vision development.
  accommodation, 162
  anatomy, 161-164
  astigmatism, 165
  axial length, 161-163
  cardinal points, 162-163
  depth of focus, 162
  emmetropization, 163-164
  eye movements of others, monitoring,
    166-167
  face recognition, 164-166
  line orientation receptors, 166
  monitoring other's eye movements,
    166-167
  movement, recognizing, 167
  neural processing, 164, 165f
  physiology, 164-167
  recognizing faces, 164-166
  recognizing movements, 167
  retinal receptors, 164
  social seeing, 167
Young-Helmholtz hypothesis, 579, 582

Z

Zonula occludens, 53
Zonular fork, 205, 206f
Zonules
  accommodation, 202f, 203-207, 208f,
    209-212
  lens, 118, 119f, 136-137
  presbyopia, 216-220
Zygomatic nerve, 31f
Zygomaticofacial artery, 10f
Zygomaticotemporal artery, 10f